NURSING SKILLS

CHIPPEWA VALLEY TECHNICAL COLLEGE

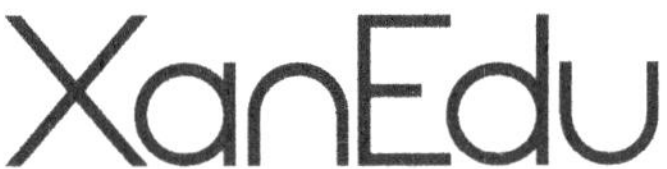

Printed in the United States of America

ISBN 13: 978-1-73491-413-9

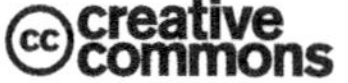

XanEdu
4750 Venture Drive, Suite 400
Ann Arbor, MI 48108
800-562-2147
www.xanedu.com

CONTENTS

INTRODUCTION

This open access *Nursing Skills* textbook includes physical assessments routinely performed by entry-level registered nurses[1,2,3] and basic nursing skills performed by licensed practical nurses.[4] It is based on the Wisconsin Technical College System (WTCS) statewide nursing curriculum for the Nursing Skills course (543-102), the 2019 NCLEX-RN Test Plan,[5] the 2020 NCLEX-PN Test Plan,[6] and the Wisconsin Nurse Practice Act.[7] Learning activities are included to encourage the student to engage in critical thinking and apply the nursing process while analyzing assessment findings.

The project is supported by a $2.5 million Open Resources for Nursing (Open RN) grant from the Department of Education and is licensed under CC-BY 4.0 creative commons license. This free book is available online and can also be downloaded in multiple formats for offline use. The online version is required for interaction with the adaptive learning activities included in each chapter.

The following video provides a quick overview of how to navigate the online version.

Interactive Activity

An interactive or media element has been excluded from this version of the text. You can view it online here: https://wtcs.pressbooks.pub/nursingskills/?p=4

This book references information contained in the free electronic versions of the Open RN *Nursing Skills*, Open RN *Nursing Pharmacology*, and Open RN *Nursing Fundamentals* textbooks. These books can be accessed at the following URLs:

- Open RN Nursing Skills: https://wtcs.pressbooks.pub/nursingskills
- Open RN Nursing Pharmacology: https://wtcs.pressbooks.pub/pharmacology
- Open RN Nursing Fundamentals: https://wtcs.pressbooks.pub/nursingfundamentals

---

1 NCSBN. (n.d.). *2019 NCLEX-RN test plan.* https://www.ncsbn.org/2019_RN_TestPlan-English.htm

2 Giddens, J. F. (2007). A survey of physical examination techniques performed by RNs: Lessons for nursing education. *Journal of Nursing Education, 46*(2), 83-87. https://doi.org/10.3928/01484834-20070201-09

3 Giddens, J. F. & Eddy, L. (2009). A survey of physical examination skills taught in undergraduate nursing programs: Are we teaching too much? *Journal of Nursing Education, 48*(1), 24-29. https://doi.org/10.3928/01484834-20090101-05

4 NCSBN. (2019). *NCLEX-PN examination: Test plan for the national council licensure examination for practical nurses.* https://www.ncsbn.org/2020_NCLEXPN_TestPlan-English.pdf

5 NCSBN. (n.d.). *2019 NCLEX-RN test plan.* https://www.ncsbn.org/2019_RN_TestPlan-English.htm

6 NCSBN. (2019). *NCLEX-PN examination: Test plan for the national council licensure examination for practical nurses.* https://www.ncsbn.org/2020_NCLEXPN_TestPlan-English.pdf

7 Wisconsin State Legislature. (2018). *Chapter 6: Standards of practice for registered nurses and licensed practical nurses.* Board of Nursing. https://docs.legis.wisconsin.gov/statutes/statutes/441

PREFACE

This *Nursing Skills* textbook is an open educational resource with a *CC-BY 4.0* license developed for entry-level undergraduate nursing students. It is aligned with the Wisconsin Technical College System (WTCS) statewide nursing curriculum for the Nursing Skills course (543-102) that describes techniques for obtaining a health history and performing a basic physical assessment using a body systems approach. It also includes evidence-based clinical skills with related mathematical calculations and conversions.

Online learning activities are provided in each chapter using the free H5P software platform (https://h5p.org/). This textbook has also been uploaded to LibreTexts (https://libretexts.org/) for easy remixing by faculty. The project is supported by a $2.5 million Open Resources for Nursing (Open RN) grant from the Department of Education to create five free, open source nursing textbooks. However, this content does not necessarily represent the policy of the Department of Education, and you should not assume endorsement by the federal government.

More information about the Open RN grant can be found at cvtc.edu/OpenRN. The first textbook of the Open RN textbook series, *Nursing Pharmacology*, received an OE Award for Excellence from OE Global. For more information, visit the 2020 OE Awards for Excellence site.

Feedback

Please use this survey to provide constructive feedback or report any errors https://cvtc.az1.qualtrics.com/jfe/form/SV_54PkuNI7Qb0ipJb.

ABOUT THIS BOOK

Editors

- Kimberly Ernstmeyer, MSN, RN, CNE, CHSE, APNP-BC
- Dr. Elizabeth Christman, DNP, RN, CNE

Graphics Editor

- Nic Ashman, MLIS, Librarian, Chippewa Valley Technical College

Developing Authors

Developing authors remixed existing open educational resources and developed new content based on evidence-based sources:

- Mallory Bohling, MSN, RN, Blackhawk Technical College
- Dr. Elizabeth Christman, DNP, RN, CNE, Chippewa Valley Technical College/Southern New Hampshire University
- Nicole Drees, MSN, RN, Northeast Wisconsin Technical College
- Kim Ernstmeyer, MSN, RN, CNE, CHSE, APNP-BC, Chippewa Valley Technical College
- Krista Huppert, MSN, RN, Chippewa Valley Technical College
- Erin Kupkovits, MSN, RN, Madison Area Technical College
- Dr. Tennille O'Connor, DNP, RN, CNE, Chippewa Valley Technical College/Pasco Hernando State College
- Barbara Peters, MSN, RN, Northeast Wisconsin Technical College
- Mary Pomietlo, MSN, RN, CNE, Chippewa Valley Technical College
- Rorey Pritchard, EdS, MEd, MSN, RN-BC, CNOR(E), CNE, Open RN Advisory Committee Member
- Dr. Julie Teeter, DNP, RN, CNE, Gateway Technical College

Contributors

Contributors assisted in the creation of this textbook:

- Samantha Bauer, MN, BS, RN, CNL, Madison Area Technical College
- Karrie Bruegman-May, MSN, BSN, MSOLQ, Moraine Park Technical College
- Jane Flesher, MST, Proofreader, Chippewa Valley Technical College
- Deanna Hoyord, Paramedic (retired), Human Patient Simulation Technician and Photographer, Chippewa Valley Technical College
- Lindsay Kuhlman, BSN, RN, HSHS Sacred Heart
- Theresa Meinen, MS, RRT, CHSE, Director of Clinical Education – Respiratory Therapy Program, Chippewa Valley Technical College

- Vince Mussehl, MLIS, Open RN Lead Librarian, Chippewa Valley Technical College
- Joshua Myers, Web Developer, Chippewa Valley Technical College
- Jody Myhre-Oechsle, MS, CPhT, Chippewa Valley Technical College
- Matthew Pomietlo, Technology Education Student, UW-Stout
- Meredith Pomietlo, Retail Design and Marketing Student, UW-Stout
- Lauren Richards, Graphics Designer, Chippewa Valley Technical College
- Celee Schuch, Nursing Student, St. Catherine University
- Dominic Slauson, Technology Professional Developer, Chippewa Valley Technical College
- Jamie Zwicky, MSN, RN, Moraine Park Technical College

Advisory Committee

The Open RN Advisory Committee consists of industry members and nursing deans and provides input for the Open RN textbooks and virtual reality scenarios:

- Jenny Bauer, MSN, RN, NPD-BC, Mayo Clinic Health System Northwest Wisconsin, Eau Claire, WI
- Gina Bloczynski, MSN, RN, Dean of Nursing, Chippewa Valley Technical College
- Angela Branum, Western Wisconsin Health
- Lisa Cannestra, Eastern Wisconsin Healthcare Alliance
- Travis Christman, MSN, RN, Clinical Director, HSHS Sacred Heart and St. Joseph's Hospitals
- Sheri Johnson, UW Population Health Institute
- Dr. Vicki Hulback, DNP, RN, Dean of Nursing, Gateway Technical College
- Jenna Julson, MSN, RN, NPD-BC, Nursing Education Specialist, Mayo Clinic Health System Northwest Wisconsin, Eau Claire, WI
- Brian Krogh, MSN, RN, Associate Dean – Health Sciences, Northeast Wisconsin Technical College
- Hugh Leasum, MBA, MSN, RN, Nurse Manager Cardiology/ICU, Marshfield Clinic Health System, Eau Claire, WI
- Pam Maxwell, SSM Health
- Mari Kay-Nobozny, NW Wisconsin Workforce Development Board
- Dr. Amy Olson, DNP, RN, Nursing Education Specialist, Mayo Clinic Health System Northwest Wisconsin, Eau Claire, WI
- Rorey Pritchard, EdS, MEd, MSN, RN-BC, CNOR(E), CNE, Senior RN Clinical Educator, Allevant Solutions, LLC
- Kelly Shafaie, MSN, RN, Associate Dean of Nursing, Moraine Park Technical College
- Dr. Ernise Watson, PhD, RN, Associate Dean of Nursing, Madison Area Technical College
- Sherry Willems, HSHS St. Vincent Hospital

Reviewers

Reviewers provided constructive feedback on the final draft of the textbook based on a rubric.

- Dr. Caryn Aleo, PhD, RN, CCRN, CEN, CNEcl, NHDP-BC, NPD-BC, Pasco-Hernando State College, New Port Richey, FL
- Dr. Kimberly Amos, PhD, MS(N), RN, CNE, Isothermal Community College, Spindale, NC
- Sara Annunziato, MSN, RN, Rockland Community College, Suffern, NY
- Megan Baldwin, MSN, RN, CNOR, MercyOne Medical Center, Des Moines, IA
- Lisa Bechard, MSN, RN, Mid-State Technical College, Wisconsin Rapids, WI
- Dr. Kim Belcik, PhD, RN-BC, CNE, Texas State University St. David's School of Nursing, Round Rock, TX
- Nancy Bonard, MSN, RN-BC, St. Joseph's College of Maine, Standish, ME
- Dr. Joan Buckley, PhD, RN, Nassau Community College, Garden City, NY
- Valerie J. Bugosh, MSN, RN, CNE, HACC, Harrisburg Area's Community College, Harrisburg, PA
- Dr. Sara I. Cano, PhD, RN, College of Southern Maryland, La Plata, MD
- Katherine Cart, MSN, RN, MAM, CEN, Blinn College, Brenham, TX
- Travis Christman, MSN, RN, HSHS Sacred Heart Hospital & St. Joseph's, Eau Claire, WI
- Dr. Andrea Dobogai, DNP, RN, Moraine Park Technical College, Fond du Lac, WI
- Stacy Svoma Doering, MAEd, RDMS, RVT, Chippewa Valley Technical College, Eau Claire, WI
- Jessica Dwork, MSN-Ed, RN, Phoenix College, Phoenix, AZ
- Dr. Kim English, RN, BScN, MN, EDD(c), Trent/Fleming School of Nursing, Peterborough & Durham Greater Toronto Area, Canada
- Dr. Rachael Farrell, EdD, MSN, RN, CNE, Howard Community College, Columbia, MD
- Kathleen Fraley, MSN, RN, St. Clair County Community College, Port Huron, MI
- Kailey Funk, MSN, RN, Madison College, Madison, WI
- Kristin Gadzinski, MSN, RN, Lakeshore Technical College, Cleveland, WI
- Amy Gatton, MSN, RN, CNE, Nicolet Area Technical College, Rhinelander, WI
- Julia Geurs, Nursing Student, St. Catherine University, St. Paul, MN
- Jillian Golde, MSN, RN, CMSRN, Vermont Technical College, Randolph, VT
- Anna Golembiewski, MSN, RN, Waukesha County Technical College, Pewaukee, WI
- Melissa Hauge, MSN, RN-BC, Madison College, Madison, WI
- Sharon Rhodes Hawkins, MPA, MSN/ed, RN, Sinclair Community College, Dayton, OH
- Lexa Hosier, Nursing Student, St. Catherine University, St. Paul, MN
- Katherine Howard, MS, RN-BC, CNE, Raritan Bay Medical Center Nursing Program at Middlesex County College, Edison, NJ
- Tracy Joosten, MSN, RN, FNP-BC, Mid-State Technical College, Wisconsin Rapids, WI

- Jenna Julson, MSN, RN, NPD-BC, Mayo Clinic Health System Northwest Wisconsin, Eau Claire, WI
- Dr. Andrew D. Kehl, DNP, MPH, APRN, RN, Vermont Technical College, Randolph, VT
- Lindsay Kuhlman, BSN, RN, HSHS Sacred Heart Hospital, Eau Claire, WI
- Dr. Colleen Kumar, PhD, RN, CNE, JFK Muhlenberg Harold B. and Dorothy A. Snyder Schools, Plainfield, NJ
- Erin Kupkovits, MSN, RN, Madison College, Madison, WI
- Dawn M. Lyon, MSN, RN, St. Clair County Community College, Port Huron, MI
- Jennifer Madkins, MSN, RNC-OB, C-EFM, CNE, Prince George's Community College, Largo, MD
- Dr. Lydia A. Massias, EdD, MS, RN, Pasco-Hernando State College, New Port Richey, FL
- Dr. Jamie Murphy, PhD, RN, State University of New York, Delhi, NY
- Jody Myhre-Oechsle, CPhT, MS, Chippewa Valley Technical College, Eau Claire, WI
- Kelly Nelson, MSN, RN, Mid-State Technical College, Wisconsin Rapids, WI
- Dr. Colleen Nevins, DNP, RN, CNE, CSU Channel Islands, Camarillo, CA
- Angela Ngo-Bigge, MSN, RN, FNP-C, Grossmont College, El Cajon, CA
- Dr. Allison A. Nicol, PhD, RN, CNE, Milwaukee Area Technical College, Milwaukee, WI
- Dr. Tennille O'Connor, DNP, RN, CNE, Pasco-Hernando State College, New Port Richey, FL
- Dr. Amy Olson, DNP, RN, Mayo Clinic Health System, Eau Claire, WI
- Dr. Grace Paul, DNP, RN, CNE, Glendale Community College, Glendale, AZ
- Barbara B. Peters, MSN, RN, Northeast Wisconsin Technical College, Niagara, WI
- Krista Polomis, MSN, RN, Nicolet College, Rhinelander, WI
- Mary A. Pomietlo, MSN, RN, CNE, University of Wisconsin-Eau Claire, Eau Claire, WI
- Dr. Regina Prusinski, DNP, APRN, CPNP-AC, FNP-BC, Otterbein University, Westerville, OH
- Jenna E. Raths, MSN, RN, Chippewa Valley Technical College, Eau Claire, WI
- Dr. Debbie Rickeard, DNP, MSN, BScN, BA, RN, CNE, CCRN, University of Windsor, Windsor, Ontario, Canada
- Ann K. Rosemeyer, MSN, RN, Chippewa Valley Technical College, Eau Claire, WI
- Callie Schlegel, Nursing Student, St. Catherine University, St. Paul, MN
- Celee Schuch, Nursing Student, St. Catherine University, St. Paul, MN
- Dr. Barbara Sinacori, PhD, RN, CNRN, CNE, Rutgers University, New Brunswick, NJ
- Dominic Slauson, MA, Chippewa Valley Technical College, Eau Claire, WI
- Jenna Sorenson, MSN, RN, CNE, Chippewa Valley Technical College, Eau Claire, WI
- Chassity Speight-Washburn, MSN, RN, CNE, Stanly Community College, Albemarle, NC
- Dr. Suzanne H. Tang, DNP, MSN, RN, FNP-BC, PHN, Rio Hondo College, Whittier, CA
- Alison L. Thompson, MSN, RN, Austin Community College, Austin, TX
- Barbara Timmons, MSN, RN, Fox Valley Technical College, Appleton, WI

- Jacquelyn R. Titus, MS, RN, Pasco-Hernando State College, New Port Richey, FL
- Jacqueline Tousignant, MSN, RN, WCC, Nicolet College, Rhinelander, WI
- Dr. Venius Turner-Gwin, DNP, RN, Jefferson State Community College, Birmingham, AL
- Amy Tyznik, MSN, RN, Moraine Park Technical College, Fond du Lac, WI
- Jennie Ver Steeg, MA, MS, MLS, Mercy College of Health Sciences/MercyOne Des Moines, Des Moines, IA
- Dr. Nancy Whitehead, PhD, APNP, RN, Milwaukee Area Technical College, Milwaukee, WI
- Dr. LaDonna Williams, DNP, RN, Lord Fairfax Community College, Warrenton, VA
- Jamie Zwicky, MSN, RN, Moraine Park Technical College, Fond du Lac, WI

Licensing/Terms of Use

Attributions

Some of the content in this textbook was adapted from the following open educational resources or materials available in the public domain. For specific citation and attribution details, please refer to the footnotes at the bottom of each page of the book.

- *Nursing Pharmacology* by *Chippewa Valley Technical College* is licensed under *CC BY 4.0.*
- *Nursing Fundamentals* by *Chippewa Valley Technical College* is licensed under *CC BY 4.0.*
- *Anatomy & Physiology* by *OpenStax* is licensed under *CC BY 4.0.* Access for free at https://openstax.org/books/anatomy-and-physiology/*pages/1-introduction*
- *Clinical Procedures for Safer Care* by *British Columbia Institute of Technology* is licensed under *CC BY 4.0.*

- *The Complete Subjective Health Assessment* by Lapum, St-Amant, Hughes, Petrie, Morrell, and Mistry is licensed under *CC BY 4.0*.
- *Human Development Life Span* by *Overstreet* is licensed under *CC BY 4.0*.
- *StatPearls* by *StatPearls Publishing* is licensed under *CC BY 4.0*.
- *Vital Sign Measurement Across the Lifespan – 1st Canadian Edition* by Ryerson University is licensed under *CC BY 4.0*.
- *Anatomy and Physiology* by *Boundless* is licensed under *CC BY-SA 4.0*.
- *The Scholarship of Writing in Nursing Education: 1st Canadian Edition* by Lapum, St-Amant, Hughes, Tan, Bogdan, Dimaranan, Frantzke, and Savicevic is licensed under *CC BY-SA 4.0*.
- World Health Organization (WHO)
- Centers for Disease Control and Prevention (CDC)
- U.S. National Institutes of Health's National Heart, Lung, and Blood Institute (NHLBI)

Content that is not taken from the above OER or public domain should include the following attribution statement:

> Ernstmeyer, K., & Christman, E. (Eds.). (2021). Open RN *Nursing Skills* by Chippewa Valley Technical College is licensed under *CC BY 4.0*.

STANDARDS & CONCEPTUAL APPROACH

The Open RN *Nursing Skills* textbook is based on several external standards and uses a conceptual approach.

External Standards

American Nurses Association (ANA):

The ANA provides standards for professional nursing practice including nursing standards and a code of ethics for nurses.

- https://www.nursingworld.org/ana/about-ana/standards/

The National Council Licensure Examination for Registered Nurses: NCLEX-PN and NCLEX-RN Test Plans

The NCLEX-RN and NCLEX-PN test plans are updated every three years to reflect fair, comprehensive, current, and entry-level nursing competency.

- https://www.ncsbn.org/nclex.htm

The National League of Nursing (NLN): Competencies for Graduates of Nursing Programs

NLN competencies guide nursing curricula to position graduates in a dynamic health care arena with practice that is informed by a body of knowledge and ensures that all members of the public receive safe, quality care.

- http://www.nln.org/professional-development-programs/competencies-for-nursing-education/nln-competencies-for-graduates-of-nursing-programs

Quality and Safety Education for Nurses (QSEN) Institute: Pre-licensure Competencies

Quality and safety competencies include knowledge, skills, and attitudes to be developed in nursing pre-licensure programs. QSEN competencies include patient-centered care, teamwork and collaboration, evidence-based practice, quality improvement, safety, and informatics.

- https://qsen.org/competencies/

Wisconsin State Legislature, Administrative Code Chapter N6

The Wisconsin Administrative Code governs the Registered Nursing and Practical Nursing professions in Wisconsin.

- https://docs.legis.wisconsin.gov/code/admin_code/n/6

Healthy People 2030

Healthy People 2030 envisions a society in which all people can achieve their full potential for health and well-being across the life span. Healthy People provides objectives based on national data and includes social determinants of health.

- https://health.gov/healthypeople

Conceptual Approach

The Open RN *Nursing Skills* textbook incorporates the following concepts across all chapters.

- **Holism.** Florence Nightingale taught nurses to focus on the principles of holism including wellness and the interrelationship of human beings and their environment. This textbook encourages the application of holism by assessing the impact of developmental, emotional, cultural, religious, and spiritual influences on a patient's health status.
- **Evidence Based Practice (EBP).** Textbook content is based on current, evidence-based practices that are referenced by footnotes. To promote digital literacy, hyperlinks are provided to credible, free, online resources that supplement content. The Open RN textbooks will be updated as new EBP is established and with the release of updated NCLEX Test Plans every three years.
- **Cultural Competency.** Nurses have an ethical and moral obligation to provide culturally competent care to the patients they serve based on the ANA Code of Ethics.[1] Cultural considerations are included throughout this textbook.
- **Care Across the Life Span.** Developmental stages are addressed regarding patient assessments and procedures.
- **Health Promotion.** Focused interview questions and patient education topics are included to promote patient well-being and encourage self-care behaviors.
- **Scope of Practice.** Assessment techniques are included that have been identified as frequently performed by entry-level nurse generalists.[2, 3, 4, 5]

---

1 American Nurses Association. (2015). *Code of ethics for nurses with interpretive statements.* American Nurses Association. https://www.nursingworld.org/practice-policy/nursing-excellence/ethics/code-of-ethics-for-nurses/

2 Anderson, B., Nix, E., Norman, B., & McPike, H. D. (2014). An evidence based approach to undergraduate physical assessment practicum course development. *Nurse Education in Practice, 14*(3), 242–246. https://doi.org/10.1016/j.nepr.2013.08.007

3 Giddens, J., & Eddy, L. (2009). A survey of physical examination skills taught in undergraduate nursing programs: Are we teaching too much? *Journal of Nursing Education, 48*(1), 24–29. https://doi.org/10.3928/01484834-20090101-05

4 Giddens, J. (2007). A survey of physical assessment techniques performed by RNs: Lessons for nursing education. *Journal of Nursing Education, 46*(2), 83–87. https://doi.org/10.3928/01484834-20070201-09

5 Morrell, S., Ralph, J., Giannotti, N., Dayus, D., Dennison, S., & Bornais, J. (2019). Physical assessment skills in nursing curricula: A scoping review protocol. *JBI Database System Rev Implement Rep., 17*(6), 1086-1091. https://doi.org/10.11124/jbisrir-2017-003981.

- **Patient Safety.** Expected and unexpected findings on assessment are highlighted in tables to promote patient safety by encouraging notification of health care providers when changes in condition occur.
- **Clear and Inclusive Language.** Content is written using clear language preferred by entry-level pre-licensure nursing students to enhance understanding of complex concepts.[6] "They" is used as a singular pronoun to refer to a person whose gender is unknown or irrelevant to the context of the usage, as endorsed by APA style. It is inclusive of all people and helps writers avoid making assumptions about gender.[7]
- **Open Source Images and Fair Use.** Images are included to promote visual learning. Students and faculty can reuse open source images by following the terms of their associated *Creative Commons licensing*. Some images are included based on Fair Use as described in the "*Code of Best Practices for Fair Use and Fair Dealing in Open Education*" presented at the OpenEd20 conference. Refer to the footnotes of images for source and licensing information throughout the text.
- **Open Pedagogy.** Students are encouraged to contribute to the Open RN textbooks in meaningful ways. In this textbook, students assisted in reviewing content for clarity for an entry-level learner and also assisted in creating open source images.[8]

Supplementary Material Provided

Several supplementary resources are provided with this textbook.

- Supplementary, free videos to promote student understanding of concepts and procedures
- Sample documentation for assessments and procedures
- Online learning activities with formative feedback
- Critical thinking questions that encourage application of content to patient scenarios
- Free downloadable versions for offline use

An affordable print version of this textbook is published by XanEdu and is available on Amazon and in college bookstores. It has been reported that over 65% of students prefer a print version of their textbooks.[9]

---

6 Verkuyl, M., Lapum, J., St-Amant, O., Bregstein, J., & Hughes, M. (2020). Healthcare students' use of an e-textbook open educational resource on vital sign measurement: A qualitative study. *Open Learning: The Journal of Open, Distance and e-Learning.* https://doi.org/10.1080/02680513.2020.1835623

7 American Psychological Association (2021). *Singular "They"*. https://apastyle.apa.org/style-grammar-guidelines/grammar/singular-they

8 The Open Pedagogy Notebook by Steel Wagstaff is licensed under CC BY 4.0. Access for free at http://openpedagogy.org/

9 Verkuyl, M., Lapum, J., St-Amant, O., Bregstein, J., & Hughes, M. (2020). Healthcare students' use of an e-textbook open educational resource on vital sign measurement: A qualitative study. *Open Learning: The Journal of Open, Distance and e-Learning.* https://doi.org/10.1080/02680513.2020.1835623

Chapter 1

General Survey

1.1 GENERAL SURVEY INTRODUCTION

My Notes

Learning Objectives

- Perform a general survey assessment, including vital signs, ability to communicate, appropriateness of behaviors and responses, general mobility, and basic nutritional and fluid status
- Modify assessment techniques to reflect variations across the life span, cultural values and beliefs, and gender expression
- Document actions and observations
- Recognize and report significant deviations from norms

"Learn to see, learn to hear, learn to feel, learn to smell, and know that by practice alone can you become expert."[1]

This quote provides a good description of learning how to perform a general survey assessment. A **general survey assessment** is a component of a patient assessment that observes the entire patient as a whole.

General surveys begin with the initial patient contact and continue throughout the helping relationship. In this instance, observation includes using all five senses to gather cues. Nurses begin assessing patients from the moment they meet them, noting their appearance, posture, gait, verbal communication, nonverbal communication, and behaviors. Cues obtained during a general survey assessment are used to guide additional focused assessments in areas of concern.

Introduction to the Nursing Process

Before discussing the components of a general survey, it is important to understand how assessment fits under the standards for professional nursing practice established by the American Nurses Association (ANA). These standards are the foundation of the nursing profession and include duties that all registered nurses, regardless of role or specialty, are expected to perform competently.[2] There are six components of the nursing process: Assessment, Diagnosis, Outcomes Identification, Planning, Implementation, and Evaluation. See Figure 1.1[3] for an illustration of the nursing process. The mnemonic ADOPIE is an easy way to remember the ANA Standards and the nursing process. The nursing process is a continuous, cyclic process that is constantly adapting to the patient's current health status. This textbook contains several chapters pertaining to techniques used during the assessment phase of the nursing process. Read more about the "Nursing Process" in the Open RN *Nursing Fundamentals* textbook.

---

1 Dallas Hall, W. (1990). Chapter 209: An overview of the general examination. In Walker, H. K., Hall, W. D., Hurst, J. W. (Eds.), *Clinical methods: The history, physical, and laboratory examinations* (3rd ed.). Butterworths. https://www.ncbi.nlm.nih.gov/books/NBK706/

2 American Nurses Association. (2015). *Nursing: Scope and standards of practice* (3rd ed.). American Nurses Association.

3 "The Nursing Process" by Kim Ernstmeyer at Chippewa Valley Technical College is licensed under CC BY 4.0. Access for free at https://drive.google.com/file/d/1uGaETRU2QdwAha_abX0woJpilIFZxF64/view?usp=sharing

My Notes

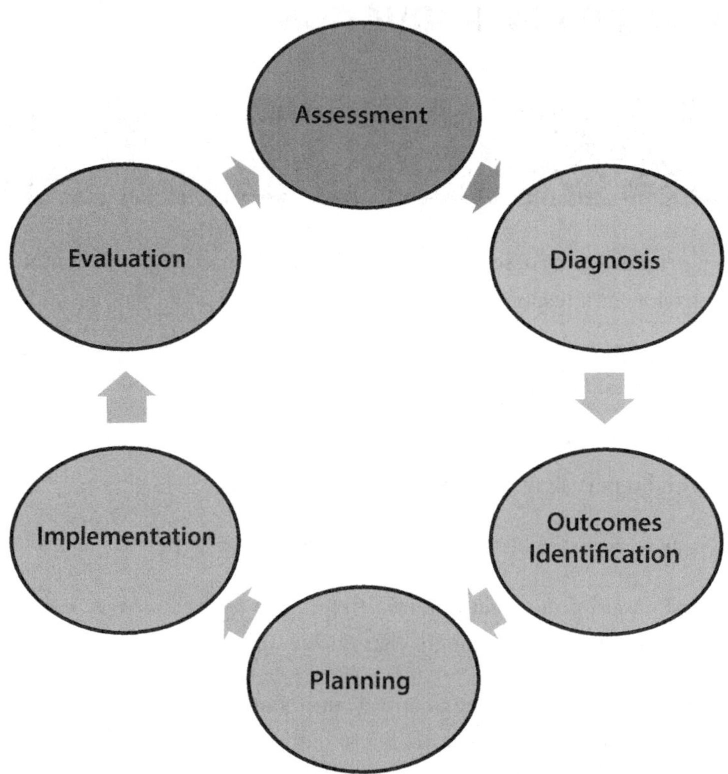

Figure 1.1 Nursing Process

Assessment

According to the ANA, assessment includes collecting "pertinent data, including but not limited to, demographics, social determinants of health, health disparities, and physical, functional, psychosocial, emotional, cognitive, sexual, cultural, age-related, environmental, spiritual/transpersonal, and economic assessments in a systematic, ongoing process with compassion and respect for the inherent dignity, worth, and unique attributes of every person."[4]

Patient data is considered either subjective or objective, and it can be collected from multiple sources.

Subjective Assessment Data

Subjective data is information obtained from the patient and/or family members and offers important cues from their perspectives. When documenting subjective data, it should be in quotation marks and start with verbiage such as, "The patient reports . . ." or "The patient's wife states . . ." It is vital for the nurse to establish rapport with a patient to obtain accurate, valuable subjective data regarding the mental, emotional, and spiritual aspects of their condition.

Example. An example of documented subjective data obtained from a patient assessment is, *"The patient reports pain severity of 2 on a 1-10 scale."* Additionally, if you create an inference, then that data is considered subjective. For example, documenting an inference, such as *"The patient appears anxious,"* is subjective data.

---

4 American Nurses Association. (2015). *Nursing: Scope and standards of practice* (3rd ed.). American Nurses Association.

My Notes

There are two types of subjective information, primary and secondary. **Primary data** is information provided directly by the patient. Patients are the best source of information about their bodies and feelings, and the nurse who actively listens to a patient will often learn valuable information while also promoting a sense of well-being. Information collected from a family member, chart, or other sources is known as **secondary data**.

Family members can provide important information, especially for infants and children or when the patient is unable to speak for themselves.

Objective Assessment Data

Objective data is anything that you can observe through your senses of hearing, sight, smell, and touch while assessing the patient. Objective data is reproducible, meaning another person can easily obtain the same data. Examples of objective data are vital signs, physical examination findings, and laboratory results.

Example. An example of documented objective data is, *"The patient's radial pulse is 58 and regular, and their skin feels warm and dry."*

Sources of Assessment Data

Assessment data is collected in three ways: during a focused interview, during physical examination, or while reviewing laboratory and diagnostic test results.

Interviewing

Interviewing includes asking the patient questions, listening, and observing verbal and nonverbal communication. Reviewing the chart prior to interviewing the patient eliminates redundancy in the interview process and allows the nurse to hone in on the most significant areas of concern or need for clarification. However, if information in the chart does not make sense or is incomplete, the nurse should use the interview process to verify data with the patient.

When beginning an interview, it may be helpful to start with questions related to the patient's medical diagnoses to gather information about how they have affected the patient's functioning, relationships, and lifestyle. Listen carefully and ask for clarification when something isn't clear to you. Patients may not volunteer important information because they don't realize it is important for their care. By using critical thinking and active listening, you may discover valuable cues that are important to provide safe, quality nursing care. Sometimes nursing students can feel uncomfortable with having difficult conversations or asking personal questions because of generational or other differences. Don't shy away from asking about information that is important to know for safe patient care. Most patients will be grateful that you cared enough to ask and listen.

Be alert and attentive to how the patient answers questions, as well as when they do not answer a question. Nonverbal communication and body language can be cues to important information that requires further investigation. A keen sense of observation is important. To avoid making inappropriate inferences, the nurse should validate any cues. For example, a nurse may make an inference that a patient is depressed when the patient avoids making eye contact during an interview. However, upon further questioning, the nurse may discover that the patient's cultural background believes direct eye contact to be disrespectful and this is why they are avoiding eye contact. Read more information about communicating with patients in the "Communication" chapter of the Open RN *Nursing Fundamentals* book.

My Notes

Physical Examination

Physical examination is a systematic data collection method of the body that uses the techniques of inspection, auscultation, palpation, and percussion. **Inspection** is the observation of a patient's anatomical structures. **Auscultation** is listening to sounds, such as heart, lung, and bowel sounds, created by organs using a stethoscope. **Palpation** is the use of touch to evaluate organs for size, location, or tenderness. **Percussion** is an advanced physical examination technique where body parts are tapped with fingers to determine their size and if fluid is present. See Figure 1.2[5] for an image of a nurse performing a physical examination.

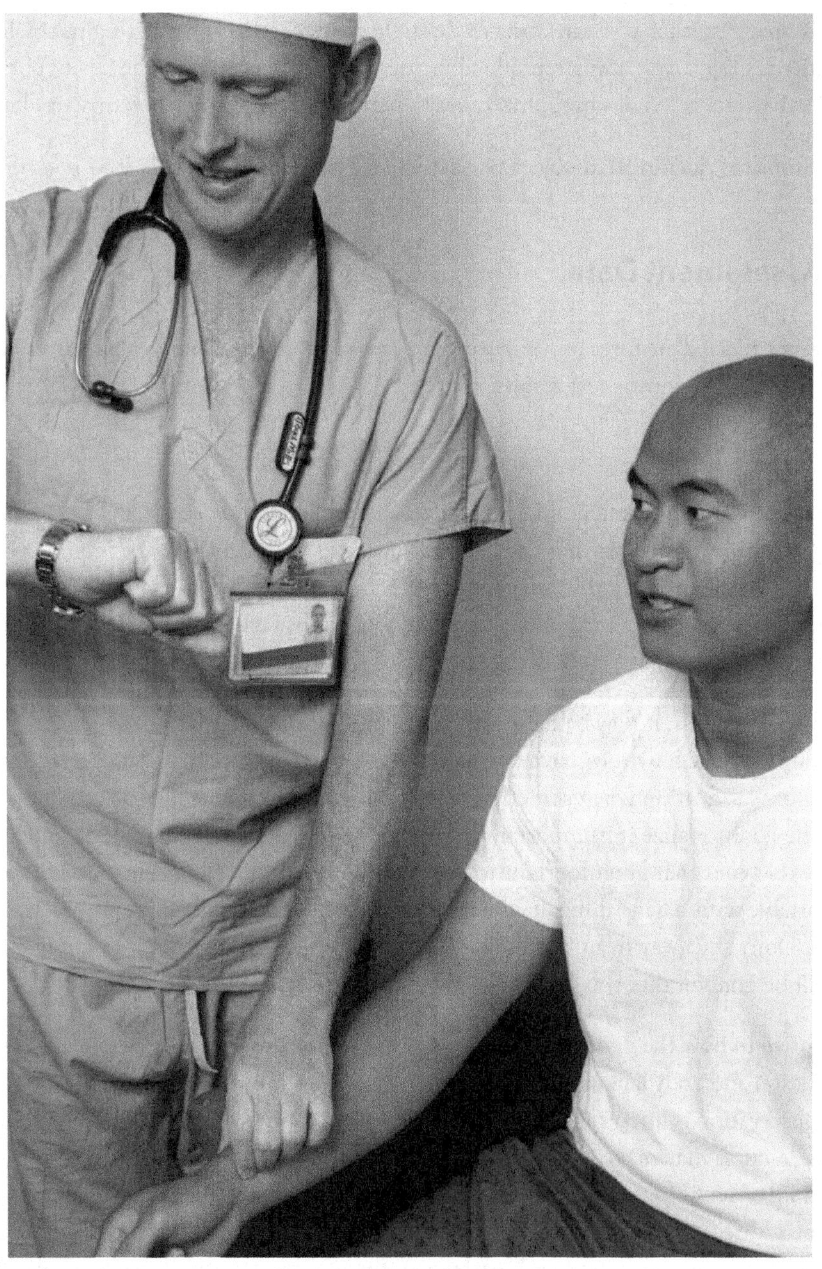

Figure 1.2 Physical Examination

5 "13394660711603.jpg" by CDC/ Amanda Mills is in the Public Domain. Access for free at http://www.publicdomainfiles.com/show_file.php?id=13394660711603

Registered Nurses (RNs) complete a physical examination and analyze the findings as part of the nursing process. Collection of physical examination data can be delegated to Licensed Practical Nurses/Licensed Vocational Nurses (LPNs/LVNs), or measurements such as vital signs and weight may be delegated to Unlicensed Assistive Personnel (UAP) when it is appropriate to do so. However, the RN remains responsible for analyzing the findings.

Assessment data is documented in the patient's electronic medical record (EMR), an electronic version of the patient's medical chart.

Reviewing Laboratory and Diagnostic Test Results

Reviewing laboratory and diagnostic test results is an important component of the assessment phase of the nursing process and provides relevant and useful information related to the needs of the patient.

Understanding how normal and abnormal results affect patient care is important when implementing the nursing care plan and administering prescriptions. Read more about interpreting laboratory and diagnostic testing results based on nursing concepts in the Open RN *Nursing Fundamentals* textbook.

My Notes

1.2 INITIATING PATIENT INTERACTION

Before every patient interaction, the nurse must perform hand hygiene and consider the use of additional personal protective equipment, introduce themselves, and identify the patient using two different identifiers. It is also important to provide a culturally safe space for interaction and to consider the developmental stage of the patient.

Hand Hygiene and Infection Prevention

Before initiating care with a patient, hand hygiene is required and a risk assessment should be performed to determine the need for personal protective equipment (PPE). This is important for protection of both patient and nurse.

Hand Hygiene

Using hand hygiene is a simple but effective way to prevent infection when performed correctly and at the appropriate times when providing patient care. See Figure 1.3.[1] for an image about hand hygiene from the Centers for Disease Control (CDC).[2] Use the hyperlinks provided below to read more information and watch a video about effective handwashing. Key points from the CDC about hand hygiene include the following:[3]

- In general, hand sanitizers are as effective as washing with soap and water and are less drying to the skin. When using hand sanitizer, use enough gel to cover both hands and rub for approximately 20 seconds, coating all surfaces of both hands until your hands feel dry. Go directly to the patient without putting your hands into pockets or touching anything else.[4]
- Be sure to wash with soap and water if your hands are visibly soiled or the patient has diarrhea from suspected or confirmed *C. Difficile* (C-diff).
- Clean all areas of the hands including the front and back, the fingertips, the thumbs, and between fingers.
- Gloves are not a substitute for cleaning your hands. Wash your hands after removing gloves.
- Hand hygiene should be performed at these times:
    - Immediately before touching a patient
    - Before performing an aseptic task (e.g., placing an indwelling device) or handling invasive medical devices
    - Before moving from working on a soiled body site to a clean body site on the same patient
    - After contact with blood, body fluids, or contaminated surfaces
    - Immediately after glove removal
    - When leaving the area after touching a patient or their immediate environment

---

1 "Animated-Logo-Clean-Hands-Count" by Centers for Disease Control and Prevention is licensed under CC0. Access for free at https://www.cdc.gov/handhygiene/campaign/index.html

2 Centers for Disease Control and Prevention. (2019, April 29). *Hand hygiene.* https://www.cdc.gov/handhygiene/index.html

3 Centers for Disease Control and Prevention. (2019, April 29). *Hand hygiene.* https://www.cdc.gov/handhygiene/index.html

4 Centers for Disease Control and Prevention. (2019, April 29). *Hand hygiene.* https://www.cdc.gov/handhygiene/index.html

My Notes

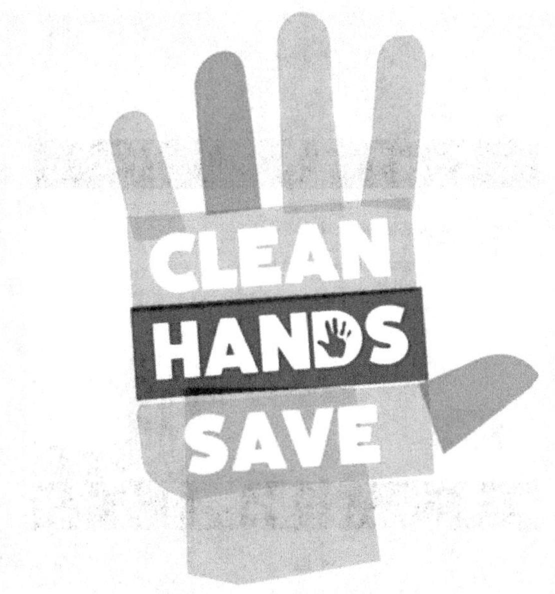

Figure 1.3 Hand Hygiene

Checklists for performing handwashing and using hand sanitizer are located in Appendix A.

Visit the Center for Disease Control and Prevention's website to read more about "Hand Hygiene in Healthcare Settings" (https://www.cdc.gov/handhygiene/index.html).

Download a factsheet from the Center for Disease Control and Prevention called "Clean Hands Count" (https://www.cdc.gov/handhygiene/pdfs/Provider-Factsheet-508.pdf).

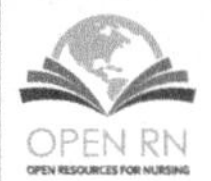

My Notes

Video Reviews of Hand Hygiene

Clean Hands Count[5]

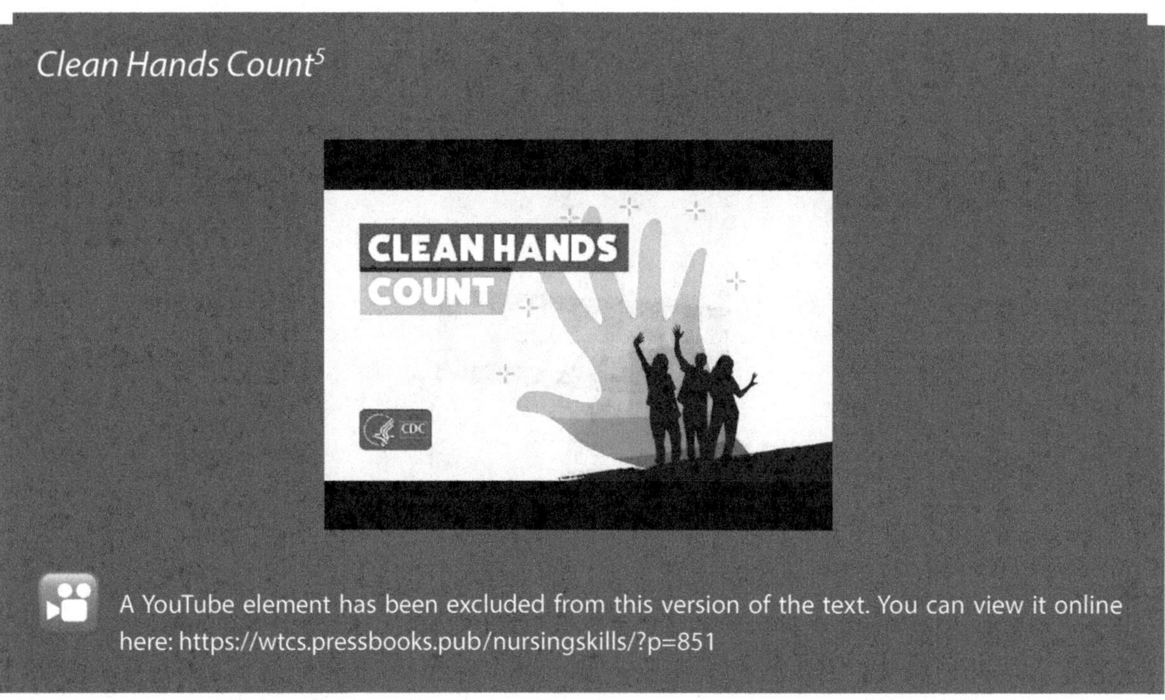

A YouTube element has been excluded from this version of the text. You can view it online here: https://wtcs.pressbooks.pub/nursingskills/?p=851

Hand Washing Technique[6]

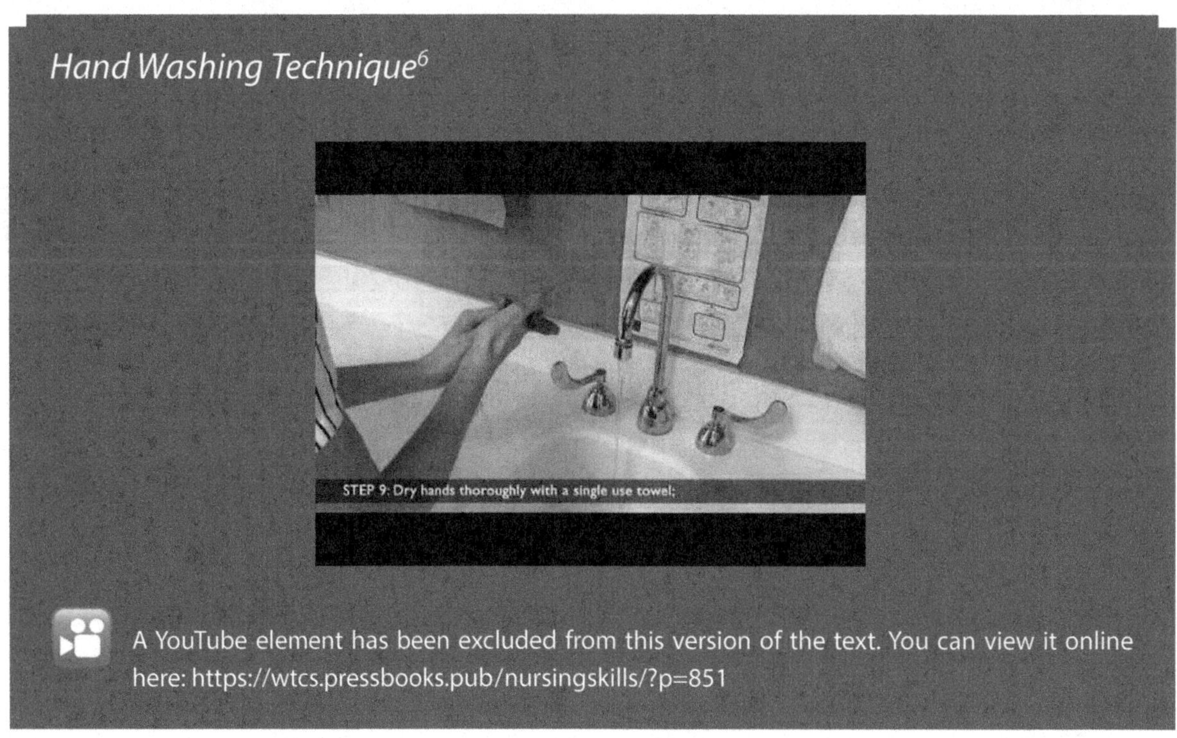

A YouTube element has been excluded from this version of the text. You can view it online here: https://wtcs.pressbooks.pub/nursingskills/?p=851

5 Centers for Disease Control and Prevention. (2017, May 5). *Clean hands count*. [Video]. YouTube. All rights reserved. https://youtu.be/MzkNSzqmUSY

6 Johns Hopkins Medicine. (2019, March 26). *Hand-washing steps using the WHO technique*. [Video]. YouTube. All rights reserved. https://youtu.be/IisgnbMfKvI

My Notes

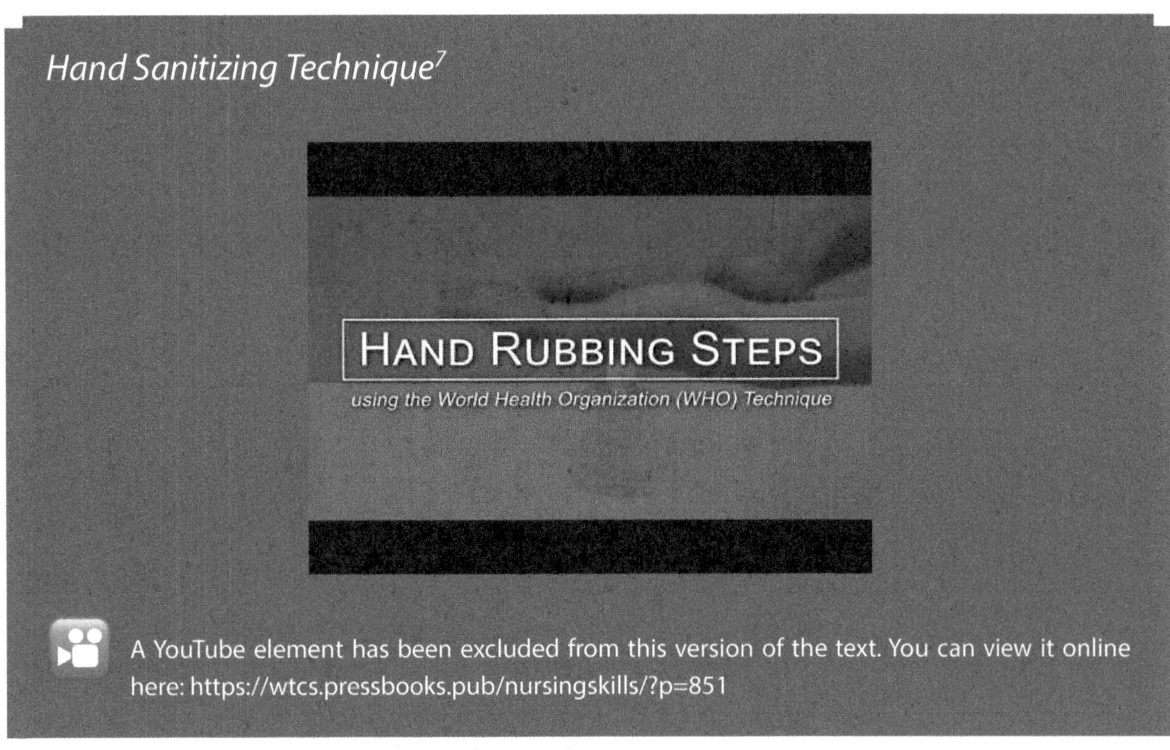

Hand Sanitizing Technique[7]

A YouTube element has been excluded from this version of the text. You can view it online here: https://wtcs.pressbooks.pub/nursingskills/?p=851

Check your knowledge with this learning activity.

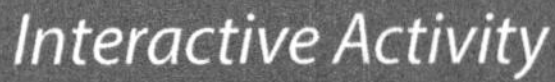

Interactive Activity

An interactive or media element has been excluded from this version of the text. You can view it online here: https://wtcs.pressbooks.pub/nursingskills/?p=851

Personal Protective Equipment (PPE)

Medical asepsis is a term used to describe measures to prevent the spread of infection in health care agencies. Performing hand hygiene at appropriate times during patient care and applying gloves when there is potential risk to body fluids are examples of using medical asepsis. Additional precautions are implemented by health care team members when a patient has, or is suspected of having, an infectious disease. These additional precautions are called **personal protective equipment (PPE)** and are based on how an infection is transmitted, such as by contact, droplet, or airborne routes. Personal protective equipment (PPE) includes gowns, eyewear, face shields, and masks. PPE is used along with environmental controls, such as surface cleaning and disinfecting to prevent

7 Johns Hopkins Medicine. (2019, May 8). *Hand rubbing steps using the WHO technique.* [Video]. YouTube. All rights reserved. https://youtu.be/B3eq5fLzAOo

My Notes

the transmission of infection.[8] See Figure 1.4[9] for an image of health care team members applying PPE. These precautions are further discussed in the "Aseptic Technique" chapter. For the purpose of this chapter, be sure to perform a general risk assessment before entering a patient's room and apply the appropriate PPE as needed. This risk assessment includes:

- Is there signage posted on the patient's door that contact, droplet, or airborne precautions are in place? If so, follow the instructions provided.
- Does this patient have a confirmed or suspected infection or communicable disease?
- Will your face, hands, skin, mucous membranes, or clothing be potentially exposed to blood or body fluids by spray, coughing, or sneezing?

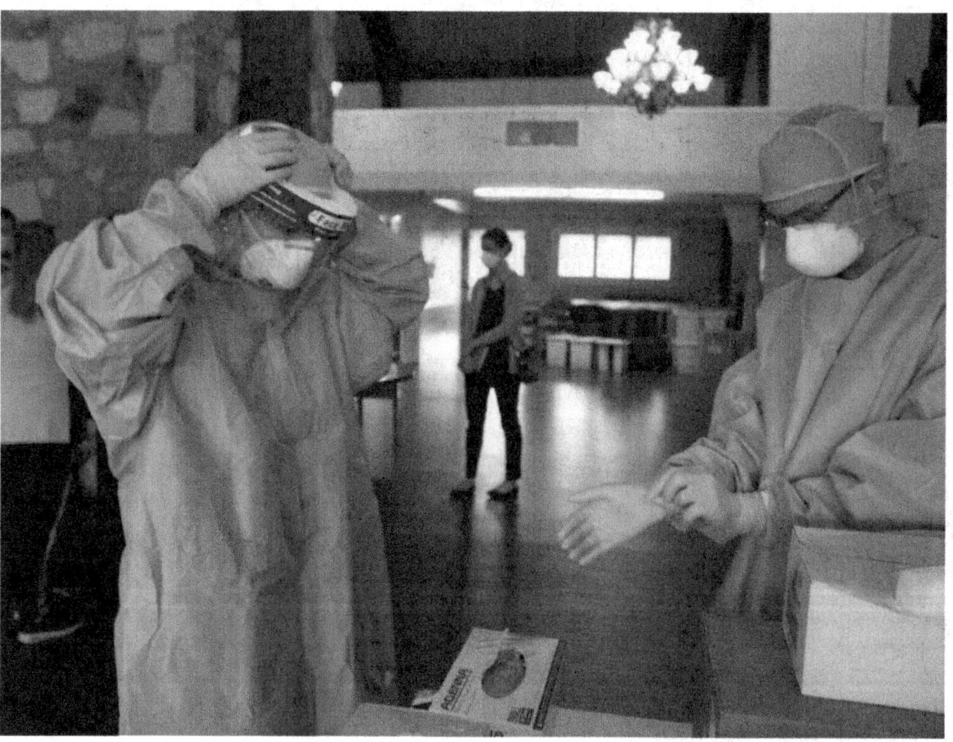

Figure 1.4 Application of Personal Protective Equipment

Introducing Oneself

When initiating care with patients, it is essential to first provide privacy, and then introduce yourself and explain what will be occurring. Providing privacy means taking actions such as talking with the patient privately in a room with the door shut. A common framework used for introductions during patient care is **AIDET**, a mnemonic for Acknowledge, Introduce, Duration, Explanation, and Thank You.[10]

8 This work is a derivative of Clinical Procedures for Safer Patient Care by British Columbia Institute of Technology licensed under CC BY 4.0. Access for free at https://opentextbc.ca/clinicalskills/front-matter/introduction-edit-this-version/

9 "Pennsylvania_National_Guard_(49923831732).jpg" by The National Guard is in the Public Domain. Access for free at https://commons.wikimedia.org/wiki/File:Pennsylvania_National_Guard_(49923831732).jpg

10 Huron. (n.d.). *AIDET patient communication.* https://www.studergroup.com/aidet

My Notes

- **Acknowledge:** Greet the patient by the name documented in their medical record. Make eye contact, smile, and acknowledge any family or friends in the room. Ask the patient their preferred way of being addressed (for example, "Mr. Doe," "Jonathon," or "Johnny") and their preferred pronouns (i.e., he/him, she/her or they/them), as appropriate.
- **Introduce:** Introduce yourself by your name and role. For example, "I'm John Doe and I am a nursing student working with your nurse to take care of you today."
- **Duration:** Estimate a time line for how long it will take to complete the task you are doing. For example, "I am here to obtain your blood pressure, heart rate, and oxygen saturation levels. This should take about 5 minutes."
- **Explanation:** Explain step by step what to expect next and answer questions. For example, "I will be putting this blood pressure cuff on your arm and inflating it. It will feel as if it is squeezing your arm for a few moments."
- **Thank You:** At the end of the encounter, thank the patient and ask if anything is needed before you leave. In an acute or long-term care setting, ensure the call light is within reach and the patient knows how to use it. If family members are present, thank them for being there to support the patient as appropriate. For example, "Thank you for taking time to talk with me today. Is there anything I can get for you before I leave the room? Here is the call light (Place within reach). Press the red button if you would like to call the nurse."

For more information about AIDET, visit "AIDET Patient Communication." https://www.studergroup.com/aidet

Patient Identification

Before performing assessments, obtaining vital signs, or providing care, patients must be properly identified using two identifiers.

First identifier:

- Ask the patient to state their name and date of birth. If they have an armband, compare the information they are stating to the information on the armband and verify they match. See Figure 1.5[11] for an image of an armband.
- If the patient doesn't have an armband, confirm the information they are stating to information provided in the chart.
- If the patient is unable to state their name and date of birth, scan their armband or ask another staff member or family member to identify them.

Confirm first identifier with a different second identifier:

- Scan the wristband.
- Compare the name and date of birth to the patient's chart.
- Ask staff to verify the patient in a long-term care setting.

11 "barcode_clinic_fist_hand_healthcare_hospital_identification_identity-1517387.jpg" by rawpixel.com is licensed under CC0. Access for free at https://pxhere.com/sv/photo/1517387

My Notes

- Compare the picture on the medication administration record (MAR) to the patient.
- If present, ask a family member to confirm the patient's name.

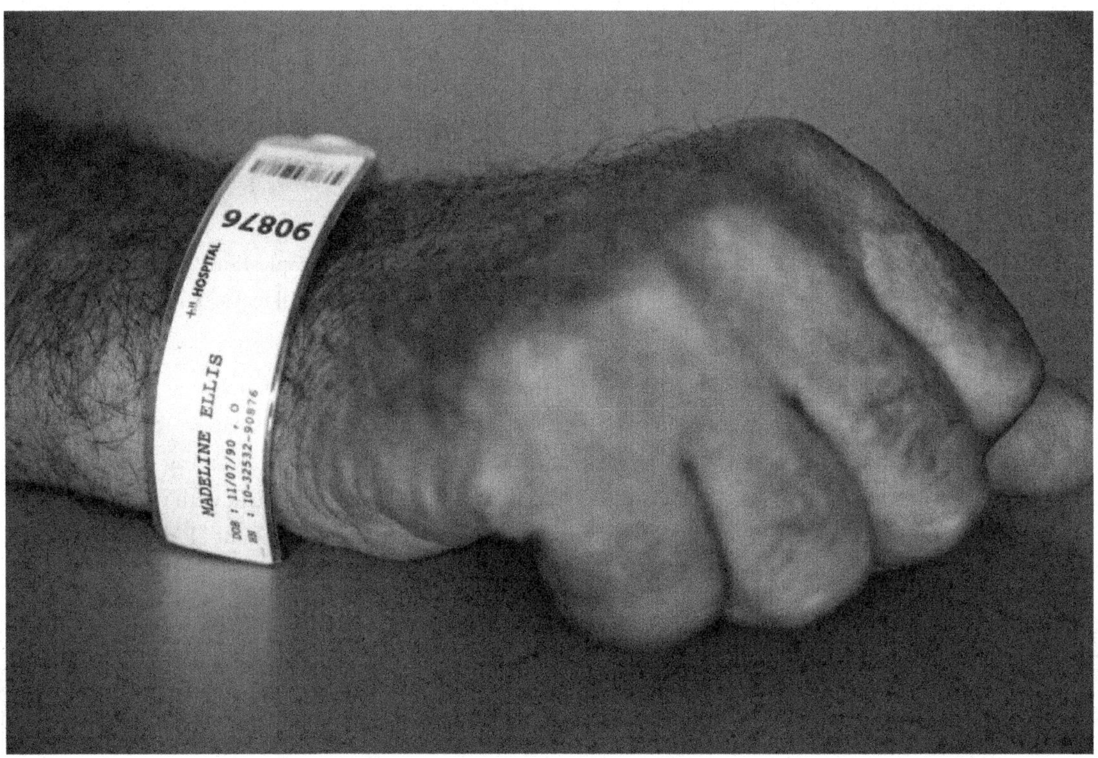

Figure 1.5 Patient Identification Armband

Cultural Safety

When initiating patient interaction, it is important to establish cultural safety. **Cultural safety** refers to the creation of safe spaces for patients to interact with health professionals without judgment or discrimination. See Figure 1.6[12] for an image representing cultural safety. Recognizing that you and all patients bring a cultural context to interactions in a health care setting is helpful when creating cultural safe spaces. If you discover you need more information about a patient's cultural beliefs to tailor your care, use an open-ended question that allows the patient to share what they believe to be important. For example, you may ask, "I am interested in your cultural background as it relates to your health. Can you share with me what is important about your cultural background that will help me care for you?"[13]

For more information about caring for diverse patients, visit the "Diverse Patients" chapter in the Open RN *Nursing Fundamentals* textbook.

12 "MODEL OF MULTINATIONAL UNITY" by Margherita Marchetti is licensed under CC0 Access for free at https://pixy.org/99952/

13 This work is a derivative of The Complete Subjective Health Assessment by Lapum, St-Amant, Hughes, Petrie, Morrell, & Mistry and is licensed under CC BY 4.0. Access for free at

My Notes

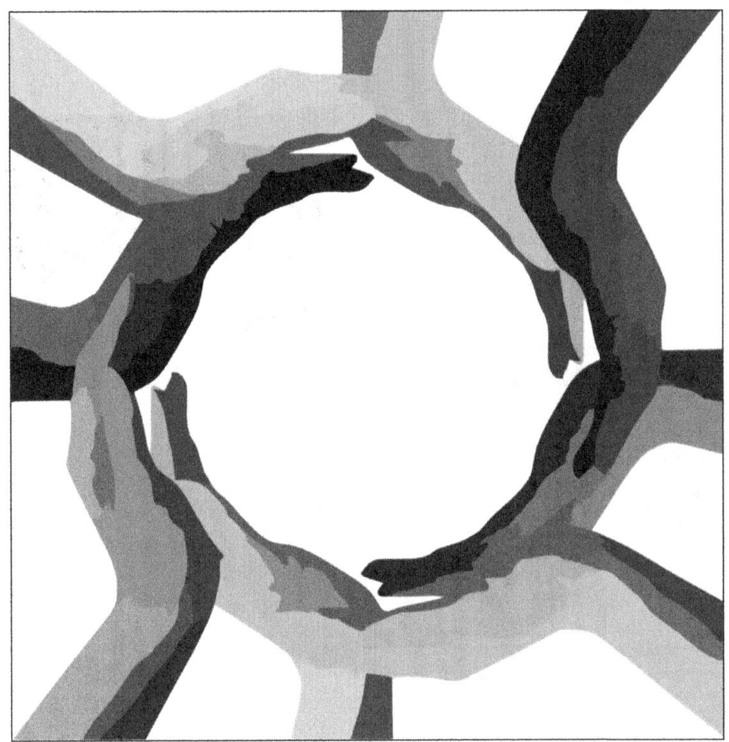

Figure 1.6 Cultural Safety Creates Safe Spaces for Everyone

Adapting to Variations Across the Life Span

It is important to adapt your interactions with patients in accordance their **developmental stage**. Developmentalists break the life span into nine stages[14]:

- Prenatal Development
- Infancy and Toddlerhood
- Early Childhood
- Middle Childhood
- Adolescence
- Early Adulthood
- Middle Adulthood
- Late Adulthood
- Death and Dying

A brief overview of the characteristics of each stage of human development is provided in Table 1.2. When caring for infants, toddlers, children, and adolescents, parents or guardians are an important source of information, and family dynamics should be included as part of the general survey assessment. When caring for older adults

14 This work is a derivative of Human Development Life Span by Laura Overstreet and is licensed under CC BY 4.0. Access for free at https://socialsci.libretexts.org/Bookshelves/Human_Development/Book%3A_Human_Development_Life_Span_(Overstreet)

My Notes

or those who are dying, other family members may be important to include in the general survey assessment. See Figure 1.7[15] for an image representing patients in various developmental stages of life.

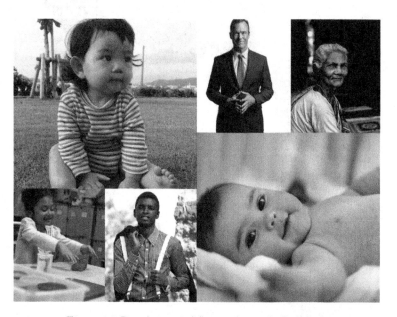

Figure 1.7 Developmental Stages Across the Life Span

Visit the *Human Development Life Span* e-book at LibreTexts to read additional information about human development across the life span (https://socialsci.libretexts.org/Bookshelves/Human_Development/Book%3A_Human_Development_Life_Span_(Overstreet)).

15 "pexels-photo-1556706.jpeg" by Daniel Reche is licensed under CC0 Access for free at https://www.pexels.com/photo/baby-lying-on-pink-bed-1556706/; "kids-1675964_960_720.jpg" by auntmasako is licensed under CC0. Access for free at https://pixabay.com/de/photos/kinder-kleinkind-m%C3%A4dchen-h%C3%BCbsch-1675964/; "100312-F-6448T-001.JPG" by U.S. Air Force photo/Senior Airman Timothy Taylor is licensed under CC0. Access for free at https://www.jbcharleston.jb.mil/News/Article/235563/jb-chs-school-age-program-receives-accreditation/; "smart-3479338_1280.jpg" by malcolmbeldon4 is licensed under CC0. Access for free at https://pixabay.com/photos/smart-young-adult-3479338/; "Business man" by Tim Engle is licensed under CC BY-NC 2.0. Access for free at https://www.flickr.com/photos/thefoto/49435874813/in/photolist-2ijtMgc-FcrirQ-7JYac9-yzqbbA-fQ6o6S-ftA52-a793kf-9Qd4Tm-aB8QzC-bBKJXm-cwkjLd-mQSvr-6RoWiG-85WsN7-3zGJuf-5cE1XK-6RjTAZ-519rRz-aB8Q3G-LhqCV-4Czd3M-6RoWo7-rtmk6-89ouFB-c1NKPN-izVYe-9ZAeyz-NEV6H-okgku7-TX5Xzw-9LgQx-2JHnws-zgAuJu-72XjXX-RvbSHq-s12ipq-2g7HoWX-9hv2jV-9sciZB-Kj2tfm-83iWnD-2jo9wy7-rRpuZt-2isWTUy-GWCVtS-2juw9oj-SqJx85-qMVkUX-2jwjG6E-2ibHr8e; "Portrait of an old woman in front of her home" by Nithi Anand is licensed under CC BY 2.0. Access for free at https://www.flickr.com/photos/nithiclicks/37595441820/in/photostream/

My Notes

Table 1.2 Variations Across the Life Span	
Stage of Development	**Common Characteristics**
Prenatal Development	Conception occurs and development begins. All major structures of the body are forming and the health of the mother is of primary concern. Understanding nutrition, teratogens (environmental factors that can lead to birth defects), and labor and delivery are primary concerns for the mother.
Infancy and Toddlerhood	The first year and a half to two years of life are ones of dramatic growth and change. A newborn with a keen sense of hearing but very poor vision is transformed into a walking, talking toddler within a relatively short period of time. Caregivers are also transformed from someone who manages feeding and sleep schedules to a constantly moving guide and safety inspector for a mobile, energetic child.
Early Childhood	Early childhood is also referred to as the preschool years, consisting of the years that follow toddlerhood and precede formal schooling. As a three- to five-year-old, the child is busy learning language, gaining a sense of self and greater independence, and beginning to learn the workings of the physical world. This knowledge does not come quickly however, and preschoolers may have initially interesting conceptions of size, time, space, and distance, such as fearing that they may go down the drain if they sit at the front of the bathtub. A toddler's fierce determination to do something may give way to a four-year-old's sense of guilt for doing something that brings the disapproval of others.
Middle Childhood	The ages of six through eleven comprise middle childhood, and much of what children experience at this age is connected to their involvement in the early grades of school. Their world becomes filled with learning and testing new academic skills, assessing one's abilities and accomplishments, and making comparisons between self and others. Schools compare students and make these comparisons public through team sports, test scores, and other forms of recognition. Growth rates slow down and children are able to refine their motor skills at this point in life. Children begin to learn about social relationships beyond the family through interaction with friends and fellow students.
Adolescence	The World Health Organization defines adolescence as a person between the age of 10 and 19. Adolescence is a period of dramatic physical change marked by an overall physical growth spurt and sexual maturation, known as puberty. It is also a time of cognitive change as the adolescent begins to think of new possibilities and to consider abstract concepts such as love, fear, and freedom. Adolescents have a sense of invincibility that puts them at greater risk of injury from high-risk behaviors such as car accidents, drug and alcohol abuse, or contracting sexually transmitted infections that can have lifelong consequences or result in death.
Early Adulthood	The twenties and thirties are often thought of as early adulthood. It is a time of physiological peak but also highest risk for involvement in violent crimes and substance abuse. It is a time of focusing on the future and putting a lot of energy into making choices that will help one earn the status of a full adult in the eyes of others. Love and work are primary concerns at this stage of life.

My Notes

Stage of Development	Common Characteristics
Middle Adulthood	The late thirties through the mid-sixties is referred to as middle adulthood. This is a period in which aging processes that began earlier become more noticeable but also a time when many people are at their peak of productivity in love and work. It can also be a time of becoming more realistic about possibilities in life previously considered and of recognizing the difference between what is possible and what is likely to be achieved in their lifetime.
Late Adulthood	This period of the life span has increased over the last 100 years. For nurses, patients in this period are referred to as "**older adults.**" The term "young old" is used to describe people between 65 and 79, and the term "old old" is used for those who are 80 and older. One of the primary differences between these groups is that the young old are very similar to midlife adults because they are still working, still relatively healthy, and still interested in being productive and active. The "old old" may remain productive, active, and independent, but risks of the heart disease, lung disease, cancer, and cerebral vascular disease (i.e., strokes) increase substantially for this age group. Issues of housing, health care, and extending active life expectancy are only a few of the topics of concern for this age group. A better way to appreciate the diversity of people in late adulthood is to go beyond chronological age and examine whether a person is experiencing optimal aging (when they are in very good health for their age and continue to have an active, stimulating life), normal aging (when the changes in health are similar to most of those of the same age), or impaired aging (when more physical challenges and diseases occur compared to others of the same age).
Death and Dying	Death is the final stage of life. Dying with dignity allows an individual to make choices about treatment, say goodbyes, and take care of final arrangements. When caring for patients who are actively dying, nurses can advocate for care that allows that person to die with dignity according to their wishes.

1.3 VITAL SIGNS

My Notes

Vital signs are typically obtained prior to performing a physical assessment. Vital signs include temperature recorded in Celsius or Fahrenheit, pulse, respiratory rate, blood pressure, and oxygen saturation using a pulse oximeter. See Figure 1.8[1] for an image of a nurse obtaining vital signs. Obtaining vital signs may be delegated to unlicensed assistive personnel (UAP) for stable patients, depending on the state's nurse practice act, agency policy, and appropriate training. However, the nurse is always accountable for analyzing the vital signs and instituting appropriate follow-up for out-of-range findings. See "Appendix A" to review a checklist for obtaining vital signs.

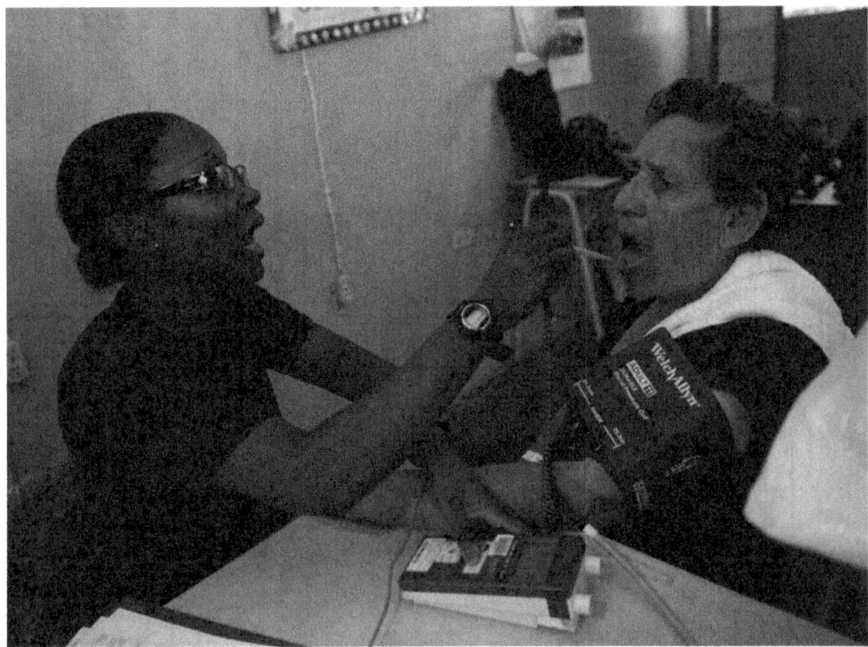

Figure 1.8 Obtaining Vital Signs

The order of obtaining vital signs is based on the patient and their situation. Health care professionals often place the pulse oximeter probe on the patient while proceeding to obtain their pulse, respirations, blood pressure, and temperature. However, in some situations this order is modified based on the urgency of their condition. For example, if a person loses consciousness, the assessment begins with checking their carotid pulse to determine if cardiopulmonary resuscitation (CPR) is required.[2]

1 "US Navy 110714-N-RM525-060 Hospitalman Seckisiesha Isaac, from New York, prepares to take a woman's temperature at a pre-screening vital signs stat.jpg" by U.S. Navy photo by Mass Communication Specialist 2nd Class Jonathen E. Davis is licensed under CC0. Access for free at https://commons.wikimedia.org/wiki/File:US_Navy_110714-N-RM525-060_Hospitalman_Seckisiesha_Isaac,_from_New_York,_prepares_to_take_a_woman%27s_temperature_at_a_pre-screening_vital_signs_stat.jpg

2 Vital Sign Measurement Across the Lifespan by Ryerson University is licensed under CC BY-SA 4.0. Access for free at https://med.libretexts.org/Bookshelves/Nursing/Book%3A_Vital_Sign_Measurement_Across_the_Lifespan_(Lapum_et_al.)

My Notes

Temperature

Accurate temperature measurements provide information about a patient's health status and guide clinical decisions. Methods of measuring body temperature vary based on the patient's developmental age, cognitive functioning, level of consciousness, and health status, as well as agency policy. Common methods of temperature measurement include oral, tympanic, axillary, and rectal routes. It is important to document the route used to obtain a patient's temperature because of normal variations in temperature in different locations of the body. Body temperature is typically measured and documented in health care agencies in degrees Celsius (ºC).[3]

Oral Temperature

Normal oral temperature is 35.8 – 37.3ºC (96.4 – 99.1ºF). An oral thermometer is shown in Figure 1.9.[4] The device has blue coloring, indicating it is an oral or axillary thermometer, as opposed to a rectal thermometer that has red coloring. Oral temperature is reliable when it is obtained close to the sublingual artery.[5]

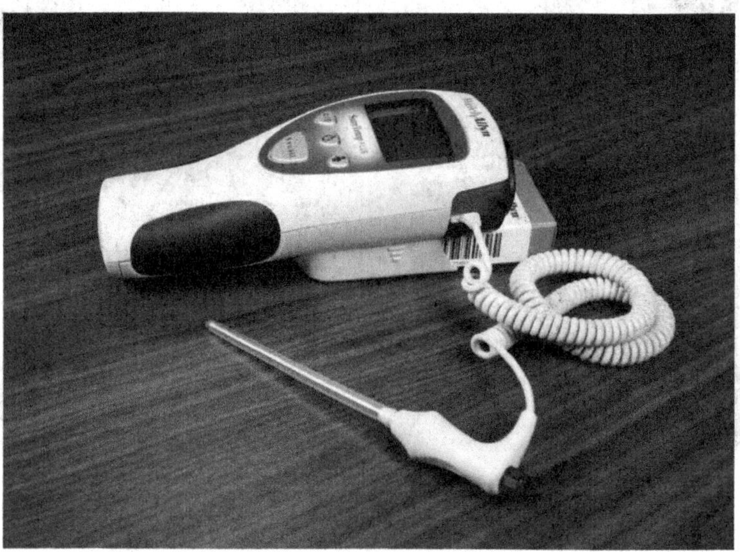

Figure 1.9 Oral Thermometer

Technique

Remove the probe from the device and slide a probe cover (from the attached box) onto the oral thermometer without touching the probe cover with your hands. Place the thermometer in the posterior sublingual pocket under the tongue, slightly off-center. Instruct the patient to keep their mouth closed but not bite on the thermometer. Leave the thermometer in place for as long as is indicated by the device manufacturer. The thermometer

---

3 Vital Sign Measurement Across the Lifespan by Ryerson University is licensed under CC BY-SA 4.0. Access for free at https://med.libretexts.org/Bookshelves/Nursing/Book%3A_Vital_Sign_Measurement_Across_the_Lifespan_(Lapum_et_al.)

4 "Thermometer-oral-768x548.jpg" by British Columbia Institute of Technology is licensed under CC BY 4.0. Access for free at https://med.libretexts.org/Bookshelves/Nursing/Book%3A_Vital_Sign_Measurement_Across_the_Lifespan_(Lapum_et_al.)/02%3A_Temperature/2.17%3A_Oral_Temperature

5 Vital Sign Measurement Across the Lifespan by Ryerson University is licensed under CC BY-SA 4.0. Access for free at https://med.libretexts.org/Bookshelves/Nursing/Book%3A_Vital_Sign_Measurement_Across_the_Lifespan_(Lapum_et_al.)

My Notes

typically beeps within a few seconds when the temperature has been taken. Read the digital display of the results. Discard the probe cover in the garbage (without touching the cover) and place the probe back into the device.[6] See Figure 1.10[7] of an oral temperature being taken.

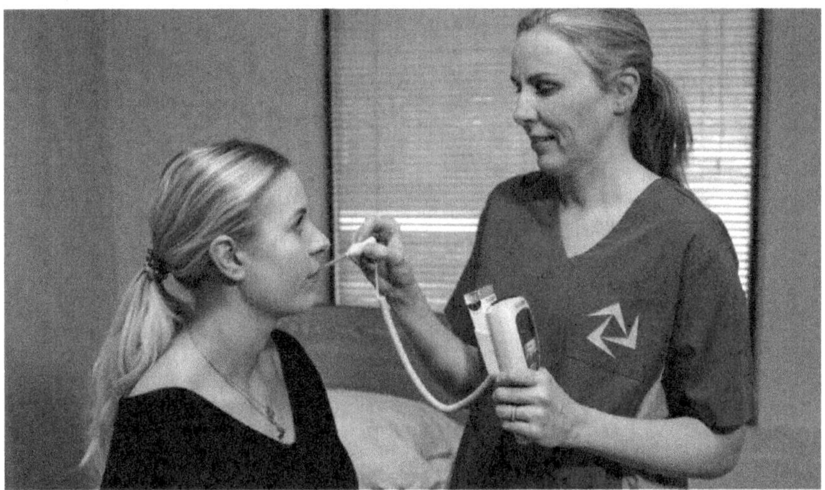

Figure 1.10 Oral Temperature

Some factors can cause an inaccurate measurement using the oral route. For example, if the patient recently consumed a hot or cold food or beverage, chewed gum, or smoked prior to measurement, a falsely elevated or decreased reading may be obtained. Oral temperature should be taken 15 to 25 minutes following consumption of a hot or cold beverage or food or 5 minutes after chewing gum or smoking.[8]

Tympanic Temperature

The tympanic temperature is typically 0.3 – 0.6°C higher than an oral temperature. It is an accurate measurement because the tympanic membrane shares the same vascular artery that perfuses the hypothalamus (the part of the brain that regulates the body's temperature). See Figure 1.11[9] of a tympanic thermometer. The tympanic method should not be used if the patient has a suspected ear infection.[10]

6 Vital Sign Measurement Across the Lifespan by Ryerson University is licensed under CC BY-SA 4.0. Access for free at https://med.libretexts.org/Bookshelves/Nursing/Book%3A_Vital_Sign_Measurement_Across_the_Lifespan_(Lapum_et_al.)

7 "Oral-Temperature-Wide-768x512.jpg" by British Columbia Institute of Technology is licensed under CC BY 4.0. Access for free at https://med.libretexts.org/Bookshelves/Nursing/Book%3A_Vital_Sign_Measurement_Across_the_Lifespan_(Lapum_et_al.)/02%3A_Temperature/2.17%3A_Oral_Temperature

8 Vital Sign Measurement Across the Lifespan by Ryerson University is licensed under CC BY-SA 4.0. Access for free at https://med.libretexts.org/Bookshelves/Nursing/Book%3A_Vital_Sign_Measurement_Across_the_Lifespan_(Lapum_et_al.)

9 "Tympanic-Thermometer.jpg" by British Columbia Institute of Technology is licensed under CC BY 4.0. Access for free at https://med.libretexts.org/Bookshelves/Nursing/Book%3A_Vital_Sign_Measurement_Across_the_Lifespan_(Lapum_et_al.)/02%3A_Temperature/2.18%3A_Tympanic_Temperature

10 Vital Sign Measurement Across the Lifespan by Ryerson University is licensed under CC BY-SA 4.0. Access for free at https://med.libretexts.org/Bookshelves/Nursing/Book%3A_Vital_Sign_Measurement_Across_the_Lifespan_(Lapum_et_al.)

My Notes

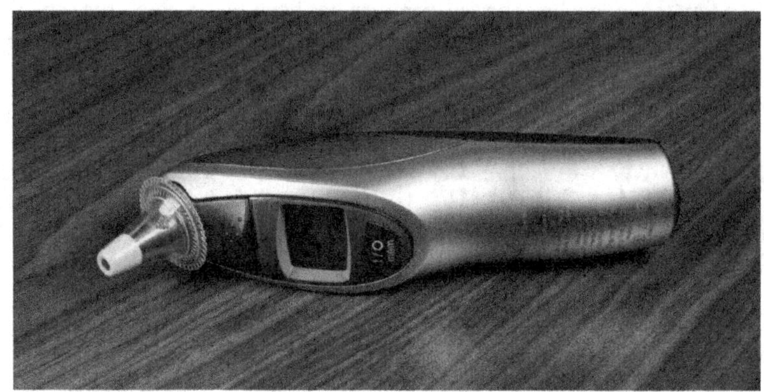

Figure 1.11 Tympanic Thermometer

Technique

Remove the tympanic thermometer from its holder and place a probe cover on the thermometer tip without touching the probe cover with your hands. Turn the device on. Ask the patient to keep their head still. For an adult or older child, gently pull the helix (outer ear) up and back to visualize the ear canal. For an infant or child under age 3, gently pull the helix down. Insert the probe just inside the ear canal but never force the thermometer into the ear. The device will beep within a few seconds after the temperature is measured. Read the results displayed, discard the probe cover in the garbage (without touching the cover), and then place the device back into the holder.[11] See Figure 1.12[12] for an image of a tympanic temperature being taken.

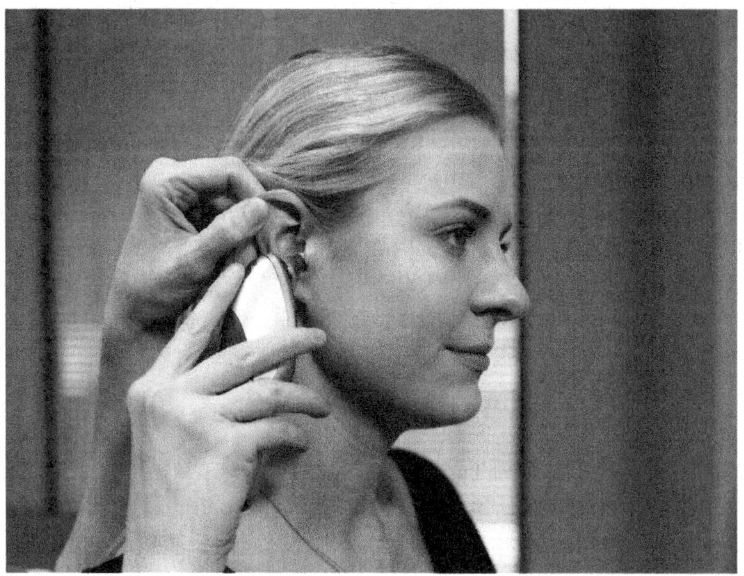

Figure 1.12 Tympanic Temperature

---

11 Vital Sign Measurement Across the Lifespan by Ryerson University is licensed under CC BY-SA 4.0. Access for free at https://med.libretexts.org/Bookshelves/Nursing/Book%3A_Vital_Sign_Measurement_Across_the_Lifespan_(Lapum_et_al.)

12 "Tympanic-Temperature-Correct-2.jpg" by British Columbia Institute of Technology is licensed under CC BY 4.0. Access for free at https://med.libretexts.org/Bookshelves/Nursing/Book%3A_Vital_Sign_Measurement_Across_the_Lifespan_(Lapum_et_al.)/02%3A_Temperature/2.18%3A_Tympanic_Temperature

Axillary Temperature

My Notes

The axillary method is a minimally invasive way to measure temperature and is commonly used in children. It uses the same electronic device as an oral thermometer (with blue coloring). However, the axillary temperature can be as much as 1°C lower than the oral temperature.[13]

Technique

Remove the probe from the device and place a probe cover (from the attached box) on the thermometer without touching the cover with your hands. Ask the patient to raise their arm and place the thermometer probe in their armpit on bare skin as high up into the axilla as possible. The probe should be facing behind the patient. Ask the patient to lower their arm and leave the device in place until it beeps, usually about 10–20 seconds. Read the displayed results, discard the probe cover in the garbage (without touching the cover), and then place the probe back into the device. See Figure 1.13[14] for an image of an axillary temperature.[15]

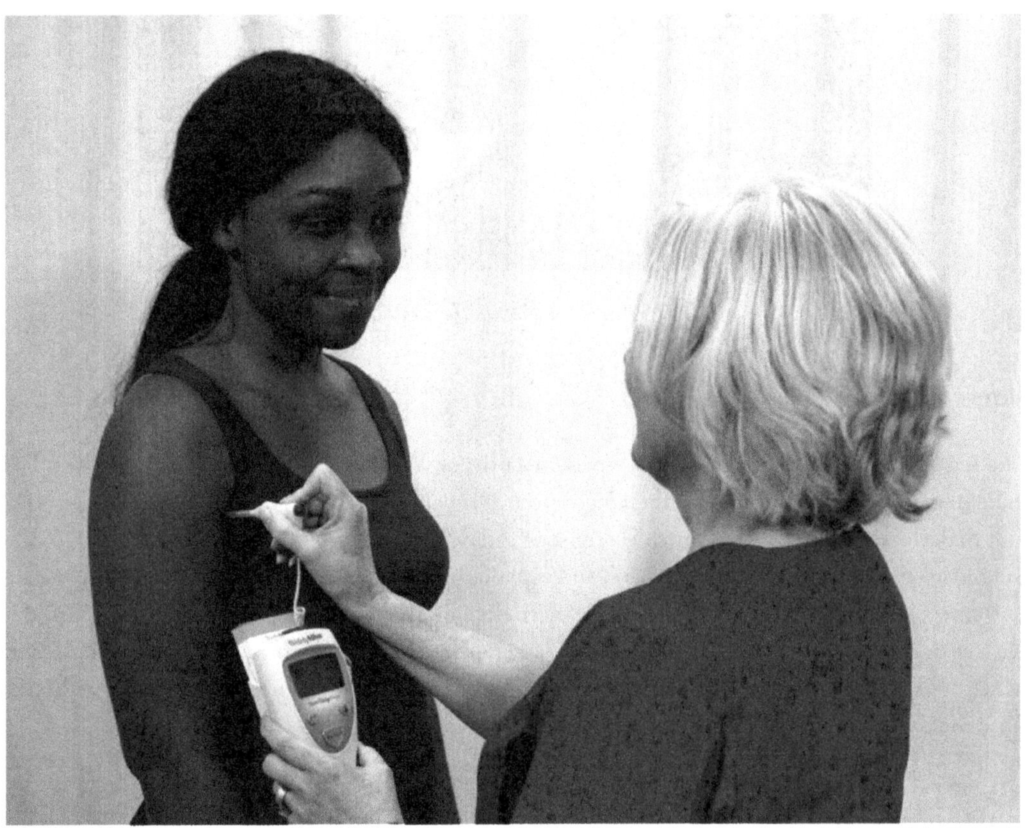

Figure 1.13 Axillary Temperature

13 Vital Sign Measurement Across the Lifespan by Ryerson University is licensed under CC BY-SA 4.0. Access for free at https://med.libretexts.org/Bookshelves/Nursing/Book%3A_Vital_Sign_Measurement_Across_the_Lifespan_(Lapum_et_al.)

14 "Axilla-Temperature-1-768x596.jpg" by British Columbia Institute of Technology is licensed under CC BY 4.0. Access for free at https://med.libretexts.org/Bookshelves/Nursing/Book%3A_Vital_Sign_Measurement_Across_the_Lifespan_(Lapum_et_al.)/02%3A_Temperature/2.19%3A_Axillary_Temperature

15 Vital Sign Measurement Across the Lifespan by Ryerson University is licensed under CC BY-SA 4.0. Access for free at https://med.libretexts.org/Bookshelves/Nursing/Book%3A_Vital_Sign_Measurement_Across_the_Lifespan_(Lapum_et_al.)

My Notes

Rectal Temperature

Measuring rectal temperature is an invasive method. Some sources suggest its use only when other methods are not appropriate. However, when measuring infant temperature, it is considered a gold standard because of its accuracy. The rectal temperature is usually 1°C higher than oral temperature. A rectal thermometer has red coloring to distinguish it from an oral/axillary thermometer.[16] See Figure 1.14[17] for an image of a rectal thermometer.

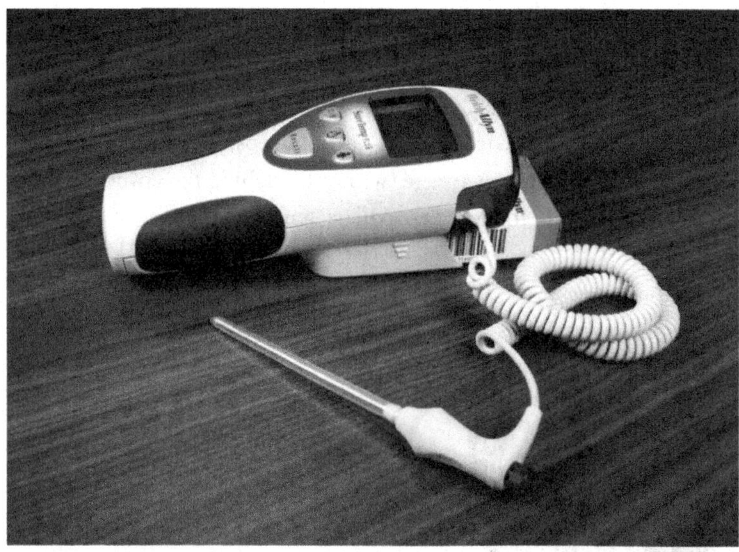

Figure 1.14 Rectal Thermometer

Technique

Before taking a rectal temperature, ensure the patient's privacy. Wash your hands and put on gloves. For infants, place them in a supine position and raise their legs upwards toward their chest. Parents may be encouraged to hold the infant to decrease movement and provide a sense of safety. When taking a rectal temperature in older children and adults, assist them into a side lying position and explain the procedure. Remove the probe from the device and place a probe cover (from the attached box) on the thermometer. Lubricate the cover with a water-based lubricant, and then gently insert the probe 2–3 cm inside the anus or less, depending on the patient's size.[18] Remove the probe when the device beeps. Read the result and then discard the probe cover in the trash can without touching it. Cleanse the device as indicated by agency policy. Remove gloves and perform hand hygiene.

---

16 Vital Sign Measurement Across the Lifespan by Ryerson University is licensed under CC BY-SA 4.0. Access for free at https://med.libretexts.org/Bookshelves/Nursing/Book%3A_Vital_Sign_Measurement_Across_the_Lifespan_(Lapum_et_al.)

17 "Thermometer-rectal-768x479.jpg" by British Columbia Institute of Technology is licensed under CC BY4.0. Access for free at https://med.libretexts.org/Bookshelves/Nursing/Book%3A_Vital_Sign_Measurement_Across_the_Lifespan_(Lapum_et_al.)/02%3A_Temperature/2.20%3A_Rectal_Temperature

18 Vital Sign Measurement Across the Lifespan by Ryerson University is licensed under CC BY-SA 4.0. Access for free at https://med.libretexts.org/Bookshelves/Nursing/Book%3A_Vital_Sign_Measurement_Across_the_Lifespan_(Lapum_et_al.)

My Notes

See Table 1.3a for normal temperature ranges for various routes.

Table 1.3 Normal Temperature Ranges[19]	
Method	**Normal Range**
Oral	35.8 – 37.3°C
Axillary	34.8 – 36.3°C
Tympanic	36.1 – 37.9°C
Rectal	36.8 – 38.2°C

19 Vital Sign Measurement Across the Lifespan by Ryerson University is licensed under CC BY-SA 4.0. Access for free at https://med.libretexts.org/Bookshelves/Nursing/Book%3A_Vital_Sign_Measurement_Across_the_Lifespan_(Lapum_et_al.)

My Notes

Interactive Activity

An interactive or media element has been excluded from this version of the text. You can view it online here: https://wtcs.pressbooks.pub/nursingskills/?p=859

Pulse refers to the pressure wave that expands and recoils arteries when the left ventricle of the heart contracts. It is palpated at many points throughout the body. The most common locations to assess pulses as part of vital sign measurement include radial, brachial, carotid, and apical areas as indicated in Figure 1.15.[20]

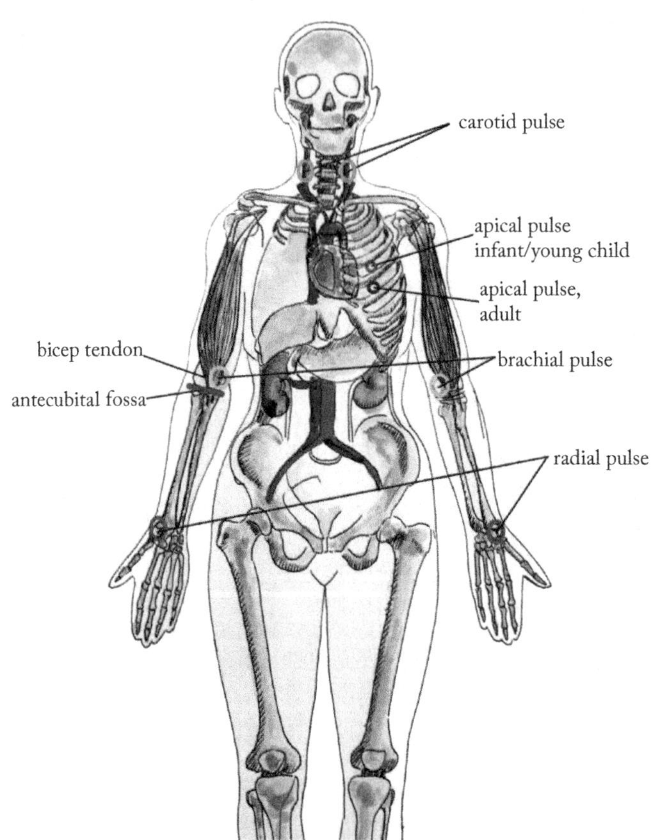

Figure 1.15 Common Pulse Assessment Locations

Pulse is measured in beats per minute. The normal adult pulse rate (heart rate) at rest is 60–100 beats per minute with different ranges according to age. See Table 1.3b for normal heart rate ranges by age. It is important to consider each patient situation when analyzing if their heart rate is within normal range. Begin by reviewing their documented baseline heart rate. Consider other factors if the pulse is elevated, such as the presence of pain or

20 "Radial-brachial-carotid-and-apical-pulse-final-930x1024.jpg" by British Columbia Institute of Technology is licensed under CC BY 4.0. Access for free at https://med.libretexts.org/Bookshelves/Nursing/Book%3A_Vital_Sign_Measurement_Across_the_Lifespan_(Lapum_et_al.)/03%3A_Pulse_and_Respiration/3.15%3A_What_is_Pulse%3F

crying in an infant. It is best to document the assessment when a patient is resting and comfortable, but if this is not feasible, document the circumstances surrounding the assessment and reassess as needed.[21]

Table 1.3b Normal Temperature Range	
Age Group	**Heart Rate**
Preterm	120 – 180
Newborn (0 to 1 month)	100 – 160
Infant (1 to 12 months)	80 – 140
Toddler (1 to 3 years)	80 – 130
Preschool (3 to 5 years)	80 – 110
School Age (6 to 12 years)	70 – 100
Adolescents (13 to 18 years) and Adults	60 – 100

Pulse Characteristics

When assessing pulses, the characteristics of rhythm, rate, force, and equality are included in the documentation.

Pulse Rhythm

A normal pulse has a regular rhythm, meaning the frequency of the pulsation felt by your fingers is an even tempo with equal intervals between pulsations. For example, if you compare the palpation of pulses to listening to music, it follows a constant beat at the same tempo that does not speed up or slow down. Some cardiovascular conditions, such as atrial fibrillation, cause an irregular heart rhythm. If a pulse has an irregular rhythm, document if it is "regularly irregular" (e.g., three regular beats are followed by one missed and this pattern is repeated) or if it is "irregularly irregular" (e.g., there is no rhythm to the irregularity).[22]

Pulse Rate

The pulse rate is counted with the first beat felt by your fingers as "One." It is considered best practice to assess a patient's pulse for a full 60 seconds, especially if there is an irregularity to the rhythm.[23]

---

21 Vital Sign Measurement Across the Lifespan by Ryerson University is licensed under CC BY-SA 4.0. Access for free at https://med.libretexts.org/Bookshelves/Nursing/Book%3A_Vital_Sign_Measurement_Across_the_Lifespan_(Lapum_et_al.)

22 Vital Sign Measurement Across the Lifespan by Ryerson University is licensed under CC BY-SA 4.0. Access for free at https://med.libretexts.org/Bookshelves/Nursing/Book%3A_Vital_Sign_Measurement_Across_the_Lifespan_(Lapum_et_al.)

23 Vital Sign Measurement Across the Lifespan by Ryerson University is licensed under CC BY-SA 4.0. Access for free at https://med.libretexts.org/Bookshelves/Nursing/Book%3A_Vital_Sign_Measurement_Across_the_Lifespan_(Lapum_et_al.)

My Notes

Pulse Force

The pulse force is the strength of the pulsation felt on palpation. Pulse force can range from absent to bounding. The volume of blood, the heart's functioning, and the arteries' elastic properties affect a person's pulse force.[24] Pulse force is documented using a four-point scale:

- 3+: Full, bounding
- 2+: Normal/strong
- 1+: Weak, diminished, thready
- 0: Absent/nonpalpable

If a pulse is absent, a Doppler ultrasound device is typically used to verify perfusion of the limbs. The Doppler is a handheld device that allows the examiner to hear the whooshing sound of the pulse. This device is also commonly used when assessing peripheral pulses in the lower extremities, such as the dorsalis pedis pulse or the posterior tibial pulse. See the following hyperlink to a video demonstrating the use of a Doppler device.

Video Review of Using a Doppler Ultrasound Device to Assess a Pulse[25]:

"Doppler Device – How to"

Pulse Equality

Pulse equality refers to a comparison of the pulse forces on both sides of the body. For example, a nurse often palpates the radial pulse on a patient's right and left wrists at the same time and compares if the pulse forces are equal. However, the carotid pulses should never be palpated at the same time because this can decrease blood flow to the brain. Pulse equality provides data about medical conditions such as peripheral vascular disease and arterial obstruction.[26]

---

24 Vital Sign Measurement Across the Lifespan by Ryerson University is licensed under CC BY-SA 4.0. Access for free at https://med.libretexts.org/Bookshelves/Nursing/Book%3A_Vital_Sign_Measurement_Across_the_Lifespan_(Lapum_et_al.)

25 Ryerson University. (2018, March 21). *Doppler device - How to.* [Video]. YouTube. All rights reserved. https://youtu.be/cn3aA0G1mgc

26 Vital Sign Measurement Across the Lifespan by Ryerson University is licensed under CC BY-SA 4.0. Access for free at https://med.libretexts.org/Bookshelves/Nursing/Book%3A_Vital_Sign_Measurement_Across_the_Lifespan_(Lapum_et_al.)

Radial Pulse

My Notes

Use the pads of your first three fingers to gently palpate the radial pulse. The pads of the fingers are placed along the radius bone on the lateral side of the wrist (i.e., the thumb side). Fingertips are placed close to the flexor aspect of the wrist (i.e., where the wrist meets the hand and bends). See Figure 1.16[27] for correct placement of fingers in obtaining a radial pulse. Press down with your fingers until you can feel the pulsation, but not so forcefully that you are obliterating the wave of the force passing through the artery. Note that radial pulses are difficult to palpate on newborns and children under the age of five, so the brachial or apical pulses are typically obtained in this population.[28]

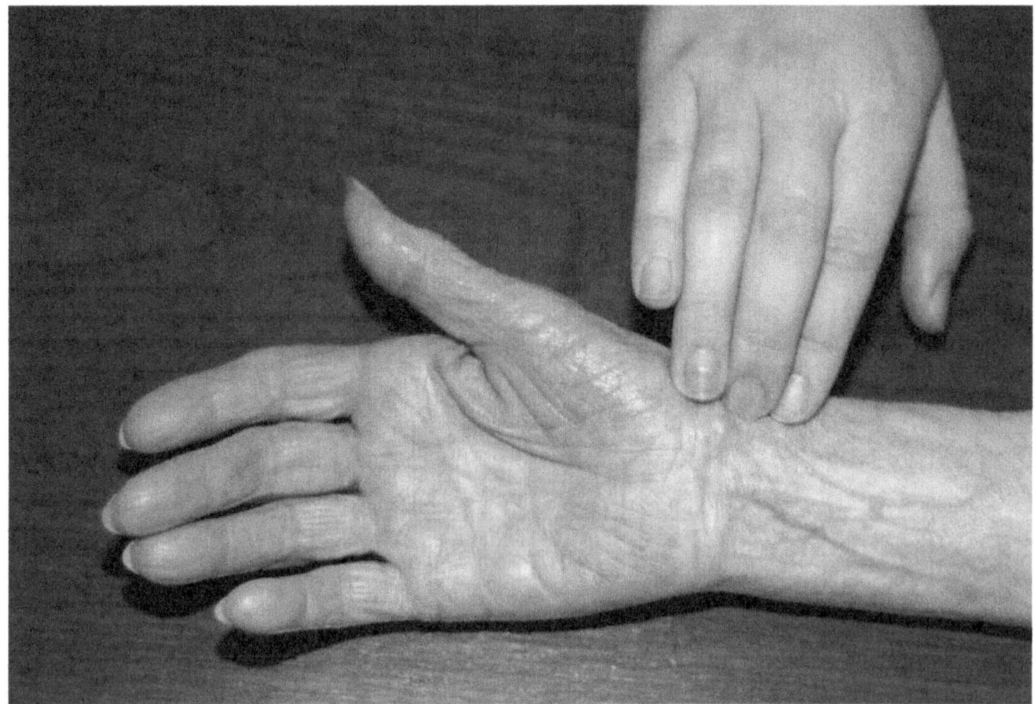

Figure 1.16 Radial Pulse

Carotid Pulse

The carotid pulse is typically palpated during medical emergencies because it is the last pulse to disappear when the heart is not pumping an adequate amount of blood.[29]

---

27 "Radial-pulse-correct.jpg" by British Columbia Institute of Technology is licensed under CC BY 4.0. Access for free at https://med.libretexts.org/Bookshelves/Nursing/Book%3A_Vital_Sign_Measurement_Across_the_Lifespan_(Lapum_et_al.)/03%3A_Pulse_and_Respiration/3.18%3A_Radial_Pulse

28 Vital Sign Measurement Across the Lifespan by Ryerson University is licensed under CC BY-SA 4.0. Access for free at https://med.libretexts.org/Bookshelves/Nursing/Book%3A_Vital_Sign_Measurement_Across_the_Lifespan_(Lapum_et_al.)

29 Vital Sign Measurement Across the Lifespan by Ryerson University is licensed under CC BY-SA 4.0. Access for free at https://med.libretexts.org/Bookshelves/Nursing/Book%3A_Vital_Sign_Measurement_Across_the_Lifespan_(Lapum_et_al.)

My Notes

Technique

Locate the carotid artery medial to the sternomastoid muscle, between the muscle and the trachea, in the middle third of the neck. With the pads of your three fingers, gently palpate one carotid artery at a time so as not to compromise blood flow to the brain. See Figure 1.17[30] for correct placement of fingers in a seated patient.[31]

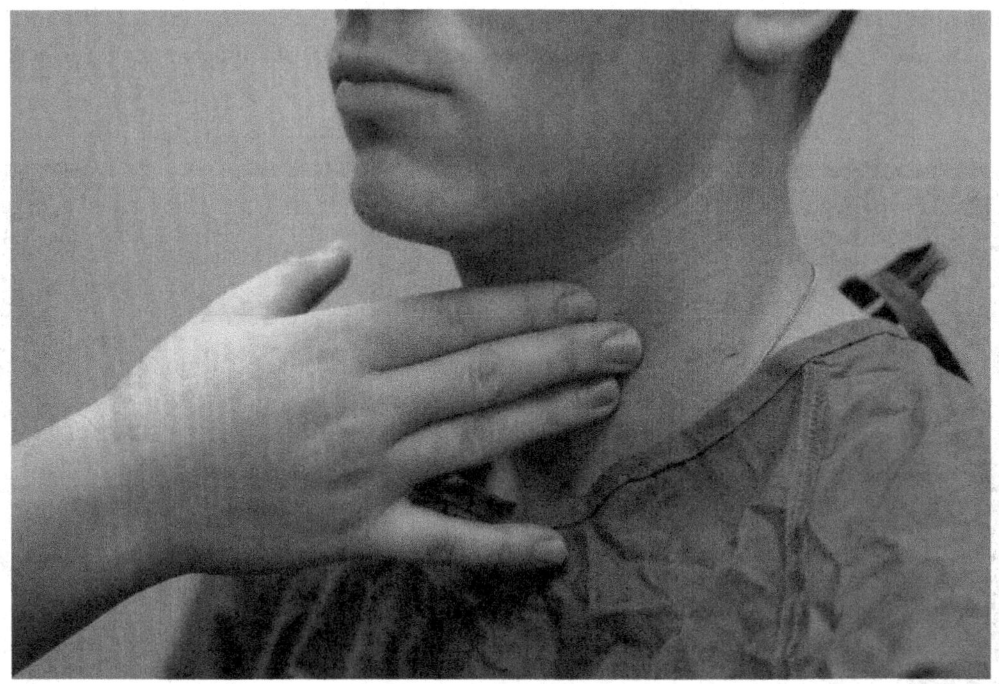

Figure 1.17 Carotid Pulse

Brachial Pulse

A brachial pulse is typically assessed in infants and children because it can be difficult to feel the radial pulse in these populations. If needed, a Doppler ultrasound device can be used to obtain the pulse.

Technique

The brachial pulse is located by feeling the bicep tendon in the area of the antecubital fossa. Move the pads of your three fingers medially from the tendon about 1 inch (2 cm) just above the antecubital fossa. It can be helpful to hyperextend the patient's arm to accentuate the brachial pulse so that you can better feel it. You may need to move

30 "Carotid-pulse-768x511.jpg" by British Columbia Institute of Technology is licensed under CC BY 4.0. Access for free at https://med.libretexts.org/Bookshelves/Nursing/Book%3A_Vital_Sign_Measurement_Across_the_Lifespan_(Lapum_et_al.)/03%3A_Pulse_and_Respiration/3.19%3A_Carotid_Pulse

31 Vital Sign Measurement Across the Lifespan by Ryerson University is licensed under CC BY-SA 4.0. Access for free at https://med.libretexts.org/Bookshelves/Nursing/Book%3A_Vital_Sign_Measurement_Across_the_Lifespan_(Lapum_et_al.)

My Notes

your fingers around slightly to locate the best place to accurately feel the pulse. You typically need to press fairly firmly to palpate the brachial pulse.[32] See Figure 1.18[33] for correct placement of fingers along the brachial artery.

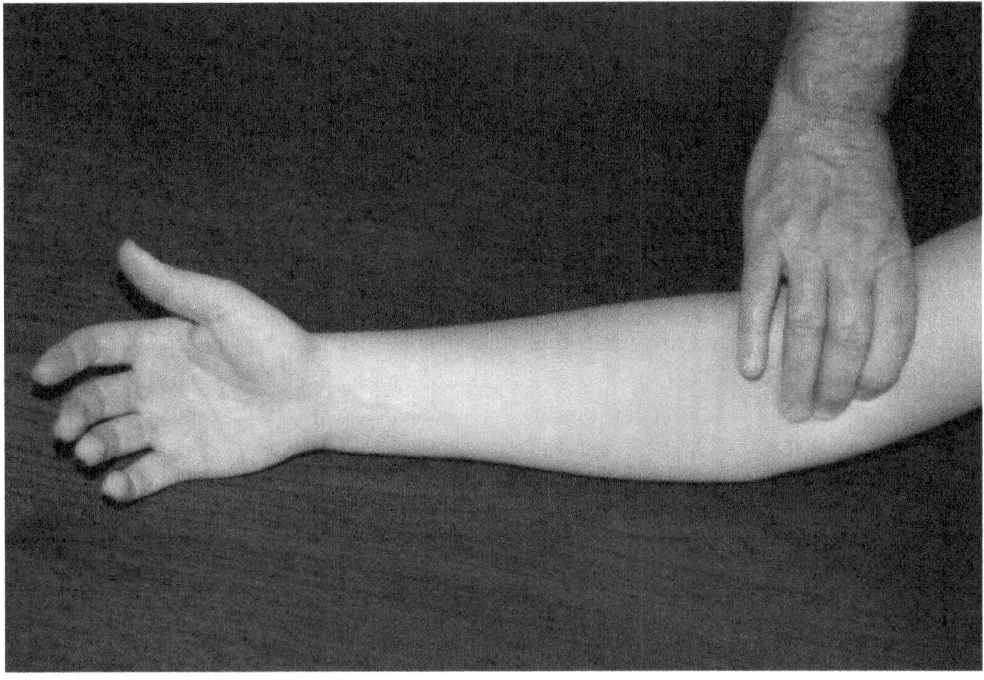

Figure 1.18 Brachial Pulse

Apical Pulse

The apical pulse rate is considered the most accurate pulse and is indicated when obtaining assessments prior to administering cardiac medications. It is obtained by listening with a stethoscope over a specific position on the patient's chest wall. Read more about listening to the apical pulse and other heart sounds in the "Cardiovascular Assessment" chapter.

Interactive Activity

An interactive or media element has been excluded from this version of the text. You can view it online here: https://wtcs.pressbooks.pub/nursingskills/?p=859

---

32 Vital Sign Measurement Across the Lifespan by Ryerson University is licensed under CC BY-SA 4.0. Access for free at https://med.libretexts.org/Bookshelves/Nursing/Book%3A_Vital_Sign_Measurement_Across_the_Lifespan_(Lapum_et_al.)

33 "Brachial-pulse.jpg" by British Columbia Institute of Technology is licensed under CC BY 4.0. Access for free at https://med.libretexts.org/Bookshelves/Nursing/Book%3A_Vital_Sign_Measurement_Across_the_Lifespan_(Lapum_et_al.)/03%3A_Pulse_and_Respiration/3.20%3A_Brachial_Pulse

My Notes

Respiratory Rate

Respiration refers to a person's breathing and the movement of air into and out of the lungs. Inspiration refers to the process causing air to enter the lungs, and expiration refers to the process causing air to leave the lungs. A respiratory cycle (i.e., one breath while measuring respiratory rate) is one sequence of inspiration and expiration.[34]

When obtaining a respiratory rate, the respirations are also assessed for quality, rhythm, and rate. The quality of a person's breathing is normally relaxed and silent. However, loud breathing, nasal flaring, or the use of accessory muscles in the neck, chest, or intercostal spaces indicate respiratory distress. People experiencing respiratory distress also often move into a tripod position, meaning they are leaning forward and placing their arms or elbows on their knees or on a bedside table. If a patient is demonstrating new signs of respiratory distress as you are obtaining their vital signs, it is vital to immediately notify the health care provider or follow agency protocol.

Respirations normally have a regular rhythm in children and adults who are awake. A regular rhythm means that the frequency of the respiration follows an even tempo with equal intervals between each respiration. However, newborns and infants commonly exhibit an irregular respiratory rhythm.

Normal respiratory rates vary based on age. The normal resting respiratory rate for adults is 10–20 breaths per minute, whereas infants younger than one year old normally have a respiratory rate of 30–60 breaths per minute. See Table 1.3c for ranges of normal respiratory rates by age. It is also important to consider factors such as sleep cycle, presence of pain, and crying when assessing a patient's respiratory rate.[35]

Read more about assessing a patient's respiratory status in the "*Respiratory Assessment*" chapter.

Table 1.3c Normal Respiratory Rate by Age[36]

Age	Normal Range
Newborn to one month	30 – 60
One month to one year	26 – 60
1-10 years of age	14 – 50
11-18 years of age	12 – 22
Adult (ages 18 and older)	10 – 20

34 Vital Sign Measurement Across the Lifespan by Ryerson University is licensed under CC BY-SA 4.0. Access for free at https://med.libretexts.org/Bookshelves/Nursing/Book%3A_Vital_Sign_Measurement_Across_the_Lifespan_(Lapum_et_al.)

35 Vital Sign Measurement Across the Lifespan by Ryerson University is licensed under CC BY-SA 4.0. Access for free at https://med.libretexts.org/Bookshelves/Nursing/Book%3A_Vital_Sign_Measurement_Across_the_Lifespan_(Lapum_et_al.)

36 Vital Sign Measurement Across the Lifespan by Ryerson University is licensed under CC BY-SA 4.0. Access for free at https://med.libretexts.org/Bookshelves/Nursing/Book%3A_Vital_Sign_Measurement_Across_the_Lifespan_(Lapum_et_al.)

My Notes

Oxygen Saturation

A patient's oxygenation status is routinely assessed using pulse oximetry, referred to as SpO2. SpO2 is an estimated oxygenation level based on the saturation of hemoglobin measured by a pulse oximeter. Because the majority of oxygen carried in the blood is attached to hemoglobin within the red blood cells, SpO2 estimates how much hemoglobin is "saturated" with oxygen. The target range of SpO2 for an adult is 94-98%. For patients with chronic respiratory conditions, such as chronic obstructive pulmonary disease (COPD), the target range for SpO2 is often lower at 88% to 92%. Although SpO2 is an efficient, noninvasive method to assess a patient's oxygenation status, it is an estimate and not always accurate. For example, if a patient is severely anemic and has a decreased level of hemoglobin in the blood, the SpO2 reading is affected. Decreased peripheral circulation can also cause a misleading low SpO2 level.

A pulse oximeter includes a sensor that measures light absorption of hemoglobin. See Figure 1.19[37] for an image of a pulse oximeter. The sensor can be attached to the patient using a variety of devices. For intermittent measurement of oxygen saturation, a spring-loaded clip is attached to a patient's finger or toe. However, this clip is too large for use on newborns and young children; therefore, for this population, the sensor is typically taped to a finger or toe. An earlobe clip is another alternative for patients who cannot tolerate the finger or toe clip or have a condition, such as vasoconstriction and poor peripheral perfusion, that could affect the results.

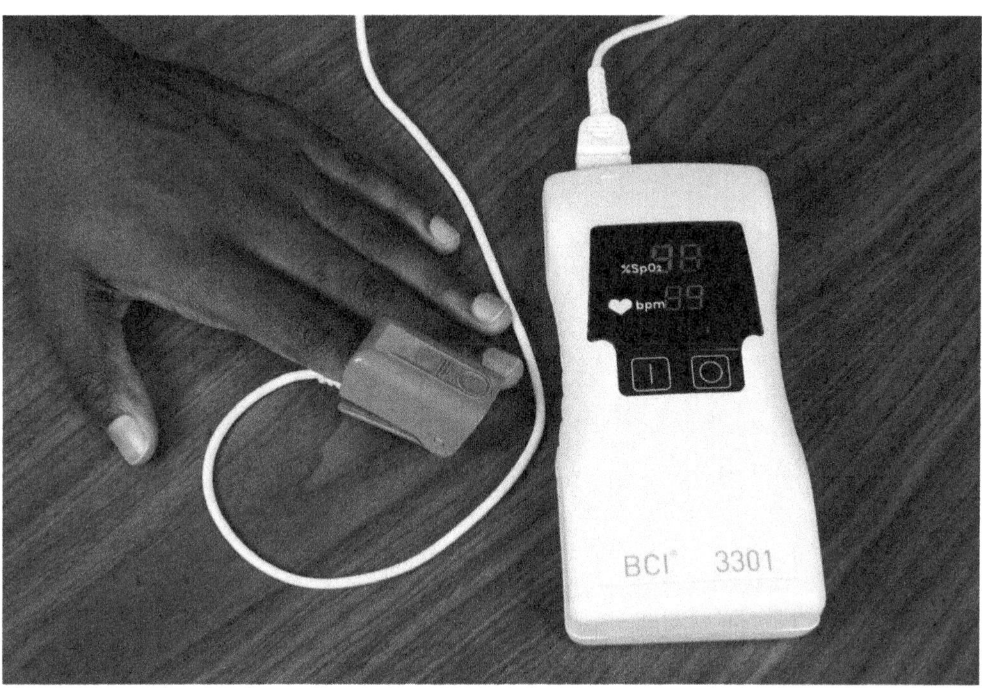

Figure 1.19 Pulse Oximeter

The target range of SpO2 for an adult is 94-98%. For patients with chronic respiratory conditions, such as chronic obstructive pulmonary disease (COPD), the target range for SpO2 is often lower at 88% to 92%.

Read more about pulse oximetry in the "Oxygen Therapy" chapter.

---

37 "02-Sat-Apparatus-1-1-1024x682.jpg" by British Columbia Institute of Technology is licensed under CC BY 4.0. Access for free at https://med.libretexts.org/Bookshelves/Nursing/Book%3A_Vital_Sign_Measurement_Across_the_Lifespan_(Lapum_et_al.)/04%3A_Oxygen_Saturation/4.09%3A_How_is_Oxygen_Saturation_Measured%3F

My Notes

Technique

Nail polish or artificial nails can affect the absorption of light waves from the pulse oximeter and decrease the accuracy of the SpO2 measurement when using a probe clipped on the finger. An alternative sensor that does not use the finger should be used for these patients or the nail polish should be removed. If a patient's hands or feet are cold, it is helpful to clip the sensor to the earlobe or tape it to the forehead.

Blood Pressure

Read information about how to accurately obtain blood pressure measurement in the "Blood Pressure" chapter.

Interpreting Results

After obtaining a patient's vital signs, it is important to immediately analyze the results, recognize deviations from expected normal ranges, and report deviations appropriately. As a nursing student, it is vital to immediately notify your instructor and/or collaborating nurse caring for the patient of any vital sign measurement out of normal range.

1.4 BASIC CONCEPTS

My Notes

When performing a general survey assessment, nurses use all of their senses to carefully observe the patient. They look at a patient and ask themselves, what are they seeing? They listen to a patient and ask themselves, what are they hearing, both verbally and nonverbally? They smell a patient's odors and ask themselves, is there anything unusual we need to further assess? They observe a patient's behaviors and make notes about their functioning and ability to complete daily activities according to their developmental level.

Before performing a general survey assessment, it is important to first ensure the patient is medically stable by completing a brief primary survey. After ensuring the patient is medically stable, a general survey assessment is an overall observation of a patient's general appearance, behavior, mobility, communication, nutritional, and fluid status. A general survey assessment also includes analyzing height, weight, and vital signs for values that are out of range and require additional follow-up.

Primary Survey

At the beginning of every shift or patient visit, nurses perform a brief **primary survey** to ensure their patient is medically stable. If any signs indicate patient distress, the provider is notified and emergency care is initiated. For example, changes in level of consciousness or abnormal vital signs often provide early warning signs that a patient's condition is deteriorating and prompt medical treatment is needed.[1] Mental status, airway, breathing, and circulation are also quickly assessed and emergency actions taken as needed.[2]

In a clinic setting, the patient is observed from the time they are called from the waiting room. Nurses observe a patient's gait and balance as they walk to the exam room and assess their verbal and nonverbal communication while interacting. If signs of distress are occurring, the nurse follows agency policy and either immediately calls a provider into the room or initiates emergency assistance.

Mental Status

When assessing a patient's overall mental status, it is important to compare findings to their known baseline if this information is known or available. Initially determine if a patient is responsive or unresponsive. Can you awaken them and are they responding to your questions? Are they oriented to person, place, and time, meaning can they tell you their name, location, and the day of the week? If you are concerned about a sudden change in a patient's mental status, obtain emergency assistance according to agency policy.

1 This work is a derivative of StatPearls by Toney-Butler and Unison-Pace licensed under CC BY 4.0. Access for free at https://www.ncbi.nlm.nih.gov/books/NBK545289/

2 Chemical Hazards Emergency Medical Management. (2020, April 17). *Primary and secondary survey.* National Institutes of Health. https://chemm.nlm.nih.gov/appendix8.htm

My Notes

Airway and Breathing

Determine if the patient's airway is open and if they are breathing adequately. Institute emergency care for respiratory distress as needed. See Figure 1.20[3] for an illustration of checking a patient's airway, breathing, and circulation (ABCs).

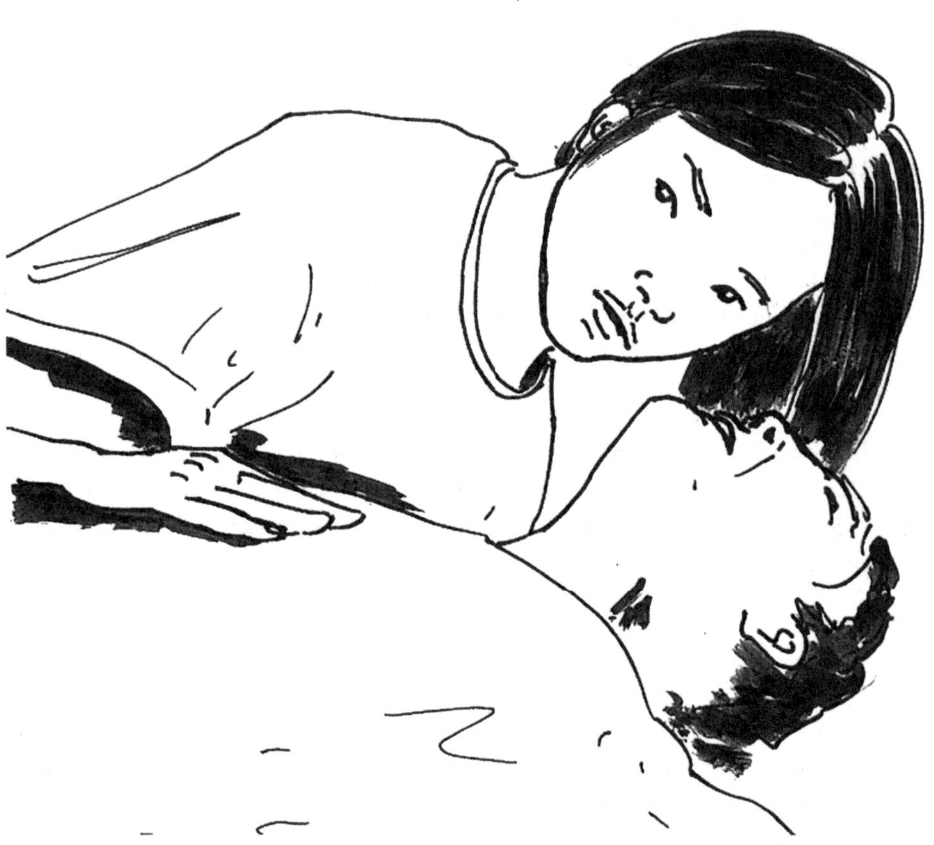

Figure 1.20 Checking a Patient's ABCs

Circulation

If a patient is not responsive, try to awaken them using a sternal rub. A sternal rub is performed by firmly rubbing one's knuckles on a patient's sternum to try to elicit a response. If they do not respond, check the carotid pulse and obtain emergency assistance as needed. Briefly observe the color and moisture of their skin. Abnormal findings such as cool, moist, pale, or bluish skin can indicate signs of shock that require emergency care.

---

3 "Checking respiratory.png" by User:Rama is licensed under CC BY-SA 3.0 FR. Access for free at https://commons.wikimedia.org/wiki/File:Checking_respiration.png

General Appearance

My Notes

After ensuring your patient is medically stable by completing a primary survey, a general survey consists of using your senses to observe a patient's general appearance, behavior, mobility, and communication. Items to consider when assessing general appearance include the following:

- **Signs of pain or distress:** Patients may exhibit signs of pain or distress that should be reported to the provider such as grimacing, moaning, or increased anxiety. Set the priorities for your focused assessments based on any signs of distress demonstrated by your patient.
- **Age:** Observe if the patient appears their stated age. Chronic disease can cause a patient to appear older than their age. Factors can occur with older adults that may influence how well the patient can participate in the assessment, such as hearing, vision, or mobility impairments.
- **Body type:** No patient is exactly the same; some patients are in good physical shape and others are not. Body type can reflect nutritional status and lifestyle choices.
- **Hygiene, grooming, and dress:** Observe the overall cleanliness of the patient's hair, face, and nails and note any odors. Odors can indicate poor hygiene or various disease states. Validate odors by performing additional focused assessments as needed. Note the appearance of the patient's clothing; is it clean and appropriate for the season? If not, findings can reflect on a patient's cognitive abilities, emotional state, and ability to complete daily activities.

Behavior

While observing the patient, note their behaviors during your interaction. Consider the following items:

- **Affect and mood:** People express their mood through facial expressions, eye contact, what they do, and what they say. Eye contact is commonly used to judge a person's mood because people who are feeling down or depressed commonly avoid eye contact. However, be aware that cultural beliefs may also affect the use of eye contact. **Affect** refers to the outward display of one's emotional state. For example, a patient with a "flat affect" refers to very few facial expressions being displayed to indicate emotion, which is often associated with depression. If the patient's mood or behavior seems inappropriate for their current situation, make a note of that as well. For example, a patient in an usually elated mood in a situation when most people would be seriously concerned can be a symptom of mental illness.
- **Family dynamics:** If other family members are accompanying the patient, note the characteristics of their interactions. **Family dynamics** are the patterns of interactions between family members that influence family structure, hierarchy, roles, values, and behaviors. Family dynamics have a strong impact on the way children see themselves, others, and their world. They can also impact the lifestyles of older adults who rely on their children for assistance in activities of daily living and health care.
- **Signs of patient abuse:** Abuse occurs in many different forms such as physical, emotional, mental, verbal, sexual, economic, or financial. Most states mandate nurses and other health care professionals to report suspected child and elder abuse to the proper authorities. Observe if your patient seems fearful, excessively quiet, or has physical signs of abuse, such as bruising or burn marks. If you suspect abuse, attempt to interview the patient alone. Promptly report your concerns according to agency policy and state mandates.

My Notes

- **Substance use disorder:** Approach your patient in a caring and nonjudgmental way, but be aware that unusual signs or behaviors can be indicators of substance use disorder. For example, if a patient's pupils are unusually dilated or constricted, this can be a sign of substance use disorder. Contact the provider with concerns about substance use disorder.

See Figure 1.21[4] of an image of a man with poor hygiene and nonverbal behavior requiring further assessment, such as disease management, medication management, and ability to complete activities of daily living.

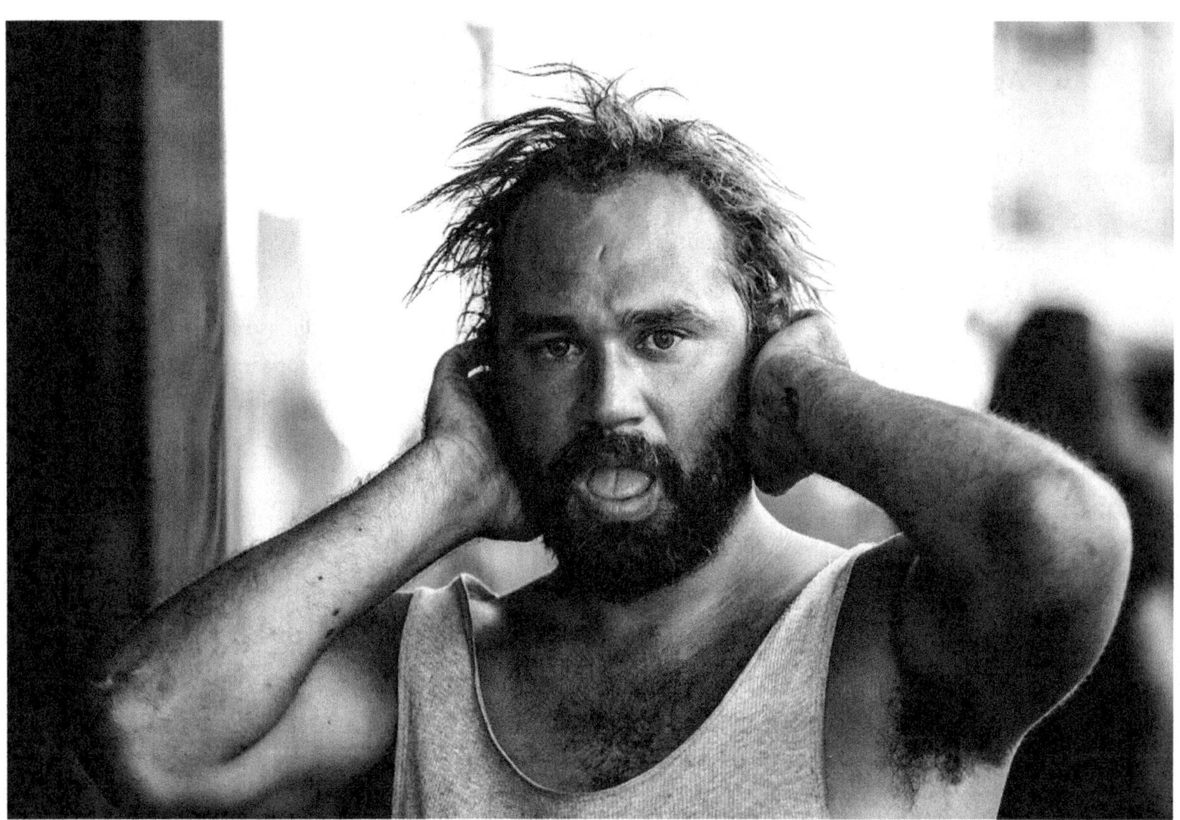

Figure 1.21 Man Requiring Additional Assessment Based on Appearance and Behavior

Mobility

Observe your patient's body movements, noting posture, gait, and range of motion.

- **Posture:** Patients with normal sitting and standing posture are upright and have a parallel alignment from the shoulders to the hips. Note if the patient is hunched, slumped, contracted, or rigid. See Figure 1.22[5] for an image of a patient with a type of slumped posture called kyphosis.

4 "Homeless man in Los Angeles(7618018076).jpg" by Alex Proimos licensed under CC BY 2.0. Access for free at https://commons.wikimedia.org/wiki/File:Homeless_man_in_Los_Angeles_(7618018076).jpg

5 "Posturalkyphosis" by Lab Science Career licensed under CC BY-NC-SA 2.0. Access for free at https://www.flickr.com/photos/lscareers/6303204058/in/photostream/

My Notes

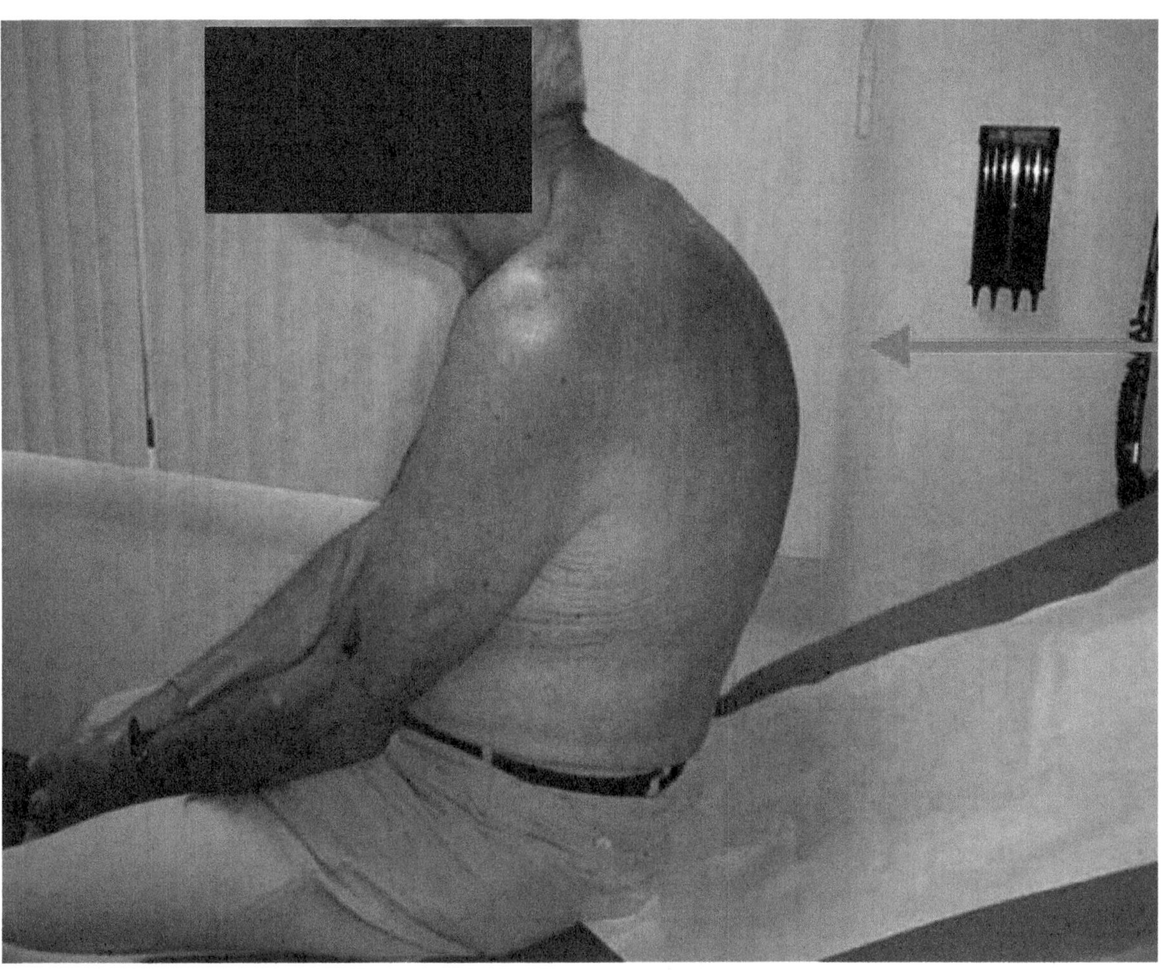

Figure 1.22 Patient with Slumped Posture

- **Gait and balance:** Observe how the patient walks or stands. Are the movements organized, coordinated, or uncoordinated? Are they able to maintain balance while standing without leaning on or touching anything? Healthy people walk with a smooth gait and arms moving freely at their sides and are able to stand unassisted. A change in gait or balance often signifies underlying health conditions and increases the risk of falling. See Figure 1.23[6] of a patient learning how to use an assistive device for an altered gait.

6 "US_Navy_071015-N-5086M-202_Retired_Marine_Corps_Cpl._Timothy_Jeffers_walks_on_his_prosthetic_legs_while_using_the_hands-free_harness_walking_gait_training_device_during_a_therapy_session_in_the_new_Comprehensive_Combat_and_Com.jpg" by U.S. Navy photo by Mass Communication Specialist 2nd Class Greg Mitchell is in the Public Domain.

My Notes

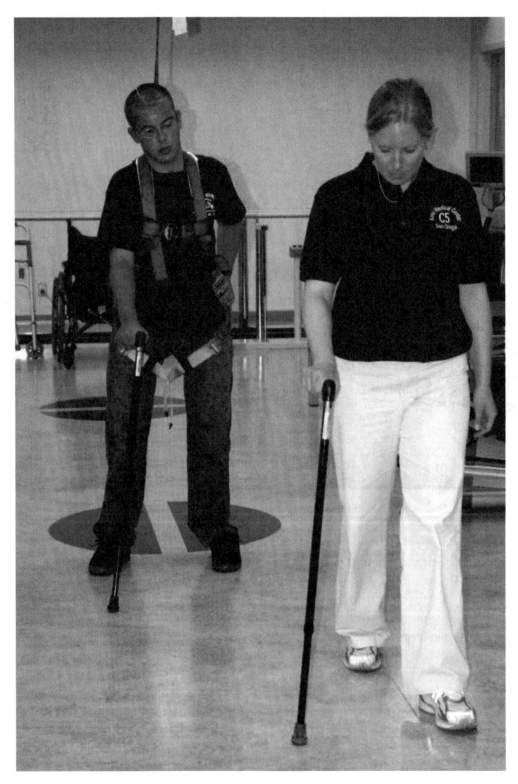

Figure 1.23 Altered Gait with Assistive Device

Range of motion and mobility: Observe the patient moving their extremities. Do extremities on the right and left sides move equally? Note any tremors or movements that are not purposeful. Are the patient's abilities appropriate for their age? Is the patient moving normally or do they have specific limitations? Does the patient use any assistive devices such as a cane or walker? Mobility is an important component in being able to care for oneself independently, so note any potential concerns for adults that may impact their ability to complete activities of daily living.

Communication

- **Speech:** Observe how your patient is speaking during your interaction. Are they speaking in an understandable tone and even pace, or is it garbled or difficult to understand? Neurological disorders can cause speech to be slow, slurred, and hard to understand. Is there an emotional component to their words? Is there a language barrier requiring an interpreter?
- **Response to commands:** Does the patient follow instructions you are providing during your assessment, or do they have difficulty in understanding or cooperating?

Nutritional Status

Visually observing the patient's overall nutritional status can provide cues for additional focused assessments related to appetite, diet, food intake, or exercise. Many factors can influence a patient's nutritional status such as financial or transportation issues, swallowing difficulties, missing teeth, or poorly fitting dentures.

Fluid Status

Observe overall fluid status. Dehydration can be indicated by dry skin, dry mucous membranes, or sunken eyes. Conversely, patients with excess fluid often have swelling or edema in their extremities and may exhibit signs of difficulty breathing.

Height, Weight, and BMI

Height and weight can be used as a guide to reflect the patient's general health. Weight is routinely assessed during all health care visits. Infants and children are measured to assess their growth and development. Hospitalized patients often have daily weights assessed to monitor for changes in their medical condition. Document findings based on agency policy. For example, in some agencies, height is documented in centimeters and weight is documented in kilograms. Recall that one inch is equivalent to 2.5 centimeters and 1 kilogram is equivalent to 2.2 pounds.

Body Mass Index (BMI) is a standardized reference range that is used to analyze a patient's weight status and provides a representation of body fat. However, it is important to note that BMI may not be accurate for athletes with increased muscle mass, people with edema or dehydration, or older adults who have lost a significant amount of muscle mass. See a BMI table in Figure 1.24.[7] To use the BMI table, find the height in inches in the left column, move across the row to closest weight, and then read the BMI where the column and row intersect. For example, a person who is 5' 9" tall is 69 inches. If the patient weighs 155 pounds, the BMI is 23. BMI indicating a healthy weight is between 18.5 to 24.9.

BMI can also be calculated using the formula of BMI = kg/m^2 (weight in kilograms divided by height in meters squared).

---

7 This work is a derivative of U.S. National Institutes of Health's National Heart, Lung, and Blood Institute (NHLBI). https://www.wikidoc.org/index.php/File:BMIReferenceChart.jpg licensed under CC BY-SA 3.0. Access for free at https://www.wikidoc.org/index.php/File:BMIReferenceChart.jpg

My Notes

The following classifications are used based on a person's BMI:

Underweight: Below 18.5 kg/m2

Healthy weight: 18.6 to 24.9 kg/m2

Overweight: 25 to 29.9 kg/m2

Obesity: Over 30 kg/m2 to 34.9 kg/m2

Extreme obesity: Over 35 kg/m2

BODY MASS INDEX (BMI)

BMI	19	20	21	22	23	24	25	26	27	28	29	30	31	32	33	34	35
Height (inches)	Body Weight (pounds)																
58	91	96	100	105	110	115	119	124	129	134	138	143	148	153	158	162	167
59	94	99	104	109	114	119	124	128	133	138	143	148	153	158	163	168	173
60	97	102	107	112	118	123	128	133	138	143	148	153	158	163	168	174	179
61	100	106	111	116	122	127	132	137	143	148	153	158	164	169	174	180	185
62	104	109	115	120	126	131	136	142	147	153	158	164	169	175	180	186	191
63	107	113	118	124	130	135	141	146	152	158	163	169	175	180	186	191	197
64	110	116	122	128	134	140	145	151	157	163	169	174	180	186	192	197	204
65	114	120	126	132	138	144	150	156	162	168	174	180	186	192	198	204	210
66	118	124	130	136	142	148	155	161	167	173	179	186	192	198	204	210	216
67	121	127	134	140	146	153	159	166	172	178	185	191	198	204	211	217	223
68	125	131	138	144	151	158	164	171	177	184	190	197	203	210	216	223	230
69	128	135	142	149	155	162	169	176	182	189	196	203	209	216	223	230	236
70	132	139	146	153	160	167	174	181	188	195	202	209	216	222	229	236	243
71	136	143	150	157	165	172	179	186	193	200	208	215	222	229	236	243	250
72	140	147	154	162	169	177	184	191	199	206	213	221	228	235	242	250	258
73	144	151	159	166	174	182	189	197	204	212	219	227	235	242	250	257	265
74	148	155	163	171	179	186	194	202	210	218	225	233	241	249	256	264	272
75	152	160	168	176	184	192	200	208	216	224	232	240	248	256	264	272	279
76	156	164	172	180	189	197	205	213	221	230	238	246	254	263	271	279	287

Source: Chart derived from the U.S. National Institute of Health's National Heart, Lung, and Blood Institute (NHLBI)

Figure 1.24 Body Mass Index

Establish a trusting, nonjudgmental relationship with your patient. Use a calm voice and do not appear rushed. Provide them with your undivided attention, and use all of your senses when interacting to pick up on important cues related to their current health status.

Life Span Considerations During a General Survey Assessment

Children

When performing a general survey on a child, be aware of their developmental stages to establish expectations for normal findings. Use a calm and gentle tone to establish trust. Demonstrations on dolls or stuffed animals before performing procedures are often helpful. Be aware that the parents of toddlers and school-aged children will likely provide most of the information during an assessment.

Adolescents

My Notes

Adolescents may refrain from sharing important information related to their care in front of their parents, especially regarding high-risk behaviors such as smoking, alcohol or drug use, sexual activity, or suicidal thoughts. It is often helpful to allow time to interview the adolescent privately, in addition to gathering information when the parent is present.

Older Adults

Recognize normal changes associated with aging when performing a general survey. If your patient wears glasses or hearing aids, be sure they are in place before asking questions. You may need to allow for extra time for your assessment, depending on the abilities of your patient. If an older adult is unable to communicate effectively, nurses may also consult a variety of sources such as family members and electronic medical records for more information.

Cultural Adaptations During a General Survey Assessment

Adapt your communication during a general survey assessment to your patient's cultural beliefs and values. For example, some individuals believe that direct eye contact with authorities is considered disrespectful and avoid eye contact. Other individuals may nod to indicate they are listening but this does not mean they are in agreement with what you are saying. Some patients prefer that a same sex individual perform care. For additional details about caring for diverse patients, see the "Diverse Patients" chapter in the Open RN *Nursing Fundamentals* textbook.

My Notes

1.5 EXPECTED VERSUS UNEXPECTED FINDINGS

Table 1.5 compares expected and unexpected findings when performing a general survey assessment. These findings are included in documentation regarding the general survey assessment.

Table 1.5 Expected Versus Unexpected Findings on General Survey Assessment

Assessment	Expected Findings	Unexpected Findings (notify provider if a new finding*)
Signs of distress	No signs of distress	Unresponsive, difficulty breathing, confused, moaning, or grimacing
Mood and appearance	Calm and cooperative Responds appropriately to questions Appears stated age	Mood is depressed, anxious, or agitated Signs of suspected substance use disorder are present, such as the scent of alcohol
Orientation	Alert and oriented to person, place, and time	Unable to provide name, location, or day
Hygiene	Well groomed. Clothing is appropriate for weather	Unkempt appearance or inappropriate clothing according to the weather
Family dynamics	Family members demonstrate mutual respect, trust, and caring	Family members communicate in an unfriendly, disrespectful, or hostile manner Signs of suspected abuse are present
Speech and communication	Speech is clear and understandable; patient follows instructions appropriately	Speech is garbled or difficult to understand; unable to respond appropriately to questions or follow commands
Range of motion	Moves all extremities equally bilaterally with good posture	New facial drooping or altered/unequal movement of extremities
Mobility	Gait is smooth and even and can maintain balance without assistance. If present, assistive devices are used appropriately and this is documented	Gait is shuffling, staggering, or limping. Balance is impaired; assistive devices like a cane or walker are not used appropriately
Nutrition	BMI within normal range	BMI out of range. Unexplained weight loss or gain has occurred
Fluid status	Moist mucous membranes	Dry skin and dry mucous membranes; sunken eyes in adults; sunken fontanel in infants
CRITICAL CONDITIONS to report immediately:		Newly unresponsive or altered mental status; difficulty breathing; vital signs out of range; skin is cool, clammy, or cyanotic

1.6 SAMPLE DOCUMENTATION

My Notes

Sample Documentation of Expected Findings

Mrs. Smith is a 65-year-old patient who appears her stated age. She is calm, cooperative, alert, and oriented x 3. She is well-groomed and her clothing is clean and appropriate for the weather. Her speech is clear and understandable, and she follows instructions appropriately. Mrs. Smith moves all extremities equally bilaterally with good posture. Her gait is smooth and she maintains balance without assistance. Her skin is warm and her mucous membranes are moist. She is 5'4" and she weighs 143 with a BMI of 24 in the normal weight category. Her vital signs were BP 120/70, pulse 74 and regular, respiratory rate 14, temperature 36.8 Celsius, and pulse oximetry was 98% on room air.

Sample Documentation of Unexpected Findings

Mrs. Smith is a 65-year-old patient who appears older than her stated age. She appears slightly agitated during the interview. She is oriented to person only and denies pain. She is wearing a heavy winter coat on a warm summer day and has an unclean body odor. She is slow to respond to questions and does not follow commands. She seems to neglect the use of her right arm. Her gait is shuffled with stooped posture but has no assistive devices. She is 5'4" and weighs 102 pounds with a BMI of 17.5 in the underweight category. Her vital signs were 186/55, pulse 102 and irregular, respiratory rate 22, temperature 38.1 Celsius, and pulse oximetry was 88%.

My Notes

1.7 CHECKLIST FOR GENERAL SURVEY

Use this checklist to perform a "General Survey." Checklists for hand washing, using hand sanitizer, and obtaining vital signs are included in "Appendix A."

Steps

Disclaimer: Always review and follow agency policy regarding this specific skill.

1. Knock, enter the room, greet the patient, and provide for privacy.
2. Introduce yourself, your role, the purpose of your visit, and an estimate of the time it will take.
3. Perform hand hygiene.
4. Ask the patient their legal name and date of birth for the first identifier. Verify information provided in their chart or wristband, if present. Use one of the following for the second identifier:
    - Scan wristband
    - Compare name/DOB to MAR
    - Ask staff to verify patient (in settings where wristbands are not worn)
    - Compare picture on MAR to patient
5. Address patient needs (pain, toileting, glasses/hearing aids) prior to starting assessment. Note if the patient has signs of distress such as difficulty breathing or chest pain. If signs are present, defer general survey and obtain emergency assistance per agency policy.
6. Explain the procedure to the patient; ask if he/she has any questions. Obtain an interpreter as needed if English is not the patient's primary language.
7. Pause and explain to the instructor what you would purposefully observe and assess during a general survey assessment.
8. Upon completion of the survey, thank the patient and ask if anything is needed.
9. Ensure five safety measures before leaving the room:
    - CALL LIGHT: Within reach
    - BED: Low and locked (in lowest position and brakes on)
    - SIDE RAILS: Secured
    - TABLE: Within reach
    - ROOM: Risk-free for falls (scan room and clear any obstacles)
10. Perform hand hygiene and clean stethoscope.
11. Follow agency policy for reporting findings outside of normal range.
12. Document the assessment.

1.8 LEARNING ACTIVITIES

My Notes

Learning Activities

(Answers to "Learning Activities" can be found in the "Answer Key" at the end of the book. Answers to interactive activity elements will be provided within the element as immediate feedback.)

Maria is working on a medical surgical unit and receives a direct admission from the internal medicine clinic. She arrives at the patient's room to complete the initial admission assessment. All of the following conditions are found.

Of these conditions, which of the following should be reported immediately to the health care provider.

a. Patient ambulates with assistance of wheeled walker.
b. Patient's BMI is outside of the normal range.
c. Patient appears unkempt and has strong body odor.
d. Patient is experiencing increased difficulty breathing.

Interactive Activity

An interactive or media element has been excluded from this version of the text. You can view it online here: https://wtcs.pressbooks.pub/nursingskills/?p=876

Interactive Activity

An interactive or media element has been excluded from this version of the text. You can view it online here: https://wtcs.pressbooks.pub/nursingskills/?p=876

Interactive Activity

An interactive or media element has been excluded from this version of the text. You can view it online here: https://wtcs.pressbooks.pub/nursingskills/?p=876

My Notes

I GLOSSARY

Affect: Outward display of one's emotional state. A "flat" affect with little display of emotion is associated with depression.

AIDET: Mnemonic for introducing oneself in health care that includes Acknowledge, Introduce, Duration, Explanation, and Thank You.[1]

BMI: A standardized reference range to gauge a patient's weight status.

Cultural safety: The creation of safe spaces for patients to interact with health professionals without judgment, racial reductionism, racialization, or discrimination.

Developmental stages: A person's life span can be classified into nine categories of development, including Prenatal Development, Infancy and Toddlerhood, Early Childhood, Middle Childhood, Adolescence, Early Adulthood, Middle Adulthood, Late Adulthood, and Death and Dying.

Family dynamics: Patterns of interactions between family members that influence family structure, hierarchy, roles, values, and behaviors.

General survey assessment: A component of a patient assessment that observes the entire patient as a whole. Observation includes using all five senses to gather cues that provide a guideline for additional focused assessments in areas of concern.

Medical asepsis: Measures to prevent the spread of infection in health care agencies.

Older adults: People over the age of 65.

Personal Protective Equipment (PPE): Includes gowns, eyewear, face shields, and masks, along with environmental controls, to prevent the transmission of infection for patients who are diagnosed or suspected of having an infectious disease.

Primary survey: A brief observation at the start of a shift or visit to verify the patient is stable by assessing mental status, airway, breathing, and circulation.

---

1. Huron. (n.d.). *AIDET patient communication*. https://www.studergroup.com/aidet

Chapter 2

Health History

2.1 HEALTH HISTORY INTRODUCTION

My Notes

Learning Objectives

- Establish a therapeutic nurse-patient relationship
- Use effective verbal and nonverbal communication techniques
- Collect health history data
- Modify assessment techniques to reflect variations across the life span and cultural variations
- Document actions and observations
- Recognize and report significant deviations from norms

"'Sickness' is what is happening to the patient. Listen to them."[1]

The profession of **nursing** is defined by the American Nurses Association as "the protection, promotion, and optimization of health and abilities, prevention of illness and injury, facilitation of healing, alleviation of suffering through the diagnosis and treatment of human response, and advocacy in the care of individuals, families, groups, communities, and populations."[2] Simply put, nurses treat human responses to health problems and/or life processes. Nurses look at each person holistically, including emotional, spiritual, psychosocial, and physical health needs. They also consider problems and issues that the person experiences as a part of a family and a community. To collect detailed information about a patient's human response to illness and life processes, nurses perform a health history. A **health history** is part of the Assessment phase of the nursing process. It consists of using directed, focused interview questions and open-ended questions to obtain symptoms and perceptions from the patient about their illnesses, functioning, and life processes. While obtaining a health history, the nurse is also simultaneously performing a general survey. Visit the "General Survey Assessment" chapter more information.

1 Weed, L. L. (1975). *Your health care and how to manage it.* University of Vermont.

2 American Nurses Association. (2015). *Nursing: Scope and standards of practice* (3rd ed.). American Nurses Association.

My Notes

2.2 HEALTH HISTORY BASIC CONCEPTS

During a health history, the nurse collects subjective data from the patient, their caregivers, and/or family members using focused and open-ended questions. Before discussing the components of a health history, let's review some important concepts related to assessment and communicating effectively with patients.

Subjective Versus Objective Data

Obtaining a patient's health history is a component of the Assessment phase of the nursing process. Information obtained while performing a health history is called subjective data. **Subjective data** is information obtained from the patient and/or family members and can provide important cues about functioning and unmet needs requiring assistance. Subjective data is considered a **symptom** because it is something the patient reports. When documenting subjective data in a progress note, it should be included in quotation marks and start with verbiage such as, "The patient reports . . ." or "The patient's wife states . . ." An example of subjective data is when the patient reports, "I feel dizzy."

A patient is considered the **primary source** of subjective data. **Secondary sources** of data include information from the patient's chart, family members, or other health care team members. Patients are often accompanied by their care partners. **Care partners** are family and friends who are involved in helping to care for the patient. For example, parents are care partners for children; spouses are often care partners for each other, and adult children are often care partners for their aging parents.

When obtaining a health history, care partners may contribute important information related to the health and needs of the patient. If data is gathered from someone other than the patient, the nurse should document where the information is obtained.

Objective data is information observed through your senses of hearing, sight, smell, and touch while assessing the patient. Objective data is obtained during the physical examination component of the assessment process. Examples of objective data are vital signs, physical examination findings, and laboratory results. An example of objective data is recording a blood pressure reading of 140/86. Subjective data and objective data are often recorded together during an assessment. For example, the symptom the patient reports, "I feel itchy all over," is documented in association with the **sign** of an observed raised red rash located on the upper back and chest.

Addressing Barriers and Adapting Communication

It is vital to establish rapport with a patient before asking questions about sensitive topics to obtain accurate data regarding the mental, emotional, and spiritual aspects of a patient's condition. When interviewing a patient, also consider the patient's developmental status and level of understanding. Ask one question at a time and allow adequate time for the patient to respond. If the patient does not provide an answer even with additional time, try rephrasing the question in a different way for improved understanding.

If any barriers to communication exist, adapt your communication to that patient's specific needs. For more information about potential communication barriers and strategies for adapting communication, visit the "Communication" chapter in Open RN *Nursing Fundamentals.*

Cultural Safety

It is important to conduct a health history in a culturally safe manner. **Cultural safety** refers to the creation of safe spaces for patients to interact with health professionals without judgment or discrimination. Focus on factors

My Notes

related to a person's cultural background that may influence their health status. It is helpful to use an open-ended question to allow the patient to share what they believe to be important. For example, ask "I am interested in your cultural background as it relates to your health. Can you share with me what is important to know about your cultural background as part of your health care?"

If a patient's primary language is not English, it is important to obtain a medical translator, as needed, prior to initiating the health history. The patient's family member or care partner should not interpret for the patient. The patient may not want their care partner to be aware of their health problems or their care partner may not be familiar with correct medical terminology that can result in miscommunication.

My Notes

2.3 COMPONENTS OF A HEALTH HISTORY

The purpose of obtaining a health history is to gather subjective data from the patient and/or their care partners to collaboratively create a nursing care plan that will promote health and maximize functioning. A comprehensive health history is completed by a registered nurse and may not be delegated. It is typically done on admission to a health care agency or during the initial visit to a health care provider, and information is reviewed for accuracy and currency at subsequent admissions or visits.

A comprehensive health history investigates several areas:

- Demographic and biological data
- Reason for seeking health care
- Current and past medical history
- Family health history
- Functional health and activities of daily living
- Review of body systems

Each of these areas is further described in the following sections.

The "History and Physical" documentation in a patient's electronic medical record is completed by a health care provider on admission to a health care agency. It is very similar to the health history obtained by a nurse and is helpful to read when caring for a patient for an overview of their treatment plan.

2.4 DEMOGRAPHIC AND BIOLOGICAL DATA

My Notes

Demographic and biographic data includes basic characteristics about the patient, such as their name, contact information, birthdate, age, gender and preferred pronouns, allergies, languages spoken and preferred language, relationship status, occupation, and resuscitation status.[1] See Table 2.4a for sample focused questions used to gather demographic and biological data.

Table 2.4a Demographic and Biological Data

Data	Focused Interview Questions
Name **Contact Information** **Emergency Contact Information**	What is your full name? What do you prefer to be called? What is your address? What is your phone number? Whom can we contact in an emergency? What is their relationship to you? At what number can we contact them?
Birthdate and Age	What is your birthdate? What is your current age?
Gender	What is your biological gender? With what gender do you identify? What are your preferred pronouns (he/him/his, she/her/hers, them/they/theirs, etc.)?
Allergies	Do you have any allergies? How do you react to each allergen?
Preferred Language	What is your primary language that you prefer to speak? Note: If English is not their primary language, offer to obtain a medical interpreter as needed.

1 This work is a derivative of The Complete Subjective Health Assessment by Lapum, St-Amant, Hughes, Petrie, Morrell, and Mistry licensed under CC BY-SA 4.0. Access for free at https://openlibrary.ecampusontario.ca/catalogue/item/?id=df19b620-466b-4167-be67-85062048bc57

My Notes

Data	Focused Interview Questions
Relationship Status	Tell me about your relationship status. *Avoid questions that imply expected behaviors, such as: ■ Are you married? ■ Do you have a boyfriend? ■ Do you have wife?
Occupation and Education	What is your occupation? Where do you work or go to school? What is the highest level of education you have completed?
Resuscitation Status	Have you considered preferences for resuscitation if your heart stops or you stop breathing, also called CPR? Do you have any advance directives on file with a hospital or provider, such as a "Living Will" or "Power of Attorney for Health Care"? Would you like more information about advance directives?

My Notes

See Table 2.4b for a sample demographic form used during a complete health history.

Table 2.4b Sample Demographic Form[2]
Demographic Information Form Interview Date: Patient Name: Address: Emergency Contact Name: Relationship: Date of Birth: Age: Sex: Male / Female / Another Option Gender You Self-Identify With: Preferred Pronouns: Allergies: Primary Language: Interpreter needed: Yes No Relationship Status: Occupation/Education: Resuscitation Status:
Information from: Patient / Other Patient Accompanied: Yes / No Details:

2 This work is a derivative of The Complete Subjective Health Assessment by Lapum, St-Amant, Hughes, Petrie, Morrell, and Mistry licensed under CC BY-SA 4.0. Access for free at https://openlibrary.ecampusontario.ca/catalogue/item/?id=df19b620-466b-4167-be67-85062048bc57

My Notes

2.5 REASON FOR SEEKING HEALTH CARE

It is helpful to begin the health history by obtaining the reason why the patient is seeking health care in their own words. During a visit to a clinic or emergency department or on admission to a health care agency, the patient's reasons for seeking care are referred to as the **chief complaint**. After a patient has been admitted, the term **main health needs** is used to classify what the patient feels is most important at that time. Whichever term is used, it recognizes that patients are complex beings, with potentially multiple coexisting health needs, but there is often a pressing issue that requires most immediate care. This is not to suggest that other issues be ignored, but rather it allows health care team members to prioritize care and address more urgent needs first.[1] See Table 2.5a for suggested focused interview questions to use to investigate the reason a patient is seeking care based on the health care setting.

The nurse is always aware of critical assessment findings requiring immediate notification of a health care provider or the initiation of emergency care according to agency policy. For example, if a patient reports chest pain, difficulty breathing, sudden changes in vision or the ability to speak, sudden weakness or paralysis, uncontrolled bleeding, or thoughts of self-harm, the provider should immediately be notified with possible initiation of emergency care.

Table 2.5a Focused Questions for Reasons for Seeking Health Care by Setting[2]

Setting	Focused Assessment Questions	Sample Responses (Subjective Data)
Clinic Visit	Please tell me what brought you in today. Can you tell me how long this has been going on? How is this affecting you?	"I have a headache that will not go away." "I have had this headache since yesterday morning when I woke up." "I am not able to see clearly, and I feel sick to my stomach so I was not able to go to work."
Hospital Admission	Please tell me what brought you in today. Can you tell me how long this has been going on? Have you taken anything to improve the symptoms you are reporting?	"I am having chest pain and my arm hurts." "The chest pain started after I finished shoveling my driveway about an hour ago." "I took an aspirin like the commercials always say to do."

1 This work is a derivative of The Complete Subjective Health Assessment by Lapum, St-Amant, Hughes, Petrie, Morrell, and Mistry licensed under CC BY-SA 4.0. Access for free at https://openlibrary.ecampusontario.ca/catalogue/item/?id=df19b620-466b-4167-be67-85062048bc57

2 This work is a derivative of The Complete Subjective Health Assessment by Lapum, St-Amant, Hughes, Petrie, Morrell, and Mistry licensed under CC BY-SA 4.0. Access for free at https://openlibrary.ecampusontario.ca/catalogue/item/?id=df19b620-466b-4167-be67-85062048bc57

My Notes

Setting	Focused Assessment Questions	Sample Responses (Subjective Data)
Inpatient Follow-Up	Tell me what your main concerns are today since your admission.	"I am wondering how long I am going to be admitted. I need to get back to work."
	Have you noticed any improvements since you were admitted?	"I feel huge improvements. I do not feel at all like I did yesterday."
	Do you have any symptoms currently?	"I do not have any chest pain and I do not have any arm pain anymore."

Chief Complaint

After identifying the reason why the patient is seeking health care, additional focused questions are used to obtain detailed information about this concern. The mnemonic **PQRSTU** is often used to ask the patient questions in an organized fashion. See Figure 2.1[3] for an image of PQRSTU.

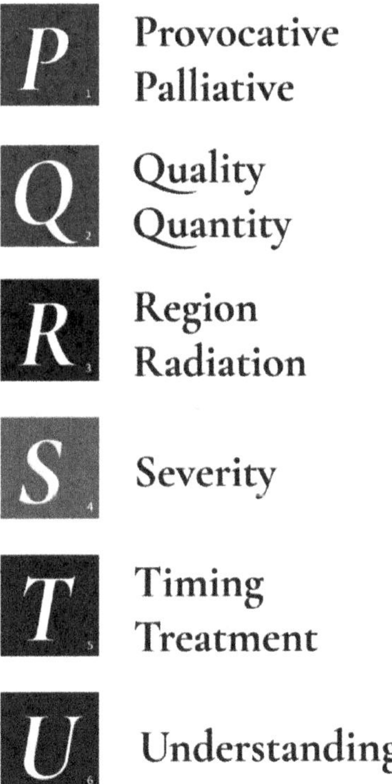

Figure 2.1 PQRSTU Mnemonic

3 This work is a derivative of The Complete Subjective Health Assessment by Lapum, St-Amant, Hughes, Petrie, Morrell, and Mistry licensed under CC BY-SA 4.0. Access for free at https://openlibrary.ecampusontario.ca/catalogue/item/?id=df19b620-466b-4167-be67-85062048bc57

My Notes

The PQRSTU mnemonic is often used to assess pain, but it can also be used to assess many other symptoms. See Table 2.5b for suggested focus questions for pain and other symptoms using the PQRSTU mnemonic.[4]

Table 2.5b Sample PQRSTU Focused Questions for Pain and Other Symptoms

PQRSTU	Questions Related to Pain	Questions Related to Other Symptoms
Provocation/ **Palliation**	What makes your pain worse? What makes your pain feel better?	What makes your breathing worse? What makes your nausea better?
Quality	What does the pain feel like? Note: You can provide suggestions for pain characteristics such as "aching," "stabbing," or "burning."	What does the dizziness feel like? Do you feel light-headed, as if you're going to faint or the room is spinning?
Region	Where exactly do you feel the pain? Does it move around or radiate elsewhere? Note: Instruct the patient to point to the pain location.	Where exactly do you feel the itching? Does it move around?
Severity	How would you rate your pain on a scale of 0 to 10, with "0" being no pain and "10" being the worst pain you've ever experienced?	How would you rate your shortness of breath on a scale of 0 to 10, with "0" being no problem and "10" being the worst breathing issues you've ever experienced?

4 This work is a derivative of The Complete Subjective Health Assessment by Lapum, St-Amant, Hughes, Petrie, Morrell, and Mistry licensed under CC BY-SA 4.0. Access for free at https://openlibrary.ecampusontario.ca/catalogue/item/?id=df19b620-466b-4167-be67-85062048bc57

My Notes

PQRSTU	Questions Related to Pain	Questions Related to Other Symptoms
Timing/ **Treatment**	When did the pain start? What were you doing when the pain started? Is the pain constant or does it come and go? If the pain is intermittent, when does it occur? How long does the pain last? Have you taken anything to help relieve the pain?	When did your breathing issues begin? What were you doing when the itching first started? Is the nausea constant or does it come and go? If the nausea is intermittent, does anything trigger it? How long did the nausea last? Have you taken anything to relieve the itching?
Understanding	What do you think is causing the pain?	What do you think is causing the itching?

While interviewing a patient about their chief complaint, use open-ended questions to allow the patient to elaborate on information that further improves your understanding of their health concerns. If their answers do not seem to align, continue to ask focused questions to clarify information. For example, if a patient states that "the pain is tolerable" but also rates the pain as a "7" on a 0-10 pain scale, these answers do not align, and the nurse should continue to use follow-up questions using the PQRSTU framework. For example, upon further questioning the patient explains they rate the pain as a "7" in their knee when participating in physical therapy exercises, but currently feels the pain is tolerable while resting in bed. This additional information will help the nurse customize interventions for effective treatment.

My Notes

2.6 CURRENT AND PAST MEDICAL HISTORY

After exploring a patient's chief complaint, their current and past medical histories are reviewed to obtain a full understanding of their "human response" to medical conditions and life processes. While obtaining this information, it is also helpful to determine their understanding of the condition and its associated treatment. If a patient has a prior medical diagnosis, but is unaware of what it means or does not understand the recommended treatment, they may not be following instructions intended. For example, a patient diagnosed with "high blood pressure" may erroneously think they only need to take their medications when they feel as if their blood pressure is high, instead of daily at the recommended doses.

Categories included in past medical history include current health, medications, childhood illnesses, chronic illnesses, acute illnesses, accidents, injuries, and obstetrical health for females. **Medication reconciliation** is a comparison of a list of current medications with a previous list and is completed at every hospitalization and clinic visit. Not all categories of current and past health histories apply to every patient, so only ask questions that are relevant to the patient you are interviewing. See Table 2.6[1] for suggested focused interview questions related to current and past medical history.

Table 2.6 Sample Focused Questions for Current and Past Health History

Category	Focused Questions
Current health	What are your current goals for your health? Are there any other issues affecting your current health or the ability to complete your daily activities? Tell me more.
Medications	What are your current medications, including prescriptions, over-the-counter medications, vitamins, and herbal supplements and why are you taking them (to establish the patient's understanding of their medications)? Do you take your medications as prescribed? Note: If the response is "no" or "sometimes," follow up with an open-ended question such as, "Tell me more about the reasons for not taking the medications as prescribed."
Allergies	Do you have any allergies to medications, food, latex, or other items? If yes, what is your reaction?
Childhood illnesses	Tell me about any significant childhood illnesses that you had. Do you recall what childhood vaccines you received? When did they occur? Were you hospitalized? Did you experience any complications?

1 This work is a derivative of The Complete Subjective Health Assessment by Lapum, St-Amant, Hughes, Petrie, Morrell, and Mistry licensed under CC BY-SA 4.0. Access for free at https://openlibrary.ecampusontario.ca/catalogue/item/?id=df19b620-466b-4167-be67-85062048bc57

My Notes

Category	Focused Questions
Chronic illnesses	Tell me about any chronic illnesses you currently have or have experienced (such as cancer, cardiac or respiratory issues, diabetes, or arthritis). When were you diagnosed? Do you see a specialist for this chronic illness? If so, what is their name and location? How is this condition currently being treated? How has the chronic illness affected you? How do you cope with the illness? Have you experienced any complications or disability from this chronic illness?
Acute illnesses, surgeries, accidents, or injuries	Tell me about any acute illnesses or surgeries that you have experienced. Have you had any accidents or injuries? Did you experience any complications?
Reproductive health	For Females: When was your last menstrual period? Have you ever been pregnant? Are you pregnant now or is there any chance of being pregnant now? Tell me about your pregnancies. Were there any issues or complications?
Immunizations	If a patient's vaccination record is not included in their record: ■ Can you tell me what immunizations you have received and if you had any significant reactions? ■ When was your last flu vaccine?

My Notes

2.7 FAMILY HEALTH HISTORY

Many diseases have a genetic component. It is important to understand the risk and likelihood of a patient developing illnesses based on their family health. Ask about the health status, age, and, if applicable, cause of death of immediate blood relatives (parents, grandparents, and siblings). Questions to ask include the following:

- Tell me about the health of your blood relatives. Does anyone have diseases like cancer, heart problems, or respiratory problems?
- Have any of your blood relatives died? If so, do you know the cause of death? What age did they die?

2.8 FUNCTIONAL HEALTH AND ACTIVITIES OF DAILY LIVING

My Notes

Functional health assessment collects data related to the patient's functioning and their physical and mental capacity to participate in **Activities of Daily Living (ADLs)** and Instrumental Activities of Daily Living (IADLs). Activities of Daily Living (ADLs) are daily basic tasks that are fundamental to everyday functioning (e.g., hygiene, elimination, dressing, eating, ambulating/moving). See Figure 2.2[1] for an illustration of ADLs.

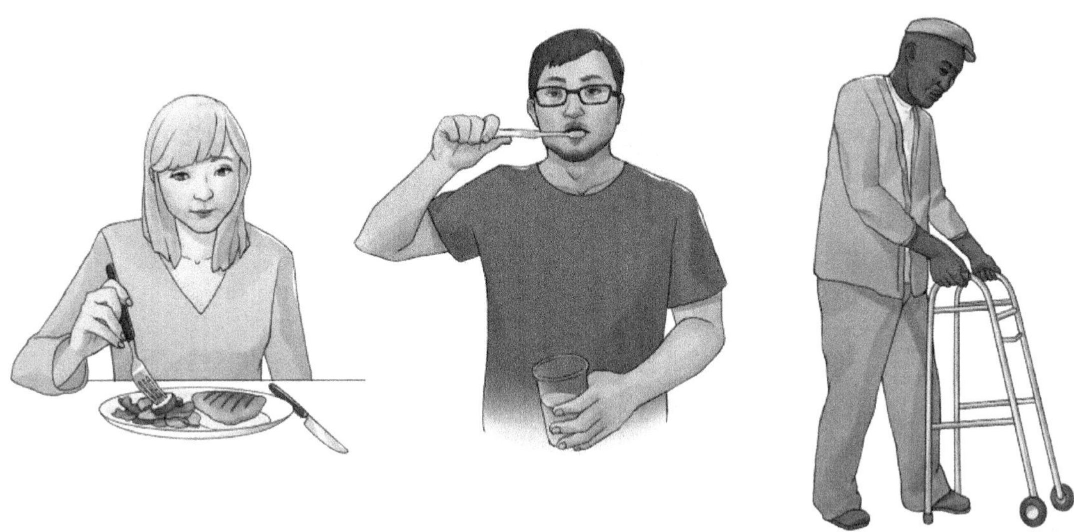

Figure 2.2 Activities of Daily Living (ADLs)

Instrumental Activities of Daily Living (IADL) are more complex daily tasks that allow patients to function independently such as managing finances, paying bills, purchasing and preparing meals, managing one's household, taking medications, and facilitating transportation. See Figure 2.3[2] for an illustration of IADLs. Assessment of IADLs is particularly important to inquire about with young adults who have just moved into their first place, as well as with older patients with multiple medical conditions and/or disabilities.

1 "ADL-1024x534.jpg" by unknown is licensed under CC BY-SA 4.0. Access for free at https://ecampusontario.pressbooks.pub/healthassessment/chapter/functional-health/

2 "iADL-1024x494.jpg" by unknown is licensed under CC BY-SA 4.0. Access for free at https://ecampusontario.pressbooks.pub/healthassessment/chapter/functional-health/

My Notes

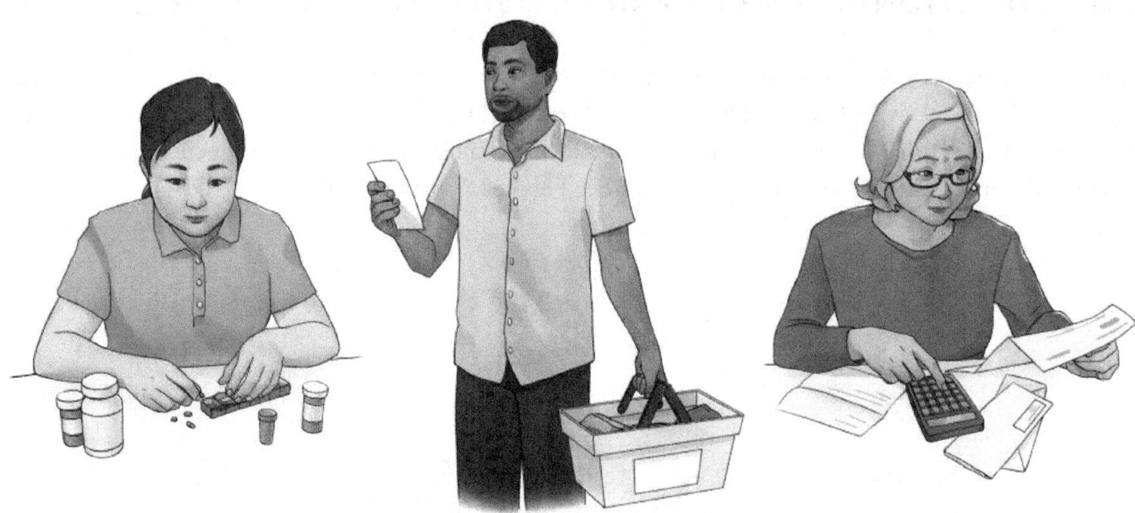

Figure 2.3 Instrumental Activities of Daily Living (IADLs)

Information obtained when assessing functional health provides the nurse a holistic view of a patient's human response to illness and life conditions. It is helpful to use an assessment framework, such as Gordon's Functional Health Patterns,[3] to organize interview questions according to evidence-based patterns of human responses. Using this framework provides the patient and their family members an opportunity to identify health-related concerns to the nurse that may require further in-depth assessment. It also verifies patient understanding of conditions so that misperceptions can be clarified. This framework includes the following categories:

- **Nutritional-Metabolic:** Food and fluid consumption relative to metabolic need
- **Elimination:** Excretion including bowel and bladder
- **Activity-Exercise:** Exercise and activity
- **Sleep-Rest:** Sleep and rest
- **Cognitive-Perceptual:** Perception and cognition
- **Role-Relationship:** Roles and relationships
- **Sexuality-Reproductive:** Reproduction and sexuality
- **Coping-Stress Tolerance:** Coping and effectiveness of managing stress
- **Value-Belief:** Values, beliefs, and goals that guide choices and decisions
- **Self-Perception and Self-Concept:** Self-concept and mood state[4]
- **Health Perception-Health Management:** A patient's perception of their health and well-being and how it is managed. This is an umbrella category of all the categories above and underlies performing a health history.

---

3 Gordon, M. (2008). *Assess notes nursing: Nursing assessment and diagnostic reasoning for clinical practice.* F. A. Davis Company.

4 Gordon, M. (2008). *Assess notes nursing: Nursing assessment and diagnostic reasoning for clinical practice.* F.A. Davis Company.

The functional health section can be started by saying, "I would like to ask you some questions about factors that affect your ability to function in your day-to-day life. Feel free to share any health concerns that come to mind during this discussion." Focused interview questions for each category are included in Table 2.8. Each category is further described below.

My Notes

Nutrition

The nutritional category includes, but is not limited to, food and fluid intake, usual diet, financial ability to purchase food, time and knowledge to prepare meals, and appetite. This is also an opportune time to engage in health promotion discussions about healthy eating. Be aware of signs for malnutrition and obesity, especially if rapid and excessive weight loss or weight gain have occurred.

Life Span Considerations

When assessing nutritional status, the types of questions asked and the level of detail depend on the developmental age and health of the patient. Family members may also provide important information.

- **Infants:** Ask parents about using breast milk or formula, amount, frequency, supplements, problems, and introductions of new foods.
- **Pregnant women:** Include questions about the presence of nausea and vomiting and intake of folic acid, iron, omega-3 fatty acids, vitamin D, and calcium.
- **Older adults or patients with disabling illnesses:** Inquire about the ability to purchase and cook their food, decreased sense of taste, ability to chew or swallow foods, loss of appetite, and enough fiber and nutrients.[5]

For more information about nutrition, visit the "Nutrition" chapter in Open RN *Nursing Fundamentals.*

Elimination

Elimination refers to the removal of waste products through the urine and stool. Health care professionals refer to urinating as **voiding** and stool elimination as having a bowel movement. Familiar terminology may need to be used with patients, such as "pee" and "poop." Constipation commonly occurs in hospitalized patients, so it is important to assess the date of their last bowel movement and monitor the frequency, color, and consistency of their stool. Assess urine concentration, frequency, and odor, especially if concerned about urinary tract infection, incontinence, or infection. Findings that require further investigation include **dysuria** (pain or difficulty upon urination), blood in the stool, **melena** (black, tarry stool), constipation, diarrhea, or excessive laxative use.[6]

5 This work is a derivative of The Complete Subjective Health Assessment by Lapum, St-Amant, Hughes, Petrie, Morrell, and Mistry licensed under CC BY-SA 4.0. Access for free at https://openlibrary.ecampusontario.ca/catalogue/item/?id=df19b620-466b-4167-be67-85062048bc57

6 This work is a derivative of The Complete Subjective Health Assessment by Lapum, St-Amant, Hughes, Petrie, Morrell, and Mistry licensed under CC BY-SA 4.0. Access for free at https://openlibrary.ecampusontario.ca/catalogue/item/?id=df19b620-466b-4167-be67-85062048bc57

My Notes

Life Span Considerations

When assessing elimination, the types of questions asked and the level of detail depends on the developmental age and health of the patient.

Toddlers: Ask parents or guardians about toilet training. Toilet training takes several months, occurs in several stages, and varies from child to child. It is influenced by culture and depends on physical and emotional readiness, but most children are toilet trained between 18 months and three years.

Older Adults: Constipation and incontinence are common symptoms associated with aging. Additional focused questions may be required to further assess these issues.[7]

For more information about elimination, visit the "Elimination" chapter in Open RN *Nursing Fundamentals.*

Mobility, Activity, and Exercise

Mobility refers to a patient's ability to move around (e.g., sit up, sit down, stand up, walk). Activity and exercise refer to informal and/or formal activity (e.g., walking, swimming, yoga, strength training). In addition to assessing the amount of exercise, it is also important to assess activity because some people may not engage in exercise but have an active lifestyle (e.g., walk to school or work in a physically demanding job).

Findings that require further investigation include insufficient aerobic exercise and identified risks for falls.[8]

Life Span Considerations

Mobility and activity depend on developmental age and a patient's health and illness status. With infants, it is important to assess their ability to meet specific developmental milestones at each well-baby visit. Mobility can become problematic for patients who are ill or are aging and can result in self-care deficits. Thus, it is important to assess how a patient's mobility is affecting their ability to perform ADLs and IADLs.[9]

For more information, visit the "Mobility" chapter in Open RN *Nursing Fundamentals.*

Sleep and Rest

The sleep and rest category refers to a patient's pattern of rest and sleep and any associated routines or sleeping medications used. Although it varies for different people and their life circumstances, obtaining eight hours of

---

7 This work is a derivative of The Complete Subjective Health Assessment by Lapum, St-Amant, Hughes, Petrie, Morrell, and Mistry licensed under CC BY-SA 4.0. Access for free at https://openlibrary.ecampusontario.ca/catalogue/item/?id=df19b620-466b-4167-be67-85062048bc57

8 This work is a derivative of The Complete Subjective Health Assessment by Lapum, St-Amant, Hughes, Petrie, Morrell, and Mistry licensed under CC BY-SA 4.0. Access for free at https://openlibrary.ecampusontario.ca/catalogue/item/?id=df19b620-466b-4167-be67-85062048bc57

9 This work is a derivative of The Complete Subjective Health Assessment by Lapum, St-Amant, Hughes, Petrie, Morrell, and Mistry licensed under CC BY-SA 4.0. Access for free at https://openlibrary.ecampusontario.ca/catalogue/item/?id=df19b620-466b-4167-be67-85062048bc57

sleep every night is a general guideline. Findings that require further investigation include disruptive sleep patterns and reliance on sleeping pills or other sedative medications.[10]

Life Span Considerations

Older Adults: Disruption in sleep patterns can be especially troublesome for older adults. Assessing sleep patterns and routines will contribute to collaborative interventions for improved rest.[11]

For more information, visit the "Sleep and Rest" chapter in Open RN *Nursing Fundamentals.*

Cognitive and Perceptual

The cognitive and perceptual category focuses on a person's ability to collect information from the environment and use it in reasoning and other thought processes. This category includes the following:

- Adequacy of vision, hearing, taste, touch, feeling, and smell
- Any assistive devices used
- Pain level and pain management
- Cognitive functional abilities, such as orientation, memory, reasoning, judgment, and decision-making[12]

If a patient is experiencing pain, it is important to perform an in-depth assessment using the PQRSTU method described in the "Reason for Seeking Health Care" section of this chapter. It is also helpful to use evidence-based assessment tools when assessing pain, especially for patients who are unable to verbally describe the severity of their pain. See Figure 2.4[13] for an image of the Wong-Baker FACES tool that is commonly used in health care.

---

10 This work is a derivative of The Complete Subjective Health Assessment by Lapum, St-Amant, Hughes, Petrie, Morrell, and Mistry licensed under CC BY-SA 4.0. Access for free at https://openlibrary.ecampusontario.ca/catalogue/item/?id=df19b620-466b-4167-be67-85062048bc57

11 This work is a derivative of The Complete Subjective Health Assessment by Lapum, St-Amant, Hughes, Petrie, Morrell, and Mistry licensed under CC BY-SA 4.0. Access for free at https://openlibrary.ecampusontario.ca/catalogue/item/?id=df19b620-466b-4167-be67-85062048bc57

12 Gordon, M. (2008). Assess notes nursing: Nursing assessment and diagnostic reasoning for clinical practice. F.A. Davis Company.

13 Wong-Baker FACES Foundation (2020). Wong-Baker FACES® Pain Rating Scale.

My Notes

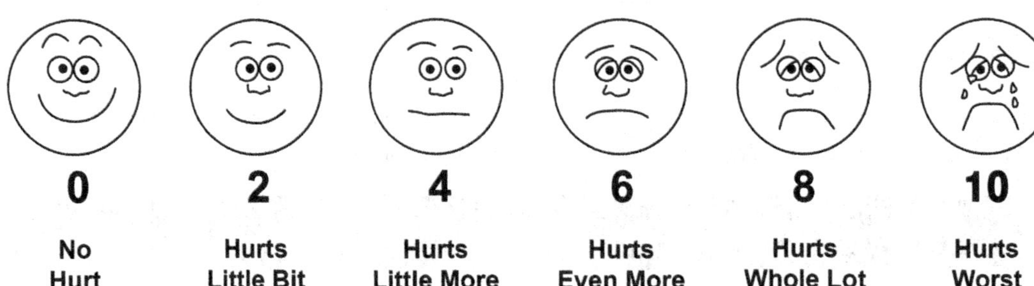

Figure 2.4 The Wong-Baker FACES Pain Rating Scale. Used with permission from http://www.WongBakerFACES.org.

Life Span Considerations

Older Adults: Older adults are especially at risk for problems in the cognitive and perceptual category. Be alert for cues that suggest deficits are occurring that have not been previously diagnosed.

Roles – Relationships

Quality of life is greatly influenced by the roles and relationships established with family, friends, and the broader community. Roles often define our identity. For example, a patient may describe themselves as a "mother of an 8 year old." This category focuses on roles and relationships that may be influenced by health-related factors or may offer support during illness.[14] Findings that require further investigation include indications that a patient does not have any meaningful relationships or has "negative" or abusive relationships in their lives.

Life Span Considerations

Be sensitive to cues when assessing individuals with any of the following characteristics: isolation from family and friends during crisis, language barriers, loss of a significant person or pet, loss of job, significant home care needs, prolonged caregiving, history of abuse, history of substance abuse, or homelessness.[15]

Sexuality – Reproduction

Sexuality and sexual relations are an aspect of health that can be affected by illness, aging, and medication. This category includes a person's gender identity and **sexual orientation**, as well as reproductive issues. It involves a

---

14 Gordon, M. (2008). *Assess notes nursing: Nursing assessment and diagnostic reasoning for clinical practice.* F. A. Davis Company.

15 Gordon, M. (2008). *Assess notes nursing: Nursing assessment and diagnostic reasoning for clinical practice.* F. A. Davis Company.

combination of emotional connection, physical companionship (holding hands, hugging, kissing) and sexual activity that impact one's feeling of health.[16]

The Joint Commission has defined terms to use when caring for diverse patients. **Gender identity** is a person's basic sense of being male, female, or other gender.[17] **Gender expression** are characteristics in appearance, personality, and behavior that are culturally defined as masculine or feminine.[18] **Sexual orientation** is the preferred term used when referring to an individual's physical and/or emotional attraction to the same and/or opposite gender.[19] **LGBT** is an acronym standing for the lesbian, gay, bisexual, and transgender population. It is an umbrella term that generally refers to a group of people who are diverse in gender identity and sexual orientation. It is important to provide a safe environment to discuss health issues because the LGBT population experiences higher rates of smoking, alcohol use, substance abuse, HIV and other STD infections, anxiety, depression, suicidal ideation and attempts, and eating disorders as a result of stigma and marginalization.[20]

Life Span Considerations

Although sexuality is frequently portrayed in the media, individuals often consider these topics as private subjects. Use sensitivity when discussing these topics with different age groups across cultural beliefs while maintaining professional boundaries.

> For more information, read the Joint Commission's PDF Field Guide called "Advancing Effective Communication, Cultural Competence, and Patient- and Family-Centered Care for the Lesbian, Gay, Bisexual, and Transgender (LGBT) Community" (https://www.jointcommission.org/-/media/tjc/documents/resources/patient-safety-topics/health-equity/lgbtfieldguide_web_linked_verpdf.pdf).

---

16 This work is a derivative of The Complete Subjective Health Assessment by Lapum, St-Amant, Hughes, Petrie, Morrell, and Mistry licensed under CC BY-SA 4.0. Access for free at https://openlibrary.ecampusontario.ca/catalogue/item/?id=df19b620-466b-4167-be67-85062048bc57

17 The Joint Commission. (2011). *Advancing effective communication, cultural competence, and patient- and family-centered care for the lesbian, gay, bisexual, and transgender (LGBT) community: A field guide.* https://www.jointcommission.org/-/media/tjc/documents/resources/patient-safety-topics/health-equity/lgbtfieldguide_web_linked_verpdf.pdf downloaded from https://www.jointcommission.org/resources/patient-safety-topics/health-equity/#t=_Tab_StandardsFAQs&sort=relevancy

18 The Joint Commission. (2011). *Advancing effective communication, cultural competence, and patient-and family-centered care for the lesbian, gay, bisexual, and transgender (LGBT) community: A field guide.* https://www.jointcommission.org/-/media/tjc/documents/resources/patient-safety-topics/health-equity/lgbtfieldguide_web_linked_verpdf.pdf downloaded from https://www.jointcommission.org/resources/patient-safety-topics/health-equity/#t=_Tab_StandardsFAQs&sort=relevancy

19 The Joint Commission. (2011). *Advancing effective communication, cultural competence, and patient- and family-centered care for the lesbian, gay, bisexual, and transgender (LGBT) community: A field guide.* https://www.jointcommission.org/-/media/tjc/documents/resources/patient-safety-topics/health-equity/lgbtfieldguide_web_linked_verpdf.pdf downloaded from https://www.jointcommission.org/resources/patient-safety-topics/health-equity/#t=_Tab_StandardsFAQs&sort=relevancy

20 The Joint Commission. (2011). *Advancing effective communication, cultural competence, and patient-and family-centered care for the lesbian, gay, bisexual, and transgender (LGBT) community: A field guide.* https://www.jointcommission.org/-/media/tjc/documents/resources/patient-safety-topics/health-equity/lgbtfieldguide_web_linked_verpdf.pdf downloaded from https://www.jointcommission.org/resources/patient-safety-topics/health-equity/#t=_Tab_StandardsFAQs&sort=relevancy

My Notes

Coping-Stress Tolerance

Individuals experience stress that can lead to dysfunction if not managed in a healthy manner. Throughout life, healthy and unhealthy coping strategies are learned. Coping strategies are behaviors used to manage anxiety. Effective strategies control anxiety and lead to problem-solving but ineffective strategies can lead to abuse of food, tobacco, alcohol, or drugs.[21] Nurses teach and reinforce effective coping strategies.

Substance Use and Abuse

Alcohol, tobacco products, marijuana, and drugs are often used as ineffective coping strategies. It is important to use a nonjudgmental approach when assessing a patient's use of substances so they do not feel stigmatized. Substance abuse can affect people of all ages. Make a distinction between use and abuse as you assess frequency of use and patterns of behavior. Substance abuse often causes disruption in everyday function (e.g., loss of employment, deterioration of relationships, or precarious living circumstances) because of dependence on a substance. Action is needed if patients indicate that they have a problem with substance use or show signs of dependence, addiction, or binge drinking.[22]

Life Span Considerations

Some individuals are at increased risk for problems with coping strategies and stress management. Be sensitive to cues when assessing individuals with characteristics such as uncertainty in medical diagnosis or prognosis, financial problems, marital problems, poor job fit, or few close friends and family members.[23]

Value-Belief

This category includes values and beliefs that guide decisions about health care and can also provide strength and comfort to individuals. It is common for a person's spirituality and values to be influenced by religious faith. A **value** is an accepted principle or standard of an individual or group. A **belief** is something accepted as true with a sense of certainty.

Spirituality is a way of living that comes from a set of values and beliefs that are important to a person. The Joint Commission asks health care professionals to respect patients' cultural and personal values, beliefs, and preferences and accommodate patients' rights to religious and other spiritual services.[24] When performing an assessment, use open-ended questions to allow the patient to share values and beliefs they believe are important. For example, ask, "I am interested in your spiritual and religious beliefs and how they relate to your health. Can you share with me any spiritual beliefs or religious practices that are important to you during your stay?"

For more information about assessing and providing for patients' spiritual needs, visit the "Spirituality" chapter in Open RN *Nursing Fundamentals*.

---

21 Gordon, M. (2008). *Assess notes nursing: Nursing assessment and diagnostic reasoning for clinical practice.* F. A. Davis Company.

22 This work is a derivative of The Complete Subjective Health Assessment by Lapum, St-Amant, Hughes, Petrie, Morrell, and Mistry licensed under CC BY-SA 4.0. Access for free at https://openlibrary.ecampusontario.ca/catalogue/item/?id=df19b620-466b-4167-be67-85062048bc57

23 Gordon, M. (2008). *Assess notes nursing: Nursing assessment and diagnostic reasoning for clinical practice.* F. A. Davis Company.

24 The Joint Commission. (2018). *The source, 16*(1). https://store.jcrinc.com/assets/1/14/ts_16_2018_01.pdf

Self-Perception and Self-Concept

My Notes

The focus of this category is on the subjective thoughts, feelings, and attitudes of a patient about themself. **Self-concept** refers to all the knowledge a person has about themself that makes up who they are (i.e., their identity). **Self-esteem** refers to a person's self-evaluation of these items as being worthy or unworthy. **Body image** is a mental picture of one's body related to appearance and function. It is best to assess these items toward the end of the interview because you will have already collected data that contributes to an understanding of the patient's self-concept. Factors that influence a patient's self-concept vary from person to person and include elements of life they value, such as talents, education, accomplishments, family, friends, career, financial status, spirituality, and religion.[25] The self-perception and self-concept category also focuses on feelings and mood states such as happiness, anxiety, hope, power, anger, fear, depression, and control.[26]

Life Span Considerations

Some individuals are at risk for problems with self-perception and self- concept. Be sensitive to cues when assessing individuals with characteristics such as uncertainty regarding a medical diagnosis or surgery, significant personal loss, history of abuse or neglect, loss of body part or function, or history of substance abuse.[27]

Violence and Trauma

There are many types of violence that a person may experience, including neglect or physical, emotional, mental, sexual, or financial abuse. You are legally mandated to report suspected cases of child abuse or neglect, as well as suspected cases of elder abuse. At any time, if you or the patient is in immediate danger, follow agency policy and procedure. Trauma results from violence or other distressing events in a life. Collaborative intervention with the patient is required when violence and trauma are identified. People respond in different ways to trauma. It is important to use a trauma-informed approach when caring for patients who have experienced trauma. For example, a patient may respond to the traumatic situation in a way that seems unfitting (such as with laughter, ambivalence, or denial). This does not mean the patient is lying but can be a symptom of trauma. To reduce the effects of trauma, it is important to implement collaborative interventions to support patients who have experienced trauma.[28]

Loss of Body Part

A person can have negative feelings or perceptions about the characteristics, function, or limits of a body part as a result of a medical condition, surgery, trauma, or mental condition. Pay attention to cues, such as neglect of a body part or negative comments about a body part, and use open-ended questions to obtain additional information.

---

25 This work is a derivative of The Complete Subjective Health Assessment by Lapum, St-Amant, Hughes, Petrie, Morrell, and Mistry licensed under CC BY-SA 4.0. Access for free at https://openlibrary.ecampusontario.ca/catalogue/item/?id=df19b620-466b-4167-be67-85062048bc57

26 Gordon, M. (2008). *Assess notes nursing: Nursing assessment and diagnostic reasoning for clinical practice.* F. A. Davis Company.

27 Gordon, M. (2008). *Assess notes nursing: Nursing assessment and diagnostic reasoning for clinical practice.* F. A. Davis Company.

28 This work is a derivative of The Complete Subjective Health Assessment by Lapum, St-Amant, Hughes, Petrie, Morrell and Mistry licensed under CC BY-SA 4.0. Access for free at https://openlibrary.ecampusontario.ca/catalogue/item/?id=df19b620-466b-4167-be67-85062048bc57

My Notes

Mental Health

Mental health is frequently underscreened and unaddressed in health care. The mental health of all patients should be assessed, even if they appear well or state they have no mental health concerns so that any changes in condition are quickly noticed and treatment implemented. Mental health includes emotional and psychological symptoms that can affect a patient's day-to-day ability to function. The World Health Organization (2014) defines **mental health** as "a state of well-being in which every individual realizes their own potential, can cope with normal stresses of life, can work productively and fruitfully, and is able to make a contribution to their community."[29] Mental illness includes conditions diagnosed by a health care provider, such as depression, anxiety, addiction, schizophrenia, post-traumatic stress disorder, and others. Mental illness can disrupt everyday functioning and affect a person's employment, education, and relationships.

It is helpful to begin this component of a mental health assessment with a statement such as, "Mental health is an important part of our lives, so I ask all patients about their mental health and any concerns or questions they may have."[30] Be attentive of critical findings that require intervention. For example, if a patient talks about feeling hopeless or depressed, it is important to screen for suicidal thinking. Begin with an open-ended question, such as, "Have you ever felt like hurting yourself?" If the patient responds with a "Yes," then progress with specific questions that assess the immediacy and the intensity of the feelings. For example, you may say, "Tell me more about that feeling. Have you been thinking about hurting yourself today? Have you put together a plan to hurt yourself?" When assessing for suicidal thinking, be aware that a patient most at risk is someone who has a specific plan about self-harm and can specify how and when they will do it. They are particularly at risk if planning self-harm within the next 48 hours. The age of the patient is not a factor in this determination of risk. If you believe the patient is at high risk, do not leave the patient alone. Collaborate with them regarding an immediate plan for emergency care.[31]

Health Perception-Health Management

Health perception-health management is an umbrella term encompassing all of the categories described above, as well as environmental health.

Environmental Health

Environmental health refers to the safety of a patient's physical environment, also called a social determinant of health. Examples of environmental health include, but are not limited to, exposure to violence in the home or community; air pollution; and availability of grocery stores, health care providers, and public transportation. Findings that require further investigation include a patient living in unsafe environments.[32]

---

29 This work is a derivative of The Complete Subjective Health Assessment by Lapum, St-Amant, Hughes, Petrie, Morrell and Mistry licensed under CC BY-SA 4.0. Access for free at https://openlibrary.ecampusontario.ca/catalogue/item/?id=df19b620-466b-4167-be67-85062048bc57

30 This work is a derivative of The Complete Subjective Health Assessment by Lapum, St-Amant, Hughes, Petrie, Morrell, and Mistry licensed under CC BY-SA 4.0. Access for free at https://openlibrary.ecampusontario.ca/catalogue/item/?id=df19b620-466b-4167-be67-85062048bc57

31 This work is a derivative of The Complete Subjective Health Assessment by Lapum, St-Amant, Hughes, Petrie, Morrell, and Mistry licensed under CC BY-SA 4.0. Access for free at https://openlibrary.ecampusontario.ca/catalogue/item/?id=df19b620-466b-4167-be67-85062048bc57

32 This work is a derivative of The Complete Subjective Health Assessment by Lapum, St-Amant, Hughes, Petrie, Morrell, and Mistry licensed under CC BY-SA 4.0. Access for free at https://openlibrary.ecampusontario.ca/catalogue/item/?id=df19b620-466b-4167-be67-85062048bc57

My Notes

See Table 2.8 for sample focused questions for all categories related to functional health.[33]

Begin this section by saying, "I would like to ask you some questions about factors that affect your ability to function in your day-to-day life. Feel free to share any health concerns that come to mind during this discussion."

Table 2.8 Focused Interview Questions for Functional Health Categories[34]	
Category	**Focused Questions**
Nutrition	Tell me about your diet. What foods do you usually eat? What fluids do you usually drink every day? What have you eaten in the last 24 hours? Is this typical of your usual eating pattern? Tell me about your appetite. Have you had any changes in your appetite? Do you have any goals related to your nutrition? Do you have any financial concerns about purchasing food? Are you able to prepare the meals you want to eat?
Elimination	When was your last bowel movement? Do you have any problems with constipation, diarrhea, or incontinence? Do you take laxatives or stool softeners? Do you have any problems urinating, such as frequent urination or burning on urination? Do you ever experience leaking or dribbling of urine?

33 This work is a derivative of The Complete Subjective Health Assessment by Lapum, St-Amant, Hughes, Petrie, Morrell, and Mistry licensed under CC BY-SA 4.0. Access for free at https://openlibrary.ecampusontario.ca/catalogue/item/?id=df19b620-466b-4167-be67-85062048bc57

34 This work is a derivative of The Complete Subjective Health Assessment by Lapum, St-Amant, Hughes, Petrie, Morrell, and Mistry licensed under CC BY-SA 4.0. Access for free at https://openlibrary.ecampusontario.ca/catalogue/item/?id=df19b620-466b-4167-be67-85062048bc57

My Notes

Category	Focused Questions
Mobility, Activity, and Exercise	Tell me about your ability to move around. Do you have any problems sitting up, standing up, or walking? Do you use any mobility aids (e.g., cane, walker, wheelchair)? Tell me about the activity and/or exercise in which you engage. What type? How frequent? For how long?
Sleep and Rest	Tell me about your sleep routine. How many hours of sleep do you usually get? Do you feel rested when you awaken? Do you do anything to wind down before you go to bed (e.g., watch TV, read)? Do you take any sleeping medication? Do you take any naps during the day?
Cognitive and Perceptual	Are you having any pain? Note: If present, use the PQRSTU method to further assess pain. Are you having any issues with seeing, hearing, smelling, tasting, or feeling things? Have you noticed any changes in memory or problems concentrating? Have you noticed any changes in the ability to make decisions? What is the easiest way for you to learn (e.g., written materials, explanations, or learning-by-doing)?
Roles and Relationships	Tell me about the most influential relationships in your life with family and friends. How do these relationships influence your day-to-day life, health, and illness? Who are the people with whom you talk to when you require support or are struggling in your life? Do you have family or others dependent on you? Have you had any recent losses of someone important to you, a pet, or a job? Do you feel safe in your current relationship?

My Notes

Category	Focused Questions
Sexuality-Reproduction	The expression of love and caring in a sexual relationship and creation of family are often important aspects in a person's life. Do you have any concerns about your sexual health? Tell me about the ways that you ensure your safety when engaging in intimate and sexual practices.
Coping-Stress	Tell me about the stress in your life. Have you experienced a recent loss in your life that has impacted you? How do you cope with stress?
Values-Belief	I am interested in your spiritual and religious beliefs and how they relate to your health. Can you share with me any spiritual beliefs or religious practices that are important to you?
Self-Perception and Self-Concept	Tell me what makes you who you are. How would you describe yourself? Have you noticed any changes in how you view your body or the things you can do? Are these a problem for you? Have you found yourself feeling sad, angry, fearful, or anxious? What helps you to feel better when this happens? Have you ever used any tobacco products (e.g., cigarettes, pipes, vaporizers, hookah)? If so, how much? How much alcohol do you drink every week? Have you used cannabis products? If so, how often do you use them? Have you ever used drugs or prescription drugs that were not prescribed for you? If so, what type? Have you ever felt you had a problem with any of these substances because they affected your daily life? If so, tell me more. Do you want to quit any of these substances? Many patients have experienced violence or trauma in their lives. Have you experienced any violence or trauma in your life? How has it affected you? Would you like to talk with someone about it?

My Notes

Category	Focused Questions
Health Perception – Health Management	Tell me about how you take care of yourself and manage your home. Have you had any falls in the past six months? Do you have enough finances to pay your bills and purchase food, medications, and other needed items? Do you have any current or future concerns about being able to function independently? Tell me about where you live. Do you have any concerns about safety in your home or neighborhood? Tell me about any factors in your environment that may affect your health. Do you have any concerns about how your environment is affecting your health?

2.9 REVIEW OF BODY SYSTEMS

My Notes

A body system review asks focused questions related to overall health status and body systems such as cardiac, respiratory, neurological, gastrointestinal, urinary, and musculoskeletal systems. See “Chapter Resources A” for a sample health history form that contains brief questions according to body systems. Nurses often incorporate review of system questions into the physical examination of each system. For example, while listening to bowel sounds in the abdomen, a nurse often inquires about the patient’s bowel pattern. Additional focused assessment questions related to each body system are found in each assessment chapter of this book.

My Notes

2.10 SAMPLE DOCUMENTATION

Information obtained during a health history interview is typically documented on agency-specific forms. See "Chapter Resources A" for a sample health history form used for documentation purposes. Additional information collected that is not included on the form should be documented in an associated progress note.

2.11 CHECKLIST FOR OBTAINING A HEALTH HISTORY

My Notes

Use the checklist below to review the steps for completion of "Obtaining a Health History."

Steps

Disclaimer: Always review and follow agency policy regarding this specific skill.

1. Gather supplies: health history agency form.
2. Knock, enter the room, greet the patient, and provide for privacy.
3. Perform safety steps:
    - Perform hand hygiene.
    - Check the room for transmission-based precautions.
    - Introduce yourself, your role, the purpose of your visit, and an estimate of the time it will take.
    - Confirm patient ID using two patient identifiers (e.g., name and date of birth).
    - Explain the process to the patient and ask if they have any questions.
    - Be organized and systematic.
    - Use appropriate listening and questioning skills.
    - Listen and attend to patient cues.
    - Ensure the patient's privacy and dignity.
    - Assess ABCs.
4. Address patient needs (pain, toileting, glasses/hearing aids) prior to starting. Note if the patient has signs of distress such as difficulty breathing or chest pain. If signs are present, defer the health history and obtain emergency assistance per agency policy.
5. Complete a health history interview, including the following components per your instructor's instructions:
    - Demographic and Biological Data
    - Reason for Seeking Health Care
    - Current and Past Medical History
    - Family History
    - Functional Health
    - Review of Body Systems

My Notes

6. Ensure five safety measures before leaving the room:

    - CALL LIGHT: Within reach
    - BED: Low and locked (in lowest position and brakes on)
    - SIDE RAILS: Secured
    - TABLE: Within reach
    - ROOM: Risk-free for falls (scan room and clear any obstacles)

7. Document the health history findings and report any concerns according to agency policy.

2.12 LEARNING ACTIVITIES

My Notes

Learning Activities

(Answers to "Learning Activities" can be found in the "Answer Key" at the end of the book. Answers to interactive activity elements will be provided within the element as immediate feedback.)

You are admitting a patient with a new diagnosis of type 2 diabetes. During the admission assessment, you note that the patient identifies as Muslim. How could you explore the patient's cultural background to better understand how the patient's culture might influence the patient's health status and decisions?

Interactive Activity

An interactive or media element has been excluded from this version of the text. You can view it online here: https://wtcs.pressbooks.pub/nursingskills/?p=1101

Interactive Activity

An interactive or media element has been excluded from this version of the text. You can view it online here: https://wtcs.pressbooks.pub/nursingskills/?p=1101

Interactive Activity

An interactive or media element has been excluded from this version of the text. You can view it online here: https://wtcs.pressbooks.pub/nursingskills/?p=1101

My Notes

II GLOSSARY

Activities of daily living: Daily basic tasks fundamental to everyday functioning (e.g., hygiene, elimination, dressing, eating, ambulating/ moving).

Belief: Something accepted as true with a sense of certainty.[1]

Body image: A mental picture of one's body related to appearance and function.[2]

Care partners: Family and friends who are involved in helping to care for the patient.

Chief complaint: The reason a patient is seeking health care during a visit to a clinic or on admission to a health care facility.

Cultural safety: The creation of safe spaces for patients to interact with health professionals without judgment or discrimination.

Dysuria: Discomfort or pain on urinating.

Elimination: Refers to the removal of waste products through the urine and stool.

Functional health: The patient's physical and mental capacity to participate in activities of daily living (ADLs) and instrumental activities of daily living (IADLs).

Gender expression: Characteristics in appearance, personality, and behavior, culturally defined as masculine or feminine.[3]

Gender identity: One's basic sense of being male, female, or other gender.[4]

Health history: The process of using directed interview questions to obtain symptoms and perceptions about a patient's illness or life condition. The purpose of obtaining a health history is to gather subjective data from the patient and/or the patient's family so that the health care team and the patient can collaboratively create a plan that will promote health, address acute health problems, and minimize chronic health conditions.

Instrumental activities of daily living: Complex daily tasks that allow patients to function independently such as managing finances, paying bills, purchasing and preparing meals, managing one's household, taking medications, and facilitating transportation.

---

1 Gordon, M. (2008). *Assess notes nursing: Nursing assessment and diagnostic reasoning for clinical practice.* F. A. Davis Company.

2 Gordon, M. (2008). *Assess notes nursing: Nursing assessment and diagnostic reasoning for clinical practice.* F. A. Davis Company.

3 The Joint Commission. (2011). *Advancing effective communication, cultural competence, and patient-and family-centered care for the lesbian, gay, bisexual, and transgender (LGBT) community: A field guide.* https://www.jointcommission.org/-/media/tjc/documents/resources/patient-safety-topics/health-equity/lgbtfieldguide_web_linked_verpdf.pdf downloaded from https://www.jointcommission.org/resources/patient-safety-topics/health-equity/#t=_Tab_StandardsFAQs&sort=relevancy

4 The Joint Commission. (2011). A*dvancing effective communication, cultural competence, and patient- and family-centered care for the lesbian, gay, bisexual, and transgender (LGBT) community: A field guide.* https://www.jointcommission.org/-/media/tjc/documents/resources/patient-safety-topics/health-equity/lgbtfieldguide_web_linked_verpdf.pdf downloaded from https://www.jointcommission.org/resources/patient-safety-topics/health-equity/#t=_Tab_StandardsFAQs&sort=relevancy

My Notes

LGBT: An acronym standing for lesbian, gay, bisexual, and transgender and is an umbrella term that generally refers to a group of people who are diverse with regard to their gender identity and sexual orientation. There are expanded versions of this acronym.[5]

Main health care needs: Term used to classify what needs the patient feels are most important to address after admission to a health care agency.

Medication reconciliation: A comparison of a list of current medications with a previous list and is completed at every hospitalization and clinic visit.

Melena: Dark, tarry-looking stool due to the presence of digested blood.

Mental health: A state of well-being in which every individual realizes their own potential, can cope with normal stresses of life, can work productively and fruitfully, and is able to make a contribution to their community.[6]

Mobility: A patient's ability to move around (e.g., sit up, sit down, stand up, walk).

Nursing: The protection, promotion, and optimization of health and abilities, prevention of illness and injury, facilitation of healing, alleviation of suffering through the diagnosis and treatment of human response, and advocacy in the care of individuals, families, groups, communities, and population.[7]

Objective data: Information observed through your sense of hearing, sight, smell, and touch while assessing the patient.

Primary source of data: Information obtained directly from the patient.

Secondary source of data: Information from the patient's chart, family members, or other health care team members.

Self-concept: Knowledge a person has about themselves that makes up who they are (i.e., their identity).

Self-esteem: A person's self-evaluation of their self-concept as being worthy or unworthy.

Sexual orientation: The preferred term used when referring to an individual's physical and/or emotional attraction to the same and/or opposite gender.[8]

Sign: Objective data found by the nurse or health care provider when assessing a patient.

Spirituality: A way of living that comes from a set of meanings, values, and beliefs that are important to a person.[9]

Subjective data: Information obtained from the patient and/or family members that offers important cues from their perspectives.

Symptom: Subjective data that the patient reports, such as "I feel dizzy."

---

5 The Joint Commission. (2011). *Advancing effective communication, cultural competence, and patient-and family-centered care for the lesbian, gay, bisexual, and transgender (LGBT) community: A field guide.* https://www.jointcommission.org/-/media/tjc/documents/resources/patient-safety-topics/health-equity/lgbtfieldguide_web_linked_verpdf.pdf downloaded from https://www.jointcommission.org/resources/patient-safety-topics/health-equity/#t=_Tab_StandardsFAQs&sort=relevancy

6 This work is a derivative of The Complete Subjective Health Assessment by Lapum, St-Amant, Hughes, Petrie, Morrell, and Mistry licensed under CC BY-SA 4.0. Access for free at https://openlibrary.ecampusontario.ca/catalogue/item/?id=df19b620-466b-4167-be67-85062048bc57

7 American Nurses Association. (2015). *Nursing: Scope and standards of practice* (3rd ed.). American Nurses Association.

8 The Joint Commission. (2011). *Advancing effective communication, cultural competence, and patient- and family-centered care for the lesbian, gay, bisexual, and transgender (LGBT) community: A field guide.* https://www.jointcommission.org/-/media/tjc/documents/resources/patient-safety-topics/health-equity/lgbtfieldguide_web_linked_verpdf.pdf downloaded from https://www.jointcommission.org/resources/patient-safety-topics/health-equity/#t=_Tab_StandardsFAQs&sort=relevancy

9 Gordon, M. (2008). *Assess notes nursing: Nursing assessment and diagnostic reasoning for clinical practice.* F. A. Davis Company.

My Notes

Value: An accepted principle or standard of an individual or group.[10]

Voiding: Medical terminology used for urinating.

10 Gordon, M. (2008). *Assess notes nursing: Nursing assessment and diagnostic reasoning for clinical practice.* F. A. Davis Company.

CHAPTER RESOURCES A: SAMPLE HEALTH HISTORY FORM

My Notes

Please view a "Sample Health History Form" (https://docs.google.com/document/d/1cw1THqBpHKi7_IggH3FoiVy3HidVzoO1dWpzupkLL1M/edit?usp=sharing).

Chapter 3

Blood Pressure

3.1 BLOOD PRESSURE INTRODUCTION

My Notes

Learning Objectives

- Accurately measure and document blood pressure using American Heart Association standards
- Adapt the procedure to reflect variations across the life span
- Recognize and report significant deviations from blood pressure norms

The accurate measurement of blood pressure is important for ensuring patient safety and optimizing body system function. Blood pressure measurements are used by health care providers to make important decisions about a patient's care. Blood pressure measurements help providers make decisions about whether a patient needs fluids or prescription medications. It is crucial to follow the proper steps to obtain a patient's blood pressure to ensure the care team has accurate data to help make health care decisions and determine a plan of care.

My Notes

3.2 BLOOD PRESSURE BASICS

What is Blood Pressure?

A blood pressure reading is the measurement of the force of blood against the walls of the arteries as the heart pumps blood through the body. It is reported in millimeters of mercury (mmHg). This pressure changes in the arteries when the heart is contracting compared to when it is resting and filling with blood. Blood pressure is typically expressed as the reflection of two numbers, systolic pressure and diastolic pressure. The **systolic blood pressure** is the maximum pressure on the arteries during systole, the phase of the heartbeat when the ventricles contract. **Systole** causes the ejection of blood out of the ventricles and into the aorta and pulmonary arteries. The **diastolic blood pressure** is the resting pressure on the arteries during **diastole**, the phase between each contraction of the heart when the ventricles are filling with blood.[1]

Blood pressure measurements are obtained using a stethoscope and a **sphygmomanometer**, also called a blood pressure cuff. To obtain a manual blood pressure reading, the blood pressure cuff is placed around a patient's extremity, and a stethoscope is placed over an artery. For most blood pressure readings, the cuff is usually placed around the upper arm, and the stethoscope is placed over the brachial artery. The cuff is inflated to constrict the artery until the pulse is no longer palpable, and then it is deflated slowly. The American Heart Association (AHA) recommends that the blood pressure cuff be inflated at least 30 mmHg above the point at which the radial pulse is no longer palpable. The first appearance of sounds, called **Korotkoff sounds**, are noted as the systolic blood pressure reading. Korotkoff sounds are named after Dr. Korotkoff, who first discovered the audible sounds of blood pressure when the arm is constricted.[2] The blood pressure cuff continues to be deflated until Korotkoff sounds disappear. The last Korotkoff sounds reflect the diastolic blood pressure reading.[3] It is important to deflate the cuff slowly at no more than 2-3 mmHg per second to ensure that the absence of pulse is noted promptly and that the reading is accurate. Blood pressure readings are documented as systolic blood pressure/diastolic pressure, for example, 120/80 mmHg.

Abnormal blood pressure readings can signify an area of concern and a need for intervention. Normal adult blood pressure is less than 120/80 mmHg. **Hypertension** is the medical term for elevated blood pressure readings of 130/80 mmHg or higher. See Table 4.2 for blood pressure categories according to the 2017 American College of Cardiology and American Heart Association Blood Pressure Guidelines.[4] Prior to diagnosing a person with hypertension, the health care provider will calculate an average blood pressure based on two or more blood pressure readings obtained on two or more occasions.

For more information about hypertension and blood pressure medications, visit the "Cardiovascular and Renal System" chapter in Open RN *Nursing Pharmacology*.

1 This work is a derivative of Vital Sign Measurement Across the Lifespan - 1st Canadian Edition by Ryerson University licensed under CC BY 4.0. Access for free at https://pressbooks.library.ryerson.ca/vitalsign/

2 This work is a derivative of StatPearls by Campbell and Pillarisetty licensed under CC BY 4.0. Access for free at https://www.ncbi.nlm.nih.gov/books/NBK539778/

3 This work is a derivative of Clinical Procedures for Safer Patient Care by British Columbia Institute of Technology licensed under CC BY 4.0. Access for free at https://opentextbc.ca/clinicalskills/

4 American College of Cardiology. Whelton, P. K., Carey, R. M., Aronow, W. S., et al. (2018, May 7). *2017 guidelines for high blood pressure in adults.* https://www.acc.org/latest-in-cardiology/ten-points-to-remember/2017/11/09/11/41/2017-guideline-for-high-blood-pressure-in-adults

My Notes

Hypotension is the medical term for low blood pressure readings less than 90/60 mmHg.[5] Hypotension can be caused by dehydration, bleeding, cardiac conditions, and the side effects of many medications. Hypotension can be of significant concern because of the potential lack of perfusion to critical organs when blood pressures are low. **Orthostatic hypotension** is a drop in blood pressure that occurs when moving from a lying down (supine) or seated position to a standing (upright) position. When measuring blood pressure, orthostatic hypotension is defined as a decrease in blood pressure by at least 20 mmHg systolic or 10 mmHg diastolic within three minutes of standing. When a person stands, gravity moves blood from the upper body to the lower limbs. As a result, there is a temporary reduction in the amount of blood in the upper body for the heart to pump, which decreases blood pressure. Normally, the body quickly counteracts the force of gravity and maintains stable blood pressure and blood flow. In most people, this transient drop in blood pressure goes unnoticed. However, some patients with orthostatic hypotension can experience light-headedness, dizziness, or fainting. This is a significant safety concern because of the increased risk of falls and injury, particularly in older adults.[6]

Table 4.2 Blood Pressure Categories[7]

Blood Pressure Category	Systolic mm Hg (upper #)	Diastolic mm Hg (lower #)
Normal	< 120	< 80
Stage 1	130-139	80-89
Stage 2	At least 140	At least 90
Hypertensive Crisis	> 180	> 120

View Ahmend Alzawi's Korotkoff Sounds video on YouTube.[8]

5 National Heart, Lung, and Blood Institute. (n.d.). *Low blood pressure*. https://www.nhlbi.nih.gov/health-topics/low-blood-pressure

6 U.S. National Library of Medicine. (2020, June 23). *Orthostatic hypotension*. https://ghr.nlm.nih.gov/condition/orthostatic-hypotension

7 American College of Cardiology. Whelton, P. K., Carey, R. M., Aronow, W. S., et al. (2018, May 7). *2017 guidelines for high blood pressure in adults*. https://www.acc.org/latest-in-cardiology/ten-points-to-remember/2017/11/09/11/41/2017-guideline-for-high-blood-pressure-in-adults

8 Alzawi, A. (2015, November 19). *Korotkoff+Blood+Pressure+Sights+and+Sounds SD*. [Video]. YouTube. All rights reserved. https://youtu.be/UfCr_wUepxo

My Notes

Equipment to Measure Blood Pressure

Manual Blood Pressure

A sphygmomanometer, commonly called a blood pressure cuff, is used to measure blood pressure while Korotkoff sounds are auscultated using a stethoscope. See Figure 3.1[9] for an image of a sphygmomanometer.

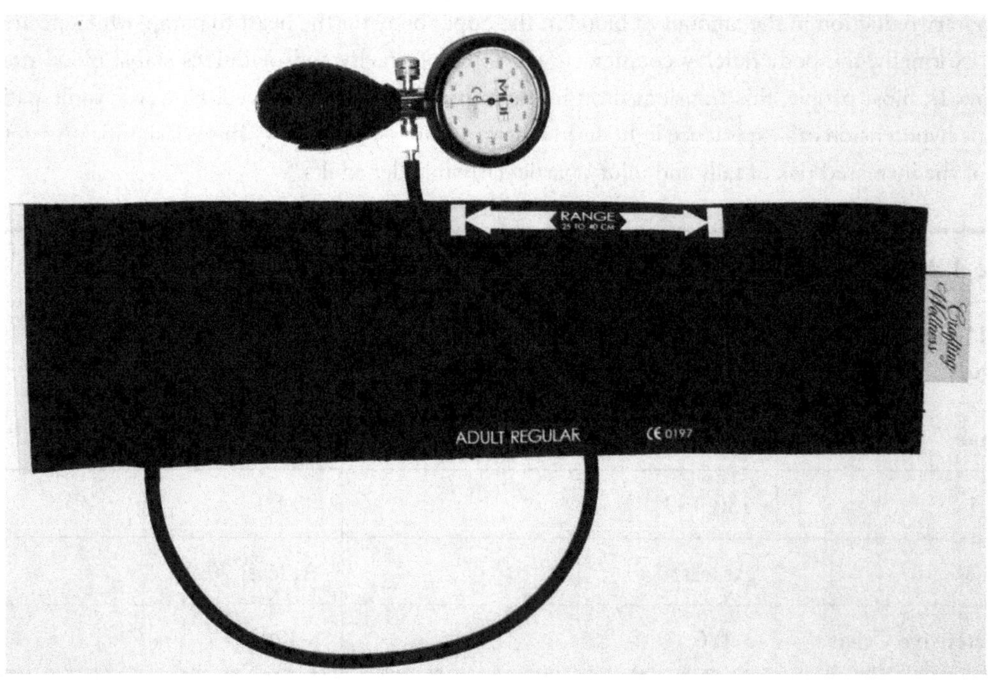

Figure 3.1 A Sphygmomanometer

There are various sizes of blood pressure cuffs. It is crucial to select the appropriate size for the patient to obtain an accurate reading. An undersized cuff will cause an artificially high blood pressure reading, and an oversized cuff will produce an artificially low reading. See Figure 3.2[10] for an image of various sizes of blood pressure cuffs ranging in size for a large adult to an infant.

---

9 "Sphygmomanometer&Cuff.JPG" by ML5 is in the Public Domain. Access for free at https://commons.wikimedia.org/wiki/File:Sphygmomanometer%26Cuff.JPG

10 "BP-Multiple-Cuff-Sizes.jpg" by British Columbia Institute of Technology (BCIT) is licensed under CC BY 4.0. Access for free at https://opentextbc.ca/vitalsign/chapter/how-is-blood-pressure-measured/

My Notes

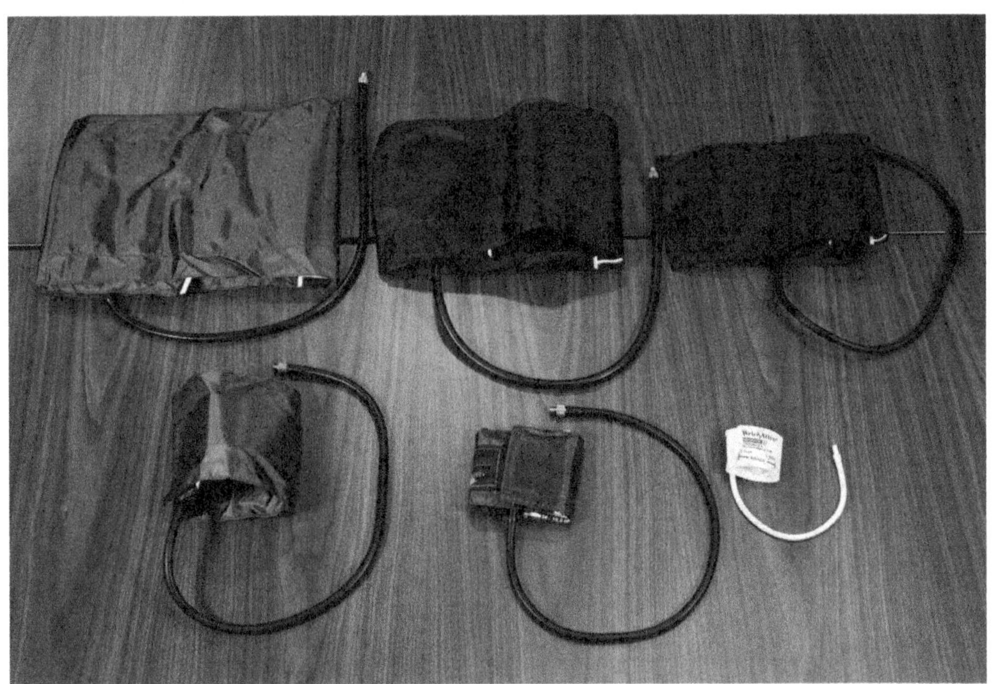

Figure 3.2 Sizes of Blood Pressure Cuffs

The width of the cuff should be 40% of the person's arm circumference, and the length of the cuff's bladder should be 80–100% of the person's arm circumference. Keep in mind that only about half of the blood pressure cuff is the bladder and the other half is cloth with a hook and loop fastener to secure it around the arm.

 **View Ryerson University's "Accurate Blood Pressure Cuff Sizing" video on YouTube.[11]**

Automatic Blood Pressure Equipment

Automatic blood pressure monitors are often used in health care settings to efficiently measure blood pressure for multiple patients or to repeatedly measure a single patient's blood pressure at a specific frequency such as every 15 minutes. See Figure 3.3[12] for an image of an automatic blood pressure monitor. To use an automatic blood pressure monitor, appropriately position the patient and place the correctly sized blood pressure cuff on their bare arm or other extremity. Press the start button on the monitor. The cuff will automatically inflate and then deflate at a rate of 2 mmHg per second. The monitor digitally displays the blood pressure reading when done. If the blood pressure reading is unexpected, it is important to follow up by obtaining a reading using a manual blood pressure cuff. Additionally, automatic blood pressure monitors should not be used if the patient has a rapid or irregular heart rhythm, such as atrial fibrillation, or has tremors as it may lead to an inaccurate reading.

---

11 Ryerson University. (2018, March 21). *Blood pressure - Accurate cuff sizing.* [Video]. YouTube. All rights reserved. https://youtu.be/uNTMwoJTfFE

12 "Automatische bloeddrukmeter (0).jpg" by Harmid is in the Public Domain. Access for free at https://commons.wikimedia.org/wiki/File:Automatische_bloeddrukmeter_(0).jpg

My Notes

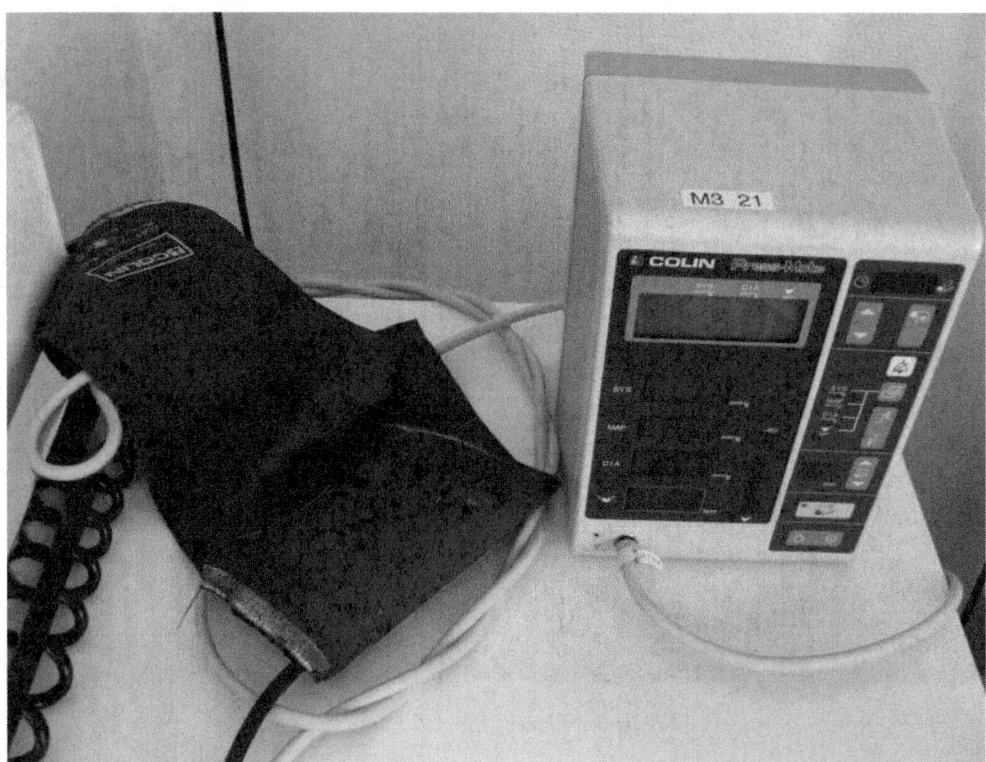

Figure 3.3 Automatic Blood Pressure Monitor

Interactive Activity

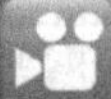 An interactive or media element has been excluded from this version of the text. You can view it online here: https://wtcs.pressbooks.pub/nursingskills/?p=485

Interactive Activity

 An interactive or media element has been excluded from this version of the text. You can view it online here: https://wtcs.pressbooks.pub/nursingskills/?p=485

3.3 BLOOD PRESSURE ASSESSMENT

My Notes

Subjective Assessment

Before taking a person's blood pressure, it is important to determine if they have a history of elevated blood pressure or if they are taking any blood pressure medication. It is helpful to establish a baseline by asking their usual blood pressure reading or reviewing previous records in their chart. It is also important to determine if there are any arm restrictions such as those due to a fistula, mastectomy, stroke, or IV line before measuring blood pressure. See Table 3.3a for sample interview questions associated with the subjective assessment of blood pressure.

Table 3.3a Interview Questions for Subjective Assessment of Blood Pressure

Interview Questions
Have you ever been diagnosed with an elevated blood pressure? ■ Please describe the treatment.
Are you currently taking any medications, herbs, or supplements for your blood pressure? ■ Please identify what you are taking.
Do you have any restrictions on taking blood pressure in your arms such as those due to a fistula or mastectomy? ■ Please describe the restrictions.
What is your usual blood pressure reading?
Do you take your blood pressure at home? ■ What time of day do your take the reading? ■ Where do you obtain the reading from (i.e., cuff location and placement)? ■ What is the range of results that you commonly receive in the home setting?
If applicable: ■ Are you experiencing any symptoms related to high or low blood pressure now, such as a severe headache, dizziness with position changes, light-headedness, or fainting episodes?

Objective Assessment

Inspection

Before obtaining a blood pressure reading, it is important to inspect and consider conditions that would prevent the use of a blood pressure cuff, such as a history of clots or presence of current clots, lymphedema, wounds, a fistula, or current IV access lines. If these conditions exist, obtain the blood pressure in an alternative extremity.

My Notes

Life Span Considerations

Children

Blood pressure measurement is not routinely performed on children under the age of 3 unless there are cardiac concerns.

Older Adults

Blood pressure measurements are sometimes difficult to hear in older adults. For patients who are clinically stable and Korotkoff sound auscultation is difficult, Doppler auscultation may be helpful.

Clinical Tips

Blood pressure assessment should be completed after the patient has rested for a minimum of five minutes. If the patient has ingested caffeine or nicotine within 30 minutes before measuring blood pressure, this should be documented with the reading.

There are times when it is difficult to auscultate Korotkoff sounds. As a result, the care team must decide what alternate measures could be performed to obtain accurate blood pressure results. For patients who are critically ill or hemodynamically unstable, an arterial line may be placed directly into an artery to measure blood pressure. This is an invasive procedure and is not used for routine monitoring.

See Table 3.3b for a comparison of expected versus unexpected findings when assessing blood pressure.

Table 3.3b Expected Versus Unexpected Findings on Blood Pressure Assessment

Assessment	Expected Findings	Unexpected Findings (Document or notify provider if this is a new finding*)
Inspection	Not applicable	Evidence of fistula, lymphadenopathy, IVs, clots, deficits from a stroke, or other restrictions from using the arm for blood pressure readings should be documented and communicated in handoff reports for continuity of care.
Auscultation	Able to identify Korotkoff sounds and blood pressure reading within expected parameters	Unable to identify Korotkoff sounds or blood pressure readings are outside of expected parameters.
Palpation	Able to palpate pulse	Unable to palpate pulse.
***CRITICAL CONDITIONS to report immediately**		Blood pressure readings are outside of expected parameters for this patient's age or the patient has symptoms associated with a blood pressure that is out of range.

3.4 SAMPLE DOCUMENTATION

My Notes

Sample Documentation of Expected Findings

Blood pressure was 120/80 mmHg on the left arm with the patient in a seated position using a manual cuff.

Sample Documentation of Unexpected Findings

Blood pressure reading was collected with routine vital signs and noted to be 160/95 in the right arm. Blood pressure was retaken in the left arm after the patient rested for 5 minutes and was 154/93. Patient reports no history of hypertension and no current blood pressure medications. Patient denies dizziness, headache, visual changes, and light-headedness. Dr. Smith was notified, and an order for furosemide 20 mg was received.

My Notes

3.5 CHECKLIST FOR MANUAL BLOOD PRESSURE

Use the checklist below to review the steps for obtaining a "Manual Blood Pressure."

Note: The two-step method includes the first step of inflating the cuff and palpating the radial pulse to estimate the systolic blood pressure before obtaining the blood pressure reading. This procedure is based on current AHA recommendations.[1]

Steps

Disclaimer: Always review and follow agency policy regarding this specific skill.

1. Gather supplies: blood pressure cuff and stethoscope. (Select an appropriately sized cuff for the patient.)
    - The width of the cuff should be 40% of the person's arm circumference, and the length of the cuff's bladder should be 80–100% of the person's arm circumference.
2. Perform safety steps:
    - Perform hand hygiene.
    - Check the room for transmission-based precautions.
    - Introduce yourself, your role, the purpose of your visit, and an estimate of the time it will take.
    - Confirm patient ID using two patient identifiers (e.g., name and date of birth).
    - Explain the process to the patient and ask if they have any questions.
    - Be organized and systematic.
    - Use appropriate listening and questioning skills.
    - Listen and attend to patient cues.
    - Ensure the patient's privacy and dignity.
    - Assess ABCs.
3. Cleanse the stethoscope and blood pressure cuff prior to placing it on the patient's skin.
4. Place the patient in a relaxed reclining or sitting position. The patient should be seated quietly for at least five minutes in a chair prior to blood pressure measurement. Ask the patient which arm they prefer to use. Be aware of conditions that contraindicate the use of an arm for blood pressure measurement, such as a previous mastectomy or the presence of a fistula. During the procedure, both feet should be on the floor and the arm should be supported at heart level.
    - Adapt the procedure to life span considerations of the patient.
5. Remove or rearrange clothing so the cuff and the stethoscope are on bare skin.

---

1 Chobanian, A. V., Bakris, G. L., Black, H. R., Cushman, W. C., Green, L. A., Izzo, J. L., Jones Jr., D. W., Materson, B. J., Oparil, S., Wright Jr., J., Roccella, E. J., & National High Blood Pressure Education Program Coordinating Committee. (2003). Seventh report of the Joint National Committee on the Prevention, Detection, Evaluation and Treatment of High Blood Pressure. *Hypertension, 42*(6), 1206-1252. https://doi.org/10.1161/01.HYP.0000107251.49515.c2

My Notes

6. Center the bladder of the blood pressure cuff over the brachial artery with the lower margin 1" above the antecubital space. Fit the cuff evenly and snugly. Palpate the brachial artery in the antecubital space.
7. Locate the radial pulse.
8. Inflate the cuff rapidly (while palpating the radial or brachial pulse) to the level at which pulsations are no longer felt and inflate the cuff 30 mmHg above the palpated pressure or the patient's usual blood pressure. Note the level and rapidly deflate the cuff; wait 30 seconds.
9. With the eartips of the stethoscope placed downward and forward, place the bell/diaphragm lightly on the brachial artery and rapidly inflate the cuff to 30 points above where the brachial or radial pulse is no longer felt.
10. Deflate the cuff gradually at a constant rate by opening the valve on the bulb (2-3 mm Hg/second) until the first Korotkoff sound is heard. Note the systolic pressure.
11. Continue to deflate the cuff slowly at 2 mm Hg/second. Note the point at which Korotkoff sounds disappear completely as the diastolic pressure.
12. Deflate the cuff completely and remove the patient's arm from the cuff.
13. Inform the patient of the blood pressure reading.
14. Cleanse the stethoscope and blood pressure cuff.
15. Perform proper hand hygiene.
16. Ensure five safety measures before leaving the room:
    - CALL LIGHT: Within reach
    - BED: Low and locked (in lowest position and brakes on)
    - SIDE RAIL: Secured
    - TABLE: Within reach
    - ROOM: Risk-free for falls (scan room and clear any obstacles)
17. Document findings and report significant deviations from norms according to agency policy.

My Notes

3.6 SUPPLEMENTARY VIDEO OF BLOOD PRESSURE ASSESSMENT

Video Review of Blood Pressure Assessment[1]

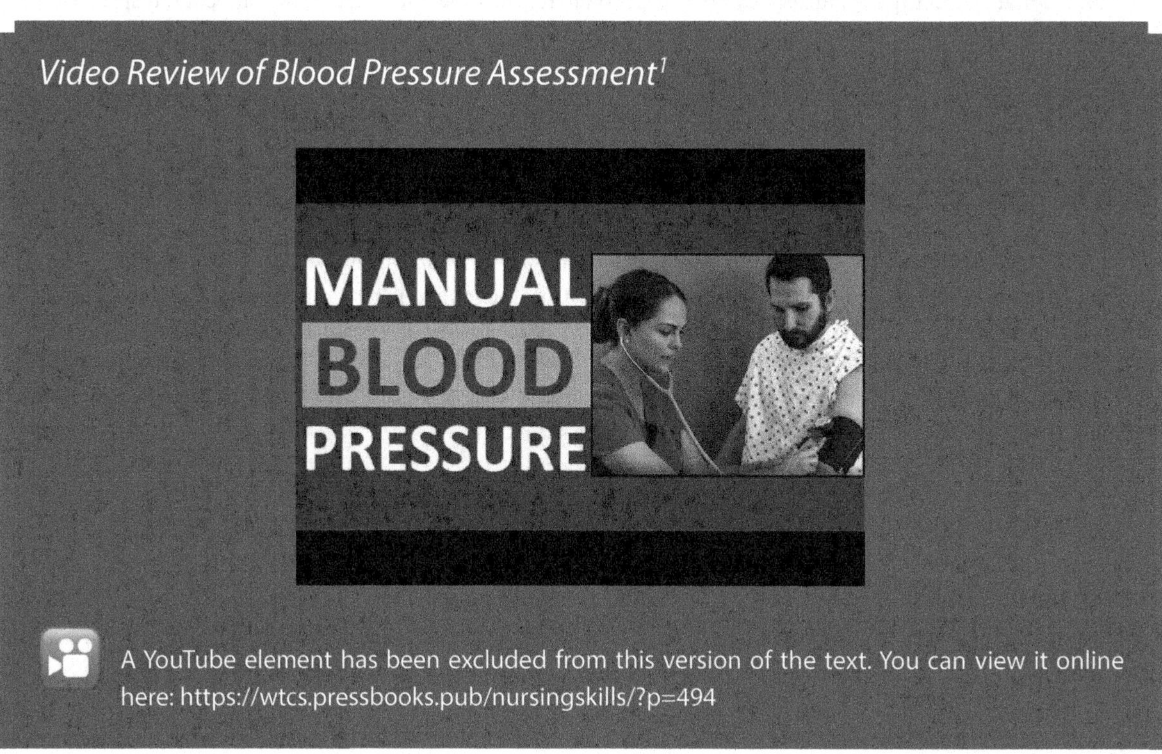

A YouTube element has been excluded from this version of the text. You can view it online here: https://wtcs.pressbooks.pub/nursingskills/?p=494

1 RegisteredNurseRN. (2019, June 4). *Blood pressure measurement: How to check blood pressure manually*. [Video]. YouTube. All rights reserved. Video used with permission. https://youtu.be/UGOoeqSo_ws

3.7 LEARNING ACTIVITIES

My Notes

Learning Activities

(Answers to "Learning Activities" can be found in the "Answer Key" at the end of the book. Answers to interactive activity elements will be provided within the element as immediate feedback.)

You are a nurse assigned to help with blood pressure screenings at the local senior center. What elements must be considered when selecting equipment and location of blood pressure assessment?

Interactive Activity

An interactive or media element has been excluded from this version of the text. You can view it online here: https://wtcs.pressbooks.pub/nursingskills/?p=496

Interactive Activity

An interactive or media element has been excluded from this version of the text. You can view it online here: https://wtcs.pressbooks.pub/nursingskills/?p=496

Interactive Activity

An interactive or media element has been excluded from this version of the text. You can view it online here: https://wtcs.pressbooks.pub/nursingskills/?p=496

My Notes

III GLOSSARY

Diastole: The phase between each contraction of the heart when the ventricles are filling with blood.

Diastolic blood pressure: The resting pressure of blood on the arteries between each cardiac contraction.

Hypertension: Elevated blood pressure over 130/80 mmHg in an adult.

Hypotension: Decreased blood pressure less than 90/60 mmHg in an adult.

Korotkoff sounds: The audible sounds of blood pressure named after Dr. Korotkoff who discovered them.

Orthostatic hypotension: A decrease in blood pressure by at least 20 mmHg systolic or 10 mmHg diastolic within three minutes of standing from a seated or lying position.

Sphygmomanometer: A device used to measure blood pressure and is commonly referred to as a blood pressure cuff.

Systole: The phase of the heartbeat when the left ventricle contracts and pumps blood into the arteries.

Systolic blood pressure: The maximum pressure of blood on the arteries during the contraction of the left ventricle of the heart referred to as systole.

Chapter 4

Aseptic Technique

4.1 ASEPTIC TECHNIQUE INTRODUCTION

My Notes

Learning Objectives

- Perform appropriate hand hygiene
- Use standard precautions
- Use category-specific, transmission-based precautions
- Maintain a sterile field and equipment
- Apply and safely remove sterile gloves and personal protective equipment
- Dispose of contaminated wastes appropriately

According to the Centers for Disease Control and Prevention (CDC), over 2 million patients in America contract a healthcare-associated infection, and 99,000 patients die from a healthcare-associated infection every year.[1] **Healthcare-associated infections** (HAIs) are unintended and often preventable infections caused by care received in a health care setting. Healthcare-associated infections can be prevented by consistently following standard precautions and transmission-based precautions outlined by the CDC (2020). Standard precautions are used when caring for all patients and include performing appropriate **hand hygiene**; wearing **personal protective equipment** when indicated; implementing category-specific transmission precautions; encouraging respiratory hygiene; and following environmental infection control measures, including handling of sharps, laundry, and hazardous waste. Additional infection control measures include the appropriate use of aseptic technique and sterile technique when performing nursing procedures to protect the patient from transmission of microorganisms.[2] Each of these strategies to keep patients and health care workers free of infection is discussed in further detail in this chapter.

---

1 The Joint Commission. (n.d.). *Hand hygiene*. https://www.centerfortransforminghealthcare.org/improvement-topics/hand-hygiene/?_ga=2.185680553.1649963228.1601313691-322773533.1571518854

2 Collins, A. S. (2008). Preventing health care-associated infections. In Hughes, R.G. (Ed.). *Patient safety and quality: An evidence-based handbook for nurses*. https://www.ncbi.nlm.nih.gov/books/NBK2683/

My Notes

4.2 ASEPTIC TECHNIQUE BASIC CONCEPTS

Standard Versus Transmission-Based Precautions

Standard Precautions

Standard precautions are used when caring for all patients to prevent health care associated infections. According to the Centers for Disease Control and Prevention (CDC), **standard precautions** are "the minimum infection prevention practices that apply to all patient care, regardless of suspected or confirmed infection status of the patient, in any setting where health care is delivered."[1] They are based on the principle that all blood, body fluids (except sweat), nonintact skin, and mucous membranes may contain transmissible infectious agents. These standards reduce the risk of exposure for the health care worker and protect the patient from potential transmission of infectious organisms.

Current standard precautions according to the CDC (2019) include the following:

1. Appropriate hand hygiene
2. Use of personal protective equipment (e.g., gloves, gowns, masks, eyewear) whenever infectious material exposure may occur
3. Appropriate patient placement and care using transmission-based precautions when indicated
4. Respiratory hygiene/cough etiquette
5. Proper handling and cleaning of environment, equipment, and devices
6. Safe handling of laundry
7. Sharps safety (i.e., engineering and work practice controls)
8. Aseptic technique for invasive nursing procedures such as parenteral medication administration[2]

Each of these standard precautions is described in more detail in the following subsections.

Transmission-Based Precautions

In addition to standard precautions, transmission-based precautions are used for patients with documented or suspected infection, or colonization, of highly-transmissible or epidemiologically-important pathogens. Epidemiologically-important pathogens include, but are not limited to, Coronavirus disease (COVID-19), *C. difficile* (C-diff), *Methicillin-resistant Staphylococcus aureus* (MRSA), *Vancomycin-resistant enterococci* (VRE), *Respiratory Syncytial Virus* (RSV), measles, and tuberculosis (TB). For patients with these types of pathogens, standard precautions are used along with specific transmission-based precautions.

There are three categories of transmission-based precautions: **contact precautions**, **droplet precautions**, and **airborne precautions**. Transmission-based precautions are used when the route(s) of transmission is (are) not

---

1 Centers for Disease Control and Prevention. (2016, January 26). *Standard precautions for all patient care.* https://www.cdc.gov/infectioncontrol/basics/standard-precautions.html

2 Centers for Disease Control and Prevention. (2016, January 26). *Standard precautions for all patient care.* https://www.cdc.gov/infectioncontrol/basics/standard-precautions.html

My Notes

completely interrupted using standard precautions alone. Some diseases, such as tuberculosis, have multiple routes of transmission so more than one transmission-based precautions category must be implemented. See Table 4.2 outlining the categories of transmission precautions with associated PPE and other precautions. When possible, patients with transmission-based precautions should be placed in a single occupancy room with dedicated patient care equipment (e.g., blood pressure cuffs, stethoscope, thermometer). Transport of the patient and unnecessary movement outside the patient room should be limited. However, when transmission-based precautions are implemented, it is also important for the nurse to make efforts to counteract possible adverse effects of these precautions on patients, such as anxiety, depression, perceptions of stigma, and reduced contact with clinical staff.

Table 4.2 Transmission-Based Precautions[3]

Precaution	Implementation	PPE and Other Precautions
Contact	Known or suspected infections with increased risk for contact transmission (e.g., draining wounds, fecal incontinence) or with epidemiologically important organisms, such as C-diff, MRSA, VRE, or RSV	■ Gloves ■ Gown ■ Dedicated equipment Note: Use only soap and water for hand hygiene in patients with *C. difficile* infection.
Droplet	Known or suspected infection with pathogens transmitted by large respiratory droplets generated by coughing, sneezing, or talking, such as influenza, coronavirus, or pertussis	■ Mask ■ Goggles or face shield
Airborne	Known or suspected infection with pathogens transmitted by small respiratory droplets, such as measles	Fit-tested N-95 respirator or PAPR ■ Airborne infection isolation room ■ Single patient room ■ Patient door closed ■ Restricted susceptible personnel room entry

View a list of transmission-based precautions used for specific medical conditions at the CDC "Guideline for Isolation Precautions."

Patient Transport

Several principles are used to guide transport of patients requiring transmission-based precautions. In the inpatient and residential settings, these principles include the following:

3 Siegel, J. D., Rhinehart, E., Jackson, M., Chiarello, L., & Healthcare Infection Control Practices Advisory Committee. (2019, July 22). *2007 guideline for isolation precautions: Preventing transmission of infectious agents in healthcare settings.* https://www.cdc.gov/infectioncontrol/guidelines/isolation/index.html

My Notes

- Limiting transport for essential purposes only, such as diagnostic and therapeutic procedures that cannot be performed in the patient's room
- Using appropriate barriers on the patient consistent with the route and risk of transmission (e.g., mask, gown, covering the affected areas when infectious skin lesions or drainage is present)
- Notifying other health care personnel involved in the care of the patient of the transmission-based precautions. For example, when transporting the patient to radiology, inform the radiology technician of the precautions.[4]

Appropriate Hand Hygiene

Hand hygiene is the single most important practice to reduce the transmission of infectious agents in health care settings and is an essential element of standard precautions.[5] Routine handwashing during appropriate moments is a simple and effective way to prevent infection. However, it is estimated that health care professionals, on average, properly clean their hands less than 50% of the time it is indicated.[6] The Joint Commission, the organization that sets evidence-based standards of care for hospitals, recently updated its hand hygiene standards in 2018 to promote enforcement. If a Joint Commission surveyor witnesses an individual failing to properly clean their hands when it is indicated, a deficiency will be cited requiring improvement by the agency. This deficiency could potentially jeopardize a hospital's accreditation status and their ability to receive payment for patient services. Therefore, it is essential for all health care workers to ensure they are using proper hand hygiene at the appropriate times.[7]

There are several evidence-based guidelines for performing appropriate hand hygiene. These guidelines include frequency of performing hand hygiene according to the care circumstances, solutions used, and technique performed. The Healthcare Infection Control Practices Advisory Committee (HICPAC) recommends health care personnel perform hand hygiene at specific times when providing care to patients. These moments are often referred to as the "**Five Moments for Hand Hygiene**."[8]

---

4 Siegel, J. D., Rhinehart, E., Jackson, M., Chiarello, L., & Healthcare Infection Control Practices Advisory Committee. (2019, July 22). *2007 guideline for isolation precautions: Preventing transmission of infectious agents in healthcare settings.* https://www.cdc.gov/infectioncontrol/guidelines/isolation/index.html

5 Siegel, J. D., Rhinehart, E., Jackson, M., Chiarello, L., & Healthcare Infection Control Practices Advisory Committee. (2019, July 22). *2007 guideline for isolation precautions: Preventing transmission of infectious agents in healthcare settings.* https://www.cdc.gov/infectioncontrol/guidelines/isolation/index.html

6 Centers for Disease Control and Prevention (2019, April 29). *Hand hygiene in healthcare settings.* https://www.cdc.gov/handhygiene/

7 The Joint Commission. (n.d.). *Update: Citing observations of hand hygiene noncompliance.* https://www.jointcommission.org/-/media/tjc/documents/standards/jc-requirements/ambulatory-care/2018/update_citing_observations_of_hand_hygiene_noncompliancepdf.pdf?db=web&hash=F89BFFFAEDA700CC2E667049D8F542B2

8 World Health Organization. (n.d.). *My 5 moments of hand hygiene.* https://www.who.int/infection-prevention/campaigns/clean-hands/5moments/en/

My Notes

See Figures 4.1[9] and 4.2[10] for an illustration and application of the five moments of hand hygiene. The five moments of hand hygiene are as follows:

- Immediately before touching a patient
- Before performing an aseptic task or handling invasive devices
- Before moving from a soiled body site to a clean body site on a patient
- After touching a patient or their immediate environment
- After contact with blood, body fluids, or contaminated surfaces (with or without glove use)
- Immediately after glove removal

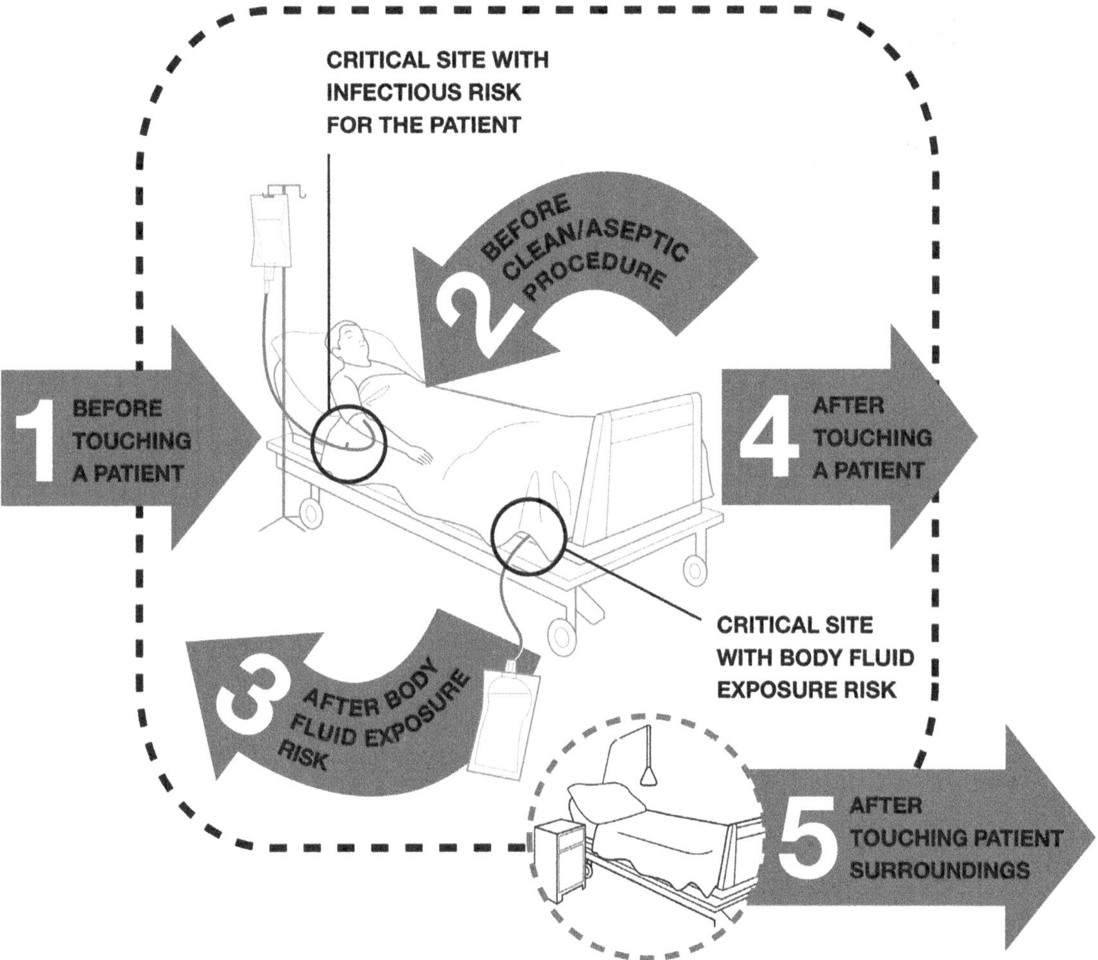

Figure 4.1 Five Moments of Hand Hygiene

9 "5Moments_Image.gif" by World Health Organization is licensed under CC BY-NC-SA 3.0 IGO. Access for free at https://www.who.int/infection-prevention/campaigns/clean-hands/5moments/en/

10 This work is derived from "Hand_Hygiene_When_and_How_Leaflet.pdf" by World Health Organization and is licensed under CC BY-NC-SA 3.0 IGO. Access for free at https://www.who.int/infection-prevention/tools/hand-hygiene/workplace_reminders/en/

My Notes

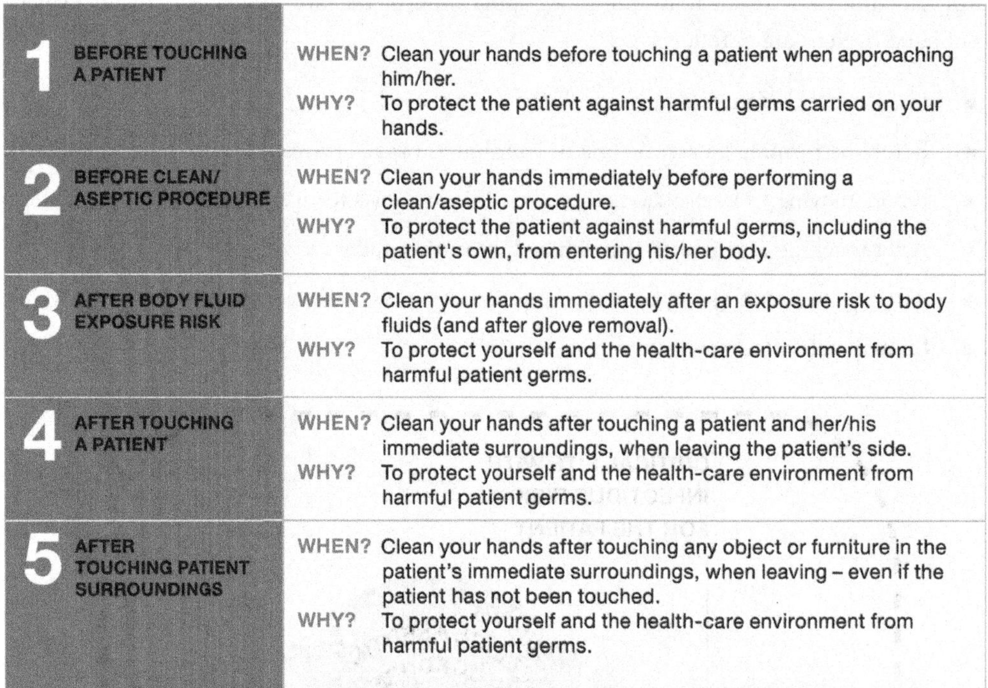

1 BEFORE TOUCHING A PATIENT
WHEN? Clean your hands before touching a patient when approaching him/her.
WHY? To protect the patient against harmful germs carried on your hands.
2 BEFORE CLEAN/ ASEPTIC PROCEDURE
WHEN? Clean your hands immediately before performing a clean/aseptic procedure.
WHY? To protect the patient against harmful germs, including the patient's own, from entering his/her body.
3 AFTER BODY FLUID EXPOSURE RISK
WHEN? Clean your hands immediately after an exposure risk to body fluids (and after glove removal).
WHY? To protect yourself and the health-care environment from harmful patient germs.
4 AFTER TOUCHING A PATIENT
WHEN? Clean your hands after touching a patient and her/his immediate surroundings, when leaving the patient's side.
WHY? To protect yourself and the health-care environment from harmful patient germs.
5 AFTER TOUCHING PATIENT SURROUNDINGS
WHEN? Clean your hands after touching any object or furniture in the patient's immediate surroundings, when leaving – even if the patient has not been touched.
WHY? To protect yourself and the health-care environment from harmful patient germs.

Figure 4.2 Five Moments of Hand Hygiene Expanded

When performing hand hygiene, washing with soap and water, or an approved alcohol-based hand rub solution that contains at least 60% alcohol, may be used. Unless hands are visibly soiled, an alcohol-based hand rub is preferred over soap and water in most clinical situations due to evidence of improved compliance. Hand rubs are also preferred because they are generally less irritating to health care workers' hands. However, it is important to recognize that alcohol-based rubs do not eliminate some types of germs, such as *Clostridium difficile* (C-diff).

When using the alcohol-based handrub method, the CDC recommends the following steps. See Figure 4.3[11] for a handrub poster created by the World Health Organization.

- **Apply** product to the palm of one hand in an amount that will cover all surfaces.
- **Rub** hands together, covering all the surfaces of the hands, fingers, and wrists until the hands are dry. Surfaces include the palms and fingers, between the fingers, the backs of the hands and fingers, the fingertips, and the thumbs.
- The process should take about 20 seconds, and the solution should be dry.[12]

---

11 This work is derived from "Hand_Hygiene_When_and_How_Leaflet.pdf" by World Health Organization and is licensed under CC BY-NC-SA 3.0 IGO. Access for free at https://www.who.int/infection-prevention/tools/hand-hygiene/workplace_reminders/en/

12 Centers for Disease Control and Prevention (2019, April 29). *Hand hygiene in healthcare settings.* https://www.cdc.gov/handhygiene/

My Notes

How to Handrub?

RUB HANDS FOR HAND HYGIENE! WASH HANDS WHEN VISIBLY SOILED

Duration of the entire procedure: 20-30 seconds

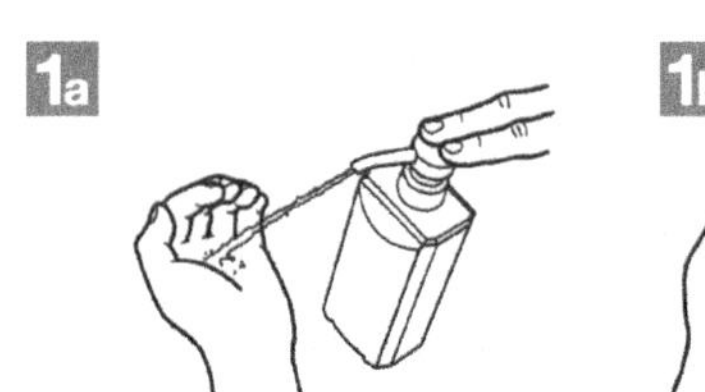

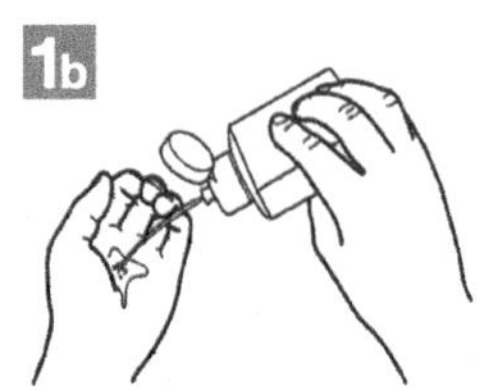

Apply a palmful of the product in a cupped hand, covering all surfaces;

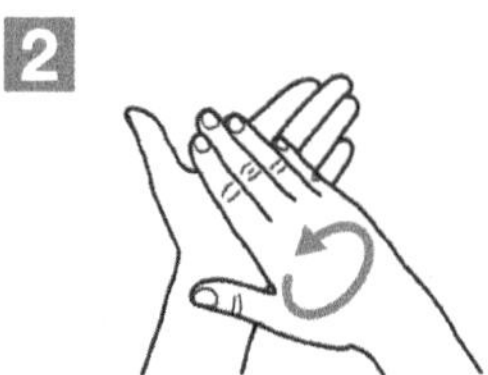

Rub hands palm to palm;

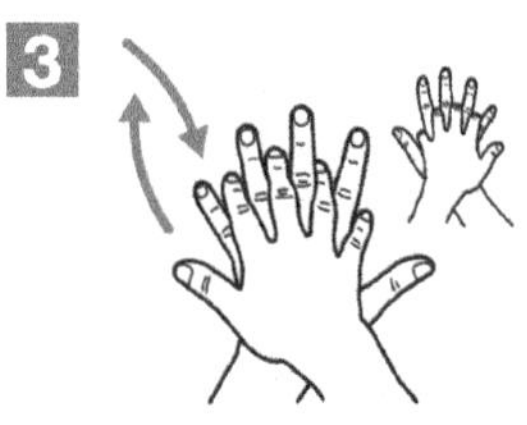

Right palm over left dorsum with interlaced fingers and vice versa;

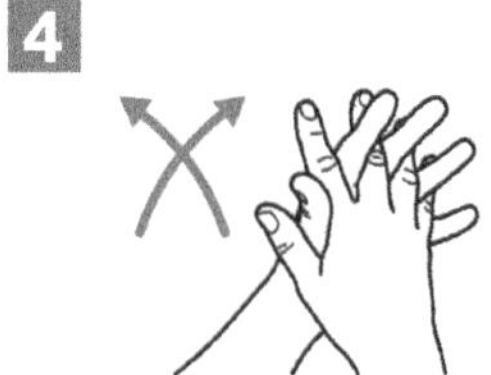

Palm to palm with fingers interlaced;

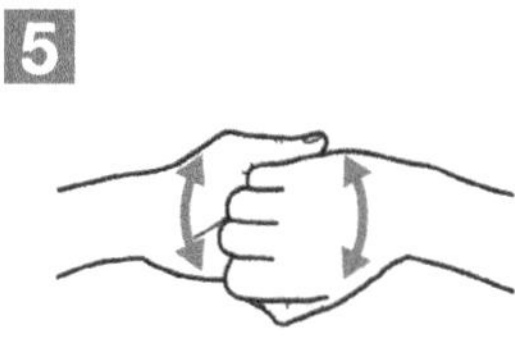

Backs of fingers to opposing palms with fingers interlocked;

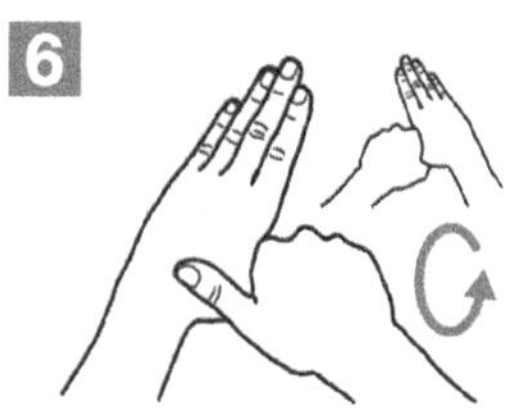

Rotational rubbing of left thumb clasped in right palm and vice versa;

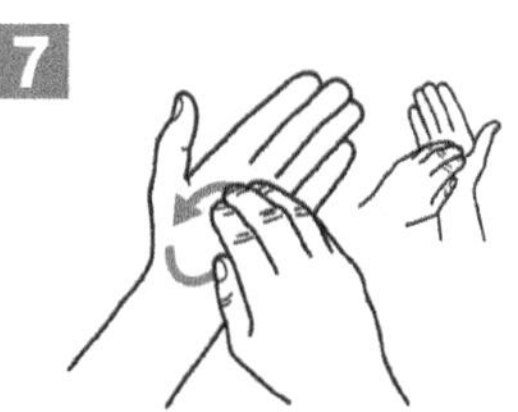

Rotational rubbing, backwards and forwards with clasped fingers of right hand in left palm and vice versa;

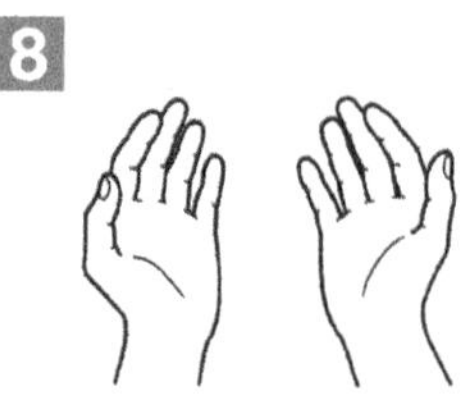

Once dry, your hands are safe.

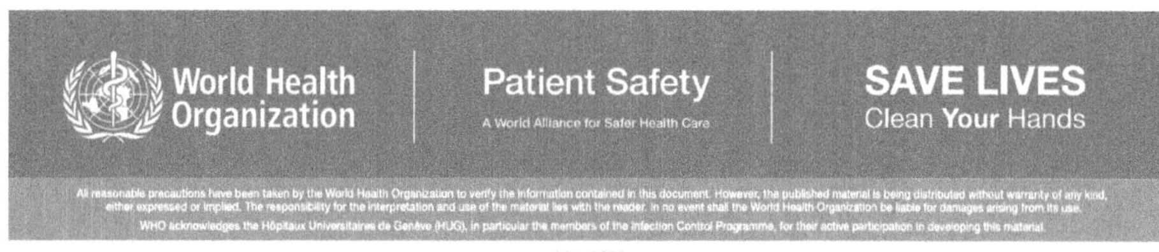

May 2009

Figure 4.3 WHO Handrub Poster

My Notes

When washing with soap and water, the CDC recommends using the following steps. See Figure 4.4[13] for an image of a handwashing poster created by the World Health Organization.

- **Wet** hands with warm or cold running water and apply facility-approved soap.
- **Lather** hands by rubbing them together with the soap. Use the same technique as the handrub process to clean the palms and fingers, between the fingers, the backs of the hands and fingers, the fingertips, and the thumbs.
- **Scrub** thoroughly for at least 20 seconds.
- **Rinse** hands well under clean, running water.
- **Dry** the hands using a clean towel or disposable toweling.
- **Use** a clean paper towel to shut off the faucet.[14]

13 "How_To_HandWash_Poster.pdf" by World Health Organization is licensed under CC BY-NC-SA 3.0 IGO. Access for free at https://www.who.int/infection-prevention/campaigns/clean-hands/5moments/en/

14 Centers for Disease Control and Prevention (2019, April 29). *Hand hygiene in healthcare settings.* https://www.cdc.gov/handhygiene/

My Notes

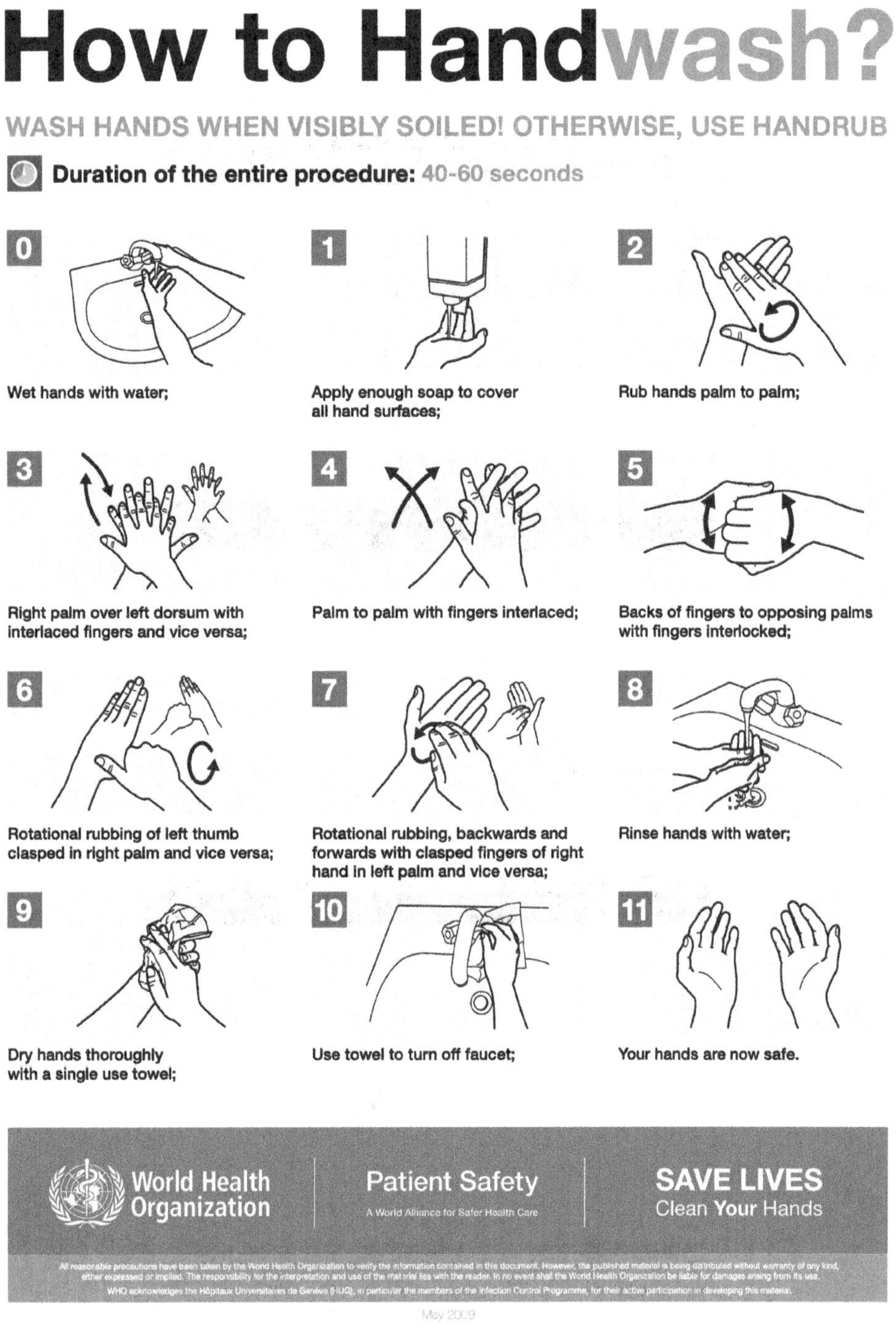

How to Handwash?

WASH HANDS WHEN VISIBLY SOILED! OTHERWISE, USE HANDRUB

Duration of the entire procedure: 40-60 seconds

0 Wet hands with water;

1 Apply enough soap to cover all hand surfaces;

2 Rub hands palm to palm;

3 Right palm over left dorsum with interlaced fingers and vice versa;

4 Palm to palm with fingers interlaced;

5 Backs of fingers to opposing palms with fingers interlocked;

6 Rotational rubbing of left thumb clasped in right palm and vice versa;

7 Rotational rubbing, backwards and forwards with clasped fingers of right hand in left palm and vice versa;

8 Rinse hands with water;

9 Dry hands thoroughly with a single use towel;

10 Use towel to turn off faucet;

11 Your hands are now safe.

World Health Organization | Patient Safety A World Alliance for Safer Health Care | **SAVE LIVES** Clean **Your** Hands

May 2009

Figure 4.4 WHO Handwashing Poster

By performing hand hygiene at the proper moments and using appropriate techniques, you will ensure your hands are safe and you are not transmitting infectious organisms to yourself or others.

My Notes

Video Reviews of Handwashing

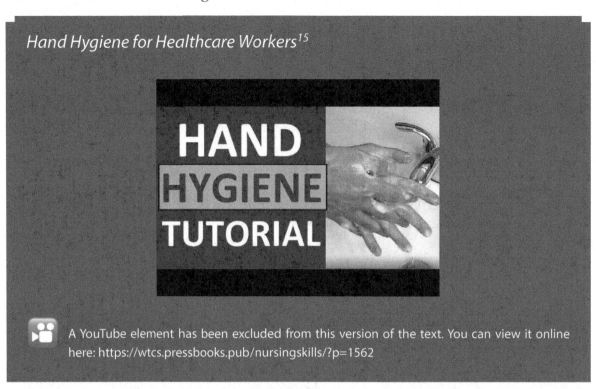

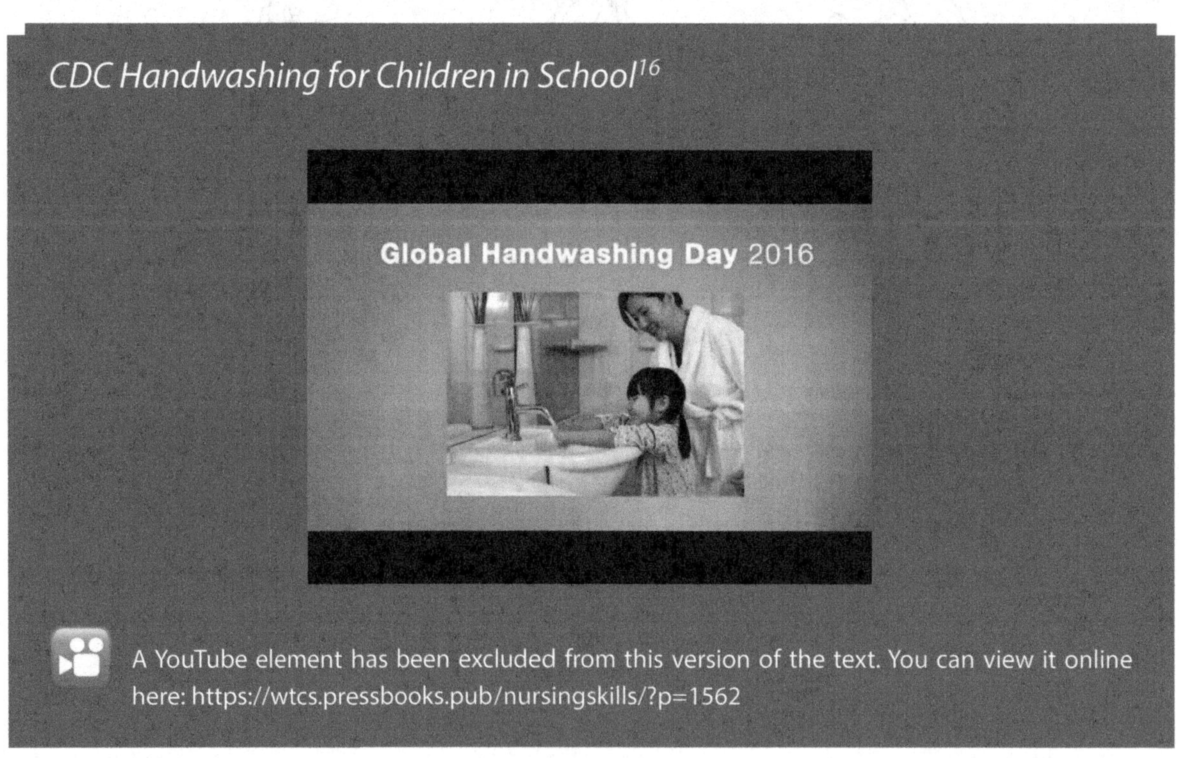

---

15 RegisteredNurseRN. (2018, December 1). *Hand hygiene for healthcare workers / Hand washing soap and water technique nursing skill.* [Video]. YouTube. All rights reserved. Video used with permission. https://youtu.be/G5-Rp-6FMCQ

16 Centers for Disease Control and Prevention. (2016, October 17). *YouTube live handwashing presentation.* [Video]. YouTube. All rights reserved. https://youtu.be/LWmok9avzr4

For more information about hand hygiene recommendations, use the following links:

My Notes

WHO "Guidelines on Hand Hygiene" (https://www.who.int/infection-prevention/publications/hand-hygiene-2009/en/)

WHO "Hand Hygiene" brochure (https://www.who.int/gpsc/5may/Hand_Hygiene_When_and_How_Leaflet.pdf?ua=1)

CDC "Hand Hygiene in Healthcare Settings" (https://www.cdc.gov/handhygiene/index.html)

Joint Commission on "Hand Hygiene" (https://www.centerfortransforminghealthcare.org/improvement-topics/hand-hygiene/?_ga=2.185680553.1649963228.1601313691-322773533.1571518854)

Personal Protective Equipment (PPE)

Personal Protective Equipment (PPE) includes gloves, gowns, face shields, goggles, and masks used to prevent the spread of infection to and from patients and health care providers. Depending on the anticipated exposure, PPE may include the use of gloves, a fluid-resistant gown, goggles or a face shield, and a mask or respirator. When used for a patient with transmission-based precautions, PPE supplies are typically stored in an isolation cart next to the patient's room, and a card is posted on the door alerting staff and visitors to precautions needed before entering the room.

Gloves

Gloves protect both patients and health care personnel from exposure to infectious material that may be carried on the hands. Gloves are used to prevent contamination of health care personnel hands during activities such as the following:

- anticipating direct contact with blood or body fluids, mucous membranes, nonintact skin, and other potentially infectious material
- having direct contact with patients who are colonized or infected with pathogens transmitted by the contact route, such as *Vancomycin- resistant enterococci* (VRE), *Methicillin-resistant Staphylococcus aureus* (MRSA), and *Respiratory Syncytial Virus* (RSV)
- handling or touching visibly or potentially contaminated patient care equipment and environmental surfaces[17]

Nonsterile disposable medical gloves for routine patient care are made of a variety of materials, such as latex, vinyl, and nitrile. Many people are allergic to latex, so be sure to check for latex allergies for the patient and other health care professionals. See Figure 4.5[18] for an image of nonsterile medical gloves in various sizes in a

17 Centers for Disease Control and Prevention (2016, January 26). *Standard precautions for all patient care.* https://www.cdc.gov/infectioncontrol/basics/standard-precautions.html

18 "Surgery Centre Accriditation.jpg" by Accredia is licensed under CC BY-SA 4.0. Access for free at https://commons.m.wikimedia.org/wiki/File:Surgery_Centre_Accriditation.jpg

My Notes

health care setting. At times, gloves may need to be changed when providing care to a single patient to prevent cross-contamination of body sites. It is also necessary to change gloves if the patient interaction requires touching portable computer keyboards or other mobile equipment that is transported from room to room. Discarding gloves between patients is necessary to prevent transmission of infectious material. Gloves must not be washed for subsequent reuse because microorganisms cannot be reliably removed from glove surfaces and continued glove integrity cannot be ensured.[19]

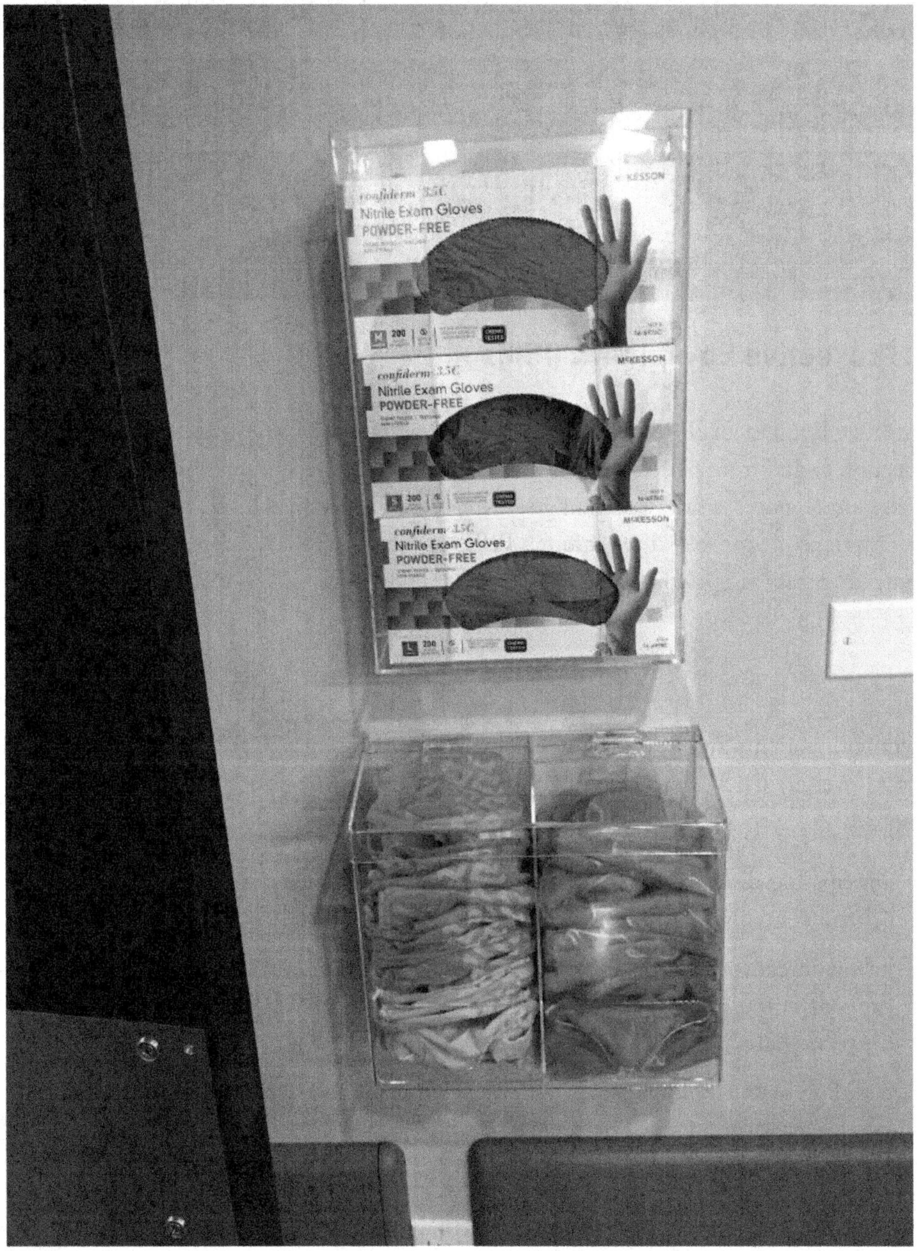

Figure 4.5 Non-Sterile Medical Gloves

19 Siegel, J. D., Rhinehart, E., Jackson, M., Chiarello, L., & Healthcare Infection Control Practices Advisory Committee. (2019, July 22). *2007 guideline for isolation precautions: Preventing transmission of infectious agents in healthcare settings.* https://www.cdc.gov/infectioncontrol/guidelines/isolation/index.html

When gloves are worn in combination with other PPE, they are put on last. Gloves that fit snugly around the wrist should be used in combination with isolation gowns because they will cover the gown cuff and provide a more reliable continuous barrier for the arms, wrists, and hands.

My Notes

Gloves should be removed properly to prevent contamination. See Figure 4.6[20] for an illustration of properly removing gloves. Hand hygiene should be performed following glove removal to ensure the hands will not carry potentially infectious material that might have penetrated through unrecognized tears or contaminated the hands during glove removal. One method for properly removing gloves includes the following steps:

- Grasp the outside of one glove near the wrist. Do not touch your skin.
- Peel the glove away from your body, pulling it inside out.
- Hold the removed glove in your gloved hand.
- Put your fingers inside the glove at the top of your wrist and peel off the second glove.
- Turn the second glove inside out while pulling it away from your body, leaving the first glove inside the second.
- Dispose of the gloves safely. Do not reuse.
- Perform hand hygiene immediately after removing the gloves.[21]

---

20 "poster-how-to-remove-gloves.pdf" by Centers for Disease Control and Prevention is in the *Public Domain*. Access for free at https://www.cdc.gov/vhf/ebola/resources/posters.html

21 Siegel, J. D., Rhinehart, E., Jackson, M., Chiarello, L., & Healthcare Infection Control Practices Advisory Committee. (2019, July 22). *2007 guideline for isolation precautions: Preventing transmission of infectious agents in healthcare settings.* https://www.cdc.gov/infectioncontrol/guidelines/isolation/index.html

My Notes

How to Remove Gloves

To protect yourself, use the following steps to take off gloves

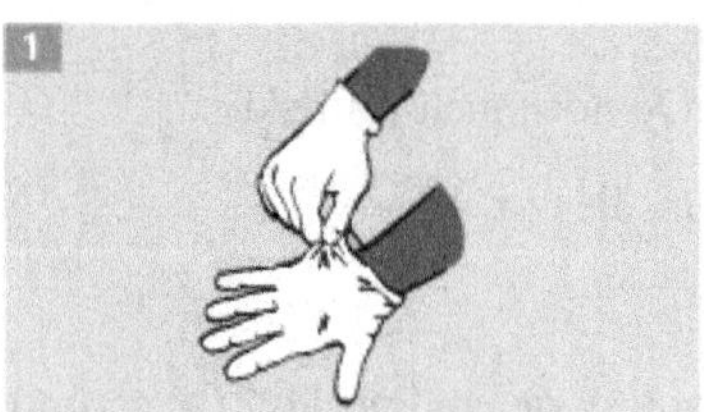

Grasp the outside of one glove at the wrist. Do not touch your bare skin.

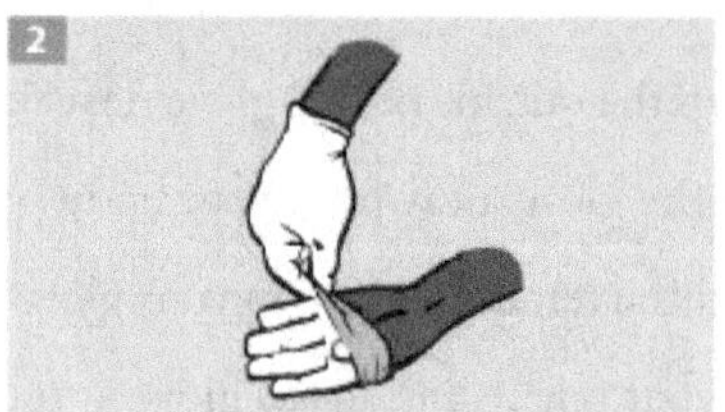

Peel the glove away from your body, pulling it inside out.

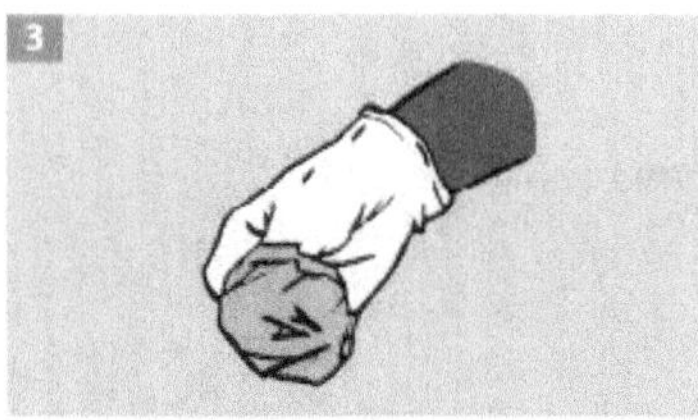

Hold the glove you just removed in your gloved hand.

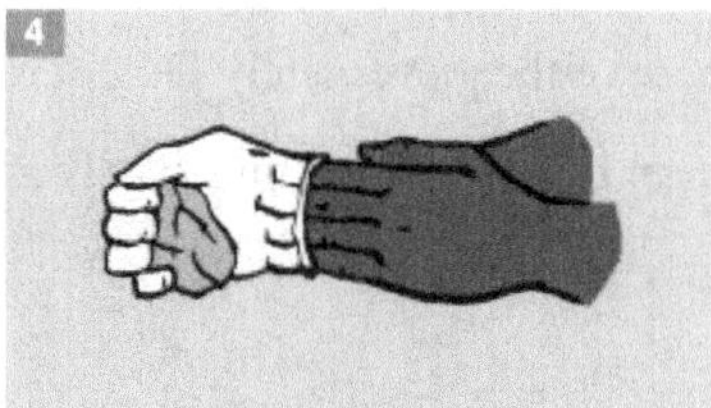

Peel off the second glove by putting your fingers inside the glove at the top of your wrist.

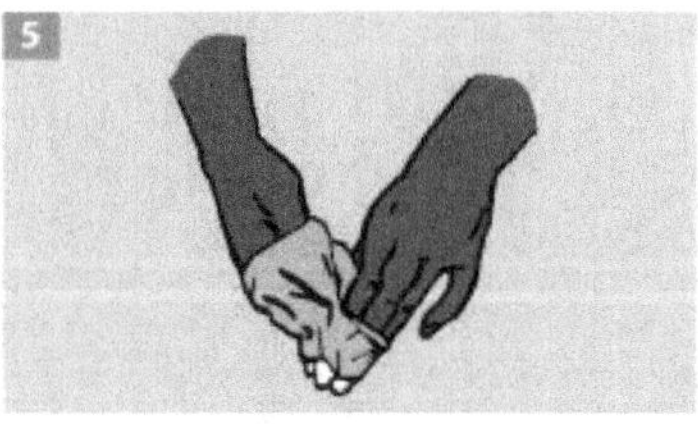

Turn the second glove inside out while pulling it away from your body, leaving the first glove inside the second.

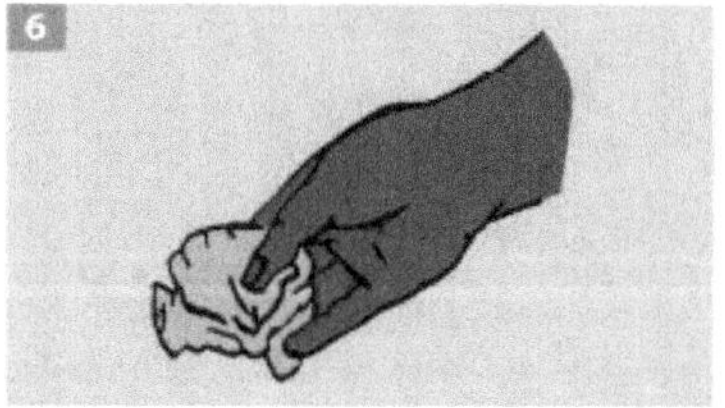

Dispose of the gloves safely. Do not reuse the gloves.

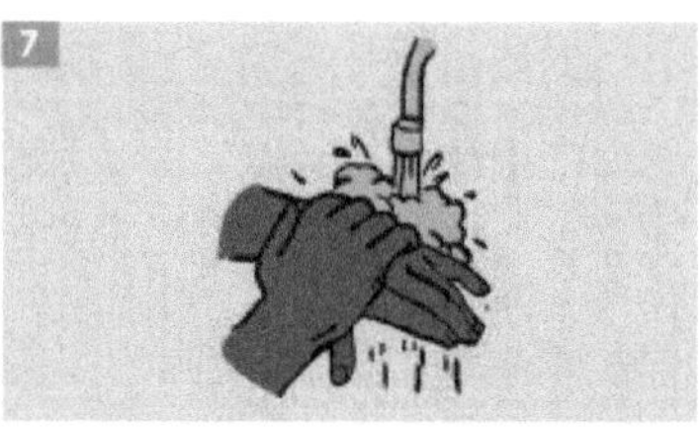

Clean your hands immediately after removing gloves.

Adapted from Workers' Compensation Board of B.C.

CS 254759-A

Figure 4.6 Proper Removal of Gloves to Prevent Contamination

My Notes

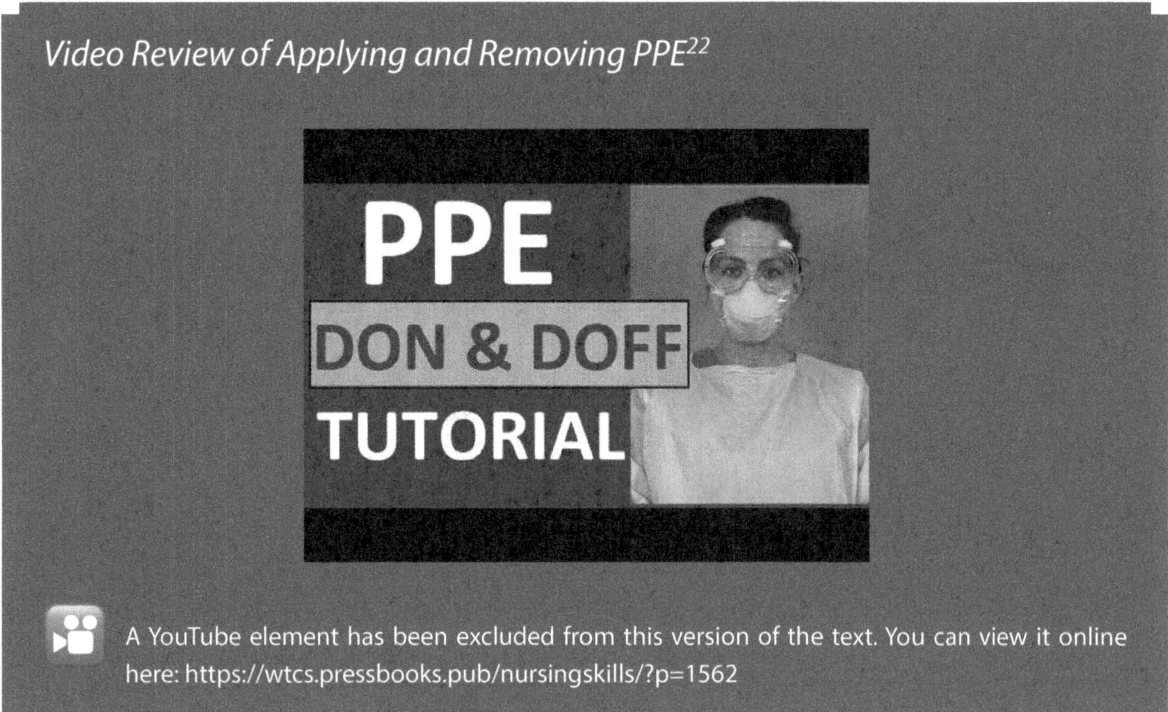

Video Review of Applying and Removing PPE[22]
PPE
DON & DOFF
TUTORIAL
A YouTube element has been excluded from this version of the text. You can view it online here: https://wtcs.pressbooks.pub/nursingskills/?p=1562

Gowns

Isolation gowns are used to protect the health care worker's arms and exposed body areas and to prevent contamination of their clothing with blood, body fluids, and other potentially infectious material. Isolation gowns may be disposable or washable/reusable. See Figure 4.7[23] for an image of a nurse wearing an isolation gown along with goggles and a respirator. When using standard precautions, an isolation gown is worn only if contact with blood or body fluid is anticipated. However, when contact transmission-based precautions are in place, donning of both gown and gloves upon room entry is indicated to prevent unintentional contact of clothing with contaminated environmental surfaces.

Gowns are usually the first piece of PPE to be donned. Isolation gowns should be removed before leaving the patient room to prevent possible contamination of the environment outside the patient's room. Isolation gowns should be removed in a manner that prevents contamination of clothing or skin. The outer, "contaminated," side of the gown is turned inward and rolled into a bundle, and then it is discarded into a designated container to contain contamination. See more information about putting on and removing PPE in the subsection below.[24]

---

22 RegisteredNurseRN. (2020, May 29). *PPR training video: Donning and doffing PPE nursing skills.* [Video]. YouTube. All rights reserved. Video used with permission. https://youtu.be/iwvnA_b9Q8Y

23 "U.S. Navy Doctors, Nurses and Corpsmen Treat COVID Patients in the ICU Aboard USNS Comfort (49825651378).jpg" by *Navy Medicine* is in the Public Domain. Access for free at https://commons.wikimedia.org/wiki/File:U.S._Navy_Doctors,_Nurses_and_Corpsmen_Treat_COVID_Patients_in_the_ICU_Aboard_USNS_Comfort_(49825651378).jpg

24 Siegel, J. D., Rhinehart, E., Jackson, M., Chiarello, L., & Healthcare Infection Control Practices Advisory Committee. (2019, July 22). *2007 guideline for isolation precautions: Preventing transmission of infectious agents in healthcare settings.* https://www.cdc.gov/infectioncontrol/guidelines/isolation/index.html

My Notes

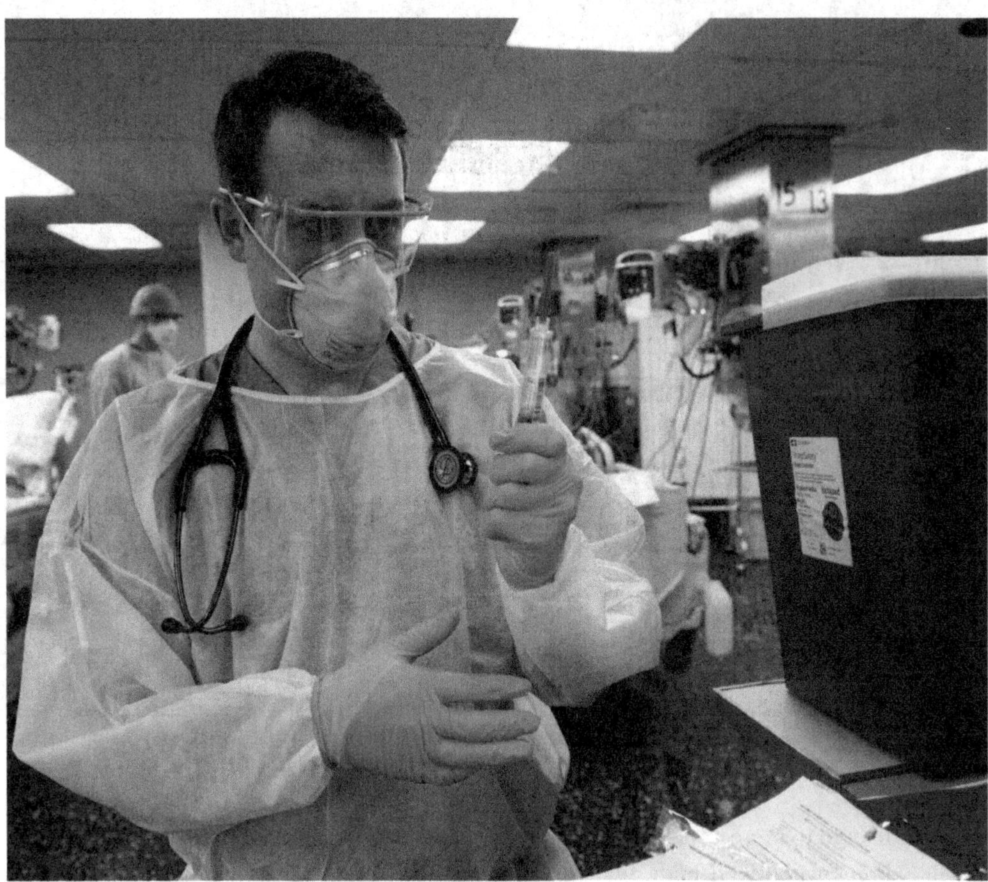

Figure 4.7 Isolation Gown

Masks

The mucous membranes of the mouth, nose, and eyes are susceptible portals of entry for infectious agents. Masks are used to protect these sites from entry of large infectious droplets. See Figure 4.8[25] for an image of nurse wearing a surgical mask. Masks have three primary purposes in health care settings:

- Used by health care personnel to protect them from contact with infectious material from patients (e.g., respiratory secretions and sprays of blood or body fluids), consistent with standard precautions and droplet transmission precautions
- Used by health care personnel when engaged in procedures requiring sterile technique to protect patients from exposure to infectious agents potentially carried in a health care worker's mouth or nose
- Placed on coughing patients to limit potential dissemination of infectious respiratory secretions from the patient to others in public areas (i.e., respiratory hygiene)[26]

25 "USNS Comfort (T-AH 20) Performs Surgery (49803007781).jpg" by Navy Medicine is in the Public Domain. Access for free at https://commons.wikimedia.org/wiki/File:USNS_Comfort_(T-AH_20)_Performs_Surgery_(49803007781).jpg

26 Siegel, J. D., Rhinehart, E., Jackson, M., Chiarello, L., & Healthcare Infection Control Practices Advisory Committee. (2019, July 22). *2007 guideline for isolation precautions: Preventing transmission of infectious agents in healthcare settings.* https://www.cdc.gov/infectioncontrol/guidelines/isolation/index.html

My Notes

Masks may be used in combination with goggles or a face shield to provide more complete protection for the face. Masks should not be confused with respirators used during airborne transmission-based precautions to prevent inhalation of small, aerosolized infectious droplets.[27]

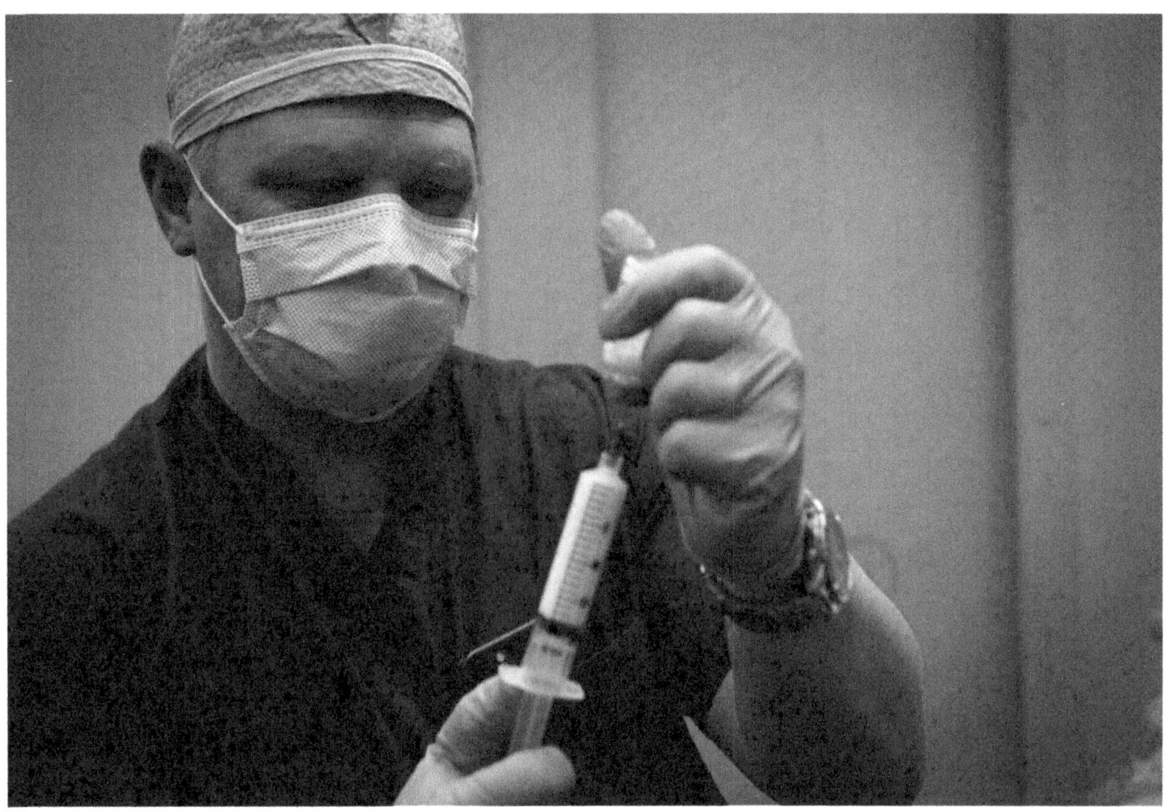

Figure 4.8 Surgical Mask

It is important to properly wear and remove masks to avoid contamination. See Figure 4.9[28] for CDC face mask recommendations for health care personnel.

27 Siegel, J. D., Rhinehart, E., Jackson, M., Chiarello, L., & Healthcare Infection Control Practices Advisory Committee. (2019, July 22). *2007 guideline for isolation precautions: Preventing transmission of infectious agents in healthcare settings.* https://www.cdc.gov/infectioncontrol/guidelines/isolation/index.html

28 "fs-facemask-dos-donts.pdf" by Centers for Disease Control and Prevention is in the Public Domain. Access for free at https://www.cdc.gov/coronavirus/2019-ncov/hcp/using-ppe.html

My Notes

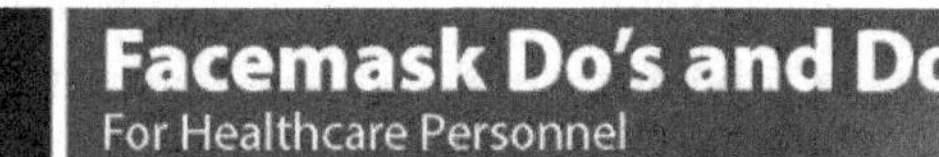

When putting on a facemask

Clean your hands and put on your facemask so it fully covers your mouth and nose.

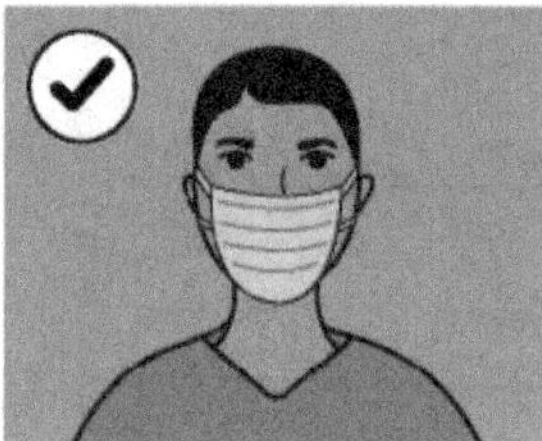

DO secure the elastic bands around your ears.

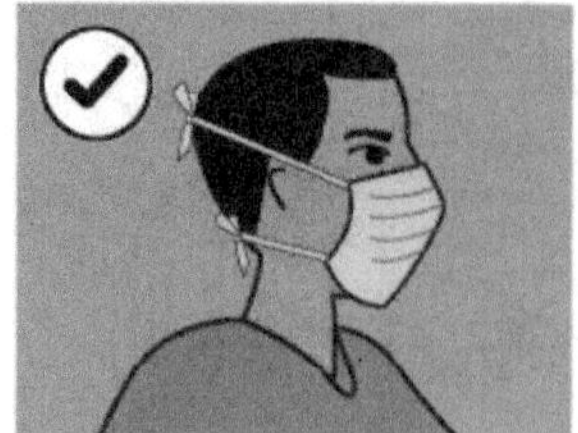

DO secure the ties at the middle of your head and the base of your head.

When wearing a facemask, don't do the following:

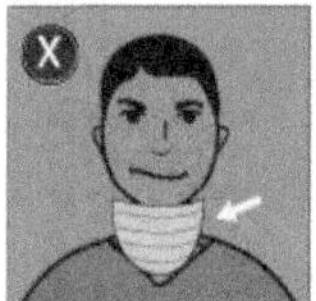

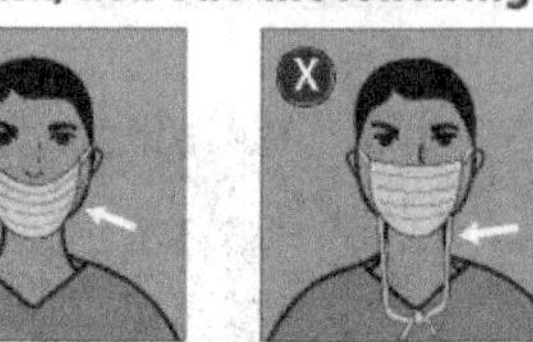

DON'T wear your facemask under your nose or mouth.

DON'T allow a strap to hang down. **DON'T** cross the straps.

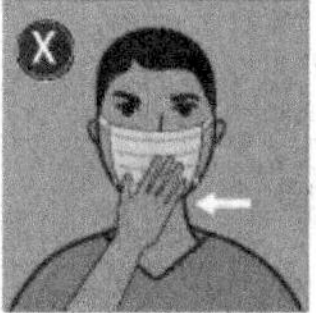

DON'T touch or adjust your facemask without cleaning your hands before and after.

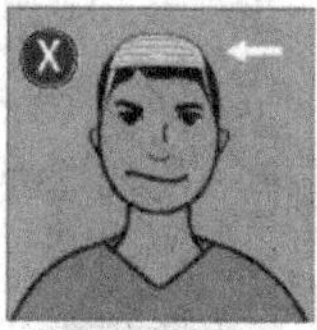

DON'T wear your facemask on your head.

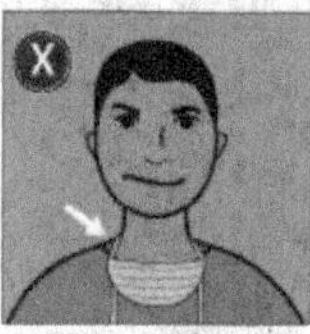

DON'T wear your facemask around your neck.

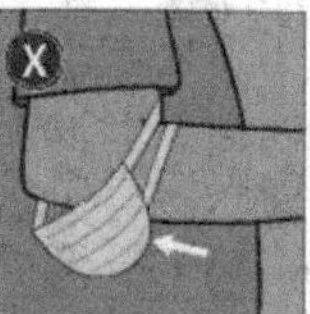

DON'T wear your facemask around your arm.

When removing a facemask

Clean your hands and remove your facemask touching only the straps or ties.

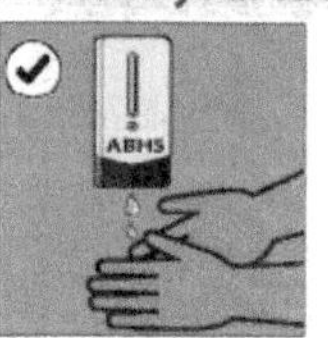

DO leave the patient care area, then clean your hands with alcohol-based hand sanitizer or soap and water.

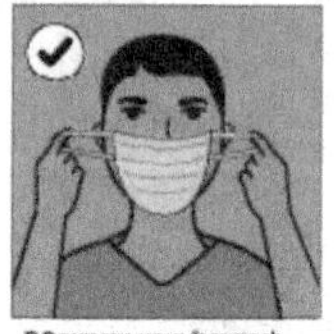

DO remove your facemask touching ONLY the straps or ties, throw it away*, and clean your hands again.

*If implementing limited-reuse: Facemasks should be carefully folded so that the outer surface is held inward and against itself to reduce contact with the outer surface during storage. Folded facemasks can be stored between uses in a clean, sealable paper bag or breathable container.

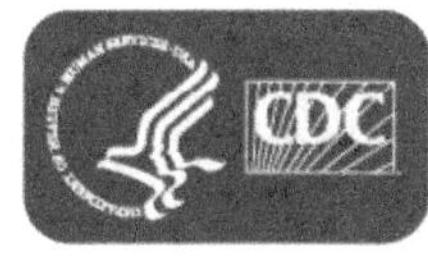

Additional information is available about how to safely put on and remove personal protective equipment, including facemasks: https://www.cdc.gov/coronavirus/2019-ncov/hcp/using-ppe.html.

cdc.gov/coronavirus

Figure 4.9 CDC Face Mask Recommendations

Goggles/Face Shields

My Notes

Eye protection chosen for specific work situations (e.g., goggles or face shields) depends upon the circumstances of exposure, other PPE used, and personal vision needs. Personal eyeglasses are not considered adequate eye protection. See Figure 4.10[29] for an image of a health care professional wearing a face shield along with a N95 respirator.

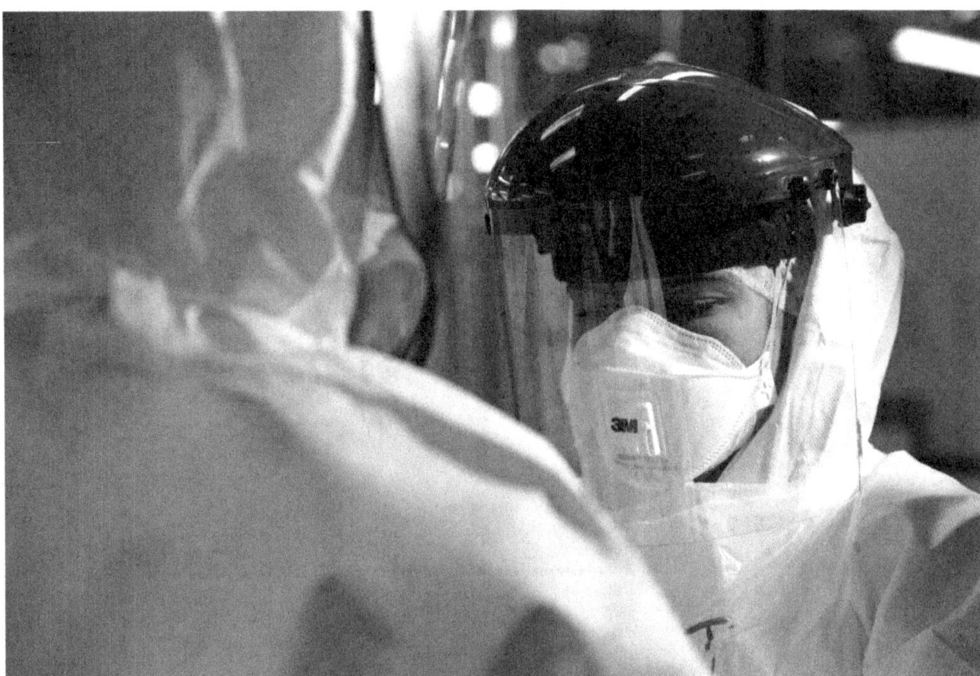

Figure 4.10 Face Shield and a N95 Respirator

Respirators and PAPRs

Respiratory protection used during airborne transmission precautions requires the use of special equipment. Traditionally, a fitted respirator mask with N95 or higher filtration has been worn by health care professionals to prevent inhalation of small airborne infectious particles. A user-seal check (formerly called a "fit check") should be performed by the wearer of a respirator each time a respirator is donned to minimize air leakage around the facepiece.

A newer piece of equipment used for respiratory protection is the powered air-purifying respirator (PAPR). A PAPR is an air-purifying respirator that uses a blower to force air through filter cartridges or canisters into the breathing zone of the wearer. This process creates an air flow inside either a tight-fitting facepiece or loose-fitting

---

29 "Checking Personal Protective Equipment (PPE) in the fight against Ebola" by DFID - UK Department for International Development is licensed under CC BY 2.0. Access for free at https://www.flickr.com/photos/dfid/15650272810/in/photolist-pHmjS4-pFfxeU-oLuzxj-qMMZQZ-pyN4Vz-nfVDH4-qvwAs8-qMXaBP-qMXaDH-qvs51C-qwb4oa-q6cKqu-pQXQXY-pK9Y7L-ok6kJE-qG9VwM-oeqdE5-pQXJRQ-pTnngY-pGtNvA-phn5z9-oerYA8-p58esM-oKTyND-pSaMep-pB1uJR-q6bu3C-p7Dtef-pFmdgn-rgh5wA-oCVKH6-ozymNw-ovCUoB-oxEVMp-oxFbgp-ovHMjj-ptBqy5-pCYRsM-qG5LkW-pQVQQe-pQU8yE-q8qC6s-q6bRs1-q8i1qg-q8hfKa-pjN2vu-p58ewV-pQTq2G-q9KMMf-ifc7sk

My Notes

hood or helmet, providing a higher level of protection against aerosolized pathogens, such as COVID-19, than a N95 respirator. See Figure 4.11[30] for an example of PAPR in use.

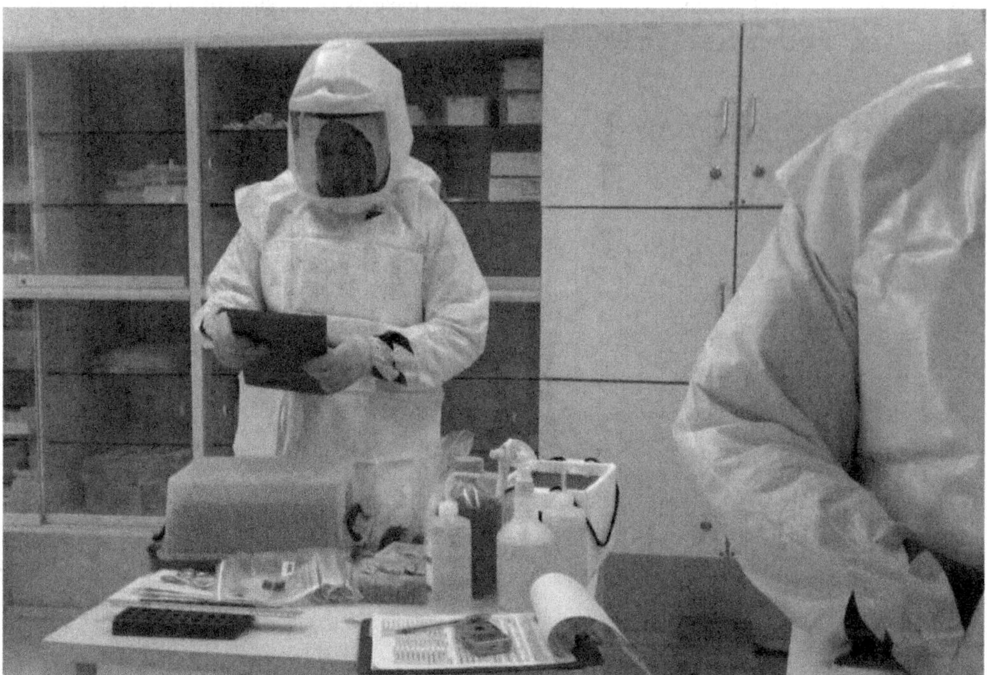

Figure 4.11 PAPR In Use

The CDC currently recommends N95 or higher level respirators for personnel exposed to patients with suspected or confirmed tuberculosis and other airborne diseases, especially during aerosol-generating procedures such as respiratory-tract suctioning.[31] It is important to apply, wear, and remove respirators appropriately to avoid contamination. See Figure 4.12[32] for CDC recommendations when wearing disposable respirators.

---

30 "PAPRs_in_use_01.jpg" by *Ca.garcia.s* is licensed under CC BY-SA 4.0. Access for free at https://commons.wikimedia.org/wiki/File:PAPRs_in_use_01.jpg

31 Siegel, J. D., Rhinehart, E., Jackson, M., Chiarello, L., & Healthcare Infection Control Practices Advisory Committee. (2019, July 22). *2007 guideline for isolation precautions: Preventing transmission of infectious agents in healthcare settings.* https://www.cdc.gov/infectioncontrol/guidelines/isolation/index.html

32 "fs-respirator-on-off.pdf" by Centers for Disease Control and Prevention is in the Public Domain. Access for free at https://www.cdc.gov/coronavirus/2019-ncov/hcp/using-ppe.html

My Notes

Respirator On / Respirator Off

When you put on a disposable respirator

Position your respirator correctly and check the seal to protect yourself from COVID-19.

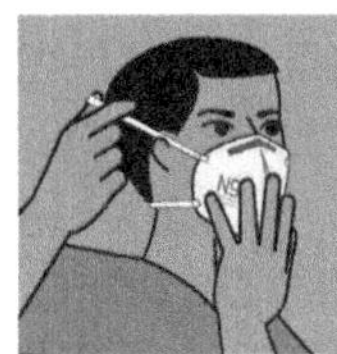

Cup the respirator in your hand. Hold the respirator under your chin with the nose piece up. The top strap (on single or double strap respirators) goes over and rests at the top back of your head. The bottom strap is positioned around the neck and below the ears.

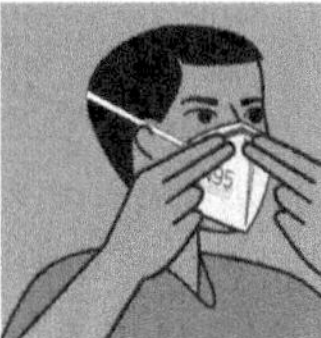

Place your fingertips from both hands at the top of the metal nose clip (if present). Slide fingertips down both sides of the metal strip to mold the nose area to the shape of your nose.

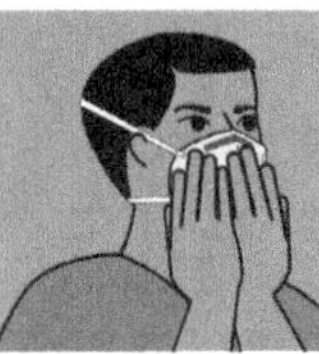

Place both hands over the respirator, take a quick breath in to check the seal. Breathe out. If you feel a leak when breathing in or breathing out, there is not a proper seal.

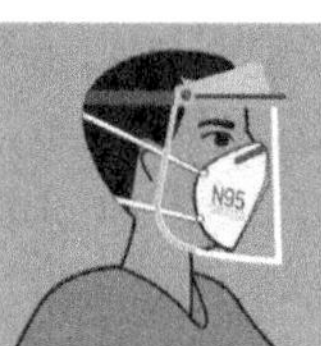

Select other PPE items that do not interfere with the fit or performance of your respirator.

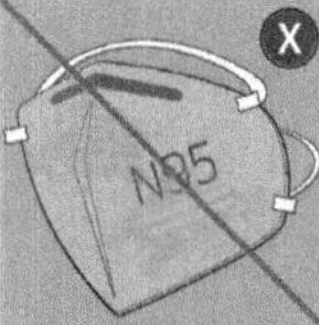

Do not use a respirator that appears damaged or deformed, no longer forms an effective seal to the face, becomes wet or visibly dirty, or if breathing becomes difficult.

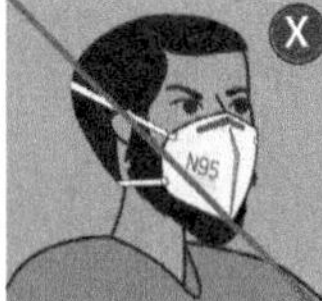

Do not allow facial hair, jewelry, glasses, clothing, or anything else to prevent proper placement or to come between your face and the respirator.

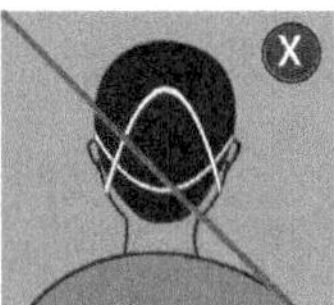

Do not crisscross the straps.

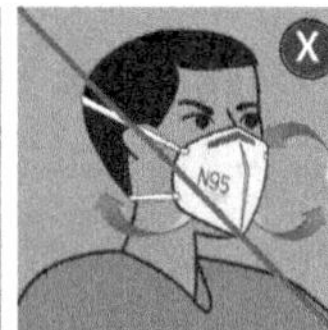

Do not wear a respirator that does not have a proper seal. If air leaks in or out, ask for help or try a different size or model.

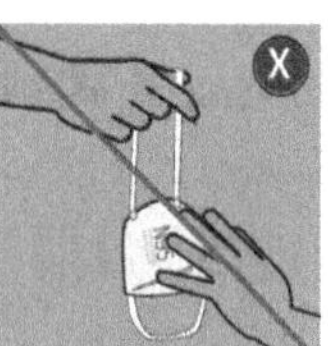

Do not touch the front of the respirator during or after use! It may be contaminated.

When you take off a disposable respirator

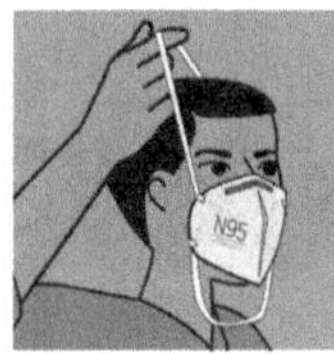

Remove by pulling the bottom strap over back of head, followed by the top strap, without touching the respirator.

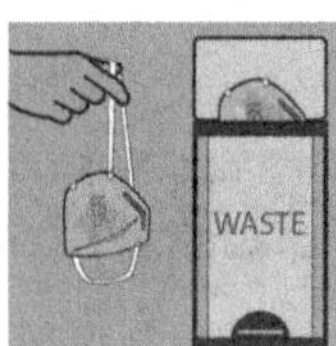

Discard in a waste container.

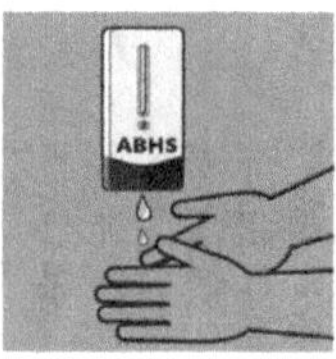

Clean your hands with alcohol-based hand sanitizer or soap and water.

Employers must comply with the OSHA Respiratory Protection Standard, 29 CFR 1910.134, which includes medical evaluations, training, and fit testing.

Additional information is available about how to safely put on and remove personal protective equipment, including respirators: https://www.cdc.gov/coronavirus/2019-ncov/hcp/using-ppe.html

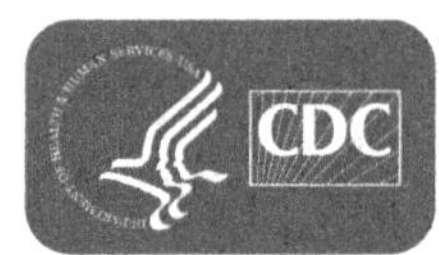

cdc.gov/coronavirus

Figure 4.12 CDC Recommendations for Wearing Disposable Respirators

How to Put On (Don) PPE Gear

Follow agency policy for donning PPE according to transmission-based precautions. More than one donning method for putting on PPE may be acceptable. The CDC recommends the following steps for donning PPE:[33]

- Identify and gather the proper PPE to don. Ensure the gown size is correct.

33 Centers for Disease Control and Prevention. (2020, August 19). *Using personal protective equipment (PPE)*. https://www.cdc.gov/coronavirus/2019-ncov/hcp/using-ppe.html

My Notes

- Perform hand hygiene using hand sanitizer.
- Put on the isolation gown. Tie all of the ties on the gown. Assistance may be needed by other health care personnel to tie back ties.
- Based on specific transmission-based precautions and agency policy, put on a mask or N95 respirator. The top strap should be placed on the crown (top) of the head, and the bottom strap should be at the base of the neck. If the mask has loops, hook them appropriately around your ears. Masks and respirators should extend under the chin, and both your mouth and nose should be protected. Perform a user-seal check each time you put on a respirator. If the respirator has a nosepiece, it should be fitted to the nose with both hands, but it should not be bent or tented. Masks typically require the nosepiece to be pinched to fit around the nose, but do not pinch the nosepiece of a respirator with one hand. Do not wear a respirator or mask under your chin or store it in the pocket of your scrubs between patients.
- Put on a face shield or goggles when indicated. When wearing an N95 respirator with eye protection, select eye protection that does not affect the fit or seal of the respirator and one that does not affect the position of the respirator. Goggles provide excellent protection for the eyes, but fogging is common. Face shields provide full-face coverage.
- Put on gloves. Gloves should cover the cuff (wrist) of the gown.
- You may now enter the patient's room.

Video Reviews of PPE Use

How to Put On a Respirator[34]

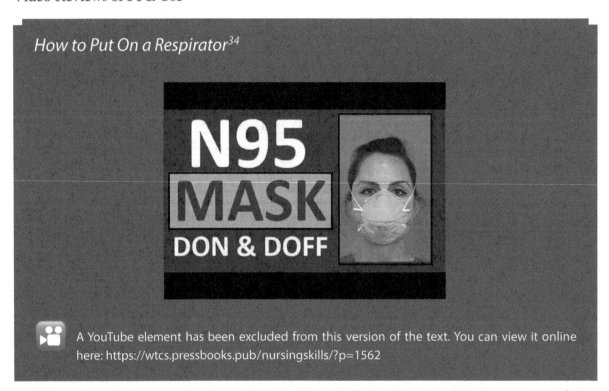

A YouTube element has been excluded from this version of the text. You can view it online here: https://wtcs.pressbooks.pub/nursingskills/?p=1562

34 RegisteredNurseRN. (2020, May 11). *N95 mask - How to wear | N95 respirator nursing skill tutorial.* [Video]. YouTube. All rights reserved. Video used with permission. https://youtu.be/i-uD8rUwG48

My Notes

Donning and Doffing PPE[35]

PPE DON & DOFF TUTORIAL

A YouTube element has been excluded from this version of the text. You can view it online here: https://wtcs.pressbooks.pub/nursingskills/?p=1562

How to Take Off (Doff) PPE Gear

More than one doffing method for removing PPE may be acceptable. Train using your agency's procedure, and practice until you have successfully mastered the steps to avoid contamination of yourself and others. There are established cases of nurses dying from disease transmitted during incorrect removal of PPE. Below are sample steps of doffing established by the CDC:[36]

- Remove the gloves. Ensure glove removal does not cause additional contamination of the hands. Gloves can be removed using more than one technique (e.g., glove-in-glove or bird beak).
- Remove the gown. Untie all ties (or unsnap all buttons). Some gown ties can be broken rather than untied; do so in a gentle manner and avoid a forceful movement. Reach up to the front of your shoulders and carefully pull the gown down and away from your body. Rolling the gown down is also an acceptable approach. Dispose of the gown in a trash receptacle. If it is a washable gown, place it in the specified laundry bin for PPE in the room.
- Health care personnel may now exit the patient room.
- Perform hand hygiene.
- Remove the face shield or goggles. Carefully remove the face shield or goggles by grabbing the strap and pulling upwards and away from head. Do not touch the front of the face shield or goggles.

---

35 RegisteredNurseRN. (2020, May 29). *PPE training video: Donning and doffing PPE nursing skill.* [Video]. YouTube. All rights reserved. Video used with permission. https://youtu.be/iwvnA_b9Q8Y

36 Centers for Disease Control and Prevention. (2020, August 19). *Using personal protective equipment (PPE).* https://www.cdc.gov/coronavirus/2019-ncov/hcp/using-ppe.html

My Notes

- Remove and discard the respirator or face mask. Do not touch the front of the respirator or face mask. Remove the bottom strap by touching only the strap and bringing it carefully over the head. Grasp the top strap and bring it carefully over the head, and then pull the respirator away from the face without touching the front of the respirator. For masks, carefully untie (or unhook ties from the ears) and pull the mask away from your face without touching the front.
- Perform hand hygiene after removing the respirator/mask. If your workplace is practicing reuse, perform hand hygiene before putting it on again.

Additional Video Reviews of PPE

Use: Putting on PPE[37]

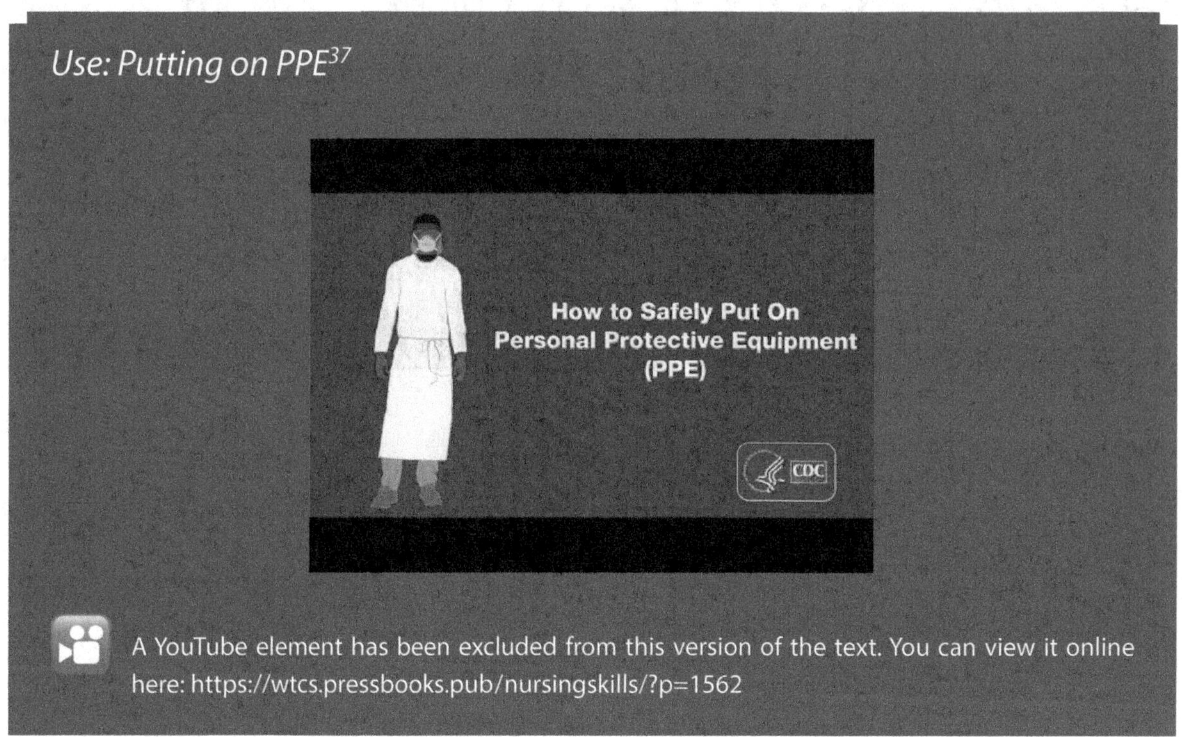

A YouTube element has been excluded from this version of the text. You can view it online here: https://wtcs.pressbooks.pub/nursingskills/?p=1562

37 Centers for Disease Control and Prevention. (2020, July 14). *Demonstration of donning (putting on) personal protective equipment (PPE).* [Video]. YouTube. All rights reserved. https://youtu.be/H4jQUBAlBrI

My Notes

Removing PPE[38]

How to Safely Take Off Personal Protective Equipment (PPE)

CDC

A YouTube element has been excluded from this version of the text. You can view it online here: https://wtcs.pressbooks.pub/nursingskills/?p=1562

Respiratory Hygiene

Respiratory hygiene is targeted at patients, accompanying family members and friends, and health care workers with undiagnosed transmissible respiratory infections. It applies to any person with signs of illness, including cough, congestion, rhinorrhea, or increased production of respiratory secretions when entering a health care facility. See Figure 4.13[39] for an example of a "Cover Your Cough" poster used in public areas to promote respiratory hygiene. The elements of respiratory hygiene include the following:

- Education of health care facility staff, patients, and visitors
- Posted signs, in language(s) appropriate to the population served, with instructions to patients and accompanying family members or friends
- Source control measures for a coughing person (e.g., covering the mouth/nose with a tissue when coughing and prompt disposal of used tissues, or applying surgical masks on the coughing person to contain secretions)
- Hand hygiene after contact with one's respiratory secretions
- Spatial separation, ideally greater than 3 feet, of persons with respiratory infections in common waiting areas when possible.[40]

---

38 Centers for Disease Control and Prevention. (2020, April 21). *Demonstration of doffing (taking off) personal protective equipment (PPE).* [Video]. YouTube. All rights reserved. https://youtu.be/PQxOc13DxvQ

39 "cycphceng.pdf" by https://www.health.state.mn.us/index.html is in the Public Domain. Access for free at https://www.health.state.mn.us/people/cyc/

40 Siegel, J. D., Rhinehart, E., Jackson, M., Chiarello, L., & Healthcare Infection Control Practices Advisory Committee. (2019, July 22). *2007 guideline for isolation precautions: Preventing transmission of infectious agents in healthcare settings.* https://www.cdc.gov/infectioncontrol/guidelines/isolation/index.html

My Notes

Health care personnel are advised to wear a mask and use frequent hand hygiene when examining and caring for patients with signs and symptoms of a respiratory infection. Health care personnel who have a respiratory infection are advised to avoid direct patient contact, especially with high-risk patients. If this is not possible, then a mask should be worn while providing patient care.[41]

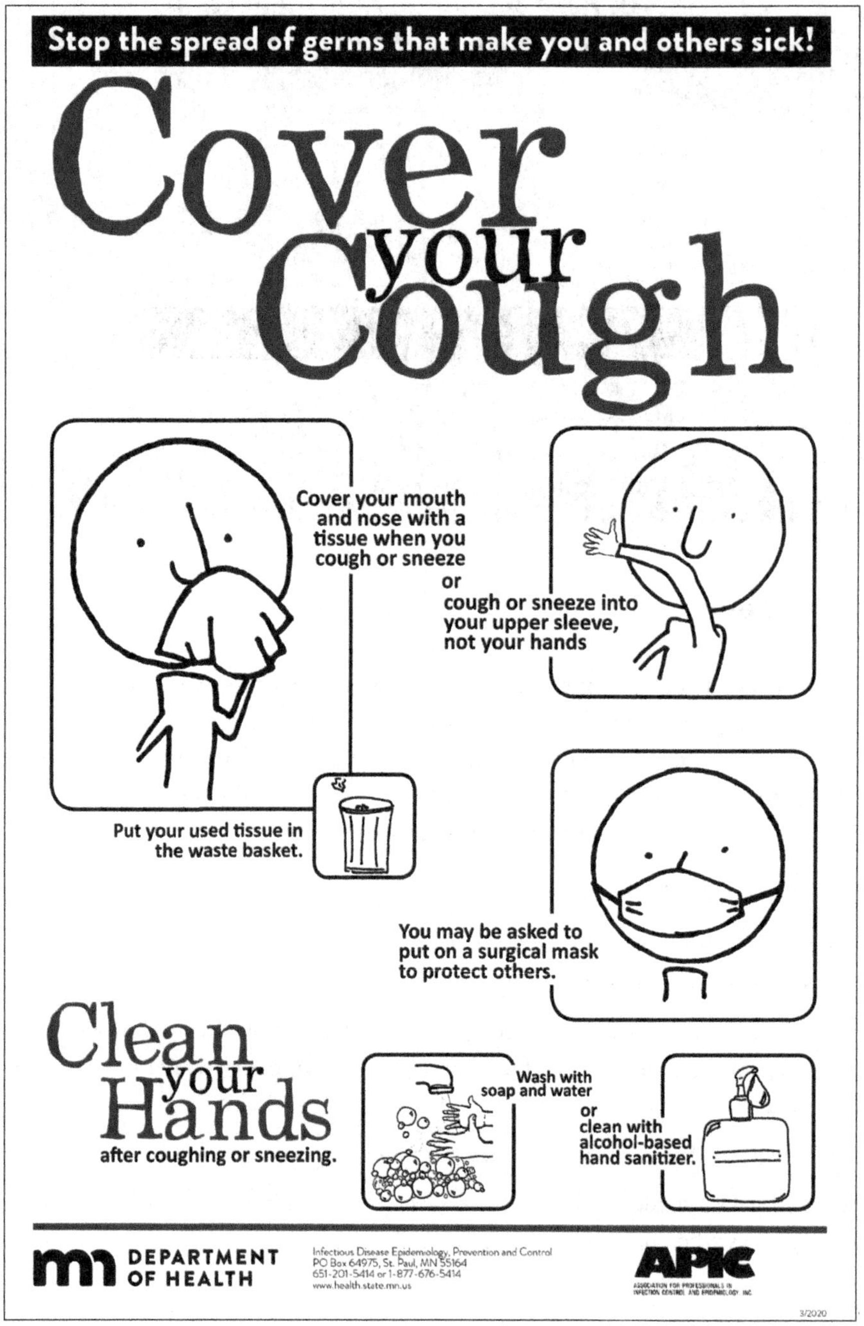

Figure 4.13 Cover Your Cough Poster

41 Siegel, J. D., Rhinehart, E., Jackson, M., Chiarello, L., & Healthcare Infection Control Practices Advisory Committee. (2019, July 22). *2007 guideline for isolation precautions: Preventing transmission of infectious agents in healthcare settings.* https://www.cdc.gov/infectioncontrol/guidelines/isolation/index.html

Environmental Measures

My Notes

Routine cleaning and disinfecting surfaces in patient-care areas are part of standard precautions. The cleaning and disinfecting of all patient-care areas are important for frequently touched surfaces, especially those closest to the patient that are most likely to be contaminated (e.g., bedrails, bedside tables, commodes, doorknobs, sinks, surfaces, and equipment in close proximity to the patient).

Medical equipment and instruments/devices must also be cleaned to prevent patient-to-patient transmission of infectious agents. For example, stethoscopes should be cleaned before and after use for all patients. Patients who have transmission-based precautions should have dedicated medical equipment that remains in their room (e.g., stethoscope, blood pressure cuff, thermometer). When dedicated equipment is not possible, such as a unit-wide bedside blood glucose monitor, disinfection after each patient's use should be performed according to agency policy.[42]

Disposal of Contaminated Waste

Medical waste requires careful disposal according to agency policy. The Occupational Safety and Health Administration (OSHA) has established measures for discarding regulated medical waste items to protect the workers who generate medical waste, as well as those who manage the waste from point of generation to disposal. Contaminated waste is placed in a leak-resistant biohazard bag, securely closed, and placed in a labeled, leakproof, puncture-resistant container in a storage area. Sharps containers are used to dispose of sharp items such as discarded tubes with small amounts of blood, scalpel blades, needles, and syringes.[43]

Sharps Safety

Injuries due to needles and other sharps have been associated with transmission of blood-borne pathogens (BBP), including hepatitis B, hepatitis C, and HIV to health care personnel. The prevention of sharps injuries is an essential element of standard precautions and includes measures to handle needles and other sharp devices in a manner that will prevent injury to the user and to others who may encounter the device during or after a procedure. The Bloodborne Pathogens Standard is a regulation that prescribes safeguards to protect workers against health hazards related to blood-borne pathogens. It includes work practice controls, hepatitis B vaccinations, hazard communication and training, plans for when an employee is exposed to a BBP, and record keeping.

When performing procedures that include needles or other sharps, dispose of these items immediately in FDA-cleared sharps disposal containers. Additionally, to prevent needlestick injuries, needles and other contaminated sharps should not be recapped. See Figure 4.14[44] for an image of a sharps disposal container. FDA-cleared sharps disposal containers are made from rigid plastic and come marked with a line that indicates when the container should be considered full, which means it's time to dispose of the container. When a sharps disposal container is about three-quarters full, follow agency policy for proper disposal of the container.

---

42 Siegel, J. D., Rhinehart, E., Jackson, M., Chiarello, L., & Healthcare Infection Control Practices Advisory Committee. (2019, July 22). *2007 guideline for isolation precautions: Preventing transmission of infectious agents in healthcare settings.* https://www.cdc.gov/infectioncontrol/guidelines/isolation/index.html

43 Centers for Disease Control and Prevention. (2015, November 5). *Background I. Regulated medical waste.* https://www.cdc.gov/infectioncontrol/guidelines/environmental/background/medical-waste.html#i3

44 "Sharps-Containers.jpg" by Federal Drug Administration (FDA) is in the Public Domain. Access for free at https://www.fda.gov/medical-devices/safely-using-sharps-needles-and-syringes-home-work-and-travel/sharps-disposal-containers

My Notes

If you are stuck by a needle or other sharps or are exposed to blood or other potentially infectious materials in your eyes, nose, mouth, or on broken skin, immediately flood the exposed area with water and clean any wound with soap and water. Report the incident immediately to your instructor or employer and seek immediate medical attention according to agency and school policy.

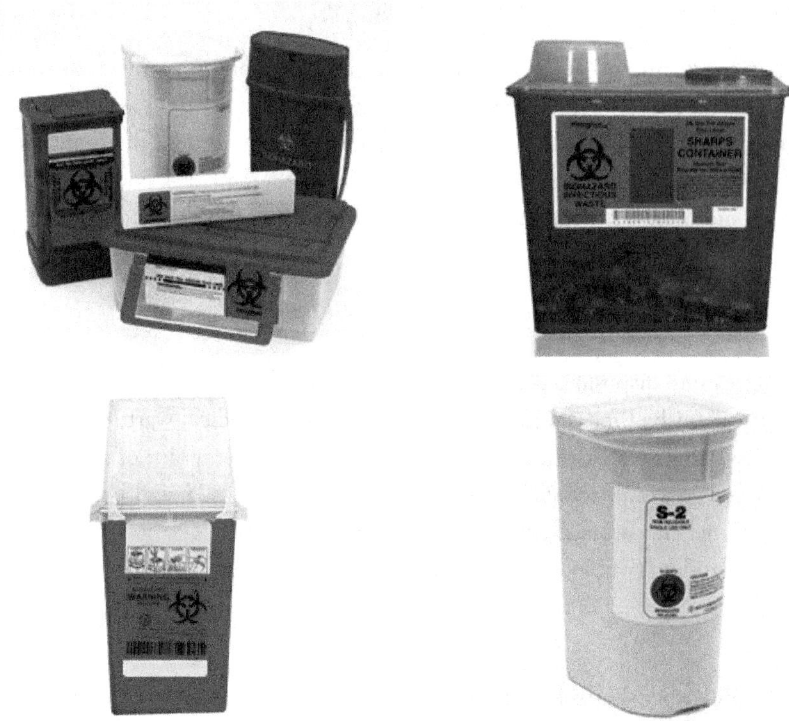

Figure 4.14 Sharps Disposal Containers

Textiles and Laundry

Soiled textiles, including bedding, towels, and patient or resident clothing may be contaminated with pathogenic microorganisms. However, the risk of disease transmission is negligible if they are handled, transported, and laundered in a safe manner. Follow agency policy for handling soiled laundry using standard precautions. Key principles for handling soiled laundry are as follows:

- Do not shake items or handle them in any way that may aerosolize infectious agents.
- Avoid contact of one's body and personal clothing with the soiled items being handled.
- Place soiled items in a laundry bag or designated bin in the patient's room before transporting to a laundry area. When laundry chutes are used, they must be maintained to minimize dispersion of aerosols from contaminated items.[45]

---

45 Siegel, J. D., Rhinehart, E., Jackson, M., Chiarello, L., & Healthcare Infection Control Practices Advisory Committee. (2019, July 22). *2007 guideline for isolation precautions: Preventing transmission of infectious agents in healthcare settings.* https://www.cdc.gov/infectioncontrol/guidelines/isolation/index.html

4.3 ASEPTIC TECHNIQUE

My Notes

In addition to using standard precautions and transmission-based precautions, **aseptic technique** (also called medical asepsis) is the purposeful reduction of pathogens to prevent the transfer of microorganisms from one person or object to another during a medical procedure. For example, a nurse administering parenteral medication or performing urinary catheterization uses aseptic technique. When performed properly, aseptic technique prevents contamination and transfer of pathogens to the patient from caregiver hands, surfaces, and equipment during routine care or procedures. The word "aseptic" literally means an absence of disease-causing microbes and pathogens. In the clinical setting, aseptic technique refers to the purposeful prevention of microbe contamination from one person or object to another. These potentially infectious, microscopic organisms can be present in the environment, on an instrument, in liquids, on skin surfaces, or within a wound.

There is often misunderstanding between the terms aseptic technique and sterile technique in the health care setting. Both **asepsis** and sterility are closely related, and the shared concept between the two terms is removal of harmful microorganisms that can cause infection. In the most simplistic terms, asepsis is creating a protective barrier from pathogens, whereas **sterile technique** is a purposeful attack on microorganisms.

Sterile technique (also called surgical asepsis) seeks to eliminate every potential microorganism in and around a sterile field while also maintaining objects as free from microorganisms as possible. It is the standard of care for surgical procedures, invasive wound management, and central line care. Sterile technique requires a combination of meticulous hand washing, creation of a sterile field, using long-lasting antimicrobial cleansing agents such as Betadine, donning sterile gloves, and using sterile devices and instruments.

Principles of Aseptic Non-Touch Technique

Aseptic non-touch technique (ANTT) is the most commonly used aseptic technique framework in the health care setting and is considered a global standard. There are two types of ANTT: surgical-ANTT (sterile technique) and standard-ANTT.

Aseptic non-touch technique starts with a few concepts that must be understood before it can be applied. For all invasive procedures, the "ANTT-approach" identifies key parts and key sites throughout the preparation and implementation of the procedure. A **key part** is any sterile part of equipment used during an aseptic procedure, such as needle hubs, syringe tips, needles, and dressings. A **key site** is any nonintact skin, potential insertion site, or access site used for medical devices connected to the patients. Examples of key sites include open wounds and insertion sites for intravenous (IV) devices and urinary catheters.

ANTT includes four underlying principles to keep in mind while performing invasive procedures:

- Always wash hands effectively.
- Never contaminate key parts.
- Touch non-key parts with confidence.
- Take appropriate infective precautions.

Preparing and Preventing Infections Using Aseptic Technique

When planning for any procedure, careful thought and preparation of many infection control factors must be considered beforehand. While keeping standard precautions in mind, identify anticipated key sites and key parts to the procedure. Consider the degree to which the environment must be managed to reduce the risk of infection,

My Notes

including the expected degree of contamination and hazardous exposure to the clinician. Finally, review the expected equipment needed to perform the procedure and the level of key part or key site handling. See Table 4.3 for an outline of infection control measures when performing a procedure.

Table 4.3 Infection Control Measures When Performing Procedures

Infection Control Measure	Key Considerations	Examples
Environmental control	■ Recognize and avoid risks in the environment that may increase risk of infection.	■ Ensure clean bed linens. ■ Monitor patient lines that are near or across work areas. ■ Clean surfaces before establishing a work area. ■ Keep food and personal items away from working areas.
Hand hygiene	■ Perform hand hygiene frequently and during key moments. (Review the "Five Key Moments" under the "Appropriate Hand Hygiene" section.)	■ Scrub with soap solution and water for 20-30 seconds. ■ Use alcohol-based rub until dry, unless hands are visibly soiled or the patient has C-diff.
Personal protective equipment (PPE)	■ Select sterile or clean gloves based on the need to touch key parts or key sites directly. ■ Gloves do not replace the need for hand hygiene.	■ Gloves (sterile or clean, based on the procedure) ■ Mask or respirator ■ Protective eyewear, goggles, or face shield ■ Gown (sterile or clean, whichever is appropriate)
Aseptic field management	Determine level of aseptic field needed and how it will be managed before the procedure begins: ■ **General aseptic field**: Key parts and sites are easily protected. Sterile field does not need to be set up and managed as a key part. ■ **Critical aseptic field**: Key parts and sites are large, numerous, or not easily protected using non-touch technique. Sterile field needs to be established before and managed during procedure.	General aseptic field: IV irrigation Dry dressing changes Critical aseptic field: Urinary catheter placement Central line dressing change Sterile dressing change

My Notes

Infection Control Measure	Key Considerations	Examples
Non-touch technique	■ Handling key parts only at the time needed to assemble or use in procedure ■ Handling syringes away from the hub ■ Applying bandages by the edges away from key parts that will contact key sites	■ Handling key parts only at the time needed to assemble or use in procedure ■ Handling syringes away from the hub ■ Applying bandages by the edges away from key parts that will contact key sites
Sequencing	■ Order of procedure requires planning to be efficient, logical, and safe. ■ Practicing guidelines give direction as to optimal order from preparation to completion.	■ Generally, follow "clean to dirty" standards, working from least to most contaminated key parts and sites.

Use of Gloves and Sterile Gloves

There are two different levels of medical-grade gloves available to health care providers: clean (exam) gloves and sterile (surgical) gloves. Generally speaking, clean gloves are used whenever there is a risk of contact with body fluids or contaminated surfaces or objects. Examples include starting an intravenous access device or emptying a urinary catheter collection bag. Alternatively, sterile gloves meet FDA requirements for sterilization and are used for invasive procedures or when contact with a sterile site, tissue, or body cavity is anticipated. Sterile gloves are used in these instances to prevent transient flora and reduce resident flora contamination during a procedure, thus preventing the introduction of pathogens. For example, sterile gloves are required when performing central line dressing changes, insertion of urinary catheters, and during invasive surgical procedures. See Figure 4.15[1] for images of a nurse opening and removing sterile gloves from packaging.

See the "Checklist for Applying and Removing Sterile Gloves" for details on how to apply sterile gloves.

1 "Book-pictures-2015-199-001-300x241.jpg," "Book-pictures-2015-215.jpg," and "Book-pictures-2015-219.jpg" by British Columbia Institute of Technology are licensed under CC BY 4.0. Access for free at https://opentextbc.ca/clinicalskills/chapter/sterile-gloving/

My Notes

Video Review of Applying Sterile Gloves[2]

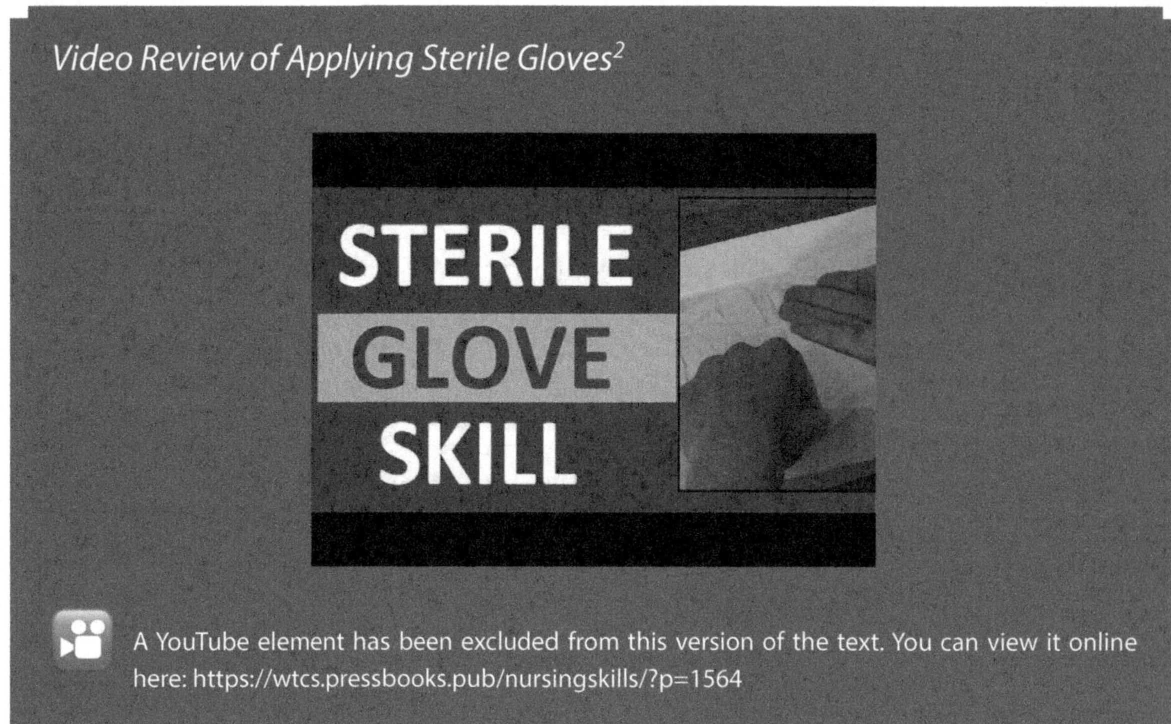

A YouTube element has been excluded from this version of the text. You can view it online here: https://wtcs.pressbooks.pub/nursingskills/?p=1564

2 RegisteredNurseRN. (2017, April 28). *Sterile gloving nursing technique | Don/donning sterile gloves tips.* [Video]. YouTube. All rights reserved. Video used with permission. https://youtu.be/lumZOF-METc

My Notes

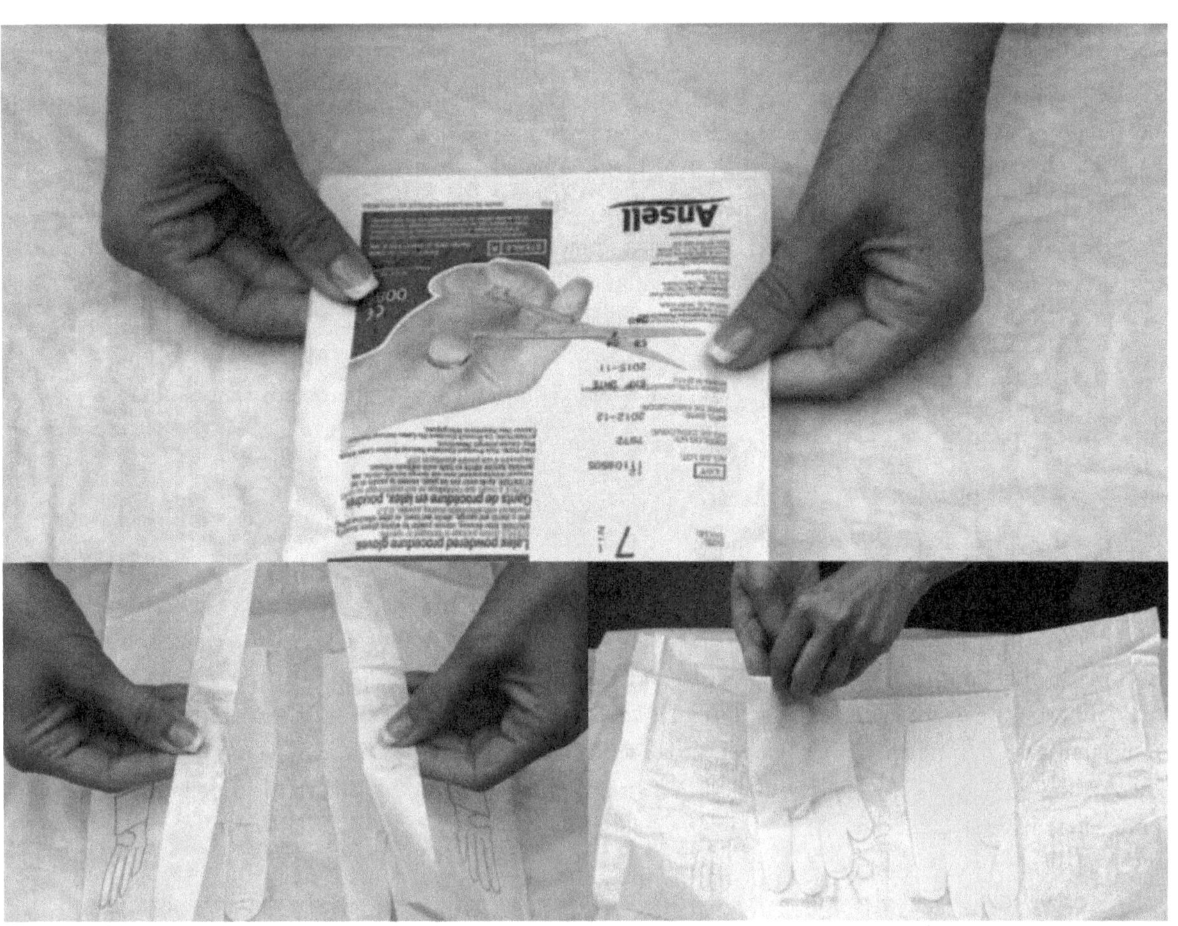

Figure 4.15 Sterile Gloves

My Notes

4.4 STERILE FIELDS

A sterile field is established whenever a patient's skin is intentionally punctured or incised, during procedures involving entry into a body cavity, or when contact with nonintact skin is possible (e.g., surgery or trauma). Surgical asepsis requires adherence to strict principles and intentional actions to prevent contamination and to maintain the sterility of specific parts of a sterile field during invasive procedures. Creating and maintaining a sterile field is foundational to aseptic technique and encompasses practice standards that are performed immediately prior to and during a procedure to reduce the risk of infection, including the following:

- Handwashing
- Using sterile barriers, including drapes and appropriate personal protective equipment
- Preparing the patient using an approved antimicrobial product
- Maintaining a sterile field
- Using aseptically safe techniques

There are basic principles of asepsis that are critical to understand and follow when creating and maintaining a sterile field. The most basic principle is to allow only sterile supplies within the sterile field once it is established. This means that prior to using any supplies, exterior packaging must be checked for any signs of damage, such as previous exposure to moisture, holes, or tears. Packages should not be used if they are expired or if sterilization indicators are not the appropriate color. Sterile contents inside packages are dispensed onto the sterile field using the methods outlined below. See Figure 4.16[1] for an image of a nurse dispensing sterile supplies from packaging onto an established sterile field.

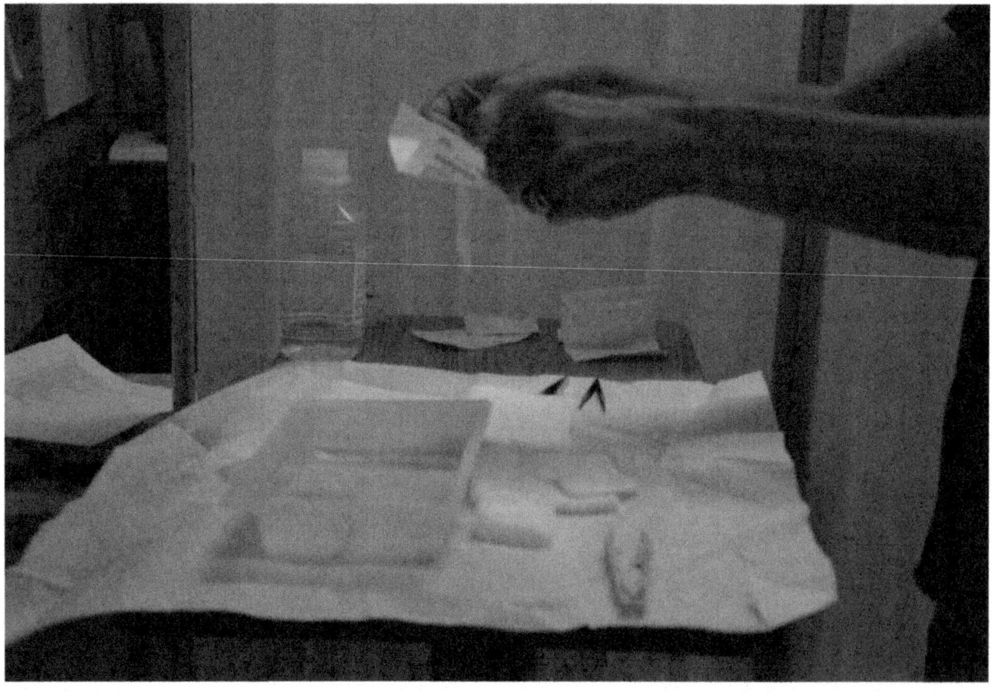

Figure 4.16 Dispensing Sterile Supplies onto a Sterile Field

---

1 "DSC_0319-1024x678.jpg" by British Columbia Institute of Technology is licensed under CC BY 4.0. Access for free at https://opentextbc.ca/clinicalskills/chapter/sterile-gloving/

When establishing and maintaining a sterile field, there are other important principles to strictly follow:

- Disinfect any work surfaces and allow to them thoroughly dry before placing any sterile supplies on the surface.
- Be aware of areas of sterile fields that are considered contaminated:
    - Any part of the field within 1 inch from the edge.
    - Any part of the field that extends below the planar surface (i.e., a drape hanging down below the tray tabletop).
    - Any part of the field below waist level or above shoulder level.
    - Any supplies or field that you have not directly monitored (i.e., turned away from the sterile field or walked out of the room).
    - Within 1 inch of any visible holes, tears, or moisture wicked from an unsterile area.
- When handling sterile kits and trays:
    - Sterile kits and trays generally have an outer protective wrapper and four inner flaps that must be opened aseptically.
    - Open sterile kits away from your body first, touching only the very edge of the opening flap.
    - Using the same technique, open each of the side flaps one at a time using only one hand, being careful not to allow your body or arms to be directly above the opened drape. Take care not to allow already-opened corners to flip back into the sterile area again.
    - Open the final flap toward you, being careful to not allow any part of your body to be directly over the field. See Figure 4.17[2] for images of opening the flaps of a sterile kit.
    - If you must remove parts of the sterile kit (i.e., sterile gloves), reach into the sterile field with the elbow raised, using only the tips of the fingers before extracting. Pay close attention to where your body and clothing are in relationship to the sterile field to avoid inadvertent contamination.

2 "Book-pictures-2015-700.jpg," "Book-pictures-2015-706.jpg," "Book-pictures-2015-708.jpg," and "Book- pictures-2015 -709.jpg" by British Columbia Institute of Technology are licensed under CC BY 4.0. Access for free at https://opentextbc .ca/clinicalskills/chapter/sterile-gloving/

My Notes

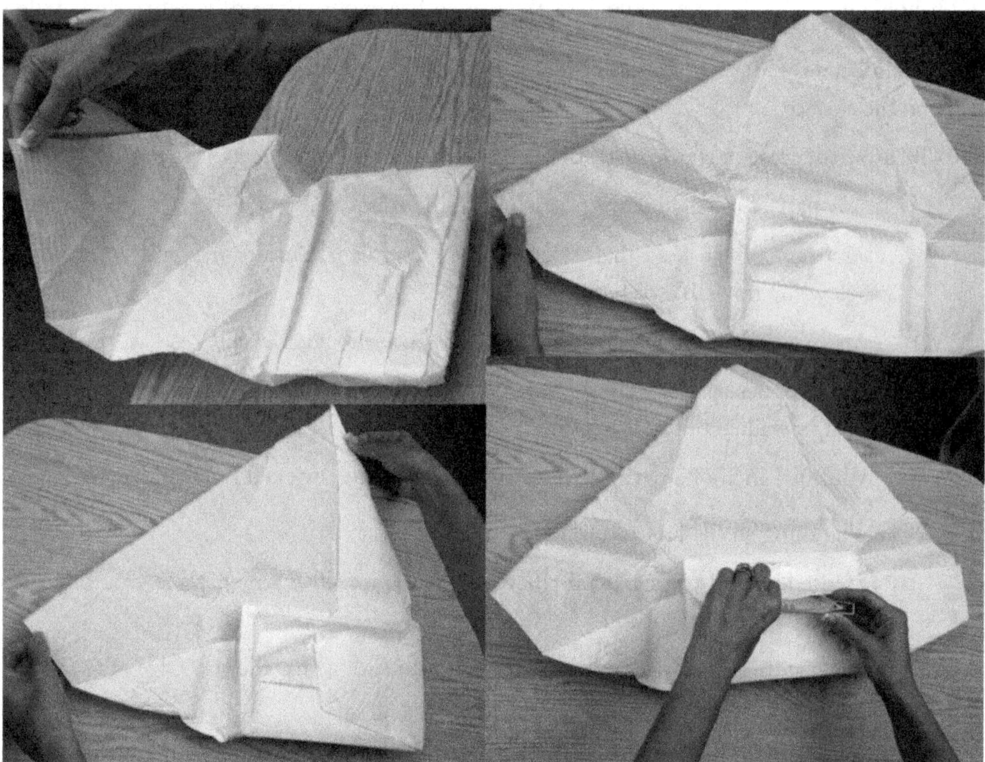

Figure 4.17 Opening a Sterile Kit

- When dispensing sterile supplies onto a sterile field:
    - Before dispensing sterile supplies to a sterile field, do not allow sterile items to touch any part of the outer packaging once it is opened, including the former package seal.
    - Heavy or irregular items should be opened and held, allowing a second person with sterile gloves to transfer them to the sterile field.
    - Wrapped sterile items should be opened similarly to a sterile kit. Tuck each flap securely within your palm, and then open the flap away from your body first. Then open each side flap; secure the flap in the palm one at a time and open. Finally, open the flap (closest to you) toward you, while also protecting the other opened flaps from springing back onto the wrapped item.
    - Peel pouches (i.e., gloves, gauze, syringes, etc.) can be opened by firmly grasping each side of the sealed edge with the thumb side of each hand parallel to the seal and pulling carefully apart.
    - Drop items from six inches away from the sterile field.
    - Sterile solutions should be poured into a sterile bowl or tray from the side of the sterile field and not directly over it. Use only sealed, sterile, unexpired solutions when pouring onto a sterile field. Solution should be held six inches away from the field as it is being poured. Avoid splashing solutions because this allows wicking and transfer of microbes. After pouring of solution stops, it should not be restarted because the edge is considered

My Notes

contaminated. See Figure 4.18[3] of an image of a nurse pouring sterile solution into a receptacle in a sterile field before the procedure begins.

- Don sterile gloves away from the sterile field to avoid contaminating the sterile field.

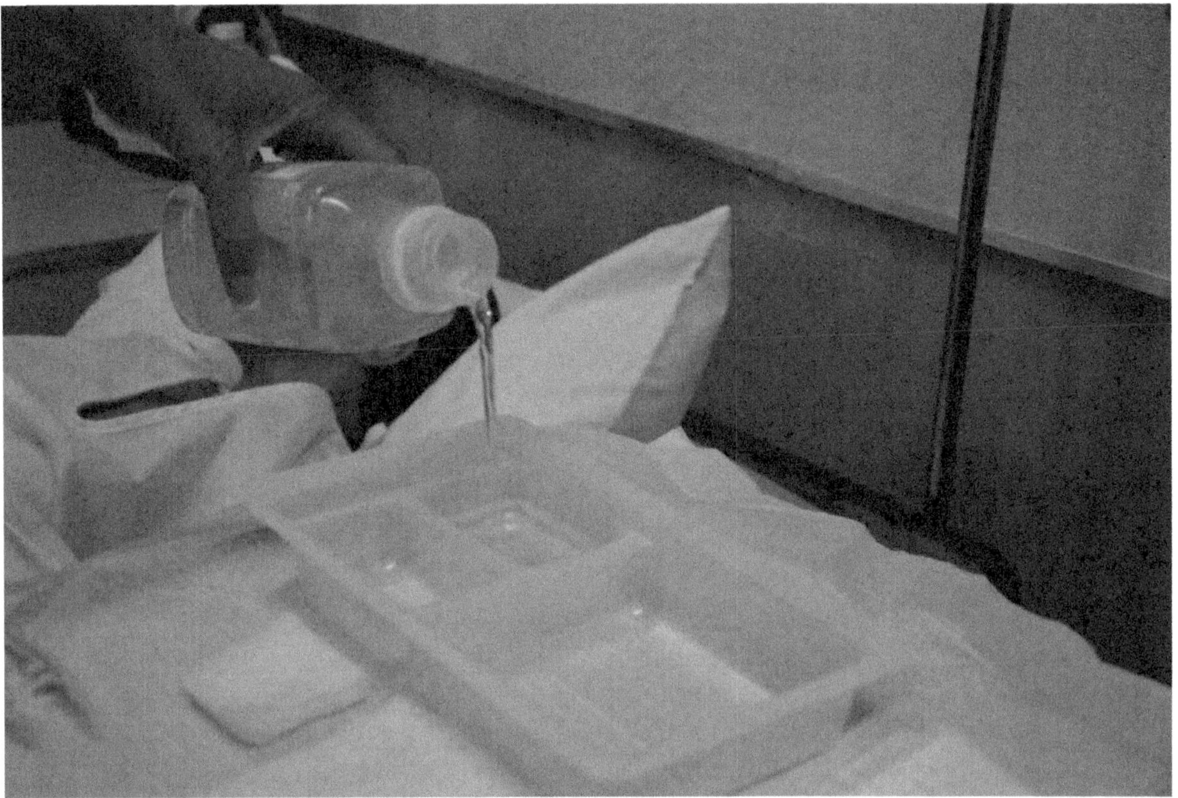

Figure 4.18 Pouring Sterile Solution

3 "DSC_0313.jpg" by British Columbia Institute of Technology is licensed under CC BY 4.0. Access for free at https://opentextbc.ca/clinicalskills/chapter/sterile-gloving/

My Notes

4.5 CHECKLIST FOR HAND HYGIENE WITH SOAP AND WATER

Use the checklist below to review the steps for completion of "Hand Hygiene with Soap and Water."

Steps

Disclaimer: Always review and follow agency policy regarding this specific skill.

1. Remove jewelry according to agency policy; push your sleeves above your wrists.
2. Turn on the water and adjust the flow so that the water is warm. Wet your hands thoroughly, keeping your hands and forearms lower than your elbows. Avoid splashing water on your uniform.
3. Apply a palm-sized amount of hand soap.
4. Perform hand hygiene using plenty of lather and friction for at least 15 seconds:
    - Rub hands palm to palm
    - Back of right and left hand (fingers interlaced)
    - Palm to palm with fingers interlaced
    - Rotational rubbing of left and right thumbs
    - Rub your fingertips against the palm of your opposite hand
    - Rub wrists
    - Repeat sequence at least 2 times
    - Keep fingertips pointing downward throughout
5. Clean under your fingernails with disposable nail cleaner (if applicable).
6. Wash for a minimum of 20 seconds.
7. Keep your hands and forearms lower than your elbows during the entire washing.
8. Rinse your hands with water, keeping your fingertips pointing down so water runs off your fingertips. Do not shake water from your hands.
9. Do not lean against the sink or touch the inside of the sink during the hand-washing process.
10. Dry your hands thoroughly from your fingers to wrists with a paper towel or air dryer.
11. Dispose of the paper towel(s).
12. Use a new paper towel to turn off the water.
13. Dispose of the paper towel.

4.6 CHECKLIST FOR HAND HYGIENE WITH ALCOHOL-BASED HAND SANITIZER

My Notes

Use the checklist below to review the steps for completion of "Hand Hygiene with Alcohol-Based Hand Sanitizer."

Steps

Disclaimer: Always review and follow agency policy regarding this specific skill.

1. Gather supplies (antiseptic hand rub).
2. Remove jewelry according to agency policy; push your sleeves above your wrists.
3. Apply enough product into the palm of one hand and enough to cover your hands thoroughly, per product directions.
4. Rub your hands together, covering all surfaces of your hands and fingers with antiseptic until the alcohol is dry (a minimum of 30 seconds):
    - Rub hands palm to palm
    - Back of right and left hand (fingers interlaced)
    - Palm to palm with fingers interlaced
    - Rotational rubbing of left and right thumbs
    - Rub your fingertips against the palm of your opposite hand
    - Rub your wrists
5. Repeat hand sanitizing sequence a minimum of two times.
6. Repeat hand sanitizing sequence until the product is dry.

My Notes

4.7 CHECKLIST FOR PERSONAL PROTECTIVE EQUIPMENT (PPE)

Use the checklist below to review the steps for completion of "Applying and Removing Personal Protective Equipment."[1]

Steps

Disclaimer: Always review and follow agency policy regarding this specific skill.

1. Check the provider's order for the type of precautions.
2. Ensure that all supplies are available before check-off begins: isolation cart, gowns, gloves, mask, eye/face shields, shoes, and head cover.
3. Perform hand hygiene.
4. Apply PPE in the correct order:
    - 1st (GOWN): Gown should cover all outer garments. Pull the sleeves down to the wrists, and tie at neck & waist.
    - 2nd (MASK/RESPIRATOR): Apply surgical mask or N95 respirator if indicated by transmission-based precaution. Fit the mask around the nose and chin, securing bands around ears or tie straps at top of head and base of neck.
    - 3rd (EYE PROTECTION): Apply goggles/face shield if indicated for patient condition or transmission-based precautions.
    - 4th (CLEAN GLOVES): Pull on gloves to cover the wrist of the gown.
5. Remove PPE in the correct order:
    - 1st REMOVE GLOVES: REMEMBER: GLOVE TO GLOVE; SKIN TO SKIN. Do not touch contaminated gloves to your skin. Take off the contaminated glove with your gloved hand, wrapping the contaminated glove in the palm of your gloved hand. Take off the glove with your bare hand to the skin of your wrist, moving inside of the glove to remove the contaminated glove inside out over the other glove. Note: If the gown is tied in front, untie it prior to removing your glove.
    - 2nd REMOVE GOWN: Untie all ties (or unsnap all buttons). Some gown ties can be broken rather than untied. Do so in a gentle manner, avoiding a forceful movement. Reach up to the shoulders and carefully pull the gown down and away from the body. Rolling the gown down is an acceptable approach. Dispose in trash receptacle.
    - 3rd PERFORM HAND HYGIENE.
    - 4th REMOVE FACE SHIELD or GOGGLES: Carefully remove face shield or goggles by grabbing the strap and pulling upwards and away from head. Do not touch the front of face shield or goggles.

---

1 Centers for Disease Control and Prevention. (2020, August 19). *Using personal protective equipment (PPE)*. https://www.cdc.gov/coronavirus/2019-ncov/hcp/using-ppe.html

My Notes

- 5th REMOVE MASK or RESPIRATOR: Do not touch the front of the face shield or goggles.
    - Respirator: Remove the bottom strap by touching only the strap and bringing it carefully over the head. Grasp the top strap and bring it carefully over the head, and then pull the respirator away from the face without touching the front of the respirator.
    - Face mask: Carefully untie (or unhook from the ears) and pull it away from the face without touching the front.
- 6th PERFORM HAND HYGIENE after removing the mask.

My Notes

4.8 CHECKLIST FOR APPLYING AND REMOVING STERILE GLOVES

Use the checklist below to review the steps for completion of "Applying and Removing Sterile Gloves."

Steps

Disclaimer: Always review and follow agency policy regarding this specific skill.

1. Gather the supplies: hand sanitizer and sterile gloves.
2. Perform hand hygiene.
3. Open the sterile gloves on a dry, flat, clean work surface.
4. Remove the outer package by separating and peeling apart the sides of the package.
5. Grasp the inner package and lay it on a clean, dry, flat surface at waist level.
6. Open the top flap away from your body; open the bottom flap toward your body.
7. Open the side flaps without contaminating the inside of the wrapper or allowing it to close.
8. With your nondominant hand, use your thumb and index finger to only grasp the inside surface of the cuff of the glove for your dominant hand.
9. Lift out the glove, being careful to not touch any surfaces and holding the glove no more than 12-18" above the table without contaminating the sterile glove; carefully pull the glove over your hand.
10. Use your nondominant, nonsterile hand to grasp the flap of the package, and hold the package steady. With the sterile glove on your dominant hand, hold 4 fingers together of the gloved hand to reach in the outer surface of the cuff of the sterile glove, reaching under the folded cuff and with the thumb outstretched to not touch the second sterile glove. Lift the glove off the package without breaking sterility.
11. While holding the fingers of the nondominant hand outstretched and close together, tuck your thumb into the palm, and use the sterile dominant hand to pull the second sterile glove over the fingers of the nondominant hand.
12. After the second sterile glove is on, interlock the fingers of your sterile gloved hands, being careful to keep your hands above your waist.
13. Do not touch the inside of the package or the sterile part of the gloves with your bare hands during the process.
14. Maintain sterility throughout the procedure of donning sterile gloves.

Removing Sterile Gloves

1. Grasp the outside of one cuff with the other gloved hand. Avoid touching your skin.
2. Pull the glove off, turning it inside out and gather it in the palm of the gloved hand.
3. Tuck the index finger of your bare hand inside the remaining glove cuff and peel the glove off inside out and over the previously removed glove.

My Notes

4. Dispose of contaminated wastes appropriately.

5. Perform hand hygiene.

My Notes

4.9 ASEPSIS LEARNING ACTIVITIES

Learning Activities

(Answers to "Learning Activities" can be found in the "Answer Key" at the end of the book. Answers to interactive activity elements will be provided within the element as immediate feedback.)

You are caring for an elderly male patient who is experiencing urinary retention. The provider has just ordered an intermittent catheterization for the patient based on the results of a recent bladder scan of 375 mL. You gather the equipment and enter the patient's room. Based on the five moments of hand hygiene, describe the instances in which you will sanitize your hands when working with the patient and performing the intermittent catheterization.

Based upon the information provided, which clinical scenarios require the use of soap and water (versus alcohol- based hand scrubs) for proper hand sanitization?

a. Entry into patient's room with no contact precautions
b. Patient on ***Clostridium Difficile*** (C-Diff) contact precautions
c. Prior to Foley catheter insertion for a patient with no contact precautions
d. Hands are visibly soiled

Interactive Activity

An interactive or media element has been excluded from this version of the text. You can view it online here: https://wtcs.pressbooks.pub/nursingskills/?p=1570

Interactive Activity

An interactive or media element has been excluded from this version of the text. You can view it online here: https://wtcs.pressbooks.pub/nursingskills/?p=1570

IV GLOSSARY

My Notes

Airborne precautions: Infection prevention and control interventions to be used in addition to standard precautions for diseases spread by airborne transmission, such as measles and tuberculosis.

Asepsis: A state of being free of disease-causing microorganisms.

Aseptic non-touch technique: A standardized technique, supported by evidence, to maintain asepsis and standardize practice.

Aseptic technique (medical asepsis): The purposeful reduction of pathogen numbers while preventing microorganism transfer from one person or object to another. This technique is commonly used to perform invasive procedures, such as IV starts or urinary catheterization.

Contact precautions: Infection prevention and control interventions to be used in addition to standard precautions for diseases spread by contact with the patient, their body fluids, or their surroundings, such as C-diff, MRSA, VRE, and RSV.

Doff: To take off or remove personal protective equipment, such as gloves or a gown.

Don: To put on equipment for personal protection, such as gloves or a gown.

Droplet precautions: Infection prevention and control interventions to be used in addition to standard precautions; used for diseases spread by large respiratory droplets such as influenza, COVID-19, or pertussis.

Five moments of hand hygiene: Hand hygiene should be performed during the five moments of patient care: immediately before touching a patient; before performing an aseptic task or handling invasive devices; before moving from a soiled body site to a clean body site on a patient; after touching a patient or their immediate environment; after contact with blood, body fluids, or contaminated surfaces (with or without glove use); and immediately after glove removal.

Hand hygiene: A way of cleaning one's hands to substantially reduce the number of pathogens and other contaminants (e.g., dirt, body fluids, chemicals, or other unwanted substances) to prevent disease transmission or integumentary harm, typically using soap, water, and friction. An alcohol-based hand rub solution may be appropriate hand hygiene for hands not visibly soiled.

Healthcare-Associated Infections (HAIs): Unintended infections caused by care received in a health care setting.

Key part: Any sterile part of equipment used during an aseptic procedure, such as needle hubs, syringe tips, dressings, etc.

Key site: The site contacted during an aseptic procedure, such as nonintact skin, a potential insertion site, or an access site used for medical devices connected to the patients. Examples of key sites include the insertion or access site for intravenous (IV) devices, urinary catheters, and open wounds.

Personal Protective Equipment (PPE): Personal protective equipment, such as gloves, gowns, face shields, goggles, and masks, used to prevent transmission of disease from patient to patient, patient to health care provider, and health care provider to patient.

Standard precautions: The minimum infection prevention practices that apply to all patient care, regardless of suspected or confirmed infection status of the patient, in any setting where health care is delivered.

Sterile technique (surgical asepsis): Techniques used to eliminate every potential microorganism in and around a sterile field while maintaining objects and areas as free from microorganisms as possible. This technique is the standard of care for surgical procedures, invasive wound management, and central line care.

Chapter 5

Math Calculations

5.1 MATH CALCULATIONS INTRODUCTION

My Notes

Learning Objectives

- Accurately perform calculations using decimals, fractions, percentages, ratios, and/or proportions
- Convert between the metric and household systems
- Use military time
- Use dimensional analysis
- Accurately solve calculations related to conversions, dosages, liquid concentrations, reconstituted medications, weight-based medications, and intravenous infusions and evaluate final answer to ensure safe medication administration

The Institute of Medicine (IOM) has estimated that the average hospitalized patient experiences at least one medication error each day. Nurses are the last step in the medication administration process before the medication reaches the patient, so they bear the final responsibility to ensure the medication is safe. To safely prepare and administer medications, the nurse performs a variety of mathematical calculations, such as determining the number of tablets, calculating the amount of solution, and setting the rate of an intravenous infusion.[1]

Dosage calculation in clinical practice is more than just solving a math problem. Nurses must perform several tasks during drug calculations, such as reading drug labels for pertinent information, determining what information is needed to set up the math calculation, performing the math calculations, and then critically evaluating the answer to determine if it is within a safe dosage range for that specific patient. Finally, the nurse selects an appropriate measurement device to accurately measure the calculated dose or set the rate of administration.[2] This chapter will explain how to perform these tasks related to dosage calculations using authentic problems that a nurse commonly encounters in practice.

---

1 Institute of Medicine. (2007). *Preventing medication errors.* The National Academies Press. https://doi.org/10.17226/11623

2 Ozimek, D. (2019). *Teaching dosage calculations: Strategies for narrowing the theory-practice gap* [Webinar]. The University of Texas at Austin Charles A. Dana Center. https://www.utdanacenter.org/our-work/higher-education/collaborations/math-for-nurses

My Notes

5.2 MATH BASIC CONCEPTS

Measuring Devices

Depending on the type and amount of medication that is being administered, there are several devices used for measuring and administering medications.

A **medication cup** that is composed of plastic or paper is used to hold and dispense oral medications to a patient. A paper cup is used to administer nonliquid medications, such as tablets or capsules. A plastic medication cup is used to dispense both liquid and nonliquid medications, and calibrated cups are also used to measure liquid medications prior to administration. Calibrated medication cups have labelled measurements such as ounces (oz), cubic centimeters (cc), milliliters (mL), teaspoons (tsp), and tablespoons (Tbs). See Figure 5.1[1] for an image of a calibrated medication cup.

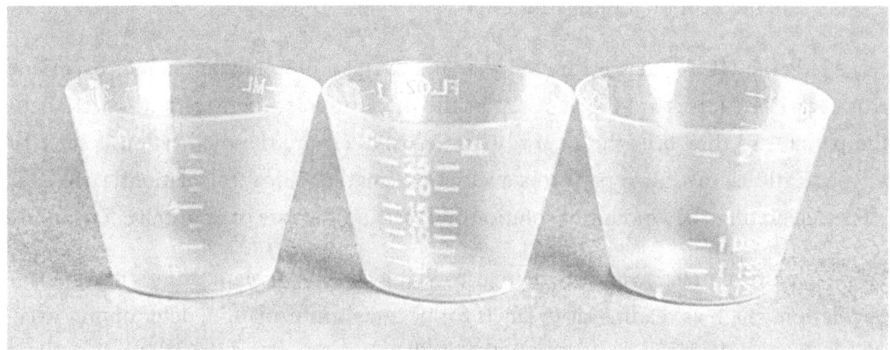

Figure 5.1 Medication Cups

Oral syringes are used to administer liquid medications via the oral route, especially to children, because they allow for precise measurement of small doses. See Figure 5.2[2] for an image of an oral syringe. Oral syringes have different tips than syringes used for injections.

1 "Medication Cups" by Deanna Hoyord, Chippewa Valley Technical College is licensed under CC BY 4.0. Access for free at https://drive.google.com/file/d/1eRvEXjJlEurr_Hwpri47HI27fAV8SBTh/view?usp=sharing

2 "Oral Syringes 3I3A0820.jpg" by Deanna Hoyord, Chippewa Valley Technical College is licensed under CC BY 4.0. Access for free at https://drive.google.com/file/d/1mSPygd---4Do690n5tLEQfwbAUmYonfU/view?usp=sharing

My Notes

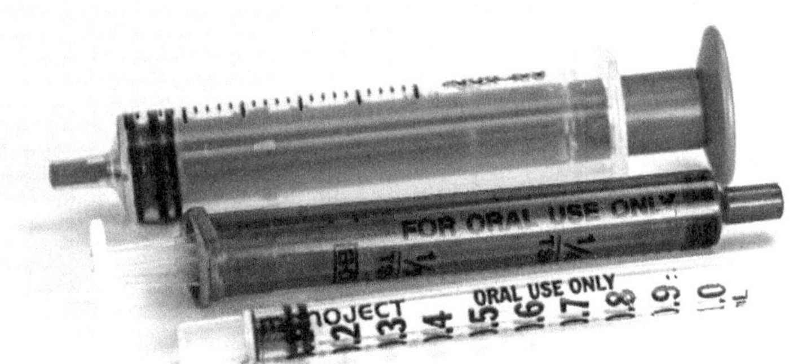

Figure 5.2 Oral Syringes

Syringes are used when administering medications through the parenteral route (i.e., intradermally, subcutaneously, intramuscularly, or intravenously). Syringes used for injections are available in many sizes and are selected by the nurse based on the type of injection and the type of medication administered. Common syringe sizes range from 1 mL to 60 mL. See Figure 5.3[3] for an image comparing various sizes of syringes. Syringes are calibrated based on the volume they hold. For example, a 1-mL syringe is calibrated in hundredths and a 3-mL syringe is calibrated in tenths. Syringes that hold larger volumes, such as 5-, 10-, and 12-mL syringes are usually calibrated in fifths (two tenths). Large syringes, such as 60-mL syringes, are calibrated in whole numbers.

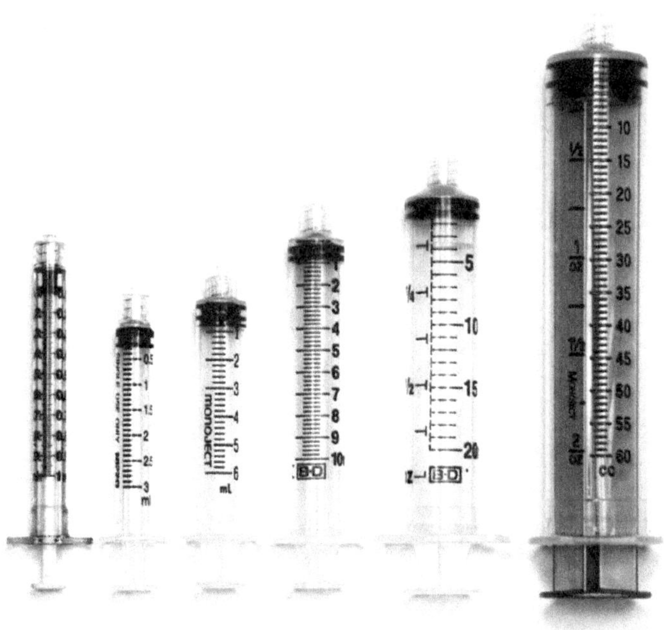

Figure 5.3 Various Sizes of Syringes

3 "Syringes 3I3A0446.jpg" by Deanna Hoyord, Chippewa Valley Technical College is licensed under CC BY 4.0. Access for free at https://drive.google.com/file/d/1zuWMuY1s41uADPIksge49qZFrCoKr6Ww/view?usp=sharing

My Notes

Special syringes are used to administer insulin and are calibrated in units. See Figure 5.4[4] for an image of an insulin syringe. Insulin syringes are easily identified by a standard orange cap.

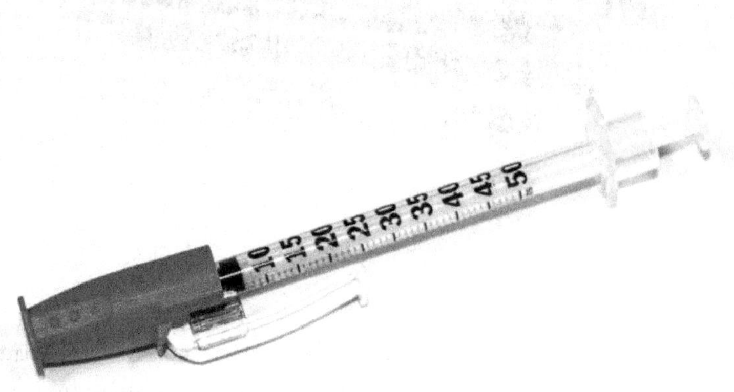

Figure 5.4 Insulin Syringe

4 "Insulin Syringe 3I3A0783.jpg" by Deanna Hoyord, Chippewa Valley Technical College is licensed under CC BY 4.0. Access for free at https://drive.google.com/file/d/1aL5h5h4J1E7BKP5gJz_103536Jtxest_/view?usp=sharing

5.3 MILITARY TIME

My Notes

Military time is a method of measuring the time based on the full 24 hours of the day rather than two groups of 12 hours indicated by AM and PM. It is also referred to as using a 24-hour clock. Using military time is the standard method used to indicate time for medication administration. The use of military time reduces potential confusion that may be caused by using AM and PM and also avoids potential duplication when giving scheduled medications. For example, instead of stating medication is due at 7 AM and 7 PM, it is documented on the medication administration record (MAR) as due at 0700 and 1900. See Figure 5.5[1] for an example clock and Table 5.3 for a military time conversion chart.

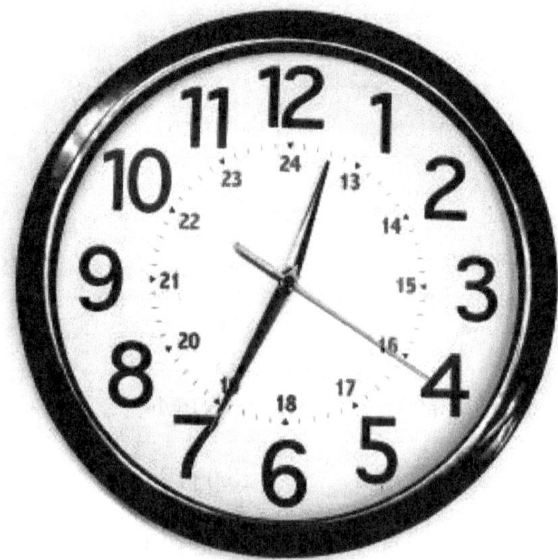

Figure 5.5 Military Time Clock

- Conversion of an AM time to military time simply involves removing the colon and adding a zero to the time. For example, 6:30 AM becomes 0630.
- Conversion of a PM time to military time involves removing the colon and adding 1200 to the time. For example, 7:15 PM becomes 1915.

1 "Military Time Clock 3I3A0711.jpg" by Deanna Hoyord, Chippewa Valley Technical College is licensed under CC BY 4.0. Access for free at https://drive.google.com/file/d/17pBmGrortEnvCup9s6wpIMHv6K-NdQNY/view?usp=sharing

My Notes

Table 5.3 Military Time Conversion Chart			
Normal Time	**Military Time**	**Normal Time**	**Military Time**
12:00 AM	0000	12:00 PM	1200
1:00 AM	0100	1:00 PM	1300
2:00 AM	0200	2:00 PM	1400
3:00 AM	0300	3:00 PM	1500
4:00 AM	0400	4:00 PM	1600
5:00 AM	0500	5:00 PM	1700
6:00 AM	0600	6:00 PM	1800
7:00 AM	0700	7:00 PM	1900
8:00 AM	0800	8:00 PM	2000
9:00 AM	0900	9:00 PM	2100
10:00 AM	1000	10:00 PM	2200
11:00 AM	1100	11:00 PM	2300

Practice Problems: Military Time

Practice converting military time using the following problems. *The answers are found in the Answer Key (Math Calculations Chapter section) at the end of the book.*

1. A patient has a medication scheduled for 1930. What time does this indicate? Include AM or PM.
2. As you prepare to administer a PRN dose of pain medication, you notice the previous dose was administered at 0030. What time does this indicate? Include AM or PM.
3. You administer medication to a patient at 9 AM. How should this be documented in military time?
4. You administer medication to a patent at 10 PM. How should this be documented in military time?

5.4 EQUIVALENCIES

My Notes

The nurse performs a variety of calculations in the clinical setting including intake and output conversions, weight conversions, dosages, volumes, and rates. The metric system is typically used when documenting and performing calculations in the clinical setting. Dosages may be calculated and converted into micrograms (mcg), milligrams (mg), milliequivalents (mEq), and grams (gm); volumes may be calculated in cubic centimeters (cc), milliliters (mL), and liters (L); and rates may be calculated in drops per minute (gtt/min), milliliters per hour (mL/hr), or units per hour (units/hr). Each of these types of calculations will be described in the following sections. Let's begin by discussing equivalencies.

Equivalency is a mathematical term that refers to two values or quantities that are the same amount. For example, one cup is equivalent to eight ounces. Nurses must memorize common household and metric equivalents to perform drug calculations and convert quantities easily.

Household Equivalencies

The household system of measurement is familiar to patients and includes drops, teaspoons, tablespoons, ounces, cups, and pounds. See Table 5.4a for common household measurement conversions and abbreviations that must be memorized by nurses.

Table 5.4a Common Household Conversions

Measurement and Abbreviation	Common Conversions
drop (gtt)	15 -20 gtt = 1 mL
teaspoon (tsp)	1 tsp = 5 mL
tablespoon (Tbs)	1 Tbs = 3 tsp = 15 mL
ounce (oz)	1 oz = 30 mL
pound (lb)	1 lb = 16 oz
cup (C)	1 C = 8 oz = 240 mL
pint (pt)	1 pt = 2 C
quart (qt)	1 qt = 4 C
gallon (gal)	1 gal = 4 qt

Metric Equivalencies

The metric system is organized by units of 10. The basic units of measurement in the metric system include meter for length, liter for volume, and gram for weight. The decimal point is easily moved either to the right or left with

My Notes

multiplication or division in units of 10. For example, there are 1,000 mL in 1 liter, and 0.5 liters is the same as 500 mL. See Table 5.4b for a metric equivalency chart.

When converting to a smaller unit, the decimal moves to the right.

→→→→→→→→→→

When converting to a larger unit, the decimal moves to the left.

←←←←←←←←←←

Table 5.4b Common Metric Equivalencies in Health Care						
Kilo- **1000 units**	**Hecto-** **100 units**	**Deca-** **10 units**	**1** **Unit**	**Deci-** **0.1 units**	**Centi-** **0.01 units**	**Milli-** **0.001 units**

Nurses often need to convert household measurements to metric equivalents or vice versa. See Table 5.4c for common metric conversions that nurses must memorize.

Table 5.4c Common Metric Conversions in Health Care

Metric Measurement	Common Conversions
1 kilogram (kg)	1 kg = 2.2 pounds = 1000 mg
1 centimeter (cm)	1 in = 2.54 cm = 25.4 mm
37 degrees Celsius	97.8 degrees F
1 liter	1000 mL = 1000 cc
1 gram	1000 mg
1 mg	1000 mcg

Video Reviews of Metric Conversions

My Notes

Conversions: Metric Table[1]

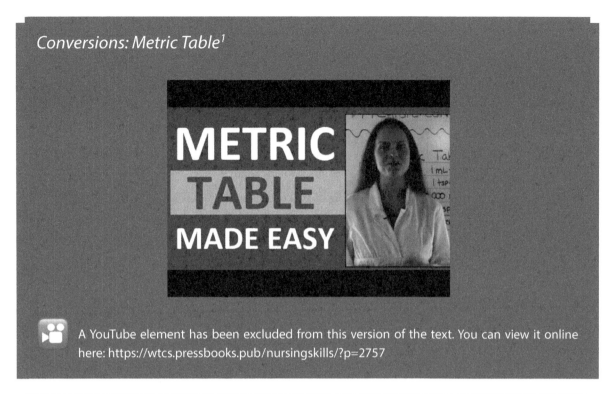

A YouTube element has been excluded from this version of the text. You can view it online here: https://wtcs.pressbooks.pub/nursingskills/?p=2757

Metric Conversions[2]

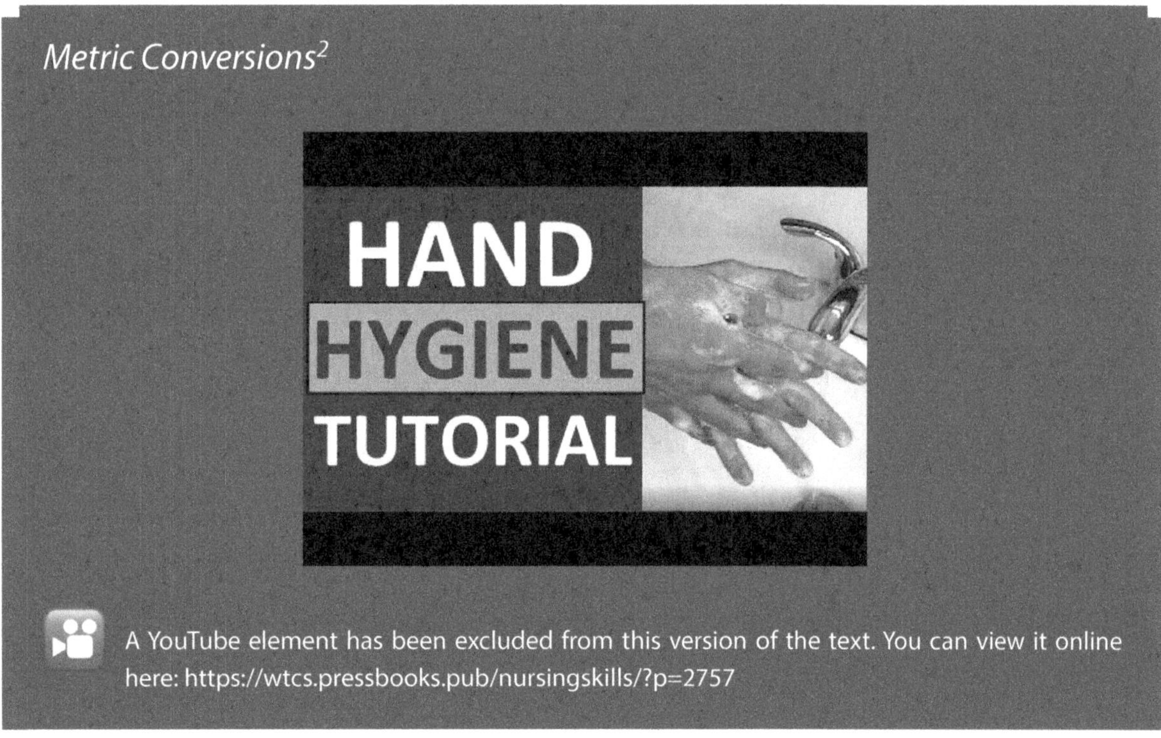

A YouTube element has been excluded from this version of the text. You can view it online here: https://wtcs.pressbooks.pub/nursingskills/?p=2757

---

1 RegisteredNurseRN. (2015, February 4). *What is the metric table for nursing calculations?* [Video]. YouTube. All rights reserved. Video used with permission. https://youtu.be/aGMLRnWGanM

2 RegisteredNurseRN. (2015, February 5). *Metric conversions made easy | How solve in metric conversions w/ dimensional analysis (Vid 1).* [Video]. YouTube. All rights reserved. Video used with permission. https://youtu.be/0N6SmKVWZdI

My Notes

Other Measurements

The nurse encounters other miscellaneous measurements in practice, such as:

- **Units (U):** Units are used in insulin and heparin dosages.
- **International Units (IU):** International units are used for vitamins, such as Vitamin D 600 IU.
- **Milliequivalents (mEq):** Milliequivalents are used in electrolyte replacement, such as Potassium 40 mEq.
- **Percentages:** Percentages are used in intravenous (IV) fluids, such as 0.9% Normal Saline IV fluid, meaning 9 g of NaCl are diluted in 1000 mL water.
- **Ratios:** Ratios are used in medications such as Epinephrine 1:1000, meaning 1 gram of Epinephrine is diluted in 1000 mL of fluid (equivalent to 1 mg/mL).

Practice Problems: Household and Metric Equivalents

Practice converting household and metric equivalents using the following problems and referencing Tables 5.4a-c. The answers are found in the Answer Key ("Math Calculations" chapter section) at the end of the book.

1. A prescription for a child is written as 1 teaspoon every 4 hours. How many milliliters (mL) will you draw up in an oral syringe?
2. A patient's prescription states to administer one ounce of medication. How many milliliters will you measure in the medication cup?
3. A patient's prescription states to administer 0.5 grams of medication. How many milligrams will you administer?
4. A baby weighs 3.636 kilograms. How many grams does this convert to?
5. A patient's pupils are 7 mm in size. How many centimeters does this convert to?

5.5 ROUNDING

My Notes

Follow agency policy according to rounding. When performing calculations, do not round until calculating the final answer. Dosages of oral liquid medications for adults are typically rounded to the tenth for doses over 1 mL, with 0.05 and above rounding up and 0.04 and lower rounding down. For example, 17.276 rounds to 17.3, and 17.248 rounds to 17.2. For doses less than 1 mL, the dosage is rounded to the hundredth. For example, 0.0467 rounds to 0.05.

For pediatric patients, it is important to be as precise as possible to avoid medication errors. Oral liquid medications less than 1 mL should be rounded to the hundredth. For example, 0.276 rounds to 0.28, and 0.243 rounds to 0.24.

When rounding, it is also important to use critical thinking to evaluate your final answer. For example, a drop cannot be administered as a fraction of a drop, so drops are rounded to the nearest whole number.

Avoiding Medication Errors with Decimals

There are two very important standards of practice for documenting decimals to avoid medication errors:[1]

- Use leading zeros for decimals (i.e., use 0.6 mg)
- Do not use trailing zeros (i.e., do not use 6.0 mg)

Practice Problems: Rounding

Practice rounding using the following problems. *The answers are found in the Answer Key (Math Caculations Chapter) at the end of the book.*

1. Round the liquid dose for an adult that is calculated as 6.5349.
2. Round the liquid dose for a child that is calculated as 6.5349.
3. Round the liquid dose for an adult that is calculated as 5.479.
4. Round the liquid dose for a child that is calculated as 5.479.
5. Round the liquid dose for an adult that is calculated as 0.1947.
6. Round the liquid dose for a child that is calculated as 0.1947.
7. Round the liquid dose for an adult that is calculated as 0.1968.
8. Round the liquid dose for a child that is calculated as 0.1968.

1 Saljoughian, M. (2020). Avoiding medication errors. *U.S. Pharmacist, 45*(10). https://www.uspharmacist.com/article/avoiding-medication-errors

My Notes

5.6 USING DIMENSIONAL ANALYSIS

A common method used to perform calculations with different units of measurement is called dimensional analysis. **Dimensional analysis** is a problem-solving technique where measurements are converted to equivalent units of measure by multiplying a given unit of measurement by a fractional form of 1 to obtain the desired unit of administration. This method is also referred to as creating proportions that state equivalent ratios. Equivalencies described in Section 5.7 are used to set up ratios with the fractional form of 1 to achieve the desired unit the problem is asking for. The units of measure that must be eliminated to solve the problem are set up on the diagonal so that they can be cancelled out. Lines are drawn during the problem-solving process to show that cancellation has occurred.[1]

When setting up a dosage calculation using dimensional analysis, it is important to begin by identifying the goal unit to be solved. After the goal unit is set, the remainder of the equation is set up using fractional forms of 1 and equivalencies to cancel out units to achieve the goal unit. It is important to understand that when using this problem-solving method, the numerator and denominator are interchangeable because they are expressing a relationship.[2] Let's practice using dimensional analysis to solve simple conversion problems of ounces to milliliters in Section 5.7 "Conversions" to demonstrate the technique.

Video Review of Dimensional Analysis[3]

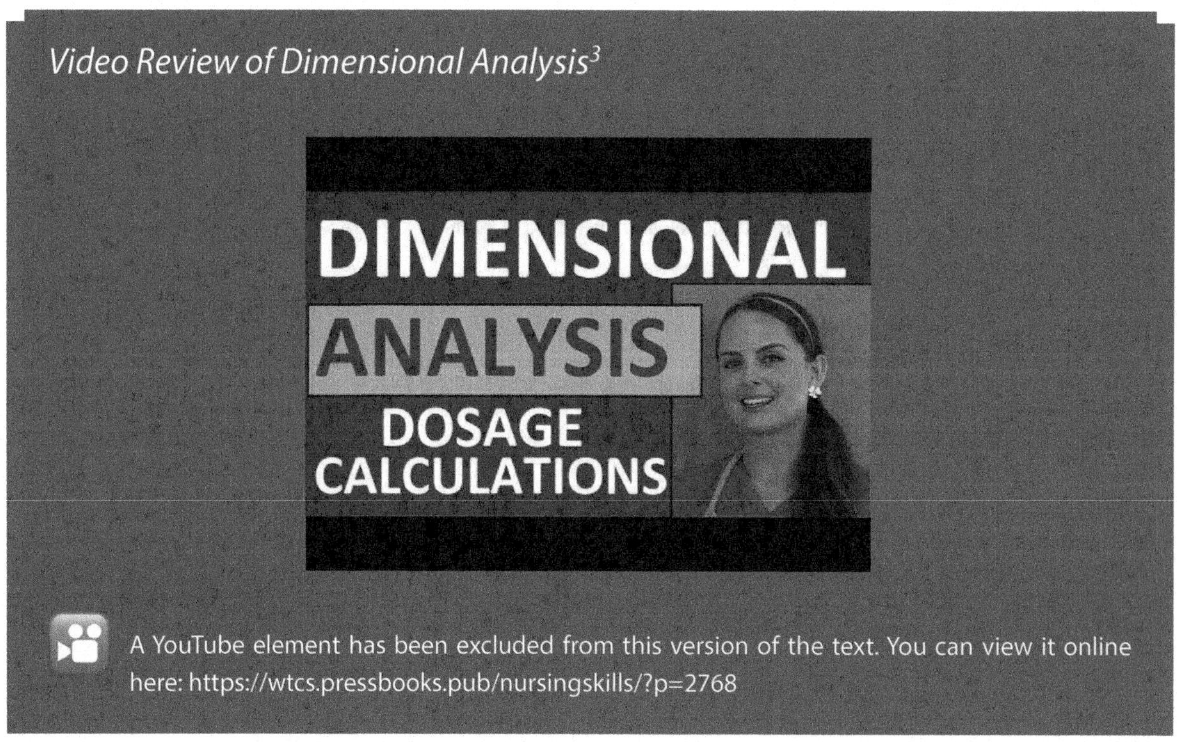

A YouTube element has been excluded from this version of the text. You can view it online here: https://wtcs.pressbooks.pub/nursingskills/?p=2768

1 Esser, P. (2019). *Dimensional analysis in nursing*. Southwest Technical College. https://swtcmathscience.wixsite.com/swtcmath/dimensional-analysis-in-nursing

2 Esser, P. (2019). *Dimensional analysis in nursing*. Southwest Technical College. https://swtcmathscience.wixsite.com/swtcmath/dimensional-analysis-in-nursing

3 RegisteredNurseRN. (2015, February 4). *Dimensional analysis for nursing & nursing students for dosage calculations nursing school.* [Video]. YouTube. All rights reserved. Used with permission. https://youtu.be/6dyM2puXbgc

5.7 CONVERSIONS

My Notes

Ounces to Milliliters

When caring for patients, nurses often need to convert between ounces and milliliters. Although these equivalencies are typically memorized, let's start with a simple problem of converting ounces to milliliters to demonstrate the technique of dimensional analysis.

Practice Problem #1: Ounces to Millileters

A patient drank an 8 ounce can of juice. The nurse must document the intake in milliliters. How many milliliters of juice did the patient drink?

Here is an example of how to solve this conversion problem using dimensional analysis.

1. Identify the unit being solved for as the goal. In this example, we want to convert the patient's oral intake from ounces to milliliters, so we are solving for milliliters (mL):

$$mL = ?$$

2. Set up the numerator in the first fraction to match the desired unit to be solved. In this case, we want to know how many milliliters should be documented, so mL is placed in the numerator. To complete the fraction, we add information already known. In this example, we know that 30 mL is equivalent to 1 ounce, so 30 mL is added to the numerator and 1 ounce is added to the denominator:

$$mL = \frac{30\ mL}{1\ ounce}$$

3. Add the second fraction to the equation. When using dimensional analysis, fractions are set up so the same units are diagonal from each other so they cancel each other out, leaving the desired unit. For this problem, the second fraction is set up to include ounces in the numerator so that it will cancel out ounces in the denominator of the first fraction. "8" is then added to the numerator because we know from the problem that the patient consumed 8 ounces. "1" is then added to the denominator because the purpose of the second fraction is to cancel out units:

$$ml = \frac{30\ mL}{1\ ounce}\ x\ \frac{8\ ounces}{1}$$

4. Cancel out similar units that are diagonal to each other. After canceling out ounces, we are left with our desired units of mL:

$$mL = \frac{30\ mL}{1\ \cancel{ounce}}\ x\ \frac{8\ \cancel{ounces}}{1}$$

My Notes

5. Multiply across the numerators and then multiply across the denominators:

$$mL = \frac{30\ mL}{1\ \cancel{ounce}}\ x\ \frac{8\ \cancel{ounces}}{1} = \frac{30\ mL\ x\ 8}{1\ x\ 1\ =\ 1} = 240\ mL$$

6. Divide the numerator by the denominator to get the final answer with the desired goal unit:

$$\frac{240\ mL}{1} = 240\ mL$$

Practice Problem #2: Ounces to Millileters

In a similar manner, dimensional analysis can be used to calculate a patient's total liquid intake on their meal tray. See Figure 5.6[1] for an example of a patient's meal tray in a hospital setting.

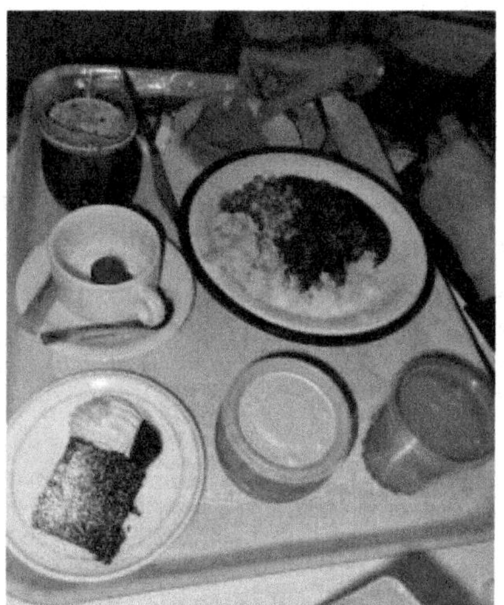

Figure 5.6 Meal Tray

Sample scenario: Your patient consumed 8 ounces of coffee, 4 ounces of orange juice, and 4 ounces of milk. How many milliliters of intake will you document?

Calculate using dimensional analysis.

1 "Hospital Meal" by *Michael Coghlin* is licensed under CC BY-SA 2.0. Access for free at https://www.flickr.com/photos/mikecogh/7393655810/in/photolist-cgmqhj-2eCwWSo-23HjV3g-2bspuTk-ft9AkM-feEZsG-9oTcJ9-8RN15F-e9Niu8-rPVue6-231b3qf-NCMjB2-24kec1w-ajQokX-2eZt6SZ-LD4vbJ-QsxFBm-MUnLLB-24kfuLS-28nDVY3-oKyJZt-4WnrN7-2fBRZcU-Rucd3T-DFAxMU-6D4331-255Vj5K-25dio1V-qJyKhs-FU16qL-2dMae5e-DruaZ7-29GD9RY-dZKQL5-9F4tf-MG47wg-5ubNrL-bEkiyK-7eKQBA-ap24s8-kNkPjh-awC3GY-MHQyFh-P7e8Rd-in1b87-7DMMaw-BckTza-ejM6LK-cBYxzG-ia8BCz

My Notes

1. Add up the total intake in ounces:

$$8 + 4 + 4 = 16\ ounces$$

2. Start by identifying mL as the goal unit for which you are solving. In this case, we want to know the number of milliliters:

$$mL = ?$$

3. Create the first fraction by matching milliliters in the numerator. Then, using known equivalency that 30 mL is equal to 1 ounce, place 30 in the numerator and 1 ounce in the denominator:

$$mL = \frac{30\ ml}{1\ ounce}$$

4. Create the second fraction to cross out units. You know you want to cross out ounces, so place ounces in the numerator. Then, add the known amount of ounces consumed, which was 16:

$$mL = \frac{30\ mL}{1\ ounce}\ x\ \frac{16\ ounces}{1}$$

5. Multiply across the numerators and then the denominators. Divide the numerator by the denominator of 1 for the final answer in mL:

$$mL = \frac{30\ mL}{1\ \cancel{ounce}}\ x\ \frac{16\ \cancel{ounces}}{1} = 30\ x\ 16 = 480\ mL$$

My Notes

Video Review of Calculating Intake and Output[2]

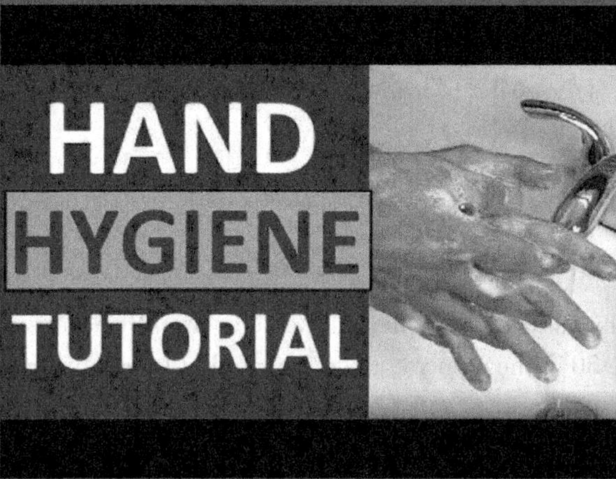

A YouTube element has been excluded from this version of the text. You can view it online here: https://wtcs.pressbooks.pub/nursingskills/?p=2774

Pounds to Kilograms

Converting pounds to kilograms is typically memorized as an equivalency, but let's practice using the technique of dimensional analysis.

Sample problem: The patient entered their weight as 137 pounds on their intake form. Convert the patient's weight to kilograms to document it in the electronic medical record. Round your answer to the nearest tenth.

Calculate using dimensional analysis.

1. Start by identifying kg as the goal unit for which you are solving. Then, set up the first fraction so that the numerator matches the goal unit of kg. For the denominator, add 2.2 lbs because the known equivalency is 1 kg is equivalent to 2.2 pounds. Set up the second fraction with pounds in the numerator so that pounds will cross out diagonally to eliminate this unit. Then, add the patient's known weight (137 lb) in the numerator, with 1 in the denominator because the function of this fraction is to cross out units. Multiply across the numerators and then the denominators. Finally, divide the final fraction to solve the problem.

$$kg = \frac{1\ kg}{2.2\ \cancel{lb}}\ x\ \frac{137\ \cancel{lb}}{1} = \frac{137\ kg}{2.2} = 62.2727 = 62.3\ kg$$

Review the following modules within *SWTC's Dimensional Analysis in Nursing* page for more information about solving tablet problems.
Modules 1.0 – 1.4

2 RegisteredNurseRN. (2018, February 26). *Intake and output nursing calculation practice problems NCLEX review (CNA, LPN, RN) I and O.* [Video]. YouTube. All rights reserved. Video used with permission. https://youtu.be/a6ovyZIs9tg

5.8 TABLET DOSAGE

My Notes

When tablets are prescribed for a patient, the dosage of the tablets supplied is often different from the prescription, and nurses must calculate the number of tablets to administer. Dimensional analysis can be used to calculate the number of tablets to administer. Let's practice using dimensional analysis using a practice problem.

Practice Problem: Tablet Dosage

Jane Doe recently had her prescription changed by her provider from Carvedilol 6.25 mg twice daily to Carvedilol 25 mg once daily. Jane shows you her prescription bottle (see Figure 5.7[1]) and asks, "How many pills can I take every day so I can use up what I have before purchasing another refill?" How many 6.25 mg tablets will you instruct Jane to take based on the new prescribed dose of Carvedilol 25 mg once daily?

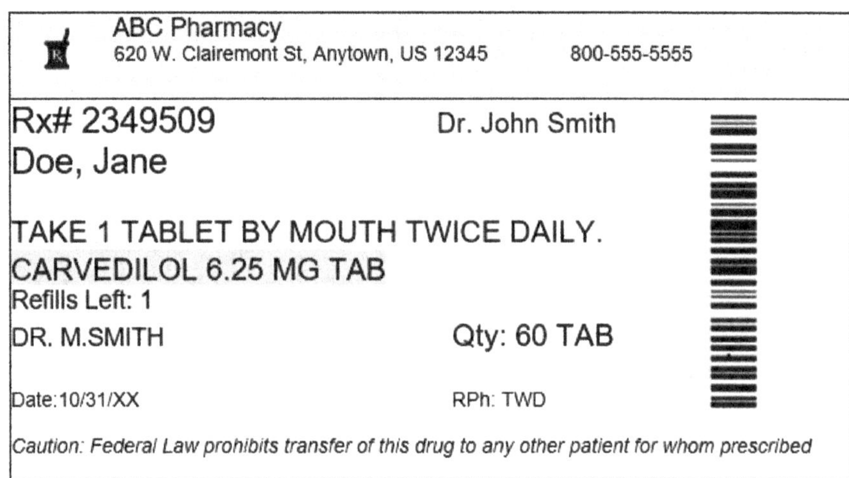

Figure 5.7 Prescription Bottle of Carvedilol

Solve this question by using dimensional analysis.

1. Start by identifying the goal unit for which you are solving, which is a tablet (tab) in this scenario:

$$Tab \ =$$

2. Set up the first fraction with tab in the numerator to match the goal unit. From the prescription bottle, we know that one of the supplied tablets has a concentration of 6.25 mg, so plug in 1 in the numerator and 6.25 mg in the denominator:

$$Tab \ = \ \frac{1 \ tab}{6.25 \ mg}$$

---

1 "Carvedilol Rx Bottle Label Fig. 5.PNG" by Jody Myhre-Oechsle, Chippewa Valley Technical College, Open RN is licensed under CC BY 4.0. Access for free at https://drive.google.com/file/d/1HN12jb9ybypOmmPG1nq6_saEhyj9KTDa/view?usp=sharing

My Notes

3. Set up the second fraction with the intent to cross out mg, so place mg in the numerator. By reviewing the prescription, we know the new dosage prescribed is 25 mg, so plug in 25 in the numerator, and 1 in the denominator to cross off units:

$$Tab = \frac{1\ tab}{6.25\ mg}\ x\ \frac{25\ mg}{1}$$

4. Cross out mg diagonally:

$$Tab = \frac{1\ tab}{6.25\ \cancel{mg}}\ x\ \frac{25\ \cancel{mg}}{}$$

5. Multiply across the numerators and denominators, and then divide the final fraction to solve the problem:

$$Tab = \frac{1\ tab}{6.25\ \cancel{mg}}\ x\ \frac{25\ \cancel{mg}}{1} = 4\ tabs$$

Review the following modules within *SWTC's Dimensional Analysis in Nursing* page for more information about solving tablet problems.
Modules 1.5 – 1.7

Video Reviews of Calculating Tablet and Capsule Dosages[2, 3, 4, 5]

My Notes

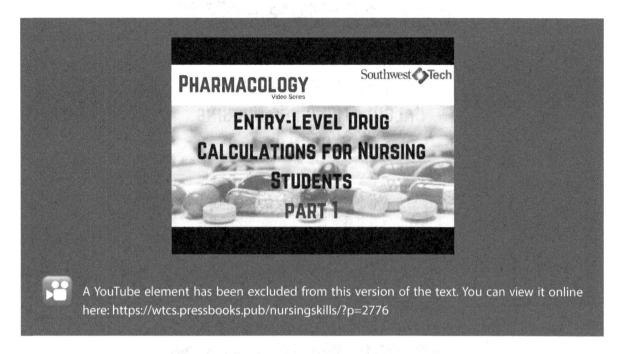

A YouTube element has been excluded from this version of the text. You can view it online here: https://wtcs.pressbooks.pub/nursingskills/?p=2776

2 Southwest Tech Math/Science Center. (2018, April 25). *Entry-level drug calculations for nursing students part 1 – Pharmacology, nursing math**. [Video]. YouTube. All rights reserved. Video used with permission. https://youtu.be/HDmRmoi929U

3 Southwest Tech Math/Science Center. (2018, April 25). *Entry-level drug calculations for nursing students part 5 – Pharmacology, nursing math**. [Video]. YouTube. All rights reserved. Video used with permission. https://youtu.be/taMmPMVDzC0

4 Southwest Tech Math/Science Center. (2018, April 25). *Entry-level drug calculations for nursing students part 6 – Pharmacology, nursing math**. [Video]. YouTube. All rights reserved. Video used with permission. https://youtu.be/vAY1xd2Y9kc

5 Southwest Tech Math/Science Center. (2018, April 25). *Entry-level drug Calculations for nursing students part 7 – Pharmacology, nursing math**. [Video]. YouTube. All rights reserved. Video used with permission. https://youtu.be/XN1Die8jTE

My Notes

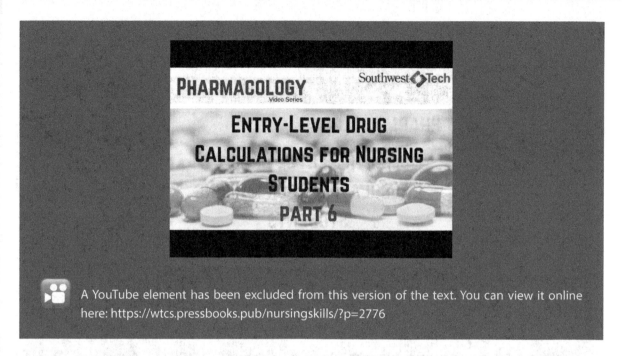

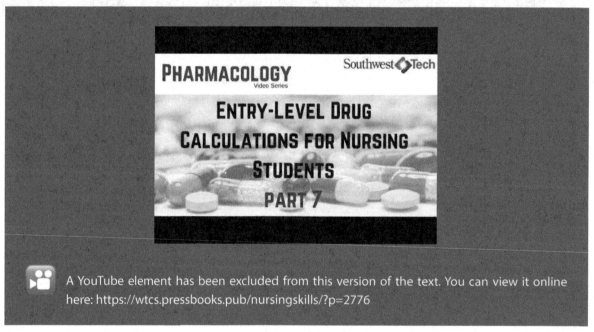

A YouTube element has been excluded from this version of the text. You can view it online here: https://wtcs.pressbooks.pub/nursingskills/?p=2776

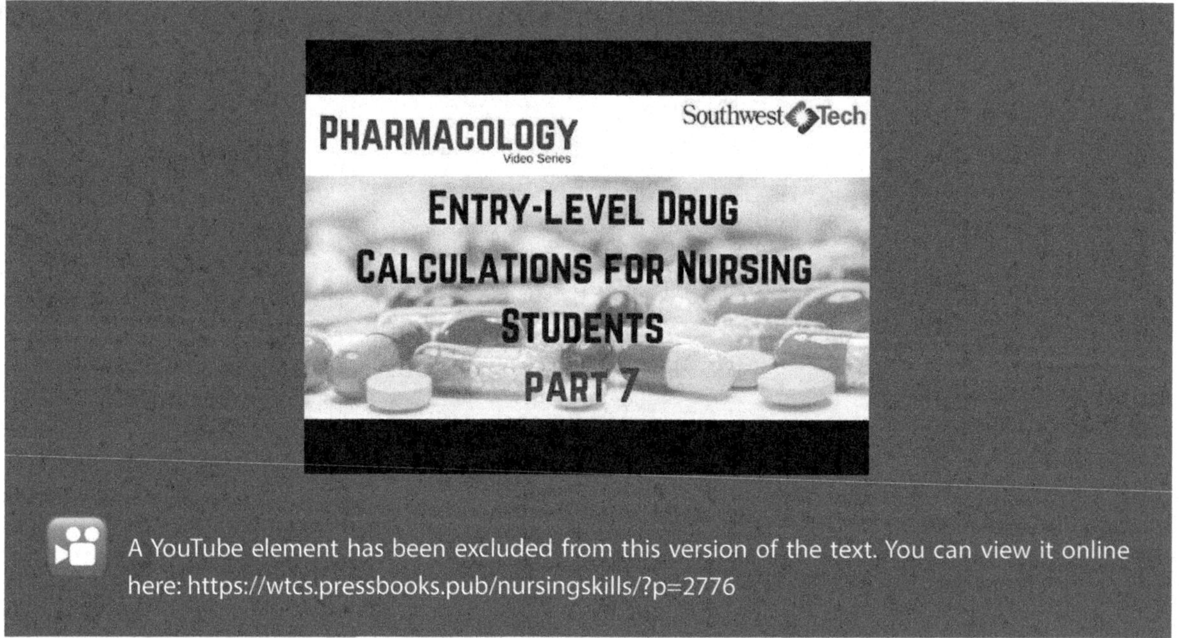

A YouTube element has been excluded from this version of the text. You can view it online here: https://wtcs.pressbooks.pub/nursingskills/?p=2776

Please practice tablet dosage calculations with the following interactive learning activity.

Interactive Activity

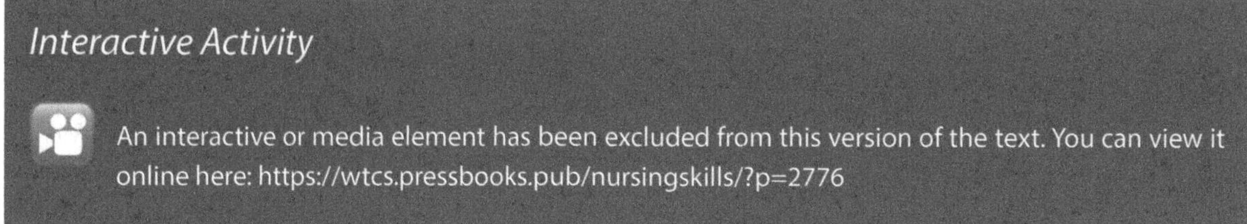

An interactive or media element has been excluded from this version of the text. You can view it online here: https://wtcs.pressbooks.pub/nursingskills/?p=2776

5.9 LIQUID CONCENTRATIONS

My Notes

Medications can also be supplied in liquid instead of tablets or capsules. Liquid concentrations are typically provided in milligrams (mg) per a given number of milliliters (mL). The nurse must calculate how many milliliters (mL) to administer based on the prescribed dose in milligrams (mg). Let's practice using dimensional analysis to solve how much liquid medication to administer based on the prescription and the medication supplied.

Practice Problem: Liquid Concentrations

John Smith has been prescribed Phenergan as needed every 4-6 hours for nausea and vomiting. John is feeling nauseated and is requesting another dose of Phenergan. It has been 8 hours since the last dose was given. How many mL will you administer?

Provider Order: Phenergan 12.5 mg IV PRN every 4 to 6 hours for nausea and vomiting.

Medication Supplied: See Figure 5.8[1] for an image of the label of the drug as it is supplied.

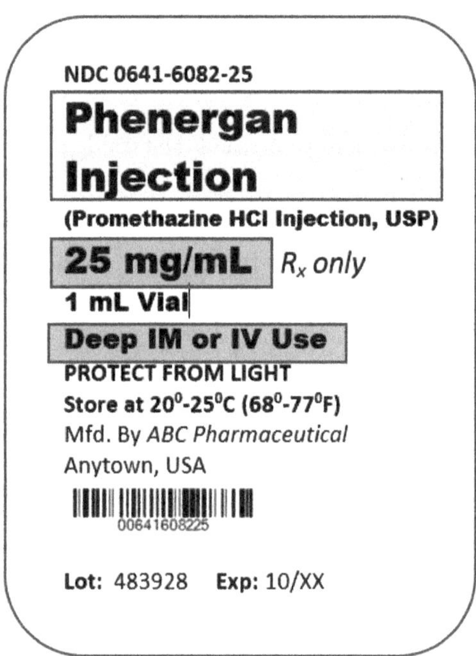

Figure 5.8 Phenergan Medication Label

Solve this question by using dimensional analysis.

1. Start by identifying mL as the goal unit for which you are solving because you need to know how many mL of medication to administer:

$$mL =$$

1 "Phenergan Label Fig. 8.PNG" by Jody Myhre-Oechsle, Chippewa Valley Technical College, Open RN is licensed under CC BY 4.0. Access for free at https://drive.google.com/file/d/1C61JIbqbyk4_vvCE8ZqxkJloc6_Eg4UU/view?usp=sharing

My Notes

2. Set up the first fraction with mL in the numerator to match the goal unit. In this problem, we know from the drug label that 1 mL contains 25 mg of medication, so plug in 1 in numerator and 25 mg in the denominator:

$$mL = \frac{1\ mL}{25\ mg}$$

3. Set up the second fraction to cross out mg, so place mg in the numerator. We know from the order that the new dosage prescribed is 12.5 mg, so plug in 12.5 next to mg in the numerator and 1 in the denominator to cross off units:

$$mL = \frac{1\ mL}{25\ mg} = x = \frac{12.5\ mg}{1}$$

4. Cross out mg diagonally:

$$mL = \frac{1\ mL}{25\ \cancel{mg}}\ x\ \frac{12.5\ \cancel{mg}}{1}$$

5. Multiply across the numerators and denominators, and then divide the final fraction to solve the problem:

$$mL = \frac{1\ mL}{25\ \cancel{mg}}\ x\ \frac{12.5\ \cancel{mg}}{1} = \frac{12.5\ mL}{25} = 0.5\ mL$$

My Notes

Video Reviews of How to Use Dimensional Analysis to Calculate Oral Medication Dosages[2, 3, 4, 5]

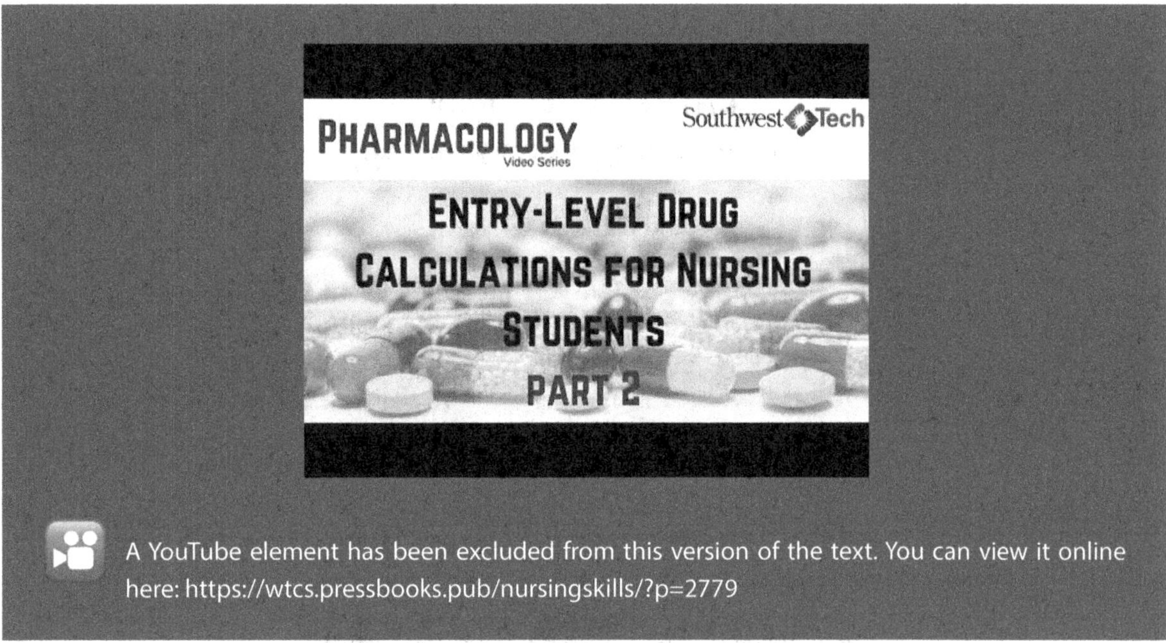

A YouTube element has been excluded from this version of the text. You can view it online here: https://wtcs.pressbooks.pub/nursingskills/?p=2779

2 Southwest Tech Math/Science Center. (2018, April 25). *Entry-level drug calculations for nursing students part 2 – Pharmacology, nursing math**. [Video]. YouTube. All rights reserved. Video used with permission. https://youtu.be/VHHpGeu9sNw

3 Southwest Tech Math/Science Center. (2018, April 25). *Entry-level drug calculations for nursing students part 4 – Pharmacology, nursing math**. [Video]. YouTube. All rights reserved. Video used with permission. https://youtu.be/f6bpA3usjkI

4 RegisteredNurseRN. (2015, February 21). *Dosage calculations | Nursing drug calculations | Oral medications problems nursing school (Video 3)*. [Video]. YouTube. All rights reserved. Video used with permission. https://youtu.be/*zZ3M747ChrQ*

5 RegisteredNurseRN. (2018, April 25). *Weight-based calculations | Drug medication calculations by weight nursing students (Video 6)*. [Video]. YouTube. All rights reserved. Video used with permission. https://youtu.be/*F_LfMcRT8aY*

My Notes

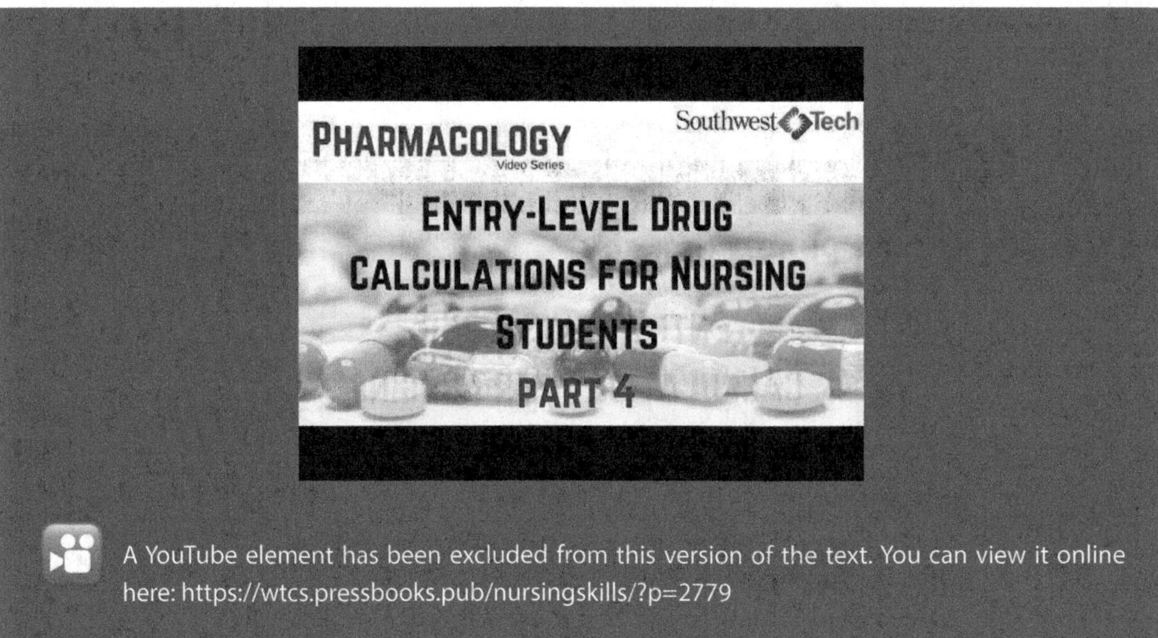

A YouTube element has been excluded from this version of the text. You can view it online here: https://wtcs.pressbooks.pub/nursingskills/?p=2779

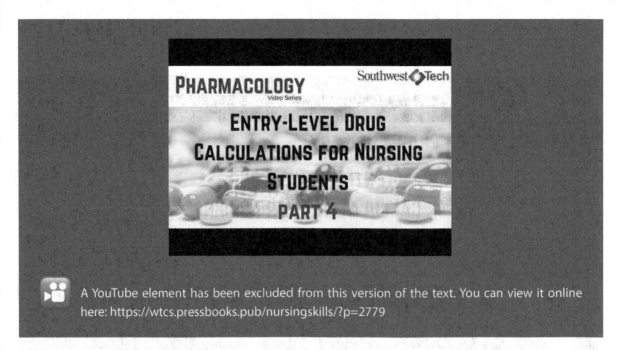

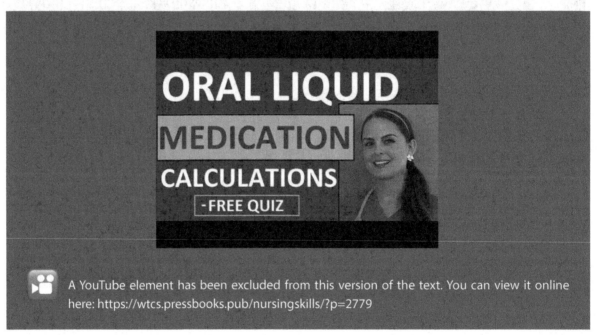

A YouTube element has been excluded from this version of the text. You can view it online here: https://wtcs.pressbooks.pub/nursingskills/?p=2779

My Notes

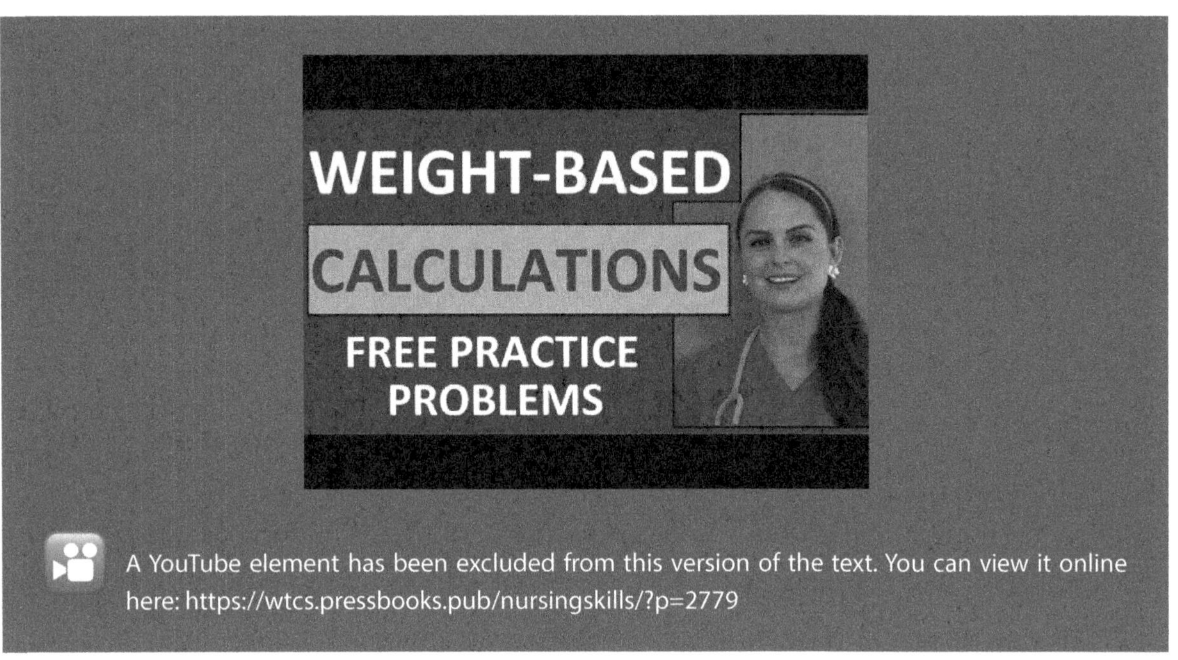

A YouTube element has been excluded from this version of the text. You can view it online here: https://wtcs.pressbooks.pub/nursingskills/?p=2779

 **Review the following modules within *SWTC's Dimensional Analysis in Nursing* page for more information about solving liquid problems.**
Modules 1.8 – 1.9

Please practice liquid dosing calculations with the following interactive learning activity.

Interactive Activity

An interactive or media element has been excluded from this version of the text. You can view it online here: https://wtcs.pressbooks.pub/nursingskills/?p=2779

My Notes

5.10 RECONSTITUTED MEDICATION

In the previous section, we calculated medication doses that were provided in a liquid form in a given concentration. Medications are also commonly supplied in dry form, such as powders or crystals, that must be reconstituted with fluid before they are administered parenterally by injection. **Reconstitution** is the process of adding a liquid diluent to a dry ingredient to make a specific concentration of liquid. See Figure 5.9[1] for an example of a vial of medication that requires reconstitution. When reconstituting medications, it is important to follow the reconstitution instructions carefully so the medication is prepared in the correct concentration. When calculating the dosage of reconstituted medication to administer to the patient, the amount of fluid used to dilute the medication must also be considered. Let's practice using dimensional analysis to determine how much of a reconstituted medication should be administered.

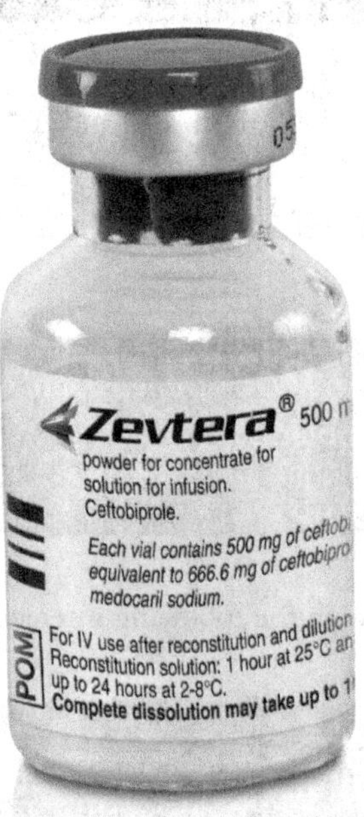

Figure 5.9 Dry Medication Requiring Reconstitution

Practice Problem: Reconstituted Medication

Patient Information:

Name: Liam Vang, DOB: 04/04/19xx, Age 8, Allergies: NKDA, Weight: 60 kg

Provider Order: Cefazolin 500 mg IM every 8 hours

Medication Supplied: See Figure 5.10[2] for the drug label of the medication as it is supplied.

---

1 "Zevtera 1Vial UK(3)(1) (29608654394).jpg" by Mohamd Ghani is licensed under CC BY-SA 2.0. Access for free at https://commons.wikimedia.org/wiki/File:Zevtera_1Vial_UK(3)(1)_(29608654394).jpg

2 "Cefazolin Label Fig. 9.PNG" by Jody Myhre-Oechsle, Chippewa Valley Technical College, Open RN is licensed under CC BY 4.0. Access for free at https://drive.google.com/file/d/1dhCaUjxBiguZhASER0DWYPbG74osm-Ip/view?usp=sharing

My Notes

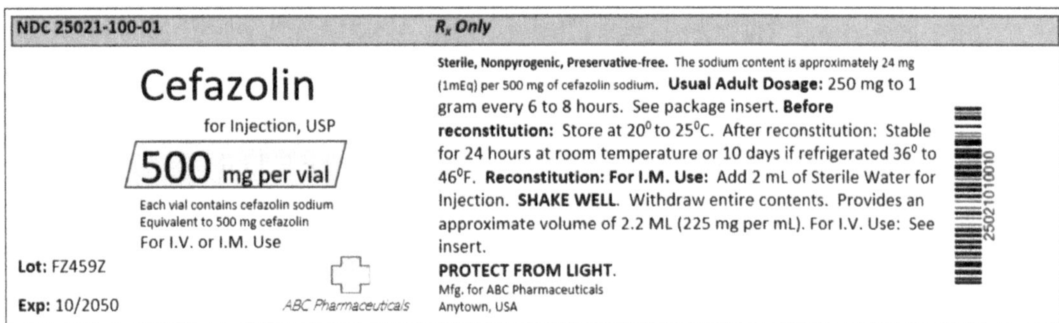

Figure 5.10 Drug Label of Cefazolin

1. Start by reading the order and the drug label. Liam has an order to receive 500 mg of Cefazolin. The vial of medication in powder form states there are 500 mg per vial. The powder must be reconstituted before it can be administered. The reconstitution instructions on the label state to add 2 mL of sterile water to the vial to reconstitute the powder into a liquid form for injection. The label states that after the powder is reconstituted with the 2 mL of diluent, the concentration of fluid will be 225 mg/mL. See a close-up image of reconstitution instructions in Figure 5.11.[3]

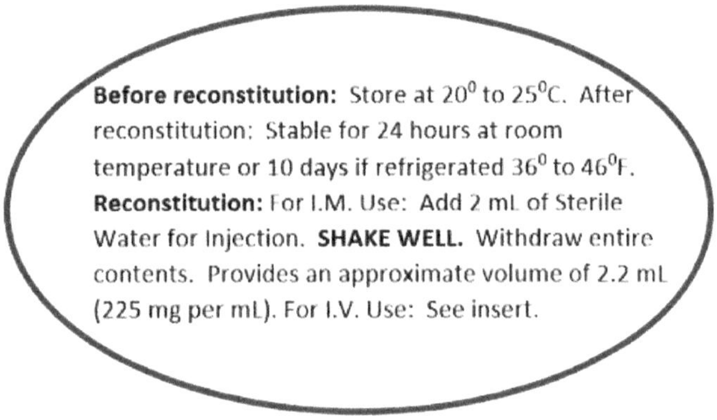

Before reconstitution: Store at 20° to 25°C. After reconstitution: Stable for 24 hours at room temperature or 10 days if refrigerated 36° to 46°F. **Reconstitution:** For I.M. Use: Add 2 mL of Sterile Water for Injection. **SHAKE WELL.** Withdraw entire contents. Provides an approximate volume of 2.2 mL (225 mg per mL). For I.V. Use: See insert.

Figure 5.11 Reconstitution Instructions

When setting up the problem, we need to identify the correct information to include in the equation. There are several numbers we may be tempted to try to incorporate into our equation, such as 500 mg per vial, 2 mL diluent, and approximate volume of 2.2 mL. These are numbers specific to the reconstitution process. However, keep in mind that our final goal is to calculate the number of mL of fluid to administer after the medication is reconstituted, so this will be the goal unit. The other piece of important information that the drug label states is that the reconstituted medication will provide a concentration of 225 mg/mL.

3 "Reconstitution Instructions.png" by Jody Myhre-Oechsle, Chippewa Valley Technical College, Open RN is licensed under CC BY 4.0. Access for free at https://drive.google.com/file/d/17u4QdPc8bu9baO_pkNOStN4caEHHmHba/view?usp=sharing

My Notes

2. Start by identifying the goal unit for which you are solving, which is mL to administer as an injection:

$$mL = ?$$

3. Set up the first fraction by matching the numerator to the goal unit of mL. In this problem, we know from the drug label that the known concentration of the reconstituted medication is 225 mg per mL, so add 1 mL to the numerator and 225 mg to the denominator:

$$mL = \frac{1\ mL}{225\ mg}$$

4. Set up the second fraction with mg in the numerator with the intent to cross off mg diagonally. Look at the given information to determine how it relates to mg. The order tells us to give Liam 500 mg of the medication. Plug in 500 in the numerator of the second fraction with one in the denominator so that mg will cross off diagonally:

$$mL = \frac{1\ mL}{225\ mg} \quad x \quad \frac{500\ mg}{1}$$

5. Cross off units diagonally. Multiply across the numerators and the denominators, and then divide the final fraction for the answer in mL:

$$mL = \frac{1\ mL}{225\ \cancel{mg}} \quad x \quad \frac{500\ \cancel{mg}}{1} \quad = \quad \frac{500\ mL}{225} \quad = \quad 2.2222\ mL$$

6. Because the patient is a child, round to hundredth for the final answer:

2.22 mL

Video Reviews of Using Dimensional Analysis to Calculate Reconstitution[4, 5]

My Notes

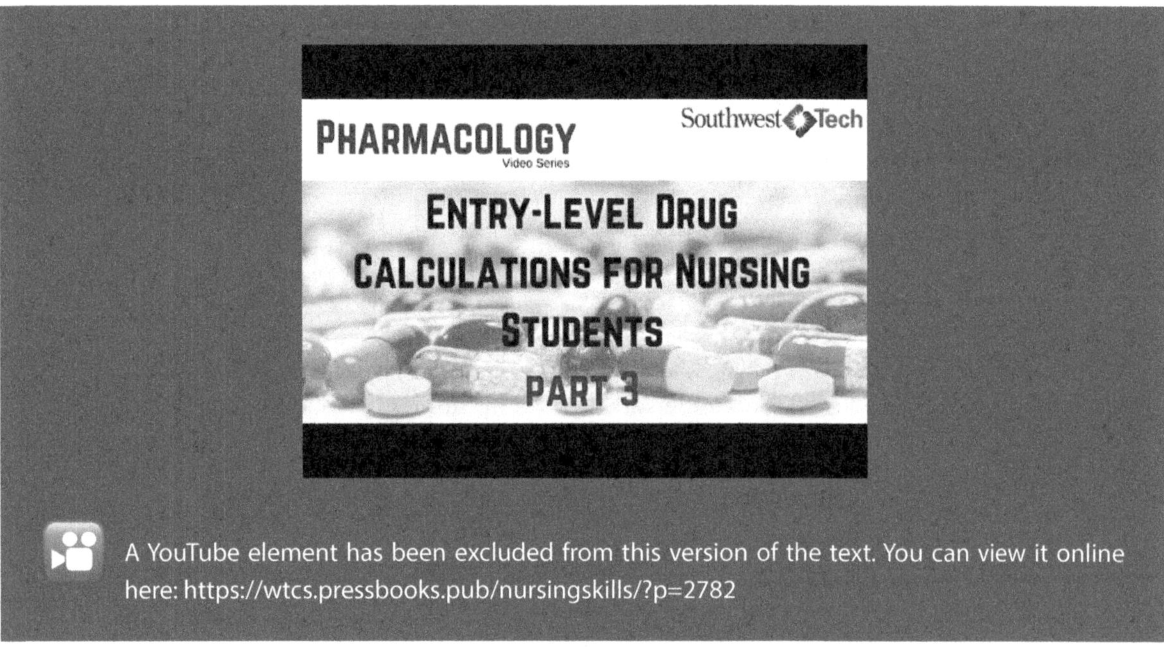

A YouTube element has been excluded from this version of the text. You can view it online here: https://wtcs.pressbooks.pub/nursingskills/?p=2782

Please practice medication reconstitution calculations with the following interactive learning activity.

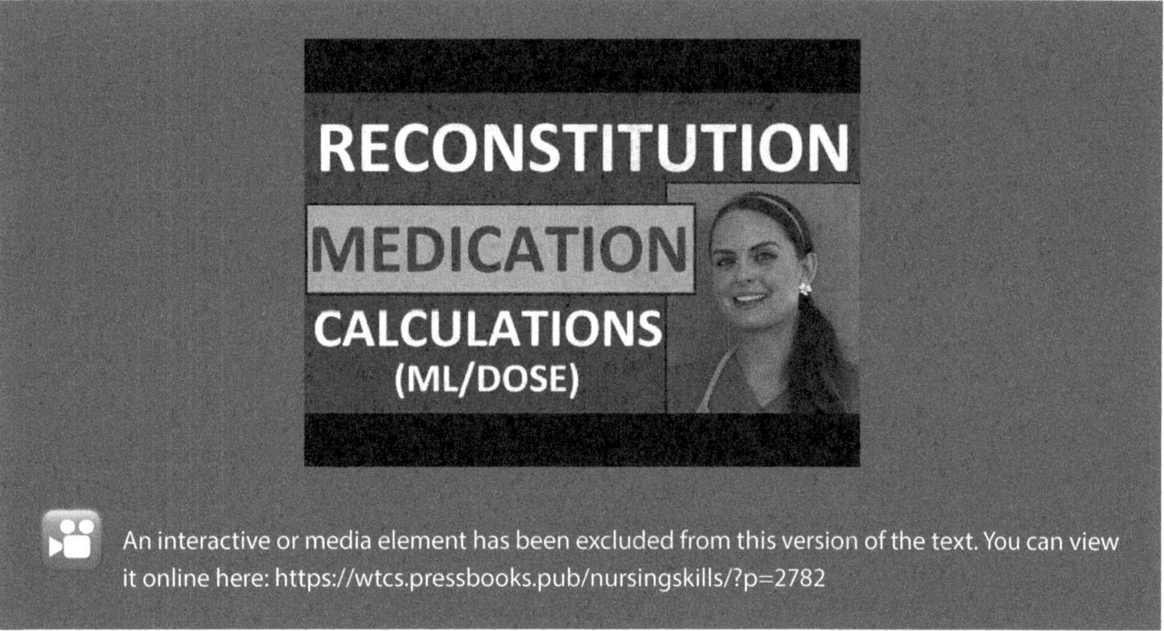

An interactive or media element has been excluded from this version of the text. You can view it online here: https://wtcs.pressbooks.pub/nursingskills/?p=2782

---

4 Southwest Tech Math/Science Center. (2018, April 25). *Entry-level drug calculations for nursing students part 3 – Pharmacology, nursing math**. [Video]. YouTube. All rights reserved. Video used with permission. https://youtu.be/g9nqo-aZuHE

5 RegisteredNurseRN. (2015, October 7). *Dosage calculations made easy | Reconstitution calculation medication problems nursing students (10).* [Video]. YouTube. All rights reserved. Video used with permission. https://youtu.be/TK3ZAaMuhYk

5.11 WEIGHT-BASED CALCULATIONS

Liquid medications are often prescribed based on the patient's weight. Dimensional analysis can be used to determine the amount of liquid medication the patient will receive based on their weight, the provider order, and the concentration of medication supplied.

Practice Problem: Weight-Based Calculations

Patient Information:

Name: Aidan Smith, DOB: 5/09/20xx, Age 4, Allergies: NKDA, Weight: 22 pounds

Provider Order: Tylenol 15mg/kg PO every 4-6 hours for pain or fever

Medication Supplied: See Figure 5.12[1] for the drug label of the medication supplied.

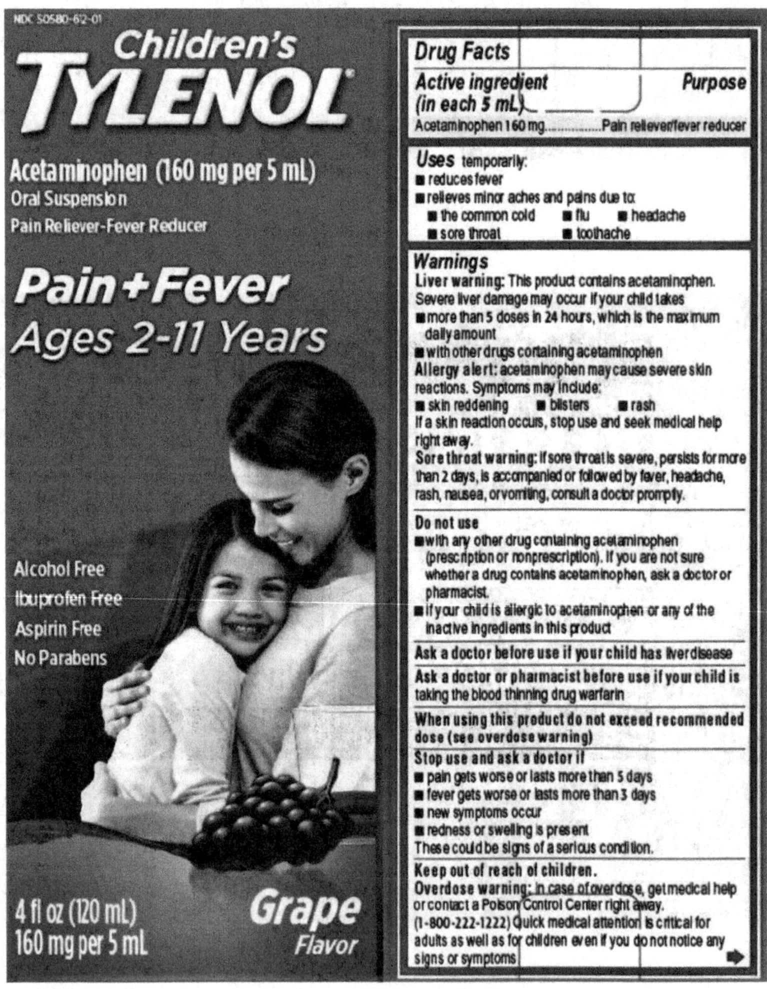

Figure 5.12 Acetaminophen

---

1 This work is a derivative of tylenol-01.jpg, courtesy of the U.S.National Library of Medicine. This image is included on the basis of Fair Use. Access for free at https://dailymed.nlm.nih.gov/dailymed/drugInfo.cfm?setid=d8aa3b1a-5f63-49db-998c-35cd11bd733f

My Notes

Aidan had his last dose of Tylenol eight hours ago and now has a fever of 38 degrees Celsius. Calculate the amount of Tylenol you will prepare and administer to Aidan using dimensional analysis.

1. Review the medication label. We see that acetaminophen (Tylenol) is supplied in a concentration of 160 mg in 5 mL.

2. Set up the equation by starting with the goal unit for which we are solving, which, in this case, is milliliters of liquid medication to administer:

$$mL = ?$$

3. Set up the first fraction by matching the numerator to mL. Plug in the known amount of mL from the drug label, which is 5. Add 160 mg to the denominator because the medication supplied has a known concentration amount of 160 mg in 5 mL:

$$mL = \frac{5\ mL}{160\ mg}$$

4. Create the second fraction with the intent to cross out units by placing mg in the numerator. Look for other important information in the problem related to mg. The prescription is for 15 mg of acetaminophen (Tylenol) for each kg of weight. Add 15 the numerator and 1 kg in the denominator because 15 mg of Tylenol are ordered for every 1 kg of patient weight:

$$mL = \frac{5\ mL}{160\ \cancel{mg}}\ x\ \frac{15\ \cancel{mg}}{1\ kg}$$

5. Create the third fraction with the intent to cross out kg, so place kg in the numerator. Look for important information in the problem related to kg. The patient's chart tells us their weight is 22 pounds. Add 1 kg to the numerator and then place 2.2 lb (based on a known equivalency) in the denominator:

$$mL = \frac{5\ mL}{160\ \cancel{mg}}\ x\ \frac{15\ \cancel{mg}}{1\ kg}\ x\ \frac{1\ kg}{2.2\ lb}$$

6. Place lb in the numerator of the fourth fraction with the intent to cross out pounds. Look at the information provided and see that the patient weighs 22 pounds. Add 22 pounds in the numerator and 1 in the denominator with the intent to cross off units:

$$mL = \frac{5\ mL}{160\ \cancel{mg}}\ x\ \frac{15\ \cancel{mg}}{1\ kg}\ x\ \frac{1\ \cancel{kg}}{2.2\ lb}\ x\ \frac{22\ lb}{1} =$$

7. Cancel out units diagonally:

$$mL = \frac{5\ mL}{160\ \cancel{mg}}\ x\ \frac{15\ \cancel{mg}}{1\ kg}\ x\ \frac{1\ \cancel{kg}}{2.2\ \cancel{lb}}\ x\ \frac{22\ \cancel{lb}}{1} =$$

My Notes

8. After canceling out similar units, we are left with mL, our goal unit, so we can complete the calculation. Multiply across the numerators and the denominators, and then divide the final fraction for the answer:

$$mL = \frac{5\ mL\ x\ 15\ x\ 1\ x\ 22 =}{160\ x\ 1\ x\ 2.2\ x\ 1\ =} \frac{1650\ mL}{352} = \frac{1650\ mL}{352} = 4.6875\ mL$$

9. Round your final answer. Because the patient is a child, round the final answer to the hundredth, so the final answer is 4.69 mL.

Review the following module within *SWTC's Dimensional Analysis in Nursing Page* for more information about solving weight-based problems.
Modules 1.12

Please practice weight-based calculations with the interactive learning activity below.

Interactive Activity

An interactive or media element has been excluded from this version of the text. You can view it online here: https://wtcs.pressbooks.pub/nursingskills/?p=2785

5.12 SAFE DOSAGE RANGE

My Notes

When administering calculated liquid medication, it is important to double-check that the dosage administered is within a safe range. Safe ranges of dosages are provided in drug reference materials. Medication errors often occur in children, who have smaller ranges of safe dosage than adults due to their smaller weight.

When verifying that a dosage is within a safe range based on a patient's weight, begin by completing the dosage calculation. Then, calculate the low and high ends of the safe dosage range. Finally, verify that the calculated dose is within this range.

Practice Problem: Safe Dosage Range

Declan is an 8-month-old infant who weighs 7 kg. He has been prescribed acetaminophen 100 mg every 4-6 hours PO for a fever. The recommended dosage range for infants is 10-15 mg/kg/dose. Calculate the acceptable dosage range for Declan and determine if the prescribed dose is safe.

1. Calculate the low end of the safe dosage. Start by identifying the goal unit. For this problem we want to know the dose in milligrams:

$$mg = ?$$

2. To set up the problem, match the numerator in the first fraction to the desired unit to be solved, which in this case is mg. Based on information known from the problem, we know that the recommended low dose is 10 mg per kg, so add 1 kg to the denominator:

$$mg = \frac{10\ mg}{1\ kg}$$

3. Create the second fraction with the intent to cross out units. Place kg in the numerator. Look to the problem for information related to kg. We know that Declan weighs 7 kg, so place 7 in the numerator and 1 in the denominator with the intent to cross off units:

$$mg = \frac{10\ mg}{1\ kg}\ x\ \frac{7\ kg}{1}$$

4. Cross off units. Multiply across the numerators and then the denominators, and then divide the final fraction for the final low dose answer in mg:

$$mg = \frac{10\ mg}{1\ \cancel{kg}}\ x\ \frac{7\ \cancel{kg}}{1} = \frac{70}{1} = 70\ mg\ (low\ dose)$$

My Notes

5. Calculate the high dose. Set up a similar equation, but this time using the high dose information of 15 mg per kg:

$$mg = \frac{15\ mg}{1\ \cancel{kg}}\ x\ \frac{7\ \cancel{kg}}{1} = \frac{105}{1} = 105\ mg\ (high\ dose)$$

6. Based on the calculations, the safe dosage range for Declan is 70 mg – 105 mg. Compare the prescribed dose to the low- and high-dose range calculations to determine if it is safe. Declan was prescribed 100 mg. It falls within the calculated safe dosage range of 70 – 105 mg, so, yes, this is a safe dose for Declan.

Video Review of Safe Pediatric Dosage Calculations[1]

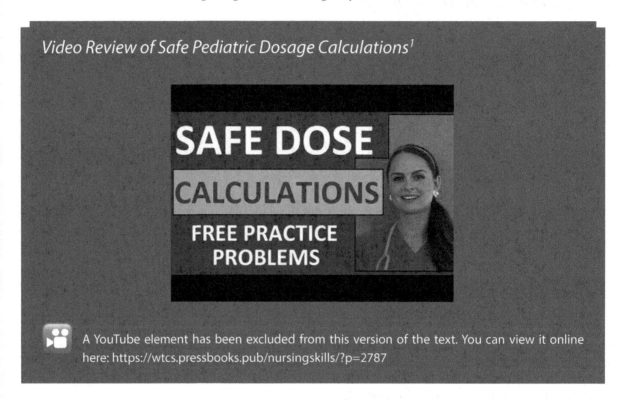

A YouTube element has been excluded from this version of the text. You can view it online here: https://wtcs.pressbooks.pub/nursingskills/?p=2787

Please practice dosage range calculations with the interactive activity below.

Interactive Activity

An interactive or media element has been excluded from this version of the text. You can view it online here: https://wtcs.pressbooks.pub/nursingskills/?p=2787

1 RegisteredNurseRN. (2016, September 13). *Safe dose dosage range pediatric calculations nursing drug math (Video 7).* [Video]. YouTube. All rights reserved. Video used with permission. https://youtu.be/QRdIVGaQf7Q

5.13 INTRAVENOUS INFUSIONS

So far in this chapter, we have practiced using dimensional analysis to determine dosage calculations for medications given orally and parenterally (by injection). Medications can also be administered intravenously (IV). There are two methods for administering intravenous medications: infusion pump or gravity using IV drip tubing.

In the United States, intravenous medications are most commonly administered via an infusion pump for patient safety. When an infusion pump is used to administer IV medications, it is typically programmed by the nurse in milliliters per hour (mL/hour). However, situations may occur when an infusion pump is not available, so the nurse must also know how to calculate drip rates using IV drip tubing to administer a medication by gravity. There are different types of IV drip tubing, and each type provides a specific number of drops of medication per milliliter.

As we perform math calculations related to IV medication administration, we are ultimately ensuring that our patients are receiving the correct dose over the correct period of time to avoid adverse effects from too-rapid or too-slow intravenous administration. Specific math calculations for IV infusion by gravity and IV infusion by pump are further described in the following sections.

My Notes

5.14 IV INFUSION BY GRAVITY

IV drip tubing comes in a variety of sizes called drop factors. The **drop factor** is the number of drops in one mL of solution using gravity IV tubing. The drop factor is printed on the IV tubing package. **Macrodrip tubing** includes tubing with drop factors of 10, 15, or 20 drops per mililiter and is typically used to deliver general IV solutions to adults. **Microdrip tubing** includes tubing with a drop factor of 60 drops per milliliter. It is typically used to deliver precise amounts of medication in small drops to children and infants. See Figure 5.13[1] for an image of macrodrip and microdrip tubing.

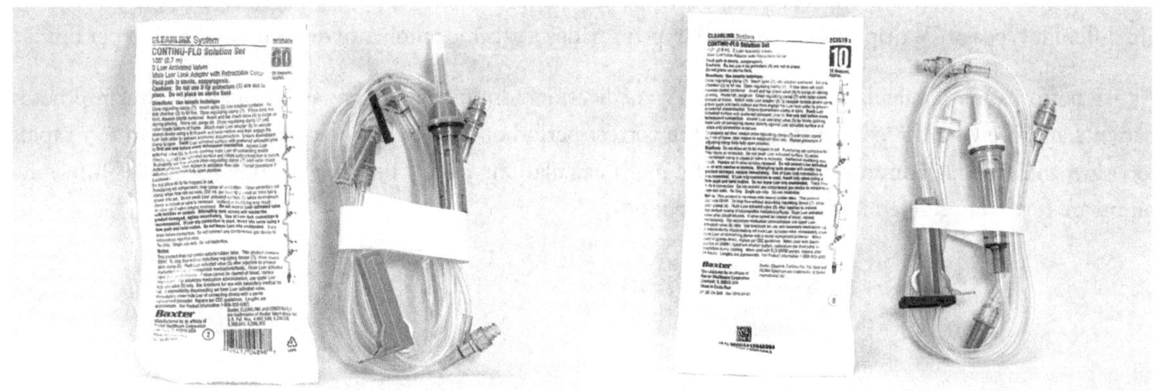

Figure 5.13 Macrodrip and Microdrip IV Tubing

1 "Microdrip Tubing" and "Macrodrip Tubing" by Deanna Hoyord, Chippewa Valley Technical College HPS Lab is licensed under CC BY 4.0. Access for free at https://drive.google.com/file/d/1Kt2jH1iQ_Ck2EKITOPTSfVbX2nfpwTAs/view?usp=sharing and https://drive.google.com/file/d/15TCV2jvzl7Jvk9COXW3b8-WslDEzeGDR/view?usp=sharing

Video Review of Micro Tubing Drip

My Notes

Chamber[2]

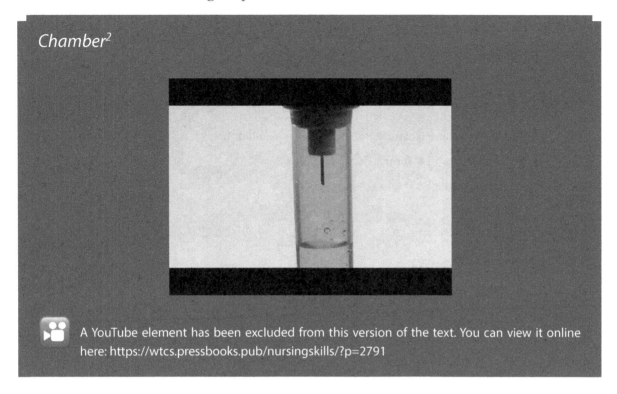

A YouTube element has been excluded from this version of the text. You can view it online here: https://wtcs.pressbooks.pub/nursingskills/?p=2791

In the sample problems below, you will be calculating the number of drops needed per minute to achieve the quantity of fluid to be used per hour in the provider order.

2 Open RN Project. (2020, December 9). Micro Tubing Drip Chamber Video. [Video]. YouTube. Licensed under CC BY 3.0. https://youtu.be/reH50eHpmSQ_

My Notes

Practice Problem: IV Infusion (Example 1)

Let's practice calculating the rate of IV infusion by gravity using macrodrip tubing.

Patient Information:

Name: Elaina Dimas, DOB: 12/09/19xx, Age 6, Allergies: NKDA, Weight: 15 kg

Diagnosis: Dehydration

Provider Order: 0.9% Sodium Chloride 500 mL IV bolus over four hours

Fluid Supplied: See Figure 5.14[3] for the IV fluid supplied.

Tubing Supplied: See Figure 5.15[4] for IV tubing supplied.

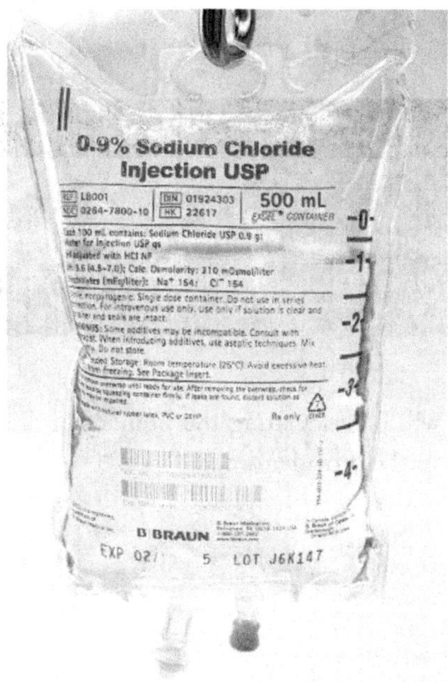

Figure 5.14 0.9% Sodium Chloride in 500 mL

3 "0.9% Sodium Chloride 500 ml" by Deanna Hoyord, Chippewa Valley Technical College HPS Lab is licensed under CC BY 4.0. Access for free at https://drive.google.com/file/d/1t8fi6aWHDh91l69XbeNlEUpDj3eOS9-B/view?usp=sharing

4 "Microdrip Tubing" by Deanna Hoyord, Chippewa Valley Technical College is licensed under CC BY 4.0. Access for free at https://drive.google.com/file/d/1Kt2jH1iQ_Ck2EKITOPTSfVbX2nfpwTAs/view?usp=sharing

My Notes

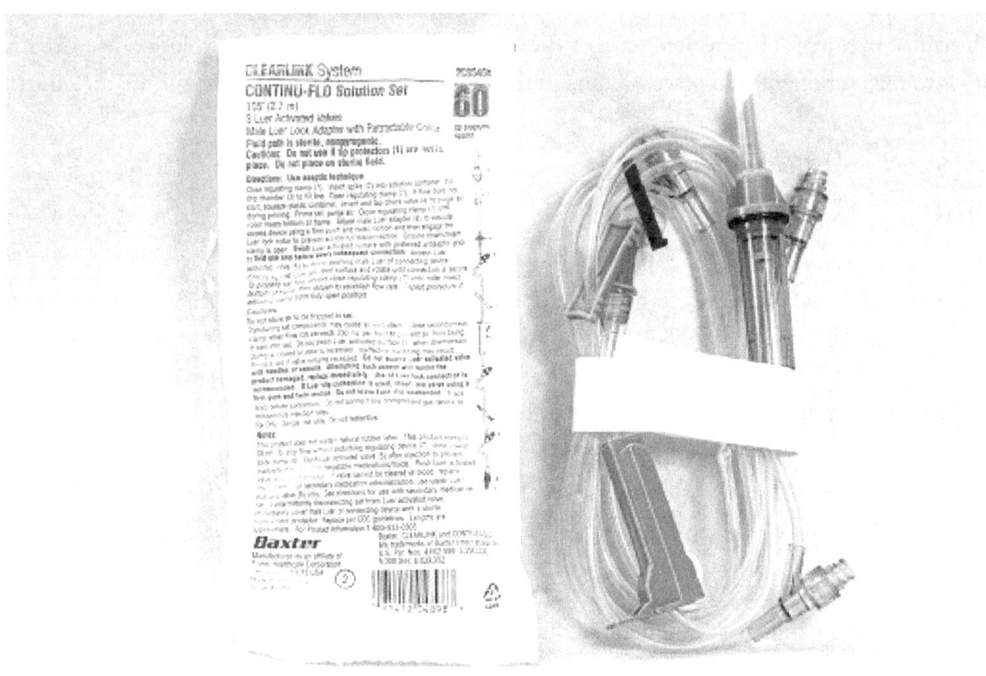

Figure 5.15 Microdrip Tubing

Solve using dimensional analysis.

1. To set up the problem, begin by identifying the goal unit(s) for which we are solving. When calculating infusion rates by gravity, we need to calculate how many drops (gtts) of the solution will be infused each minute. This will allow us to count the actual drops dripping from the tubing and regulate the rate so the volume of infusion is delivered in the time ordered. Set up the problem by identifying the goal unit to solve, but instead of solving for one unit, we will be solving for two units: drops (gtts) and minutes:

$$\frac{gtts}{min} = ?$$

2. Set up the first fraction by matching drops (gtts) in the numerator to the goal unit. Review the tubing provided to determine how many drops per minute are administered with this type of tubing. In this example, the tubing is labelled as 60 gtts/mL. Plug in 60 in the numerator for how many drops are administered by the tubing in 1 mL, and then add 1 mL to the denominator:

$$\frac{gtts}{min} = \frac{60\ gtts}{1\ mL}$$

My Notes

3. Set up the second fraction with the intent to cross off mL, so place mL in the numerator. Look for information provided in the problem related to mL. The prescription is for 500 mL of solution over four hours. Plug in 500 into the numerator, and place 4 hours in the denominator, and then cross off the mL units:

$$\frac{gtts}{min} = \frac{60\ gtts}{1\ \cancel{mL}}\ x\ \frac{500\ \cancel{mL}}{4\ hours}$$

4. Calculate the minutes to achieve our goal unit of drops per minute. Create the third fraction with hour in the numerator with the intent to cross off hour units. Using equivalencies, we know that 1 hour is equivalent to 60 minutes, so plug in 60 minutes in the denominator. Cancel out hours. Evaluate if we have reached our goal units. This equation now matches the goal of units/min and can be solved:

$$\frac{gtts}{min} = \frac{60\ gtts}{1\ \cancel{mL}}\ x\ \frac{500\ \cancel{mL}}{4\ \cancel{hours}}\ x\ \frac{1\ \cancel{hour}}{60\ min}$$

5. Multiply across the numerators and denominators, and then divide the final fraction.

$$\frac{gtts}{min} = \frac{60\ gtts}{1\ \cancel{mL}}\ x\ \frac{500\ \cancel{mL}}{4\ \cancel{hours}}\ x\ \frac{1\ \cancel{hour}}{60\ min} = \frac{60\ gtts\ x\ 500\ x\ 1}{1\ x\ 4\ x\ 60\ min} = 125\ gtts/min$$

6. The final answer is 125 drops/minute.

My Notes

Practice Problem: IV Infusion (Example 2)

Let's practice a second problem using different types of IV drip tubing and a different time to be infused.

Patient Information:

Name: Amber Gomez, DOB: 08/26/19xx, Age 26, Allergies: NKDA, Weight: 50 kg

Provider Order: Lactated Ringers 250 mL IV bolus over 2 hours

Fluid Supplied: See Figure 5.16[5] for the fluid supplied.

Tubing Supplied: See Figure 5.17[6] for the tubing available.

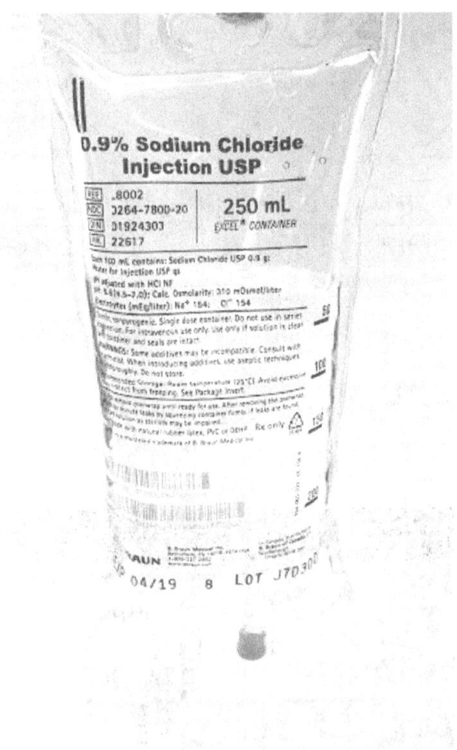

Figure 5.16 0.9% Normal Saline 250 mL

5 "0.9% Sodium Chloride 250 ml" by Deanna Hoyord, Chippewa Valley Technical College HPS Lab is licensed under CC BY 4.0. Access for free at https://drive.google.com/file/d/1yiGiKB7K35VL6m8H4xi_wC_f8KMux8H2/view?usp=sharing

6 "Macrodrip Tubing" by Deanna Hoyord, Chippewa Valley Technical College is licensed under CC BY 4.0. Access for free at https://drive.google.com/file/d/15TCV2jvzl7Jvk9COXW3b8-WslDEzeGDR/view?usp=sharing

My Notes

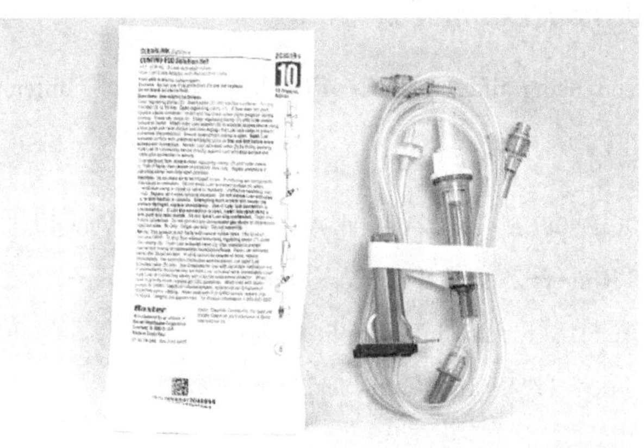

Figure 5.17 Macrodrip Tubing

Solve using dimensional analysis:

$$\frac{gtts}{min} \; x \; \frac{10 \; gtts}{1 \; \cancel{mL}} \; x \; \frac{250 \; \cancel{mL}}{2 \; \cancel{hour}} \; x \; \frac{1 \; \cancel{hour}}{60 \; min} = \frac{10 \; gtts \; x \; 250 \; x \; 1}{1 \; x \; 2 \; x \; 60 \; min} = 20.83 \; gtts/min$$

Round drops to the nearest whole number for a final answer of 21 drops/minute.

Video Review of Solving IV Drip Factor Problems[7]

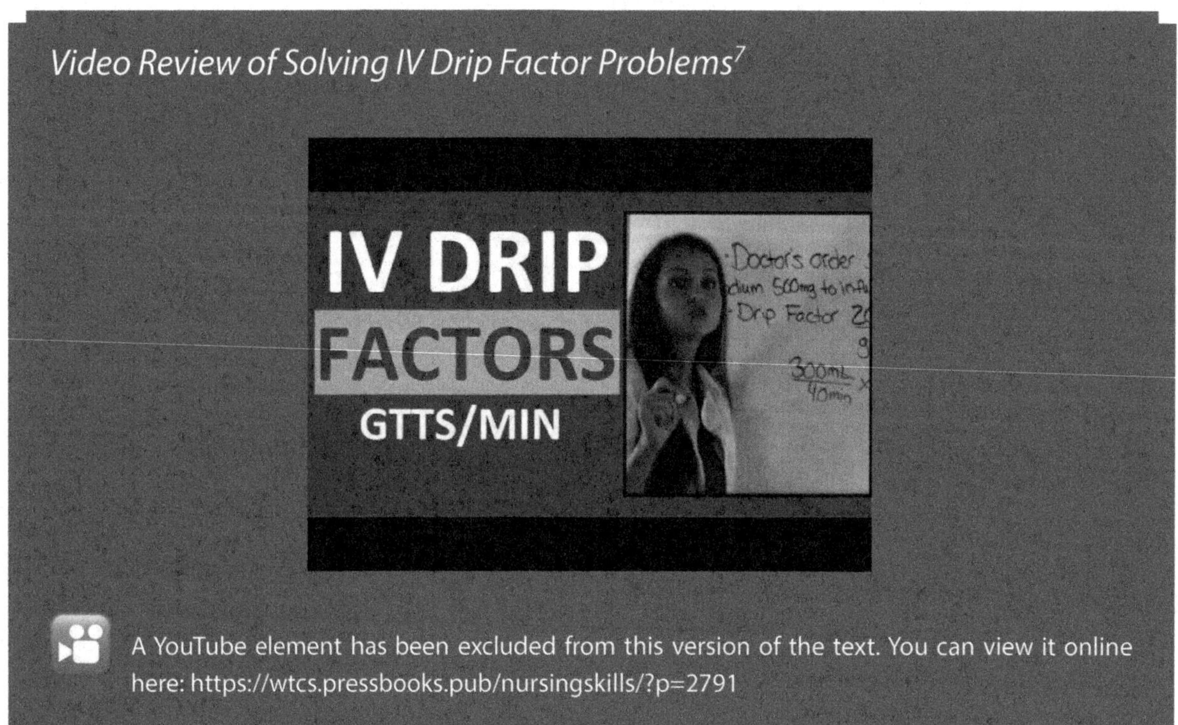

A YouTube element has been excluded from this version of the text. You can view it online here: https://wtcs.pressbooks.pub/nursingskills/?p=2791

7 RegisteredNurseRN. (2015, September 28). *Dosage calculations for nursing students on IV drip rate factors made easy (Video 4)*. [Video]. YouTube. All rights reserved. Video used with permission. https://youtu.be/W5VIc6f0fBA

Review the following module within *SWTC's Dimensional Analysis in Nursing* page for more information about solving drop rates.
Module 1.11

My Notes

Please practice flow rate calculations with the interactive activity below.

Interactive Activity

An interactive or media element has been excluded from this version of the text. You can view it online here: https://wtcs.pressbooks.pub/nursingskills/?p=2791

5.15 IV INFUSION BY PUMP

Intravenous (IV) infusion pumps are the second method used to administer intravenous medications and fluids. See Figure 5.18[1] for an image of an IV pump. Infusion pumps provide an additional safeguard by using a pump to provide an exact amount of fluid per hour to prevent medications from being inadvertently administered too slowly or too quickly. While IV pumps are intended to improve patient safety, the nurse is still responsible for safely setting up the pump. The flow rate using IV pumps is typically calculated in mL/hour. There are many different types of infusion pumps, so the nurse should become familiar with the pumps used at the clinical agency and seek assistance when working with unfamiliar equipment. For additional information about IV infusions, see the "IV Therapy Management" chapter.

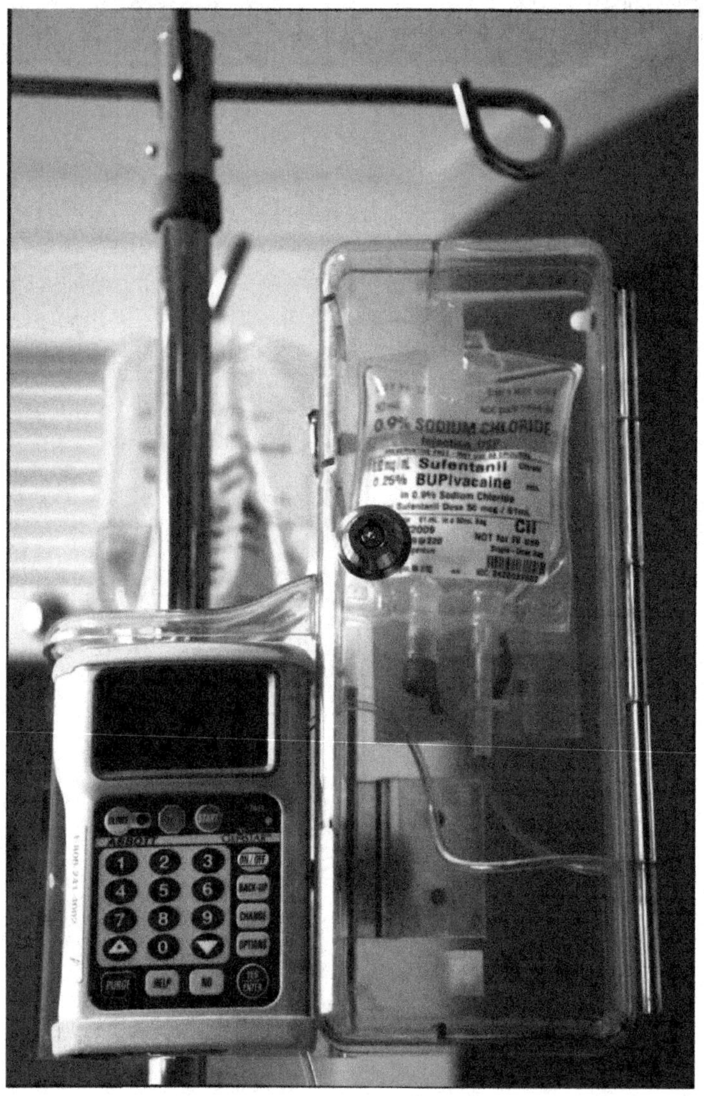

Figure 5.18 IV Infusion Pump

---

1 EDK Pump 1.jpg" by Daniel Schwen is licensed under CC BY-SA 3.0. Access for free at https://commons.wikimedia.org/wiki/File:EDK_Pump_1.jpg

Practice Problem: Infusion by Pump (Example 1)

My Notes

Let's use the same information from the problem for the patient named Amber Gomez in the "IV Infusion by Gravity" subsection, but instead we will calculate the rate of infusion using an IV infusion pump.

Name: Amber Gomez, DOB: 08/26/19xx, Age 26, Allergies: NKDA, Weight: 50 kg

Provider Order: Lactated Ringers 200 mL IV bolus over 2 hours

1. Start by identifying the goal units for which you are solving, which is mL per hour:

$$\frac{mL}{hour} = ?$$

2. Set up the first fraction by matching mL in the numerator. Look at the known information in the problem related to mL. The prescription is to administer 200 mL IV bolus over 2 hours, so put 200 mL in the numerator and 2 hours in the denominator:

$$\frac{mL}{hour} = \frac{200\ mL}{2\ hours}$$

3. Because the units match the goal unit of mL/hour, divide the numerator by the denominator for the final answer:

$$\frac{mL}{hour} = \frac{200\ mL}{2\ hours} = 100\ mL/hr$$

Practice Problem: Infusion by Pump (Example 2)

Let's practice another problem calculating flow rate via IV infusion pump, but this time the prescription states the rate in minutes instead of hours.

Patient Information:

Name: Ashley Hanson, DOB: 09/29/19xx, Age 21, Allergies: NKDA Diagnosis: Dehydration

Provider Order: Lactated Ringers 100 mL IV bolus over 30 minutes

1. Start by setting the goal units being solved. In this case, the pump will still be set for mL per hour:

$$\frac{mL}{hour} = ?$$

My Notes

2. Set up the first fraction by matching the numerator to mL. Look for additional information in the problem related to mL. The order states that 100 mL should be administered over 30 minutes. Place 100 mL in the numerator and 30 minutes in the denominator:

$$\frac{mL}{Hr} = \frac{100\ mL}{30\ minutes}$$

3. Because the pump will be set in mL/hour, convert minutes to hours. Add a second fraction with the intent of crossing off minutes. Place minutes in the numerator so the units will cross out diagonally. Using the known equivalency of 60 minutes in an hour, plug in 60 minutes in the numerator and 1 hour in the denominator. Cross off units diagonally. Multiple across the numerators and the denominators, and then divide for the final answer in mL/hr:

$$\frac{mL}{Hr} = \frac{100\ mL}{30\ \cancel{minutes}} = \frac{60\ \cancel{minutes}}{1\ hour} = \frac{100\ mL\ x\ 60}{30\ x\ 1\ hour} = \frac{6000\ mL}{30\ hour} = 200\ mL/hr$$

Video Reviews of Calculating IV Infusion Rates

IV Infusion[2]

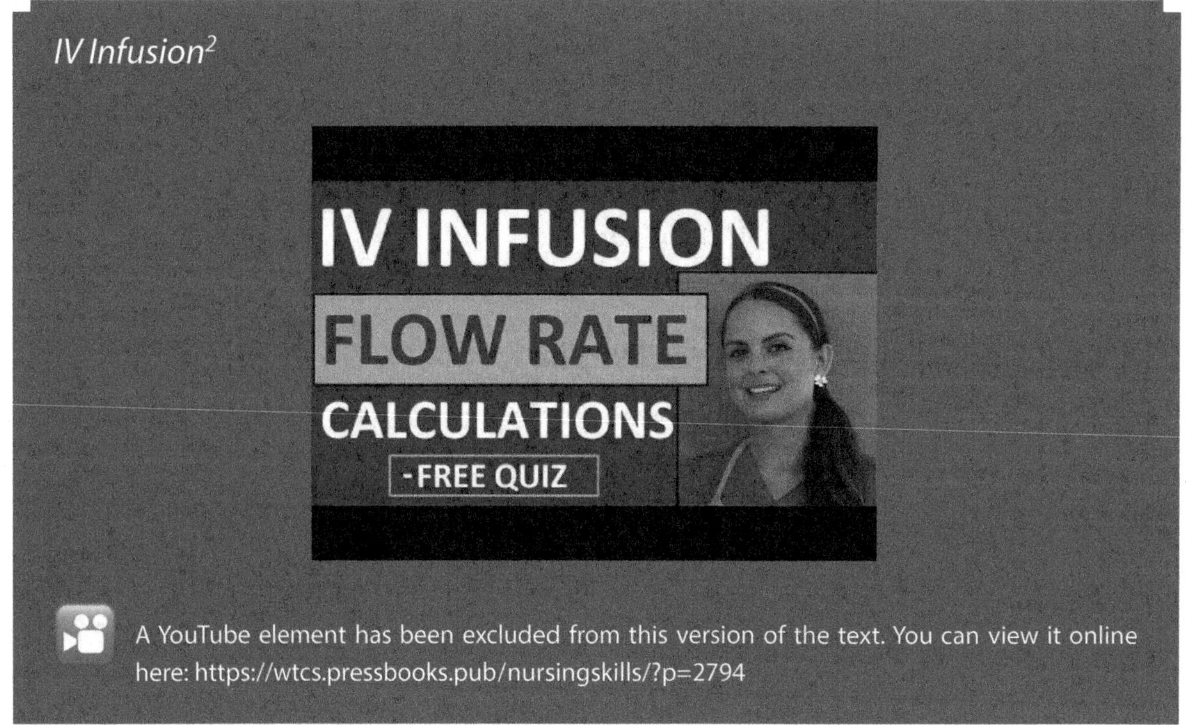

A YouTube element has been excluded from this version of the text. You can view it online here: https://wtcs.pressbooks.pub/nursingskills/?p=2794

2 RegisteredNurseRN. (2015, September 30). *Dosage calculations for nursing students made easy on IV infusion rate calculations (Video 5)*. [Video]. YouTube. All rights reserved. Video used with permission. https://youtu.be/rRN3DifaMWo

My Notes

IV Bolus Calculations[3]

A YouTube element has been excluded from this version of the text. You can view it online here: https://wtcs.pressbooks.pub/nursingskills/?p=2794

Review the following module within *SWTC's Dimensional Analysis in Nursing* page for more information about solving weight-based problems.
Module 1.10

Please practice flow rate by infusion pump calculations below.

Interactive Activity

An interactive or media element has been excluded from this version of the text. You can view it online here: https://wtcs.pressbooks.pub/nursingskills/?p=2794

3 RegisteredNurseRN. (2015, February 9). *Dosage calculations | Nursing drug calculations | IV medications problems nursing school (Vid 2)*. [Video]. YouTube. All rights reserved. Video used with permission. https://youtu.be/N9gZVo_Sc60

5.16 IV COMPLETION TIME

In addition to calculating IV flow rates, nurses also commonly calculate when an infusion will be completed so they will know when to discontinue the infusion or hang another IV bag. Let's practice calculating how long it will take an IV infusion to complete.

Practice Problem: IV Completion Time (Example 1)

Patient Information:

Name: Amanda Parks, DOB: 09/29/19xx, Allergies: NKDA, Weight: 70 kg

Provider Order: 0.9% Sodium Chloride IV at 75 mL/hr

Fluid Supplied: See Figure 5.19[1] for the IV fluid bag supplied.

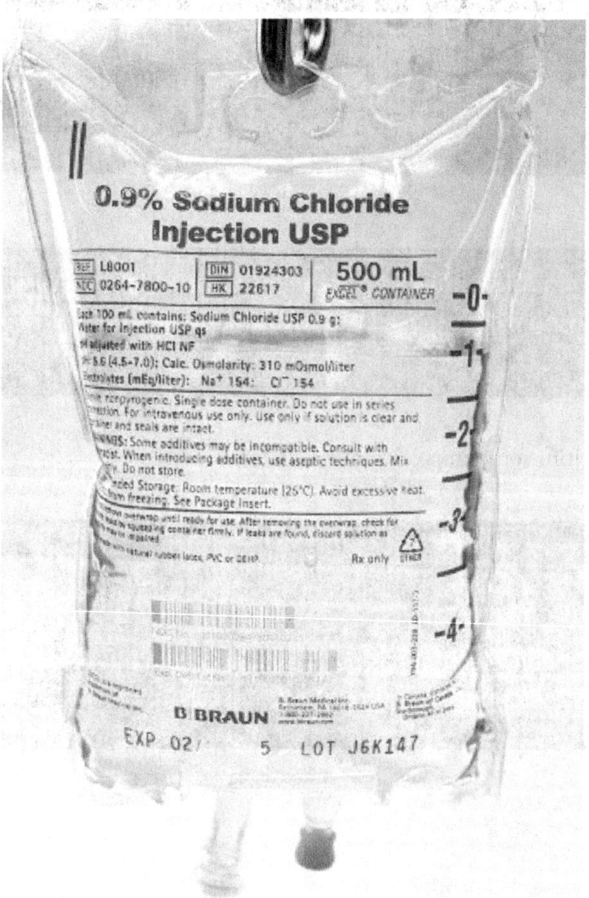

Figure 5.19 0.9% Normal Saline in 500 mL

1 "0.9% Sodium Chloride in 500 ml" by Deanna Hoyord, Chippewa Valley Technical College is licensed under CC BY 4.0. Access for free at https://drive.google.com/file/d/1t8fi6aWHDh91l69XbeNlEUpDj3eOS9-B/view?usp=sharing

My Notes

1. Begin by setting up the goal unit being solved for, which is an hour:

$$Hour = ?$$

2. Set up the first fraction by matching the numerator to hour. Look at the information in the problem related to hours. The order states the IV should be administered at 75 mL per hour, so add 75 mL to the denominator:

$$Hour = \frac{1\ hour}{75\ mL}$$

3. Set up the second fraction with the intent to cancel out mL, so add mL to the numerator of the second fraction. Look at the information in the problem related to mL. By looking at the bag, we know there are 500 mL to infuse, so plug in 500 in the numerator and place 1 in the denominator with the intent to cross out units:

$$Hour = \frac{1\ hour}{75\ \cancel{mL}}\ x\ \frac{500\ \cancel{mL}}{1}$$

4. Cross off units then multiply across the numerators and denominators. Divide the final fraction for the final answer:

$$Hour = \frac{1\ hour}{75\ \cancel{mL}}\ x\ \frac{500\ \cancel{mL}}{1} = \frac{1\ hour\ x\ 500}{75\ x\ 1} = \frac{500\ hour}{75} = 6.666667\ hours$$

5. When performing calculations related to time, it is important to remember that anything after the decimal is a portion of an hour and needs to be converted to minutes. To finish the answer, multiply 60 minutes X 0.6667 = 40.02 minutes. The final answer is the infusion will be completed in 6 hours and 40 minutes.

Practice Problem: IV Completion Time (Example 2)

Now let's add a start time to the above problem and calculate what time the infusion will end. We determined that the IV infusion will take 6.6667 hours to infuse 500 mL at 75 mL/hr.

Let's assume the infusion started at 0800.

1. Add the total infusion time to the start time of the infusion, so add 6 hours to the start time of 0800. Use military time and put a "0" before the six for 6 hours:

$$0800 + 0600 = 1400$$

2. Add the minutes to the time:

$$1400 + 40 = 1440$$

3. Answer: Our infusion will be complete at 1440.

My Notes

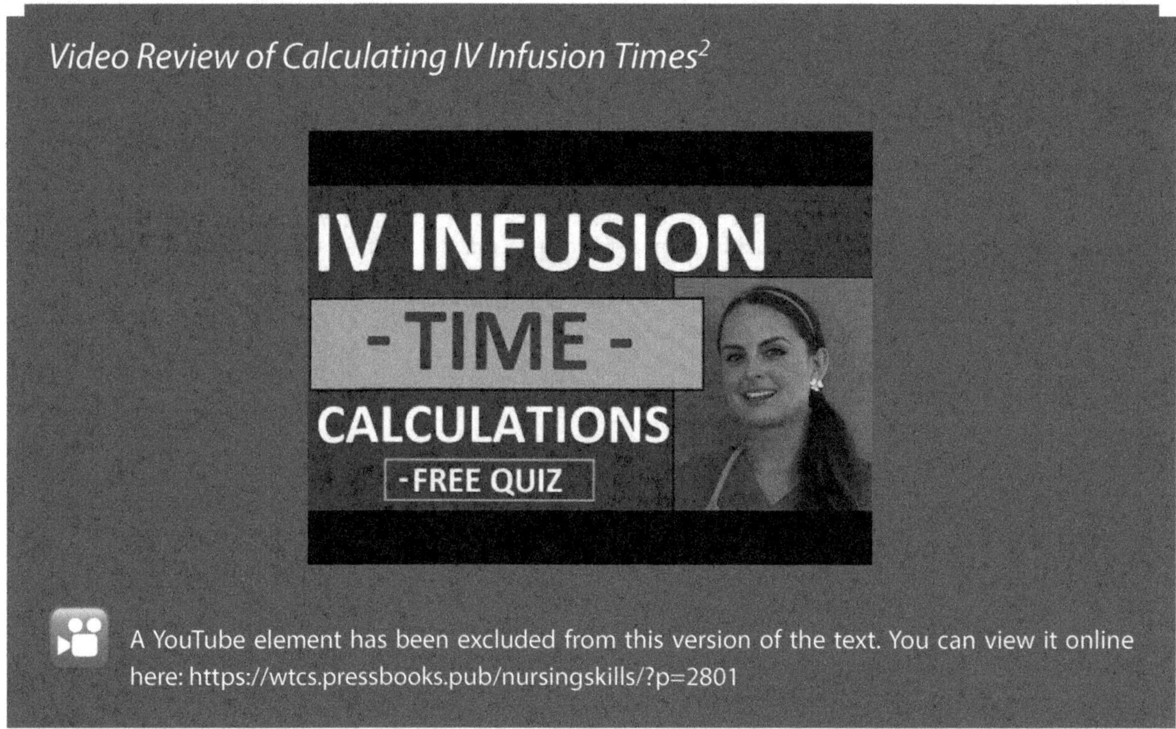

Please practice IV completion rates with the interactive learning activity below.

Interactive Activity

An interactive or media element has been excluded from this version of the text. You can view it online here: https://wtcs.pressbooks.pub/nursingskills/?p=2801

2 RegisteredNurseRN. (2015, February 21). *IV infusion time calculations nursing | Dosage calculations practice for nursing student (Vid 9)*. [Video]. YouTube. All rights reserved. Video used with permission. https://youtu.be/QPAeGgVkxBY

5.17 MULTI-STEP CALCULATIONS

My Notes

Sometimes multi-step calculations are required, especially for medications used in critical care. There are many different ways to solve multi-step calculations, so it is important to select a method that works for you that is consistently accurate. Let's practice a multi-step calculation for a medication supplied in mg/mL but is prescribed based on micrograms (mcg) per kilogram (kg) per minute, and the patient's weight is provided in pounds.

Practice Problem: Multi-Step Calculations

Patient Information:

Name: Ideen Hanson, DOB: 09/29/19xx, Allergies: NKDA, Weight: 180 lbs

Diagnosis: Hypertension

Provider Order: Begin initial infusion of Nipride at 0.5 mcg/kg/min

Medication Supplied: See Figure 5.20[1] for the drug label of the medication supplied.

Figure 5.20 Nipride Label

Problem: What rate (in mL/hr) should the nurse set the pump to begin the infusion?

1. Set up the goal units to solve for, which is mL/hr.

$$\frac{mL}{hr} =$$

2. Review the problem. The prescription is based on mcg/kg/min. Having three elements can create confusion when setting up the equation using dimensional analysis, so it can be easier to eliminate one element by doing some preliminary steps. First convert the patient weight to kilograms (kg) by dividing 180 pounds/2.2= 81.8181 kg. Now multiplying the micrograms (mcg) ordered by weight in kg to determine the amount of medication to administer per minute: 81.8181 x 0.5 mcg = 40.9090 mcg/ minute. Use this information as you set up your problem.

---

1 "Nipride Label" by Jody Myhre-Oechsle, Chippewa Valley Technical College, Open RN is licensed under CC BY 4.0. Access for free at https://drive.google.com/file/d/1FZT5OvrsT_29LRL4rqjcQwgZughRVDkB/view?usp=sharing

My Notes

3. Start by identifying the unit you are solving for, which is mL/hour. Then set up the first fraction. Match the numerator to mL. Look to the problem for information related to mL. On the drug label, we see that 50 mg of Nipride is supplied in 250 mL of D5W. Plug in 250 in the numerator, and then 50 mg in the denominator:

$$mL = \frac{250\ mL}{50\ mg}$$

4. Set up the second fraction with the intent to cross off mg by placing 1 mg in the numerator. Based on the known equivalency that 1000 mcg are equal to 1 mg, place 1000 mcg in the denominator:

$$mL = \frac{250\ mL}{50\ mg}\ x\ \frac{1\ mg}{1000\ mcg}$$

5. Cross off mg diagonally. Set up the third equation with the intent to cross off mcg by placing it in the numerator. Plug in the information previously calculated, which was 40.9090 mcg/minute:

$$mL = \frac{250\ mL}{50\ \cancel{mg}}\ x\ \frac{1\ \cancel{mg}}{1000\ mcg}\ x\ \frac{40.9090\ mcg}{1\ min}$$

6. Cross off mcg diagonally. Set up the fourth fraction with the intent to cross off minutes. Based on the known equivalency of 60 minutes in 1 hour, plug in 60 in the numerator and 1 hour in the denominator:

$$mL = \frac{250\ mL}{50\ \cancel{mg}}\ x\ \frac{1\ \cancel{mg}}{1000\ \cancel{mcg}}\ x\ \frac{40.9090\ \cancel{mcg}}{1\ min}\ x\ \frac{60\ min}{1\ hour} = 12.2727$$

7. Cross off min diagonally. Review the equation to ensure the goal unit has been met. It has been met, so multiply across the numerators and the denominators, and then divide the final fraction:

$$\frac{mL}{Hr}\ x\ \frac{250\ mL}{50\ \cancel{mg}}\ x\ \frac{1\ \cancel{mg}}{1000\ \cancel{mcg}}\ x\ \frac{40.9090\ \cancel{mcg}}{1\ \cancel{min}}\ x\ \frac{60\ \cancel{min}}{1\ hour} = 12.2727$$

8. Depending on the agency policy and available pump settings, round to 12.27 mL/hour.

Video Reviews of Multiple-Step Calculations That Commonly Occur with Heparin and Dopamine drips

My Notes

Heparin Drip[2]

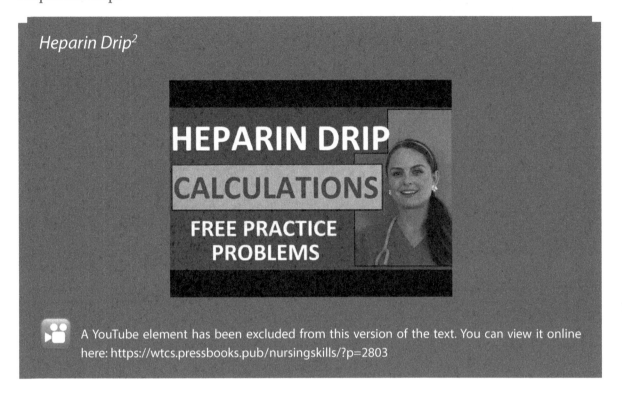

A YouTube element has been excluded from this version of the text. You can view it online here: https://wtcs.pressbooks.pub/nursingskills/?p=2803

2 RegisteredNurseRN. (2018, July 26). *Heparin drip calculation practice problems for nurses | Dosage calculations nursing.* [Video]. YouTube. All rights reserved. Video used with permission. https://youtu.be/10y4gRdnCy8

My Notes

Dopamine Drip[3]

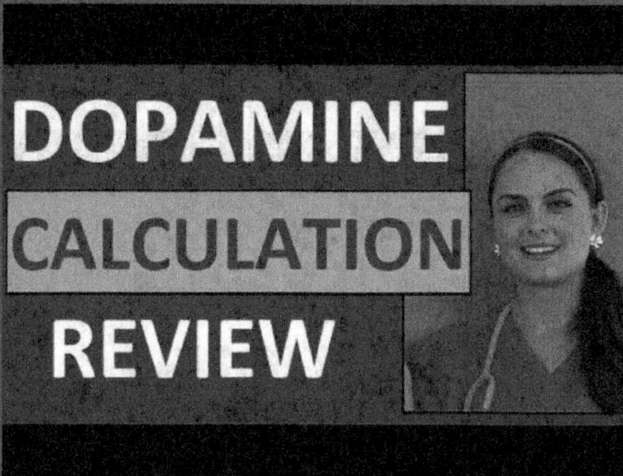

A YouTube element has been excluded from this version of the text. You can view it online here: https://wtcs.pressbooks.pub/nursingskills/?p=2803

3 RegisteredNurseRN. (2019, February 8). *Dopamine IV drip calculation & nursing considerations pharmacology implications.* [Video]. YouTube. All rights reserved. Video used with permission. https://youtu.be/R2XMro13dD0

5.18 LEARNING ACTIVITIES

My Notes

Interactive Activity

An interactive or media element has been excluded from this version of the text. You can view it online here: https://wtcs.pressbooks.pub/nursingskills/?p=3156

My Notes

V GLOSSARY

Dimensional analysis: Dimensional analysis is a problem-solving technique where measurements are converted to a different (but equivalent) unit of measure by multiplying with a fractional form of 1 to obtain a desired unit of administration.

Drop factor: The number of drops in one mL of solution when fluids or medications are administered using gravity IV tubing.

Equivalency: Two values or quantities that are the same amount. For example, one cup is equivalent to eight ounces.

Macrodrip tubing: Gravity IV tubing with drop factors of 10, 15, or 20 drops per milliliter that are typically used to deliver general IV solutions for adults.

Medication cup: A small plastic or paper cup used to dispense oral medications. Some plastic medication cups have calibration marks for measuring medication amounts.

Microdrip tubing: Gravity IV tubing with a drop factor of 60 drops per milliliter.

Military time: A method of measuring the time based on the full 24 hours of the day rather than two groups of 12 hours indicated by AM and PM.

Oral syringe: A specific type of syringe used to measure and/or administer medications via the oral route.

Reconstitution: The process of adding a liquid diluent to a dry ingredient to make a liquid in a specific concentration.

Syringe: A medical device used to administer parenteral medication into tissue or into the bloodstream. Syringes can also be used to withdraw blood or fluid.

Chapter 6

Neurological Assessment

6.1 NEUROLOGICAL ASSESSMENT INTRODUCTION

My Notes

Learning Objectives

- Perform a neurological assessment, including mental status, cranial nerves, sensory function, motor strength, cerebellar function, and reflexes
- Modify assessment techniques to reflect variations across the life span
- Document actions and observations
- Recognize and report significant deviations from norms

The neurological system is a complex and intricate system that affects all body functions. A neurological assessment includes collecting subjective and objective data through an interview and detailed physical examination of the central nervous system and the peripheral nervous system. Let's begin by reviewing the anatomy of the neurological system.

My Notes

6.2 BASIC NEUROLOGICAL CONCEPTS

When completing a neurological assessment, it is important to understand the functions performed by different parts of the nervous system while analyzing findings. For example, damage to specific areas of the brain, such as that caused by a head injury or cerebrovascular accidents (i.e., strokes), can cause specific deficits in speech, facial movements, or use of the extremities. Damage to the spinal cord, such as that caused by a motor vehicle accident or diving accident, will cause specific motor and sensory deficits according to the level where the spinal cord was damaged.

The nervous system is divided into two parts, the central nervous system and the peripheral nervous system. See Figure 6.1[1] for an image of the entire nervous system. The **central nervous system (CNS)** includes the brain and the spinal cord. The brain can be described as the interpretation center, and the spinal cord can be described as the transmission pathway. The peripheral nervous system (PNS) consists of the neurological system outside of the brain and spinal cord, including the cranial nerves that branch out from the brain and the spinal nerves that branch out from the spinal cord. The **peripheral nervous system** can be described as the communication network between the brain and the body parts. Both parts of the nervous system must work correctly for healthy body functioning.

1 "Nervous system diagram.png" by unknown is licensed under CC BY-NC-SA 3.0. Access for free at https://med.libretexts.org/Bookshelves/Nursing/Book%3A_Clinical_Procedures_for_Safer_Patient_Care_(Doyle_and_McCutcheon)/02%3A_Patient_Assessment/2.07%3A_Focused_Assessments

My Notes

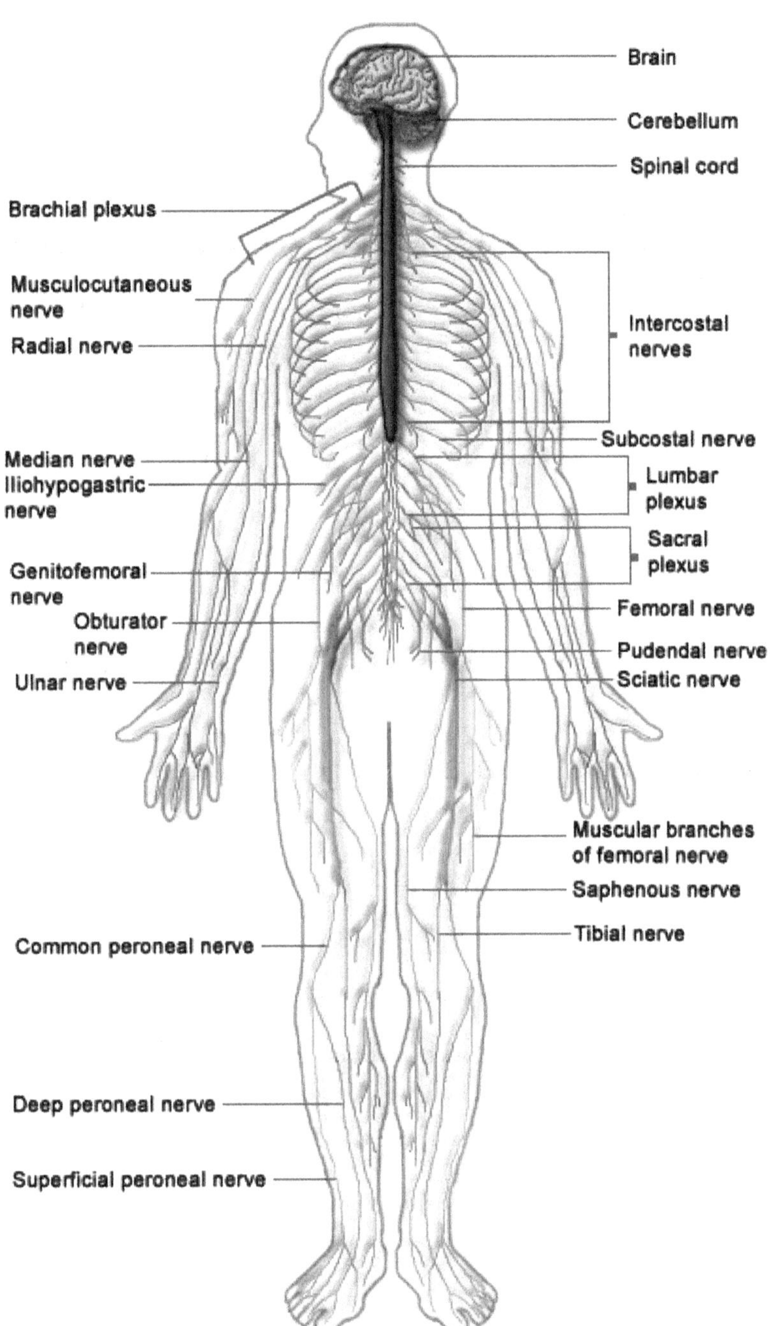

Figure 6.1 Central and Peripheral Nervous Systems

My Notes

Central Nervous System

The major regions of the brain are the cerebrum and cerebral cortex, the diencephalon, the brain stem, and the cerebellum. See Figure 6.2[2] for an illustration of the cerebellum and the lobes of the cerebrum.

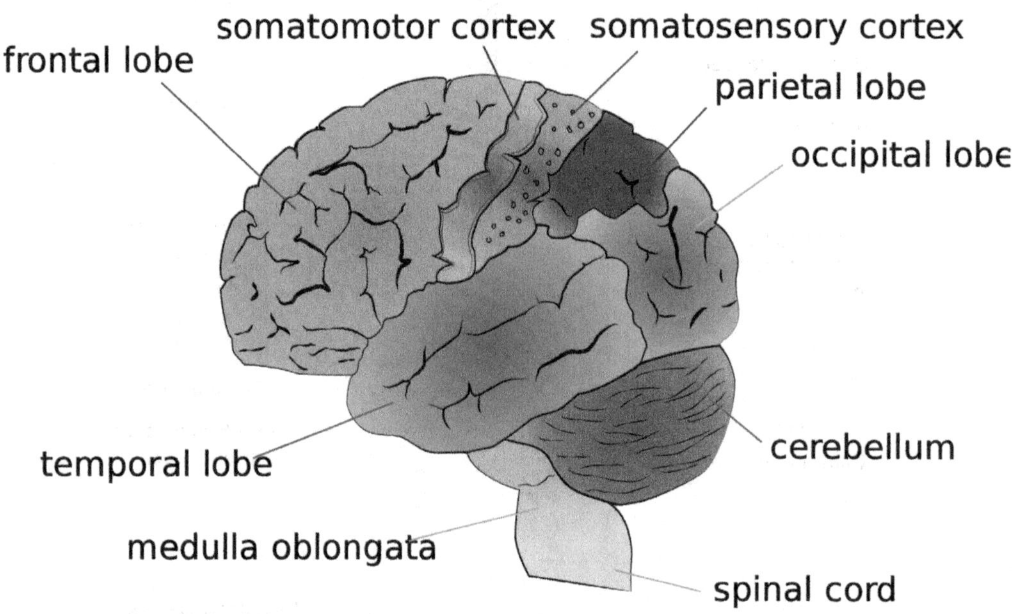

Figure 6.2 Regions of the Brain

Cerebrum and Cerebral Cortex

The largest portion of our brain is the cerebrum. The cerebrum is covered by a wrinkled outer layer of gray matter called the cerebral cortex. See Figure 6.3[3] for an image of the cerebral cortex. The cerebral cortex is responsible for the higher functions of the nervous system such as memory, emotion, and consciousness. The corpus callosum is the major pathway of communication between the right and left hemispheres of the cerebral cortex. The **cerebral cortex** is further divided into four lobes named the frontal, parietal, occipital, and temporal lobes.[4] Each lobe has specific functions.

---

2 "Cerebrum lobes.svg" by Jkwchui is licensed under CC BY-SA 3.0. Access for free at https://commons.wikimedia.org/wiki/File:Cerebrum_lobes.svg

3 "1305 CerebrumN.jpg" by OpenStax is licensed under CC BY 4.0. Access for free at https://openstax.org/books/anatomy-and-physiology/pages/13-2-the-central-nervous-system

4 This work is a derivative of Anatomy & Physiology by OpenStax and is licensed under CC BY 4.0. Access for free at https://openstax.org/books/anatomy-and-physiology/pages/1-introduction

My Notes

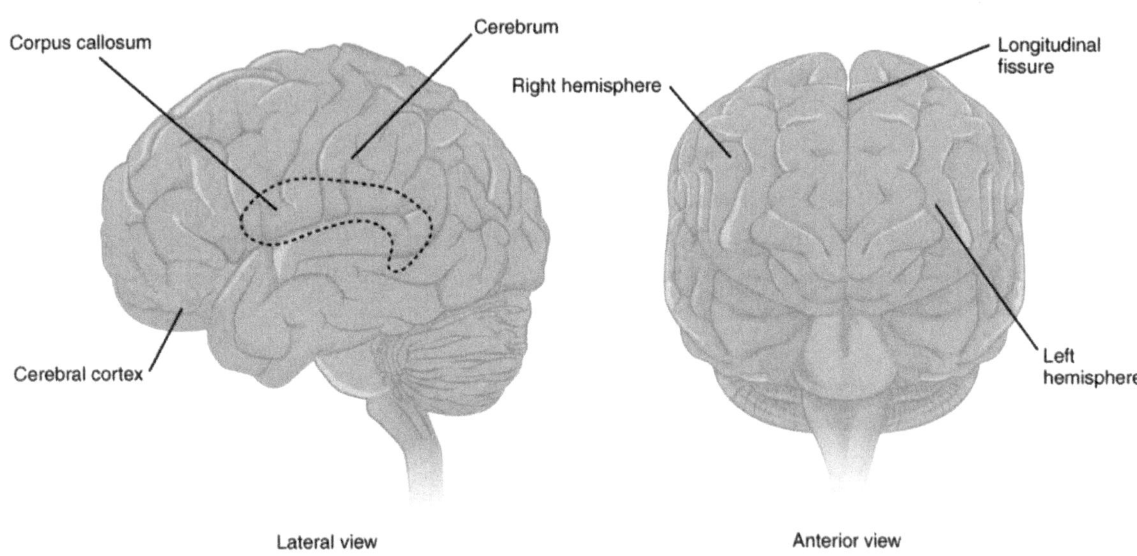

Figure 6.3 Cerebral Cortex

Frontal Lobe

The frontal lobe is associated with movement because it contains neurons that instruct cells in the spinal cord to move skeletal muscles. The anterior portion of the frontal lobe is called the prefrontal lobe, and it provides cognitive functions such as planning and problem-solving that are the basis of our personality, short-term memory, and consciousness. **Broca's area** is also located in the frontal lobe and is responsible for the production of language and controlling movements responsible for speech.[5]

Parietal Lobe

The parietal lobe processes general sensations from the body. All of the tactile senses are processed in this area, including touch, pressure, tickle, pain, itch, and vibration, as well as general senses of the body, such as **proprioception** (the sense of body position) and **kinesthesia** (the sense of movement).[6]

Temporal Lobe

The temporal lobe processes auditory information and is involved with language comprehension and production. Wernicke's area is located in the temporal lobe. Wernicke's area is involved in the comprehension of written and spoken language, and Broca's area is involved in the production of language. Because regions of the temporal lobe are part of the limbic system, memory is also an important function associated with the temporal lobe.[7] The limbic system is involved with our behavioral and emotional responses needed for survival, such as feeding, reproduction, and the fight – or – flight responses.

---

5 This work is a derivative of Anatomy & Physiology by OpenStax and is licensed under CC BY 4.0. Access for free at https://openstax.org/books/anatomy-and-physiology/pages/1-introduction

6 This work is a derivative of Anatomy & Physiology by OpenStax and is licensed under CC BY 4.0. Access for free at https://openstax.org/books/anatomy-and-physiology/pages/1-introduction

7 This work is a derivative of Anatomy & Physiology by OpenStax and is licensed under CC BY 4.0. Access for free at https://openstax.org/books/anatomy-and-physiology/pages/1-introduction

My Notes

Occipital Lobe

The occipital lobe primarily processes visual information.[8]

Diencephalon

Information from the rest of the central and peripheral nervous system is sent to the cerebrum through the diencephalon, with the exception of the olfactory nerve that connects directly to the cerebrum.[9] See Figure 6.4[10] for an illustration of the diencephalon deep within the cerebrum. The diencephalon contains the hypothalamus and the thalamus.

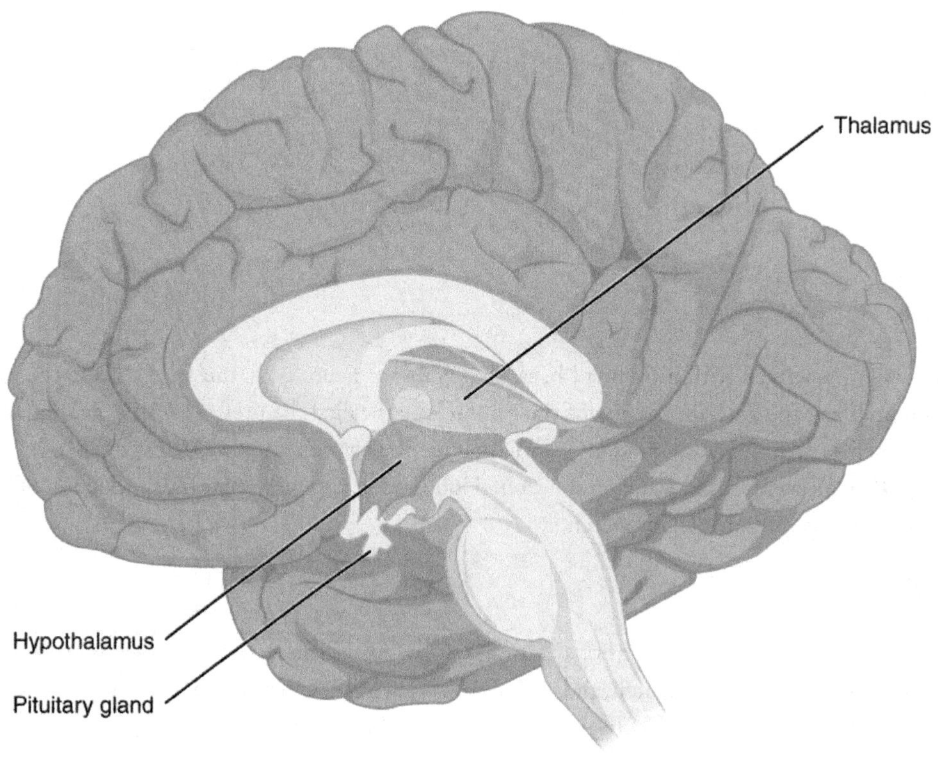

Figure 6.4 The Diencephalon Containing the Hypothalamus and the Thalamus.

The **hypothalamus** helps regulate homeostasis such as body temperature, thirst, hunger, and sleep. The hypothalamus is also the executive region in charge of the autonomic nervous system and the endocrine system through its regulation of the anterior pituitary gland. Other parts of the hypothalamus are involved in memory and emotion as part of the limbic system.[11]

---

8 This work is a derivative of Anatomy & Physiology by OpenStax and is licensed under CC BY 4.0. Access for free at https://openstax.org/books/anatomy-and-physiology/pages/1-introduction

9 This work is a derivative of Anatomy & Physiology by OpenStax and is licensed under CC BY 4.0. Access for free at https://openstax.org/books/anatomy-and-physiology/pages/1-introduction

10 "1310 Diencephalon.jpg" by OpenStax is licensed under CC BY 4.0. Access for free at https://openstax.org/books/anatomy-and-physiology/pages/13-2-the-central-nervous-system

11 This work is a derivative of Anatomy & Physiology by OpenStax and is licensed under CC BY 4.0. Access for free at https://openstax.org/books/anatomy-and-physiology/pages/1-introduction

My Notes

The **thalamus** relays sensory information and motor information in collaboration with the cerebellum. The thalamus does not just pass the information on, but it also processes and prioritizes that information. For example, the portion of the thalamus that receives visual information will influence what visual stimuli are considered important enough to receive further attention from the brain.[12]

Brain Stem

The brain stem is composed of the pons and the medulla. The pons and the medulla regulate several crucial autonomic functions in the body, including involuntary functions in the cardiovascular and respiratory systems, vasodilation, and reflexes like vomiting, coughing, sneezing, and swallowing. Cranial nerves also connect to the brain through the brain stem and provide sensory input and motor output.[13]

For more information about the functions of the autonomic nervous system, visit the "Autonomic Nervous System" chapter in the Open RN *Nursing Pharmacology* textbook.

Cerebellum

The **cerebellum** is located in the posterior part of the brain behind the brain stem and is responsible for fine motor movements and coordination. For example, when the motor neurons in the frontal lobe of the cerebral cortex send a command down the spinal cord to initiate walking, a copy of that instruction is also sent to the cerebellum. Sensory feedback from the muscles and joints, proprioceptive information about the movements of walking, and sensations of balance are sent back to the cerebellum. If the person becomes unbalanced while walking because the ground is uneven, the cerebellum sends out a corrective command to compensate for the difference between the original cerebral cortex command and the sensory feedback.[14]

Spinal Cord

The spinal cord is a continuation of the brain stem that transmits sensory and motor impulses. The length of the spinal cord is divided into regions that correspond to the level at which spinal nerves pass through the vertebrae. Immediately adjacent to the brain stem is the cervical region, followed by the thoracic, the lumbar, and finally the sacral region.[15] The spinal nerves in each of these regions innervate specific parts of the body. See more information under the "Spinal Nerves" section.

---

12 This work is a derivative of Anatomy & Physiology by OpenStax and is licensed under CC BY 4.0. Access for free at https://openstax.org/books/anatomy-and-physiology/pages/1-introduction

13 This work is a derivative of Anatomy & Physiology by OpenStax and is licensed under CC BY 4.0. Access for free at https://openstax.org/books/anatomy-and-physiology/pages/1-introduction

14 This work is a derivative of Anatomy & Physiology by OpenStax and is licensed under CC BY 4.0. Access for free at https://openstax.org/books/anatomy-and-physiology/pages/1-introduction

15 This work is a derivative of Anatomy & Physiology by OpenStax and is licensed under CC BY 4.0. Access for free at https://openstax.org/books/anatomy-and-physiology/pages/1-introduction

My Notes

Review the anatomy of the brain using the following supplementary video.

Video Review for Anatomy of the Brain[16]

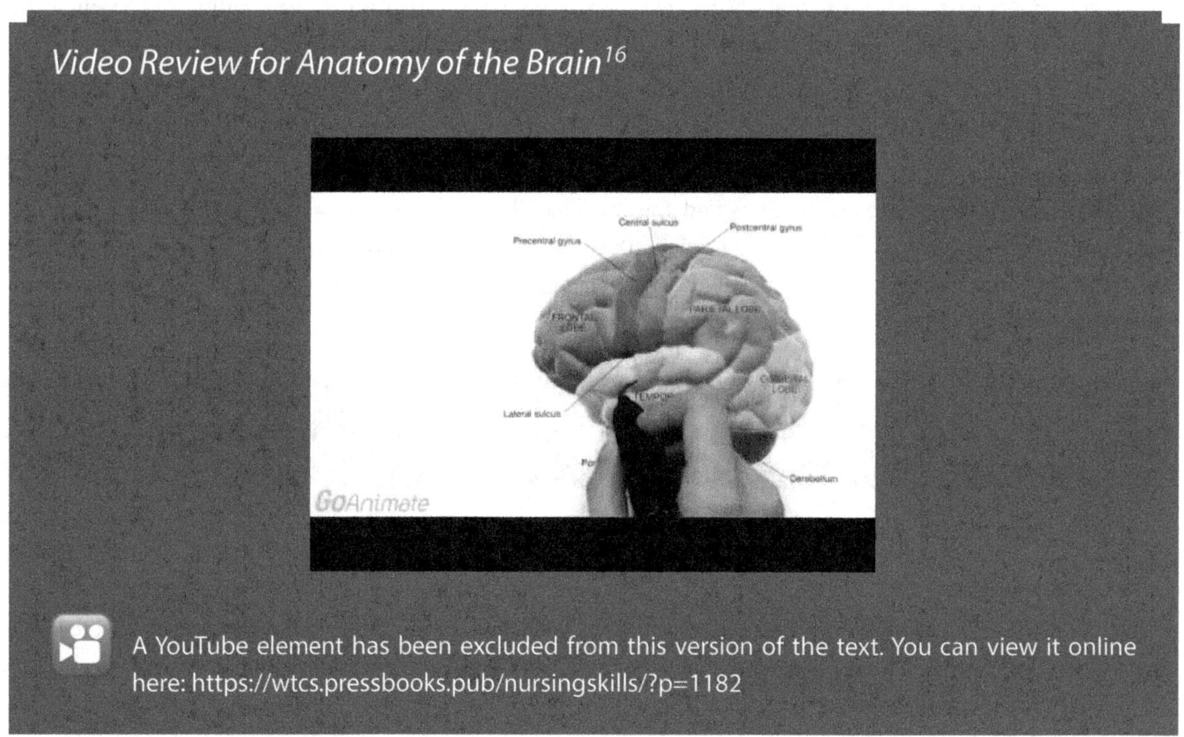

A YouTube element has been excluded from this version of the text. You can view it online here: https://wtcs.pressbooks.pub/nursingskills/?p=1182

Peripheral Nervous System

The peripheral nervous system (PNS) consists of cranial nerves and spinal nerves that exist outside of the brain, spinal cord, and autonomic nervous system. The main function of the PNS is to connect the limbs and organs to the central nervous system (CNS). Sensory information from the body enters the CNS through cranial and spinal nerves. Cranial nerves are connected directly to the brain, whereas spinal nerves are connected to the brain via the spinal cord.

Peripheral nerves are classified as sensory nerves, motor nerves, or a combination of both. **Sensory nerves** carry impulses from the body to the brain for processing. **Motor nerves** transmit motor signals from the brain to the muscles to cause movement.

Cranial Nerves

Cranial nerves are directly connected from the periphery to the brain. They are primarily responsible for the sensory and motor functions of the head and neck. There are twelve cranial nerves that are designated by Roman numerals I through XII. See Figure 6.5[17] for an image of cranial nerves. Three cranial nerves are strictly sensory

16 Forciea, B. (2015, May 12). *Anatomy and physiology: Central nervous system: Brain anatomy v2.0.* [Video]. YouTube. All rights reserved. Video used with permission. https://youtu.be/DBRdInd2-Vg

17 "1320 The Cranial Nerves.jpg" by OpenStax is licensed under CC BY 4.0. Access for free at https://openstax.org/books/anatomy-and-physiology/pages/13-4-the-peripheral-nervous-system

My Notes

nerves; five are strictly motor nerves; and the remaining four are mixed nerves.[18] A traditional mnemonic for memorizing the names of the cranial nerves is "**On Old Olympus Towering Tops A Finn And German Viewed Some Hops**," in which the initial letter of each word corresponds to the initial letter in the name of each nerve.

- The **o**lfactory nerve is responsible for the sense of smell.
- The **o**ptic nerve is responsible for the sense of vision.
- The **o**culomotor nerve regulates eye movements by controlling four of the extraocular muscles, lifting the upper eyelid when the eyes point up and for constricting the pupils.
- The **t**rochlear nerve and the **a**bducens nerve are both responsible for eye movement, but do so by controlling different extraocular muscles.
- The **t**rigeminal nerve regulates skin sensations of the face and controls the muscles used for chewing.
- The **f**acial nerve is responsible for the muscles involved in facial expressions, as well as part of the sense of taste and the production of saliva.
- The **a**ccessory nerve controls movements of the neck.
- The **v**estibulocochlear nerve manages hearing and balance.
- The **g**lossopharyngeal nerve regulates the controlling muscles in the oral cavity and upper throat, as well as part of the sense of taste and the production of saliva.
- The **v**agus nerve is responsible for contributing to homeostatic control of the organs of the thoracic and upper abdominal cavities.
- The **s**pinal accessory nerve controls the muscles of the neck, along with cervical spinal nerves.
- The **h**ypoglossal nerve manages the muscles of the lower throat and tongue.[19] Methods for assessing each of these nerves are described in the "Assessing Cranial Nerves" section.

18 This work is a derivative of Anatomy & Physiology by OpenStax and is licensed under CC BY 4.0. Access for free at https://openstax.org/books/anatomy-and-physiology/pages/1-introduction

19 This work is a derivative of Anatomy & Physiology by OpenStax and is licensed under CC BY 4.0. Access for free at https://openstax.org/books/anatomy-and-physiology/pages/1-introduction

My Notes

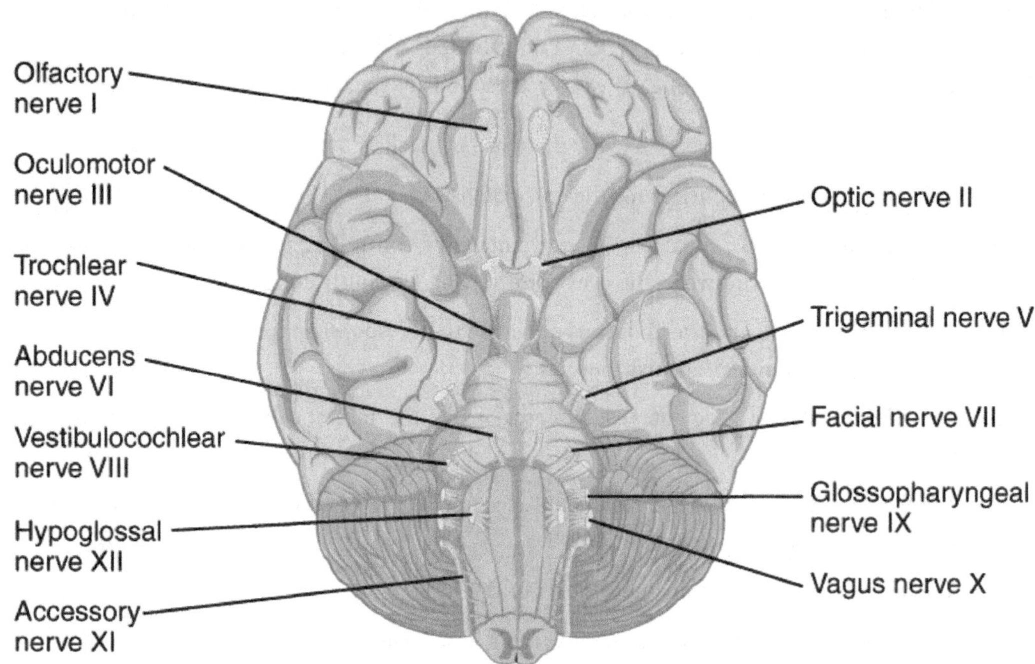

Figure 6.5 Cranial Nerves

Video Review of Cranial Nerves[20]

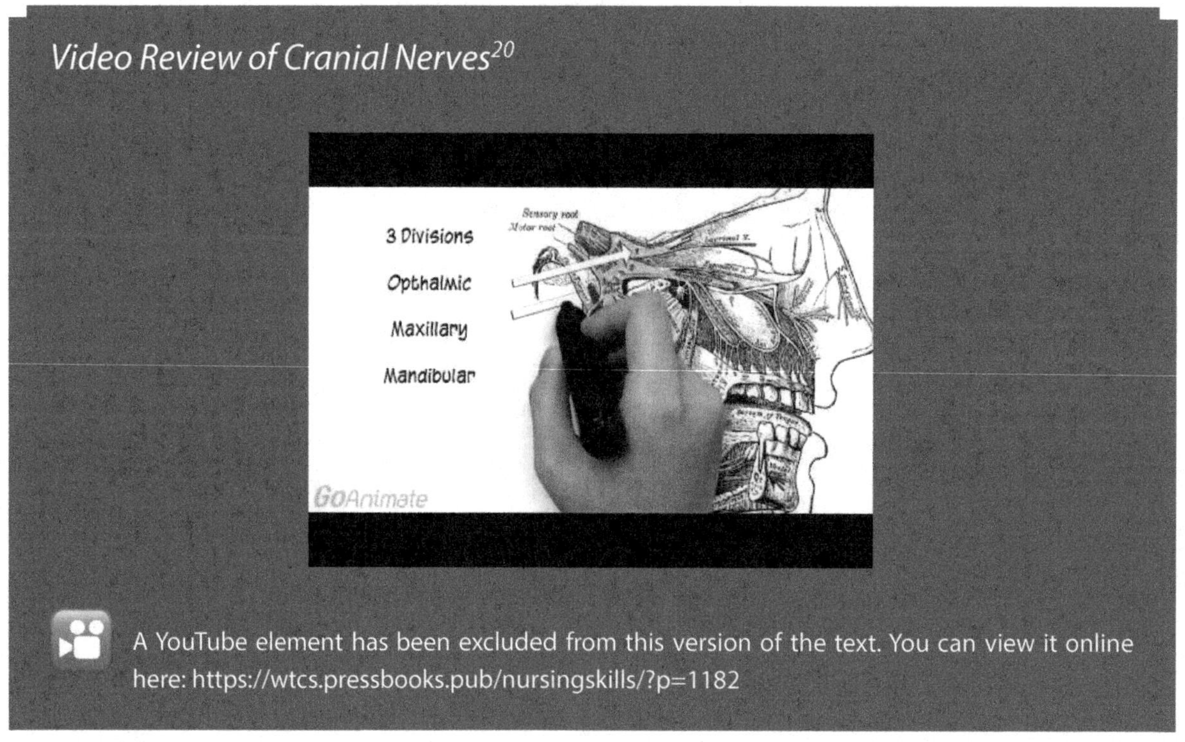

A YouTube element has been excluded from this version of the text. You can view it online here: https://wtcs.pressbooks.pub/nursingskills/?p=1182

20 Forciea, B. (2015, May 12). *Anatomy and physiology: Nervous system: Cranial nerves (v2.0).* [Video]. YouTube. All rights reserved. Video used with permission. https://youtu.be/JBEZh6CHogo

Spinal Nerves

My Notes

There are 31 spinal nerves that are named based on the level of the spinal cord where they emerge. See Figure 6.6[21] for an illustration of spinal nerves. There are eight pairs of cervical nerves designated C1 to C8, twelve thoracic nerves designated T1 to T12, five pairs of lumbar nerves designated L1 to L5, five pairs of sacral nerves designated S1 to S5, and one pair of coccygeal nerves. All spinal nerves are combined sensory and motor nerves. Spinal nerves extend outward from the vertebral column to innervate the periphery while also transmitting sensory information back to the CNS.[22]

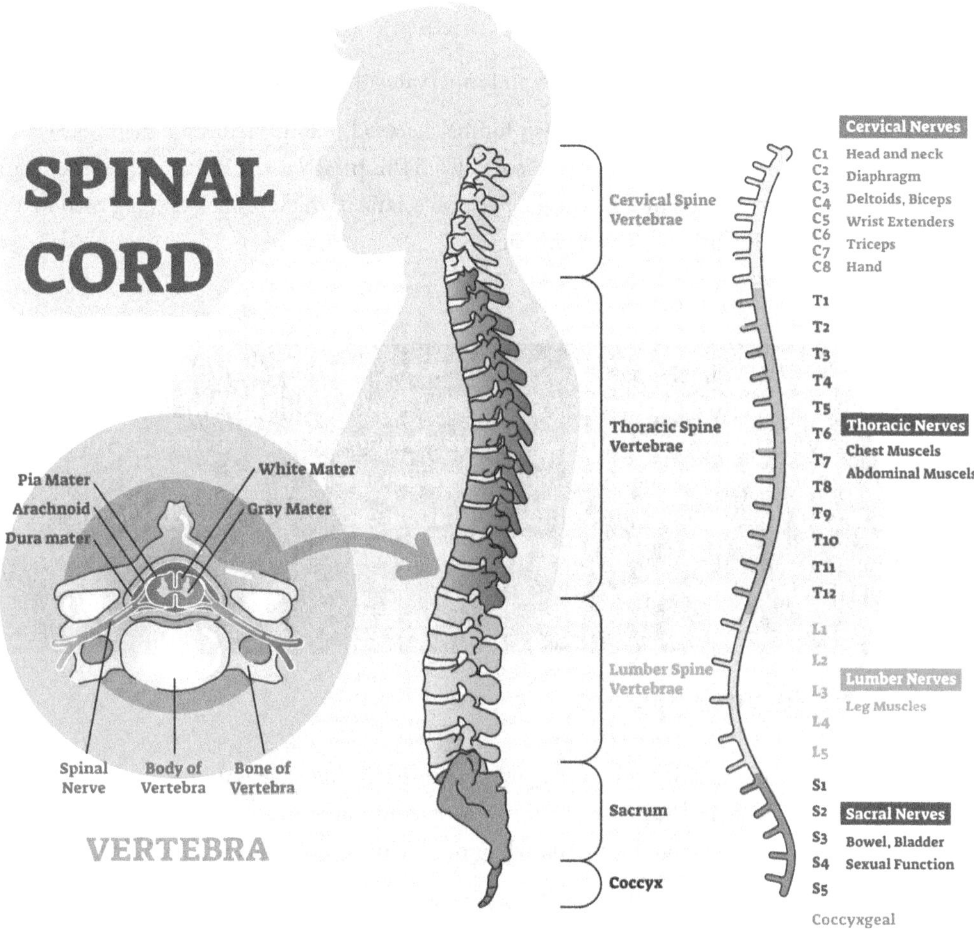

Figure 6.6 Spinal Cord and Spinal Nerves

21 "1008694237-vector.png" by *VectorMine* on *Shutterstock*. All rights reserved. Imaged used with purchased permission.

22 This work is a derivative of Anatomy & Physiology by OpenStax and is licensed under CC BY 4.0. Access for free at https://openstax.org/books/anatomy-and-physiology/pages/1-introduction

My Notes

Functions of Spinal Nerves

Each spinal nerve innervates a specific region of the body:

- C1 provides motor innervation to muscles at the base of the skull.[23]
- C2 and C3 provide both sensory and motor control to the back of the head and behind the ears.[24]
- The phrenic nerve arises from nerve roots C3, C4, and C5. This is a vital nerve because it innervates the diaphragm to enable breathing. If a patient's spinal cord is transected above C3 from an injury, then spontaneous breathing is not possible.[25]
- C5 through C8 and T1 combine to form the brachial plexus, a tangled array of nerves that serve the upper limbs and upper back.[26]
- The lumbar plexus arises from L1-L5 and innervates the pelvic region and the anterior leg.[27]
- The sacral plexus comes from the lower lumbar nerves L4 and L5 and the sacral nerves S1 to S4. The most significant systemic nerve to come from this plexus is the sciatic nerve. The sciatic nerve is associated with the painful medical condition sciatica, which is back and leg pain as a result of compression or irritation of the sciatic nerve.[28]

When a patient experiences a spinal cord injury, the degree of paralysis can be predicted by the location of the spinal cord injury. It is also important to remember when a patient has a spinal cord injury and their motor nerves are damaged, their sensory nerves may still be intact. If this occurs, the patient can still feel sensation even if they can't move the extremity. Therefore, don't assume that a paralyzed patient cannot feel pain in the affected extremity because this is not always the case.

Functions of the Nervous System

The nervous system receives information about the environment around us (sensation) and generates responses to that information (motor responses). The process of integration combines sensory perceptions and higher cognitive functions such as memories, learning, and emotion while producing a response.

---

23 This work is a derivative of Anatomy and Physiology by Boundless.com and is licensed under CC BY-SA 4.0. Access for free at https://courses.lumenlearning.com/boundless-ap/

24 This work is a derivative of Anatomy and Physiology by Boundless.com and is licensed under CC BY-SA 4.0. Access for free at https://courses.lumenlearning.com/boundless-ap/

25 This work is a derivative of Anatomy and Physiology by Boundless.com and is licensed under CC BY-SA 4.0. Access for free at https://courses.lumenlearning.com/boundless-ap/

26 This work is a derivative of Anatomy and Physiology by Boundless.com and is licensed under CC BY-SA 4.0. Access for free at https://courses.lumenlearning.com/boundless-ap/

27 This work is a derivative of Anatomy & Physiology by OpenStax and is licensed under CC BY 4.0. Access for free at https://openstax.org/books/anatomy-and-physiology/pages/1-introduction

28 This work is a derivative of Anatomy & Physiology by OpenStax and is licensed under CC BY 4.0. Access for free at https://openstax.org/books/anatomy-and-physiology/pages/1-introduction

My Notes

Sensation

Sensation is defined as receiving information about the environment. The major senses are taste, smell, touch, sight, and hearing. Additional sensory stimuli are also provided from inside the body, such as the stretch of an organ wall or the concentration of certain ions in the blood.[29]

Response

The nervous system produces a response based on the stimuli perceived by sensory nerves. For example, withdrawing a hand from a hot stove is an example of a response to a painfully hot stimulus. Responses can be classified by those that are voluntary (such as contraction of a skeletal muscle) and those that are involuntary (such as contraction of smooth muscle in the intestine). Voluntary responses are governed by the somatic nervous system, and involuntary responses are governed by the autonomic nervous system.[30]

Integration

Integration occurs when stimuli received by sensory nerves are communicated to the nervous system and the information is processed, leading to the generation of a conscious response. Consider this example of sensory integration. A batter in a baseball game does not automatically swing when they see the baseball thrown to them by the pitcher. First, the trajectory of the ball and its speed will need to be considered before creating the motor response of a swing. Then, integration will occur as the batter generates a conscious decision of whether to swing or not. Perhaps the count is three balls and one strike, and the batter decides to let this pitch go by in the hope of getting a walk to first base. Perhaps the batter is afraid to strike out and doesn't swing, or maybe the batter learned the pitcher's nonverbal cues the previous time at bat and is confident to take a swing at an anticipated fast ball. All of these considerations are included as part of the batter's integration response and the higher level functioning that occurs in the cerebral cortex.[31]

Interactive Activity

An interactive or media element has been excluded from this version of the text. You can view it online here: https://wtcs.pressbooks.pub/nursingskills/?p=1182

29 This work is a derivative of Anatomy & Physiology by OpenStax and is licensed under CC BY 4.0. Access for free at https://openstax.org/books/anatomy-and-physiology/pages/1-introduction

30 This work is a derivative of Anatomy & Physiology by OpenStax and is licensed under CC BY 4.0. Access for free at https://openstax.org/books/anatomy-and-physiology/pages/1-introduction

31 This work is a derivative of Anatomy & Physiology by OpenStax and is licensed under CC BY 4.0. Access for free at https://openstax.org/books/anatomy-and-physiology/pages/1-introduction

My Notes

6.3 NEUROLOGICAL EXAM

The neurological exam is a clinical assessment of the functioning of the central nervous system (CNS) and peripheral nervous system (PNS). See Figure 6.7[1] for an image of the anatomical underpinnings of the neurological exam. Several tests are available when performing a neurological assessment; the tests included in the assessment are selected based on the patient's medical condition and the neurological symptoms they are experiencing. The range of tests that can be included in a neurological exam include evaluation of mental status, cranial nerves, sensory functioning, motor strength, cerebellar functioning, and reflexes. The mental status exam assesses the higher cognitive functions such as memory, orientation, and language associated with the cerebrum and cerebral cortex. The cranial nerve exam tests the sensory and motor functioning of the 12 cranial nerves that connect to the diencephalon and the brain stem. The sensory response and motor strength tests evaluate functions associated with the spinal nerves. The cerebellar function tests evaluate balance, muscle tone, and coordination of voluntary movements. Deep tendon reflexes may also be used to assess the health of the nervous system.[2] Each of these components of a neurological exam is further described in the remaining sections of this chapter.

1 "1601 Anatomical Underpinnings of the Neurological Exam-02.jpg" by OpenStax is licensed under *CC BY* 3.0. Access for free at https://openstax.org/books/anatomy-and-physiology/pages/16-1-overview-of-the-neurological-exam

2 This work is a derivative of Anatomy & Physiology by OpenStax and is licensed under CC BY 4.0. Access for free at https://openstax.org/books/anatomy-and-physiology/pages/1-introduction

My Notes

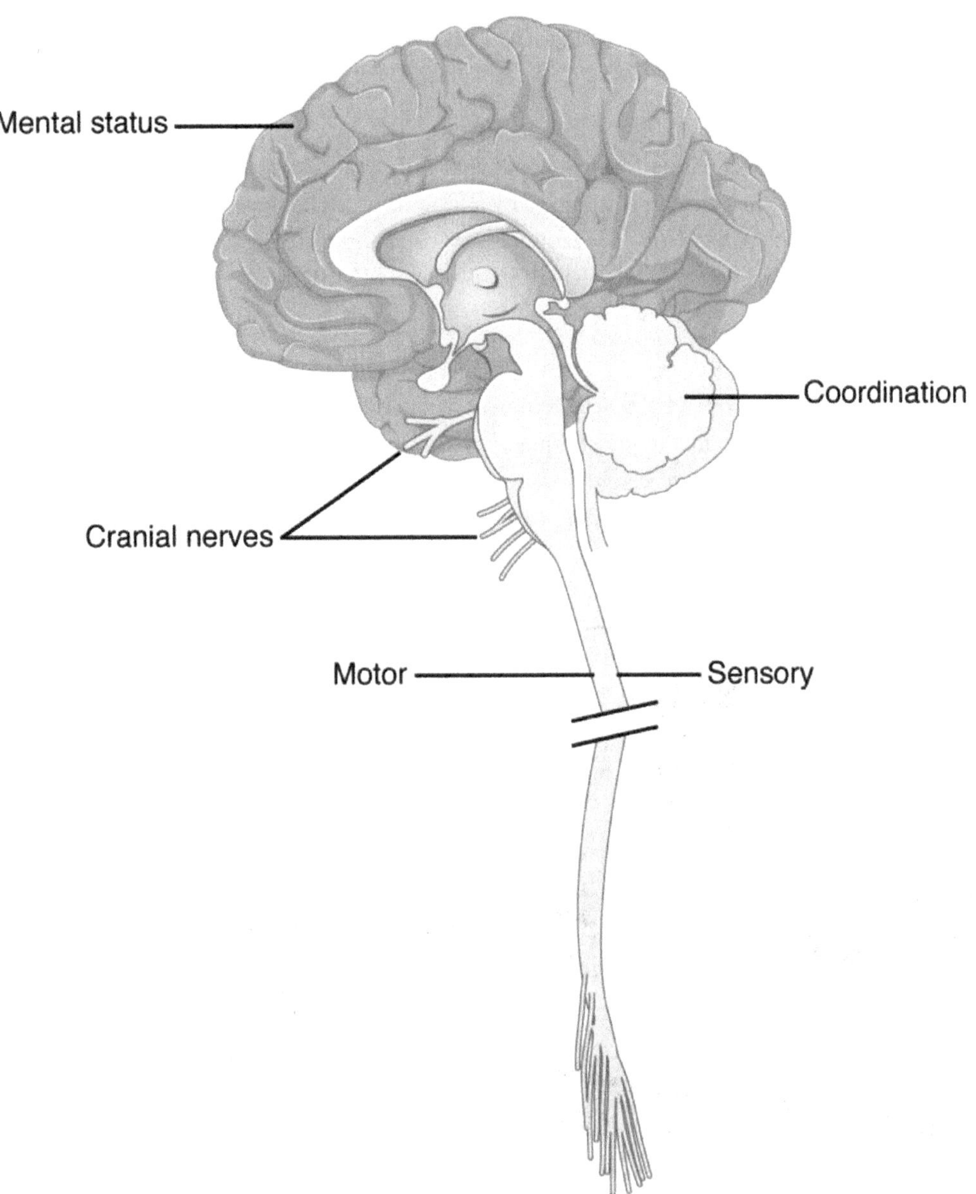

Figure 6.7 Anatomical Underpinnings of Neurological Exam

Types of Neurological Examinations

The type of neurological exam performed is based on the patient's reason for seeking care, their current medical condition, and the practice setting.

Routine Exam

Routine neurological exams performed by registered nurses during their daily clinical practice include assessing mental status and level of consciousness, pupillary response, motor strength, sensation, and gait. The Glasgow

My Notes

Coma Scale is also frequently used to objectively monitor level of consciousness in patients with neurological damage such as a head injury or cerebrovascular accident (i.e., stroke).[3]

Comprehensive

A comprehensive neurologic exam is performed on patients with a neurological concern. This exam is more extensive and may be performed in specialty settings or by advanced practice nurses. In addition to the components included in a routine neurological exam, the examiner may also assess cranial nerves, detailed cerebellar function, deep tendon reflexes, and complete a Mini-Mental State Exam (MMSE).

Periodic Reevaluation

Periodic reevaluations are performed by registered nurses when the patient has experienced an acute injury or illness causing neurological deficits that require frequent monitoring for change in condition. For example, a patient admitted to the hospital for an acute cerebrovascular accident (i.e., stroke) will have their neurological status rechecked and documented frequently according to agency policy. See Figure 6.8[4] of a nurse assessing a patient's neurological status in an intensive care unit.

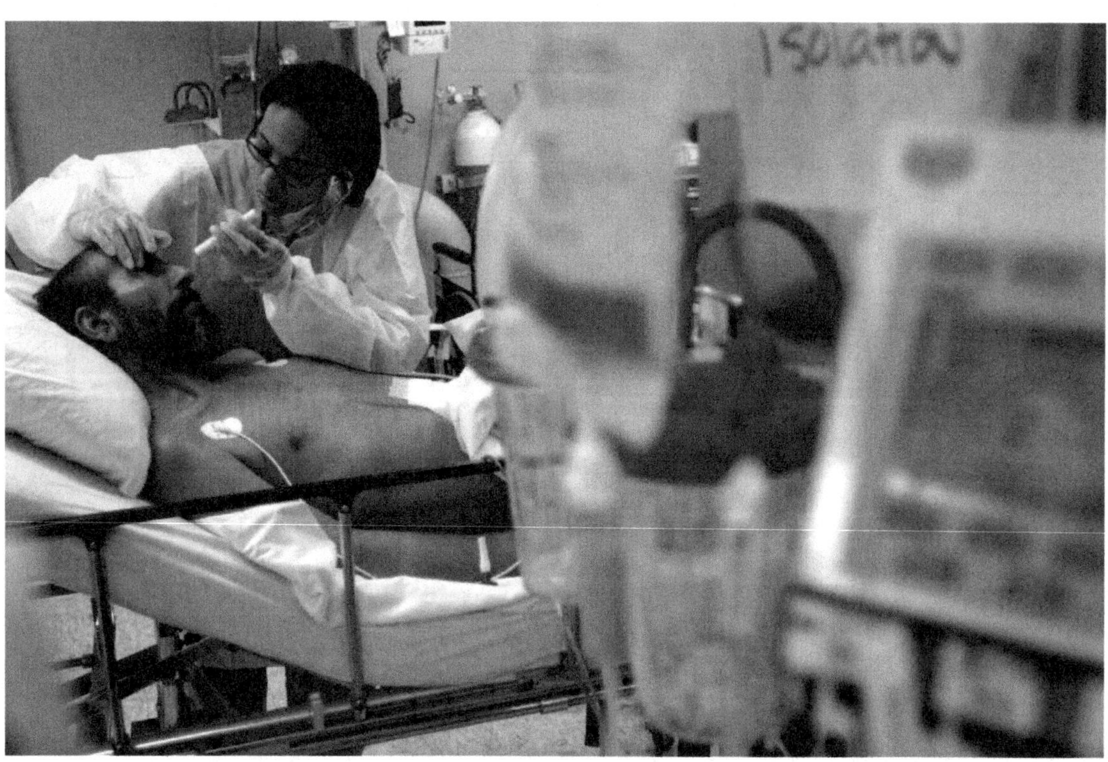

Figure 6.8 Nurse Assessing Patient's Neurological Status in ICU

---

3 Giddens, J. F. (2007). A survey of physical examination techniques performed by RNs: Lessons for nursing education. *Journal of Nursing Education, 46*(2), 83-87. https://doi.org/10.3928/01484834-20070201-09

4 "US Navy 030424-N-6967M-240 Lt. j.g. Elavonta Thomas conducts a routine check on one of the patients in the Intensive Care Units (ICU) aboard USNS Comfort (T-AH 20).jpg" by Photographer's Mate 1st Class Shane T. McCoy at U.S. Navy is in the Public Domain. Access for free at https://commons.wikimedia.org/wiki/File:US_Navy_030424-N-6967M-240_Lt._j.g._Elavonta_Thomas_conducts_a_routine_check_on_one_of_the_patients_in_the_Intensive_Care_Units_(ICU)_aboard_USNS_Comfort_(T-AH_20).jpg

6.4 ASSESSING MENTAL STATUS

My Notes

Routine assessment of a patient's mental status by registered nurses includes evaluating their level of consciousness, as well as their overall appearance, general behavior, affect and mood, general speech, and cognitive performance.[1,2] See the "General Survey Assessment" chapter for more information about an overall mental status assessment.

Level of Consciousness

Level of consciousness refers to a patient's level of arousal and alertness.[3] Assessing a patient's orientation to time, place, and person is a quick indicator of cognitive functioning. Level of consciousness is typically evaluated on admission to a facility to establish a patient's baseline status and then frequently monitored every shift for changes in condition.[4] To assess a patient's orientation status, ask, "Can you tell me your name? Where are you? What day is it?" If the patient is unable to recall a specific date, it may be helpful to ask them the day of the week, the month, or the season to establish a baseline of their awareness level.

A normal level of orientation is typically documented as, "Patient is alert and oriented to person, place, and time," or by the shortened phrase, "Alert and oriented x 3."[5] If a patient is confused, an example of documentation is, "Patient is alert and oriented to self, but disoriented to time and place."

There are many screening tools that can be used to further objectively assess a patient's mental status and cognitive impairment. Common screening tools used frequently by registered nurses to assess mental status include the Glasgow Coma Scale, the National Institutes of Health Stroke Scale (NIHSS), and the Mini-Mental State Exam (MMSE).

Glasgow Coma Scale

The Glasgow Coma Scale (GCS) is a standardized tool used to objectively assess and continually monitor a patient's level of consciousness when damage has occurred, such as after a head injury or a cerebrovascular accident (stroke). See Figure 6.9[6] for an image of the Glasgow Coma Scale. Three primary areas assessed in the GCS include eye opening, verbal response, and motor response. Scores are added from these three categories to assign a patient's level of responsiveness. Scores ranging from 15 or higher are classified as the best response, less than 8 is classified as **comatose,** and 3 or less is classified as unresponsive.

---

1 Martin, D. C. The mental status examination. In Walker, H. K., Hall, W. D., Hurst, J. W. (Eds.), *Clinical methods: The history, physical, and laboratory examinations* (3rd ed.). Butterworths. https://www.ncbi.nlm.nih.gov/books/NBK320/

2 Giddens, J. F. (2007). A survey of physical examination techniques performed by RNs: Lessons for nursing education. *Journal of Nursing Education, 46*(2), 83-87. https://doi.org/10.3928/01484834-20070201-09

3 Huntley, A. (2008). Documenting level of consciousness. *Nursing, 38*(8), 63-64. https://doi.org/10.1097/01.nurse.0000327505.69608.35

4 McDougall, G. J. (1990). A review of screening instruments for assessing cognition and mental status in older adults. *The Nurse Practitioner, 15*(11), 18–28.

5 Huntley, A. (2008). Documenting level of consciousness. *Nursing, 38*(8), 63-64. https://doi.org/10.1097/01.nurse.0000327505.69608.35

6 "glasgow-coma-scale-gcs-600w-309293585.jpg" by *joshya* on *Shutterstock*. All rights reserved. Imaged used with purchased permission.

Behaviour	Response
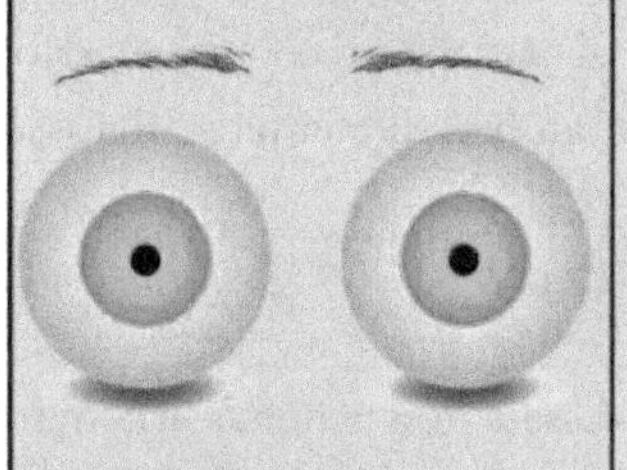 Eye Opening Response	4. Spontaneously 3. To speech 2. To pain 1. No response
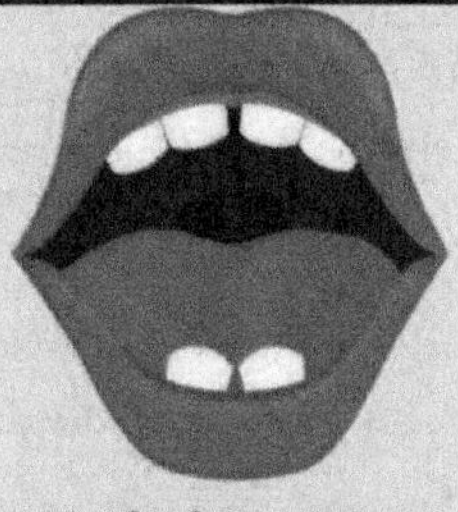 Verbal Response	5. Oriented to time, person and place 4. Confused 3. Inappropriate words 2. Incomprehensible sounds 1. No response
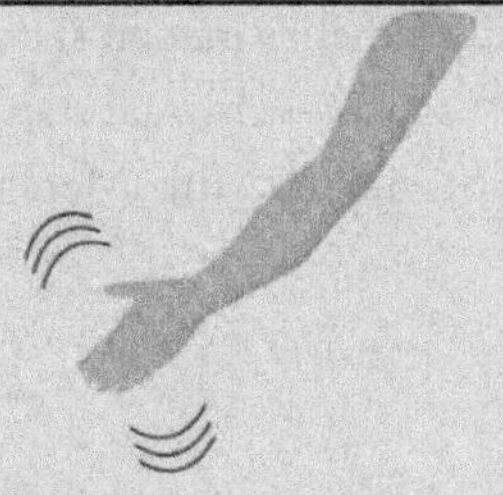 Motor Response	6. Obeys command 5. Moves to localised pain 4. Flex to withdraw from pain 3. Abnormal flexion 2. Abnormal extension 1. No response

Figure 6.9 Glasgow Coma Scale

National Institutes of Health Stroke Scale

The National Institutes of Health Stroke Scale (NIHSS) is a standardized tool that is commonly used to assess patients suspected of experiencing an acute cerebrovascular accident (i.e., stroke).[7] The three most predictive findings that occur during an acute stroke are facial drooping, arm drift/weakness, and abnormal speech. Use the following hyperlink to view the stroke scale.

A commonly used mnemonic regarding assessment of individuals suspected of experiencing a stroke is "BEFAST." BEFAST stands for **B**alance, **E**yes, **F**ace, **A**rm, and **S**peech **T**est.

- **B:** Does the person have a sudden loss of balance?
- **E:** Has the person lost vision in one or both eyes?
- **F:** Does the person's face look uneven?
- **A:** Is one arm weak or numb?
- **S:** Is the person's speech slurred? Are they having trouble speaking or seem confused?

---

7 National Institutes of Health. (n.d.). *NIH stroke scale.* https://www.stroke.nih.gov/resources/scale.htm

My Notes

- T: Time to call for assistance immediately

View the NIH Stroke Scale at the National Institutes of Health at https://www.stroke.nih.gov/resources/scale.htm

Mini-Mental Status Exam

The Mini-Mental Status Exam (MMSE) is commonly used to assess a patient's cognitive status when there is a concern of cognitive impairment. The MMSE is sensitive and specific in detecting delirium and dementia in patients at a general hospital and in residents of long-term care facilities.[8] Delirium is acute, reversible confusion that can be caused by several medical conditions such as fever, infection, and lack of oxygenation. Dementia is chronic, irreversible confusion and memory loss that impacts functioning in everyday life.

Prior to administering the MMSE, ensure the patient is wearing their glasses and/or hearing aids, if needed.[9] A patient can score up to 30 points by accurately responding and following directions given by the examiner. A score of 24-30 indicates no cognitive impairment, 18-23 indicates mild cognitive impairment, and a score less than 18 indicates severe cognitive impairment. See Figure 6.10[10] for an image of one of the questions on the MMSE regarding interlocking pentagons.

View the Mini-Mental Status Exam at www.oxfordmedicaleducation.com/geriatrics/mini-mental-state-examination-mmse

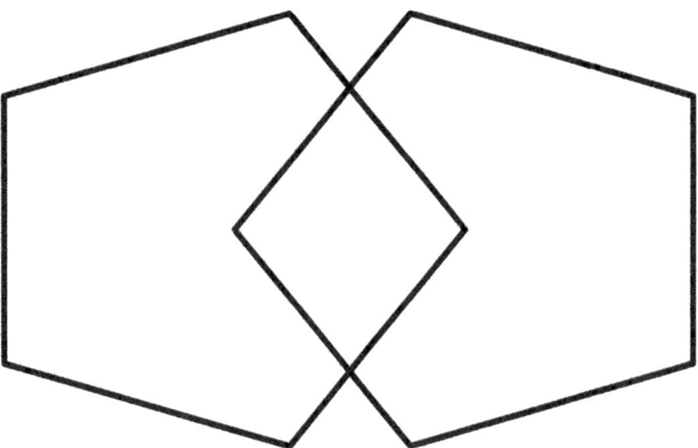

Figure 6.10 MMSE Question on Interlocking Pentagons

8 McDougall, G. J. (1990). A review of screening instruments for assessing cognition and mental status in older adults. *The Nurse Practitioner, 15*(11), 18–28.

9 Koder-Anne, D., & Klahr, A. (2010). Training nurses in cognitive assessment: Uses and misuses of the mini- mental state examination. *Educational Gerontology, 36*(10/11), 827–833. https://doi.org/10.1080/03601277.2010.485027

10 "InterlockingPentagons.svg" by Jfdwolff2 is licensed under CC BY-SA 3.0. Access for free at https://commons.wikimedia.org/wiki/File:InterlockingPentagons.svg

My Notes

6.5 ASSESSING CRANIAL NERVES

When performing a comprehensive neurological exam, examiners may assess the functioning of the cranial nerves. When performing these tests, examiners compare responses of opposite sides of the face and neck. Instructions for assessing each cranial nerve are provided below.

Cranial Nerve I – Olfactory

Ask the patient to identify a common odor, such as coffee or peppermint, with their eyes closed. See Figure 6.11[1] for an image of a nurse performing an olfactory assessment.

1 "Cranial Exam Image 11" by Meredith Pomietlo for Chippewa Valley Technical College is licensed under CC BY 4.0. Access for free at https://drive.google.com/file/d/1ln47G84bRiylffoZ8nIb2nHR89pAKlQf/view?usp=sharing

My Notes

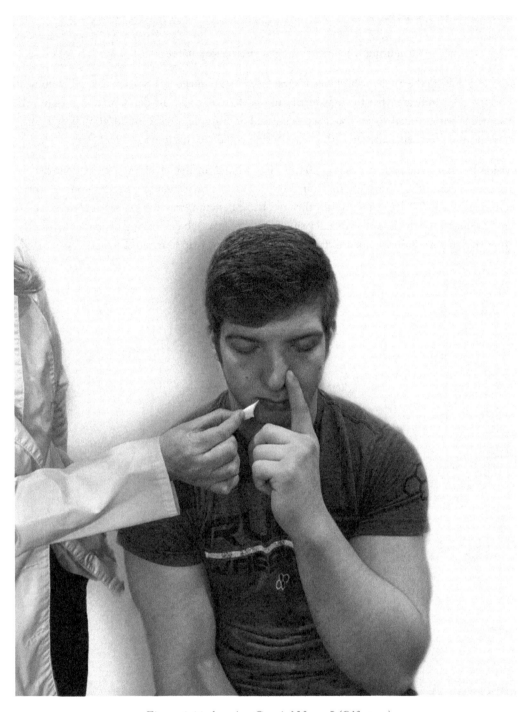

Figure 6.11 Assessing Cranial Nerve I (Olfactory)

My Notes

Cranial Nerve II – Optic

Be sure to provide adequate lighting when performing a vision assessment.

Far vision is tested using the Snellen chart. See Figure 6.12[2] for an image of a Snellen chart. The numerator of the fractions on the chart indicate what the individual can see at 20 feet, and the denominator indicates the distance at which someone with normal vision could see this line. For example, a result of 20/40 indicates this individual can see this line at 20 feet but someone with normal vision could see this line at 40 feet.

Test far vision by asking the patient to stand 20 feet away from a Snellen chart. Ask the patient to cover one eye and read the letters from the lowest line they can see.[3] Record the corresponding result in the furthermost right-hand column, such as 20/30. Repeat with the other eye. If the patient is wearing glasses or contact lens during this assessment, document the results as "corrected vision." Repeat with each eye, having the patient cover the opposite eye. Alternative charts are available for children or adults who can't read letters in English.

2 "Snellen chart.svg" by Jeff Dahl is licensed under CC BY-SA 3.0. Access for free at https://en.wikipedia.org/wiki/File:Snellen_chart.svg#file

3 Koder-Anne, D., & Klahr, A. (2010). Training nurses in cognitive assessment: Uses and misuses of the mini-mental state examination. *Educational Gerontology, 36*(10/11), 827–833. https://doi.org/10.1080/03601277.2010.485027

My Notes

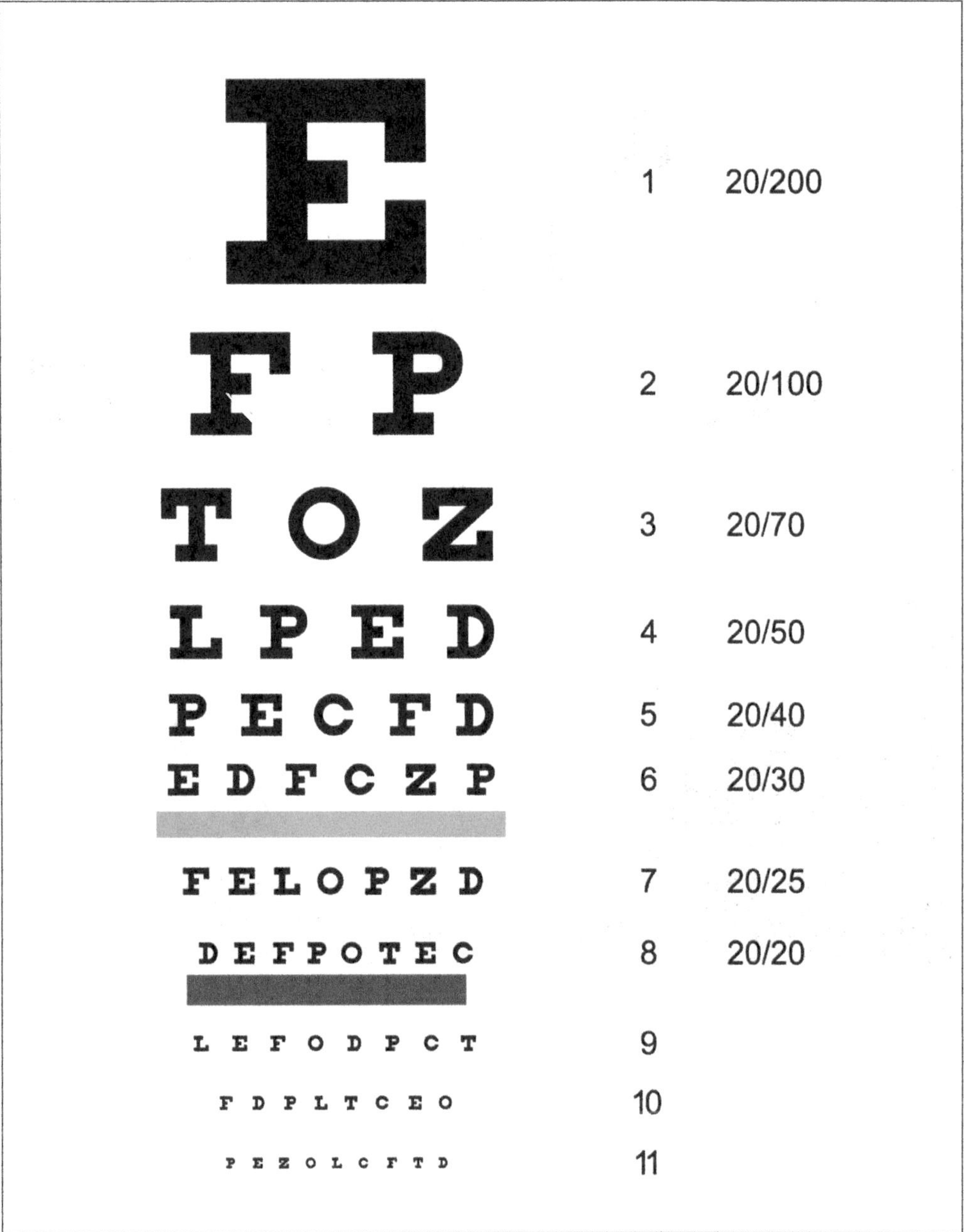

Figure 6.12 Snellen Chart

Near vision is assessed by having a patient read from a prepared card from 14 inches away. See Figure 6.13[4] for a card used to assess near vision.

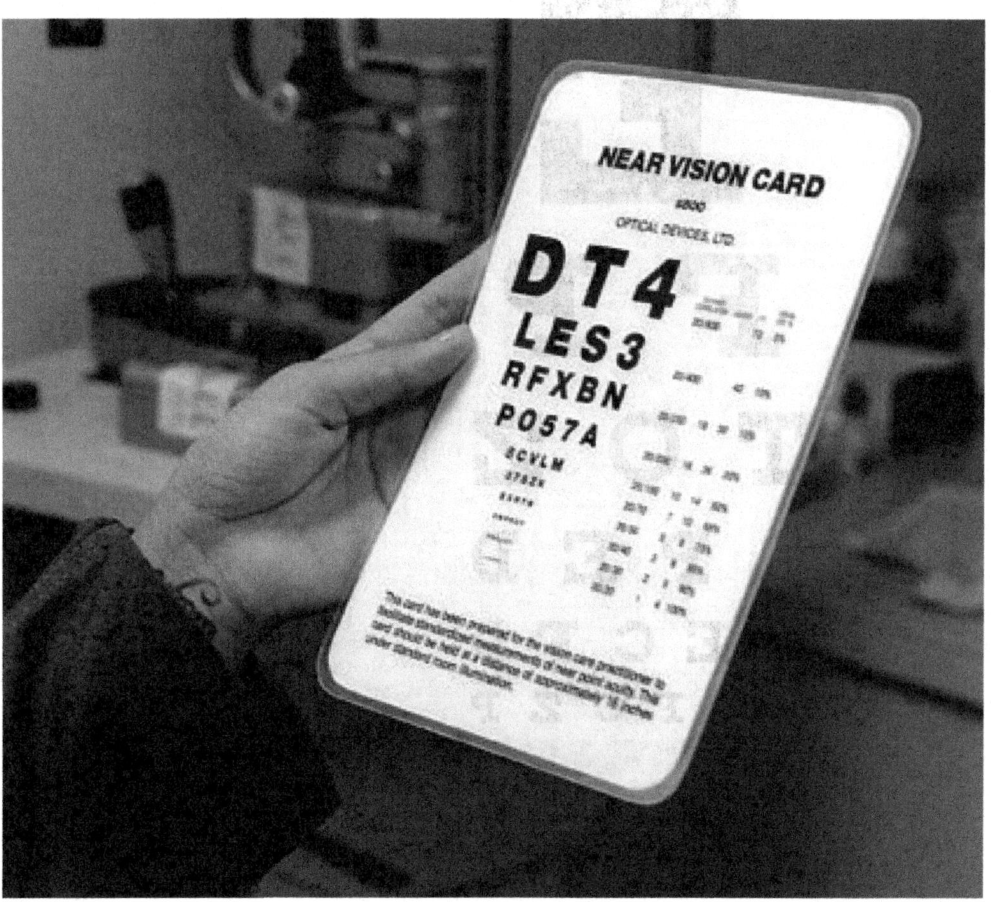

Figure 6.13 Assessing Near Vision

Cranial Nerves III, IV, and VI – Oculomotor, Trochlear, Abducens

Cranial nerves III, IV, and VI (oculomotor, trochlear, abducens nerves) are tested together.

- Test eye movement by using a penlight. Stand 1 foot in front of the patient and ask them to follow the direction of the penlight with only their eyes. At eye level, move the penlight left to right, right to left, up and down, upper right to lower left, and upper left to lower right. Watch for smooth movement of the eyes in all fields. An unexpected finding is involuntary shaking of the eye as it moves, referred to as **nystagmus**.
- Test bilateral pupils to ensure they are equally round and reactive to light and **accommodation**. Dim the lights of the room before performing this test.

4 "111012-F-ZT401-067.JPG" by Airman 1st Class Brooke P. Beers for U.S. Air Force is licensed under CC0. Access for free at https://www.pacaf.af.mil/News/Article-Display/Article/593609/keeping-sight-all-right/

My Notes

- Pupils should be round and bilaterally equal in size. The diameter of the pupils usually ranges from two to five millimeters. Emergency clinicians often encounter patients with the triad of pinpoint pupils, respiratory depression, and coma related to opioid overuse.
- Test pupillary reaction to light. Using a penlight, approach the patient from the side, and shine the penlight on one pupil. Observe the response of the lighted pupil, which is expected to quickly constrict. Repeat by shining the light on the other pupil. Both pupils should react in the same manner to light. See Figure 6.14[5] for an image of a nurse assessing a patient's pupillary reaction to light. An unexpected finding is when one pupil is larger than the other or one pupil responds more slowly than the other to light, which is often referred to as a "sluggish response."
- Test eye **convergence** and accommodation. Recall that accommodation refers to the ability of the eye to adjust from near to far vision, with pupils constricting for near vision and dilating for far vision. Convergence refers to the action of both eyes moving inward as they focus on a close object using near vision. Ask the patient to look at a near object (4-6 inches away from the eyes), and then move the object out to a distance of 12 inches. Pupils should constrict while viewing a near object and then dilate while looking at a distant object, and both eyes should move together. See Figure 6.15[6] for an image of a nurse assessing convergence and accommodation.
- The acronym PERRLA is commonly used in medical documentation and refers to, "pupils are equal, round and reactive to light and accommodation."

5 "*Cr*anial Exam Image 1" and "Pupillary Exam Image 1" by Meredith Pomietlo for Chippewa Valley Technical College are licensed under CC BY 4.0. Access for free at https://drive.google.com/file/d/1wIQwwYot62RJX-O4wq2AXysxO6YxC33a/view?usp=sharing

6 "Cranial Nerve Exam 8" and "Cranial Nerve Exam Image 3" by Meredith Pomietlo for Chippewa Valley Technical College are licensed under CC BY 4.0. Access for free at https://drive.google.com/file/d/1ccxYwIgCvq2MnEwRc0dOslVH7pQe0IhI/view?usp=sharing

My Notes

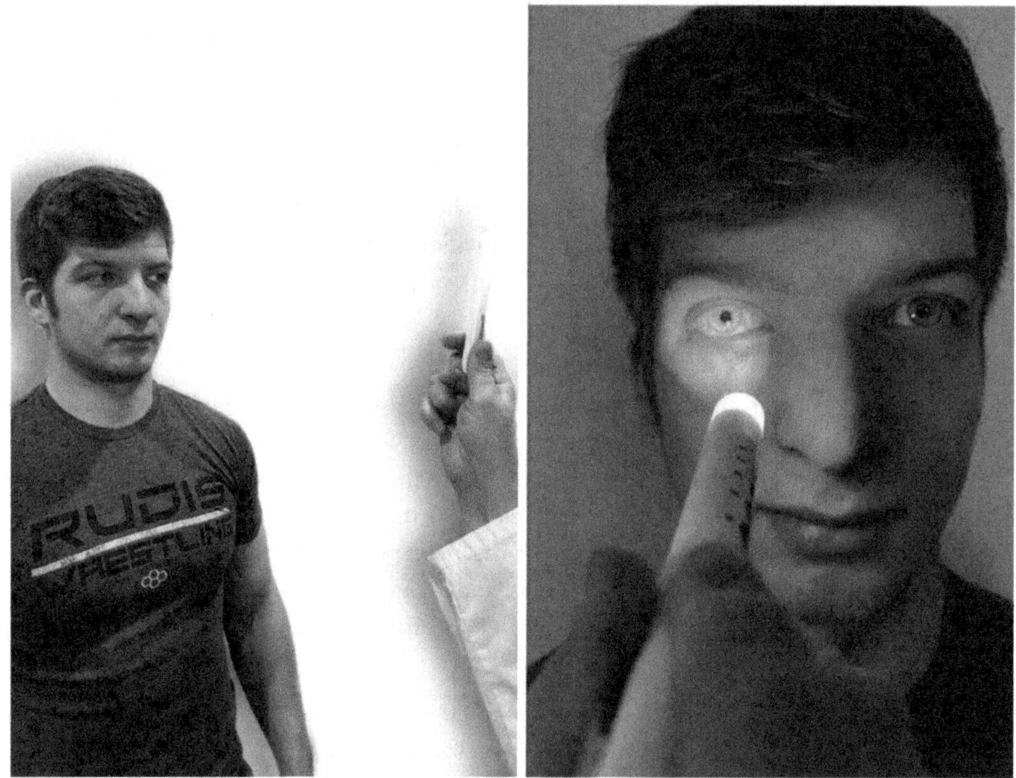

Figure 6.14 Assessing Pupillary Reaction to Light

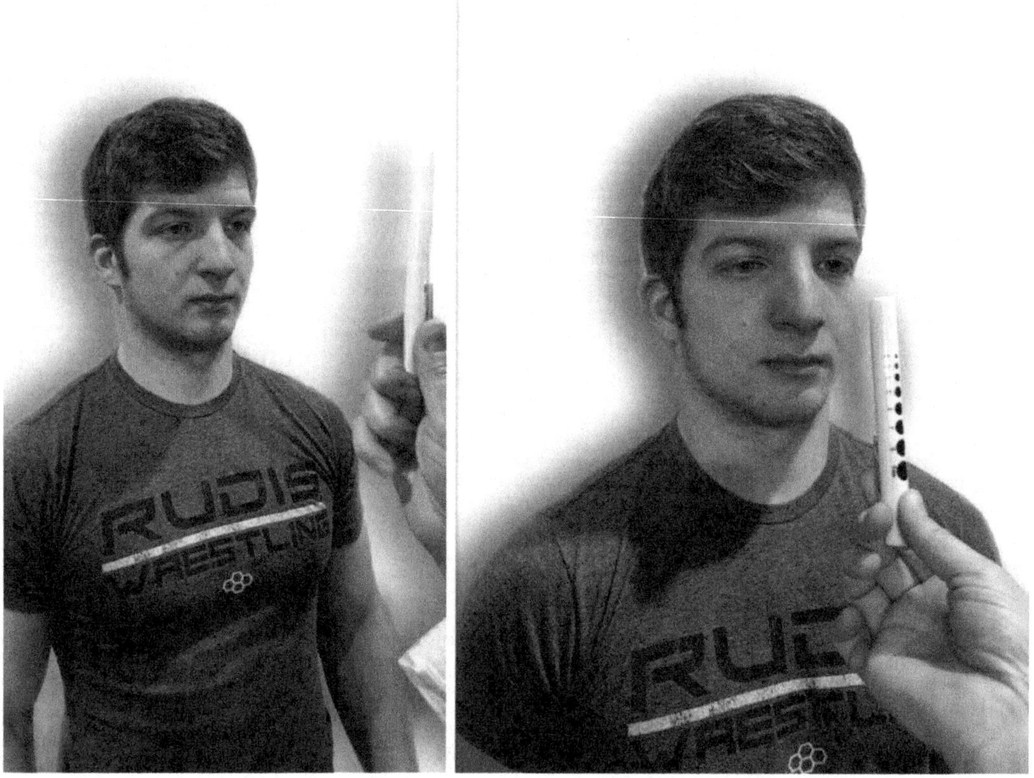

Figure 6.15 Assessing Eye Convergence and Accommodation

My Notes

Video Review for Assessment of the Cardinal Fields of Gaze[7]

6 CARDINAL FIELDS OF GAZE

A YouTube element has been excluded from this version of the text. You can view it online here: https://wtcs.pressbooks.pub/nursingskills/?p=1188

Read more details about assessing the pupillary light reflex (https://www.ncbi.nlm.nih.gov/books/NBK537180/).

7 Registered NurseRN.(2018, June 5). *Six cardinal fields of gaze nursing | Nystagmus eyes, cranial nerve 3, 4, 6, test.* [Video]. YouTube. All rights reserved. Video used with permission. https://youtu.be/lrO4pLB95p0

My Notes

Cranial Nerve V – Trigeminal

- Test sensory function. Ask the patient to close their eyes, and then use a wisp from a cotton ball to lightly touch their face, forehead, and chin. Instruct the patient to say "Now" every time they feel the placement of the cotton wisp. See Figure 6.16[8] for an image of assessing trigeminal sensory function. The expected finding is that the patient will report every instance the cotton wisp is placed. An advanced technique is to assess the corneal reflex in comatose patients by touching the cotton wisp to the cornea of the eye to elicit a blinking response.
- Test motor function. Ask the patient to clench their teeth tightly while bilaterally palpating the temporalis and masseter muscles for strength. Ask the patient to open and close their mouth several times while observing muscle symmetry. See Figure 6.17[9] for an image of assessing trigeminal motor strength. The expected finding is the patient is able to clench their teeth and symmetrically open and close their mouth.

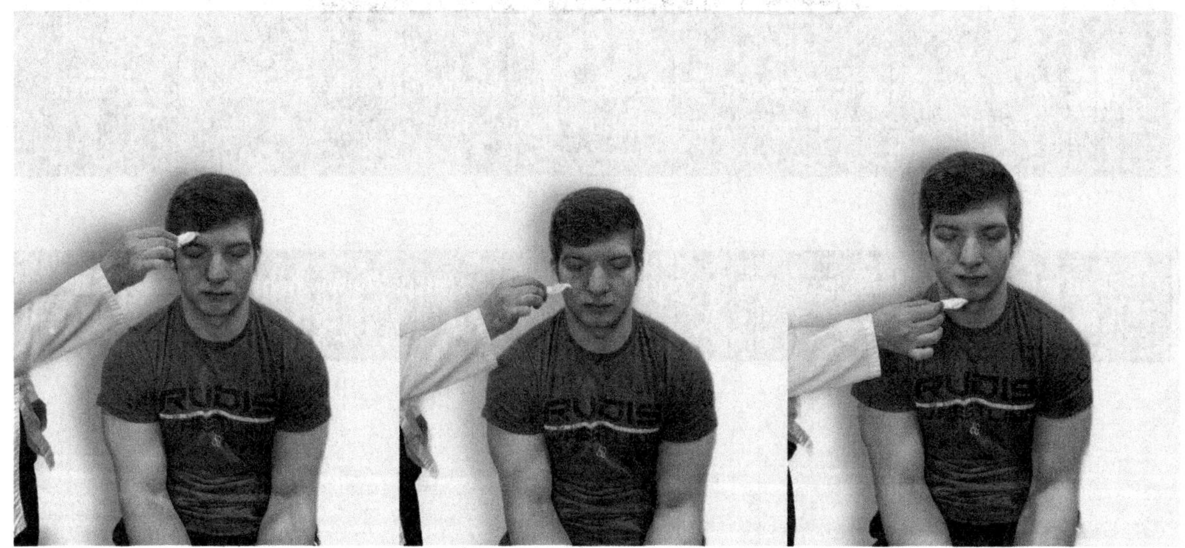

Figure 6.16 Assessing Trigeminal Sensory Function

8 "Neuro Exam Image 28," "Cranial Exam Image 12," and Neuro Exam Image 36" by Meredith Pomietlo for Chippewa Valley Technical College are licensed under CC BY 4.0. Access for free at https://drive.google.com/file/d/1uhZ9vs2sJ1mQuvcX8TdEL8C6CiS3uyc-/view?usp=sharing

9 "Cranial Exam Image 11," "Neuro Exam Image 35," and "Neuro Exam Image 4" by Meredith Pomietlo for Chippewa Valley Technical College are licensed under CC BY 4.0. Access for free at https://drive.google.com/file/d/1ln47G84bRiylffoZ8nIb2nHR89pAKlQf/view?usp=sharing

My Notes

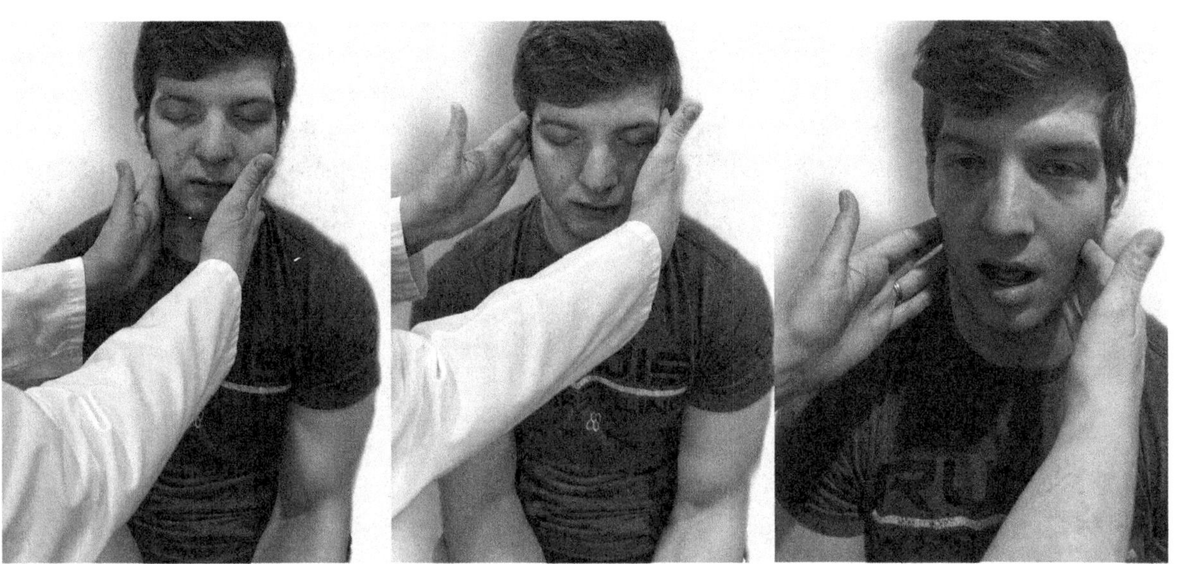

Figure 6.17 Assessing Trigeminal Motor Function

Cranial Nerve VII – Facial Nerve

- Test motor function. Ask the patient to smile, show teeth, close both eyes, puff cheeks, frown, and raise eyebrows. Look for symmetry and strength of facial muscles. See Figure 6.18[10] for an image of assessing motor function of the facial nerve.
- Test sensory function. Test the sense of taste by moistening three different cotton applicators with salt, sugar, and lemon. Touch the patient's anterior tongue with each swab separately, and ask the patient to identify the taste. See Figure 6.19[11] for an image of assessing taste.

---

10 "Cranial Exam image 15.png," "Cranial Exam Image 7.png," and "Cranial Exam Image 10.png" by Meredith Pomietlo for Chippewa Valley Technical College are licensed under CC BY 4.0. Access for free at https://drive.google.com/file/d/1o5xdSEA9D7T8IlYCV6NOKL0SNeA6rIEf/view?usp=sharing

11 "Neuro Exam Image 17.png" by Meredith Pomietlo for Chippewa Valley Technical College is licensed under CC BY 4.0. Access for free at https://drive.google.com/file/d/1xJdQdT7G7uIJK64iRGShsOTr1ZyOAyMu/view?usp=sharing

My Notes

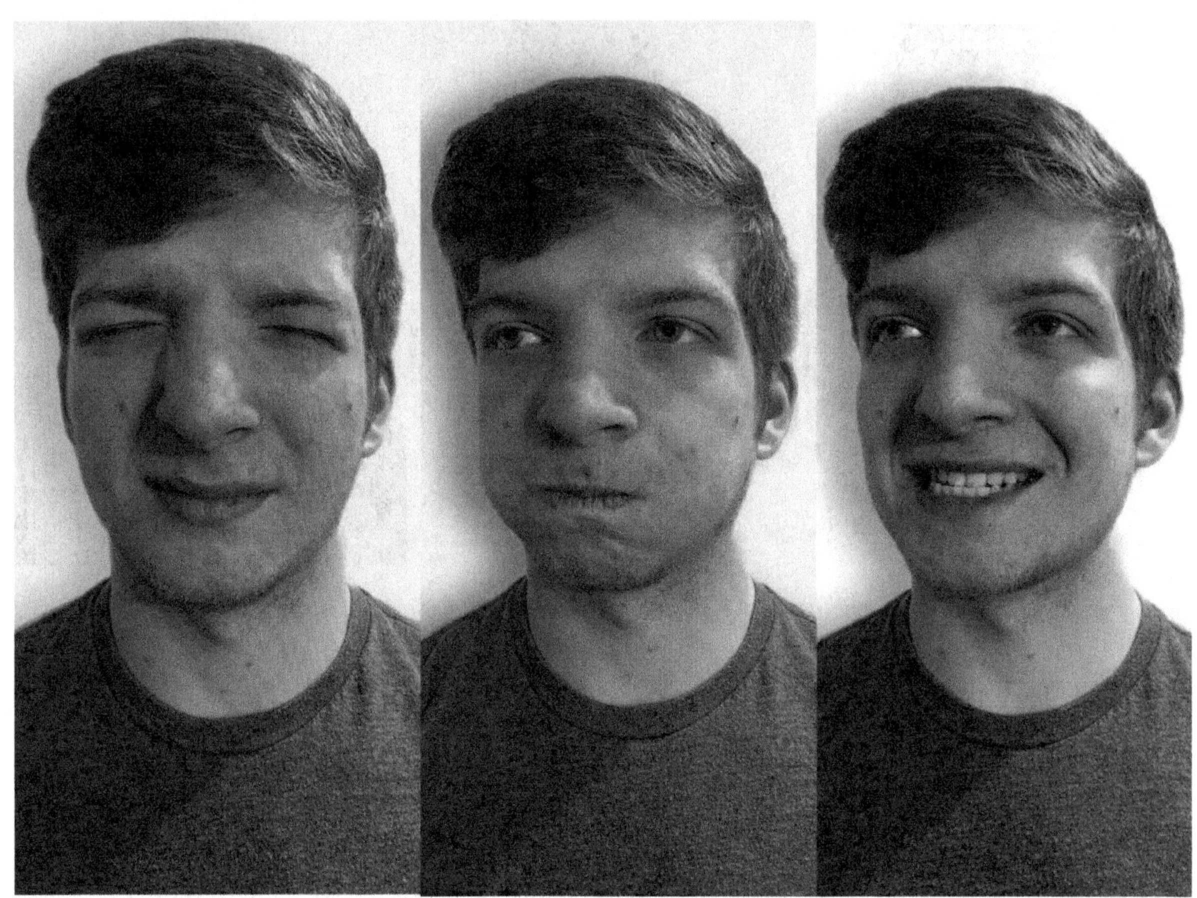

Figure 6.18 Assessing Motor Function of Facial Nerve

My Notes

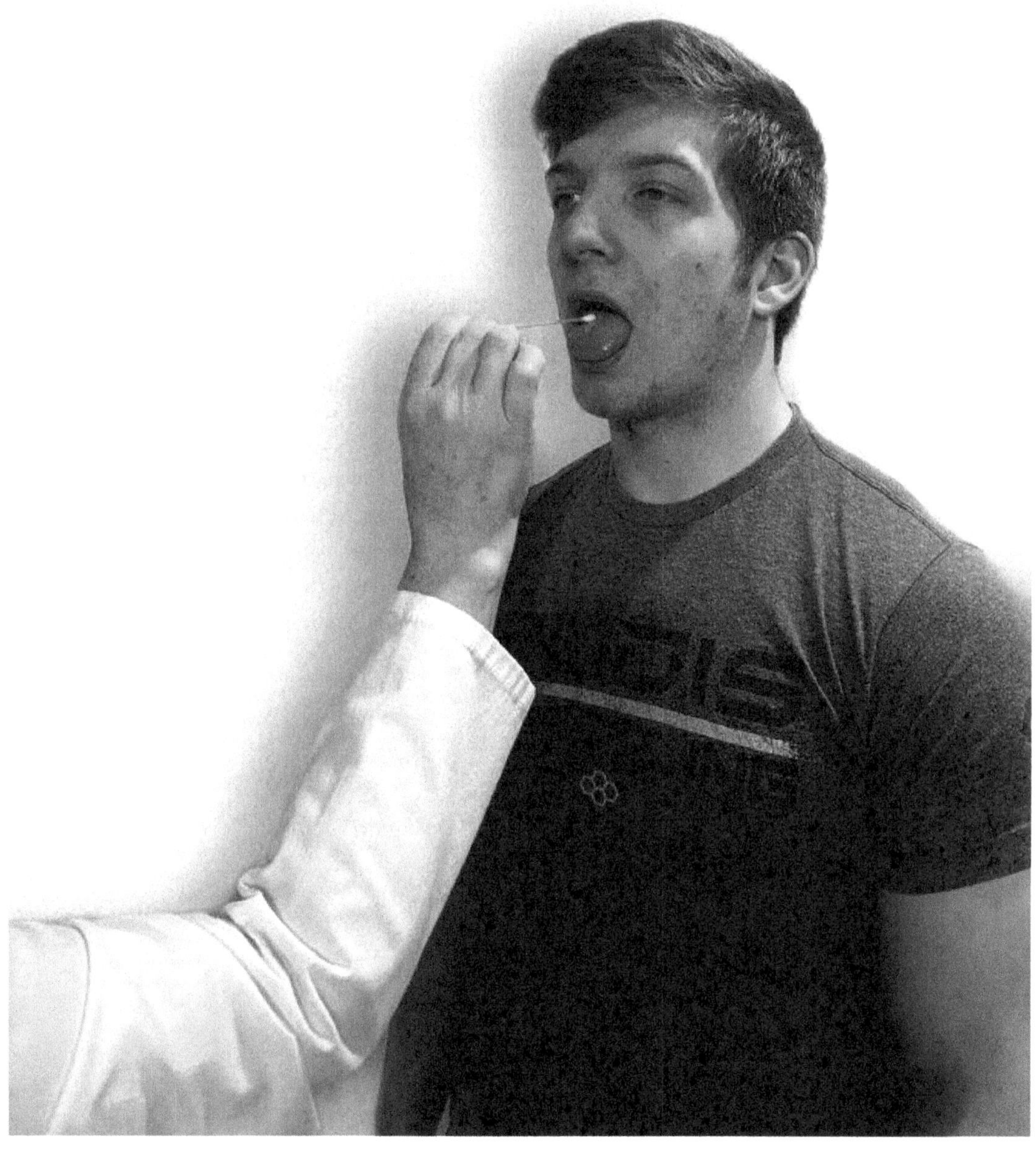

Figure 6.19 Assessing Sensory Function of Facial Nerve

My Notes

Cranial Nerve VIII – Vestibulocochlear

- Test auditory function. Perform the whispered voice test. The whispered voice test is a simple test for detecting hearing impairment if done accurately. See Figure 6.20[12] for an image assessing hearing using the whispered voice test. Complete the following steps to accurately perform this test:
    - Stand at arm's length behind the seated patient to prevent lip reading.
    - Each ear is tested individually. The patient should be instructed to occlude the non-test ear with their finger.
    - Exhale before whispering and use as quiet a voice as possible.
    - Whisper a combination of numbers and letters (for example, 4-K-2), and then ask the patient to repeat the sequence.
    - If the patient responds correctly, hearing is considered normal; if the patient responds incorrectly, the test is repeated using a different number/letter combination.
    - The patient is considered to have passed the screening test if they repeat at least three out of a possible six numbers or letters correctly.
    - The other ear is assessed similarly with a different combination of numbers and letters.
- Test balance. The Romberg test is used to test balance and is also used as a test for driving under the influence of an intoxicant. See Figure 6.21[13] for an image of the Romberg test. Ask the patient to stand with their feet together and eyes closed. Stand nearby and be prepared to assist if the patient begins to fall. It is expected that the patient will maintain balance and stand erect. A positive Romberg test occurs if the patient sways or is unable to maintain balance. The Romberg test is also a test of the body's sense of positioning (proprioception), which requires healthy functioning of the spinal cord.

12 "Whisper Test Image 1.png" by Meredith Pomietlo for Chippewa Valley Technical College is licensed under CC BY 4.0. Access for free at https://drive.google.com/file/d/1aYvKi0xI5LSNpSf_O5fdR457SX6RpDOd/view?usp=sharing

13 "Neuro Exam Image 9.png" by Meredith Pomietlo for Chippewa Valley Technical College is licensed under CC BY 4.0. Access for free at https://drive.google.com/file/d/1uBLxc54aHNbHHOvdBw_cLbITi-Znrrjl/view?usp=sharing

My Notes

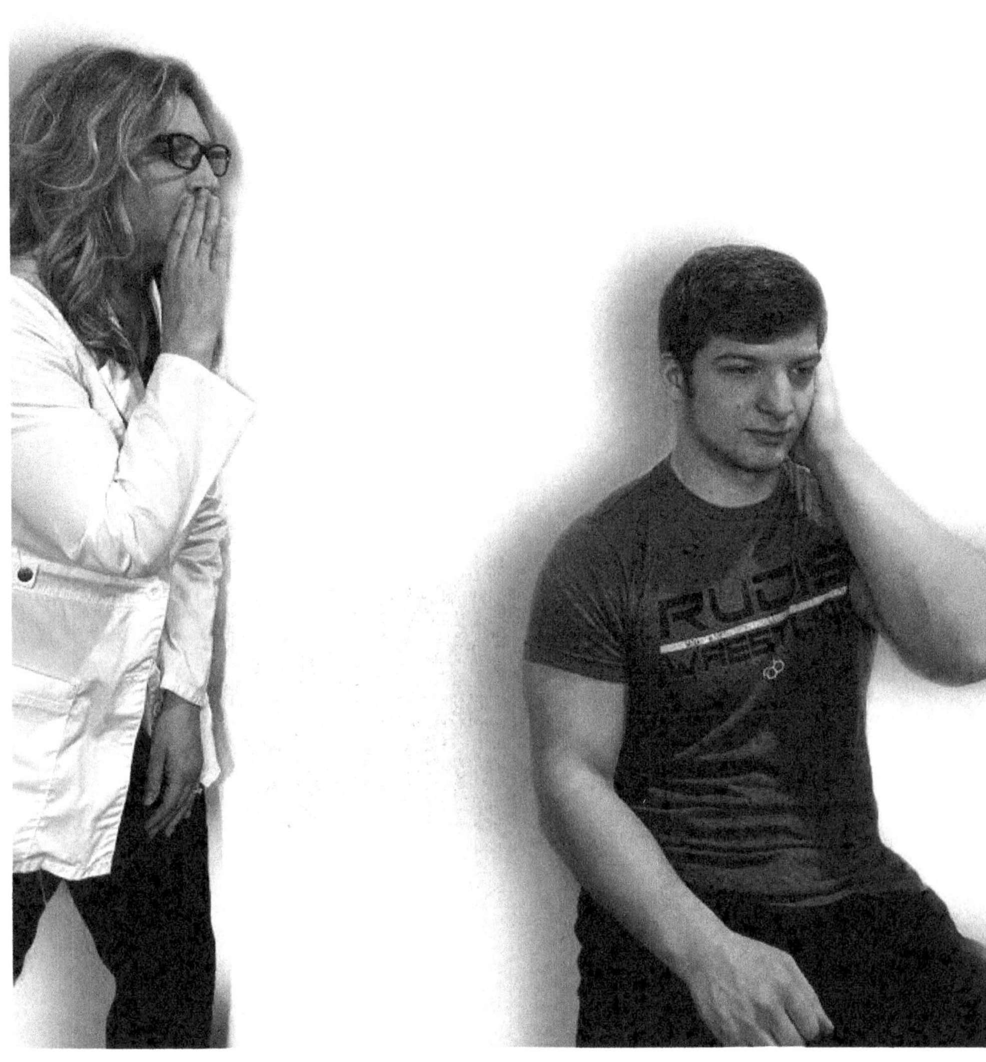

Figure 6.20 Assessing Auditory Function

My Notes

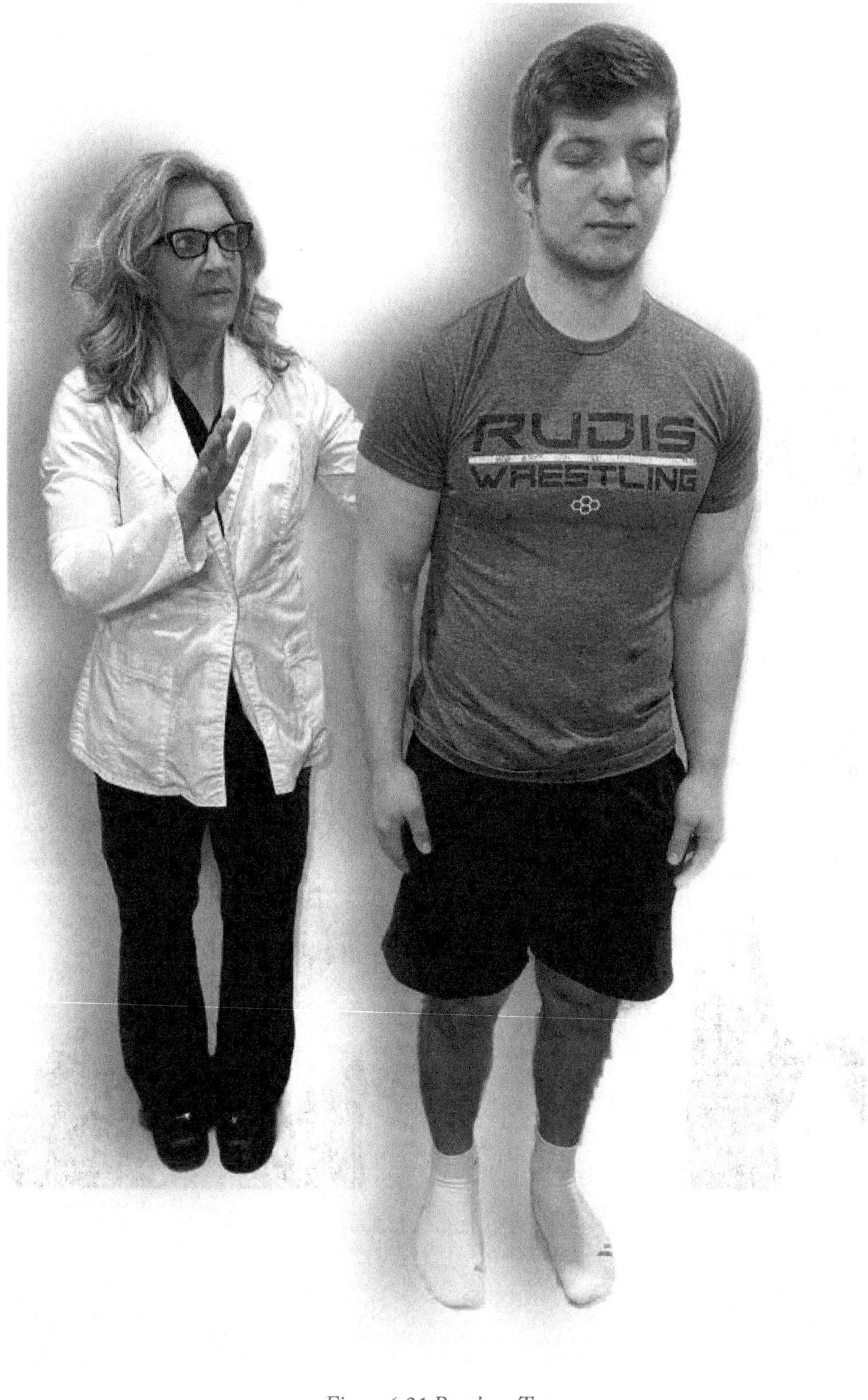

Figure 6.21 Romberg Test

Cranial Nerve IX – Glossopharyngeal

My Notes

Ask the patient to open their mouth and say "Ah" and note symmetry of the upper palate. The uvula and tongue should be in a midline position and the uvula should rise symmetrically when the patient says "Ah." (see Figure 6.22[14]).

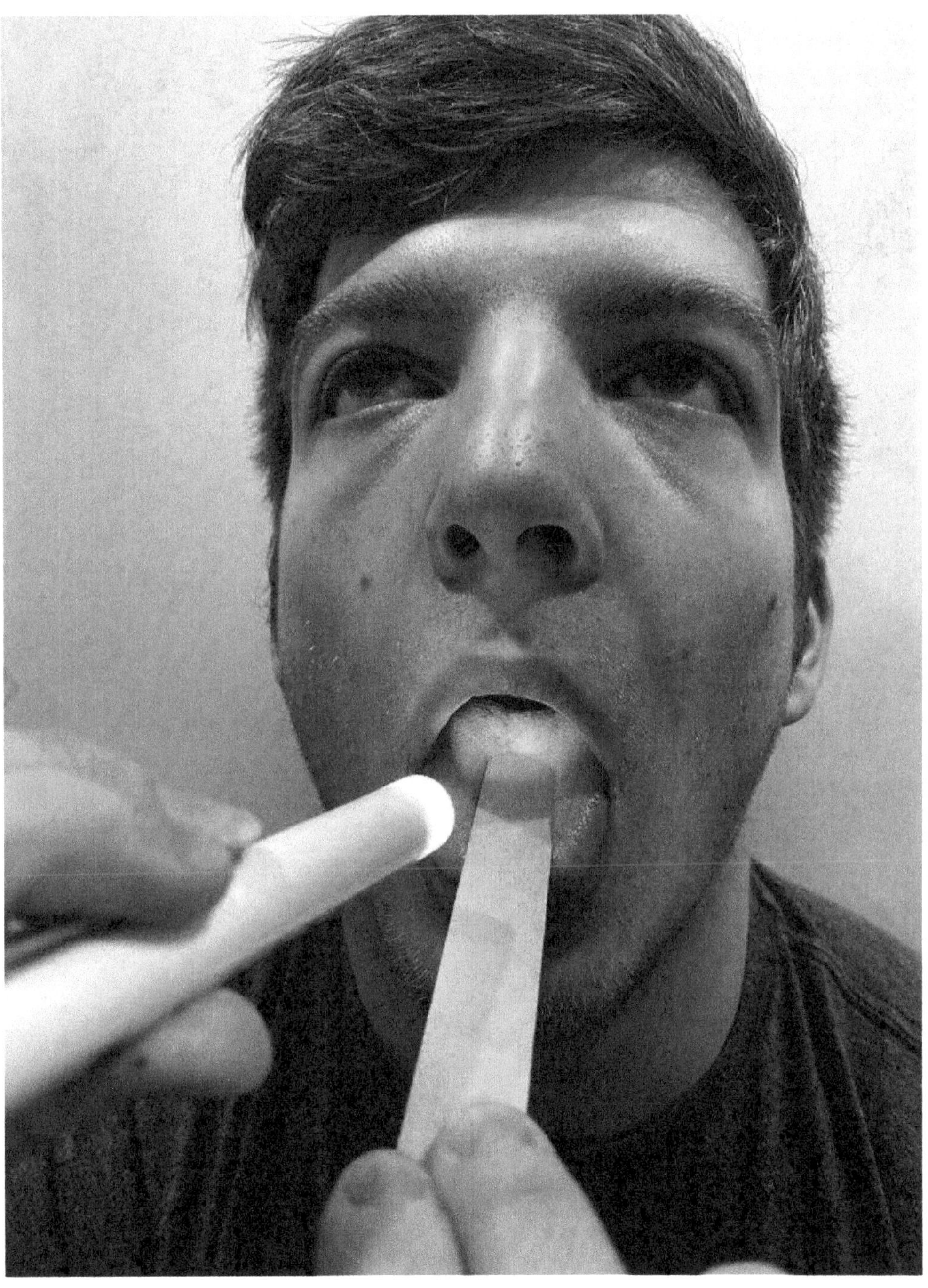

Figure 6.22 Assessing Glossopharyngeal Nerve

14 "Oral Exam Image 2.png" by Meredith Pomietlo for Chippewa Valley Technical College is licensed under CC BY 4.0. Access for free at https://drive.google.com/file/d/1-wb1lTuI92zwXVW2ikvIqjwtcVen7zis/view?usp=sharing

My Notes

Cranial Nerve X – Vagus

Use a cotton swab or tongue blade to touch the patient's posterior pharynx and observe for a gag reflex followed by a swallow. The glossopharyngeal and vagus nerves work together for integration of gag and swallowing. See Figure 6.23[15] for an image of assessing the gag reflex.

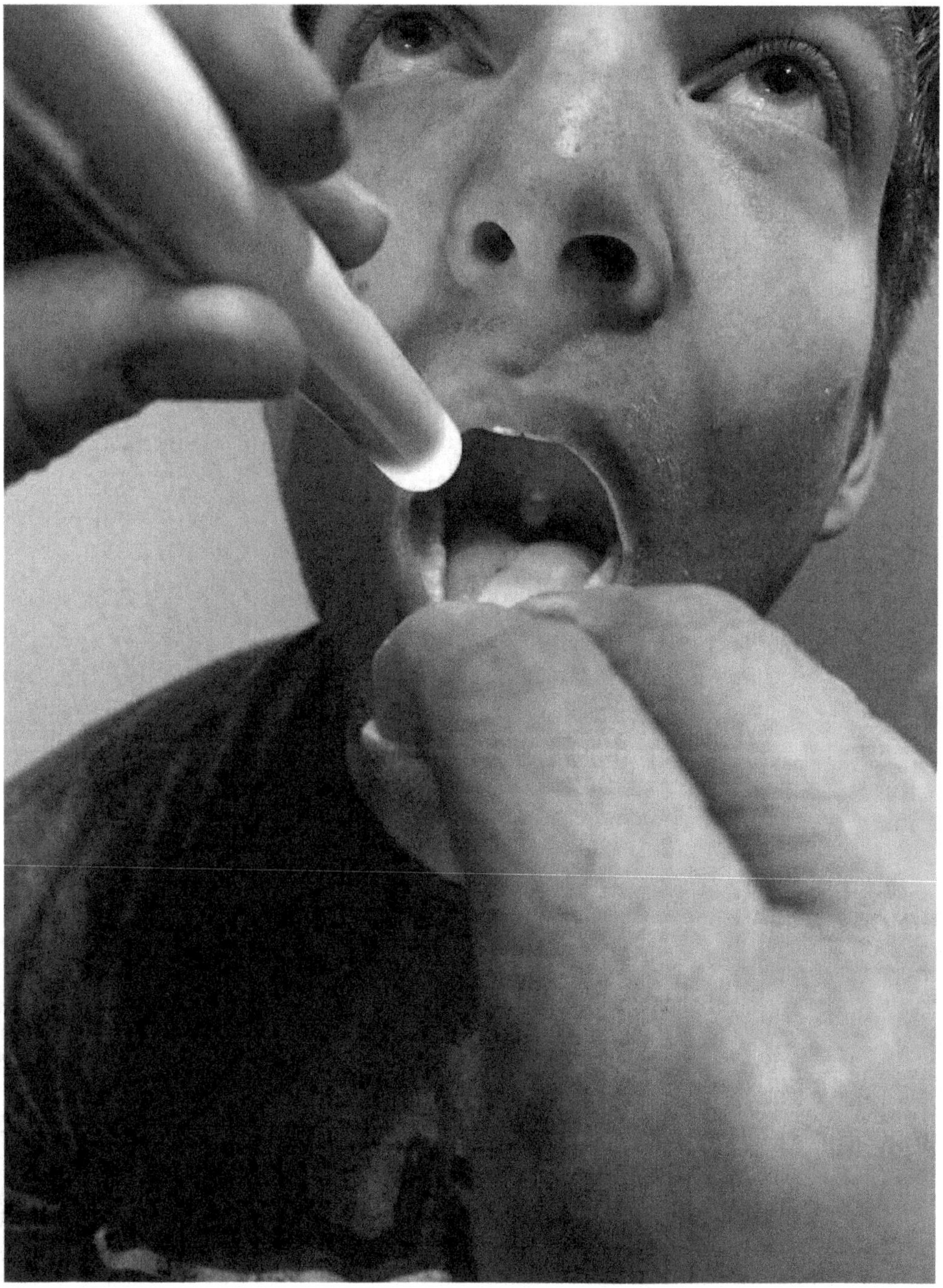

Figure 6.23 Observing the Gag Reflex

15 "Oral Exam.png" by Meredith Pomietlo for Chippewa Valley Technical College is licensed under CC BY 4.0 Access for free at https://drive.google.com/file/d/1R8sGr_5lRnYNzg3kutZc1SWqcVq8cS9C/view?usp=sharing

Cranial Nerve XI – Spinal Accessory

My Notes

Test the right sternocleidomastoid muscle. Face the patient and place your right palm laterally on the patient's left cheek. Ask the patient to turn their head to the left while resisting the pressure you are exerting in the opposite direction. At the same time, observe and palpate the right sternocleidomastoid with your left hand. Then reverse the procedure to test the left sternocleidomastoid.

Continue to test the sternocleidomastoid by placing your hand on the patient's forehead and pushing backward as the patient pushes forward. Observe and palpate the sternocleidomastoid muscles.

Test the trapezius muscle. Ask the patient to face away from you and observe the shoulder contour for hollowing, displacement, or winging of the scapula and observe for drooping of the shoulder. Place your hands on the patient's shoulders and press down as the patient elevates or shrugs the shoulders and then retracts the shoulders.[16] See Figure 6.24[17] for an image of assessing the trapezius muscle.

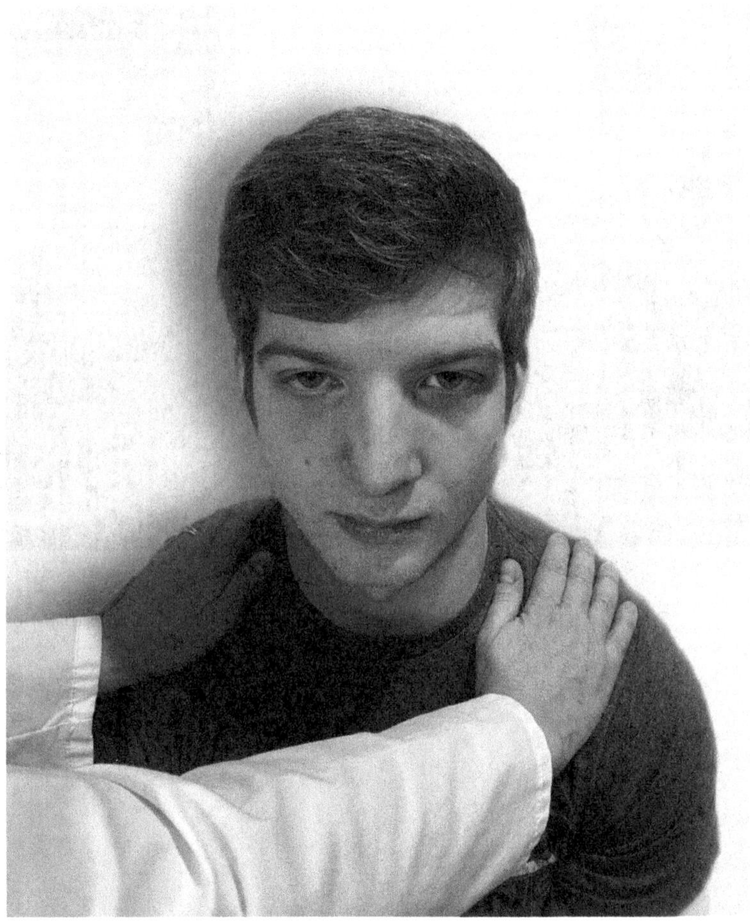

Figure 6.24 Assessing Cranial Nerve XI

16 Walker, H. K. Cranial nerve XI: The spinal accessory nerve. In Walker, H. K., Hall, W. D., Hurst, J. W. (Eds.), *Clinical methods: The history, physical, and laboratory examinations (3rd ed.).* Butterworths. https://www.ncbi.nlm.nih.gov/books/NBK387/

17 "Neuro Exam image 10" by Meredith Pomietlo for Chippewa Valley Technical College is licensed under CC BY 4.0. Access for free at https://drive.google.com/file/d/1U-b8FFMCtXcuT-CoGWupMRvp8venXgW2/view?usp=sharing

My Notes

Cranial Nerve XII – Hypoglossal

Ask the patient to protrude the tongue. If there is unilateral weakness present, the tongue will point to the affected side due to unopposed action of the normal muscle. An alternative technique is to ask the patient to press their tongue against their cheek while providing resistance with a finger placed on the outside of the cheek. See Figure 6.25[18] for an image of assessing the hypoglossal nerve.

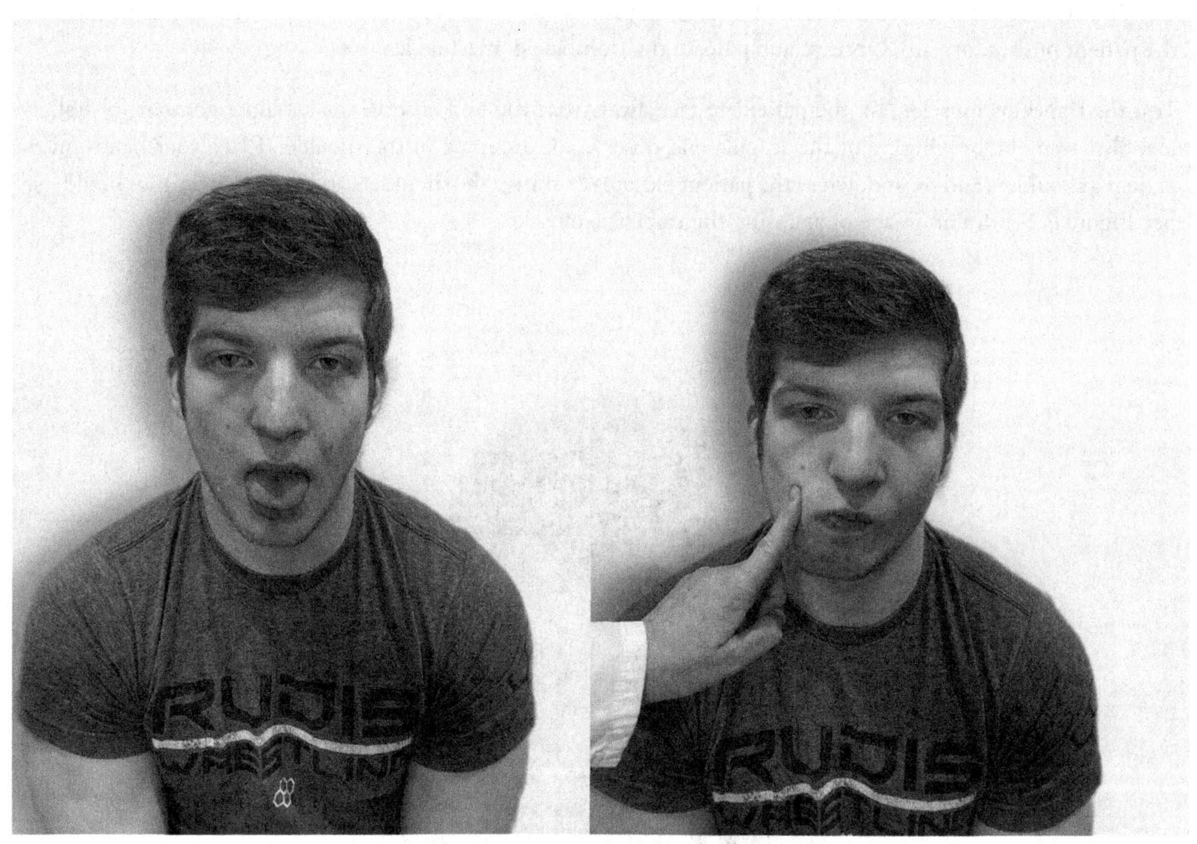

Figure 6.25 Assessing the Hypoglossal Nerve

18 "Cranial Nerve Exam Image 9.png" and "Cranial Nerve Exam Image 11.png" by Meredith Pomietlo for Chippewa Valley Technical College are licensed under CC BY 4.0. Access for free at https://drive.google.com/file/d/12O3njF-ongtVqc3K-f7-4dd7DVL6svXI/view?usp=sharing and https://drive.google.com/file/d/1wwqTCOki2nqgTfIJIqNbMYbfcE9A7ScC/view?usp=sharing

My Notes

Video Review of Cranial Nerve Assessment[19]

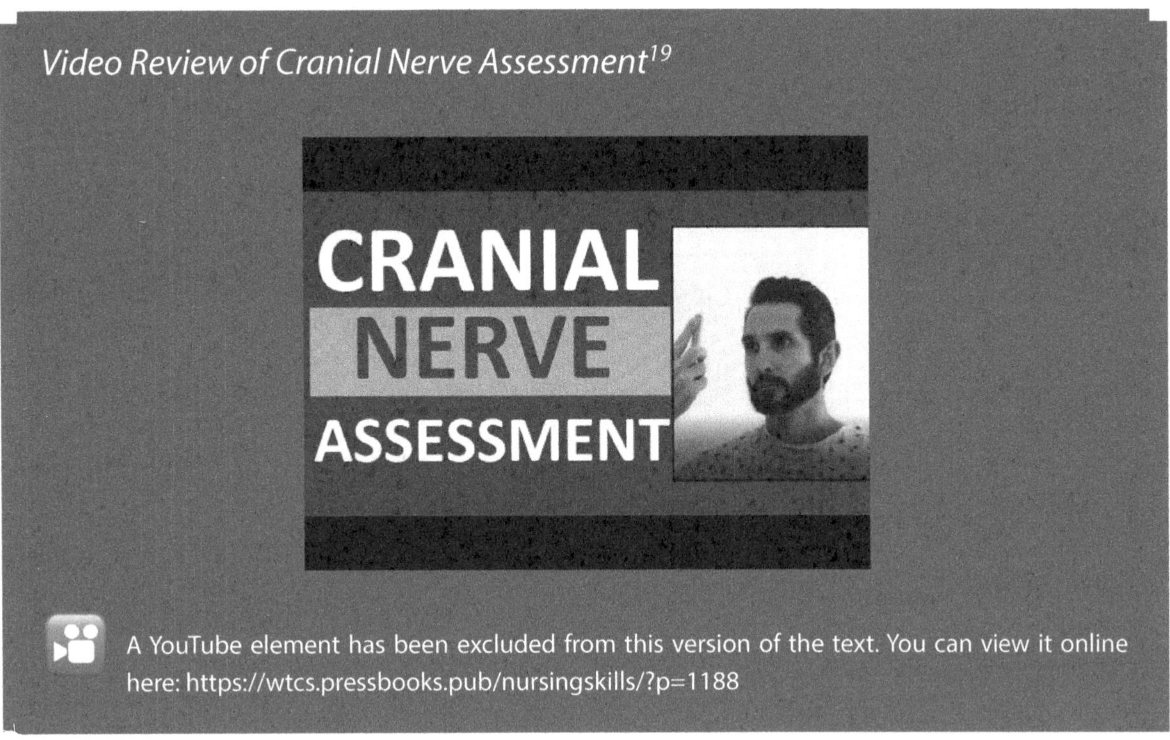

A YouTube element has been excluded from this version of the text. You can view it online here: https://wtcs.pressbooks.pub/nursingskills/?p=1188

Expected Versus Unexpected Findings

See Table 6.5 for a comparison of expected versus unexpected findings when assessing the cranial nerves.

Table 6.5 Expected Versus Unexpected Findings of an Adult Cranial Nerve Assessment

Cranial Nerve	Expected Finding	Unexpected Finding (Dysfunction)
I. Olfactory	Patient is able to describe odor.	Patient has inability to identify odors (**anosmia**).
II. Optic	Patient has 20/20 near and far vision.	Patient has decreased visual acuity and visual fields.
III. Oculomotor	Pupils are equal, round, and reactive to light and accommodation.	Patient has different sized or reactive pupils bilaterally.
IV. Trochlear	Both eyes move in the direction indicated as they follow the examiner's penlight.	Patient has inability to look up, down, inward, outward, or diagonally. **Ptosis** refers to drooping of the eyelid and may be a sign of dysfunction.

19 RegisteredNurseRN. (2018, April 8). *Cranial nerve examination nursing | Cranial nerve assessment I-XII (1-12).* [Video]. YouTube. All rights reserved. Video used with permissions. https://youtu.be/oZGFrwogx14

My Notes

Cranial Nerve	Expected Finding	Unexpected Finding (Dysfunction)
V. Trigeminal	Patient feels touch on forehead, maxillary, and mandibular areas of face and chews without difficulty.	Patient has weakened muscles responsible for chewing; absent corneal reflex; and decreased sensation of forehead, maxillary, or mandibular area.
VI. Abducens	Both eyes move in coordination.	Patient has inability to look side to side (lateral); patient reports **diplopia** (double vision).
VII. Facial	Patient smiles, raises eyebrows, puffs out cheeks, and closes eyes without difficulty; patient can distinguish different tastes.	Patient has decreased ability to taste. Patient has facial **paralysis** or asymmetry of face such as facial droop.
VIII. Vestibulocochlear (Acoustic)	Patient hears whispered words or finger snaps in both ears; patient can walk upright and maintain balance.	Patient has decreased hearing in one or both ears and decreased ability to walk upright or maintain balance.
IX. Glossopharyngeal	Gag reflex is present.	Gag reflex is not present; patient has **dysphagia**.
X. Vagus	Patient swallows and speaks without difficulty.	Slurred speech or difficulty swallowing is present.
XI. Spinal Accessory	Patient shrugs shoulders and turns head side to side against resistance.	Patient has inability to shrug shoulders or turn head against resistance.
XII. Hypoglossal	Tongue is midline and can be moved without difficulty.	Tongue is not midline or is weak.

6.6 ASSESSING SENSORY FUNCTION

My Notes

The sensory function exam tests the somatic senses, meaning those senses that are consciously perceived. Assessing sensory function includes two components, the sensory response that occurs when stimuli are perceived by afferent nerves in the peripheral nervous system and the cortical processing that occurs in the cerebral cortex of the brain.

Sensory Response

Testing of peripheral sensation begins with examining the response to light touch according to regions of the skin known as dermatomes. A **dermatome** is an area of the skin that is supplied by a single spinal nerve that sends information to the brain for processing. See Figure 6.26[1] for an illustration of color-coded dermatomes according to their associated spinal nerves. See more information about spinal nerves in the "Basic Neurological Concepts" section.

To test the sensory fields, ask the patient to close their eyes, and then gently touch the soft end of a cotton-tipped applicator on random locations of the skin according to the dermatome region. Instruct the patient to report "Now" when feeling the placement of the applicator. If a patient is unable to feel the sensation of a cotton applicator, an advanced technique is to use ice or even the prick of a pin in comatose patients.

1 "1611 Dermatomes-02.jpg" by OpenStax Anatomy and Physiology is licensed under CC BY 4.0. Access for free at https://openstax.org/books/anatomy-and-physiology/pages/16-4-the-sensory-and-motor-exams

My Notes

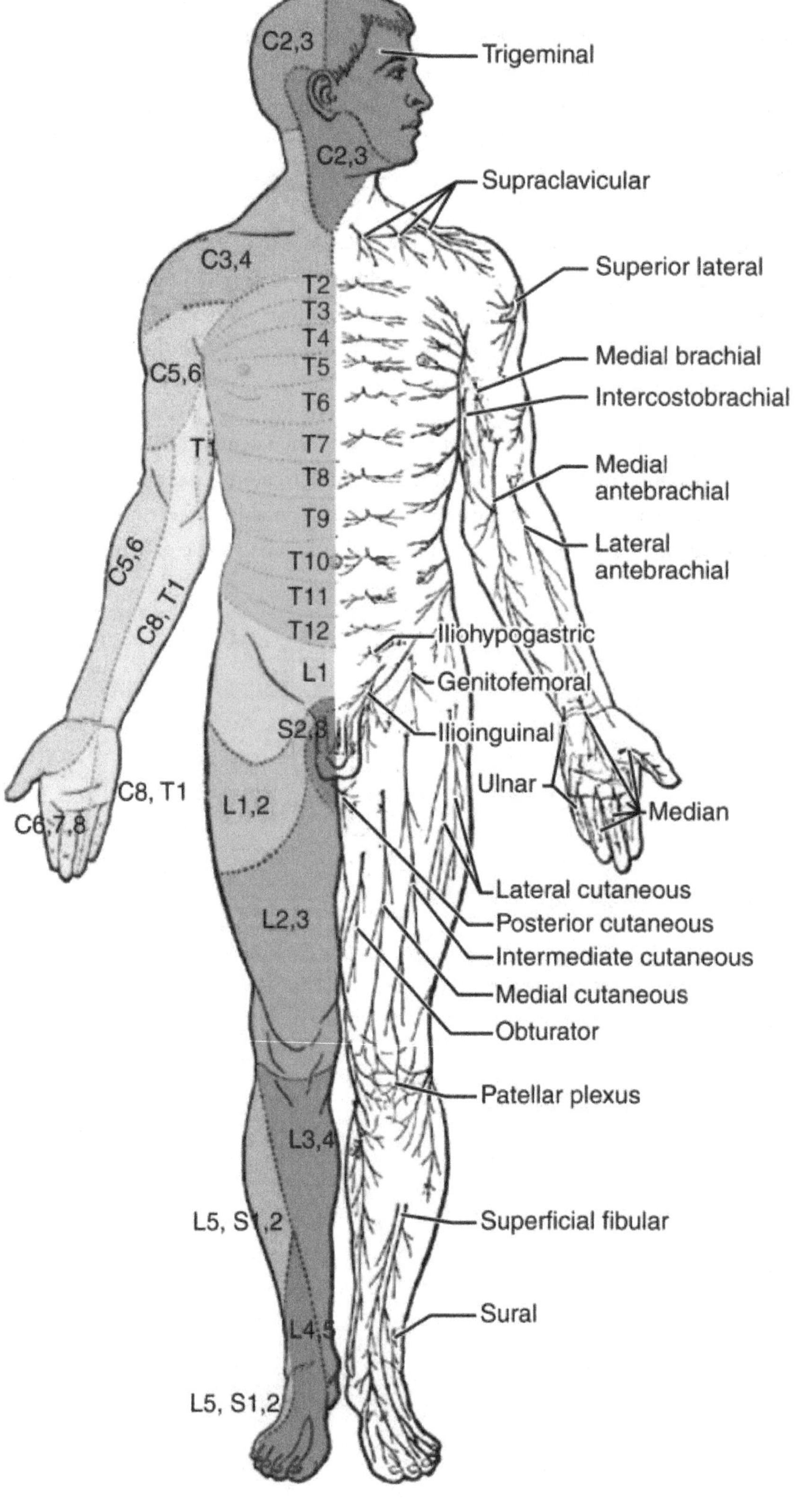

Figure 6.26 Dermatomes

My Notes

It is not necessary to test every part of the skin's surface during a routine neurological exam; testing a few distal areas with light touch is usually sufficient. In-depth testing is performed when the patient is exhibiting neurological symptoms such as motor deficits, numbness, tingling, and weakness. See Figure 6.27[2] demonstrating assessment of the sensory response.

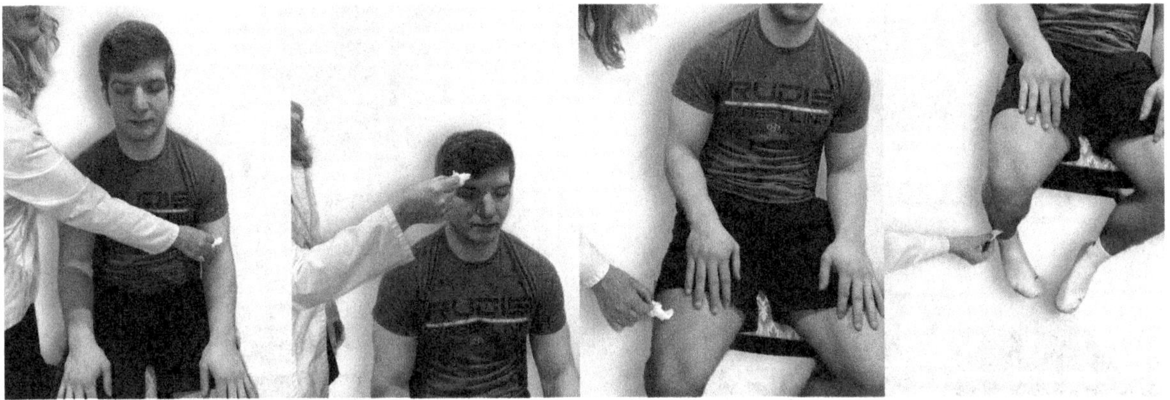

Figure 6.27 Assessing Sensory Response

Cortical Processing

Cortical processing that occurs in the cerebral cortex of the parietal lobe is assessed using stereogenesis. **Stereognosis** is the ability to perceive the physical form and identity of a familiar object such as a key or paper clip based on tactile stimuli alone.[3] The person typically uses the finger to move the object around and then correctly names the object.

To perform the stereognosis test, ask the patient to close their eyes; then place a familiar object in their hand and ask them to name it. Each hand should be tested with a different object. See Figure 6.28[4] for an image of a patient being tested for stereognosis.

Graphesthesia tests assess both cortical sensation and primary sensation. Graphesthesia is the ability to recognize a tracing on the skin while using the sensation of touch. To test graphesthesia, trace a number or letter on the patient's outstretched palm and ask them to identify it.

---

2 "Neuro Exam Image 25," "Cranial Exam Image 12," "Neuro Exam Image 26," and "Neuro Exam Image 30" by Meredith Pomietlo for Chippewa Valley Technical College are licensed under CC BY 4.0. Access for free at https://drive.google.com/file/d/141xEe5UYL7iG_4Y8GoUSjQ7siujGf4PF/view?usp=sharing, https://drive.google.com/file/d/1_3J14r_tCksJKyAUThP9n06rhI6QuGOA/view?usp=sharing, https://drive.google.com/file/d/18xHlicG_yeL4RsVswSkDtZLJVLrw4JBB/view?usp=sharing, and https://drive.google.com/file/d/1ZITMukfPAi0Urj3_KbQwjkcJYz6jg2g_/view?usp=sharing

3 This work is a derivative of StatPearls by Schermann and Tadi and is licensed under CC BY 4.0. Access for free at https://www.ncbi.nlm.nih.gov/books/NBK430685/

4 "Neuro Exam Image 8.png" and "Neuro Exam Image 31.png" by Meredith Pomietlo for Chippewa Valley Technical College are licensed under CC BY 4.0. Access for free at https://drive.google.com/file/d/1b1-pomSthDhQIQ8PFf_a0GxYGcetRuvj/view?usp=sharing and https://drive.google.com/file/d/1LuEidjvKim8NVWNgmooTFFbMCwp0KZ3-/view?usp=sharing

My Notes

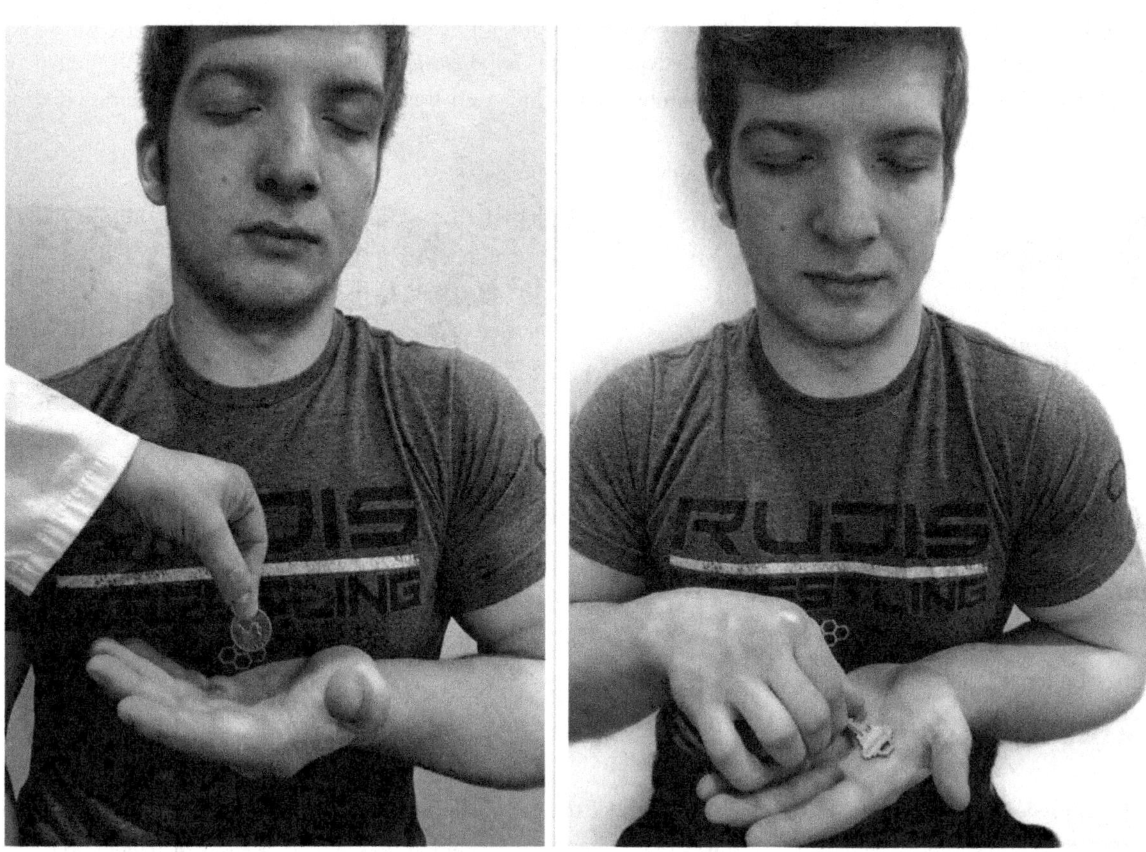

Figure 6.28 Assessing Stereognosis

6.7 ASSESSING MOTOR STRENGTH

My Notes

A brief musculoskeletal assessment is performed as part of the neurological assessment to determine the neurological stimulation of bilateral strength. Read more details about muscles and musculoskeletal assessment in the "Musculoskeletal Assessment" chapter. Unequal extremity motor strength can indicate underlying neurological disease or injury. Assessing motor strength includes comparing bilateral hand grasps, upper extremity strength, and lower extremity strength. Keep in mind that extremities on the dominant side are usually slightly stronger than the nondominant side.

Hand Grasps

To perform a hand grasp test, extend two fingers on both hands toward the patient. Ask the patient to squeeze both of your hands and compare for similar bilateral strength. See Figure 6.29[1] for an image of assessing hand grasp strength.

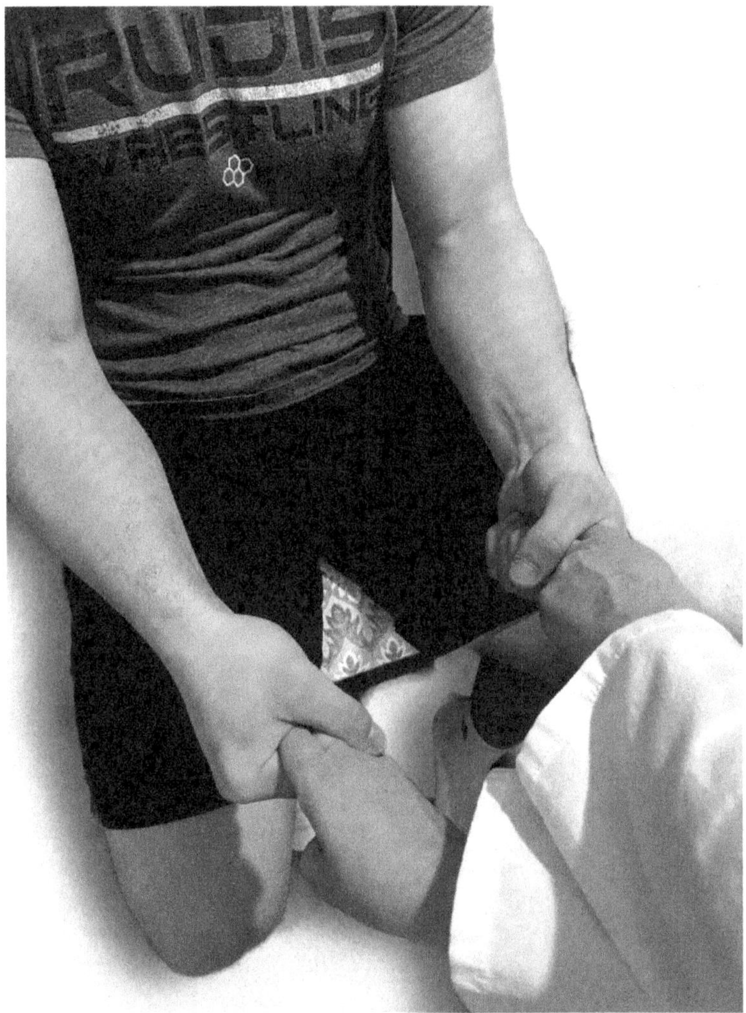

Figure 6.29 Assessing for Equal Strength in Bilateral Hand Grasps

1 "Neuro Exam Image 38.png" by Meredith Pomietlo for Chippewa Valley Technical College is licensed under CC BY 4.0. Access for free at https://drive.google.com/file/d/1D37Qu5ljGyly3xO61vqUGeQv3Zx13g9I/view?usp=sharing

My Notes

Upper Extremity Strength

To test upper extremity strength, ask the patient to extend their forearms with palms facing upwards. Place your hands on their inner forearms and ask them to pull their arms toward them while you provide resistance. An expected finding is the patient strongly bilaterally pulls against resistance with both arms.

An alternative test is to ask the patient to put their hands in the air with their palms facing you. Place your palms against theirs and ask them to push while you provide resistance. See Figure 6.30[2] for an image of assessing upper body strength.

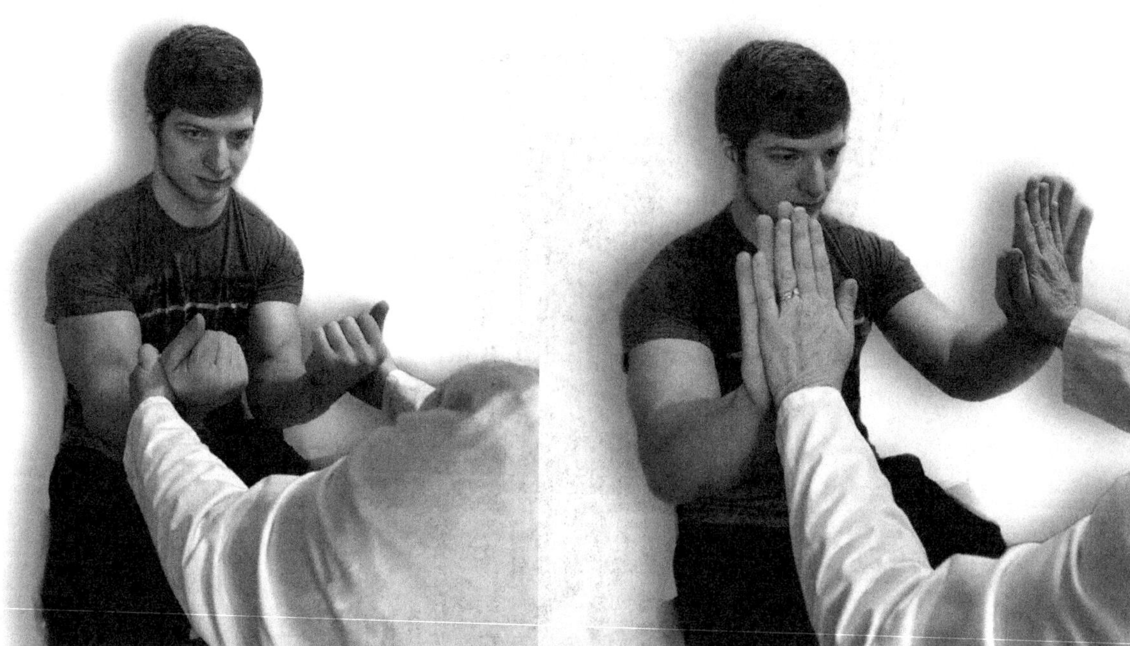

Figure 6.30 Assessing for Equal Upper Extremity Strength

Lower Body Strength

To assess lower body strength while the patient is in a seated position, place your hands behind their calves. Ask them to pull backwards with their lower legs while you provide resistance in the opposite direction.

Alternative tests are to place your hands on the patient's lower thighs and ask them to lift their legs upwards while you provide downward resistance, or place your hands on the top of their feet and ask them to pull their toes

2 "Neuro Exam Image 41.png" and "Neuro Exam Image 39.jpg" by Meredith Pomietlo for Chippewa Valley Technical College are licensed under CC BY 4.0. Access for free at https://drive.google.com/file/d/1NAeA8r9LJGl4aQf0Q40Np1YTBSSAqrYc/view?usp=sharing and https://drive.google.com/file/d/1pG7qn88mPJNwiOTUT89qQJM5RAgFbQwh/view?usp=sharing

My Notes

upwards while you provide resistance. In a similar manner, you can also place your hands on the dorsal part of their feet and ask them to press downwards "like pressing the gas pedal of a car," while providing resistance. Compare lower extremity strength on both sides. See Figure 6.31[3] for images of assessing lower extremity strength.

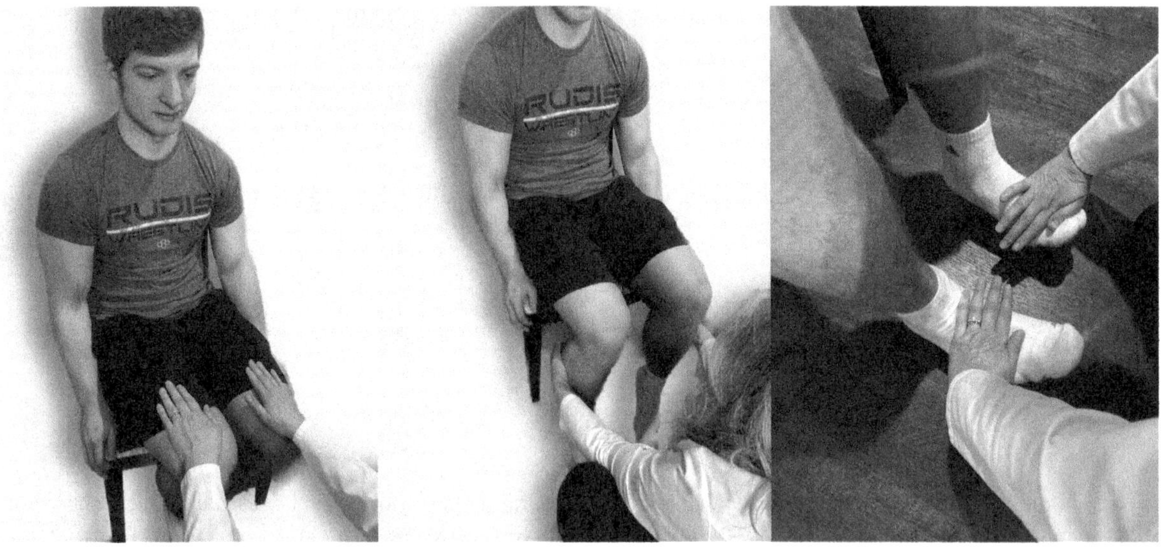

Figure 6.31 Assessing for Equal Strength in Lower Extremities

3 "Musculoskeletal Exam Image 2.png," "Neuro Exam image 6.png," and "Musculoskeletal Exam Image 7.png" by Meredith Pomietlo for Chippewa Valley Technical College are licensed under CC BY 4.0. Access for free at https://drive.google.com/file/d/1V-lF_5Y21OlehDMtYQi3qF2d5vGjgWlL/view?usp=sharing, https://drive.google.com/file/d/1OcXT2VxcOqr3TEacbj1XF7-BWTTki1ou/view?usp=sharing, and https://drive.google.com/file/d/1B4MP1eub9gLzn0vet15nd9Bw2FJ_hacA/view?usp=sharing

My Notes

6.8 ASSESSING CEREBELLAR FUNCTION

The neurological aspect of motor function is based on the activities of the cerebellum. The cerebellum is responsible for equilibrium, coordination, and the smoothness of movement. Specific tests used to evaluate cerebellar function include assessment of gait and balance, pronator drift, the finger-to-nose test, rapid alternating action, and the heel-to-shin test.

Gait and Balance

When assessing gait and balance, ask the patient to perform the following actions, using an assistive device if needed:

- Walk 10 feet, pivot, and walk back
- Look straight ahead and walk heel to toe
- Walk on tiptoes
- Walk on heels

Steps should be equal with a regular pace while arms are swinging and coordinated with walking. Balance should be maintained. A change in gait, weakness, shuffling, jerky movements, loss of balance, or incoordination of arm swing can indicate a neurological dysfunction. See Figure 6.32[1] for an image of assessing gait and balance.

When performing assessment of gait and balance, be aware that the older patient may have a mild degree of muscle weakness or decreased balance associated with aging. When feasible, obtain the patient's baseline ability and compare current findings to their baseline.

1 "Neuro Exam image 14.png," "Neuro Exam Image 19.png," "Neuro Exam image 40.png," and "Neuro Exam Image 34.png" by Meredith Pomietlo for Chippewa Valley Technical College are licensed under CC BY 4.0. Access for free at https://drive.google.com/file/d/1y7NJs3SDYBNzij7N7TlcK3PL1bDKLApN/view?usp=sharing, https://drive.google.com/file/d/1QdIjwMLfp_D_SR_1Y0n8hW0ye6GceO4l/view?usp=sharing, https://drive.google.com/file/d/1MlSv40aVyJ_um6OagqqMrSowZBqVXh9i/view?usp=sharing, and https://drive.google.com/file/d/1d_wEN13XR_RHoNP7yuEEBYbKYiPizluM/view?usp=sharing

My Notes

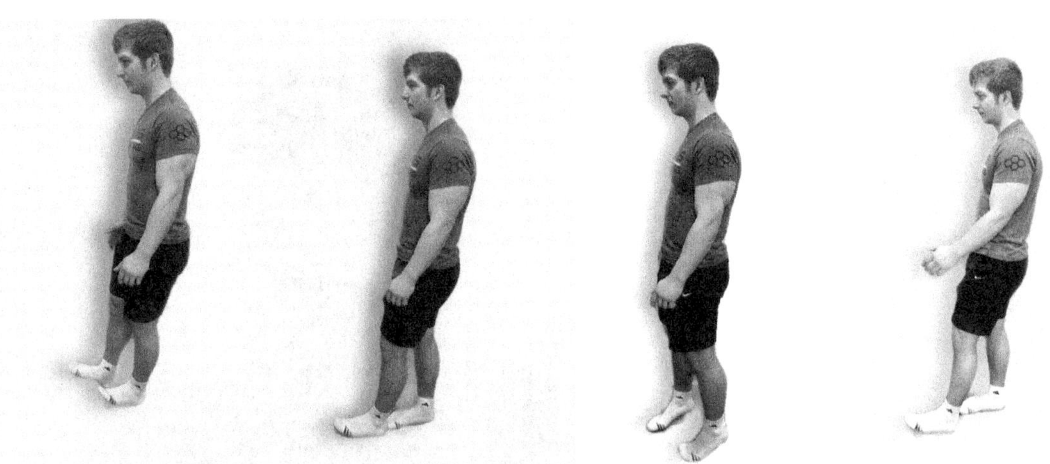

Figure 6.32 Assessing Gait and Balance

Pronator Drift

Assessing for pronator drift helps to detect mild upper limb weakness. Ask the patient to close their eyes and extend both arms at 90 degrees at shoulder level with the palms facing upwards. The patient should try to maintain this position for 20 to 30 seconds. Closing the eyes accentuates the effect because the brain is deprived of visual information about the position of the body and must rely on proprioception. **Proprioception** is the awareness of body position and movement. The expected finding is both arms will maintain this position equally. If the patient is unable to maintain the position, the result is referred to as a positive pronator drift test. Patients with weakness in one arm will not be able to keep the affected arm raised, and ultimately the palm may begin to pronate (palm facing down). In some patients, the arm may remain supinated but will drop lower than the unaffected arm.

Finger-to-Nose Test

The finger-to-nose test assesses equilibrium and coordination. Place the patient in a seated or standing position and ask them to close their eyes. Instruct the patient to extend their arms outward from the sides of the body, and then touch the tip of the nose with the right index finger and return the arm to extended position. Repeat with the left side and continue to repeat touching the nose with alternating movements by both arms.

The expected finding is the patient will smoothly touch the nose with alternating left and right index fingers and return their arms to an extended position repeatedly. An abnormal result occurs when the patient is unable to alternate fingers or demonstrates the inability to touch the nose. For example, the patient may touch the cheek or other part of the face, or movement may be clumsy with stops and restarts. See Figure 6.33[2] for an image of a finger-to-nose test.

2 "Neuro Exam Image 7.png" by Meredith Pomietlo for Chippewa Valley Technical College is licensed under CC BY 4.0. Access for free at https://drive.google.com/file/d/1wKgXQIf6aJvFVpsor_7QbVVH_pw_Ije8/view?usp=sharing

My Notes

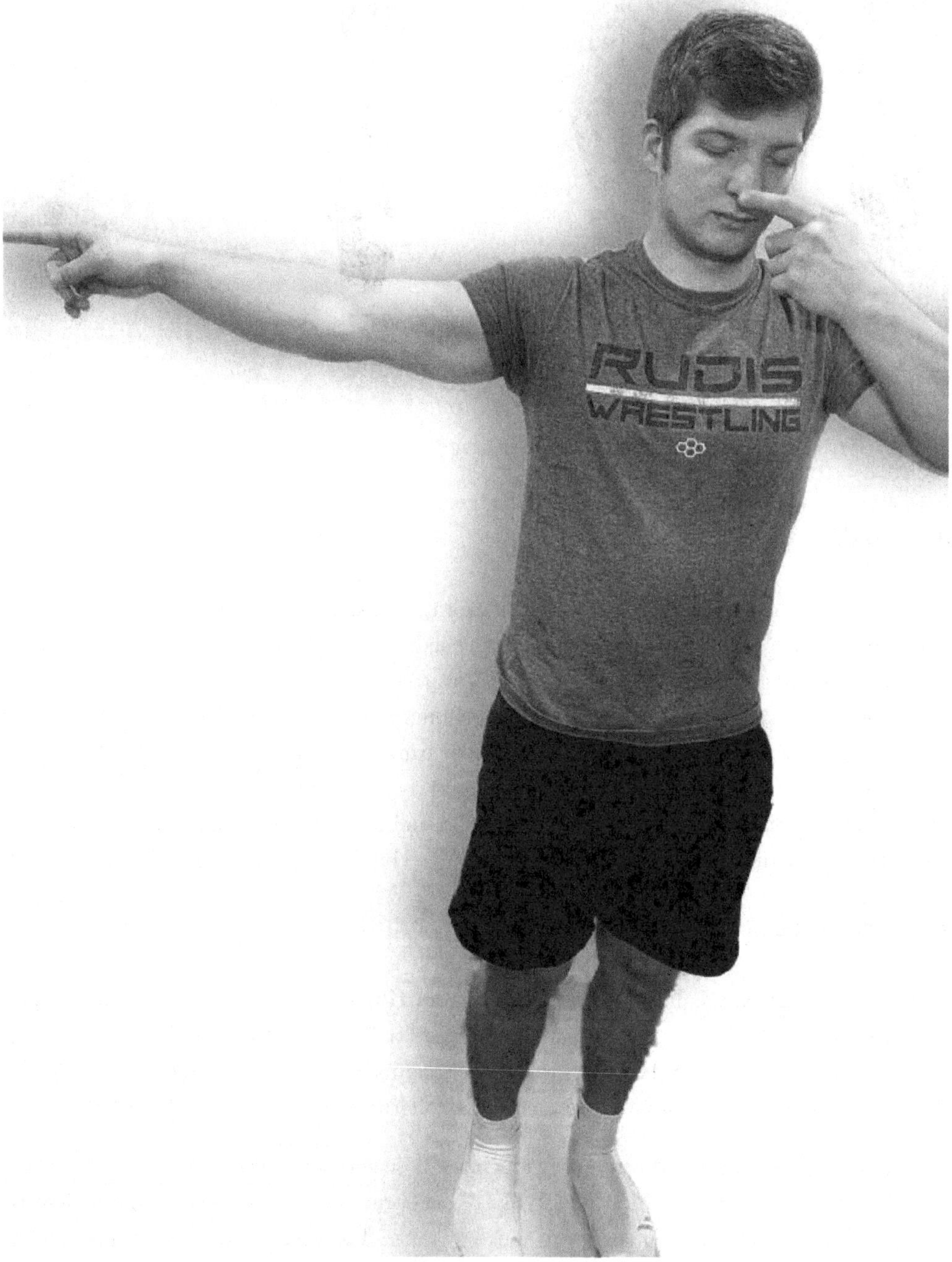

Figure 6.33 Finger-to-Nose Test

Rapid Alternating Action

To perform a rapid alternating action test, place the patient in a seated position with palms down on thighs. Ask the patient to turn their hands so their palms face upwards and then quickly return them to a downward position and repeat. Instruct the patient to alternate this movement at a fast pace. The expected finding is the rhythm, rate, and movement are smooth and coordinated as pace increases. An abnormal finding is when the patient is unable

My Notes

to alternate movements or can only do so at a slow pace. See Figure 6.34[3] for an example of the rapid alternating action test.

An alternative test is to have the patient touch the thumb to each finger on their hand in sequence and gradually increase the pace. Repeat this test on the other hand. See Figure 6.35[4] for an alternative finger touch test.

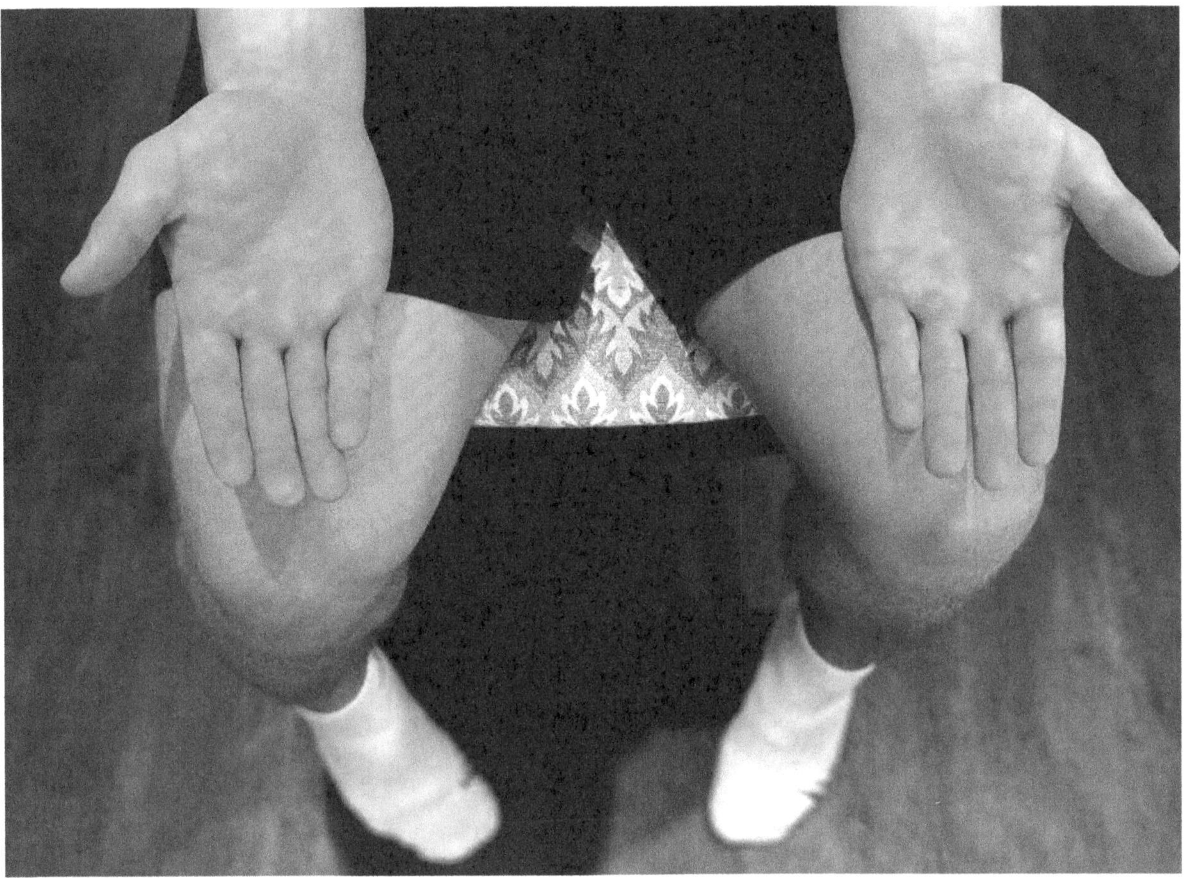

Figure 6.34 Rapid Alternating Action Test

3 "Neuro Exam Image 20.jpg" by Meredith Pomietlo for Chippewa Valley Technical College is licensed under CC BY 4.0. Access for free at https://drive.google.com/file/d/1hCihiSPRdqLv6TCFSm_dL2j3-TuDNoKY/view?usp=sharing

4 "Neuro Exam Image 15.png" by Meredith Pomietlo for Chippewa Valley Technical College is licensed under CC BY 4.0. Access for free at https://drive.google.com/file/d/1AVrPnNku_uQmNi7vcQ_5w_KuSk5Ny21H/view?usp=sharing

My Notes

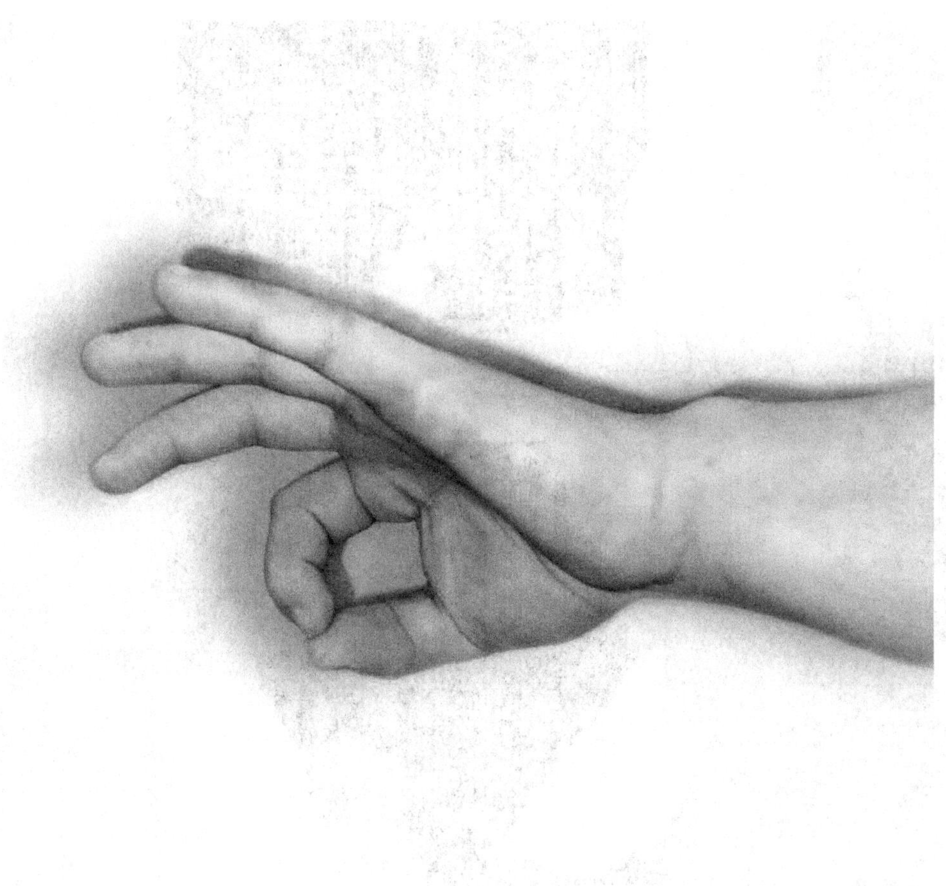

Figure 6.35 Alternative Finger Touch Test

Heel-to-Shin Test

To perform a heel-to-shin test, place the patient in a supine position. Ask the patient to place the heel of the right foot just below their left kneecap, and then slide the right heel in a straight line down the shin bone to the ankle. Ask them to repeat this procedure on the left leg. The expected action is a smooth and straight movement of both

My Notes

legs. An abnormal finding is if the heel falls off the lower leg or the patient is not able to complete the movement smoothly in a straight motion. See Figure 6.36[5] for an image of the heel-to-shin test.

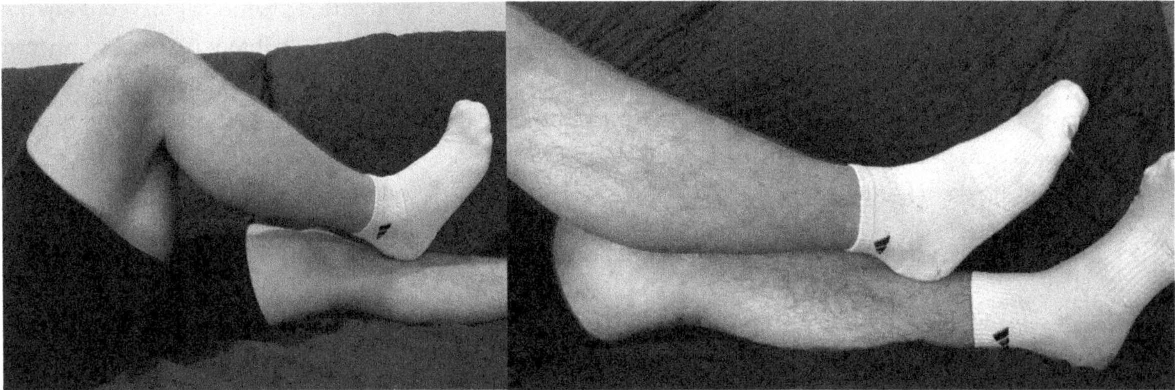

Figure 6.36 Heel-to-Shin Test

Visit Stanford Medicine 25's "Cerebellum Exam" video on YouTube for a review of cerebellar exam (https://youtu.be/Imu1kk_gOKA).

5 "Neuro Exam Image 1.png" and "Neuro Exam Image 2.png" by Meredith Pomietlo for Chippewa Valley Technical College are licensed under CC BY 4.0. Access for free at https://drive.google.com/file/d/1IgqxdX1NAxNZhVVJKytUTWvmiNFp7UMN/view?usp=sharing and https://drive.google.com/file/d/1_GqnrOEmk6HOrRPdLeYHTf7GbIw90ukG/view?usp=sharing

My Notes

6.9 ASSESSING REFLEXES

Assessment of reflexes is not typically performed by registered nurses as part of a routine nursing neurological assessment of adult patients, but it is used in nursing specialty units and in advanced practice. Spinal cord injuries, neuromuscular diseases, or diseases of the lower motor neuron tract can cause weak or absent reflexes. To perform deep reflex tendon testing, place the patient in a seated position. Use a reflex hammer in a quick striking motion by the wrist on various tendons to produce an involuntary response. Before classifying a reflex as absent or weak, the test should be repeated after the patient is encouraged to relax because voluntary tensing of the muscles can prevent an involuntary reflexive action.

Reflexes are graded from 0 to 4+, with "2+" considered normal:

- 0: Absent
- 1+: Hypoactive
- 2+: Normal
- 3+: Hyperactive without clonus
- 4+: Hyperactive with clonus (involuntary muscle contraction)

To observe assessment of deep tendon reflexes, view the following video.

View Stanford Medicine's "Assessment of Deep Tendon Reflexes" video.[1]

1 Stanford Medicine 25. (2014, March 16). *Deep tendon reflexes (Stanford medicine 25).* [Video]. YouTube. All rights reserved. https://youtu.be/0sqCIzuotWo

My Notes

Brachioradialis Reflex

The brachioradialis reflex is used to assess the cervical spine nerves C5 and C6. Ask the patient to support their arm on their thigh or on your hand. Identify the insertion of the brachioradialis tendon on the radius and briskly tap it with the reflex hammer. The reflex consists of flexion and supination of the forearm. See Figure 6.37[2] for an image of obtaining the brachioradialis reflex.

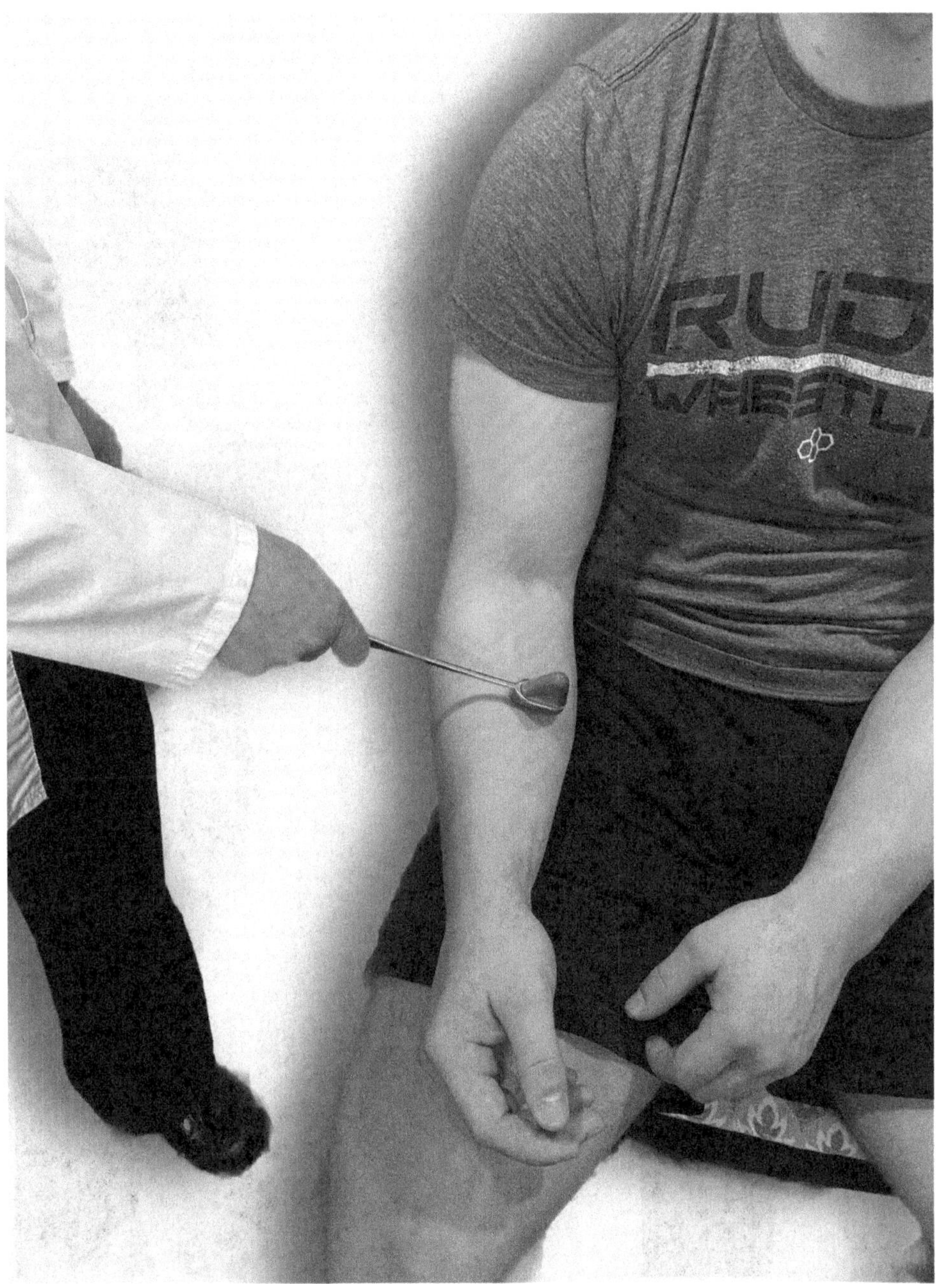

Figure 6.37 Brachioradialis Reflex

2 "Deep Reflex Exam Image 4.png" by Meredith Pomietlo for Chippewa Valley Technical College is licensed under CC BY 4.0. Access for free at https://drive.google.com/file/d/1vf3NM3peMaVHHS2cMDE4uz-oHbU8V7_b/view?usp =sharing

My Notes

Triceps Reflex

The triceps reflex assesses cervical spine nerves C6 and C7. Support the patient's arm underneath their bicep to maintain a position midway between flexion and extension. Ask the patient to relax their arm and allow it to fully be supported by your hand. Identify the triceps tendon posteriorly just above its insertion on the olecranon. Tap briskly on the tendon with the reflex hammer. Note extension of the forearm. See Figure 6.38[3] for an image of the triceps reflex exam.

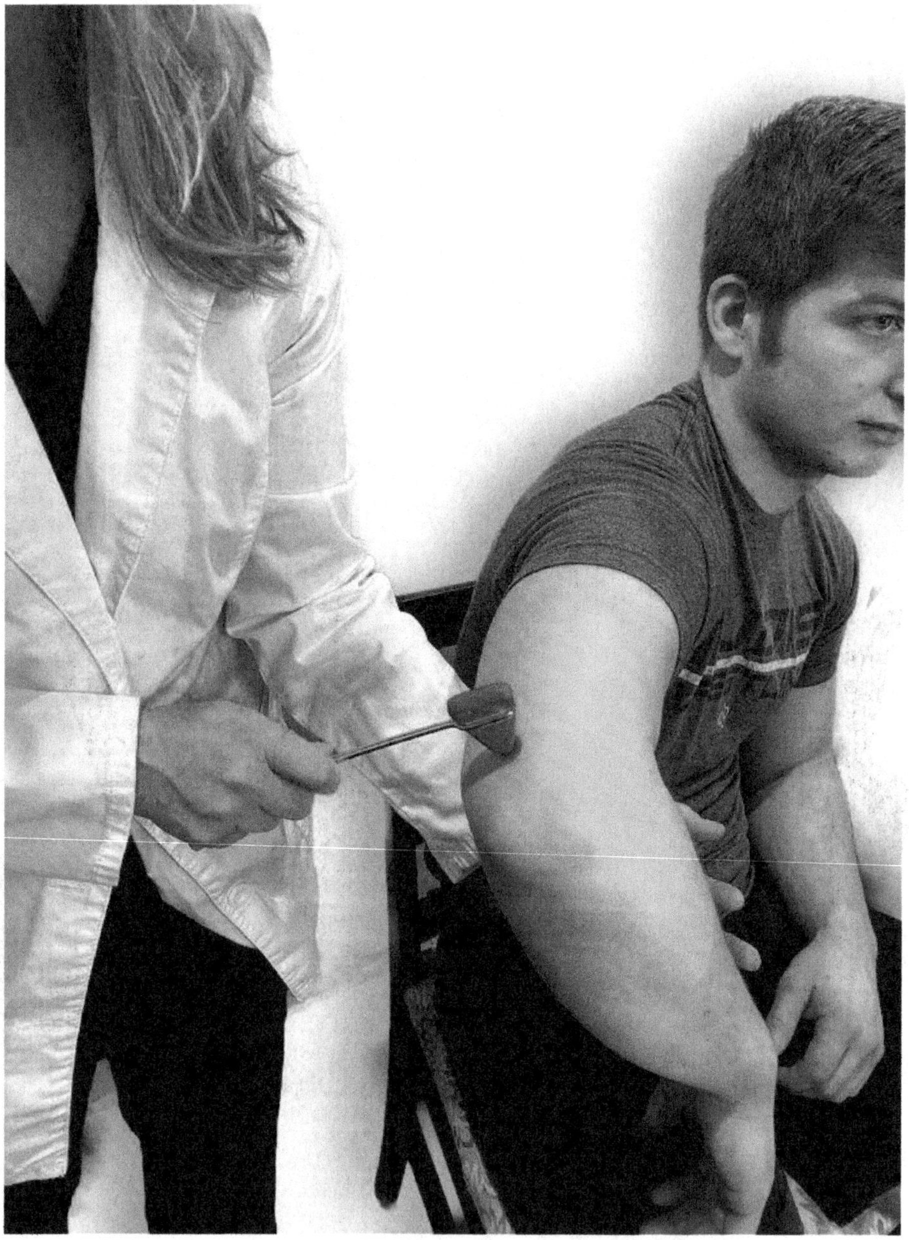

Figure 6.38 Triceps Reflex

3 "Deep Reflex Exam Image 2.png" by Meredith Pomietlo for Chippewa Valley Technical College is licensed under CC BY 4.0. Access for free at https://drive.google.com/file/d/1E6BVP9s2-5LT8xR4QwYb04l3GzvRhRiV/view?usp=sharing

Patella (Knee Jerk) Reflex

My Notes

The patellar reflex, commonly referred to as the knee jerk test, assesses lumbar spine nerves L2, L3, and L4. Ask the patient to relax the leg and allow it to swing freely at the knee. Tap the patella tendon briskly, looking for extension of the lower leg. See Figure 6.39[4] for an image of assessing a patellar reflex.

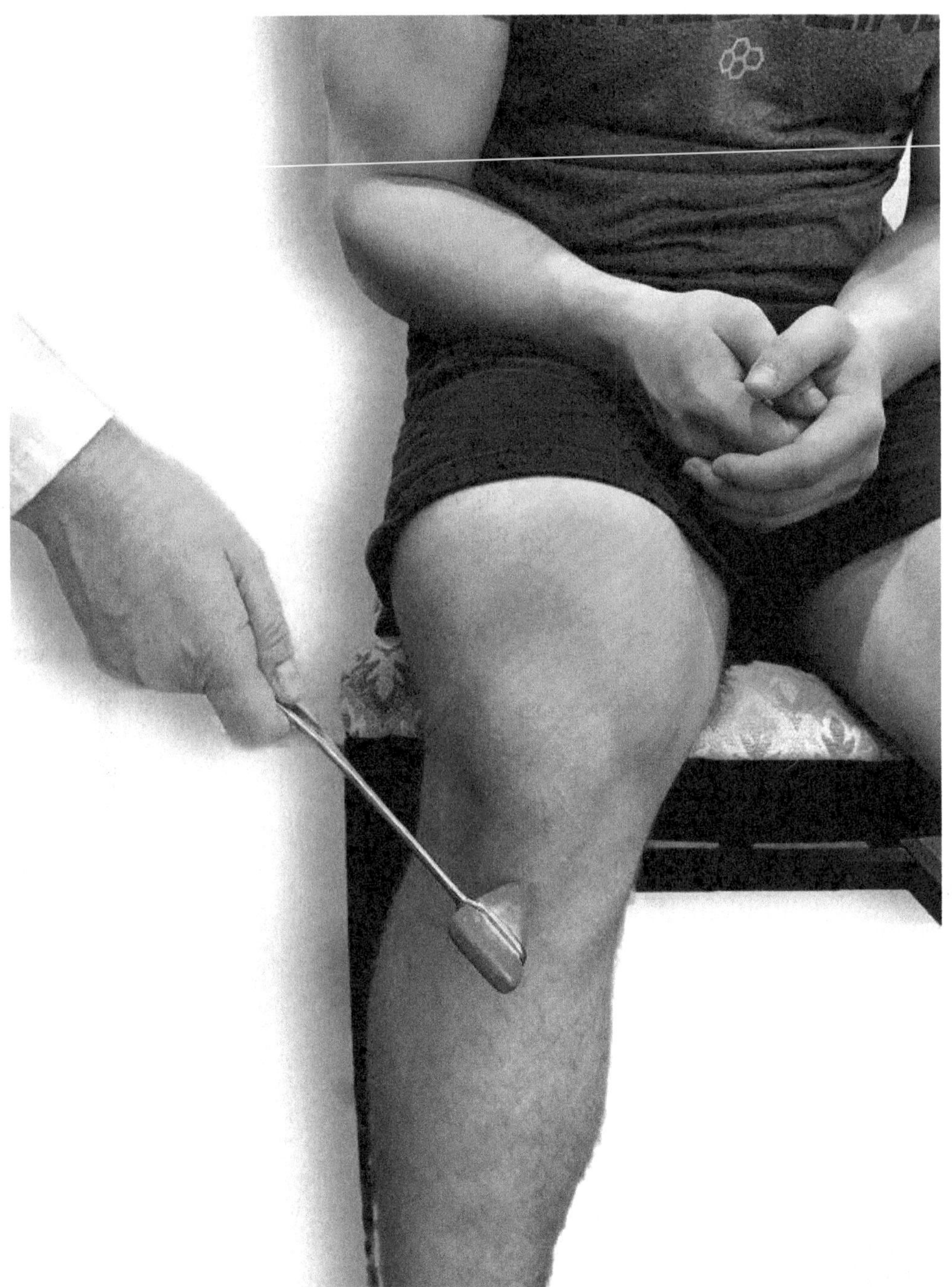

Figure 6.39 Patellar Reflex

4 "Deep Reflex Exam Image 3.jpg" by Meredith Pomietlo for Chippewa Valley Technical College is licensed under CC BY 4.0. Access for free at https://drive.google.com/file/d/1P2GVK3v4gor-ywg5Ba47-JpHfyW5ymcU/view?usp=sharing

My Notes

Plantar Reflex

The plantar reflex assesses lumbar spine L5 and sacral spine S1. Ask the patient to extend their lower leg, and then stabilize their foot in the air with your hand. Stroke the lateral surface of the sole of the foot toward the toes. Many patients are ticklish and withdraw their foot, so it is sufficient to elicit the reflex by using your thumb to stroke lightly from the sole of the foot toward the toes. If there is no response, use a blunt object such as a key or pen. The expected reflex is flexion (i.e., bending) of the great toe. An abnormal response is toe extension (i.e., straightening), also known as the Babinski reflex, which is considered abnormal after 2 years of age. See Figures 6.40 – 6.43[5,6,7,8] for images of assessing the plantar reflex.

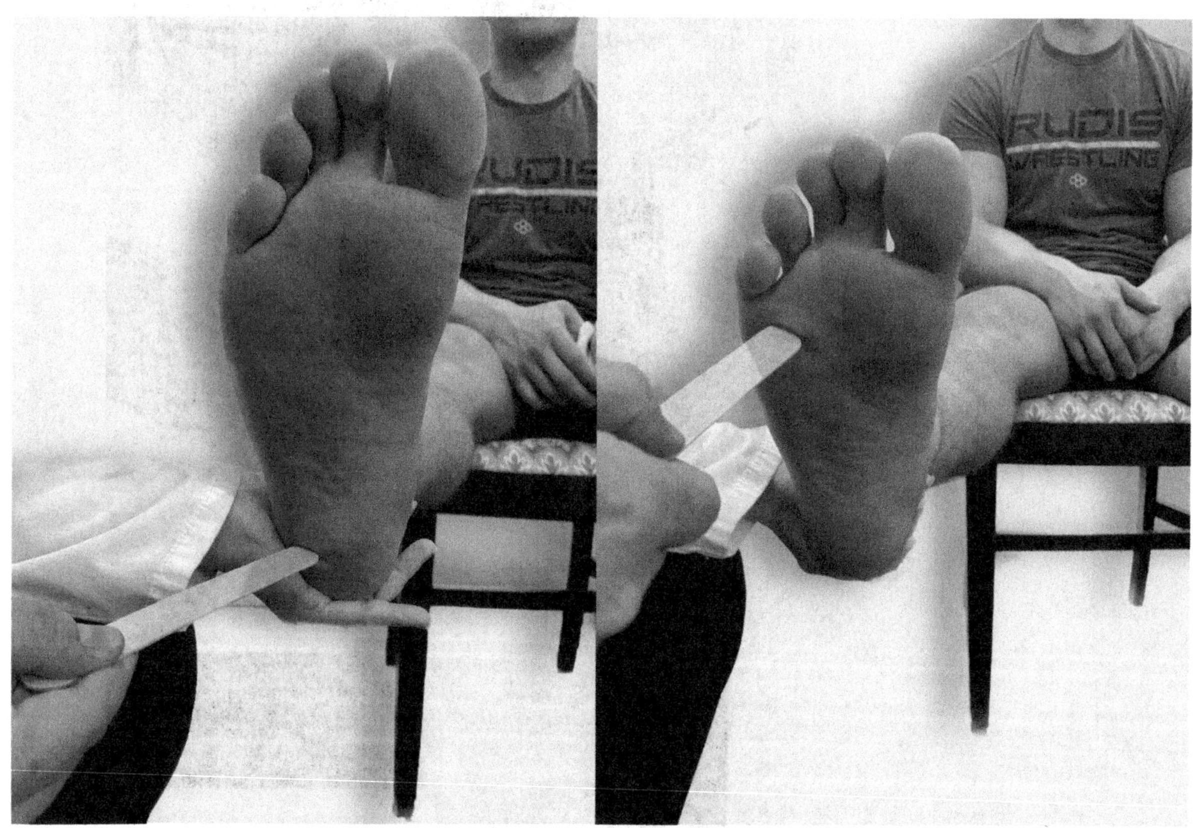

Figure 6.40 The Plantar Reflex

5 "Neuro Exam Image 23.png" and "Neuro Exam Image 21.png" by Meredith Pomietlo for Chippewa Valley Technical College are licensed under CC BY 4.0. Access for free at https://drive.google.com/file/d/1OdY6tCY3XSgmjSrow58tlONMQ6apA_NT/view?usp=sharing and https://drive.google.com/file/d/1Xe2R4dKPVyB3Y-Py9cQkZ9pSsq5qOEMN/view?usp=sharing

6 "Lawrence 1960 20.4.png" by Earl Lawrence House & Ben Pansky is in the Public Domain. Access for free at https://commons.wikimedia.org/wiki/File:Lawrence_1960_20.4.png

7 "BabinskiSign.jpg" by Medicus of Borg is in the Public Domain. Access for free at https://commons.wikimedia.org/wiki/File:BabinskiSign.jpg

8 "Babinski-newborn.jpg" by Medicus of Borg is licensed under CC BY-SA 3.0. Access for free at https://commons.wikimedia.org/wiki/File:Babinski-newborn.jpg

My Notes

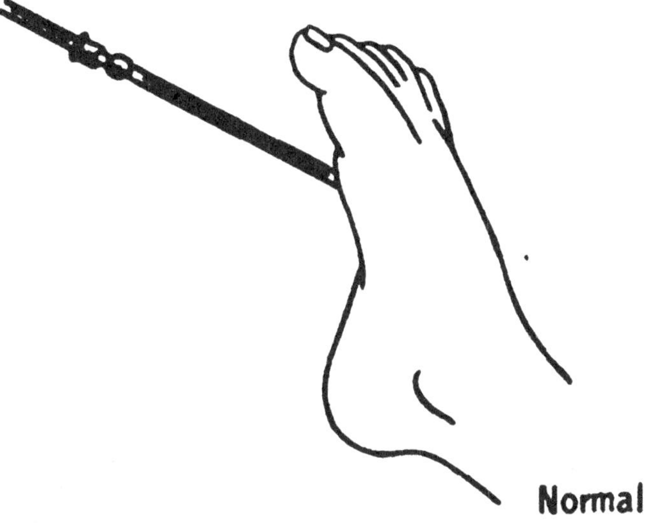

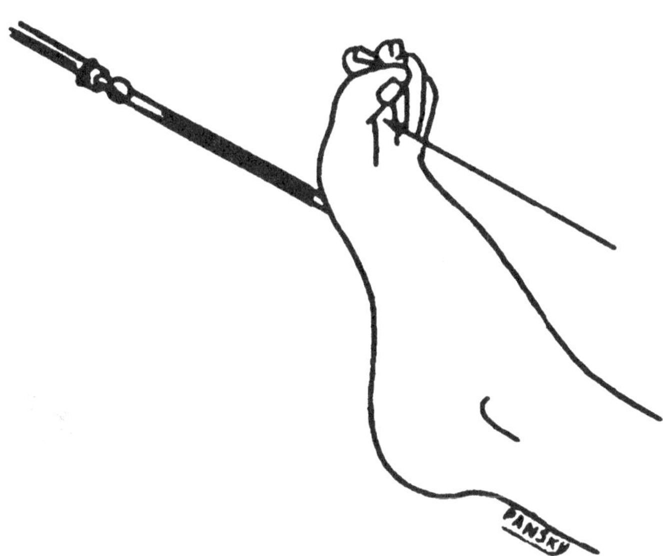

Figure 6.41 Plantar Reflex and Babinski Sign

My Notes

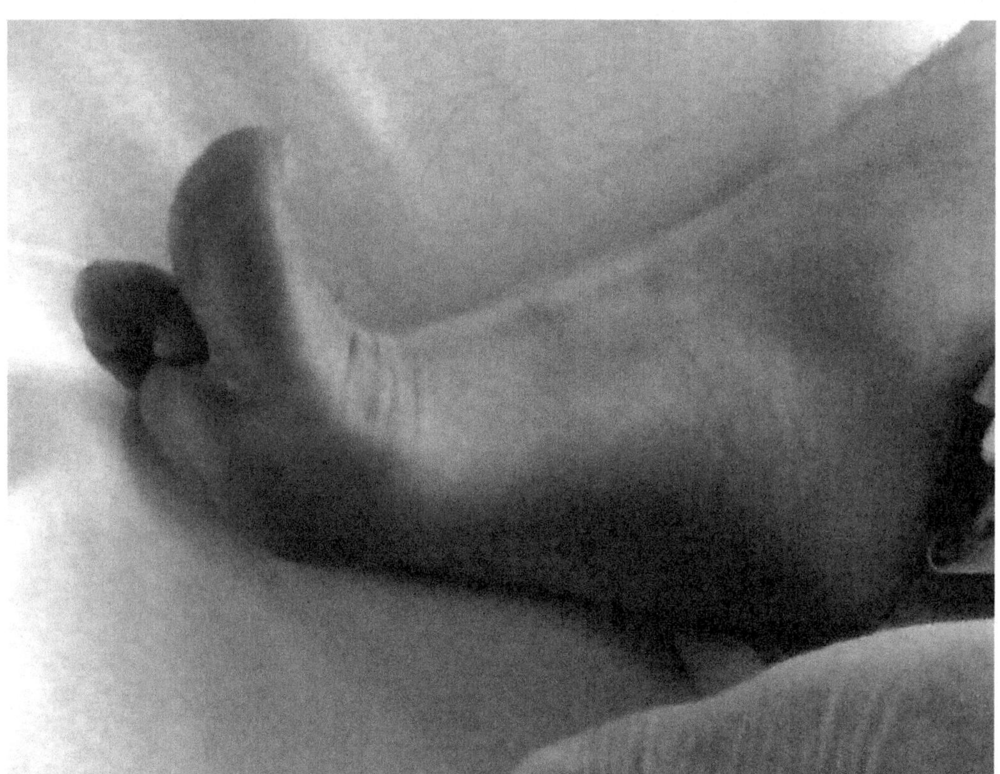

Figure 6.42 The Babinski Sign in an Adult

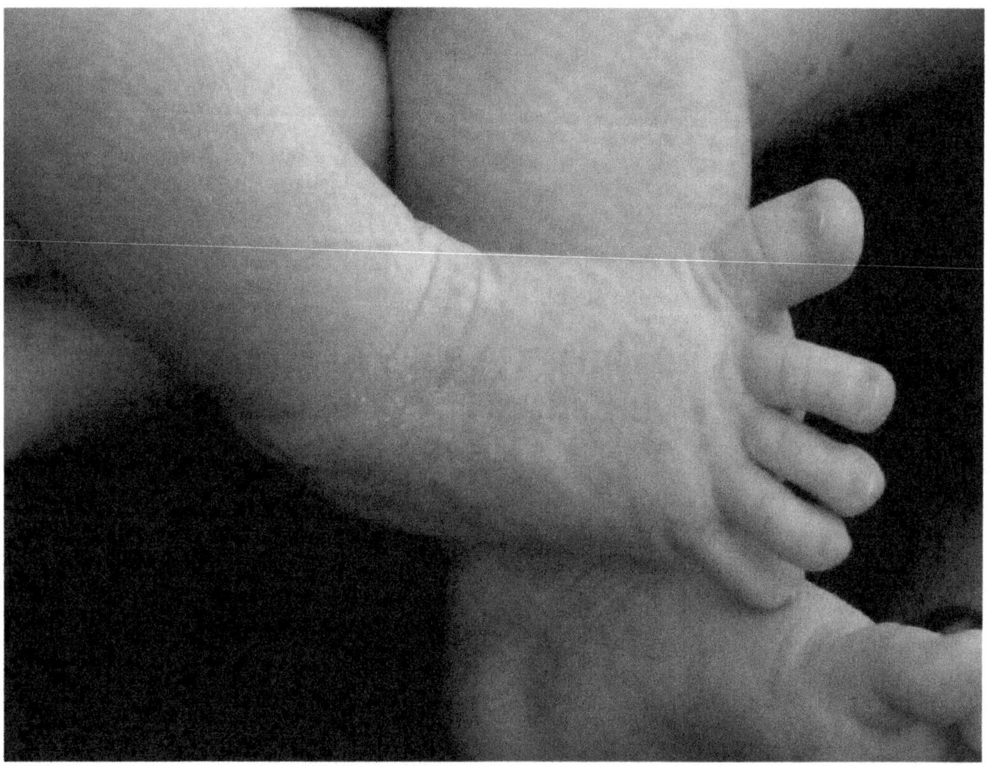

Figure 6.43 The Normal Babinski Reflex in a Newborn

My Notes

Video Reviews for Assessment of Deep Tendon Reflexes[9]

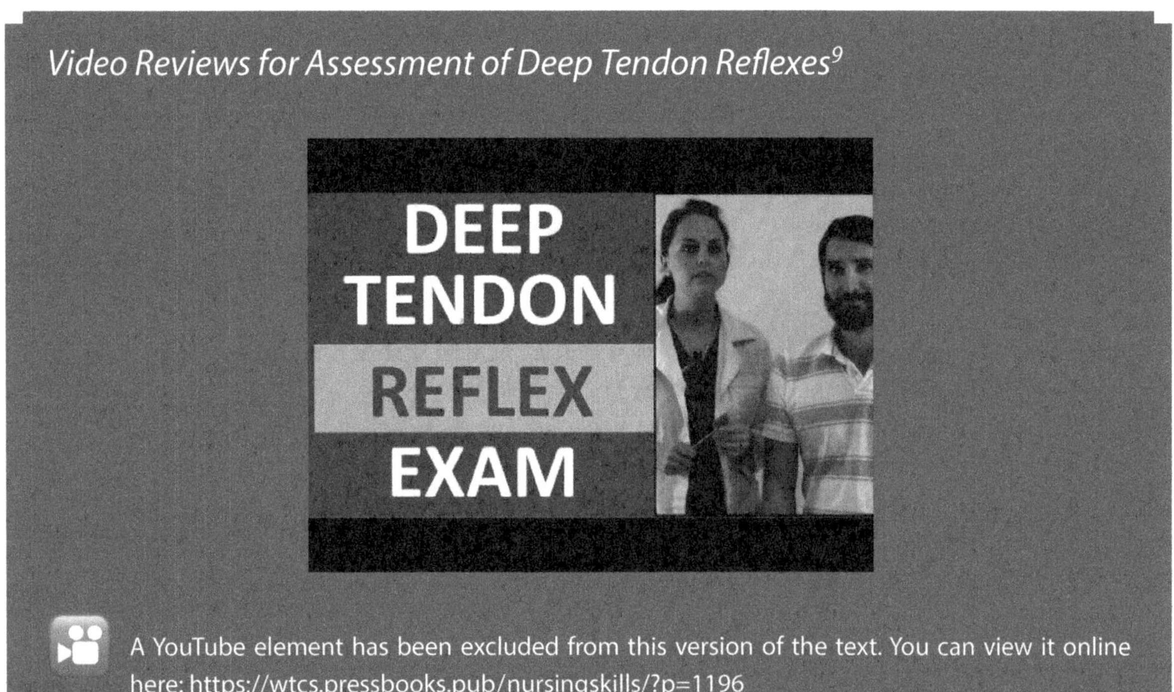

A YouTube element has been excluded from this version of the text. You can view it online here: https://wtcs.pressbooks.pub/nursingskills/?p=1196

Babinski-Plantar Reflex[10]

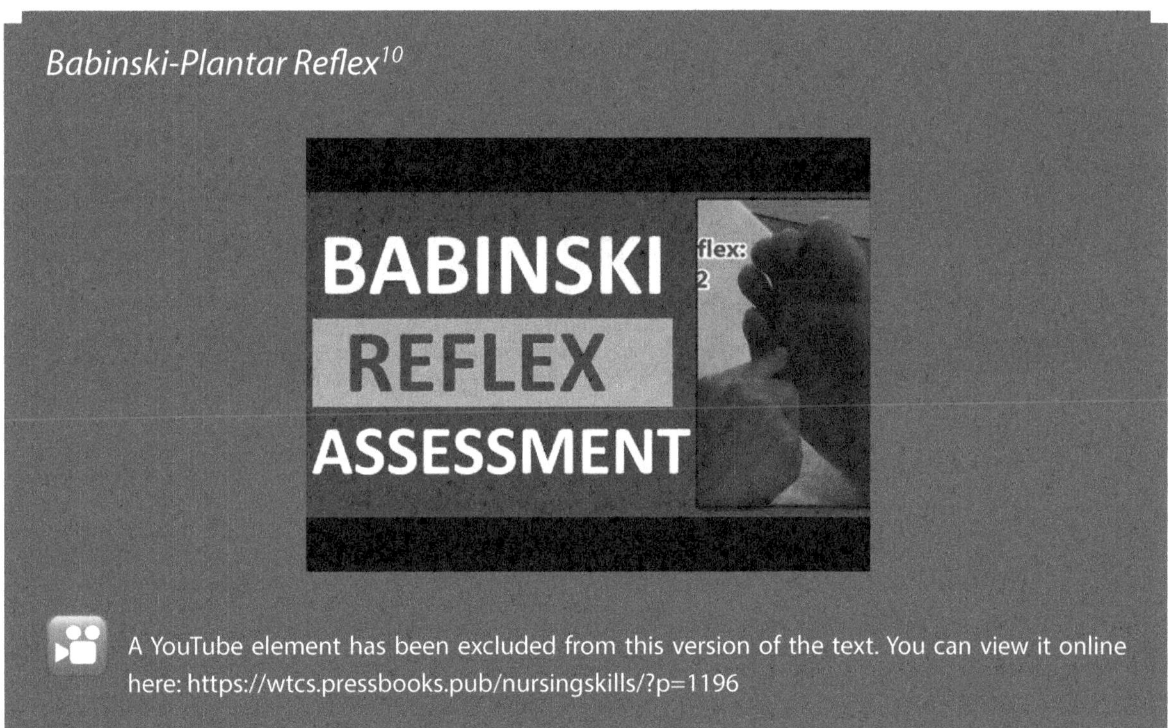

A YouTube element has been excluded from this version of the text. You can view it online here: https://wtcs.pressbooks.pub/nursingskills/?p=1196

9 RegisteredNurseRN (2016, April 1). *Deep tendon reflex examination for nursing head to toe assessment of neuro system.* [Video]. YouTube. All rights reserved. Video used with permission. https://youtu.be/eqOpNQH09pA

10 RegisteredNurseRN (2016, March 29). *Babinski reflex | Plantar reflex test | Nursing head to toe assessment.* [Video]. YouTube. All rights reserved. Video used with permission. https://youtu.be/dcJgxuLtHdg

My Notes

Newborn Reflexes

Newborn reflexes originate in the central nervous system and are exhibited by infants at birth but disappear as part of child development. Neurological disease or delayed development is indicated if these reflexes are not present at birth, do not spontaneously resolve, or reappear in adulthood. Common newborn reflexes include sucking, rooting, palmar grasp, plantar grasp, **Babinski**, Moro, and tonic neck reflexes.

Sucking Reflex

The sucking reflex is common to all mammals and is present at birth. It is linked with the rooting reflex and breastfeeding. It causes the child to instinctively suck anything that touches the roof of their mouth and simulates the way a child naturally eats. See Figure 6.44[11] for an image of the newborn sucking reflex.

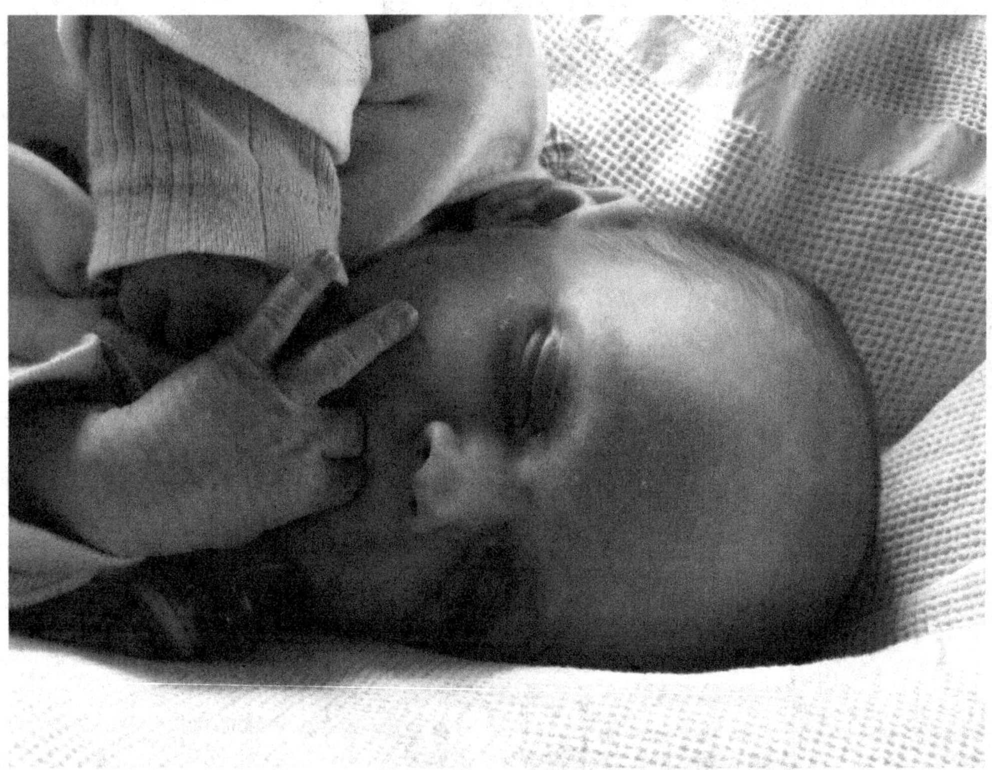

Figure 6.44 Newborn Sucking Reflex

11 "BabySuckingFingers.jpg" by Florence Devouard (anthere) is licensed under CC BY-SA 3.0. Access for free at https://commons.wikimedia.org/wiki/File:BabySuckingFingers.jpg

Rooting Reflex

The rooting reflex assists in the act of breastfeeding. A newborn infant will turn its head toward anything that strokes its cheek or mouth, searching for the object by moving its head in steadily decreasing arcs until the object is found. See Figure 6.45[12] for an image of a newborn exhibiting the rooting reflex.

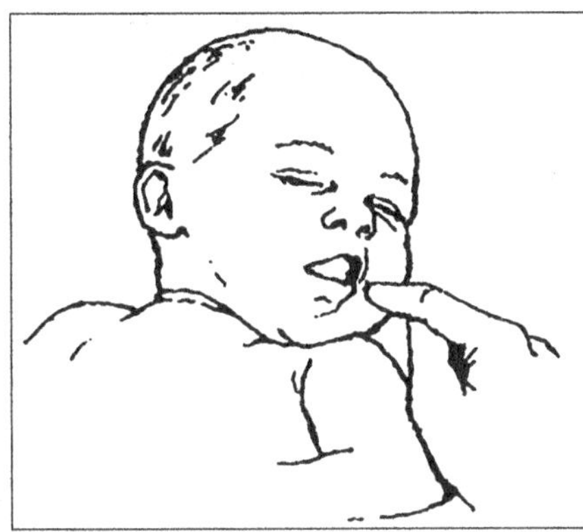

Figure 6.45 Newborn Rooting Reflex

Palmar and Plantar Grasps

When an object is placed in an infant's hand and the palm of the child is stroked, the fingers will close reflexively, referred to as the palmar grasp reflex. A similar reflexive action occurs if an object is placed on the plantar surface of an infant's foot, referred to as the plantar grasp reflex. See Figure 6.46[13] for an image of the palmar grasp reflex.

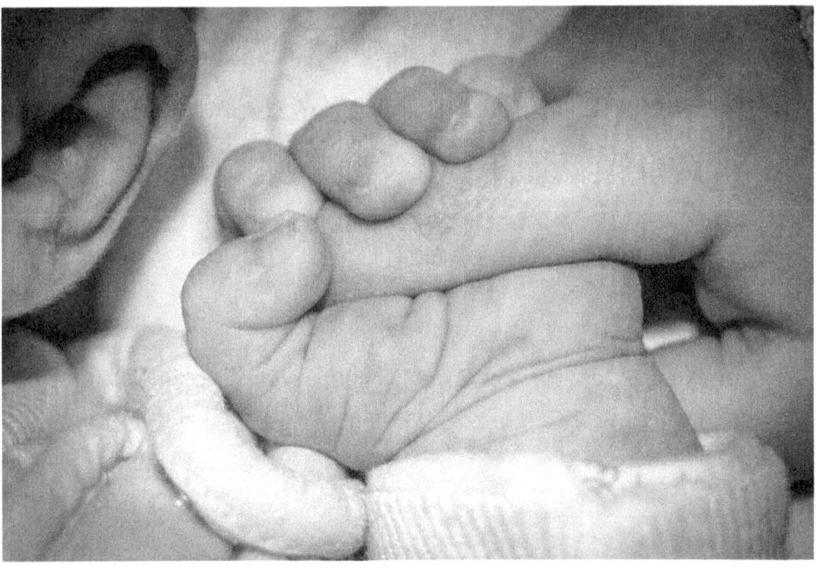

Figure 6.46 Newborn Palmer Grasp Reflex

---

12 "Rooting Reflex" by Ashley Arbuckle is licensed under CC BY 2.0. Access for free at https://www.flickr.com/photos/aarbuckle9/8416689403

13 "baby-428395_960_720.jpg" by jarmoluk is licensed under *CC0*. Access for free at https://pixabay.com/photos/baby-handle-tiny-father-family-428395/

My Notes

Moro Reflex

The Moro reflex is present at birth and is often stimulated by a loud noise. The Moro reflex occurs when the legs and head of the infant extend while the arms jerk up and out with the palms up. See Figure 6.47[14] for an image of an infant exhibiting the Moro reflex.

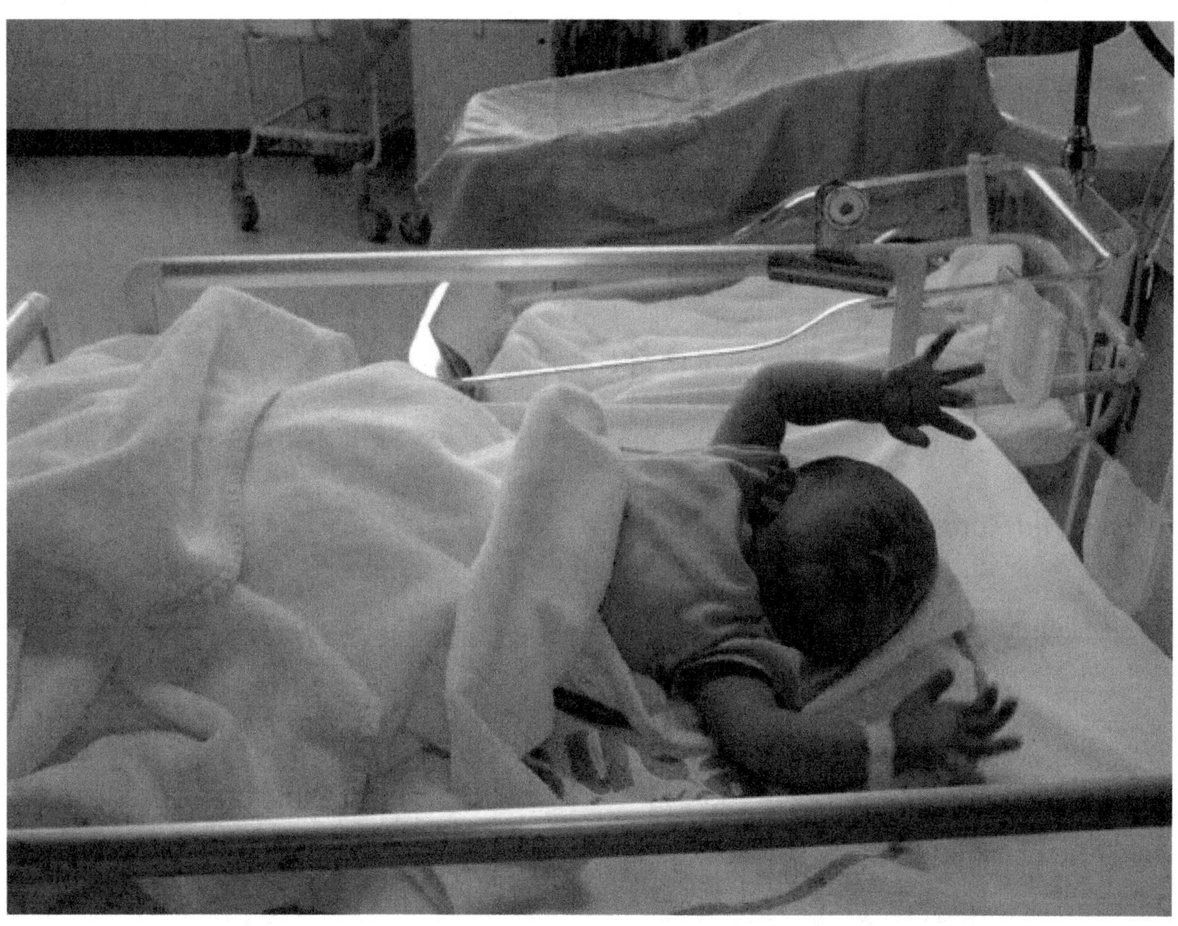

Figure 6.47 Newborn Moro Reflex

Tonic Neck Reflex

The asymmetrical tonic neck reflex, also known as the "fencing posture," occurs when the child's head is turned to the side. The arm on the same side as the head is turned will straighten and the opposite arm will bend. See Figure 6.48[15] for an image of the tonic neck reflex.

---

14 "Moro reflex.jpg" by tawamie is licensed under CC BY-SA 3.0. Access for free at https://commons.wikimedia.org/wiki/File:Moro_Reflex.JPG

15 "Asymmetrical tonic neck reflex (ATNR) in a two-week-old female.jpg" by Samuel Finlayson is licensed under CC BY-SA 4.0. Access for free at https://commons.wikimedia.org/wiki/File:Asymmetrical_tonic_neck_reflex_(ATNR)_in_a_two-week-old_female.jpg

My Notes

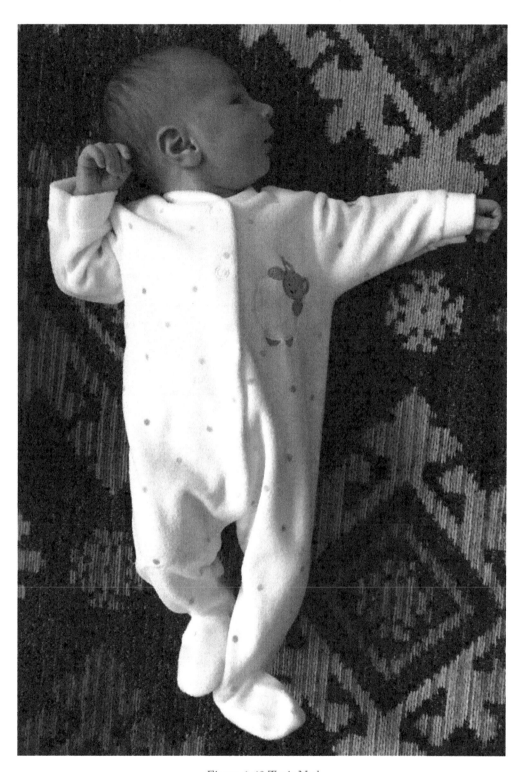

Figure 6.48 Tonic Neck

Walking-Stepping Reflex

Although infants cannot support their own weight, when the soles of their feet touch a surface, it appears as if they are attempting to walk by placing one foot in front of the other foot.

My Notes

6.10 NEUROLOGICAL ASSESSMENT

Now that we have reviewed tests included in a neurological exam, let's review components of a routine neurological assessment typically performed by registered nurses. The neurological assessment begins by collecting subjective data followed by a physical examination.

Subjective Assessment

Subjective data collection guides the focus of the physical examination. Collect data from the patient using effective communication and pay particular attention to what the patient is reporting, including current symptoms and any history of neurological illness. Ask follow-up questions related to symptoms such as confusion, headache, vertigo, seizures, recent injury or fall, weakness, numbness, tingling, difficulty swallowing (called **dysphagia**) or speaking (called **dysphasia**), or lack of coordination of body movements.[1]

See Table 6.10a for sample interview questions to use during the subjective assessment

Table 6.10a Interview Questions Related to Subjective Assessment of Neurological System

Interview Questions	Follow-up
Are you experiencing any current neurological concerns such as headache, dizziness, weakness, numbness, tingling, tremors, loss of balance, or decreased coordination? **Have you experienced any difficulty swallowing or speaking?** **Have you experienced any recent falls?**	If the patient is seeking care for an acute neurological problem, use the PQRSTU method to further evaluate their chief complaint. The PQRSTU method is described in the "Health History" chapter. Note: If critical findings of an acute neurological event are actively occurring, such as signs of a stroke, obtain emergency assistance according to agency policy.
Have you ever experienced a neurological condition such as a stroke, transient ischemic attack, seizure, or head injury?	Describe the condition(s), date(s), and treatment(s).
Are you currently taking any medications, herbs, or supplements for a neurological condition?	Please describe.

1 This work is a derivative of Clinical Procedures for Safer Patient Care by British Columbia Institute of Technology licensed under CC BY 4.0. Access for free at https://opentextbc.ca/clinicalskills/

Life Span Considerations

My Notes

Newborn

At birth, the neurologic system is not fully developed. The brain is still developing, and the newborn's anterior fontanelle doesn't close until approximately 18 months of age. The sensory and motor systems gradually develop in the first year of life. The newborn's sensory system responds to stimuli by crying or moving body parts. Initial motor activity is primitive in the form of newborn reflexes. Additional information about newborn reflexes is provided in the "Assessing Reflexes" section. As the newborn develops, so do the motor and sensory integration. Specific questions to ask parents or caregivers of infants include the following:

- Have you noticed your infant sleeping excessively or having difficulty arousing?
- Has your infant had difficulty feeding, sucking, or swallowing?

Children

Depending on the child's age and developmental level, they may answer questions independently or the child's parent/guardian may provide information. Specific questions for children include the following:

- Have you ever had a head injury or a concussion?
- Do you experience headaches? If so, how often?
- Have you had a seizure or convulsion?
- Have you noticed if your child has any problems with walking or balance?
- Have you noticed if your child experiences episodes of not being aware of their environment?

Older Adults

The aging adult experiences a general slowing in nerve conduction, resulting in a slowed motor and sensory interaction. Fine coordination, balance, and reflex activity may be impaired. There may also be a gradual decrease in cerebral blood flow and oxygen use that can cause dizziness and loss of balance. Examples of specific subjective questions for the older adult include the following:

- Have you ever had a head injury or recent fall?
- Do you experience any shaking or tremors of your hands? If so, do they occur more with rest or activity?
- Have you had any weakness, numbness, or tingling in any of your extremities?
- Have you noticed a problem with balance or coordination?
- Do you ever feel light-headed or dizzy? If so, does it occur with activity or change in position?

Educate older adults to change positions slowly, especially when standing up from a lying or sitting position. Light-headedness and loss of balance during these activities increase the risk for falls.

My Notes

Objective Assessment

The physical examination of the neurological system includes assessment of both the central and peripheral nervous systems. A routine neurological exam usually starts by assessing the patient's mental status followed by evaluation of sensory function and motor function. Comprehensive neurological exams may further evaluate cranial nerve function and deep tendon reflexes. The nurse must be knowledgeable of what is normal or expected for the patient's age, development, and condition to analyze the meaning of the data that is being collected.

Inspection

Nurses begin assessing a patient's overall neurological status by observing their general appearance, posture, ability to walk, and personal hygiene in the first few minutes of nurse-patient interaction. For additional information about obtaining an overall impression of a patient's status while performing an assessment, see the "General Survey" chapter.

Level of orientation is assessed and other standardized tools to evaluate a patient's mental status may be used, such as the Glasgow Coma Scale (GCS), NIH Stroke Scale, or Mini-Mental State Exam (MMSE). Read more information about these tools under the "Assessing Mental Status" section earlier in this chapter.

The nurse also assesses a patient's cerebellar function by observing their gait and balance. See the "Assessing Cerebellar Function" section earlier in chapter for more information.

Auscultation

Auscultation refers to the action of listening to sounds from the heart, lungs, or other organs with a stethoscope as a part of physical examination. Auscultation is not typically performed by registered nurses during a routine neurological assessment. However, advanced practice nurses and other health care providers may auscultate the carotid arteries for the presence of a swishing sound called a **bruit**. Bruits suggest interference with cerebral blood flow that can cause neurological deficits.

Palpation

Palpation during a physical examination typically refers to the use of touch to evaluate organs for size, location, or tenderness, but palpation during the neurologic physical exam involves using touch to assess sensory function and motor function. Refer to sections on "Assessing Sensory Function," "Assessing Motor Function," "Assessing Cranial Nerves," and "Assessing Reflexes" earlier in this chapter for additional information on how to perform these tests.

See Table 6.10b for a summary of expected and unexpected findings when performing an adult neurological assessment.

My Notes

Table 6.10b Expected Versus Unexpected Findings on Adult Neurological Assessment		
Assessment	**Expected Findings**	**Unexpected Findings (Document and notify provider if new finding*)**
Inspection	Alert and oriented to person, place, and time Symmetrical facial expressions Clear and appropriate speech Ability to follow instructions PERRLA (Pupils are equal, round, and reactive to light and accommodation) Cranial nerves all intact Negative Romberg test Sensory function present Cortical functioning (indicated by stereognosis) intact Good balance Coordinated gait with equal arm swing Finger-to-nose, rapid alternating arm movements, and heel-to-shin performance intact Negative pronator drift test Motor strength in upper and lower extremities equal bilaterally Deep tendon reflexes intact	Not alert and oriented to person, place, and/or time Asymmetrical facial expressions Garbled speech Inability to follow directions Pupils unequal in size or reactivity Deficits in one or more cranial nerve assessments Positive Romberg test Sensory function impaired in one or more areas Stereognosis not intact Poor balance Shuffled or asymmetrical gait with unequal arm swing Unable to complete finger-to-nose, alternating arm movement, or heel-to-shin tests Positive pronator drift test Unequal strength of upper and/or lower extremities One or more deep tendon reflexes are not reactive
Critical findings to report immediately and/or obtain emergency assistance:		Change in mental status, pupil responsiveness, facial drooping, slurred words or inability to speak, or sudden unilateral loss of motor strength

My Notes

6.11 SAMPLE DOCUMENTATION

Sample Documentation of Expected Findings

Patient denies any new onset of symptoms of headaches, dizziness, visual disturbances, numbness, tingling, or weakness. Patient is alert and oriented to person, place, and time. Dress is appropriate, well-groomed, and proper hygiene. Patient is cooperative and appropriately follows instructions during the exam. Speech is clear and facial expressions are symmetrical. Glasgow scores at 15. Gait is coordinated and erect with good balance. PERRLA, pupil size 4mm. Sensation intact in all extremities to light touch. Cranial nerves intact x 12. No deficits demonstrated on Mini-Mental Status Exam. Upper and lower extremity strength and hand grasps are 5/5 (equal with full resistance bilaterally). Follows commands appropriately. Cerebellar function intact as demonstrated through alternating hand movements and finger-to-nose test. Negative Romberg and Pronator drift. Balance is stable during heel-to-toe test. Tolerated exam without difficulty.

Sample Documentation of Unexpected Findings

Patient is alert and oriented to person, place, and time. Speech is clear; affect and facial expressions are appropriate to situation. Patient cooperative with exam and exhibits pleasant and calm behavior. Dress is appropriate, well-groomed, and proper hygiene. Posture remains erect in wheelchair, with intermittent drift to left side. History of CVA with left sided hemiplegia. Bilateral hearing aids in place with corrective lenses on. Pupils are 4mm equal and round. Reaction intact right and accommodation intact right eye. Left pupil 2mm, round nonreactive to light and accommodation. Upper extremity hand grips, nonsymmetrical due to left-sided weakness. Right hand grip and upper extremity strength strong at 4/5. Left lower extremity residual weakness, rated at 1/5, right lower extremity strength 4/5. Sensation intact to light touch bilaterally, R>L. Unable to assess Romberg and Pronator drift.

6.12 CHECKLIST FOR NEUROLOGICAL ASSESSMENT

My Notes

Begin assessing a patient's general appearance, posture, ability to walk, personal hygiene, and other general survey assessments during the first few minutes of the initial nurse-patient interaction. When asking the patient to perform specific neurological tests, it is helpful to demonstrate movements for the patient. Explain the purpose and use of any equipment used.

Use the checklist below to review the steps for completion of a routine "Neurological Assessment."

Steps

Disclaimer: Always review and follow agency policy regarding this specific skill.

1. Gather supplies: penlight. For a comprehensive neurological exam, additional supplies may be needed: Snellen chart; tongue depressor; cotton wisp or applicator; and percussion hammer; objects to touch, such as coins or paper clips; substances to smell, such as vanilla, mint, or coffee; and substances to taste such as sugar, salt, or lemon.
2. Perform safety steps:
    - Perform hand hygiene.
    - Check the room for transmission-based precautions.
    - Introduce yourself, your role, the purpose of your visit, and an estimate of the time it will take.
    - Confirm patient ID using two patient identifiers (e.g., name and date of birth).
    - Explain the process to the patient and ask if they have any questions.
    - Be organized and systematic.
    - Use appropriate listening and questioning skills.
    - Listen and attend to patient cues.
    - Ensure the patient's privacy and dignity.
    - Assess ABCs.
3. Obtain subjective assessment data related to history of neurological disease and any current neurological concerns using effective communication.
4. Assess the patient's behavior, language, mood, hygiene, and choice of dress while performing the interview. Note any hearing or visual deficits and ensure glasses and hearing aids are in place, if needed.
5. Assess level of consciousness and orientation; use Glasgow Coma Scale if appropriate.
6. (Optional) Complete Mini-Mental State Examination (MMSE), if indicated.
7. Assess for PERRLA.

My Notes

8. Assess motor strength and sensation.
    - Hand grasps
    - Upper body strength/resistance
    - Lower body strength/resistance
    - Sensation in extremities
9. Assess coordination and balance.
    - Ask the patient to walk, using an assistive device if needed, assessing gait for smoothness, coordination, and arm swing.
    - As appropriate, assess the patient's ability to tandem walk (heel to toe), walk on tiptoes, walk on heels.
    - Assess cerebellar functioning using tests such as Romberg, pronator drift, rapid alternating hand movement, fingertip-to-nose, and heel-to-shin tests.
10. (Optional) Perform a cranial nerve assessment and assess deep tendon reflexes as indicated.
11. Assist the patient to a comfortable position, ask if they have any questions, and thank them for their time.
12. Ensure five safety measures when leaving the room:
    - CALL LIGHT: Within reach
    - BED: Low and locked (in lowest position and brakes on)
    - SIDE RAILS: Secured
    - TABLE: Within reach
    - ROOM: Risk-free for falls (scan room and clear any obstacles)
13. Perform hand hygiene.
14. Document the assessment findings and report any concerns according to agency policy.

6.13 LEARNING ACTIVITIES

My Notes

Learning Activities

(Answers to "Learning Activities" can be found in the '"Answer Key'" at the end of the book. Answers to interactive activity elements will be provided within the element as immediate feedback.)

1. A male client has an impairment of cranial nerve II. Specific to this impairment, the nurse would plan to do which of the following to ensure client safety?
    a. Use loud a tone when speaking to the client
    b. Test the temperature of the shower water
    c. Check the temperature of the food prior to eating
    d. Remove obstacles when ambulating
2. The nurse is performing a mental status examination on a client with confusion. This test assesses which of the following?
    a. Cerebral function
    b. Cerebellar function
    c. Sensory function
    d. Intellectual function

Interactive Activity

An interactive or media element has been excluded from this version of the text. You can view it online here: https://wtcs.pressbooks.pub/nursingskills/?p=1206

Interactive Activity

An interactive or media element has been excluded from this version of the text. You can view it online here: https://wtcs.pressbooks.pub/nursingskills/?p=1206

My Notes

VI GLOSSARY

Accommodation: The ability of the eye to adjust from near vision to far vision. Pupils constrict at near vision and dilate at far vision.

Anosmia: Partial or complete loss of smell. This symptom can be related to underlying cranial nerve dysfunction or other nonpathological causes such as a common cold.

Babinski response: A reflex demonstrated by the fanning of toes with the great toe pointed toward the back (dorsum) of the foot. In adults, the Babinski response is considered abnormal and an indication of motor neuron disease.

Broca's area: An area located in the frontal lobe that is responsible for the production of language and controlling movements responsible for speech.

Bruit: A swishing sound heard upon auscultation.

Central nervous system: The part of the nervous system that includes the brain (the interpretation center) and the spinal cord (the transmission pathway).

Cerebellum: The part of the brain that coordinates skeletal and smooth muscle movement and maintains equilibrium and balance.

Cerebral cortex: The cerebrum is covered by a wrinkled outer layer of gray matter.

Comatose: A decreased level of consciousness with a score of less than 8 on the Glasgow Coma Scale.

Convergence: The action of both eyes moving inward as they focus on a close object using near vision.

Dermatome: An area of the skin that is supplied by a single spinal nerve.

Diplopia: Double vision (i.e., seeing two images of a single object).

Dysphagia: Difficulty swallowing.

Dysphasia: Difficulty speaking.

Hypothalamus: The autonomic control center of the brain that controls functions such as blood pressure, heart rate, digestive movement, and pain perception.

Kinesthesia: A person's sense of movement.

Level of consciousness: A patient's level of arousal and alertness, commonly assessed by asking them to report their name, current location, and time.

Motor nerves: Nerves in the peripheral nervous system that transmit motor signals from the brain to the muscles to cause movement.

Nystagmus: Involuntary, shaky eye movements.

Paralysis: The partial or complete loss of strength, movement, or control of a muscle or group of muscles within a body part that can be caused by brain or spinal injury.

Peripheral nervous system: The part of the nervous system that includes the cranial and spinal nerves.

Proprioception: A person's sense of their body position.

Ptosis: Drooping of the eyelid.

Sensation: The function of receiving information about the environment. The major senses are taste, smell, touch, sight, and hearing.

Sensory nerves: Nerves in the peripheral nervous system that carry impulses from the body to the brain for processing.

Stereognosis: The ability to perceive the physical form and identity of an object based on tactile stimuli alone.

Thalamus: Relays sensory information and motor information in collaboration with the cerebellum.

Chapter 7

Head and Neck Assessment

7.1 HEAD AND NECK ASSESSMENT INTRODUCTION

My Notes

Learning Objectives

- Perform a head and neck assessment, including the skull, face, nose, oral cavity, and neck
- Modify assessment techniques to reflect variations across the life span
- Recognize and report significant deviations from norms
- Document actions and observations

Inspection of a patient's head, neck, and oral cavity is part of the routine daily assessment performed by a registered nurse (RN) during inpatient care.[1] There are also several head and neck conditions that the RN may be the first to notice after a patient is admitted that require notification of the health care provider. Let's get started by reviewing the basic anatomy and physiology of the head and neck and common medical conditions.

1 Giddens, J. F. (2007). A survey of physical examination techniques performed by RNs: Lessons for nursing education. *Journal of Nursing Education, 46*(2), 83-87. https://doi.org/10.3928/01484834-20070201-09

My Notes

7.2 HEAD AND NECK BASIC CONCEPTS

To perform and document an accurate assessment of the head and neck, it is important to understand their basic anatomy and physiology.

Anatomy

Skull

The anterior skull consists of facial bones that provide the bony support for the eyes and structures of the face. This anterior view of the skull is dominated by the openings of the orbits, the nasal cavity, and the upper and lower jaws. See Figure 7.1[1] for an illustration of the skull. The **orbit** is the bony socket that houses the eyeball and the muscles that move the eyeball. Inside the nasal area of the skull, the nasal cavity is divided into halves by the **nasal septum** that consists of both bone and cartilage components. The **mandible** forms the lower jaw and is the only movable bone in the skull. The **maxilla** forms the upper jaw and supports the upper teeth.[2]

1 "704 Skull -01.jpg" by OpenStax College is licensed under CC BY 3.0. Access for free at https://openstax.org/books/anatomy-and-physiology/pages/7-2-the-skull

2 This work is a derivative of Anatomy & Physiology by OpenStax and is licensed under CC BY 4.0. Access for free at https://openstax.org/books/anatomy-and-physiology/pages/1-introduction

My Notes

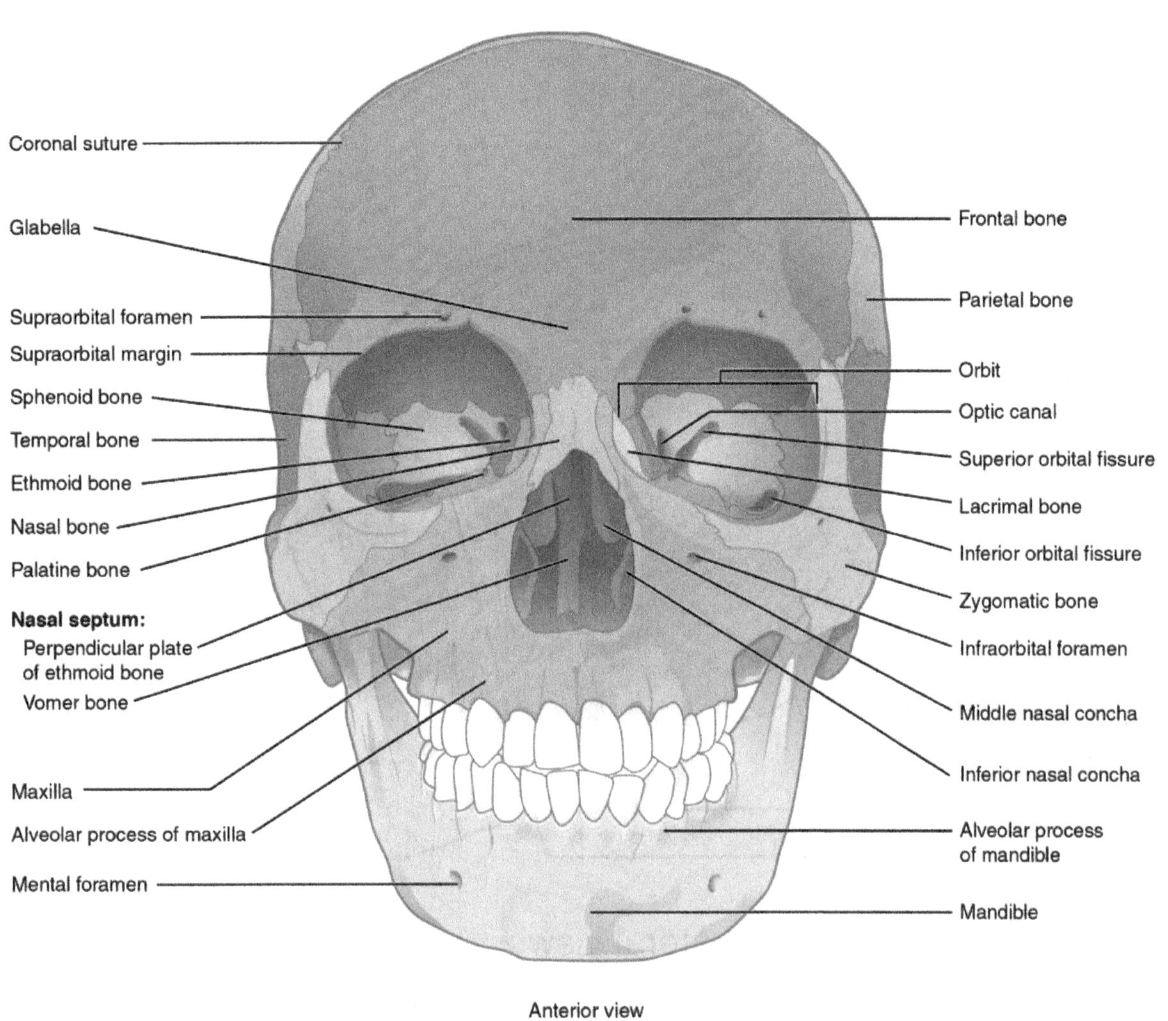
Coronal suture
Glabella
Supraorbital foramen
Supraorbital margin
Sphenoid bone
Temporal bone
Ethmoid bone
Nasal bone
Palatine bone
Nasal septum:
Perpendicular plate of ethmoid bone
Vomer bone
Maxilla
Alveolar process of maxilla
Mental foramen
Frontal bone
Parietal bone
Orbit
Optic canal
Superior orbital fissure
Lacrimal bone
Inferior orbital fissure
Zygomatic bone
Infraorbital foramen
Middle nasal concha
Inferior nasal concha
Alveolar process of mandible
Mandible
Anterior view

Figure 7.1 Skull

My Notes

The **brain case** surrounds and protects the brain that occupies the cranial cavity. See Figure 7.2[3] for an image of the brain within the cranial cavity. The brain case consists of eight bones, including the paired parietal and temporal bones plus the unpaired frontal, occipital, sphenoid, and ethmoid bones.[4]

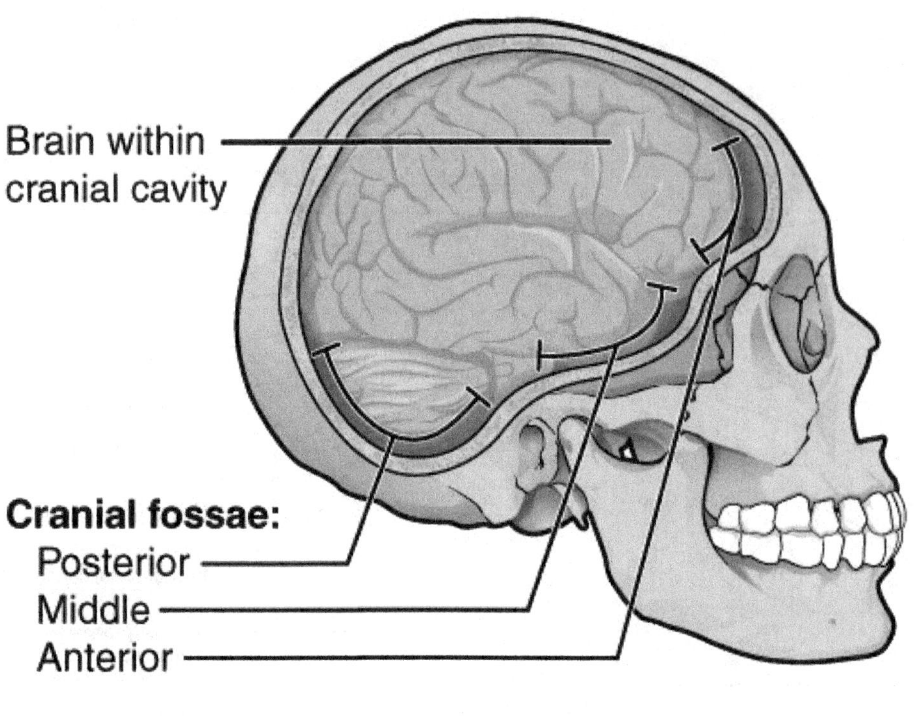

Figure 7.2 Cranial Cavity

A **suture** is an interlocking joint between adjacent bones of the skull and is filled with dense, fibrous connective tissue that unites the bones. In a newborn infant, the pressure from vaginal delivery compresses the head and causes the bony plates to overlap at the sutures, creating a small ridge. Over the next few days, the head expands, the overlapping disappears, and the edges of the bony plates meet edge to edge. This is the normal position for the remainder of the life span and the sutures become immobile.

See Figure 7.3[5] for an illustration of two of the sutures, the coronal and squamous sutures, on the lateral view of the head. The coronal suture is seen on the top of the skull. It runs from side to side across the skull and joins the frontal bone to the right and left parietal bones. The squamous suture is located on the lateral side of the skull. It unites the squamous portion of the temporal bone with the parietal bone. At the intersection of the coronal and squamous sutures is the pterion, a small, capital H-shaped suture line region that unites the frontal bone, parietal

3 This work is derivative of "727_Cranial_Fossae.jpg" by OpenStax and is licensed under CC BY 3.0. Access for free at https://openstax.org/books/anatomy-and-physiology/pages/7-2-the-skull

4 This work is a derivative of Anatomy & Physiology by OpenStax and is licensed under CC BY 4.0. Access for free at https://openstax.org/books/anatomy-and-physiology/pages/1-introduction

5 "705 Lateral View of Skull-01.jpg" by OpenStax is licensed under CC BY 3.0. Access for free at https://openstax.org/books/anatomy-and-physiology/pages/7-2-the-skull

My Notes

bone, temporal bone, and greater wing of the sphenoid bone. The pterion is an important clinical landmark because located immediately under it, inside the skull, is a major branch of an artery that supplies the brain. A strong blow to this region can fracture the bones around the pterion. If the underlying artery is damaged, bleeding can cause the formation of a collection of blood, called a **hematoma**, between the brain and interior of the skull, which can be life-threatening.[6]

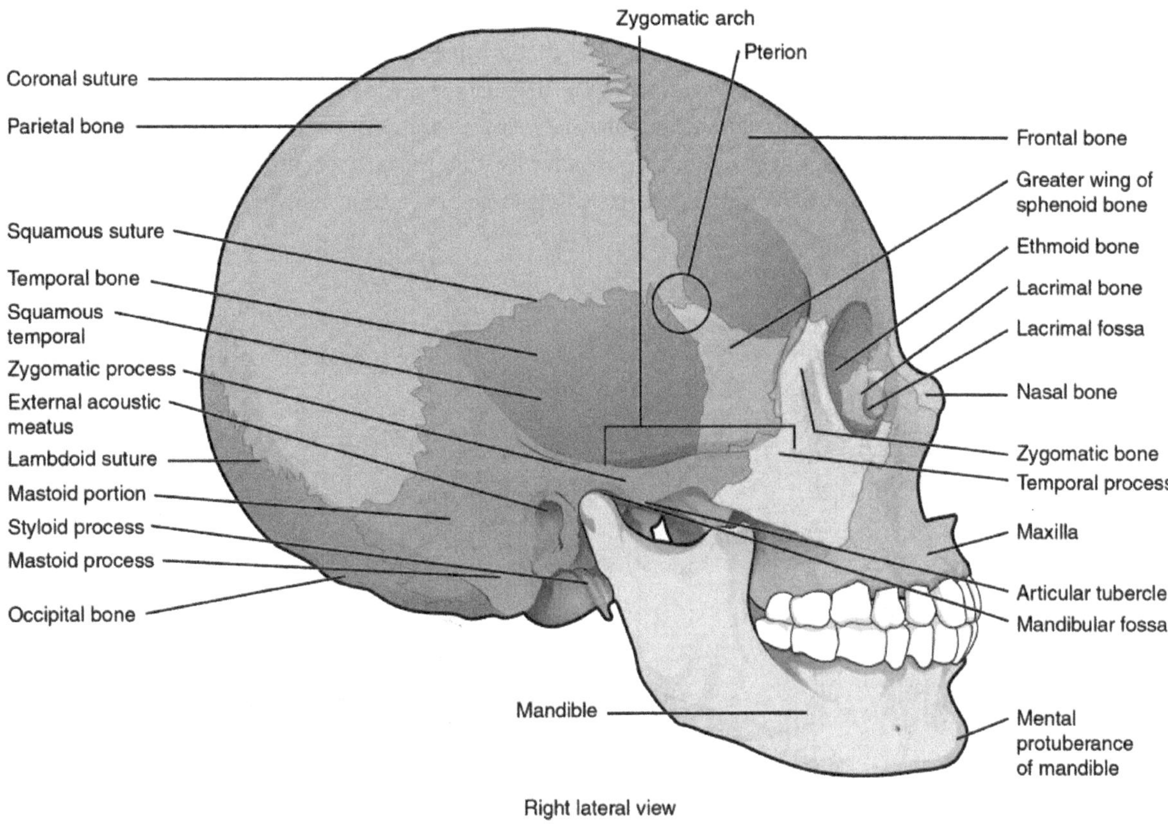

Figure 7.3 Coronal Sutures in Lateral View of Skull

6 This work is a derivative of Anatomy & Physiology by OpenStax and is licensed under CC BY 4.0. Access for free at https://openstax.org/books/anatomy-and-physiology/pages/1-introduction

My Notes

Paranasal Sinuses

The paranasal sinuses are hollow, air-filled spaces located within the skull. See Figure 7.4[7] for an illustration of the sinuses. The sinuses connect with the nasal cavity and are lined with nasal mucosa. They reduce bone mass, lightening the skull, and also add resonance to the voice. When a person has a cold or sinus congestion, the mucosa swells and produces excess mucus that often obstructs the narrow passageways between the sinuses and the nasal cavity. The resulting pressure produces pain and discomfort.[8]

Each of the paranasal sinuses is named for the skull bone that it occupies. The frontal sinus is located just above the eyebrows within the frontal bone. The largest sinus, the maxillary sinus, is paired and located within the right and left maxillary bones just below the orbits. The maxillary sinuses are most commonly involved during sinus infections. The sphenoid sinus is a single, midline sinus located within the body of the sphenoid bone. The lateral aspects of the ethmoid bone contain multiple small spaces separated by very thin, bony walls. Each of these spaces is called an ethmoid air cell.

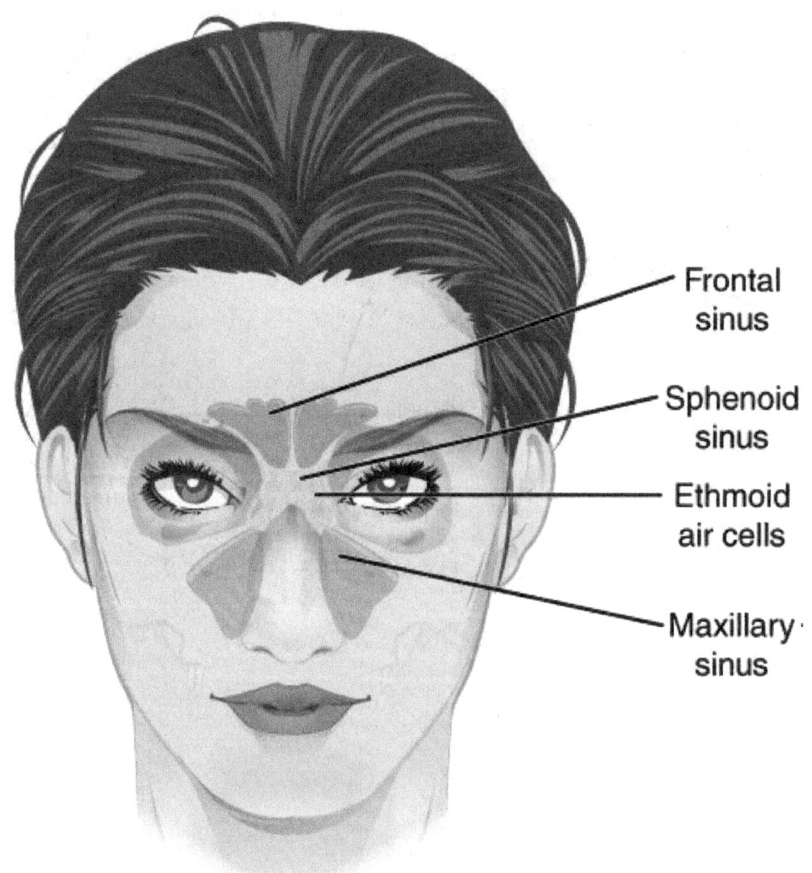

Figure 7.4 Sinuses

7 "Paranasal Sinuses ant.jpg" by OpenStax is licensed under CC BY-SA 3.0. Access for free at https://openstax.org/books/anatomy-and-physiology/pages/7-2-the-skull

8 This work is a derivative of Anatomy & Physiology by OpenStax and is licensed under CC BY 4.0. Access for free at https://openstax.org/books/anatomy-and-physiology/pages/1-introduction

Anatomy of Nose, Pharynx, and Mouth

My Notes

See Figure 7.5[9] to review the anatomy of the head and neck. The major entrance and exit for the respiratory system is through the nose. The bridge of the nose consists of bone, but the protruding portion of the nose is composed of cartilage. The **nares** are the nostril openings that open into the nasal cavity and are separated into left and right sections by the **nasal septum**. The floor of the nasal cavity is composed of the palate. The hard palate is located at the anterior region of the nasal cavity and is composed of bone. The soft palate is located at the posterior portion of the nasal cavity and consists of muscle tissue. The **uvula** is a small, teardrop-shaped structure located at the apex of the soft palate. Both the uvula and soft palate move like a pendulum during swallowing, swinging upward to close off the nasopharynx and prevent ingested materials from entering the nasal cavity.[10]

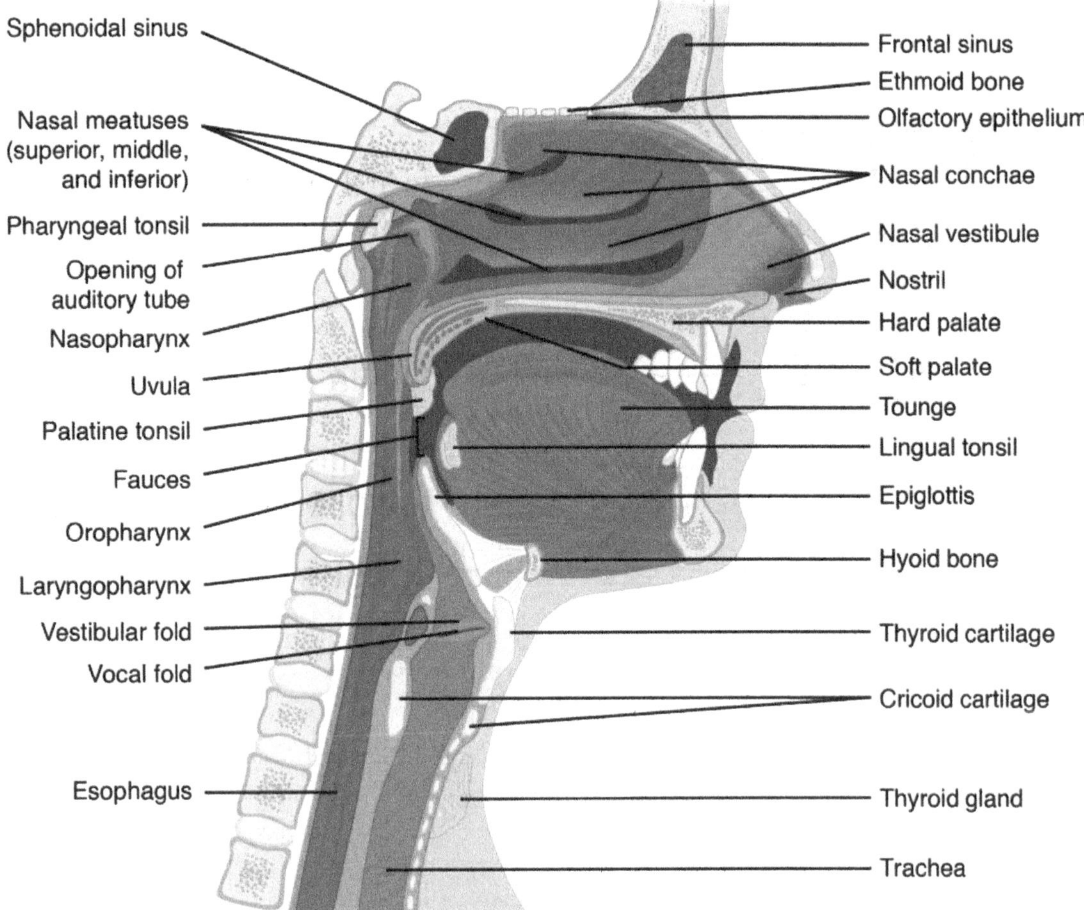

Figure 7.5 Anatomy of the Head and Neck

9 "2303 Anatomy of Nose-Pharynx-Mouth-Larynx.jpg" by OpenStax is licensed CC BY 3.0. Access for free at https://commons.wikimedia.org/wiki/File:2303_Anatomy_of_Nose-Pharynx-Mouth-Larynx.jpg

10 This work is a derivative of Anatomy & Physiology by OpenStax and is licensed under CC BY 4.0. Access for free at https://openstax.org/books/anatomy-and-physiology/pages/1-introduction

My Notes

As air is inhaled through the nose, the paranasal sinuses warm and humidify the incoming air as it moves into the pharynx. The **pharynx** is a tube-lined mucous membrane that begins at the nasal cavity and is divided into three major regions: the nasopharynx, the oropharynx, and the laryngopharynx.[11]

The **nasopharynx** serves only as an airway. At the top of the nasopharynx is the pharyngeal tonsil, commonly referred to as the adenoids. Adenoids are lymphoid tissue that trap and destroy invading pathogens that enter during inhalation. They are large in children but tend to regress with age and may even disappear.[12]

The **oropharynx** is a passageway for both air and food. The oropharynx is bordered superiorly by the nasopharynx and anteriorly by the oral cavity. The oropharynx contains two sets of tonsils, the palatine and lingual tonsils. The palatine tonsil is located laterally in the oropharynx, and the lingual tonsil is located at the base of the tongue. Similar to the pharyngeal tonsil, the palatine and lingual tonsils are composed of lymphoid tissue and trap and destroy pathogens entering the body through the oral or nasal cavities. See Figure 7.6[13] for an image of the oral cavity and oropharynx with enlarged palatine tonsils.

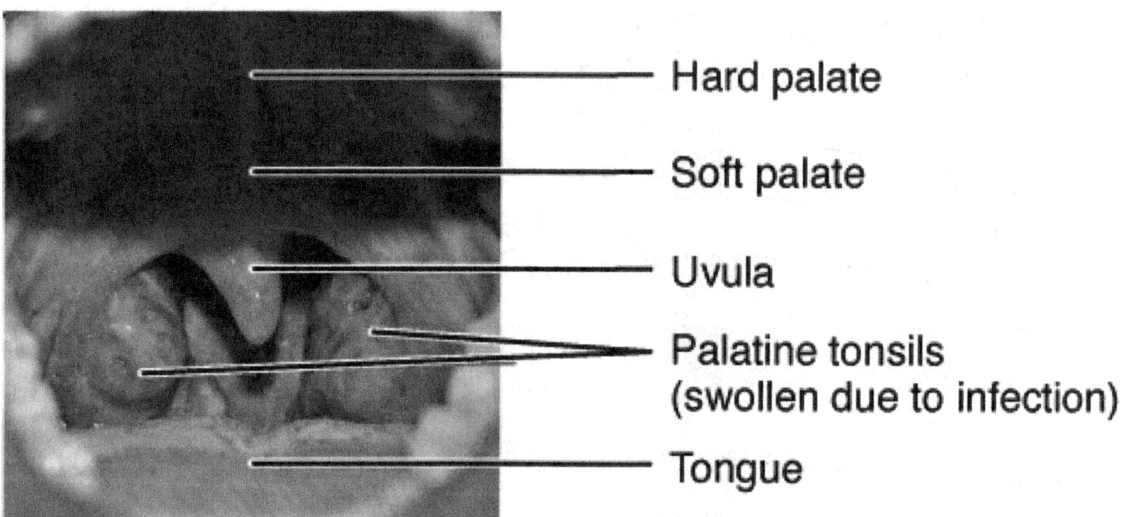

Figure 7.6 Oral Cavity and Oropharynx

The **laryngopharynx** is inferior to the oropharynx and posterior to the larynx. It continues the route for ingested material and air until its inferior end where the digestive and respiratory systems diverge. Anteriorly, the laryngopharynx opens into the larynx and posteriorly, it enters the esophagus that leads to the stomach. The **larynx** connects the pharynx to the trachea and helps regulate the volume of air that enters and leaves the lungs. It also contains the vocal cords that vibrate as air passes over them to produce the sound of a person's voice. The **trachea**

11 This work is a derivative of Anatomy & Physiology by OpenStax and is licensed under CC BY 4.0. Access for free at https://openstax.org/books/anatomy-and-physiology/pages/1-introduction

12 This work is a derivative of Anatomy & Physiology by OpenStax and is licensed under CC BY 4.0. Access for free at https://openstax.org/books/anatomy-and-physiology/pages/1-introduction

13 This work is a derivative of "2209 Location and Histology of Tonsils.jpg" by OpenStax and is licensed under CC BY 3.0 Access for free at https://openstax.org/books/anatomy-and-physiology/pages/21-1-anatomy-of-the-lymphatic-and-immune-systems

extends from the larynx to the lungs. The **epiglottis** is a flexible piece of cartilage that covers the opening of the trachea during swallowing to prevent ingested material from entering the trachea.[14]

My Notes

Muscles and Nerves of the Head and Neck

Facial Muscles

Several nerves innervate the facial muscles to create facial expressions. See Figure 7.7[15] for an illustration of nerves innervating facial muscles. These nerves and muscles are tested during a cranial nerve exam. See more information about performing a cranial nerve exam in the "Neurological Assessment" chapter.

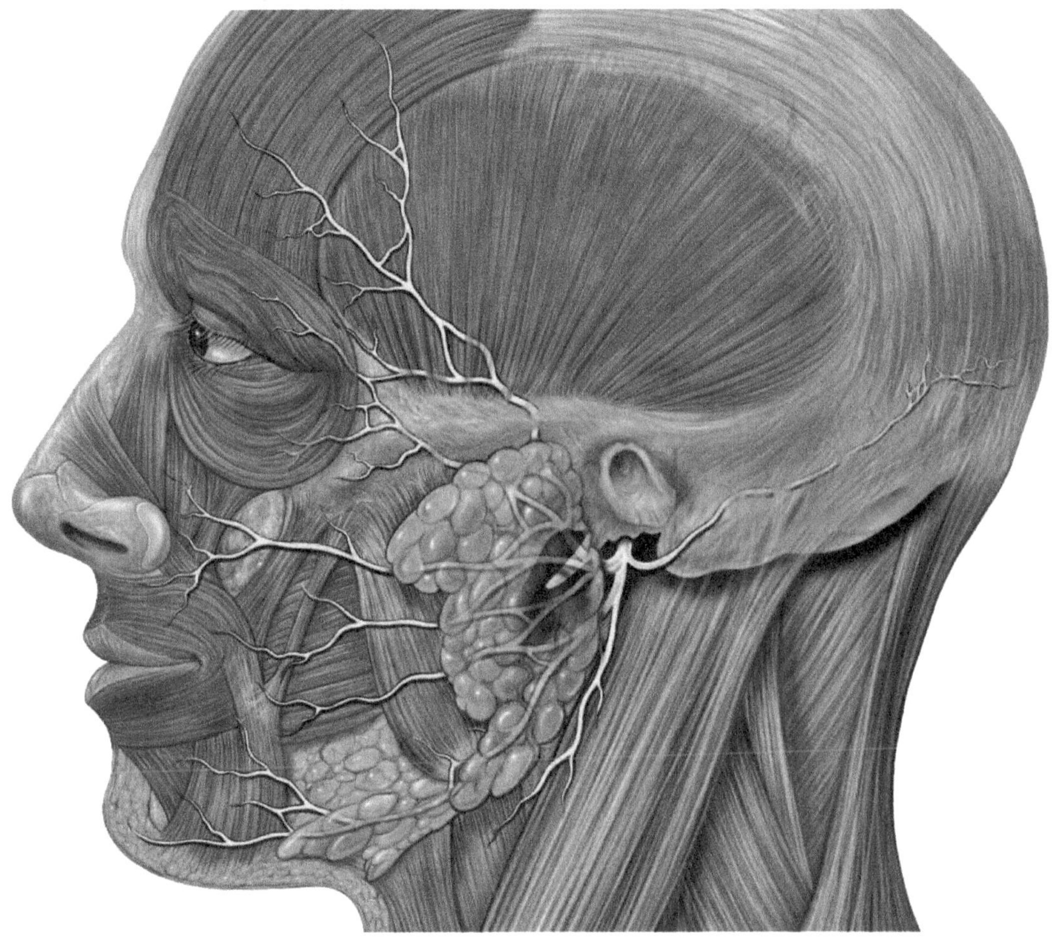

Figure 7.7 Nerve Branches Innervating Facial Muscles

14 This work is a derivative of Anatomy & Physiology by OpenStax and is licensed under CC BY 4.0. Access for free at https://openstax.org/books/anatomy-and-physiology/pages/1-introduction

15 "Head facial nerve branches.jpg" by Patrick J. Lynch, medical illustrator is licensed under CC BY 2.5. Access for free at https://commons.wikimedia.org/wiki/File:Head_facial_nerve_branches.jpg

My Notes

When a patient is experiencing a cerebrovascular accident (i.e., stroke), it is common for facial drooping to occur. **Facial drooping** is an asymmetrical facial expression that occurs due to damage of the nerve innervating a specific part of the face. See Figure 7.8[16] for an image of facial drooping occurring on the patient's right side of their face.

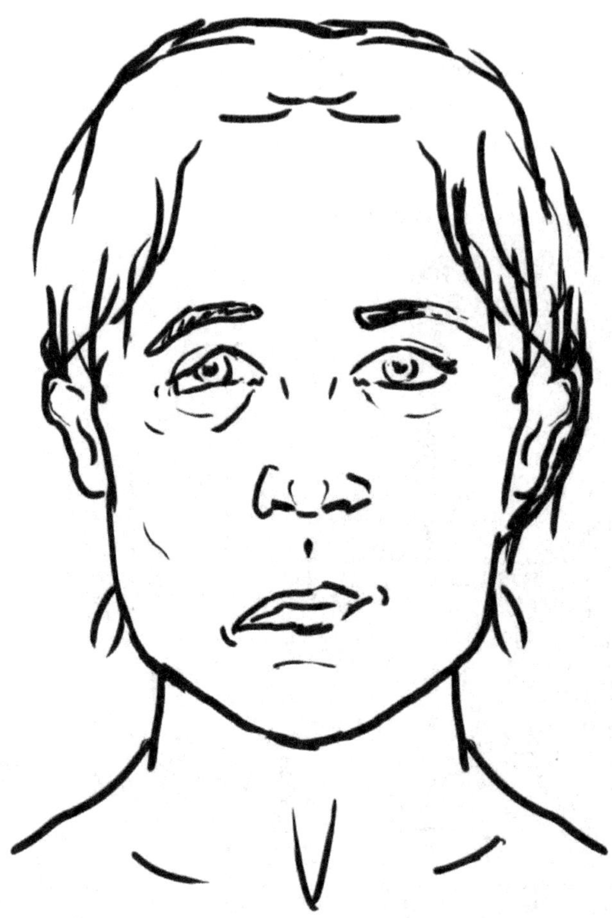

Figure 7.8 Facial Drooping

Neck Muscles

The muscles of the anterior neck assist in swallowing and speech by controlling the positions of the larynx and the hyoid bone, a horseshoe- shaped bone that functions as a solid foundation on which the tongue can move. The head, attached to the top of the vertebral column, is balanced, moved, and rotated by the neck muscles. When these muscles act unilaterally, the head rotates. When they contract bilaterally, the head flexes or extends. The major muscle that laterally flexes and rotates the head is the **sternocleidomastoid**. The **trapezius** muscle elevates the shoulders (shrugging), pulls the shoulder blades together, and tilts the head backwards. See Figure 7.9[17] for an

16 "Stroke-facial-droop.jpg" by Another-anon-artist-234 is licensed under CC0 1.0. Access for free at https://commons.wikimedia.org/wiki/File:Stroke-facial-droop.jpg

17 "1111 Posterior and Side Views of the Next.jpg" by OpenStax is licensed under CC BY 4.0. Access for free at https://openstax.org/books/anatomy-and-physiology/pages/11-3-axial-muscles-of-the-head-neck-and-back.

illustration of the sternocleidomastoid and trapezius muscles.[18] Both of these muscles are tested during a cranial nerve assessment. See more information about cranial nerve assessment in the "Neurological Assessment" chapter.

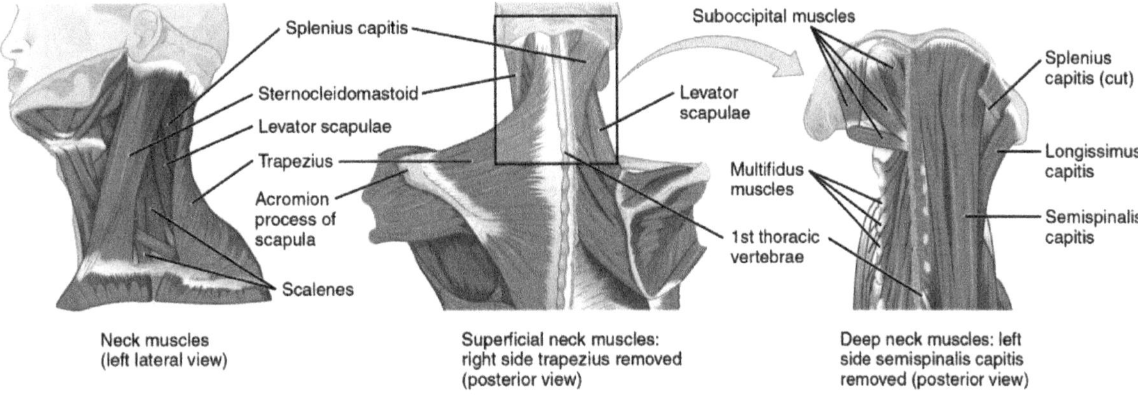

Figure 7.9 Neck Muscles

Jaw Muscles

The **masseter** muscle is the main muscle used for chewing because it elevates the mandible (lower jaw) to close the mouth. It is assisted by the temporalis muscle that retracts the mandible. The **temporalis** muscle can be felt moving by placing fingers on the patient's temple as they chew. See Figure 7.10[19] for an illustration of the masseter and temporalis muscles.[20]

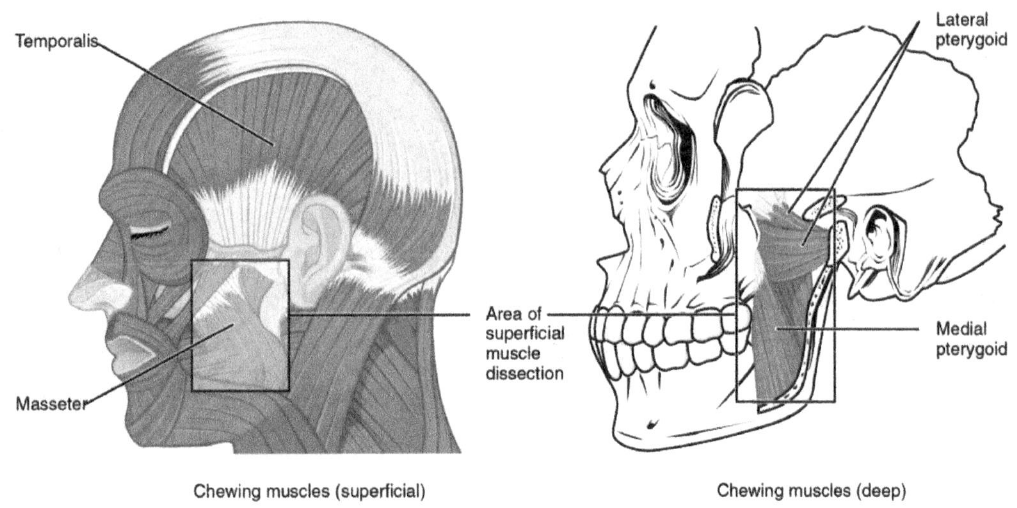

Figure 7.10 Masseter and Temporalis Muscles

18 This work is a derivative of Anatomy & Physiology by OpenStax and is licensed under CC BY 4.0. Access for free at https://openstax.org/books/anatomy-and-physiology/pages/1-introduction

19 "1108 Muscle that Move the Lower Jaw.jpg" by OpenStax is licensed under CC BY 4.0. Access for free at https://openstax.org/books/anatomy-and-physiology/pages/11-3-axial-muscles-of-the-head-neck-and-back

20 This work is a derivative of Anatomy & Physiology by OpenStax and is licensed under CC BY 4.0. Access for free at https://openstax.org/books/anatomy-and-physiology/pages/1-introduction

My Notes

Tongue Muscles

Muscles of the tongue are necessary for chewing, swallowing, and speech. Because it is so moveable, the tongue facilitates complex speech patterns and sounds.[21]

Airway and Unconsciousness

When a patient becomes unconscious and is lying supine, the tongue often moves backwards and blocks the airway. This is why it is important to open the airway when performing CPR by using a chin-thrust maneuver. See Figure 7.11[22] for an image of the tongue blocking the airway. In a similar manner, when a patient is administered general anesthesia during surgery, the tongue relaxes and can block the airway. For this reason, endotracheal intubation is performed during surgery with general anesthesia by placing a tube into the trachea to maintain an open airway to the lungs. After surgery, patients often report a sore or scratchy throat for a few days due to the endotracheal intubation.[23]

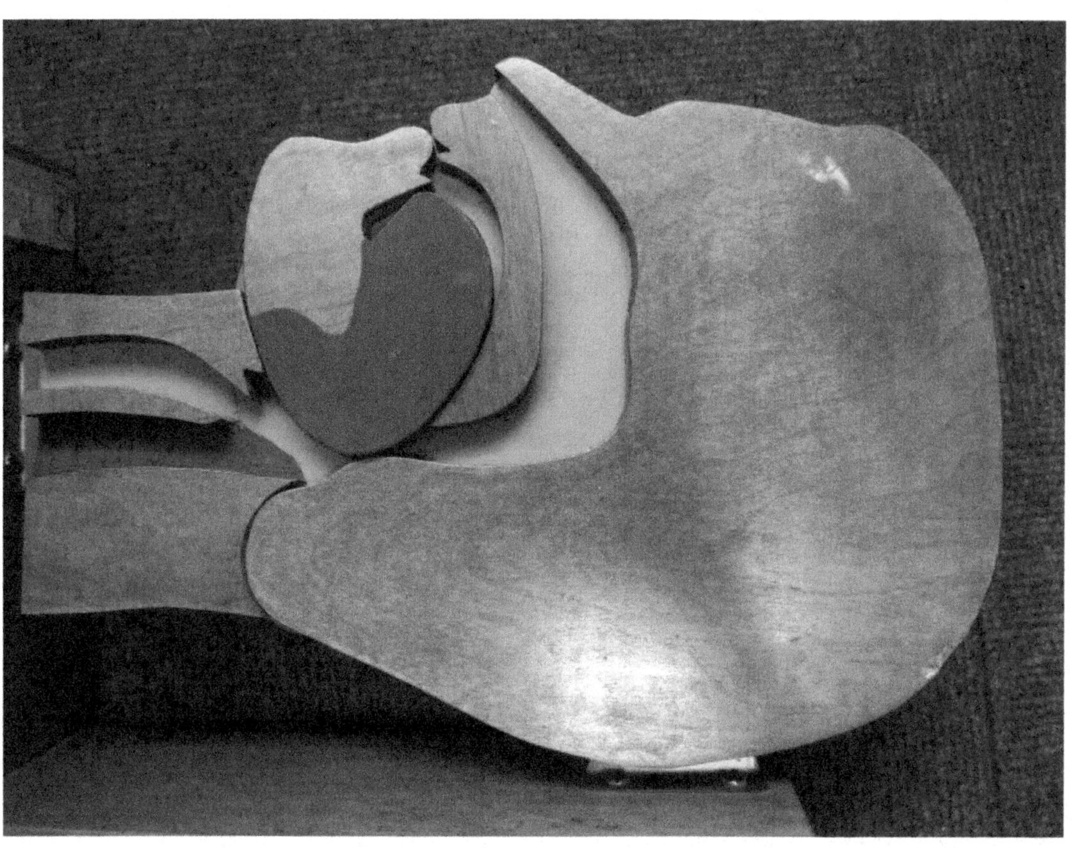

Figure 7.11 Airway Blocked by Tongue

---

21 This work is a derivative of Anatomy & Physiology by OpenStax and is licensed under CC BY 4.0. Access for free at https://openstax.org/books/anatomy-and-physiology/pages/1-introduction

22 "Airway closed in an unconscious patient because the head inflexed forward.jpg" by Dr. Lorimer is licensed under *CC BY-SA 4.0*. Access for free at https://commons.m.wikimedia.org/wiki/File:Airway_closed_in_an_unconscious_patient_because_the_head_inflexed_forward.jpg

23 This work is a derivative of Anatomy & Physiology by OpenStax and is licensed under CC BY 4.0. Access for free at https://openstax.org/books/anatomy-and-physiology/pages/1-introduction

My Notes

Swallowing

Swallowing is a complex process that uses 50 pairs of muscles and many nerves to receive food in the mouth, prepare it, and move it from the mouth to the stomach. Swallowing occurs in three stages. During the first stage, called the oral phase, the tongue collects the food or liquid and makes it ready for swallowing. The tongue and jaw move solid food around in the mouth so it can be chewed and made the right size and texture to swallow by mixing food with saliva. The second stage begins when the tongue pushes the food or liquid to the back of the mouth. This triggers a swallowing response that passes the food through the pharynx. During this phase, called the pharyngeal phase, the epiglottis closes off the larynx and breathing stops to prevent food or liquid from entering the airway and lungs. The third stage begins when food or liquid enters the esophagus and it is carried to the stomach. The passage through the esophagus, called the esophageal phase, usually occurs in about three seconds.[24]

View the following video from Medline Plus on the swallowing process: "Swallowing."[25]

Dysphagia is the medical term for swallowing difficulties that occur when there is a problem with the nerves or structures involved in the swallowing process.[26] Nurses are often the first to notice signs of dysphagia in their patients that can occur due to a multitude of medical conditions such as a stroke, head injury, or dementia. For more information about the symptoms, screening, and treatment for dysphagia, go to the "Common Conditions of the Head and Neck" section.

---

24 National Institute on Deafness and Other Communication Disorders. (2017, March 6). *Dysphagia*. https://www.nidcd.nih.gov/health/dysphagia

25 A.D.A.M. Medical Encyclopedia [Internet]. Atlanta (GA): A.D.A.M. Inc.; c1997-2021. Swallowing; [Video]. [updated 2019, July 11]. https://medlineplus.gov/ency/anatomyvideos/000126.htm

26 National Institute on Deafness and Other Communication Disorders. (2017, March 6). *Dysphagia*. https://www.nidcd.nih.gov/health/dysphagia

My Notes

Lymphatic System

The lymphatic system is the system of vessels, cells, and organs that carries excess interstitial fluid to the bloodstream and filters pathogens from the blood through **lymph nodes** found near the neck, armpits, chest, abdomen, and groin. See Figure 7.12[27] and Figure 7.13[28] for an illustration of the lymph nodes found in the head and neck regions. When a person is fighting off an infection, the lymph nodes in that region become enlarged, indicating an active immune response to infection.[29]

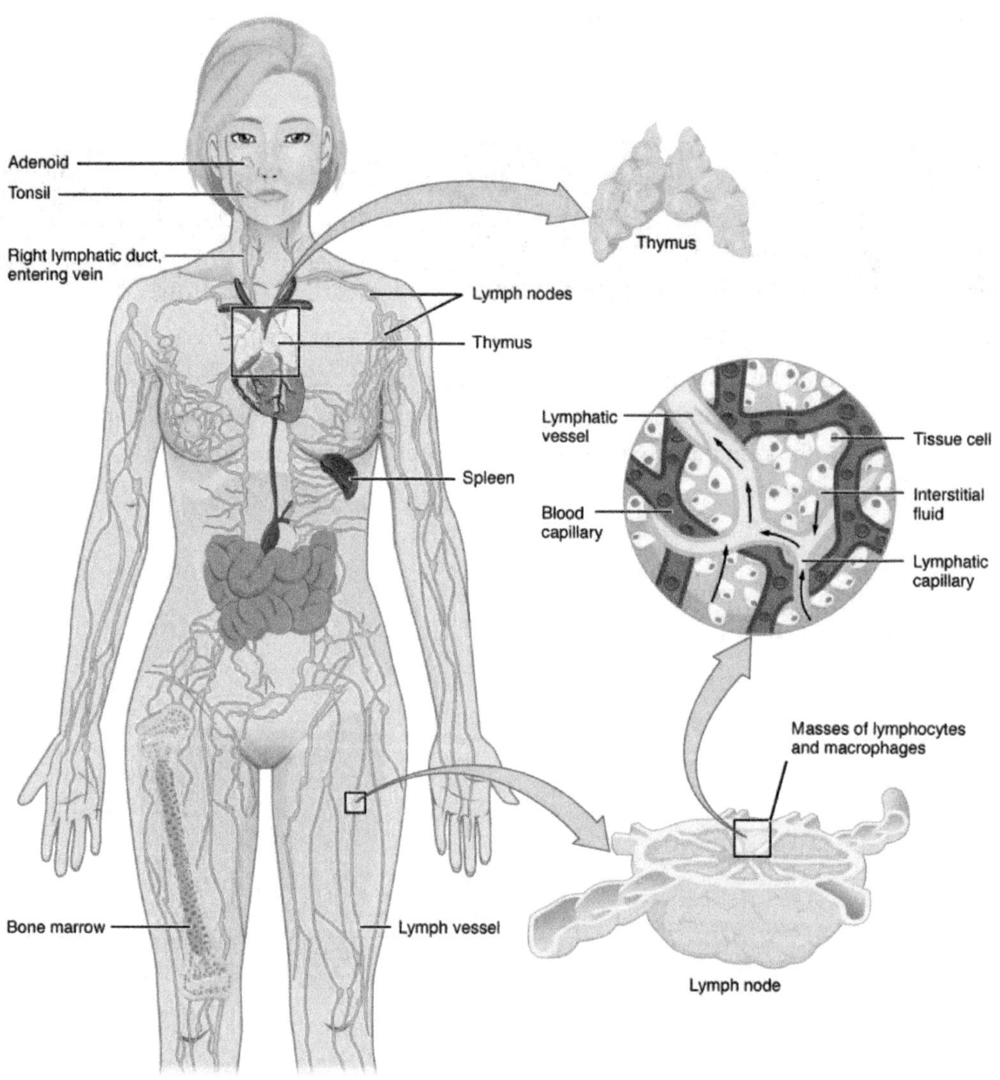

Figure 7.12 Lymphatic System

27 "2201 Anatomy of the Lymphatic System.jpg" by OpenStax College is licensed under CC BY 3.0. Access for free at https://openstax.org/books/anatomy-and-physiology/pages/21-1-anatomy-of-the-lymphatic-and-immune-systems

28 "Cervical lymph nodes and level.png" by Mikael Häggström, M.D. is licensed under CC0 1.0. Access for free at https://commons.wikimedia.org/wiki/File:Cervical_lymph_nodes_and_levels.png

29 This work is a derivative of Anatomy & Physiology by OpenStax and is licensed under CC BY 4.0. Access for free at https://openstax.org/books/anatomy-and-physiology/pages/1-introduction

My Notes

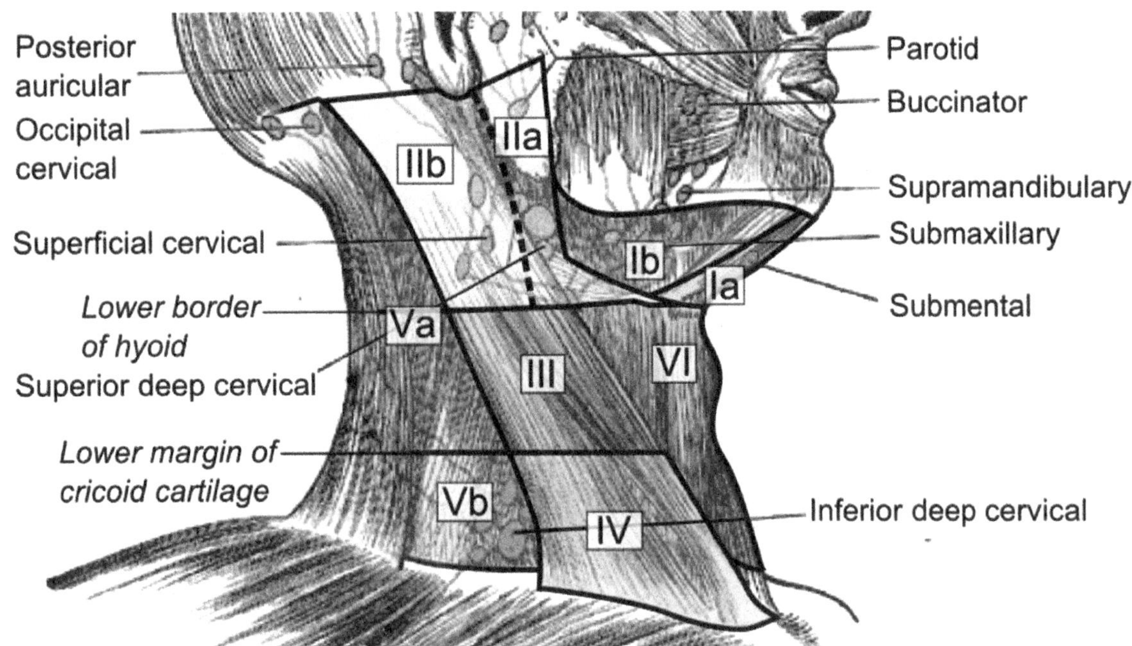

Figure 7.13 Lymph Nodes in Head and Neck

My Notes

7.3 COMMON CONDITIONS OF THE HEAD AND NECK

Headache

A headache is a common type of pain that patients experience in everyday life and a major reason for missed time at work or school. Headaches range greatly in severity of pain and frequency of occurrence. For example, some patients experience mild headaches once or twice a year, whereas others experience disabling migraine headaches more than 15 days a month. Severe headaches such as migraines may be accompanied by symptoms of nausea or increased sensitivity to noise or light. Primary headaches occur independently and are not caused by another medical condition. Migraine, cluster, and tension-type headaches are types of primary headaches. Secondary headaches are symptoms of another health disorder that causes pain-sensitive nerve endings to be pressed on or pulled out of place. They may result from underlying conditions including fever, infection, medication overuse, stress or emotional conflict, high blood pressure, psychiatric disorders, head injury or trauma, stroke, tumors, and nerve disorders such as trigeminal neuralgia, a chronic pain condition that typically affects the trigeminal nerve on one side of the cheek.[1]

Not all headaches require medical attention, but some types of headaches can signify a serious disorder and require prompt medical care. Symptoms of headaches that require immediate medical attention include a sudden, severe headache unlike any the patient has ever had; a sudden headache associated with a stiff neck; a headache associated with convulsions, confusion, or loss of consciousness; a headache following a blow to the head; or a persistent headache in a person who was previously headache free.[2]

Concussion

A **concussion** is a type of traumatic brain injury caused by a blow to the head or by a hit to the body that causes the head and brain to move rapidly back and forth. This sudden movement causes the brain to bounce around in the skull, creating chemical changes in the brain and sometimes damaging brain cells.[3] See Figure 7.14[4] for an illustration of a concussion.

---

1 National Institute of Neurological Disorders and Stroke. (2019, December 31). *Headache information page.* https://www.ninds.nih.gov/Disorders/All-Disorders/Headache-Information-Page

2 National Institute of Neurological Disorders and Stroke. (2019, December 31). *Headache information page.* https://www.ninds.nih.gov/Disorders/All-Disorders/Headache-Information-Page

3 Centers for Disease Control and Prevention. (2019, February 12). *Concussion signs and symptoms.* https://www.cdc.gov/headsup/basics/concussion_symptoms.html

4 "Concussion Anatomy.png" by Max Andrews is licensed under CC BY-SA 3.0. Access for free at https://commons.wikimedia.org/wiki/File:Concussion_Anatomy.png

My Notes

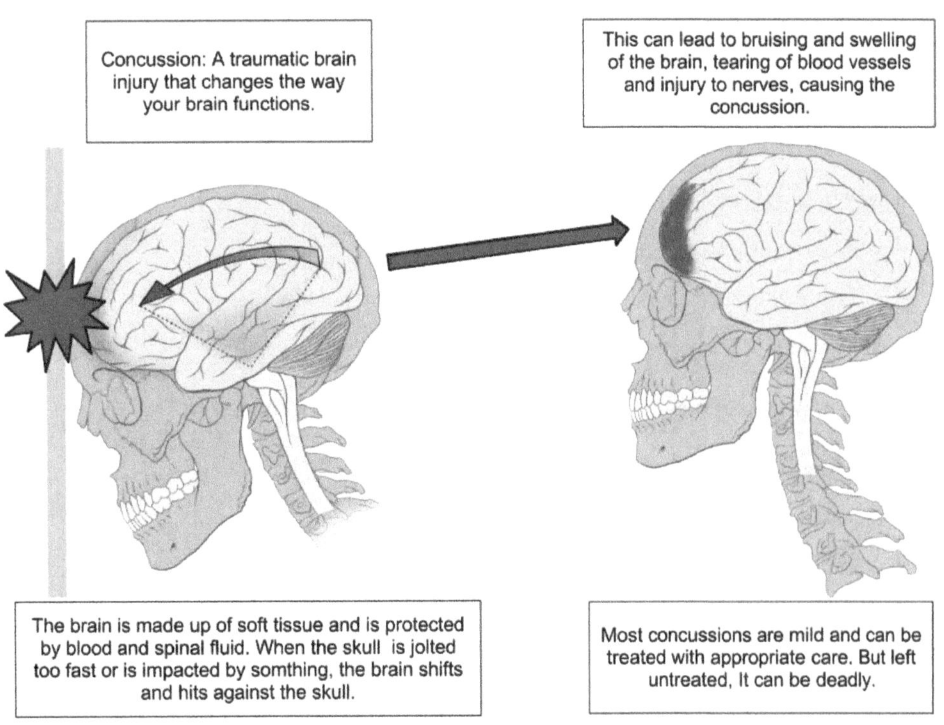

Concussion: A traumatic brain injury that changes the way your brain functions.
This can lead to bruising and swelling of the brain, tearing of blood vessels and injury to nerves, causing the concussion.
The brain is made up of soft tissue and is protected by blood and spinal fluid. When the skull is jolted too fast or is impacted by somthing, the brain shifts and hits against the skull.
Most concussions are mild and can be treated with appropriate care. But left untreated, It can be deadly.

Figure 7.14 Concussion

Video Review of Concussions[5]

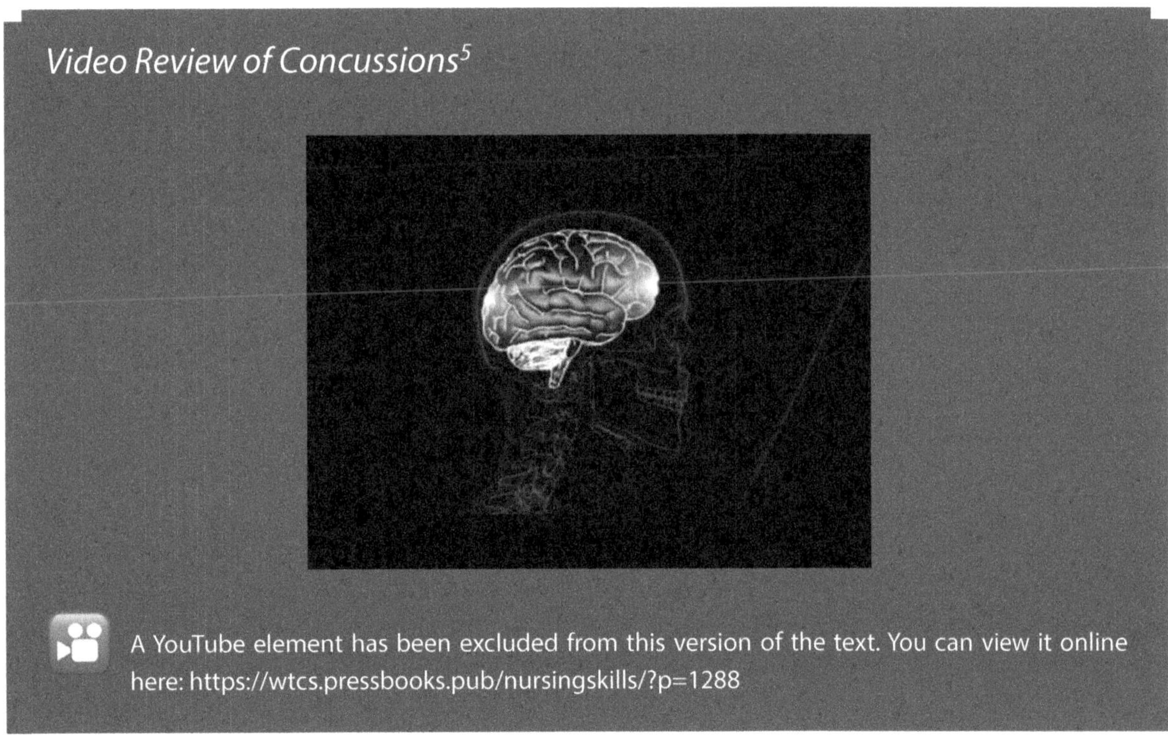

A YouTube element has been excluded from this version of the text. You can view it online here: https://wtcs.pressbooks.pub/nursingskills/?p=1288

5 Centers for Disease Control and Prevention. (2013, October 24). *What is a concussion?* [Video]. YouTube. All rights reserved. https://youtu.be/Sno_0Jd8GuA

My Notes

A person who has experienced a concussion may report the following symptoms:

- Headache or "pressure" in head
- Nausea or vomiting
- Balance problems or dizziness or double or blurry vision
- Light or noise sensitivity
- Feeling sluggish, hazy, foggy, or groggy
- Confusion, concentration, or memory problems
- Just not "feeling right" or "feeling down"[6]

The following signs may be observed in someone who has experienced a concussion:

- Can't recall events prior to or after a hit or fall
- Appears dazed or stunned
- Forgets an instruction, is confused about an assignment or position, or is unsure of the game, score, or opponent
- Moves clumsily
- Answers questions slowly
- Loses consciousness (even briefly)
- Shows mood, behavior, or personality changes[7]

Anyone suspected of experiencing a concussion should immediately be seen by a health care provider or go to the emergency department for further testing.

Read more about concussions at the following CDC webpage: "Concussion Signs and Symptoms" (https://www.cdc.gov/headsup/basics/concussion_symptoms.html)

Head Injury

Head and traumatic brain injuries are major causes of immediate death and disability. Falls are the most common cause of head injuries in young children (ages 0–4 years), adolescents (15–19 years), and the elderly (over 65 years). Strong blows to the brain case of the skull can produce fractures resulting in bleeding inside the skull. A blow to the lateral side of the head may fracture the bones of the pterion. If the underlying artery is damaged, bleeding can cause the formation of a hematoma (collection of blood) between the brain and interior of the skull. As blood accumulates, it will put pressure on the brain. Symptoms associated with a hematoma may not be apparent

6 Centers for Disease Control and Prevention. (2019, February 12). *Concussion signs and symptoms.* https://www.cdc.gov/headsup/basics/concussion_symptoms.html

7 Centers for Disease Control and Prevention. (2019, February 12). *Concussion signs and symptoms.* https://www.cdc.gov/headsup/basics/concussion_symptoms.html

My Notes

immediately following the injury, but if untreated, blood accumulation will continue to exert increasing pressure on the brain and can result in death within a few hours.[8]

See Figure 7.15[9] for an image of an epidural hematoma indicated by a red arrow associated with a skull fracture.

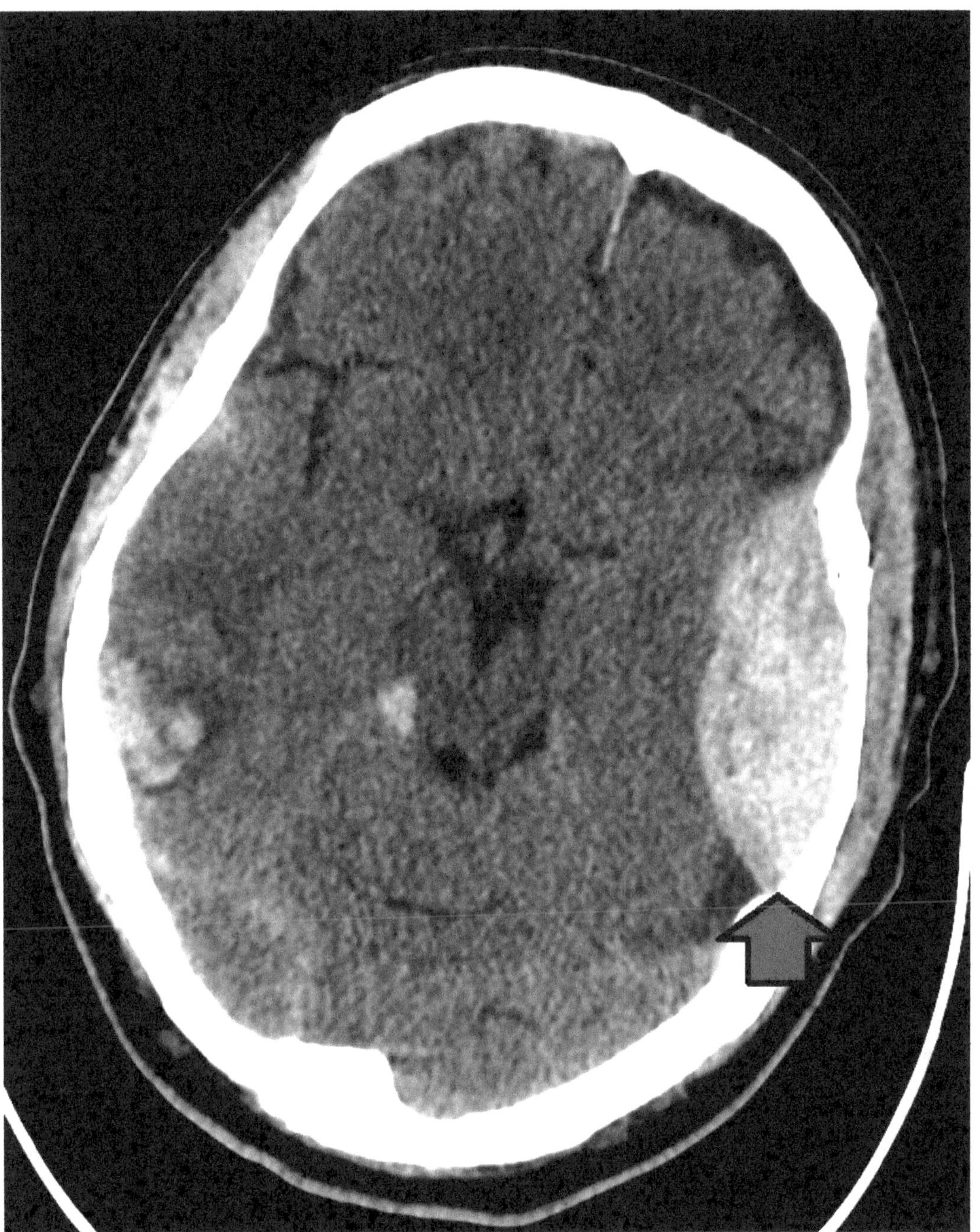

Figure 7.15 Skull Fracture and Hematoma

8 This work is a derivative of Anatomy & Physiology by OpenStax and is licensed under CC BY 4.0. Access for free at https://openstax.org/books/anatomy-and-physiology/pages/1-introduction

9 "EpiduralHeatoma.jpg" by *James Heilman, MD* is licensed under CC BY-SA 4.0. Access for free at https://commons.wikimedia.org/wiki/File:EpiduralHematoma.jpg

My Notes

Sinusitis

Sinusitis is the medical diagnosis for inflamed sinuses that can be caused by a viral or bacterial infection. When the nasal membranes become swollen, the drainage of mucous is blocked and causes pain.

There are several types of sinusitis, including these types:

- Acute Sinusitis: Infection lasting up to 4 weeks
- Chronic Sinusitis: Infection lasting more than 12 weeks
- Recurrent Sinusitis: Several episodes of sinusitis within a year

Symptoms of sinusitis can include fever, weakness, fatigue, cough, and congestion. There may also be mucus drainage in the back of the throat, called postnasal drip. Health care providers diagnose sinusitis based on symptoms and an examination of the nose and face. Treatments include antibiotics, decongestants, and pain relievers.[10]

Pharyngitis

Pharyngitis is the medical term used for infection and/or inflammation in the back of the throat (pharynx). Common causes of pharyngitis are the cold viruses, influenza, strep throat caused by group A *streptococcus*, and mononucleosis. Strep throat typically causes white patches on the tonsils with a fever and enlarged lymph nodes. It must be treated with antibiotics to prevent potential complications in the heart and kidneys. See Figure 7.16[11] for an image of strep throat in a child.

10 MedlinePlus [Internet]. Bethesda (MD): National Library of Medicine (US); [updated 2020, Aug 17]. Sinusitis; [updated 2020, Jun 10; reviewed 2016, Oct 26]; [cited 2020, Sep 4]; https://medlineplus.gov/sinusitis.html

11 "Strep throat2010.JPG" by *James Heilman, MD* is licensed under CC BY-SA 3.0. Access for free at https://commons.wikimedia.org/wiki/File:Strep_throat2010.JPG

My Notes

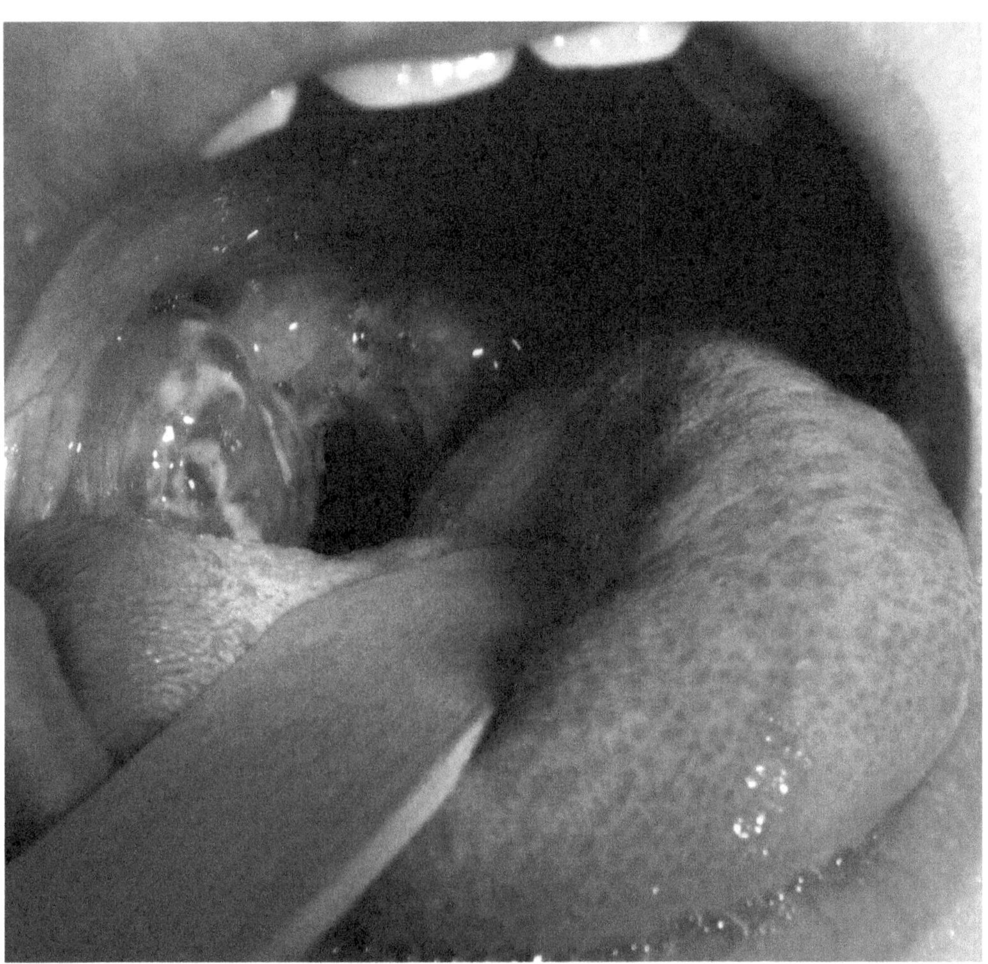

Figure 7.16 Strep Throat

If not diagnosed as strep throat, most cases of pharyngitis are caused by viruses, and the treatment is aimed at managing the symptoms. Nurses can teach patients the following ways to decrease the discomfort of a sore throat:

- Drink soothing liquids such as lemon tea with honey or ice water.
- Gargle several times a day with warm salt water made of 1/2 tsp. of salt in 1 cup of water.
- Suck on hard candies or throat lozenges.
- Use a cool-mist vaporizer or humidifier to moisten the air.
- Try over-the-counter pain medicines, such as acetaminophen.[12]

12 Centers for Disease Control and Prevention. (2020, May 1). *Disparities in oral health*. https://www.cdc.gov/OralHealth/oral_health_disparities/

My Notes

Epistaxis

Epistaxis, the medical term for a nose bleed, is a common problem affecting up to 60 million Americans each year. Although most cases of epistaxis are minor and manageable with conservative measures, severe cases can become life-threatening if the bleeding cannot be stopped.[13] See Figure 7.17[14] for an image of a severe case of epistaxis.

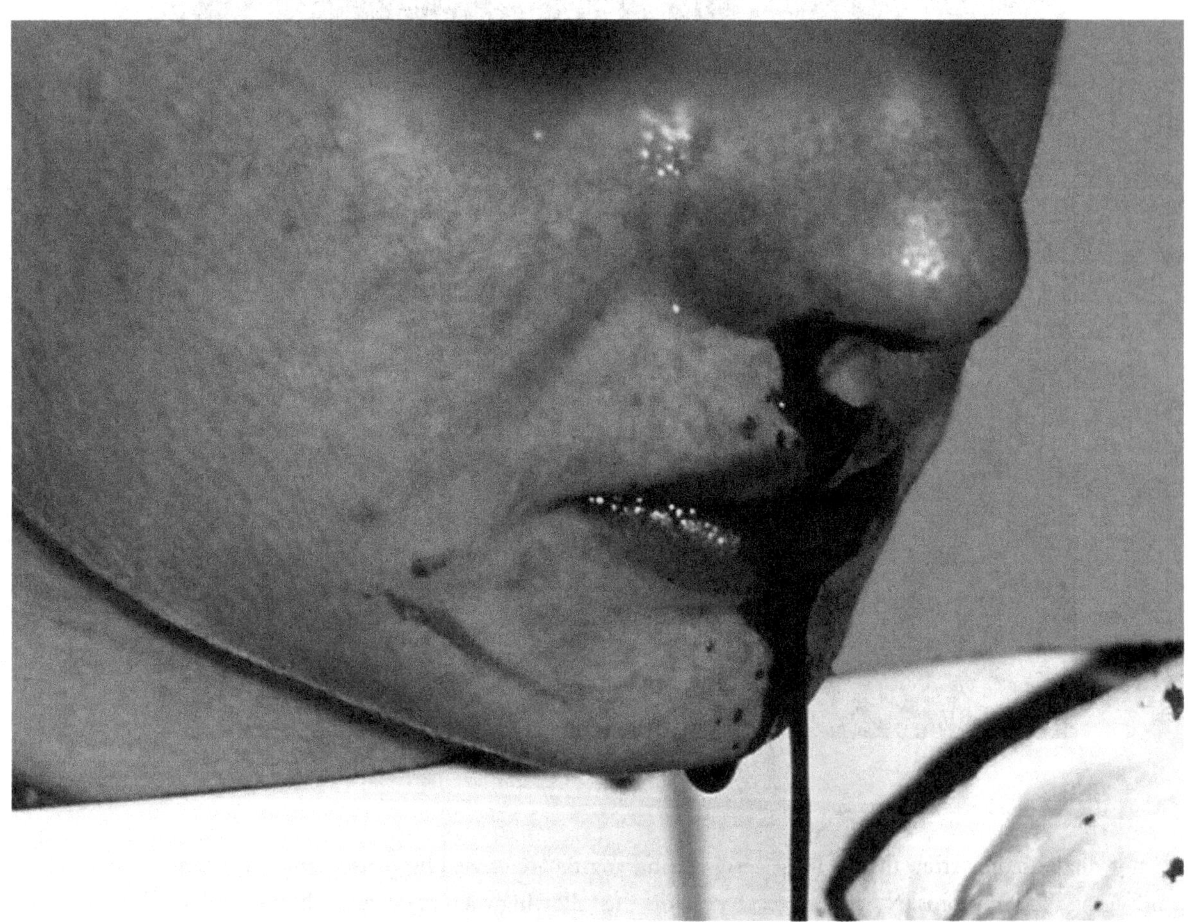

Figure 7.17 Serious Epistaxis

The most common cause of epistaxis is dry nasal membranes in winter months due to low temperatures and low humidity. Other common causes are picking inside the nose with fingers, trauma, anatomical deformity, high blood pressure, and clotting disorders. Medications associated with epistaxis are aspirin, clopidogrel, nonsteroidal anti-inflammatory drugs, and anticoagulants.[15]

13 Fatakia, A., Winters, R., & Amedee, R. G. (2010). Epistaxis: A common problem. *The Ochsner Journal, 10*(3), 176–178. https://www.ncbi.nlm.nih.gov/pmc/articles/PMC3096213/

14 "Epstaxis1.jpg" by Welleschik is licensed under CC BY-SA 3.0. Access for free at

15 Fatakia, A., Winters, R., & Amedee, R. G. (2010). Epistaxis: A common problem. *The Ochsner Journal, 10*(3), 176–178. https://www.ncbi.nlm.nih.gov/pmc/articles/PMC3096213/

My Notes

To treat a nose bleed, have the victim lean forward at the waist and pinch the lateral sides of the nose with the thumb and index finger for up to 15 minutes while breathing through the mouth.[16] Continued bleeding despite this intervention requires urgent medical intervention such as nasal packing.

Cleft Lip and Palate

During embryonic development, the right and left maxilla bones come together at the midline to form the upper jaw. At the same time, the muscle and skin overlying these bones join together to form the upper lip. Inside the mouth, the palatine processes of the maxilla bones, along with the horizontal plates of the right and left palatine bones, join together to form the hard palate. If an error occurs in these developmental processes, a birth defect of cleft lip or cleft palate may result.

Cleft lip is a common developmental defect that affects approximately 1:1,000 births, most of which are male. This defect involves a partial or complete failure of the right and left portions of the upper lip to fuse together, leaving a cleft (gap). See Figure 7.18[17] for an image of an infant with a cleft lip.

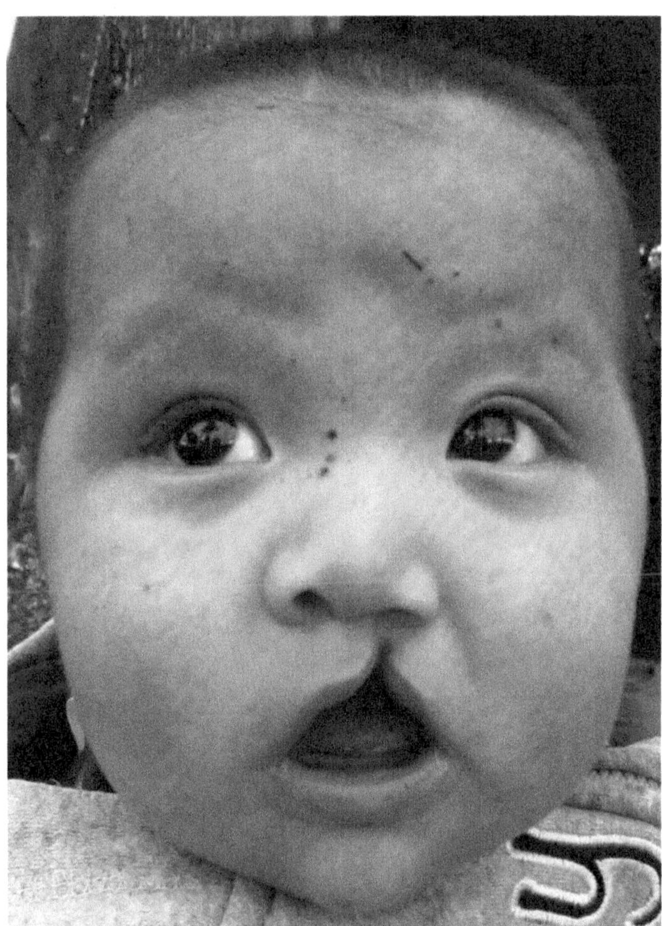

Figure 7.18 Cleft Lip

---

16 American Heart Association. (2000). Part 5: New guidelines for first aid. *Circulation, 102*(supplement 1). https://www.ahajournals.org/doi/10.1161/circ.102.suppl_1.I-77

17 "Cleftlipandpalate.JPG" by James Heilman, MD is licensed under CC BY-SA 3.0. Access for free at https://commons.wikimedia.org/wiki/File:Cleftlipandpalate.JPG

My Notes

A more severe developmental defect is a cleft palate that affects the hard palate, the bony structure that separates the nasal cavity from the oral cavity. See Figure 7.19[18] for an illustration of a cleft palate. **Cleft palate** affects approximately 1:2,500 births and is more common in females. It results from a failure of the two halves of the hard palate to completely come together and fuse at the midline, thus leaving a gap between the nasal and oral cavities. In severe cases, the bony gap continues into the anterior upper jaw where the alveolar processes of the maxilla bones also do not properly join together above the front teeth. If this occurs, a cleft lip will also be seen. Because of the communication between the oral and nasal cavities, a cleft palate makes it very difficult for an infant to generate the suckling needed for nursing, thus creating risk for malnutrition. Surgical repair is required to correct a cleft palate.[19]

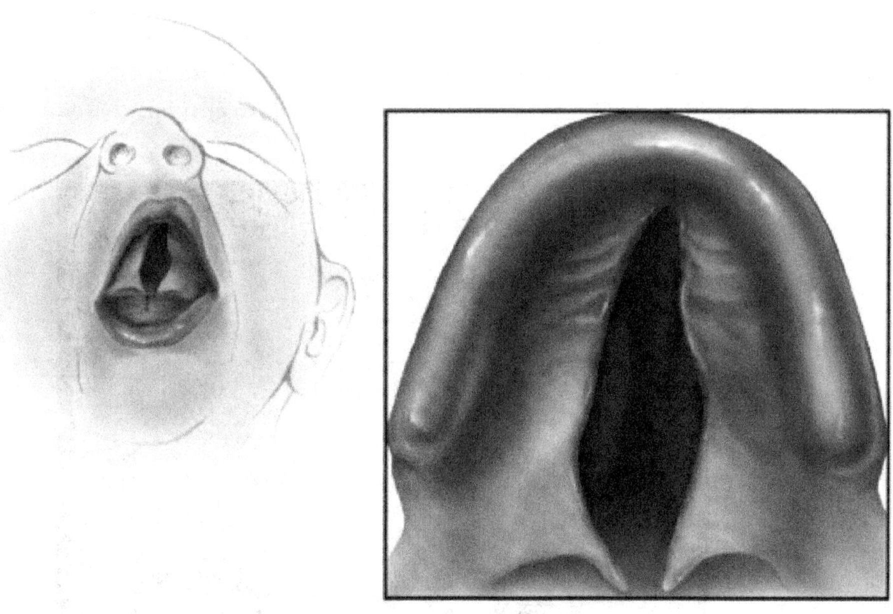

Figure 7.19 Cleft Palate

Poor Oral Health

Despite major improvements in oral health for the population as a whole, oral health disparities continue to exist for many racial, ethnic, and socioeconomic groups in the United States. Healthy People 2020, a nationwide initiative geared to improve the health of Americans, identified improved oral health as a health care goal. A growing body of evidence has also shown that periodontal disease is associated with negative systemic health consequences. Periodontal diseases are infections and inflammation of the gums and bone that surround and support the teeth. Red, swollen, and bleeding gums are signs of periodontal disease. Other symptoms of periodontal disease include bad breath, loose teeth, and painful chewing.[20] In 2020, the Centers for Disease Control and Prevention (CDC)

---

18 "Cleft palate.jpg" by Centers for Disease Control and Prevention is licensed under CC0 1.0. Access for free at https://commons.wikimedia.org/wiki/File:Cleft_palate.jpg

19 This work is a derivative of Anatomy & Physiology by OpenStax and is licensed under CC BY 4.0. Access for free at https://openstax.org/books/anatomy-and-physiology/pages/1-introduction

20 Bencosme, J. (2018). Periodontal disease: What nurses need to know. *Nursing, 48*(7), 22-27. https://doi.org/10.1097/01.nurse.0000534088.56615.e4

My Notes

reported that 42% of U.S. adults have some form of periodontitis, and almost 60% of adults aged 65 and older have periodontitis. See Figure 7.20[21] for an image of a patient with periodontal disease. Nurses may encounter patients who complain of bleeding gums, or they may discover other signs of periodontal disease during a physical assessment.

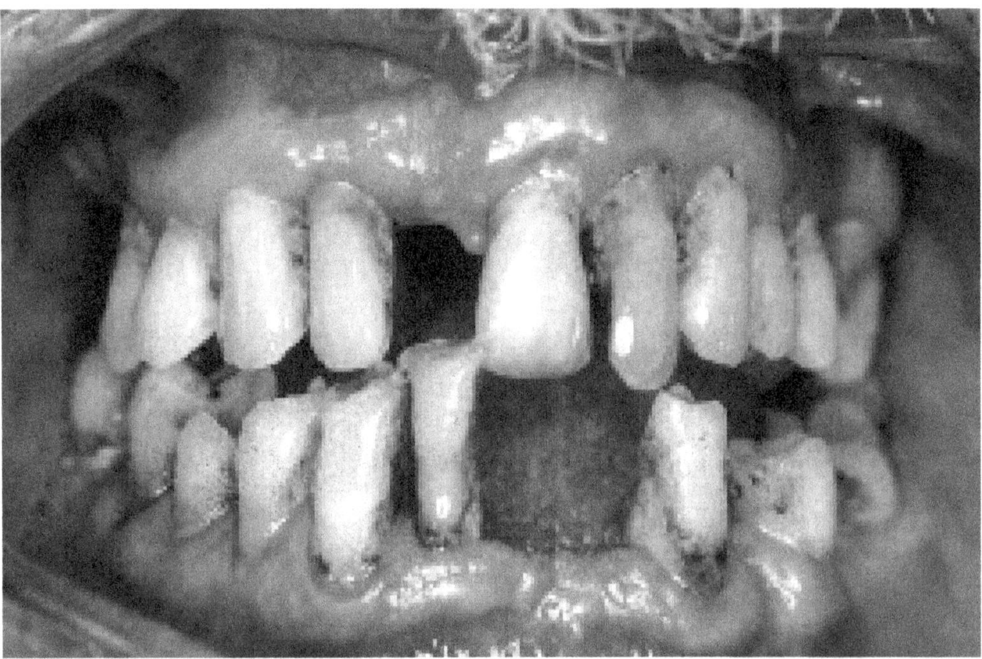

Figure 7.20 Periodontal Disease

Because many Americans lack access to oral care, it is important for nurses to perform routine oral assessment and identify needs for follow-up. If signs and/or symptoms indicate potential periodontal disease, the patient should be referred to a dental health professional for a more thorough evaluation.[22]

---

21 "Periodontal Disease.png" by Warren Schnider is licensed under CC BY-SA 4.0. Access for free at https://commons.wikimedia.org/wiki/File:Periodontal_Disease.png

22 Bencosme, J. (2018). Periodontal disease: What nurses need to know. *Nursing, 48*(7), 22-27. https://doi.org/10.1097/01.nurse.0000534088.56615.e4.

My Notes

Thrush/Candidiasis

Candidiasis is a fungal infection caused by *Candida. Candida* normally lives on the skin and inside the body without causing any problems, but it can multiply and cause an infection if the environment inside the mouth, throat, or esophagus changes in a way that encourages fungal growth.[23] See Figure 7.21[24] for an image of candidiasis.

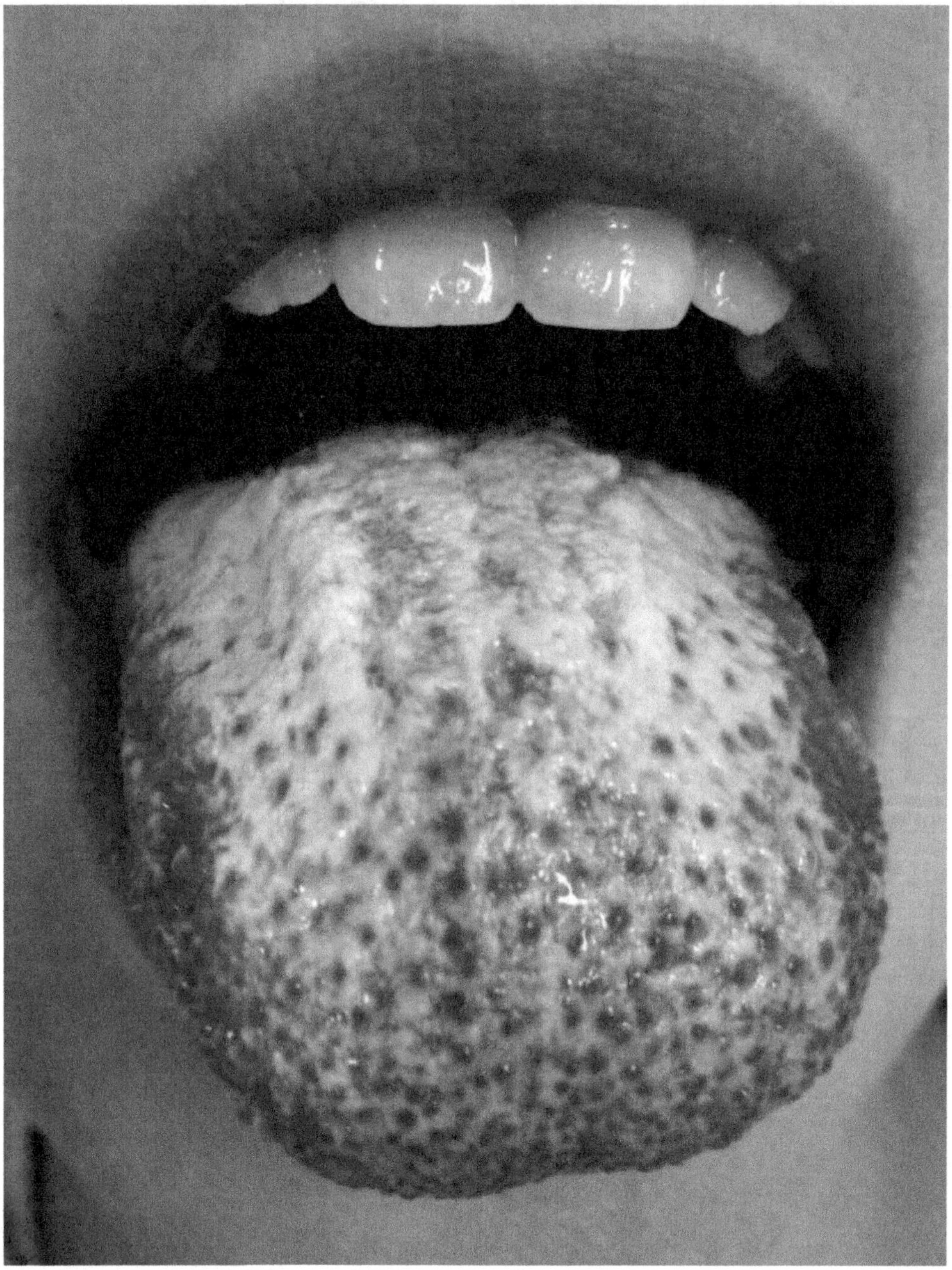

Figure 7.21 Candidiasis

23 Centers for Disease Control and Prevention. (2020, June 15). *Candida infections of the mouth, throat, and esophagus.* https://www.cdc.gov/fungal/diseases/candidiasis/thrush/index.html

24 "Human tongue infected with oral candidiasis.jpg" by James Heilman, MD is licensed under CC BY-SA 3.0. Access for free at https://commons.wikimedia.org/wiki/File:Human_tongue_infected_with_oral_candidiasis.jpg

Candidiasis in the mouth and throat can have many symptoms, including the following:

- White patches on the inner cheeks, tongue, roof of the mouth, and throat
- Redness or soreness
- Cotton-like feeling in the mouth
- Loss of taste
- Pain while eating or swallowing
- Cracking and redness at the corners of the mouth[25]

Candidiasis in the mouth or throat is common in babies but is uncommon in healthy adults. Risk factors for getting candidiasis as an adult include the following:

- Wearing dentures
- Diabetes
- Cancer
- HIV/AIDS
- Taking antibiotics or corticosteroids including inhaled corticosteroids for conditions like asthma
- Taking medications that cause dry mouth or have medical conditions that cause dry mouth
- Smoking

The treatment for mild to moderate cases of candidiasis infections in the mouth or throat is typically an antifungal medicine applied to the inside of the mouth for 7 to 14 days, such as clotrimazole, miconazole, or nystatin.

---

25 Centers for Disease Control and Prevention. (2020, June 15). *Candida infections of the mouth, throat, and esophagus*. https://www.cdc.gov/fungal/diseases/candidiasis/thrush/index.html

My Notes

"Meth Mouth"

The use of methamphetamine (i.e., meth), a strong stimulant drug, has become an alarming public health issue in the United States. A common sign of meth abuse is extreme tooth and gum decay often referred to as "Meth Mouth." See Figure 7.22[26] for an image of Meth Mouth.

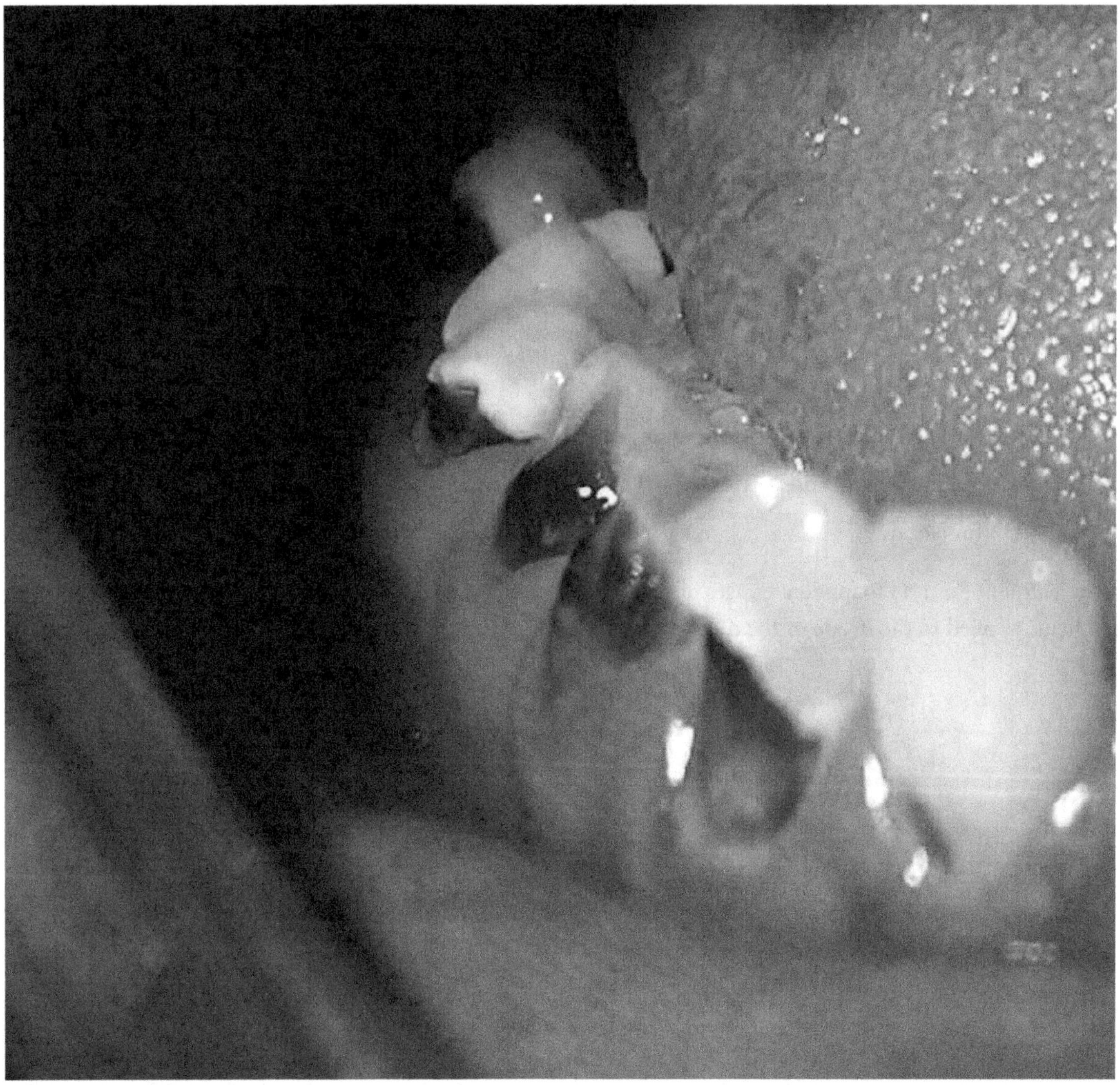

Figure 7.22 Meth Mouth

Signs of Meth Mouth include the following:

- Dry Mouth. Methamphetamines dry out the salivary glands, and the acid content in the mouth will start to destroy the enamel on the teeth. Eventually this will lead to cavities.

26 "Suspectedmethmouth09-19-05closeup.jpg" by Dozenist is licensed under CC BY-SA 3.0. Access for free at https://commons.wikimedia.org/wiki/File:Suspectedmethmouth09-19-05closeup.jpg

- Cracked Teeth. Methamphetamine can make the user feel anxious, hyper, or nervous, so they clench or grind their teeth. You may see severe wear patterns on their teeth.
- Tooth Decay. Meth users crave beverages high in sugar while they are "high." The bacteria that feed on the sugars in the mouth will secrete acid, which can lead to more tooth destruction. With meth users, tooth decay will start at the gum line and eventually spread throughout the tooth. The front teeth are usually destroyed first.
- Gum Disease. Methamphetamine users do not seek out regular dental treatment. Lack of oral health care can contribute to periodontal disease. Methamphetamines also cause the blood vessels that supply the oral tissues to shrink in size, reducing blood flow, causing the tissues to break down.
- Lesions. Users who smoke meth present with lesions and/or burns on their lips or gingival inside the cheeks or on the hard palate. Users who snort may present burns in the back of their throats.[27]

Nurses who notice possible signs of Meth Mouth should report their concerns to the health care provider, not only for a referral for dental care, but also for treatment of suspected substance abuse.

Dysphagia

Dysphagia is the medical term for difficulty swallowing that can be caused by many medical conditions. Nurses are often the first health care professionals to notice a patient's difficulty swallowing as they administer medications or monitor food intake. Early identification of dysphagia, especially after a patient has experienced a cerebrovascular accident (i.e., stroke) or other head injury, helps to prevent aspiration pneumonia.[28] **Aspiration pneumonia** is a type of lung infection caused by material from the stomach or mouth entering the lungs and can be life-threatening.

Signs of dysphagia include the following:

- Coughing during or right after eating or drinking
- Wet or gurgly sounding voice during or after eating or drinking
- Extra effort or time required to chew or swallow
- Food or liquid leaking from mouth
- Food getting stuck in the mouth
- Difficulty breathing after meals[29]

The Barnes-Jewish Hospital-Stroke Dysphagia Screen (BJH-SDS) is an example of a simple, evidence-based bedside screening tool that can be used by nursing staff to efficiently identify swallowing impairments in patients who have experienced a stroke. See internet resource below for an image of the dysphagia screening tool. The result

---

27 Maine Center for Disease Control and Prevention. (n.d.). *Meth mouth*. https://www.maine.gov/dhhs/mecdc/population-health/odh/documents/meth-mouth.pdf

28 Edmiaston, J., Connor, L. T., Steger-May, K., & Ford, A. L. (2014). A simple bedside stroke dysphagia screen, validated against videofluoroscopy, detects dysphagia and aspiration with high sensitivity. *Journal of Stroke and Cerebrovascular Diseases: The Official Journal of National Stroke Association, 23*(4), 712–716. https://doi.org/10.1016/j.jstrokecerebrovasdis.2013.06.030

29 American Speech-Language-Hearing Association. (n.d.). *Swallowing disorders in adults*. https://www.asha.org/public/speech/swallowing/Swallowing-Disorders-in-Adults/

My Notes

of the screening test is recorded as a "fail" if any of the five items tested are abnormal (Glasgow Coma Scale < 13, facial/tongue/palatal asymmetry or weakness, or signs of aspiration on the 3-ounce water test) or "pass" if all five items tested were normal. Patients with a failed screening result are placed on nothing-by-mouth (NPO) status until further evaluation is completed by a speech therapist. For more information about using the Glasgow Coma Scale, see the "Assessing Mental Status" subsection in the "Neurological Assessment" chapter.

View a PDF sample of a Nursing Bedside Swallow Screen (https://aann.org/uploads/Bedside_Swallow_Screen.pdf).

Enlarged Lymph Nodes

Lymphadenopathy is the medical term for swollen lymph nodes. In a child, a node is considered enlarged if it is more than 1 centimeter (0.4 inch) wide. See Figure 7.23[30] for an image of an enlarged cervical lymph node.

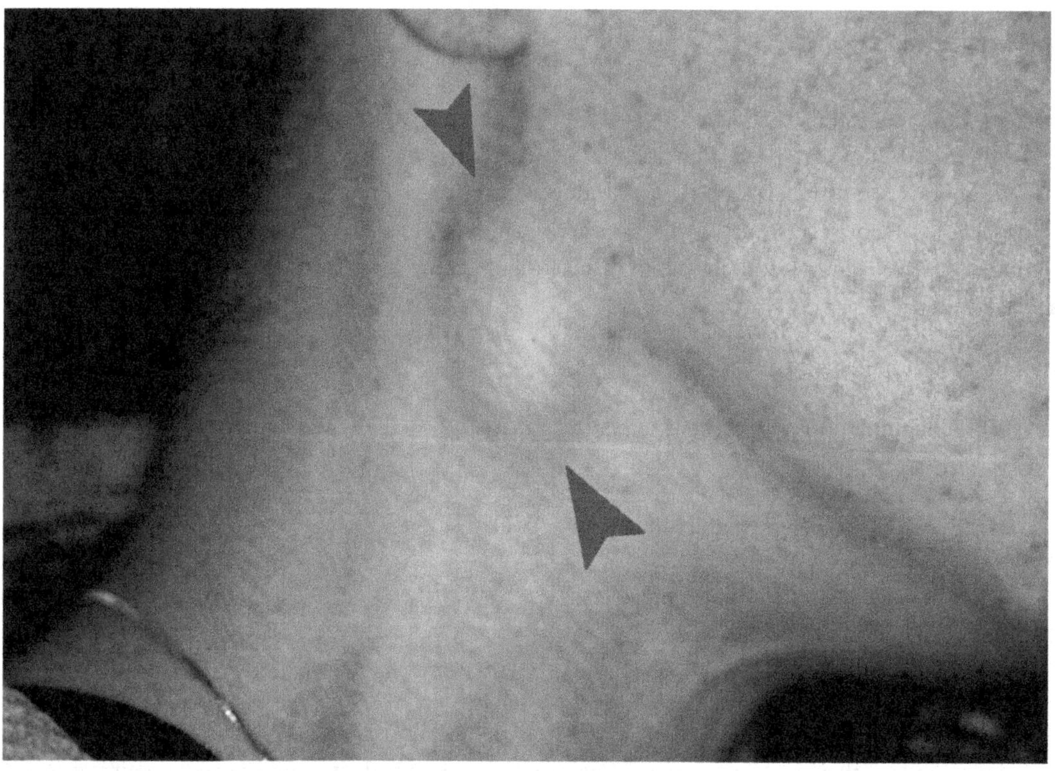

Figure 7.23 Enlarged Cervical Lymph Node

Common infections such as a cold, pharyngitis, sinusitis, mononucleosis, strep throat, ear infection, or infected tooth often cause swollen lymph nodes. However, swollen lymph nodes can also signify more serious conditions. Notify the health care provider if the patient's lymph nodes have the following characteristics:

- Do not decrease in size after several weeks or continue to get larger

---

30 "Cervical lymphadenopathy right neck.png" by Coronation Dental Specialty Group is licensed under CC BY-SA 4.0. Access for free at https://commons.wikimedia.org/wiki/File:Cervical_lymphadenopathy_right_neck.png

My Notes

- Are red and tender
- Feel hard, irregular, or fixed in place
- Are associated with night sweats or unexplained weight loss
- Are larger than 1 centimeter in diameter

The health care provider may order blood tests, a chest X-ray, or a biopsy of the lymph node if these signs occur.[31]

Thyroid

The thyroid is a butterfly-shaped gland located at the front of the neck that controls many of the body's important functions. The thyroid gland makes hormones that affect breathing, heart rate, digestion, and body temperature. If the thyroid makes too much or not enough thyroid hormone, many body systems are affected. In hypothyroidism, the thyroid gland doesn't produce enough hormone and many body functions slow down. When the thyroid makes too much hormone, a condition called hyperthyroidism, many body systems speed up.[32]

A **goiter** is an abnormal enlargement of the thyroid gland that can occur with hypothyroidism or hyperthyroidism. If you find a goiter when assessing a patient's neck, notify the health care provider for additional testing and treatment. See Figure 7.24[33] for an image of a goiter.

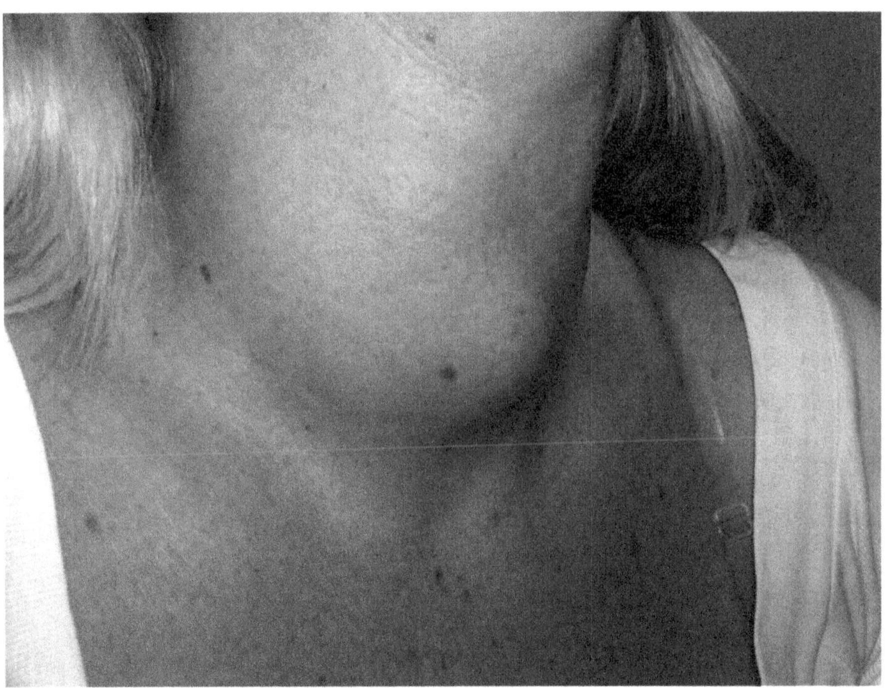

Figure 7.24 Goiter

---

31 A.D.A.M. Medical Encyclopedia [Internet]. Johns Creek (GA): Ebix, Inc., A.D.A.M.; c1997-2020. Swollen lymph nodes; [updated 2020, Aug 25; cited 2020, Sep 4]; https://medlineplus.gov/ency/article/003097.htm

32 National Institutes of Health. (2015). *Thinking about your thyroid.* https://newsinhealth.nih.gov/2015/09/thinking-about-your-thyroid

33 "Struma 00a.jpg" by Drahreg01 is licensed under CC BY-SA 3.0. Access for free at https://commons.wikimedia.org/wiki/File:Struma_001.jpg

My Notes

7.4 HEAD AND NECK ASSESSMENT

Subjective Assessment

Begin the head and neck assessment by asking focused interview questions to determine if the patient is currently experiencing any symptoms or has a previous medical history related to head and neck issues.

Table 7.4a Interview Questions for Subjective Assessment of the Head and Neck

Interview Questions	Follow-up
Have you ever been diagnosed with a medical condition related to your head such as headaches, a concussion, a stroke, or a head injury?	Please describe.
Have you ever been diagnosed with a medical condition related to your neck such a thyroid or swallowing issue?	Please describe.
Are you currently taking any medications, herbs, or supplements for headaches or for your thyroid?	Please describe.
Have you had any symptoms such as headaches, nosebleeds, nasal drainage, sinus pressure, sore throat, or swollen lymph nodes?	If yes, use the PQRSTU method to gather additional information regarding each symptom.
Specific oral assessment questions:[1] ■ **Are you having any pain, bleeding, or other problems with your teeth or gums?** ■ **Do you have any loose or sensitive teeth?** ■ **Do you experience bleeding after brushing or flossing your teeth?** ■ **Are you wearing dentures? Do they fit properly?** ■ **Are you experiencing bad breath that won't go away?** ■ **Have your eating patterns changed due to mouth pain or discomfort with chewing?**	

Life Span Considerations

Infants and Children

For infants, observe head control and muscle strength. Palpate the skull and fontanelles for smoothness. Ask the parents or guardians if the child has had frequent throat infections or a history of cleft lip or cleft palate. Observe head shape, size, and symmetry.

1 Bencosme, J. (2018). Periodontal disease: What nurses need to know. *Nursing, 48(*7), 22-27. https://doi.org/10.1097/01.nurse.0000534088.56615.e4

My Notes

Older Adults

Ask older adults if they have experienced any difficulties swallowing or chewing. Document if dentures are present. Muscle atrophy and loss of fat often cause neck shortening. Fat accumulation in the back of the neck causes a condition referred to as "Dowager's hump."

Objective Assessment

Use any information obtained during the subjective interview to guide your physical assessment.

Inspection

- Begin by inspecting the head for skin color and symmetry of facial movements, noting any drooping. If drooping is noted, ask the patient to smile, frown, and raise their eyebrows and observe for symmetrical movement. Note the presence of previous injuries or deformities.
- Inspect the nose for patency and note any nasal drainage.
- Inspect the oral cavity and ask the patient to open their mouth and say "Ah." Inspect the patient's mouth using a good light and tongue blade.
    - Note oral health of the teeth and gums.
        - If the patient wears dentures, remove them so you can assess the underlying mucosa.
        - Assess the oral mucosa for color and the presence of any abnormalities.
        - Note the color of the gums, which are normally pink. Inspect the gum margins for swelling, bleeding, or ulceration.
        - Inspect the teeth and note any missing, discolored, misshapen, or abnormally positioned teeth. Assess for loose teeth with a gloved thumb and index finger, and document halitosis (bad breath) if present.[2]
    - Assess the tongue. It should be midline and with no sores or coatings present.
    - Assess the uvula. It should be midline and should rise symmetrically when the patient says "Ah."
    - Is the patient able to swallow their own secretions? If the patient has had a recent stroke or you have any concerns about their ability to swallow, perform a brief bedside swallow study according to agency policy before administering any food, fluids, or medication by mouth.
- Inspect the neck. The trachea should be midline, and there should not be any noticeable enlargement of lymph nodes or the thyroid gland.
- Note the patient's speech. They should be able to speak clearly with no slurring or garbled words.

If any neurological concerns are present, a cranial nerve assessment may be performed. Read more about a cranial nerve assessment in the "Neurological Assessment" chapter.

---

2 Bencosme, J. (2018). Periodontal disease: What nurses need to know. *Nursing, 48*(7), 22-27. https://doi.org/10.1097/01.nurse.0000534088.56615.e4

My Notes

Auscultation

Auscultation is not typically performed by registered nurses during a routine neck assessment. However, advanced practice nurses and other health care providers may auscultate the carotid arteries for the presence of a swishing sound called a bruit.

Palpation

Palpate the neck for masses and tenderness. Lymph nodes, if palpable, should be round and movable and should not be enlarged or tender. See the figure illustrating the location of lymph nodes in the head and neck in the "Head and Neck Basic Concepts" section earlier in this chapter.

Advanced practice nurses and other health care providers palpate the thyroid for enlargement, further evaluate lymph nodes, and assess the presence of any masses.

See Table 7.4b for a comparison of expected versus unexpected findings when assessing the head and neck.

Table 7.4b Expected Versus Unexpected Findings on Adult Assessment of the Head and Neck

Assessment	Expected Findings	Unexpected Findings (to document and notify provider if new finding*)
Inspection	Skin tone is appropriate for ethnicity, and skin is dry. Facial movements are symmetrical. Nares are patent and no drainage is present. Uvula and tongue are midline. Teeth and gums are in good condition. Patient is able to swallow their own secretions. Trachea is midline. If dentures are present, there is a good fit, and the patient is able to appropriately chew food.	Skin is pale, cyanotic, or diaphoretic (inappropriately perspiring). New asymmetrical facial expressions or drooping is present. Nares are occluded or nasal drainage is present. Uvula and/or tongue is deviated to one side. White coating or lesions on the tongue or buccal membranes (inner cheeks) are present. Teeth are missing or decay is present that impacts the patient's ability to chew. After swallowing, the patient coughs, drools, chokes, or speaks in a gurgly/wet voice. Trachea is deviated to one side. Dentures have poor fit and/or the patient is unable to chew food contained in a routine diet.
Palpation	No unusual findings regarding lymph nodes is present.	Cervical lymph nodes are enlarged, tender, or non-movable. Report any concerns about lymph nodes to the health care provider.
***CRITICAL CONDITIONS to report immediately**		New asymmetry of facial expressions, tracheal deviation to one side, slurred or garbled speech, signs of impaired swallowing, coughing during or after swallowing, or a "wet" voice after swallowing.

My Notes

7.5 SAMPLE DOCUMENTATION

Sample Documentation of Expected Findings

The patient's skin tone is appropriate for ethnicity and they are not diaphoretic. Facial movements are symmetrical. Nares are patent and no drainage is present. Uvula and tongue are midline. Teeth and gums are in good condition. Patient is able to swallow without difficulty. Trachea is midline. There is no enlargement of the lymph nodes.

Sample Documentation of Unexpected Findings

The patient has a history of asthma and uses a fluticasone inhaler daily. White patches are present on the tongue and inner buccal membranes. Dr. Smith was notified at 1530 and a new order for nystatin medication was received and administered. Patient was instructed to rinse their mouth after every use of fluticasone to prevent thrush from recurring.

My Notes

7.6 CHECKLIST FOR HEAD AND NECK ASSESSMENT

Use the checklist below to review the steps for completion of a "Head and Neck Assessment."

Steps

Disclaimer: Always review and follow agency policy regarding this specific skill.

1. Gather supplies: penlight, tongue blade, and nonsterile gloves.
2. Perform safety steps:
    - Perform hand hygiene.
    - Check the room for transmission-based precautions.
    - Introduce yourself, your role, the purpose of your visit, and an estimate of the time it will take.
    - Confirm patient ID using two patient identifiers (e.g., name and date of birth).
    - Explain the process to the patient and ask if they have any questions.
    - Be organized and systematic.
    - Use appropriate listening and questioning skills.
    - Listen and attend to patient cues.
    - Ensure the patient's privacy and dignity.
    - Assess ABCs.
3. Inspect the head and facial expressions for symmetrical movement.
4. Inspect the nose with a penlight for drainage and occlusion.
5. Inspect the oral cavity for lesions, tongue position, movement of uvula, and oral health using a penlight.
6. Inspect the throat and note any enlargement of the tonsils.
7. Palpate the lymph nodes of the head and neck, including submaxillary, anterior cervical, posterior cervical, and preauricular.
8. Ask the patient to swallow their own saliva and note any signs of difficulty swallowing.
9. Assist the patient to a comfortable position, ask if they have any questions, and thank them for their time.
10. Ensure five safety measures when leaving the room:
    - CALL LIGHT: Within reach
    - BED: Low and locked (in lowest position and brakes on)
    - SIDE RAILS: Secured
    - TABLE: Within reach
    - ROOM: Risk-free for falls (scan room and clear any obstacles)

My Notes

11. Perform hand hygiene.

12. Document the assessment findings and report any concerns according to agency policy.

My Notes

7.7 SUPPLEMENTARY VIDEO ON HEAD AND NECK ASSESSMENT

Video Review of Head and Neck Assessment[1]

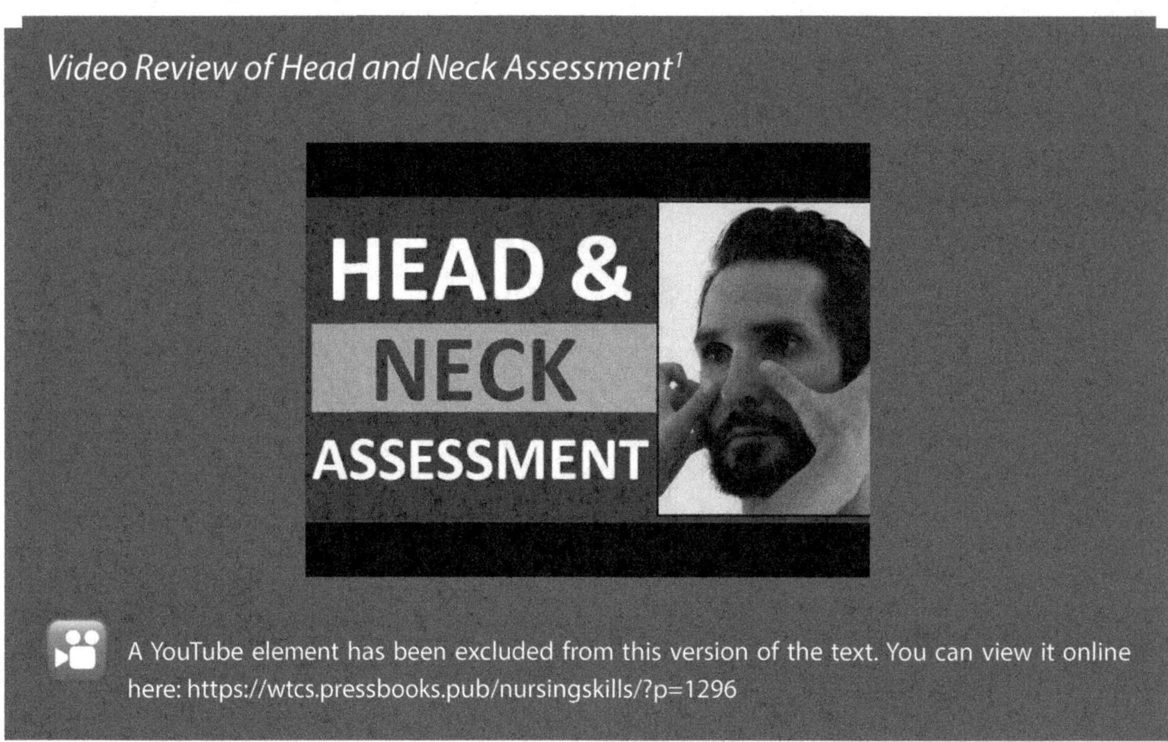

A YouTube element has been excluded from this version of the text. You can view it online here: https://wtcs.pressbooks.pub/nursingskills/?p=1296

1 RegisteredNurseRN. (2017, November 27). *Head and neck assessment nursing | Head to toe assessment of head neck ENT lymphatic cranial nerves.* [Video]. YouTube. All rights reserved. Video used with permission. https://youtu.be/MkqCjH-BlMo

7.8 LEARNING ACTIVITIES

My Notes

Learning Activities

(Answers to "Learning Activities'" can be found in the "Answer Key" at the end of the book. Answers to interactive activity elements will be provided within the element as immediate feedback.)

1. You are working as a triage nurse in a primary care clinic. You just received a phone call from a young woman who is complaining of significant discomfort related to newly diagnosed strep throat. What instructions can you provide to her to aid in symptom management in order to alleviate discomfort?
2. You are assessing a patient's head and neck and note the following findings. Which should be reported to the health care provider?
   a. Tongue is midline
   b. White patches noted on both tonsils
   c. Uvula raises when patient says "Ahhh"
   d. Speech is slurred
   e. Thyroid enlarged

Interactive Activity

An interactive or media element has been excluded from this version of the text. You can view it online here: https://wtcs.pressbooks.pub/nursingskills/?p=1298

Interactive Activity

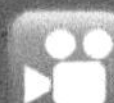

An interactive or media element has been excluded from this version of the text. You can view it online here: https://wtcs.pressbooks.pub/nursingskills/?p=1298

My Notes

VII GLOSSARY

Aspiration pneumonia: A type of lung infection caused by material from the stomach or mouth inadvertently entering the lungs that can be life-threatening.

Brain case: Eight bones that protect the brain in the cranial cavity.

Candidiasis: A fungal infection often referred to as "thrush" when it occurs in the oral cavity in children.

Cleft lip: A birth defect caused by a partial or complete failure of the right and left portions of the upper lip to fuse together, leaving a gap in the lip.

Cleft palate: A birth defect caused when two halves of the hard palate fail to completely come together and fuse at the midline, leaving a gap between them, and making it very difficult for an infant to generate the suckling needed for nursing.

Concussion: A type of traumatic brain injury caused by a bump, blow, or jolt to the head or by a hit to the body that causes the head and brain to move rapidly back and forth. This sudden movement can cause the brain to bounce around or twist in the skull, creating chemical changes in the brain and damaging brain cells.

Dysphagia: Difficulty swallowing.

Epiglottis: A flexible piece of cartilage that covers the opening of the trachea during swallowing to prevent ingested material from entering the trachea.

Epistaxis: Nosebleed.

Facial drooping: An asymmetrical facial expression that occurs due to damage of the nerve innervating a particular part of the face.

Goiter: An abnormal enlargement of the thyroid gland that can occur with hypothyroidism or hyperthyroidism.

Hematoma: Collection of blood.

Laryngopharynx: The portion of the pharynx inferior to the oropharynx and posterior to the larynx that is a passageway for ingested material and air until its inferior end where the digestive and respiratory systems diverge into the esophagus and the larynx.

Larynx: The structure connecting the pharynx to the trachea that helps regulate the volume of air that enters and leaves the lungs and contains the vocal cords.

Lymphadenopathy: Enlarged lymph nodes.

Lymph nodes: Structures in the lymphatic system that filter pathogens.

Mandible: Lower jaw bone.

Masseter: Main muscle used for chewing because it elevates the mandible to close the mouth.

Maxilla: Bone that forms the upper jaw and supports the upper teeth.

Nares: Nostril openings into the nasal cavity.

Nasal septum: Bone and cartilage that separate the nasal cavity into two compartments.

Nasopharynx: The upper region of the pharynx that connects to the nasal cavity and is a passageway for air.

Orbit: The bony socket that houses the eyeball and muscles that move the eyeball.

Oropharynx: The middle region of the pharynx bordered superiorly by the nasopharynx and anteriorly by the oral cavity that is a passageway for air and ingested material.

Pharyngitis: Infection and/or inflammation in the back of the throat (pharynx).

Pharynx: A tube lined with mucous membrane that begins at the nasal cavity and is divided into three major regions: the nasopharynx, the oropharynx, and the laryngopharynx.

Sinusitis: Inflamed sinuses caused by a viral or bacterial infection.

My Notes

Sternocleidomastoid: The major muscle that laterally flexes and rotates the head.

Suture: An interlocking joint between adjacent bones of the skull.

Temporalis: Muscle that assists in chewing by retracting the mandible. The temporalis muscle can be felt moving by placing fingers on the patient's temple as they chew.

Trachea: A tube lined with mucus membrane that carries air from the larynx to the lungs.

Trapezius: The muscle that elevates the shoulders (shrugs), pulls the shoulder blades together, and tilts the head backwards.

Uvula: A small, teardrop-shaped structure located at the apex of the soft palate that swings upward during swallowing to close off the nasopharynx and prevent ingested materials from entering the nasal cavity.

Chapter 8

Eye and Ear Assessment

8.1 EYE AND EAR ASSESSMENT INTRODUCTION

My Notes

Learning Objectives

- Perform an eye and ear assessment, including visual acuity, extraocular motion, and hearing acuity
- Modify assessment techniques to reflect variations across the life span
- Document actions and observations
- Recognize and report significant deviations from norms

The ability to see, hear, and maintain balance are important functions of our eyes and ears. Let's begin by reviewing the anatomy of the eye and ear and their common disorders.

My Notes

8.2 EYE AND EAR BASIC CONCEPTS

Anatomy of the Eye

Our sense of vision occurs due to transduction of light stimuli received through the eyes. The eyes are located within either orbit in the skull. See Figure 8.1[1] for an illustration of the eye. The eyelids, with lashes at their leading edges, help to protect the eye from abrasions by blocking particles that may land on the surface of the eye. The inner surface of each lid is a thin membrane known as the **conjunctiva**. The conjunctiva extends over the white areas of the eye called the **sclera**, connecting the eyelids to the eyeball. The **iris** is the colored part of the eye. The iris is a smooth muscle that opens and closes the **pupil**, the hole at the center of the eye that allows light to enter. The iris constricts the pupil in response to bright light and dilates the pupil in response to dim light. The **cornea** is the transparent front part of the eye that covers the iris, pupil, and anterior chamber. The cornea, with the anterior chamber and **lens**, refracts light and contributes to vision. The cornea can be reshaped by surgical procedures such as LASIK. The innermost layer of the eye is the **retina** that contains the nervous tissue and specialized cells called photoreceptors for the initial processing of visual stimuli. Two types of photoreceptors within the retina are the rods and the cones. The cones are sensitive to different wavelengths of light and provide color vision. These nerve cells of the retina leave the eye and enter the brain via the **optic nerve** (cranial nerve II).[2]

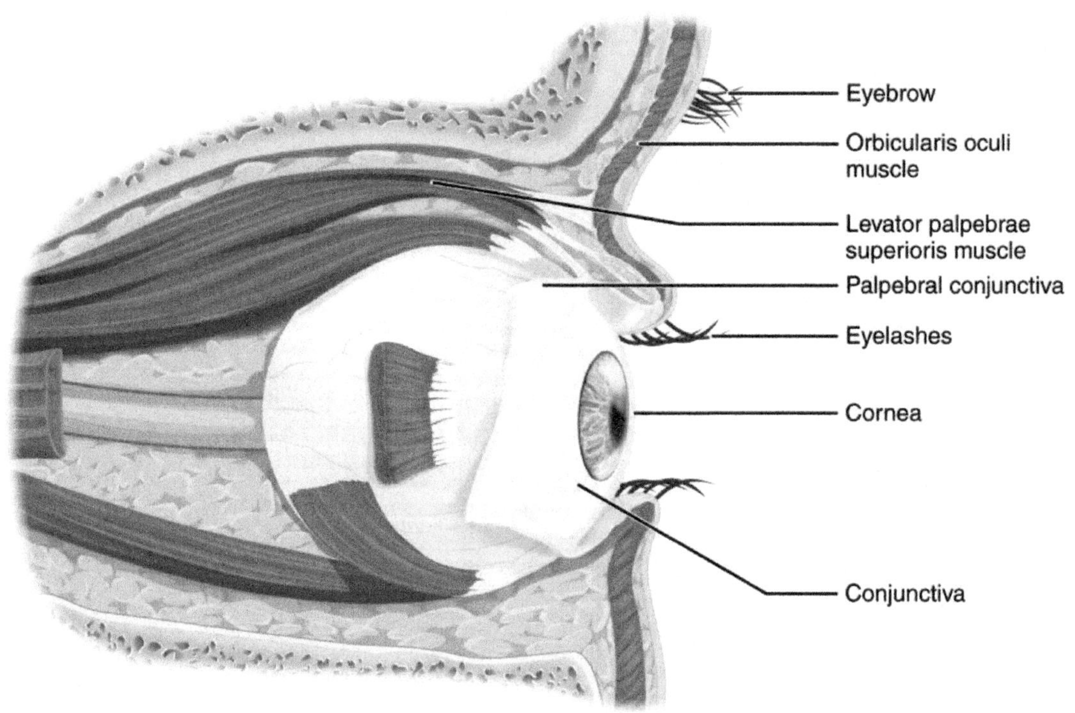

Figure 8.1 The Eye

1 "1411 Eye in The Orbit.jpg" by OpenStax College is licensed under CC BY 3.0. Access for free at https://openstax.org/books/anatomy-and-physiology/pages/14-1-sensory-perception

2 Giddens, J. (2007). A survey of physical examination techniques performed by RNs: Lessons for nursing education. *Journal of Nursing Education, 46*(2), 83-87.

My Notes

Tears are produced by the lacrimal gland that is located beneath the lateral edges of the nose. Tears flow through the **lacrimal duct** to the medial corner of the eye and flow over the conjunctiva to wash away foreign particles. Movement of the eye within the orbit occurs by the contraction of six **extraocular muscles** that originate from the bones of the orbit and insert into the surface of the eyeball. The extraocular muscles are innervated by the abducens nerve, the trochlear nerve, and the oculomotor nerve (cranial nerves III, IV, and V).[3] See the illustration of the extraocular muscles in Figure 8.2.[4]

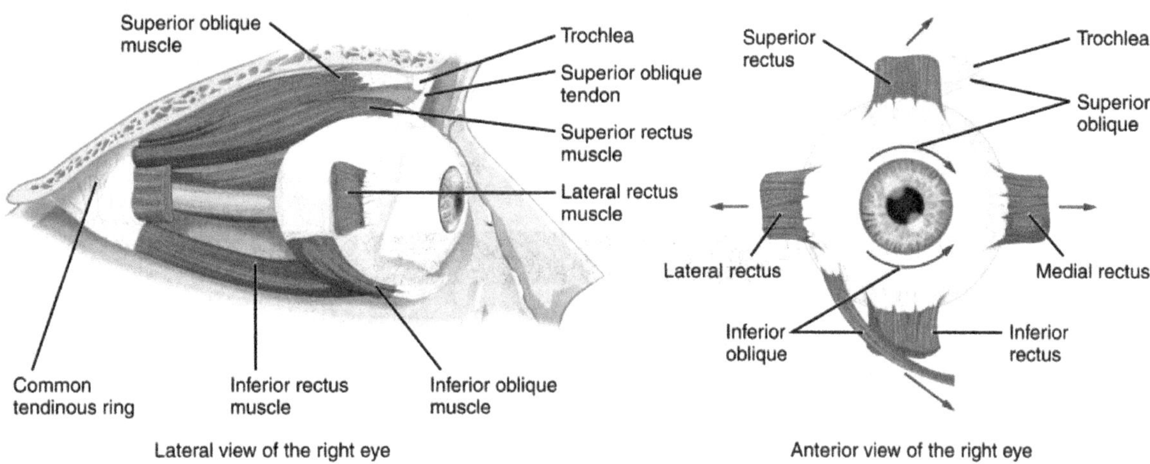

Figure 8.2 Extraocular Muscles

3 This work is a derivative of Anatomy & Physiology by OpenStax and is licensed under CC BY 4.0. Access for free at https://openstax.org/books/anatomy-and-physiology/pages/1-introduction

4 "1412 Extraocular Muscles.jpg" by OpenStax is licensed under CC BY 3.0. Access for free at https://openstax.org/books/anatomy-and-physiology/pages/14-1-sensory-perception

My Notes

Video Review for Anatomy of the Eye[5]

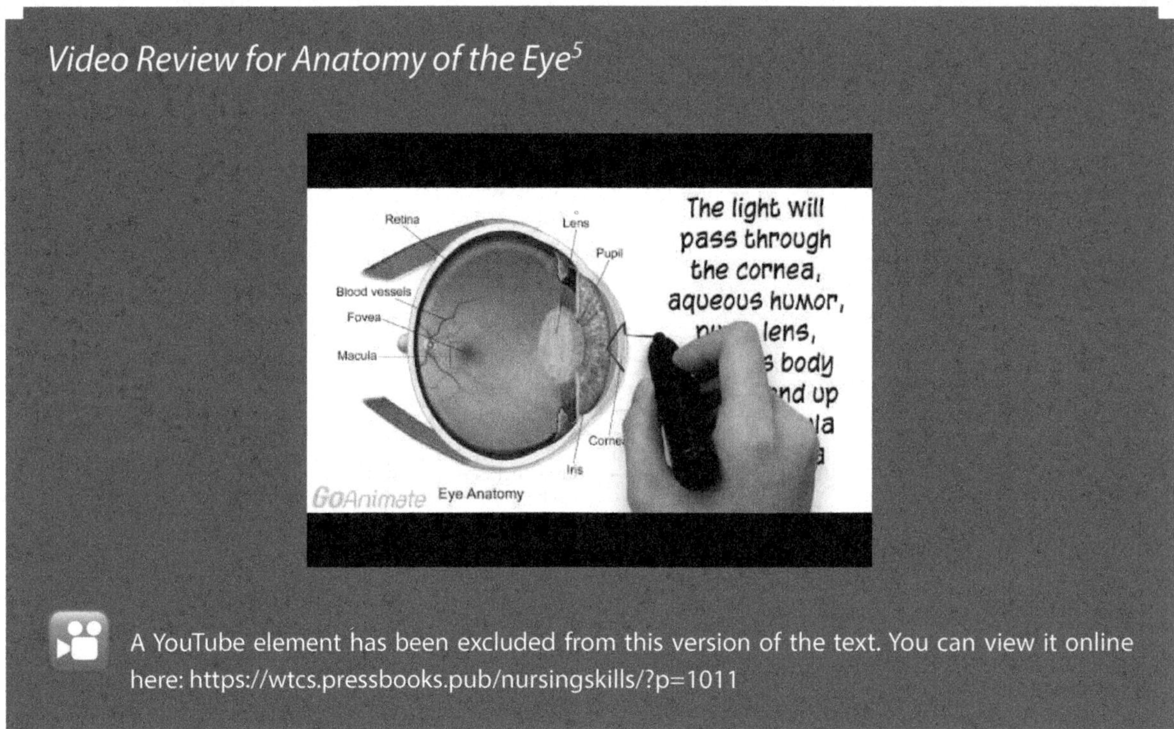

A YouTube element has been excluded from this version of the text. You can view it online here: https://wtcs.pressbooks.pub/nursingskills/?p=1011

Common Disorders of the Eye

Eye disorders that nurses commonly see in practice include myopia, presbyopia, color blindness, dry eye, conjunctivitis, styes, cataracts, macular degeneration, and glaucoma.

5 Forciea, B. (2015, May 12). *Anatomy of the eye (v2.0)*. [Video]. YouTube. All rights reserved. Video used with permission. https://youtu.be/HmKGyJUcRLw

Myopia

My Notes

Myopia is impaired vision, also known as nearsightedness that makes far-away objects look blurry. It happens when the eyeball grows too long from front to back or when there are problems with the shape of the cornea or the lens. These problems make light focus in front of the retina, instead of on it, causing blurriness. See Figure 8.3[6] for a simulated image of a person's vision with myopia. Nearsightedness usually becomes apparent between ages 6 and 14. It is corrected with glasses, contacts, or LASIK surgery.[7]

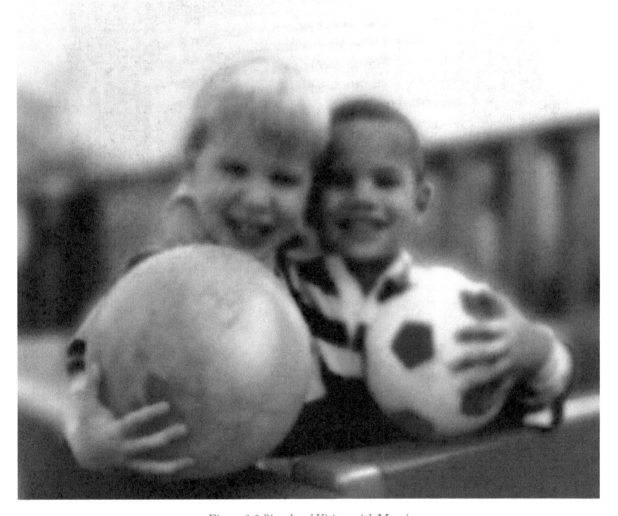

Figure 8.3 Simulated Vision with Myopia

6 "Eye disease simulation, myopia.jpg" by National Eye Institute, National Institutes of Health is in the Public Domain. Access for free at https://commons.wikimedia.org/wiki/File:Eye_disease_simulation,_myopia.jpg

7 National Eye Institute. (2019, July 9). *Types of refractive errors*. https://www.nei.nih.gov/learn-about-eye-health/eye-conditions-and-diseases/refractive-errors/types-refractive-errors#section-id-6802

My Notes

Presbyopia

Presbyopia is impaired near vision. It commonly occurs in middle-aged and older adults, making it difficult to clearly see objects up close. As people age, the lens in the eye gets harder and less flexible and stops focusing light correctly on the retina.[8] Presbyopia can be corrected with glasses and/or contacts. See Figure 8.4[9] for a simulated image of a person's vision with presbyopia.

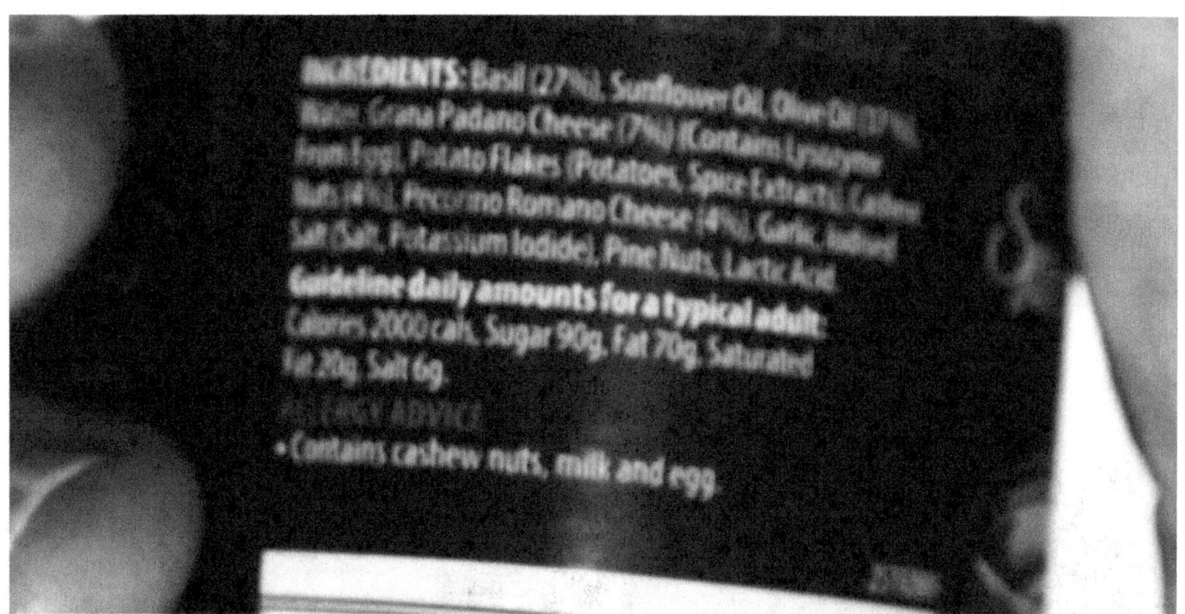

Figure 8.4 Simulated Vision with Presbyopia

Color Blindness

Color blindness makes it difficult to differentiate between certain colors. Color blindness can occur due to damage to the eye or to the brain. There's no cure for color blindness, but special glasses and contact lenses can help people differentiate between colors. Most people who have color blindness are able to use visual strategies related to color selection and don't have problems participating in everyday activities.[10]

Dry Eye

Dry eye is a very common eye condition that occurs when the eyes don't make enough tears to stay wet or the tears don't work correctly. Symptoms of dry eye include a scratchy feeling, stinging, and burning. Treatment includes over-the-counter and prescription eye drops, as well as lifestyle changes to decrease the dryness of the eyes.[11]

---

8 National Eye Institute. (2019, July 9). *Types of refractive errors*. https://www.nei.nih.gov/learn-about-eye-health/eye-conditions-and-diseases/refractive-errors/types-refractive-errors#section-id-6802

9 "Pesto ingredients - blurred.jpg" by Colin is licensed under CC BY-SA 4.0. Access for free at https://commons.wikimedia.org/wiki/File:Pesto_ingredients_-_blurred.jpg

10 National Eye Institute. (2019, July 3). *Color blindness*. https://www.nei.nih.gov/learn-about-eye-health/eye-conditions-and-diseases/color-blindness

11 National Eye Institute. (2019, July 5). *Dry eye*. https://www.nei.nih.gov/learn-about-eye-health/eye-conditions-and-diseases/dry-eye

Conjunctivitis

My Notes

Conjunctivitis is a viral or bacterial infection that causes swelling and redness in the conjunctiva and sclera. See Figure 8.5[12] for an image of conjunctivitis. The eye may feel itchy and painful with crusty yellow drainage present. Conjunctivitis is very contagious, so the nurse should educate the patient and family caregivers to wash hands frequently. Additionally, the patient should not share items like pillowcases, towels, or makeup. Bacterial conjunctivitis is treated with antibiotic eye drops.[13]

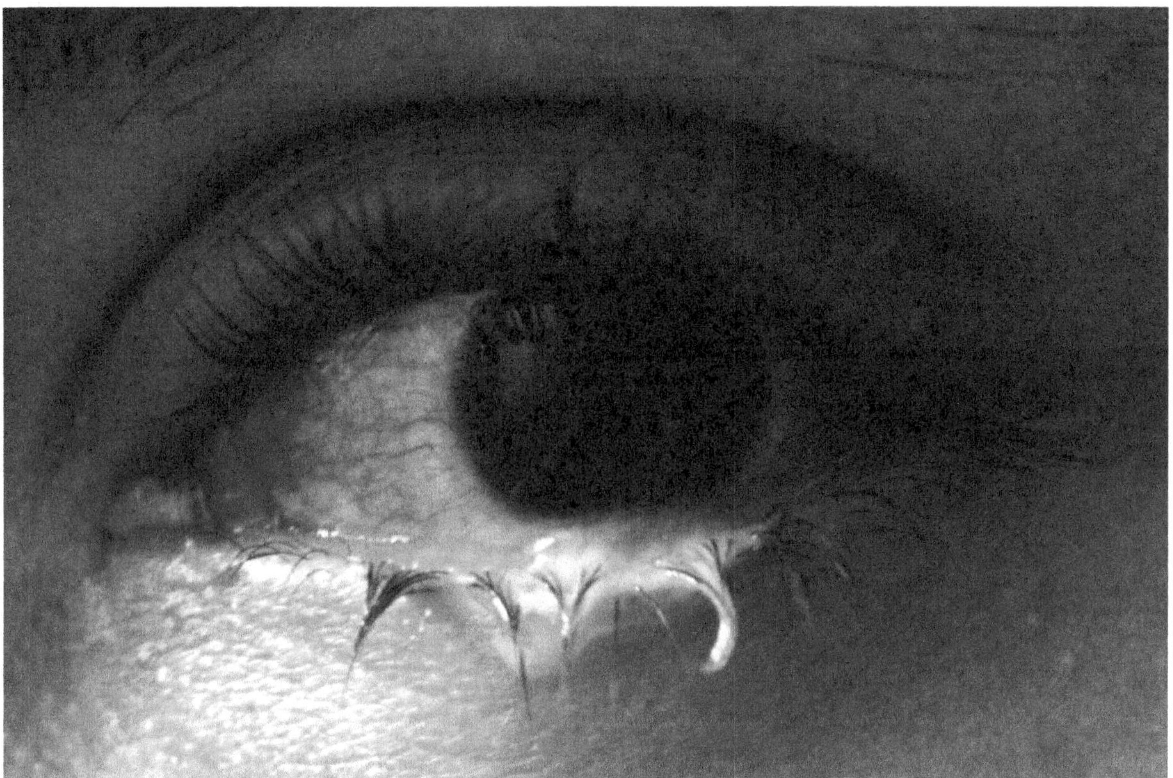

Figure 8.5 Conjunctivitis

12 "Swollen eye with conjunctivitis.jpg" by Tanalai at English Wikipedia is licensed under CC BY 3.0. Access for free at https://commons.wikimedia.org/wiki/File:Swollen_eye_with_conjunctivitis.jpg

13 National Eye Institute. (2019, July 8). *Causes of pink eye*. https://www.nei.nih.gov/learn-about-eye-health/eye-conditions-and-diseases/pink-eye/causes-pink-eye

My Notes

Stye

A stye is a bacterial infection of an oil gland in the eyelid, causing a red, tender bump at the edge of the eyelid. See Figure 8.6[14] for an image of a stye. Treatment includes applying warm compresses to the eyelid and prescription eyedrops.[15]

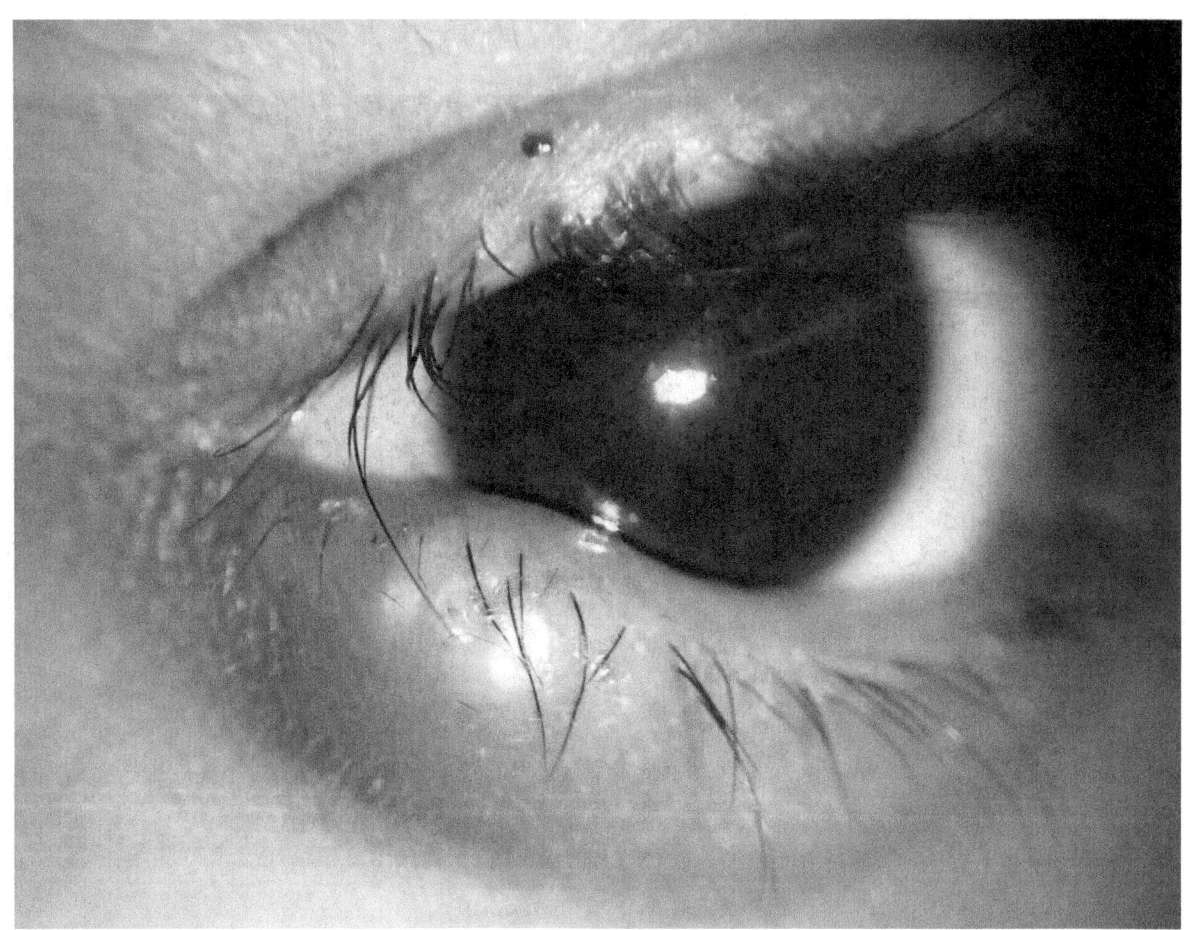

Figure 8.6 Stye

14 "External hordeolum.jpg" by Inrankabirhossain is licensed under CC BY-SA 4.0. Access for free at https://commons.wikimedia.org/wiki/File:External_hordeolum.jpg

15 National Eye Institute. (2019, July 2). Blepharitis. https://www.nei.nih.gov/learn-about-eye-health/eye-conditions-and-diseases/blepharitis

Cataracts

My Notes

A cataract is a cloudy area on the lens of the eye. Cataracts are very common in older adults. Over half of all Americans age 80 or older either have cataracts or have had surgery to remove cataracts. See Figure 8.7[16] for an image of a cataract. Cataracts develop slowly and symptoms include faded colors, blurred or double vision, halos around light, and trouble seeing at night. See Figure 8.8[17] for a simulated image of a person's vision with cataracts. Decreased vision due to cataracts may result in trouble reading and driving and increases the risk of falling. Patients often undergo surgery for cataracts. During cataract surgery, the doctor removes the clouded lens and replaces it with a new, artificial lens.[18]

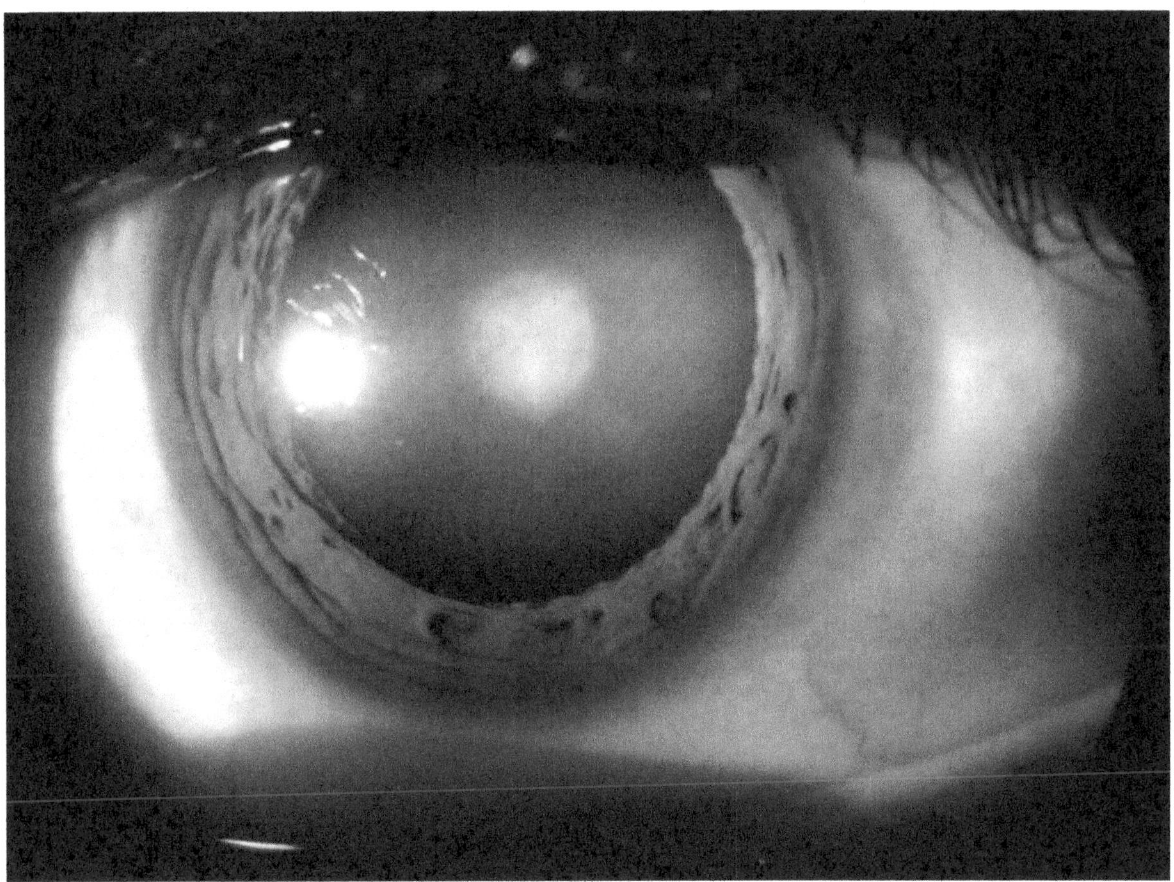

Figure 8.7 Cataracts

16 "Cataract in human eye.png" by Rakesh Ajuja, MD is licensed under CC BY-SA 3.0. Access for free at https://commons.wikimedia.org/wiki/File:Cataract_in_human_eye.png

17 "Eye disease simulation, cataract.jpg" by National Eye Institute, National Institutes of Health is in the Public Domain. Access for free at https://commons.wikimedia.org/wiki/File:Eye_disease_simulation,_cataract.jpg

18 National Eye Institute. (2019, August 3). *Cataracts.* https://www.nei.nih.gov/learn-about-eye-health/eye-conditions-and-diseases/cataracts

My Notes

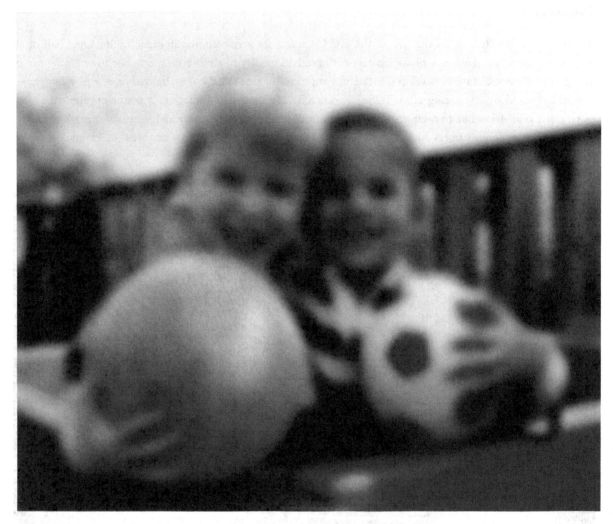

Figure 8.8 Simulated Vision with Cataracts

My Notes

Macular Degeneration

Age-related macular degeneration is a common condition that causes blurred central vision. It is the leading cause of vision loss for people 50 and older. See Figure 8.9[19] for a simulated image of a person's vision with macular degeneration. There are two types of macular degeneration: dry (nonexudative) and wet (exudative). During dry macular degeneration, cellular debris called drusen accumulates and scars the retina. In the wet (exudative) form, which is more severe, blood vessels grow behind the retina that leak exudate fluid, causing hemorrhaging and scarring. There is no treatment for dry macular degeneration, but laser therapy can be used to help treat wet (exudative) macular degeneration.[20]

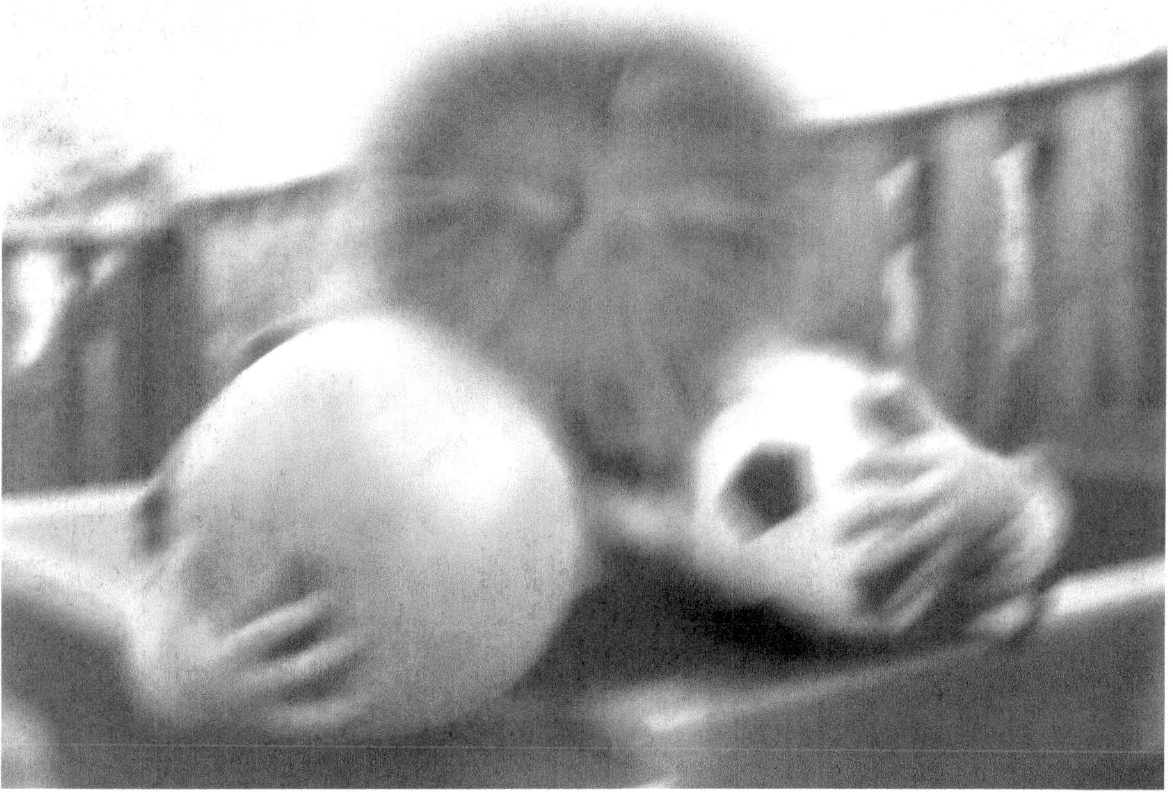

Figure 8.9 Simulated Vision with Macular Degeneration

19 "Eye disease simulation, age-related macular degeneration.jpg" by National Eye Institute, National Institutes of Health is in the Public Domain. Access for free at https://commons.wikimedia.org/wiki/File:Eye_disease_simulation,_age-related_macular_degeneration.jpg

20 National Eye Institute. (2020, August 17). *Age-related macular degeneration*. https://www.nei.nih.gov/learn-about-eye-health/eye-conditions-and-diseases/age-related-macular-degeneration

My Notes

Glaucoma

Glaucoma is a group of eye diseases that causes vision loss by damaging the optic nerve due to increased intraocular pressure. Treatment includes prescription eye drops to lower the pressure inside the eye and slow the progression of the disease. If not treated appropriately, glaucoma can cause blindness. Symptoms of glaucoma include gradual loss of peripheral vision. See Figure 8.10[21] for a simulated image of a person's vision with glaucoma. Because the loss of vision occurs so slowly, many people don't realize they have symptoms until the disease is well-progressed or it is discovered during an eye exam.[22]

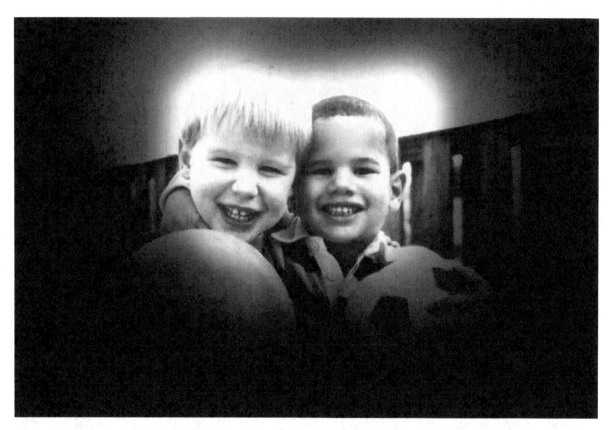

Figure 8.10 Simulated Vision with Glaucoma

Screening Tools for Eye Exams

Common screening tools used during an eye exam are the Snellen chart, a near vision chart, and Ishihara plates. Nurses working in outpatient settings or school settings use these tools when screening patients for vision problems. If a vision problem is identified, the patient is referred to an optometrist for further testing. When performing a vision assessment, be sure to provide adequate lighting.

21 "Eye disease simulation, glaucoma.jpg" by National Eye Institute, National Institutes of Health is in the Public Domain. Access for free at https://commons.wikimedia.org/wiki/File:Eye_disease_simulation,_glaucoma.jpg

22 National Eye Institute. (2020, July 28). *Glaucoma.* https://www.nei.nih.gov/learn-about-eye-health/eye-conditions-and-diseases/glaucoma

Snellen Chart

My Notes

Distant vision is tested by using the **Snellen chart**. See Figure 8.11[23] for an image of the Snellen chart. Place the patient 20 feet away from the Snellen chart. Ask them to cover one eye and read the letters from the lowest line they can see clearly. Record the corresponding fraction in the furthermost right-hand column. Repeat with the other eye. If the patient is wearing glasses or contact lens during this assessment, document the results as "corrected vision" when wearing these assistive devices.

A person with no visual impairment is documented as having 20/20 vision. A person with impaired vision has a different lower denominator of this fraction. For example, a vision measurement of 20/30 indicates the patient can see letters clearly at 20 feet that a person with normal vision can see clearly at 30 feet.[24] Alternative charts are also available for children or adults who can't read letters in English. See Figure 8.12[25] for an alternative eye chart.

---

23 "Snellen chart.jpg" by Jeff Dahl is licensed under CC BY-SA 3.0. Access for free at https://en.wikipedia.org/wiki/File:Snellen_chart.svg

24 Sue, S. (2007). Test distance vision by using a Snellen chart. *Community Eye Health, 20*(63), 52. https://www.ncbi.nlm.nih.gov/pmc/articles/PMC2040251/

25 "US Navy 070808-N-6278K-128 Hospital Corpsman 3rd Class Edward Mace, an optician attached to the Military Sealift Command (MSC) hospital ship USNS Comfort (T-AH 20), instructs a patient on how to read an eye chart.jpg" by Mass Communication Specialist 2nd Class Joan E. Kretschmer for U.S. Navy is in the Public Domain. Access for free at https://commons.wikimedia.org/wiki/File:US_Navy_070808-N-6278K-128_Hospital_Corpsman_3rd_Class_Edward_Mace,_an_optician_attached_to_the_Military_Sealift_Command_(MSC)_hospital_ship_USNS_Comfort_(T-AH_20),_instructs_a_patient_on_how_to_read_an_eye_chart.jpg

My Notes

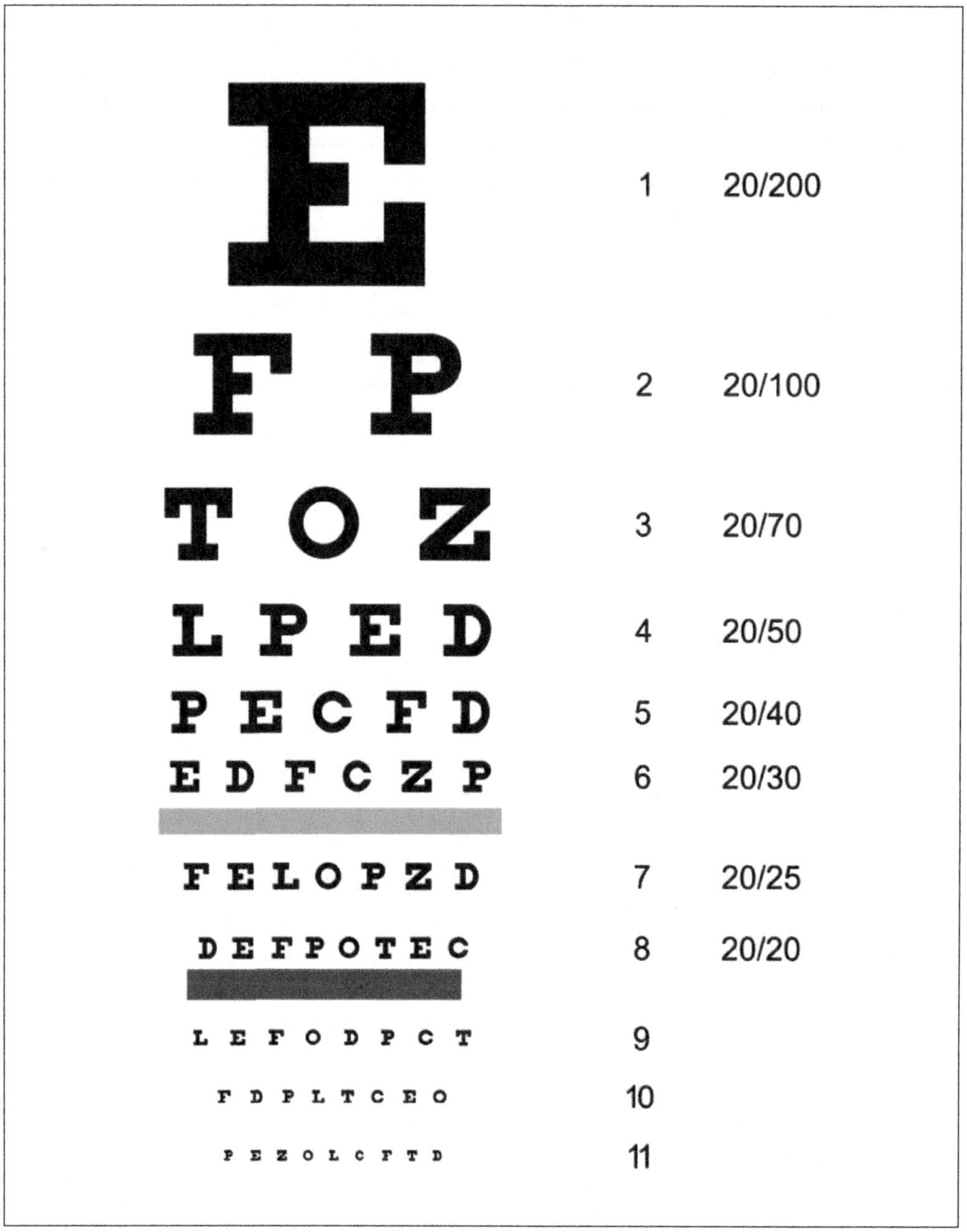

E	1	20/200
F P	2	20/100
T O Z	3	20/70
L P E D	4	20/50
P E C F D	5	20/40
E D F C Z P	6	20/30
F E L O P Z D	7	20/25
D E F P O T E C	8	20/20
L E F O D P C T	9	
F D P L T C E O	10	
P E Z O L C F T D	11	

Figure 8.11 Snellen Chart

My Notes

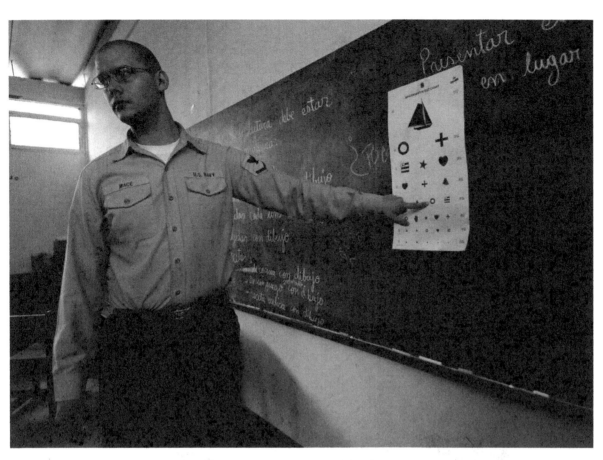

Figure 8.12 Alternative Eye Chart

My Notes

Near Vision

Near vision is assessed by having a patient read from a prepared card that is held 14 inches away from the eyes. If a card is not available, the patient can be asked to read from a newspaper as an alternative quick screening tool. See Figure 8.13[26] for an image of a prepared card used to assess near vision.

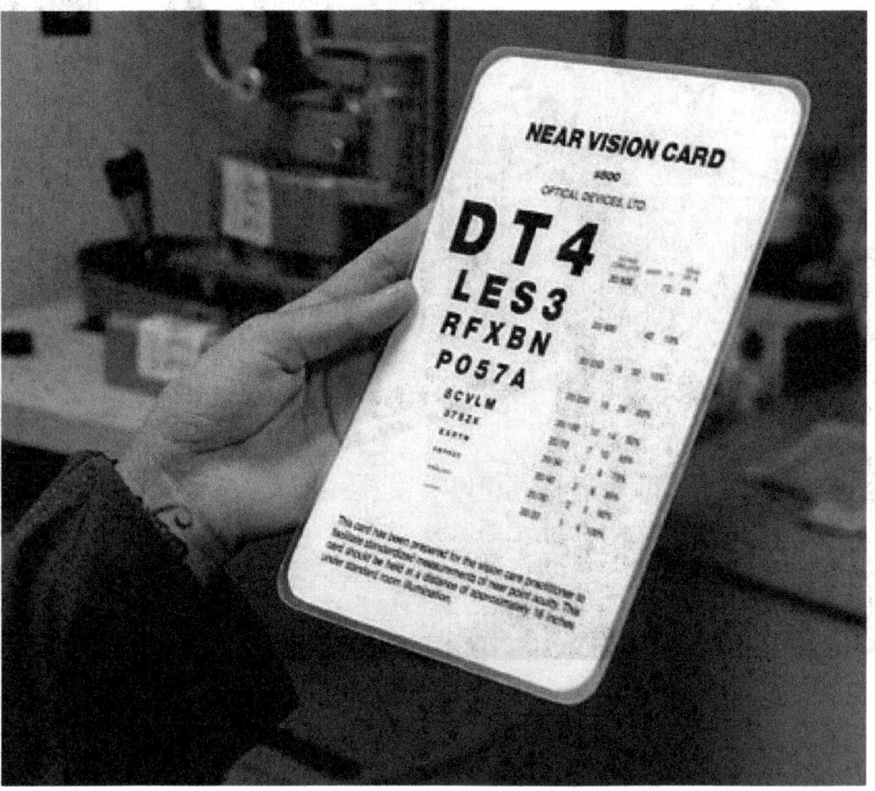

Figure 8.13 Assessing Near Vision

26 "111012-F-ZT401-067.JPG" by Airman 1st Class Brooke P. Beers for U.S. Air Force is in the Public Domain. Access for free at https://www.pacaf.af.mil/News/Article-Display/Article/593609/keeping-sight-all-right/

My Notes

Ishihara Plates

Ishihara plates are commonly used to assess color vision. Each of the colored dotted plates shows either a number or a path. See Figure 8.14[27] for an example of Ishihara plates. A person with color blindness is not able to distinguish the numbers or paths from the other colored dots on the plate.

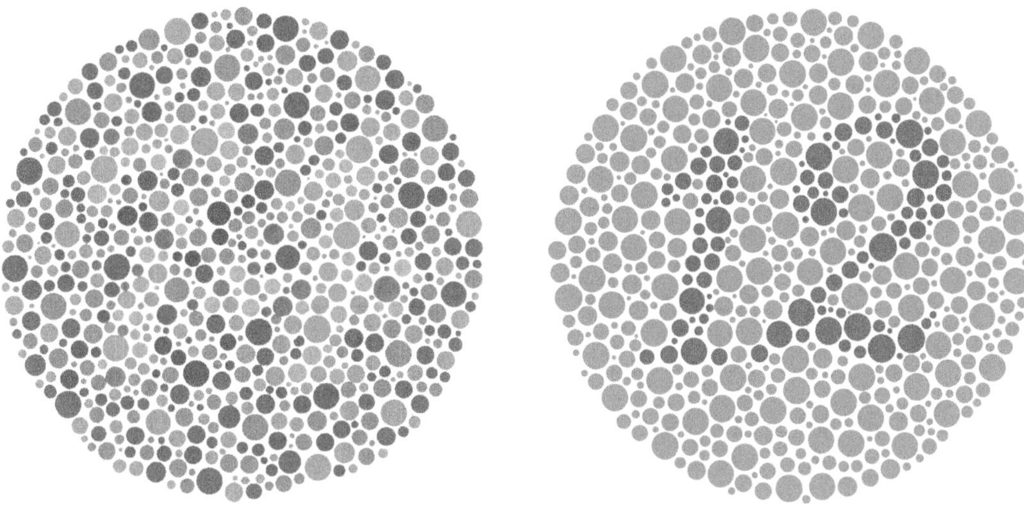

Figure 8.14 Ishihara Color Test Plates

Anatomy of the Ear

Hearing is the transduction of sound waves into a neural signal by the structures of the ear. See Figure 8.15[28] for an image of the anatomy of the ear. The large, fleshy structure on the lateral aspect of the head is known as the **auricle**. The C-shaped curves of the auricle direct sound waves toward the ear canal. At the end of the ear canal is the **tympanic membrane**, commonly referred to as the eardrum, that vibrates after it is struck by sound waves. The auricle, ear canal, and tympanic membrane are referred to as the external ear. The middle ear consists of a space with three small bones called the malleus, incus, and stapes, the Latin names that roughly translate to "hammer," "anvil," and "stirrup." The malleus is attached to the tympanic membrane and articulates with the incus. The incus, in turn, articulates with the stapes. The stapes is attached to the inner ear, where the sound waves are transduced into a neural signal. The middle ear is also connected to the pharynx through the Eustachian tube that helps equilibrate air pressure across the tympanic membrane. The Eustachian tube is normally closed but will pop open when the muscles of the pharynx contract during swallowing or yawning. The inner ear is often described as a bony labyrinth because it is composed of a series of semicircular canals. The semicircular canals have two separate regions, the cochlea and the vestibule, that are responsible for hearing and balance. The neural signals from these

---

27 This work is derivative of "Ishihara 9.png" and "Ishihara_1.png" by Shinobu Ishihara are in the Public Domain. Access for free at https://commons.wikimedia.org/wiki/File:Ishihara_9.png and https://commons.wikimedia.org/wiki/File:Ishihara_1.svg

28 "1404 The Structure of the Ear.jpg" by OpenStax is licensed under CC BY 4.0. Access for free at https://commons.wikimedia.org/wiki/File:1404_The_Structures_of_the_Ear.jpg

My Notes

two regions are relayed to the brain stem through separate fiber bundles. However, they travel together from the inner ear to the brain stem as the **vestibulocochlear nerve** (cranial nerve VIII).[29]

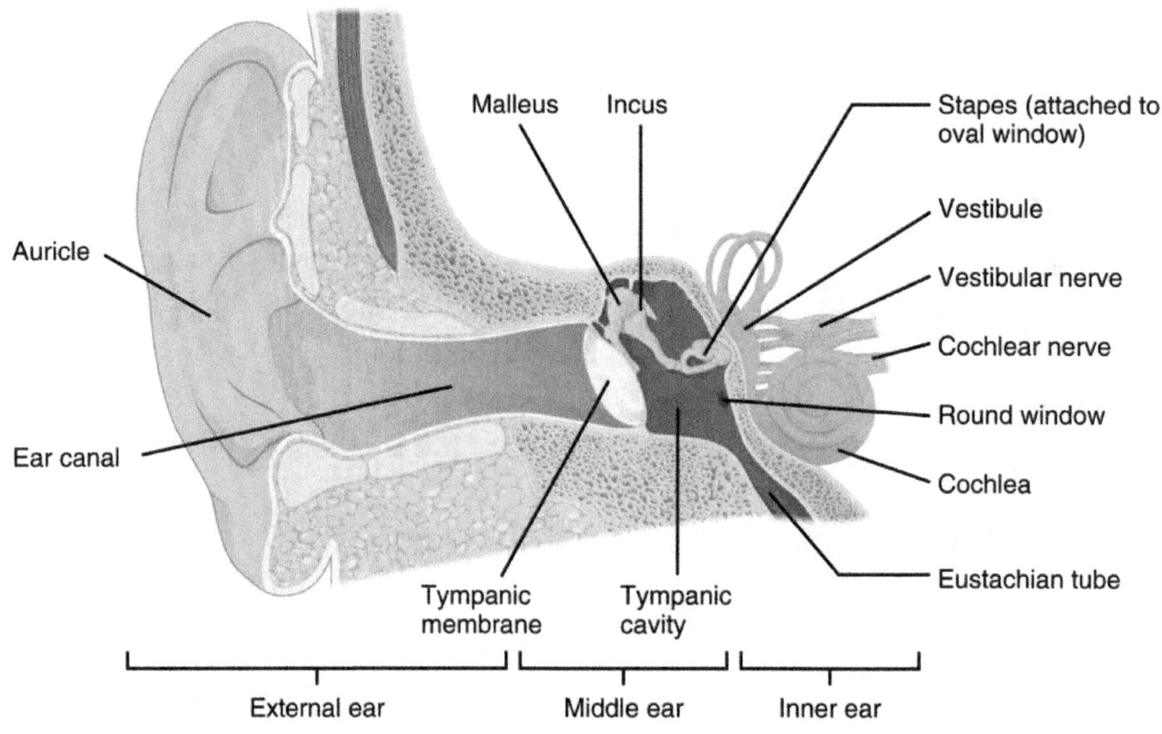

Figure 8.15 The Ear

Hearing

Sound waves cause the tympanic membrane to vibrate. This vibration is amplified as it moves across the malleus, incus, and stapes and into the cochlea. Within the inner ear, the cochlear duct contains sound-transducing neurons. As the frequency of a sound changes, different hair cells within the cochlear duct are sensitive to a particular frequency. In this manner, the cochlea separates auditory stimuli by frequency and sends impulses to the brain stem via the cochlear nerve. The cochlea encodes auditory stimuli for frequencies between 20 and 20,000 Hz, the range of sound that human ears can detect.[30]

Balance

Along with hearing, the inner ear is also responsible for the sense of balance. Semicircular canals in the vestibule have three ring-like extensions. One extension is oriented in the horizontal plane, and the other two are oriented in the vertical plane. Hair cells within the vestibule sense head position, head movement, and body motion. By comparing the relative movements of both the horizontal and vertical planes, the vestibular system can detect the direction of most head movements within three-dimensional space. However, medical conditions affecting the

29 This work is a derivative of Anatomy & Physiology by OpenStax and is licensed under CC BY 4.0. Access for free at https://openstax.org/books/anatomy-and-physiology/pages/1-introduction

30 This work is a derivative of Anatomy & Physiology by OpenStax and is licensed under CC BY 4.0. Access for free at https://openstax.org/books/anatomy-and-physiology/pages/1-introduction

My Notes

semicircular canals cause incorrect signals to be sent to the brain, resulting in a spinning type of dizziness called vertigo.

Video Review of Anatomy of the Ear[31]

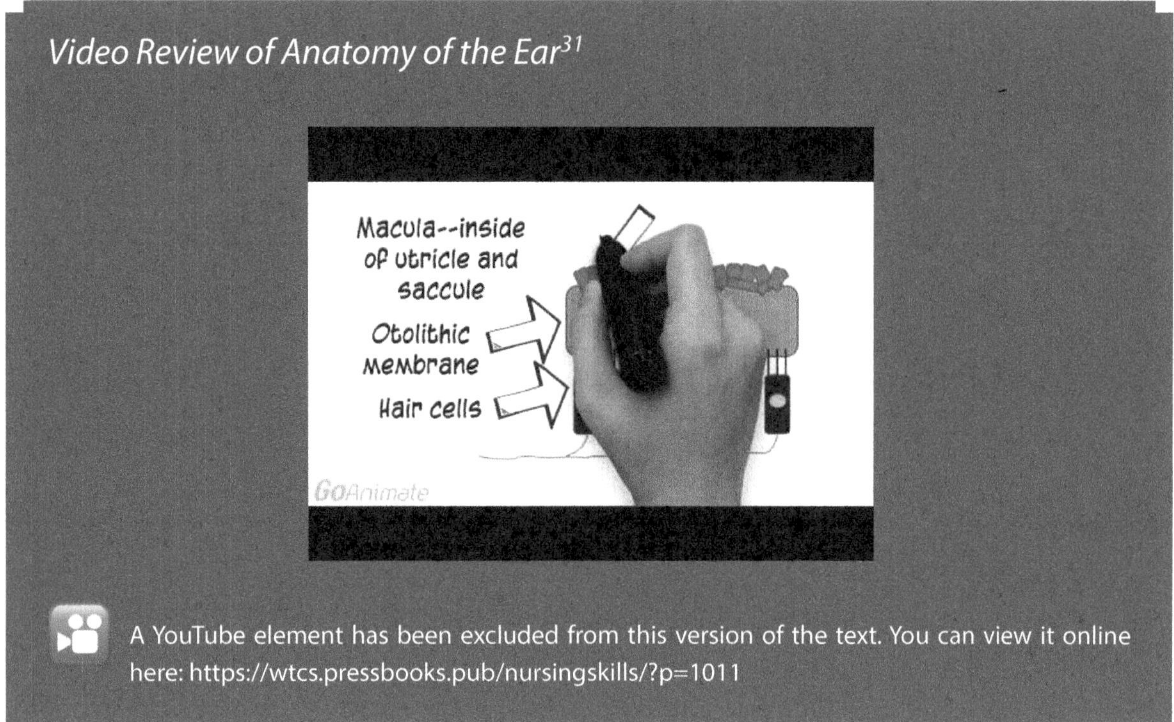

A YouTube element has been excluded from this version of the text. You can view it online here: https://wtcs.pressbooks.pub/nursingskills/?p=1011

Common Ear Disorders

Hearing Loss

Hearing loss is classified as conductive hearing loss or sensorineural hearing loss. **Conductive hearing loss** occurs when something in the external or middle ear is obstructing the transmission of sound. For example, cerumen impaction or a perforated tympanic membrane can cause conductive hearing loss. **Sensorineural hearing loss** is caused by pathology of the inner ear, cranial nerve VIII, or auditory areas of the cerebral cortex. **Presbycusis** is sensorineural hearing loss that occurs with aging due to gradual nerve degeneration. **Ototoxic medications** can also cause sensorineural hearing loss by affecting the hair cells in the cochlea.

Acute Otitis Media

Acute otitis media is the medical diagnosis for an middle ear infection. Ear infections are a common illness in the pediatric population. Children between the ages of 6 months and 2 years are more susceptible to ear infections because of the size and shape of their Eustachian tubes. Acute otitis media typically occurs after an upper respiratory infection when the Eustachian tube becomes inflamed and the middle ear fills with fluid, causing ear pain and irritability. This fluid can become infected, causing purulent fluid and low-grade fever. Acute otitis media is diagnosed by a health care provider using an otoscope to examine the tympanic membrane for bulging and purulent fluid. If not treated, acute otitis media can potentially cause perforation of the tympanic membrane. Treating early acute otitis media with antibiotics is controversial in the United States due to the effort to prevent

31 Forciea, B. (2105, May 12). *Anatomy of the ear (v2.0)*. [Video]. YouTube. All rights reserved. Video used with permission. https://youtu.be/A2ji_Vd8cuE

My Notes

antibiotic resistance. However, the treatment goals are to control pain and treat infection with antibiotics if a bacterial infection is present.[32]

Some children develop recurrent ear infections that can cause hearing loss affecting their language development. For children experiencing recurring cases, a surgery called myringotomy surgery is performed by an otolaryngologist. During myringotomy surgery, a tympanostomy tube is placed in the tympanic membrane to drain fluid from the middle ear and prevent infection from developing. If a child has a tympanostomy tube in place, it is expected to see clear fluid in their ear canal as it drains out of the tube. See Figure 8.16[33] for an image of a tympanostomy tube in the ear.[34]

32 This work is a derivative of StatPearls by Danishyar and Ashurst and is licensed under CC BY 4.0. Access for free at https://www.ncbi.nlm.nih.gov/books/NBK430685/

33 "Ear Tube.png" by BruceBlaus is licensed under CC BY-SA 4.0. Access for free at https://commons.wikimedia.org/wiki/File:Ear_Tube.png

34 This work is a derivative of StatPearls by Danishyar and Ashurst and is licensed under CC BY 4.0. Access for free at https://www.ncbi.nlm.nih.gov/books/NBK430685/

My Notes

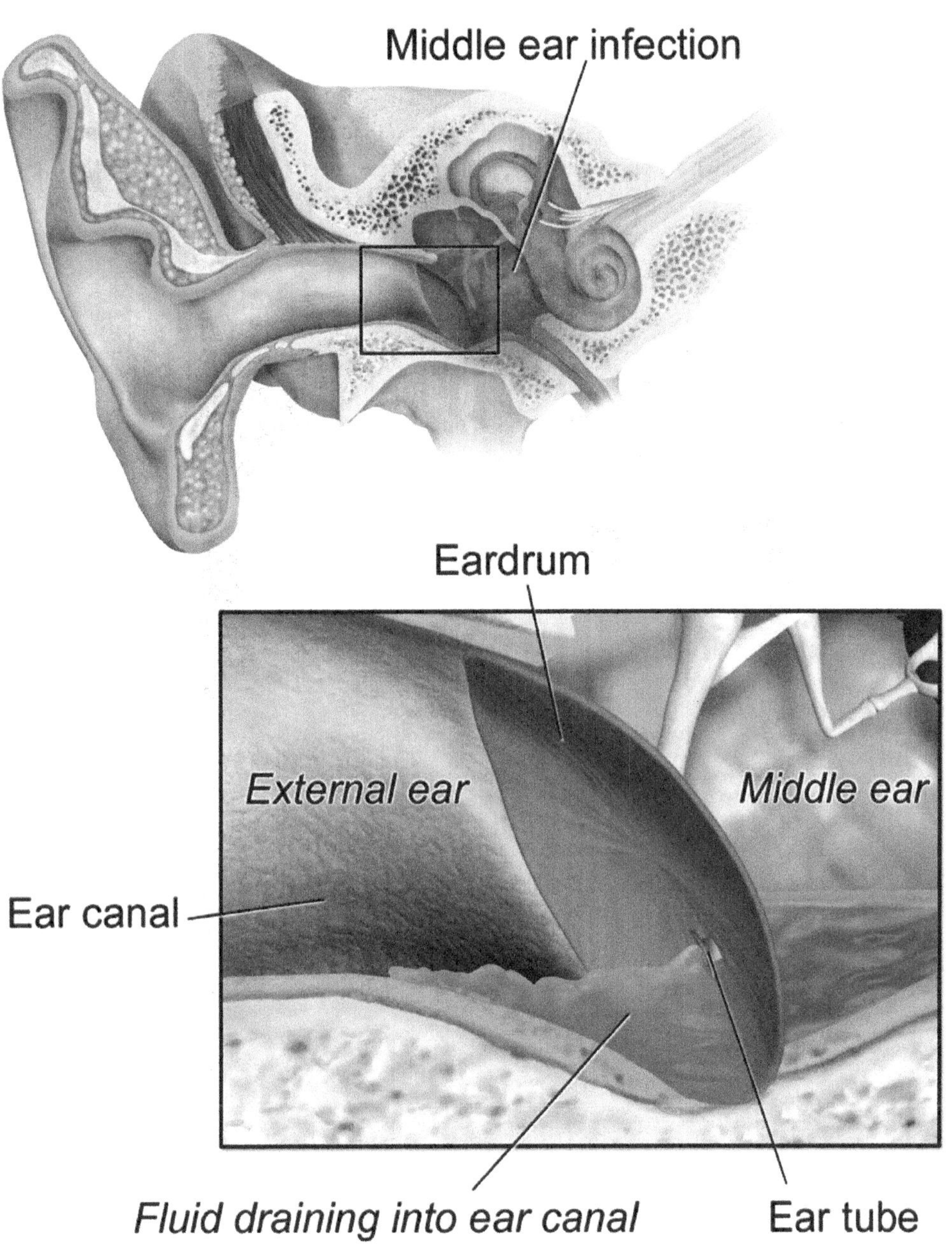

Figure 8.16 Tympanostomy Tube

My Notes

Otitis Externa

Otitis externa is the medical diagnosis for external ear inflammation and/or infection. See Figure 8.17[35] for an image of otitis externa. It is commonly known as "swimmer's ear" because it commonly occurs in swimmers, especially in summer months. Otitis externa can occur in all age groups and causes an erythematous and edematous ear canal with associated yellow, white, or grey debris. Patients often report itching in the ear canal with pain that is worsened by pulling upwards and outwards on the auricle. Otitis externa is treated with antibiotic drops placed in the ear canals.[36]

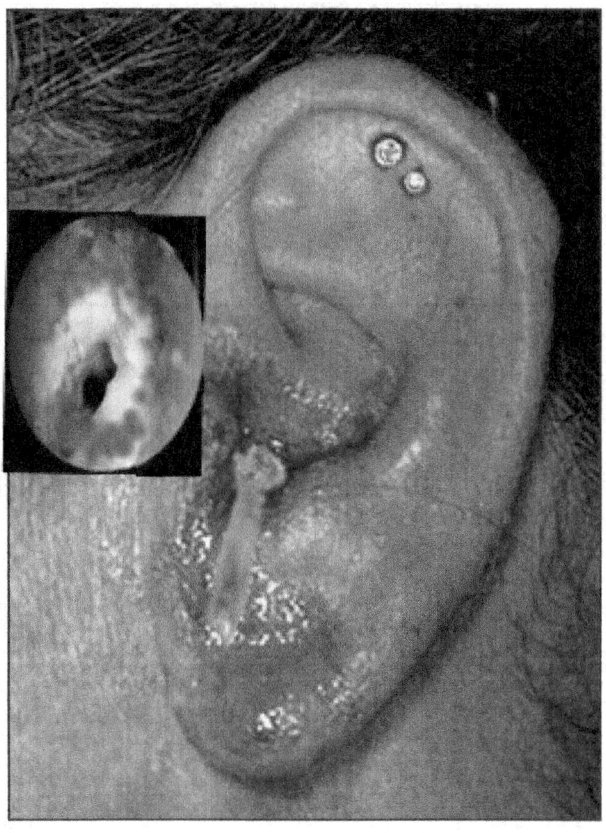

Figure 8.17 Otitis Externa

35 "Otitis externa.gif" by S. Bhjimji MD is licensed under CC BY 4.0. Access for free at https://www.ncbi.nlm.nih.gov/books/NBK556055/

36 This work is a derivative of StatPearls by Medina-Blasini and Sharman and is licensed under CC BY 4.0. Access for free at https://www.ncbi.nlm.nih.gov/books/NBK430685/

Cerumen Impaction

My Notes

Cerumen impaction refers to a buildup of earwax causing occlusion of the ear canal. This occlusion often causes symptoms such as hearing loss, ear fullness, and itching. See Figure 8.18[37] for an image of cerumen impaction.

Cerumen can be removed via irrigation of the ear canal, ear drops to dissolve the wax, or manual removal.[38] In outpatient settings, nurses often assist with ear irrigation to remove cerumen impaction according to agency policy. See Figure 8.19[39] for an image of an ear irrigation procedure.

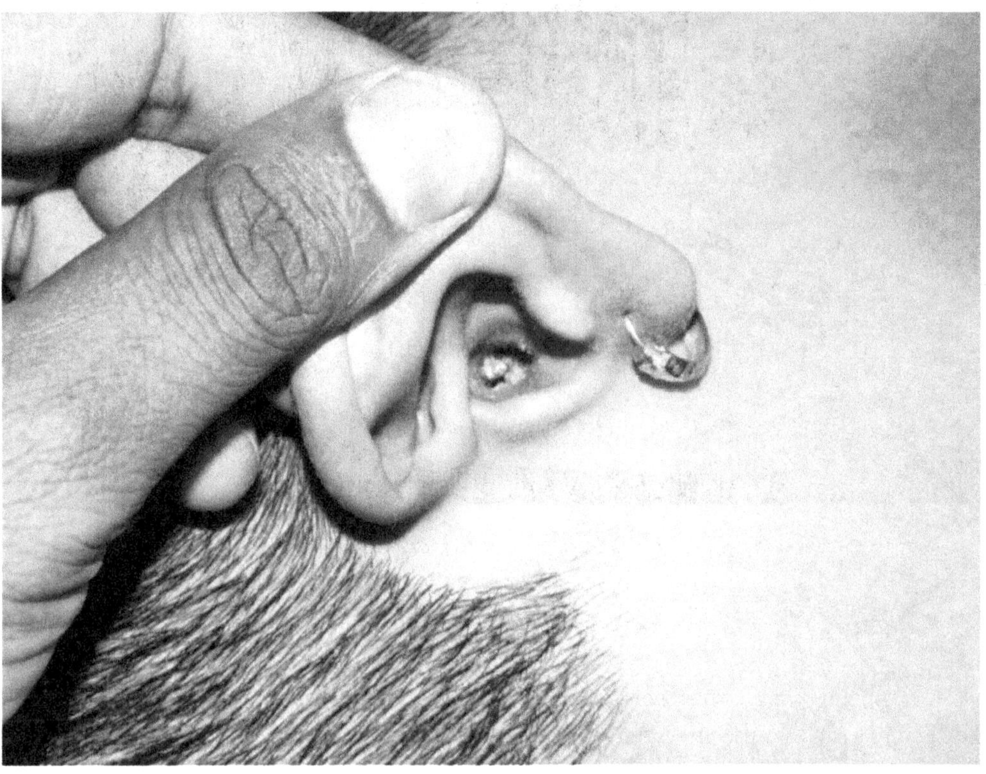

Figure 8.18 Cerumen Impaction

37 "Ear Wax.JPG" by *Anand2202* is licensed under CC BY-SA 4.0. Access for free at https://commons.wikimedia.org/wiki/File:Ear_Wax.JPG

38 This work is a derivative of StatPearls by Mankowski and Raggio and is licensed under CC BY 4.0. Access for free at https://www.ncbi.nlm.nih.gov/books/NBK430685/

39 "150915-F-GO352-025.jpg" by Staff Sgt. Jason Huddleston for U.S. Air Force is licensed under *CC0*. Access for free at https://www.59mdw.af.mil/News/Article-Display/Article/647342/photo-essay-559th-medical-group-at-a-glance/

My Notes

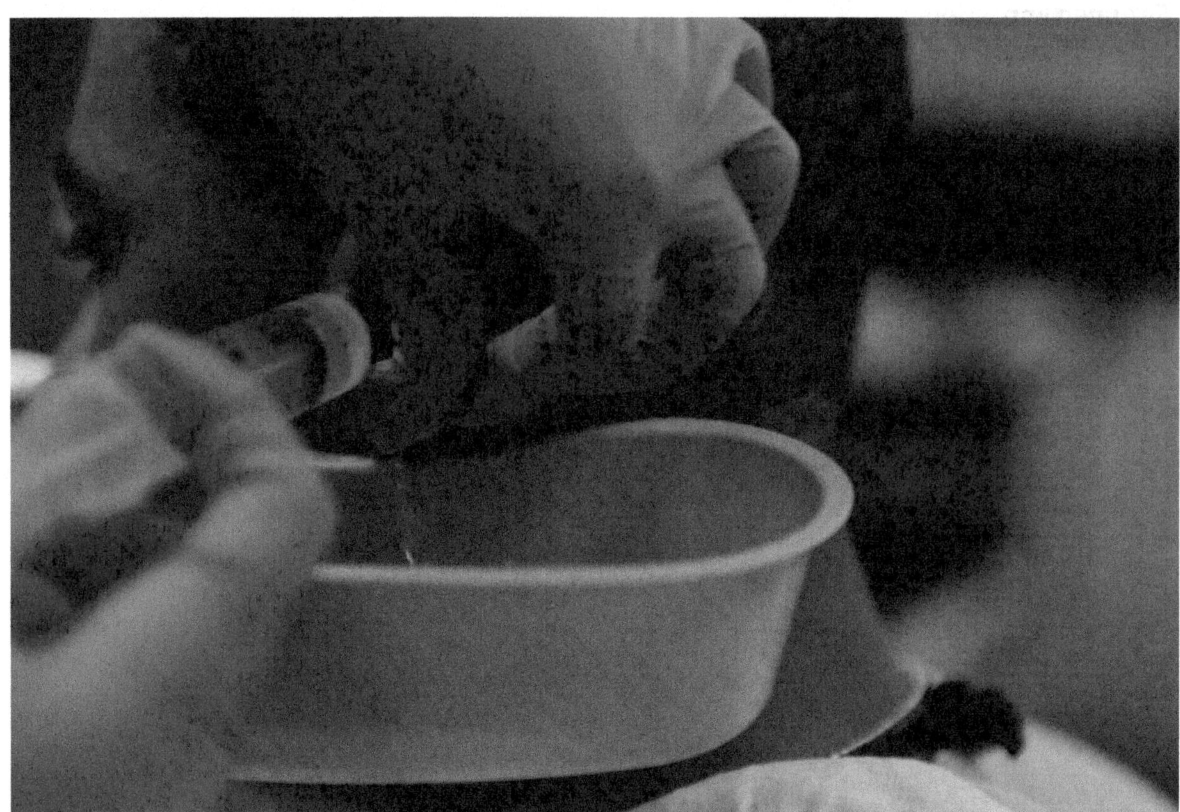

Figure 8.19 Ear Irrigation to Remove Cerumen Impaction

Tinnitus

Tinnitus is a ringing, buzzing, roaring, hissing, or whistling sound in the ears. The noise may be intermittent or continuous. Tinnitus can be caused by cerumen impaction, noise trauma, or ototoxic medications, such as diuretics or high doses of aspirin. Military personnel have a high incidence of tinnitus due to noise trauma from loud explosions and gunfire. There are no medications to treat tinnitus, but patients can be referred to an otolaryngologist for treatment such as cognitive therapy or noise masking.[40]

Vertigo

Vertigo is a type of dizziness that is often described by patients as, "the room feels as if it is spinning." Benign positional vertigo (BPV) is a common condition caused by crystals becoming lodged in the semicircular canals in the vestibule of the inner ear that send false movement signals to the brain. BPV can be treated by trained professionals using a specific set of maneuvers that guide the crystals back to the chamber where they are supposed to be in the inner ear.[41]

---

40 This work is a derivative of StatPearls by Grossan and Peterson and is licensed under CC BY 4.0. Access for free at https://www.ncbi.nlm.nih.gov/books/NBK430685/

41 Woodhouse, S. (n.d.). *Benign paraoxysmal positional vertigo (BPPV)*. Vestibular Disorders Association. https://vestibular.org/article/diagnosis-treatment/types-of-vestibular-disorders/benign-paroxysmal-positional-vertigo-bppv/

8.3 EYE AND EAR ASSESSMENT

My Notes

Now that we have reviewed the anatomy of the eyes and ears and their common disorders, let's discuss common eye and ear assessments performed by nurses.

Subjective Assessment

Nurses collect subjective information from the patient and/or family caregivers using detailed questions and pay close attention to what the patient is reporting to guide the physical exam. Focused interview questions include inquiring about current symptoms, as well as any history of eye and ear conditions. See Table 8.3a for suggested interview questions related to the eyes and ears.

Table 8.3a Suggested Interview Questions for Subjective Assessment of the Eyes and Ears

Interview Questions
Eye
Have you had any difficulty seeing or experienced blurred vision?
Do you wear glasses or contact lenses?
When was your last vision test?
Have you had any redness, swelling, watering, or discharge from the eyes?
Have you ever been diagnosed with an eye condition such as cataracts, glaucoma, or macular degeneration?
Are you currently using any medication, eye drops, or supplements for your eyes?
Ear
Have you had any trouble hearing? If so, do you wear hearing aids?
Have you had any symptoms like ringing in the ears, drainage from the ears, or ear pain?
Do you ever feel dizzy, off-balance, or like the room is spinning?
Have you ever been diagnosed with an ear condition such as an infection, tinnitus, or vertigo?
Are you currently using any medications, ear drops, or supplements for your ears?

Life Span Considerations

Pediatric

When collecting subjective data from children, information is also obtained from parents and/or legal guardians. Children aged 2-24 months commonly experience ear infections. Vision impairments may become apparent in

My Notes

school-aged children when they have difficulty seeing the board from their seats. Additional subjective data may be obtained by asking these questions:

- Have you or your child's teachers noticed your child experiencing any problems seeing or hearing?
- Has your child experienced frequent ear infections or had tubes placed in their ears? If so, have you noticed any effects on their language development?

Older Adults

The aging adult experiences a general slowing in nerve conduction. Vision, hearing, fine coordination, and balance may also become impaired. Older adults may experience presbyopia (decreased near vision), presbycusis (hearing loss), cataracts, macular degeneration, or glaucoma. They may also experience feelings of dizziness or feeling off-balance, which can result in falls. Read more about these conditions in the "Eye and Ear Basic Concepts" section earlier in this chapter.

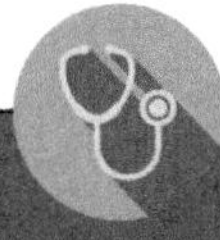

Tip: Educate all patients to have yearly eye examinations.

Objective Assessment

A routine assessment of the eyes and ears by registered nurses in inpatient and outpatient settings typically includes external inspection of eyes and ears for signs of a medical condition, as well as screening for vision and hearing problems. A vision screening test, whispered voice hearing test, and assessment of pupillary response are often included in the physical exam based on the setting.[1] Additional assessments may be performed if the patient's status warrants assessment of the cranial nerves.

Inspection

Eyes

Begin the assessment by inspecting the eyes. The sclera should be white and the conjunctiva should be pink. There should not be any drainage from the eyes. The patient should demonstrate behavioral cues indicating effective vision during the assessment.

Ears

Inspect the ears. There should not be any drainage from the ears or evidence of cerumen impaction. The patient should demonstrate behavioral cues indicating effective hearing.

1 Giddens, J. (2007). A survey of physical examination techniques performed by RNs: Lessons for nursing education. *Journal of Nursing Education, 46*(2), 83-87.

Vision Tests

My Notes

See more information about procedures for assessing vision in the "Eye and Ear Basic Concepts" section earlier in this chapter. Assess far vision using the Snellen eye chart. In outpatient settings, near vision may be assessed using a prepared card or a newspaper. Color vision may be assessed using a book containing Ishihara plates.

Hearing Test

Nurses perform a basic hearing assessment during conversation with the patient. For example, the following patient cues during normal conversation can indicate hearing loss:

- Lip-reads or watches your face and lips closely rather than your eyes
- Leans forward or appears to strain to hear what you are saying
- Moves head in a position to catch sounds with the better ear
- Misunderstands your questions or frequently asks you to repeat
- Uses an inappropriately loud voice
- Demonstrates garbled speech or distorted vowel sounds[2]

WHISPER TEST

The whispered voice test is an effective screening test used to detect hearing impairment if performed accurately. Complete the following steps to accurately perform this test:[3]

- Stand at arm's length behind the seated patient to prevent lip reading.
- Test each ear individually. The patient should be instructed to occlude the nontested ear with their finger.
- Exhale before whispering and use as quiet a voice as possible.
- Whisper a combination of numbers and letters (for example, 4-K-2), and then ask the patient to repeat the sequence.
- If the patient responds correctly, their hearing is considered normal; if the patient responds incorrectly, the test is repeated using a different number/letter combination.
- The patient is considered to have passed the screening test if they repeat at least three out of a possible six numbers or letters correctly.
- The other ear is assessed similarly with a different combination of numbers and letters.

Pupillary Response, Extraocular Movement, and Cranial Nerves

When a patient is suspected of experiencing a neurological disease or injury, their pupils are assessed to ensure they are bilaterally equal, round, and responsive to light and accommodation (PERRLA). Extraocular movement and other cranial nerves may also be assessed that affect vision, hearing, and balance. For more information about how to assess PERRLA, extraocular eye movement, and other cranial nerves, go to the "Assessing Cranial Nerves" section in the "Neurological Assessment" chapter.

---

2 Jarvis, C. (2015). *Physical examination and health assessment* (7th ed.). Saunders. p. 330.

3 Pirozzo, S., Papinczak, T., & Glasziou, P. (2003). Whispered voice test for screening for hearing impairment in adults and children: Systematic review. *BMJ (Clinical research ed.), 327*(7421), 967. https://doi.org/10.1136/bmj.327.7421.967

My Notes

See Table 8.3b for a comparison of expected versus unexpected findings when assessing the eyes and ears.

Table 8.3b Expected Versus Unexpected Findings on Eyes or Ears Assessment

Assessment	Expected Findings	Unexpected New Findings (Document and notify provider)
Inspection	**Eyes** Sclera are white. Lens is clear. Conjunctiva are pink. Eyelids do not have redness, swelling, lumps, or discharge. No drainage is present from the eyes. Patient displays behavioral cues of effective vision. Eyes appear appropriately placed in orbits. **Ears** No drainage or cerumen is present in the ear canals. Conversation includes behavioral cues of effective hearing. During the whispered voice test, the patient correctly reports at least three out of a possible six numbers or letters for both ears. Patient demonstrates good balance and a coordinated gait.	**Eyes** Yellow sclera may indicate liver dysfunction. Cloudy lens indicates cataracts. Red conjunctiva or drainage can indicate conjunctivitis. Redness or crusting on the eyelids can indicate blepharitis. A tender lump on the eye can indicate a stye. Patient displays behavioral cues indicating vision loss that is not already corrected with glasses or contacts. Sunken eyes can indicate dehydration. **Ears** Purulent drainage is present in ear canal. Cerumen impaction is present. Conversation indicates behavioral cues of uncorrected hearing loss. During the whispered voice test, the patient reports fewer than three out of a possible six numbers or letters correctly for both ears. Patient demonstrates poor balance or an uncoordinated gait.
***CRITICAL CONDITIONS to report immediately**		New and sudden problems such as vision loss, blurred vision, eye pain, red eye, ear pain, vertigo, poor balance, or gait change.

8.4 SAMPLE DOCUMENTATION

My Notes

Sample Documentation of Expected Findings

The patient reports no previous history of ear or eye conditions. Eyes have white sclera and pink conjunctiva with no drainage present. Corrected vision with glasses using Snellen chart is 20/20 bilaterally. Ear canals are clear bilaterally. Whispered voice test indicates effective hearing with the patient reporting five out six numbers correctly for both ears. Patient demonstrates good balance and coordinated gait.

Sample Documentation of Unexpected Findings

The patient reports awakening with an irritated left eye and crusty drainage but no change in vision. The sclera in the left eye is pink, the conjunctiva is red, and yellow, crusty drainage is present. The patient is able to read the newspaper without visual impairment. Dr. Smith was notified and she evaluated the patient at 1400. A new order for antibiotic eye drops was received and administered. The patient and their family members were educated to wash hands frequently to avoid contagion.

My Notes

8.5 CHECKLIST FOR EYE AND EAR ASSESSMENT

Use the checklist below to review the steps for completing an "Eye and Ear Assessment."

Steps

Disclaimer: Always review and follow agency policy regarding this specific skill.

1. Gather supplies: penlight, Ishihara plates, Snellen chart, Rosenbaum card, or a newspaper to read.
2. Perform safety steps:
    - Perform hand hygiene.
    - Check the room for transmission-based precautions.
    - Introduce yourself, your role, the purpose of your visit, and an estimate of the time it will take.
    - Confirm patient ID using two patient identifiers (e.g., name and date of birth).
    - Explain the process to the patient and ask if they have any questions.
    - Be organized and systematic.
    - Use appropriate listening and questioning skills.
    - Listen and attend to patient cues.
    - Ensure the patient's privacy and dignity.
    - Assess ABCs.
3. Use effective interview questions to collect subjective data about eye or ear eye problems.
4. Inspect the external eye. Note any unexpected findings.
5. Assess that pupils are equally round and reactive to light and accommodation (PERRLA).
6. Assess extraocular movement.
7. Inspect the external ear. Note any unexpected findings.
8. Assess distance vision acuity using the Snellen eye chart and proper technique.
9. Assess near vision acuity using a prepared card or newspaper.
10. Asses for color blindness using the Ishihara plates.
11. Assess hearing by accurately performing the whisper test.
12. Assist the patient to a comfortable position, ask if they have any questions, and thank them for their time.
13. Ensure five safety measures when leaving the room:
    - CALL LIGHT: Within reach
    - BED: Low and locked (in lowest position and brakes on)
    - SIDE RAILS: Secured

My Notes

- TABLE: Within reach
- ROOM: Risk-free for falls (scan room and clear any obstacles)

14. Perform hand hygiene.

15. Document the assessment findings. Report any concerns according to agency policy.

My Notes

8.6 SUPPLEMENTARY VIDEO ON EYE ASSESSMENT

Video Review for Eye Assessment[1]

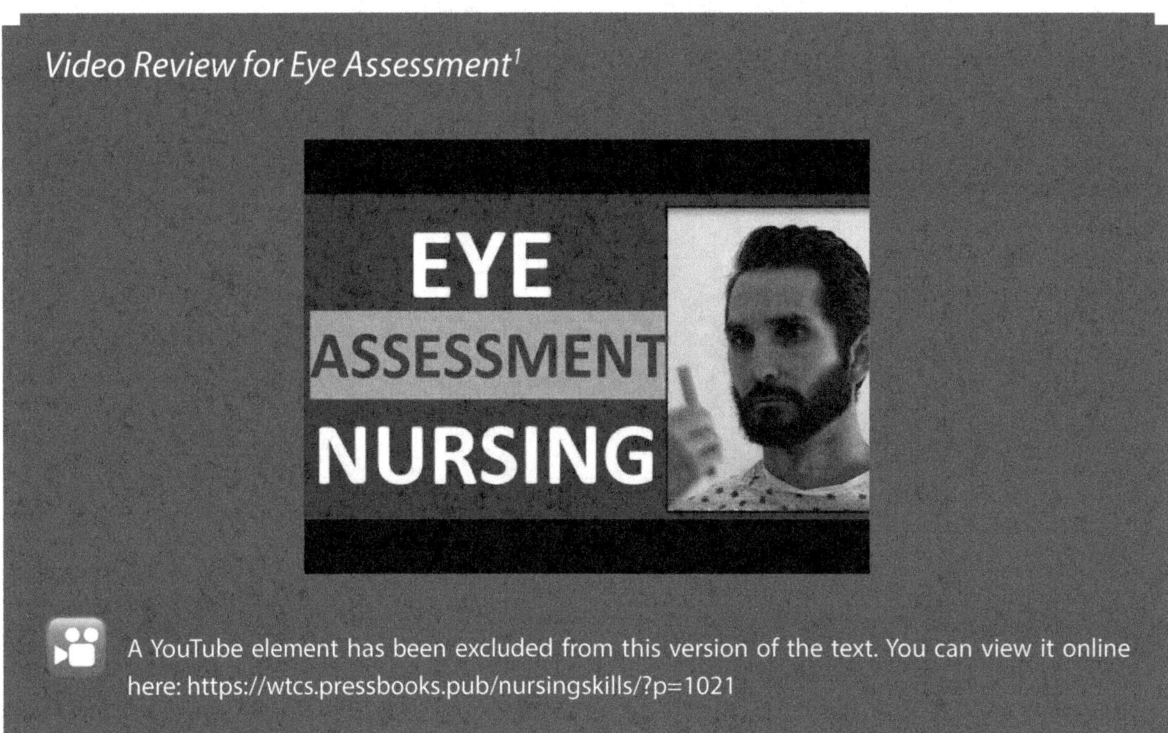

A YouTube element has been excluded from this version of the text. You can view it online here: https://wtcs.pressbooks.pub/nursingskills/?p=1021

---

1 RegisteredNurseRN. (2017, November 16). *Eye assessment nursing | How to assess eyes for head-to-toe assessment.* [Video]. YouTube. All rights reserved. Video used with permission. https://youtu.be/pgSj3l9iV6k

8.7 LEARNING ACTIVITIES

My Notes

Learning Activities

(Answers to "Learning Activities" can be found in the '"Answer Key" at the end of the book. Answers to interactive activity elements will be provided within the element as immediate feedback.)

When conducting the general survey and patient health history, a nurse can look for many assessment cues that may indicate that the patient has hearing difficulty. Describe three different cues that the nurse might identify to reflect an auditory challenge.

Interactive Activity

An interactive or media element has been excluded from this version of the text. You can view it online here: https://wtcs.pressbooks.pub/nursingskills/?p=1024

Interactive Activity

An interactive or media element has been excluded from this version of the text. You can view it online here: https://wtcs.pressbooks.pub/nursingskills/?p=1024

Interactive Activity

An interactive or media element has been excluded from this version of the text. You can view it online here: https://wtcs.pressbooks.pub/nursingskills/?p=1024

My Notes

VIII GLOSSARY

Acute otitis media: The medical diagnosis for a middle ear infection.

Auricle: The large, fleshy structure of the ear on the lateral aspect of the head.

Cerumen impaction: A buildup of earwax causing occlusion of the ear canal.

Conductive hearing loss: Hearing loss that occurs when something in the external or middle ear is obstructing the transmission of sound.

Conjunctiva: Inner surface of the eyelid.

Conjunctivitis: A viral or bacterial infection in the eye causing swelling and redness in the conjunctiva and sclera.

Cornea: The transparent front part of the eye that covers the iris, pupil, and anterior chamber.

Eustachian tube: The tube connecting the middle ear to the pharynx that helps equilibrate air pressure across the tympanic membrane.

Extraocular muscles: Six muscles that control the movement of the eye within the orbit. Extraocular muscles are innervated by three cranial nerves, the abducens nerve, the trochlear nerve, and the oculomotor nerve.

Iris: Colored part of the eye.

Lacrimal duct: Tears produced by the lacrimal gland flow through this duct to the medial corner of the eye.

Lens: An inner part of the eye that helps the eye focus.

Myopia: Impaired vision, also known as nearsightedness, that makes far-away objects look blurry.

Optic nerve: Cranial nerve II that conducts visual information from the retina to the brain.

Otitis externa: The medical diagnosis for external ear inflammation and/or infection.

Ototoxic medications: Medications that cause the adverse effect of sensorineural hearing loss by affecting the hair cells in the cochlea.

Presbycusis: Sensorineural hearing loss that occurs with aging due to gradual nerve degeneration.

Presbyopia: Impaired near vision that commonly occurs in middle-aged and older adults.

Pupil: The hole at the center of the eye that allows light to enter.

Retina: The nervous tissue and photoreceptors in the eye that initially process visual stimuli.

Sclera: White area of the eye.

Sensorineural hearing loss: Hearing loss caused by pathology of the inner ear, cranial nerve VIII, or auditory areas of the cerebral cortex.

Snellen chart: A chart used to test far vision.

Tinnitus: Ringing, buzzing, roaring, hissing, or whistling sound in the ears.

Tympanic membrane: The membrane at the end of the external ear canal, commonly called the eardrum, that vibrates after it is struck by sound waves.

Vertigo: A type of dizziness often described by patients as "the room feels as if it is spinning."

Vestibulocochlear nerve: Cranial nerve VIII that transports neural signals from the cochlea and the vestibule to the brain stem regarding hearing and balance.

Chapter 9

Cardiovascular Assessment

9.1 CARDIOVASCULAR ASSESSMENT INTRODUCTION

My Notes

Learning Objectives

- Perform a cardiovascular assessment, including heart sounds; apical and peripheral pulses for rate, rhythm, and amplitude; and skin perfusion (color, temperature, sensation, and capillary refill time)
- Identify S1 and S2 heart sounds
- Differentiate between normal and abnormal heart sounds
- Modify assessment techniques to reflect variations across the life span
- Document actions and observations
- Recognize and report significant deviations from norms

The evaluation of the cardiovascular system includes a thorough medical history and a detailed examination of the heart and peripheral vascular system.[1] Nurses must incorporate subjective statements and objective findings to elicit clues of potential signs of dysfunction. Symptoms like fatigue, indigestion, and leg swelling may be benign or may indicate something more ominous. As a result, nurses must be vigilant when collecting comprehensive information to utilize their best clinical judgment when providing care for the patient.

1 Felner, J. M. (1990). An overview of the cardiovascular system. In Walker, H. K., Hall, W. D., & Hurst, J. W. (Eds.), *Clinical methods: The history, physical, and laboratory examinations* (3rd ed., Chapter 7). Butterworths. https://www.ncbi.nlm.nih.gov/books/NBK393/

My Notes

9.2 CARDIOVASCULAR BASIC CONCEPTS

While the cardiovascular assessment most often focuses on the function of the heart, it is important for nurses to have an understanding of the underlying structures of the cardiovascular system to best understand the meaning of their assessment findings.

For more information on the cardiovascular system, visit the "Cardiovascular and Renal System" chapter in Open RN *Nursing Pharmacology*.

Specific sections include the following topics:

- "Review of Basic Concepts" for more about that anatomy and physiology of the cardiovascular system
- "Common Cardiac Disorders" for more about cardiovascular medical conditions
- "Cardiovascular Medication Classes" for more about medications used to treat common cardiovascular conditions

Video Review of Anatomy and Physiology of the Heart[1]

A YouTube element has been excluded from this version of the text. You can view it online here: https://wtcs.pressbooks.pub/nursingskills/?p=67

1 Forciea, B. (2015, May 20). *Anatomy of the heart (v2.0).* [Video]. YouTube. All rights reserved. Video used with permission. https://youtu.be/d8RSvcc8koo

9.3 CARDIOVASCULAR ASSESSMENT

My Notes

A thorough assessment of the heart provides valuable information about the function of a patient's cardiovascular system. Understanding how to properly assess the cardiovascular system and identifying both normal and abnormal assessment findings will allow the nurse to provide quality, safe care to the patient.

Before assessing a patient's cardiovascular system, it is important to understand the various functions of the cardiovascular system. In addition to the information provided in the "Review of Cardiac Basics" section, the following images provide an overview of the cardiovascular system. Figure 9.1[1] provides an overview of the structure of the heart. Note the main cardiac structures are the atria, ventricles, and heart valves. Figure 9.2[2] demonstrates blood flow through the heart. Notice the flow of deoxygenated blood from the posterior and superior vena cava into the right atria and ventricle during diastole (indicated by blue coloring of these structures). The right ventricle then pumps deoxygenated blood to the lungs via the pulmonary artery during systole. At the same time, oxygenated blood from the lungs returns to the left atria and ventricle via the pulmonary veins during diastole (indicated by red coloring of these structures) and then is pumped out to the body via the aorta during systole. Figure 9.3[3] demonstrates the conduction system of the heart. This image depicts the conduction pathway through the heart as the tissue responds to electrical stimulation. Figure 9.4[4] illustrates the arteries of the circulatory system, and Figure 9.5[5] depicts the veins of the circulatory system. The purpose of these figures is to facilitate understanding of the electrical and mechanical function of the heart within the cardiovascular system.

---

1 "Diagram of the human heart" by Wapcaplet is licensed under CC BY-SA 3.0. Access for free at https://commons.wikimedia.org/wiki/File:Diagram_of_the_human_heart_(cropped).svg

2 "Diagram of the human heart" by Wapcaplet is licensed under CC BY-SA 3.0. Access for free at https://commons.wikimedia.org/wiki/File:Diagram_of_the_human_heart_(cropped).svg

3 "2018 Conduction System of Heart.jpg" by OpenStax is licensed under *CC-BY-3.0*. Access for free at https://commons.wikimedia.org/wiki/File:2018_Conduction_System_of_Heart.jpg

4 "Arterial System en.svg" by LadyofHats, Mariana Ruiz Villarreal is in the Public Domain. Access for free at https://commons.wikimedia.org/wiki/File:Arterial_System_en.svg

5 "Venous system en.svg" by Lady of Hats Mariana Ruiz Vilarreal is in the Public Domain. Access for free at https://commons.wikimedia.org/wiki/File:Venous_system_en.svg

My Notes

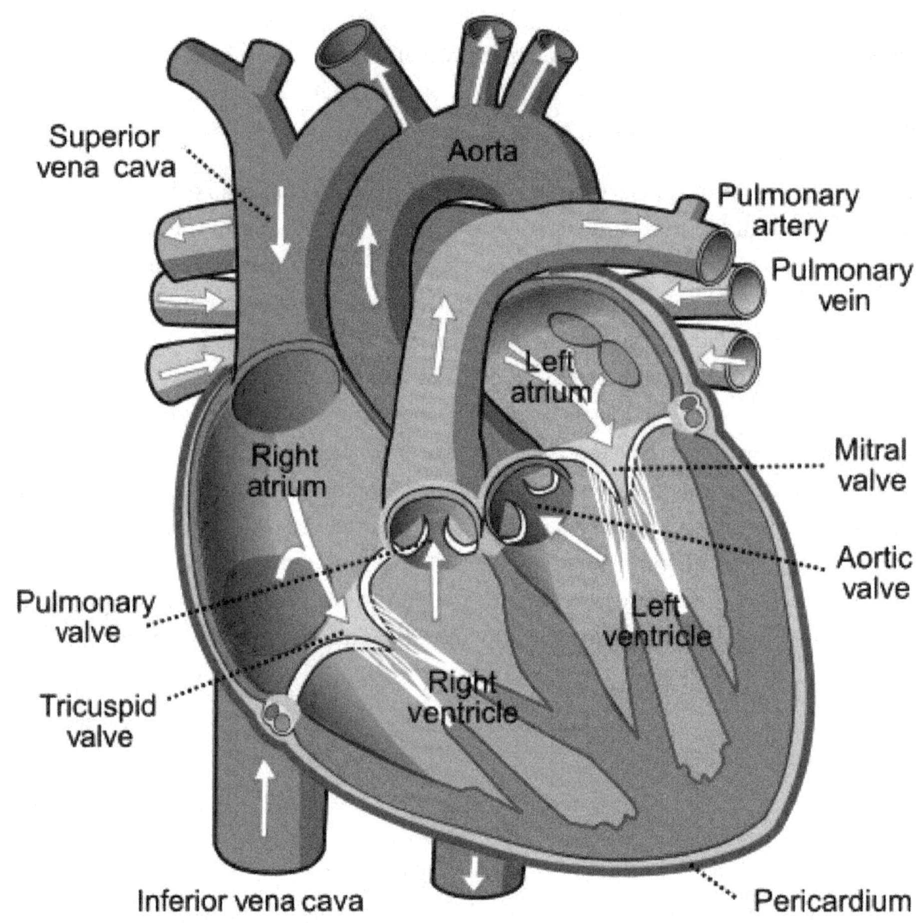

Figure 9.1 Structure of the Heart

My Notes

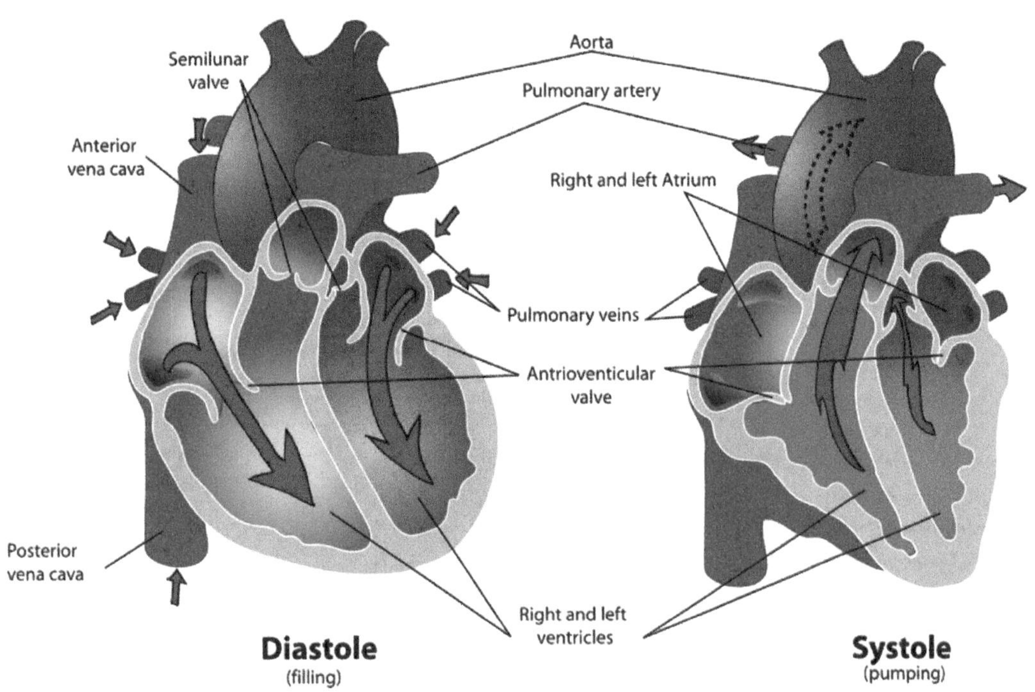

Figure 9.2 Blood Flow Through the Heart

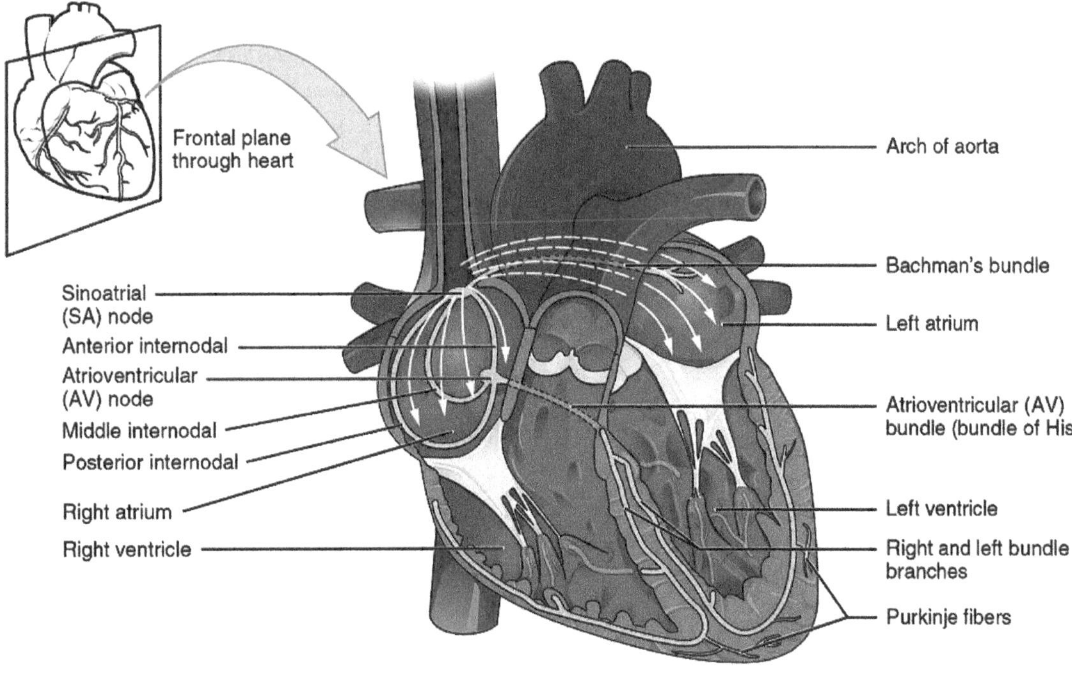

Figure 9.3 Conduction System of the Heart

My Notes

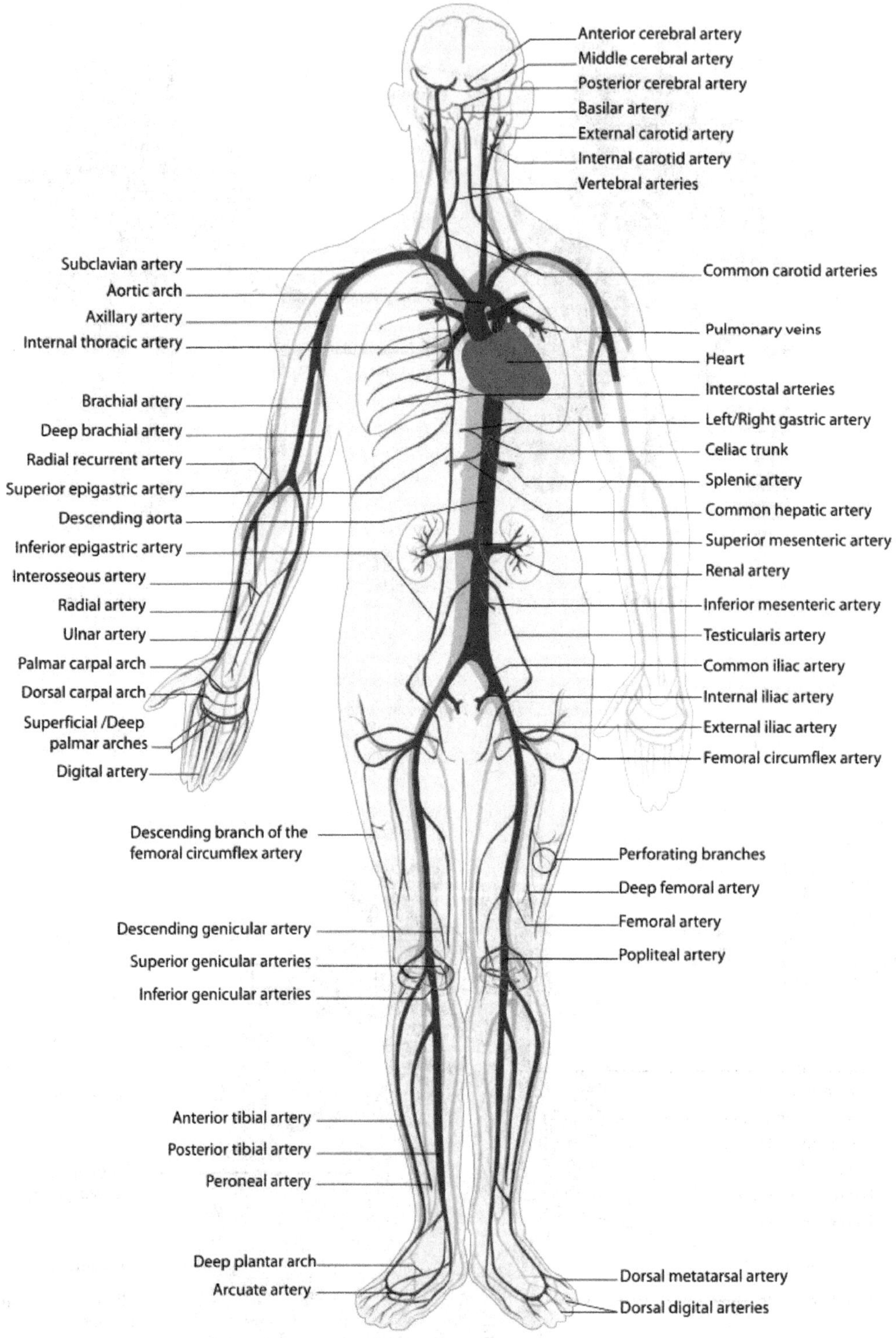

Anterior cerebral artery
Middle cerebral artery
Posterior cerebral artery
Basilar artery
External carotid artery
Internal carotid artery
Vertebral arteries
Subclavian artery
Aortic arch
Axillary artery
Internal thoracic artery
Brachial artery
Deep brachial artery
Radial recurrent artery
Superior epigastric artery
Descending aorta
Inferior epigastric artery
Interosseous artery
Radial artery
Ulnar artery
Palmar carpal arch
Dorsal carpal arch
Superficial /Deep palmar arches
Digital artery
Common carotid arteries
Pulmonary veins
Heart
Intercostal arteries
Left/Right gastric artery
Celiac trunk
Splenic artery
Common hepatic artery
Superior mesenteric artery
Renal artery
Inferior mesenteric artery
Testicularis artery
Common iliac artery
Internal iliac artery
External iliac artery
Femoral circumflex artery
Descending branch of the femoral circumflex artery
Descending genicular artery
Superior genicular arteries
Inferior genicular arteries
Anterior tibial artery
Posterior tibial artery
Peroneal artery
Deep plantar arch
Arcuate artery
Perforating branches
Deep femoral artery
Femoral artery
Popliteal artery
Dorsal metatarsal artery
Dorsal digital arteries

Figure 9.4 Circulatory System: Arteries

My Notes

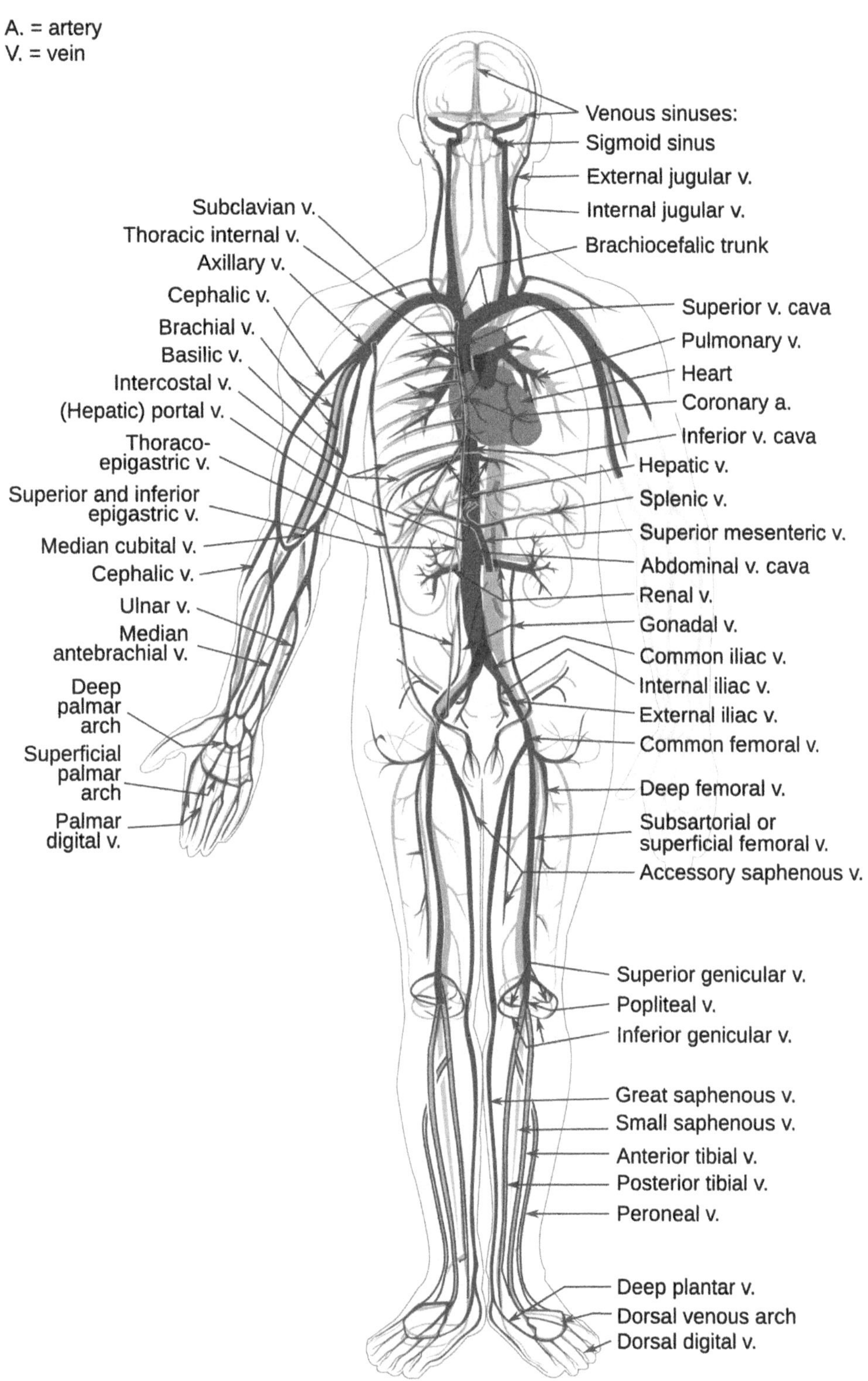
A. = artery
V. = vein
Venous sinuses:
Sigmoid sinus
External jugular v.
Internal jugular v.
Brachiocefalic trunk
Superior v. cava
Pulmonary v.
Heart
Coronary a.
Inferior v. cava
Hepatic v.
Splenic v.
Superior mesenteric v.
Abdominal v. cava
Renal v.
Gonadal v.
Common iliac v.
Internal iliac v.
External iliac v.
Common femoral v.
Deep femoral v.
Subsartorial or superficial femoral v.
Accessory saphenous v.
Superior genicular v.
Popliteal v.
Inferior genicular v.
Great saphenous v.
Small saphenous v.
Anterior tibial v.
Posterior tibial v.
Peroneal v.
Deep plantar v.
Dorsal venous arch
Dorsal digital v.
Subclavian v.
Thoracic internal v.
Axillary v.
Cephalic v.
Brachial v.
Basilic v.
Intercostal v.
(Hepatic) portal v.
Thoraco-epigastric v.
Superior and inferior epigastric v.
Median cubital v.
Cephalic v.
Ulnar v.
Median antebrachial v.
Deep palmar arch
Superficial palmar arch
Palmar digital v.

Figure 9.5. Circulatory System: Veins

My Notes

Assessing the cardiovascular system includes performing several subjective and objective assessments. At times, assessment findings are modified according to life span considerations.

Subjective Assessment

The subjective assessment of the cardiovascular and peripheral vascular system is vital for uncovering signs of potential dysfunction. To complete the subjective cardiovascular assessment, the nurse begins with a focused interview. The focused interview explores past medical and family history, medications, cardiac risk factors, and reported symptoms. Symptoms related to the cardiovascular system include chest pain, peripheral edema, unexplained sudden weight gain, shortness of breath (dyspnea), irregular pulse rate or rhythm, dizziness, or poor peripheral circulation. Any new or worsening symptoms should be documented and reported to the health care provider.

Table 9.3a outlines questions used to assess symptoms related to the cardiovascular and peripheral vascular systems. Table 9.3b outlines questions used to assess medical history, medications, and risk factors related to the cardiovascular system. Information obtained from the interview process is used to tailor future patient education by the nurse.[6, 7, 8]

---

6 This work is a derivative of Clinical Procedures for Safer Patient Care by British Columbia Institute of Technology licensed under CC BY 4.0. Access for free at https://opentextbc.ca/clinicalskills/front-matter/introduction-edit-this-version/

7 Felner, J. M. (1990). An overview of the cardiovascular system. In Walker, H. K., Hall, W. D., & Hurst, J. W. (Eds.), *Clinical methods: The history, physical, and laboratory examinations* (3rd ed., Chapter 7). Butterworths. https://www.ncbi.nlm.nih.gov/books/NBK393/

8 Scott, C. & MacInnes, J. D. (2013, September 27). Cardiac patient assessment: putting the patient first. *British Journal of Nursing, 15*(9). https://doi.org/10.12968/bjon.2006.15.9.21091

My Notes

Table 9.3a Interview Questions for Cardiovascular and Peripheral Vascular Systems[9]

Symptom	Question	Follow-Up
		Safety Note: If findings indicate current severe symptoms suggestive of myocardial infarction or another critical condition, suspend the remaining cardiovascular assessment and obtain immediate assistance according to agency policy or call 911.
Chest Pain	Have you had any pain or pressure in your chest, neck, or arm?	Review how to assess a patient's chief complaint using the PQRSTU method in the "Health History" chapter. ■ **Onset** – When did the pain start? ■ **Location** – Where is the pain? ■ **Duration** – When it occurs, how long does the pain last? Is it constant or intermittent? ■ **Characteristics** – Describe what the pain feels like (e.g., sharp, dull, heavy, etc.). ■ **Aggravating/Alleviating Factors** – What brings on the pain? What relieves the pain? ■ **Radiation** – Does the pain radiate anywhere? ■ **Treatment** – What have you used to treat the pain? ■ **Effects** – What effect has the pain had on you? ■ **Severity** – How severe is the pain from 0-10 when it occurs? ■ **Associated Symptoms** – Have you experienced any nausea or sweating with the chest pain?
Shortness of Breath **(Dyspnea)**	Do you ever feel short of breath with activity? Do you ever feel short of breath while sleeping? Do you feel short of breath when lying flat?	What level of activity elicits shortness of breath? How long does it take you to recover? Have you ever woken up from sleeping feeling suddenly short of breath (**paroxysmal nocturnal dyspnea**)? How many pillows do you need to sleep, or do you sleep in a chair (**orthopnea**)? Has this recently changed?
Edema	Have you noticed swelling of your feet or ankles? Have you noticed your rings, shoes, or clothing feel tight at the end of the day? Have you noticed any unexplained, sudden weight gain? Have you noticed any new abdominal fullness?	Has this feeling of swelling or restriction gotten worse? Is there anything that makes the swelling better (e.g., sitting with your feet elevated)? How much weight have you gained? Over what time period have you gained this weight?

9 Scott, C. & MacInnes, J. D. (2013, September 27). Cardiac patient assessment: Putting the patient first. *British Journal of Nursing, 15*(9). https://doi.org/10.12968/bjon.2006.15.9.21091

My Notes

Palpitations	Have you ever noticed your heart feels as if it is racing or "fluttering" in your chest? Have you ever felt as if your heart "skips" a beat?	Are you currently experiencing palpitations? When did palpitations start? Have you previously been treated for palpitations? If so, what treatment did you receive?
Dizziness **(Syncope)**	Do you ever feel light-headed? Do you ever feel dizzy? Have you ever fainted?	Can you describe what happened? Did you have any warning signs? Did this occur with position change?
Poor Peripheral Circulation	Do your hands or feet ever feel cold or look pale or bluish? Do you have pain in your feet or lower legs when exercising?	What, if anything, brings on these symptoms? How much activity is needed to cause this pain? Is there anything, such as rest, that makes the pain better?
Calf Pain	Do you currently have any constant pain in your lower legs?	Can you point to the area of pain with one finger?

Table 9.3b Interview Questions Exploring Cardiovascular Medical History, Medications, and Cardiac Risk Factors

Topic	Questions
Medical History	Have you ever been diagnosed with any heart or circulation conditions, such as high blood pressure, coronary artery disease, peripheral vascular disease, high cholesterol, heart failure, or valve problems? Have you had any procedures done to improve your heart function, such as ablation or stent placement? Have you ever had a heart attack or stroke?
Medications	Do you take any heart-related medications, herbs, or supplements to treat blood pressure, chest pain, high cholesterol, cardiac rhythm, fluid retention, or the prevention of clots?

My Notes

Topic	Questions
Cardiac Risk Factors	Have your parents or siblings been diagnosed with any heart conditions? ■ If yes, who has what conditions? Do you smoke or vape? ■ If yes, how many do you smoke/vape daily? ■ For how many years have you smoked/vaped? If you do not currently smoke, have you smoked in the past? ■ If yes, what did you smoke? ■ For how many years did you smoke? Are you physically active during the week? ■ How many times per week do you exercise and for how many minutes? ■ What type of exercise do you usually do? What does a typical day look like in your diet? ■ How many fruits and vegetables do you normally eat in a day? ■ Do you monitor the amount of saturated fats you eat? ■ How many times a week do you eat a meal prepared by a restaurant? ■ Do you pay attention to salt in your diet? Do you add salt to your foods before tasting it? ■ Do you have caffeine during the day? If so, how much? Do you drink alcoholic drinks? ■ How many alcoholic drinks do you have on average per day? Per week? ■ Do you drink while at work? Would you say you experience stress in your life? ■ How would you rate the amount of stress in your life from 0-10? ■ How do you cope with the stress in your life? How many hours of sleep do you normally get each day? ■ Do you have difficulty falling asleep? ■ Do you have difficulty staying asleep?

Objective Assessment

The physical examination of the cardiovascular system involves the interpretation of vital signs, inspection, palpation, and auscultation of heart sounds as the nurse evaluates for sufficient perfusion and cardiac output.

For more information about assessing a patient's oxygenation status as it relates to their cardiac output, visit the "Oxygenation" chapter in Open RN *Nursing Fundamentals*.

My Notes

Equipment needed for a cardiovascular assessment includes a stethoscope, penlight, centimeter ruler or tape measure, and **sphygmomanometer.**[10]

Evaluate Vital Signs and Level of Consciousness

Interpret the blood pressure and pulse readings to verify the patient is stable before proceeding with the physical exam. Assess the level of consciousness; the patient should be alert and cooperative.

> **As a general rule of thumb, findings of systolic blood pressure in adults less than 100, or a pulse rate less than 60 or greater than 100, require immediate follow-up. For more information on obtaining and interpreting vital signs, see the "General Survey" chapter. Keep in mind that excessive drowsiness, restlessness, or irritability can be symptoms of hypoxia.**

Inspection

- **Skin color to assess perfusion.** Inspect the face, lips, and fingertips for **cyanosis** or pallor. Cyanosis is a bluish discoloration of the skin, lips, and nail beds and indicates decreased perfusion and oxygenation. **Pallor** is the loss of color, or paleness of the skin or mucous membranes, as a result of reduced blood flow, oxygenation, or decreased number of red blood cells. Patients with light skin tones should be pink in color. For those with darker skin tones, assess for pallor on the palms, conjunctiva, or inner aspect of the lower lip.
- **Jugular Vein Distension (JVD).** Inspect the neck for JVD that occurs when the increased pressure of the superior vena cava causes the jugular vein to bulge, making it most visible on the right side of a person's neck. JVD should not be present in the upright position or when the head of bed is at 30-45 degrees.
- **Precordium for abnormalities.** Inspect the chest area over the heart (also called **precordium**) for deformities, scars, or any abnormal pulsations the underlying cardiac chambers and great vessels may produce.
- **Extremities:**
  - **Upper Extremities:** Inspect the fingers, arms, and hands bilaterally noting Color, Warmth, Movement, Sensation (CWMS). Alterations or bilateral inconsistency in CWMS may indicate underlying conditions or injury. Assess capillary refill by compressing the nail bed until it blanches and record the time taken for the color to return to the nail bed. Normal capillary refill is less than 3 seconds.[11]
  - **Lower Extremities:** Inspect the toes, feet, and legs bilaterally, noting CWMS, capillary refill, and the presence of peripheral edema, superficial distended veins, and hair distribution. Document the location and size of any skin ulcers.

---

10 Felner, J. M. (1990). An overview of the cardiovascular system. In Walker, H. K., Hall, W. D., & Hurst, J. W. (Eds.), *Clinical methods: The history, physical, and laboratory examinations* (3rd ed., Chapter 7). Butterworths. https://www.ncbi.nlm.nih.gov/books/NBK393/

11 This work is a derivative of Clinical Procedures for Safer Patient Care by British Columbia Institute of Technology licensed under CC BY 4.0. Access for free at https://opentextbc.ca/clinicalskills/front-matter/introduction-edit-this-version/

My Notes

- **Edema:** Note any presence of edema. **Peripheral edema** is swelling that can be caused by infection, thrombosis, or venous insufficiency due to an accumulation of fluid in the tissues. (See Figure 9.6[12] for an image of pedal edema.)[13]
- **Deep Vein Thrombosis (DVT):** A deep vein thrombosis (DVT) is a blood clot that forms in a vein deep in the body. DVT requires emergency notification of the health care provider and immediate follow-up because of the risk of developing a life-threatening **pulmonary embolism**.[14] Inspect the lower extremities bilaterally. Assess for size, color, temperature, and for presence of pain in the calves. Unilateral warmth, redness, tenderness, swelling in the calf, or sudden onset of intense, sharp muscle pain that increases with dorsiflexion of the foot is an indication of a deep vein thrombosis (DVT).[15] See Figure 9.7[16] for an image of a DVT in the patient's right leg, indicated by unilateral redness and edema.

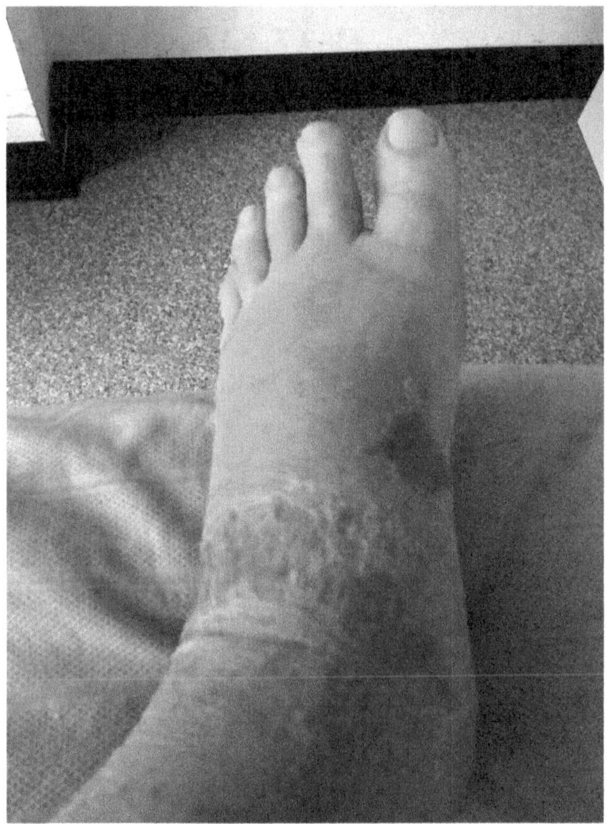

Figure 9.6 Peripheral Edema

---

12 "Swollen feet at Harefield Hospital edema.jpg" by *Ryaninuk* is licensed under CC BY-SA 4.0. Access for free at https://commons.wikimedia.org/wiki/File:Swolen_feet_at_harefield_hospital_edema.jpg

13 Simon, E. C. (2014). Leg edema assessment and management. MEDSURG Nursing, 23(1), 44-53.

14 This work is a derivative of Clinical Procedures for Safer Patient Care by British Columbia Institute of Technology licensed under CC BY 4.0. Access for free at https://opentextbc.ca/clinicalskills/front-matter/introduction-edit-this-version/

15 This work is a derivative of Clinical Procedures for Safer Patient Care by British Columbia Institute of Technology licensed under CC BY 4.0. Access for free at https://opentextbc.ca/clinicalskills/front-matter/introduction-edit-this-version/

16 "Deep vein thrombosis of the right leg.jpg" by *James Heilman, MD* is licensed under CC BY-SA 3.0. Access for free at https://commons.wikimedia.org/wiki/File:Deep_vein_thrombosis_of_the_right_leg.jpg

My Notes

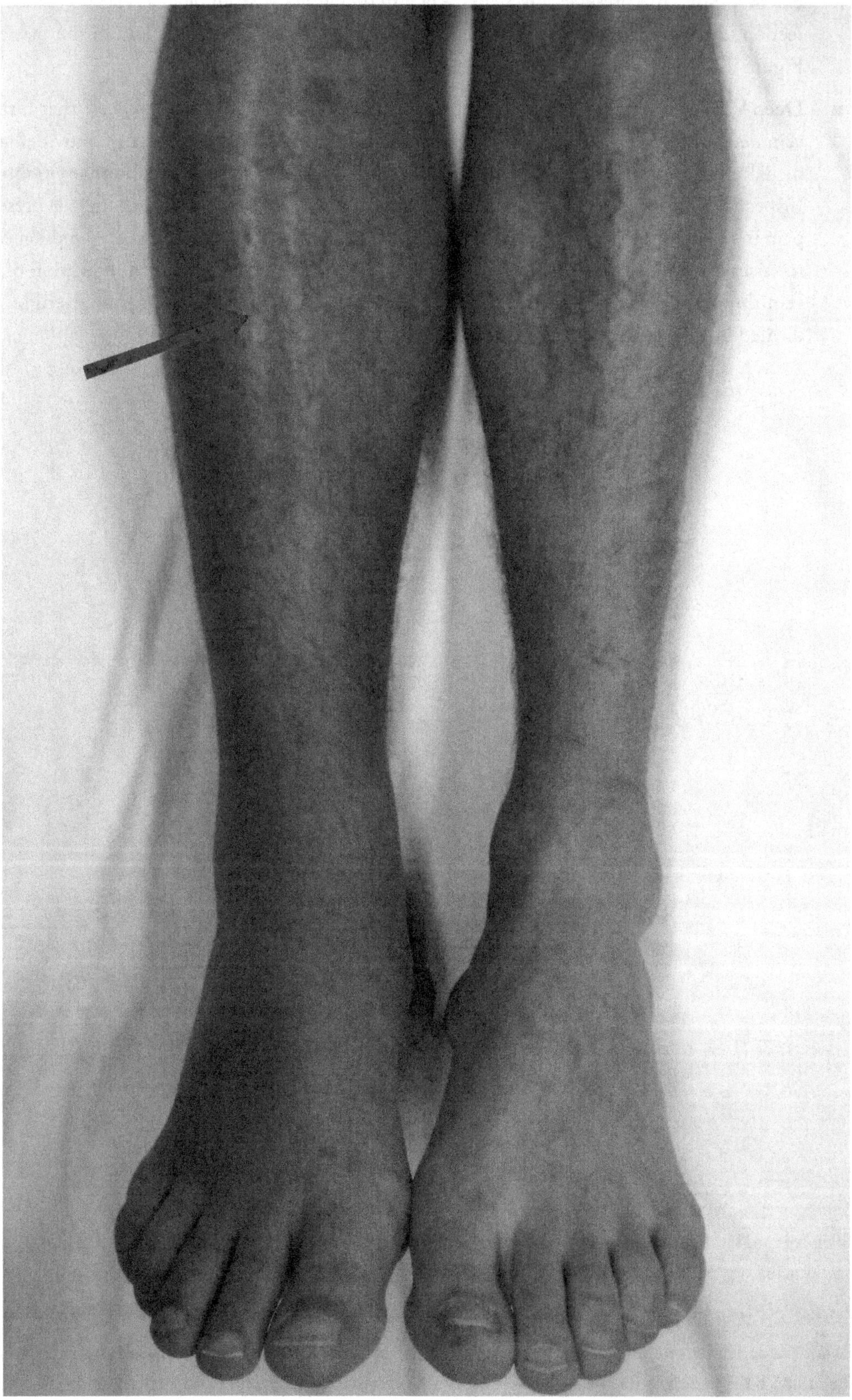

Figure 9.7 Signs of a DVT

Auscultation

My Notes

Heart Sounds

Auscultation is routinely performed over five specific areas of the heart to listen for corresponding valvular sounds. These auscultation sites are often referred to by the mnemonic "APE To Man," referring to Aortic, Pulmonic, Erb's point, Tricuspid, and Mitral areas (see Figure 9.8[17] for an illustration of cardiac auscultation areas). The aortic area is the second intercostal space to the right of the sternum. The pulmonary area is the second intercostal space to the left of the sternum. Erb's point is directly below the aortic area and located at the third intercostal space to the left of the sternum. The tricuspid (or parasternal) area is at the fourth intercostal space to the left of the sternum. The mitral (also called apical or left ventricular area) is the fifth intercostal space at the midclavicular line.

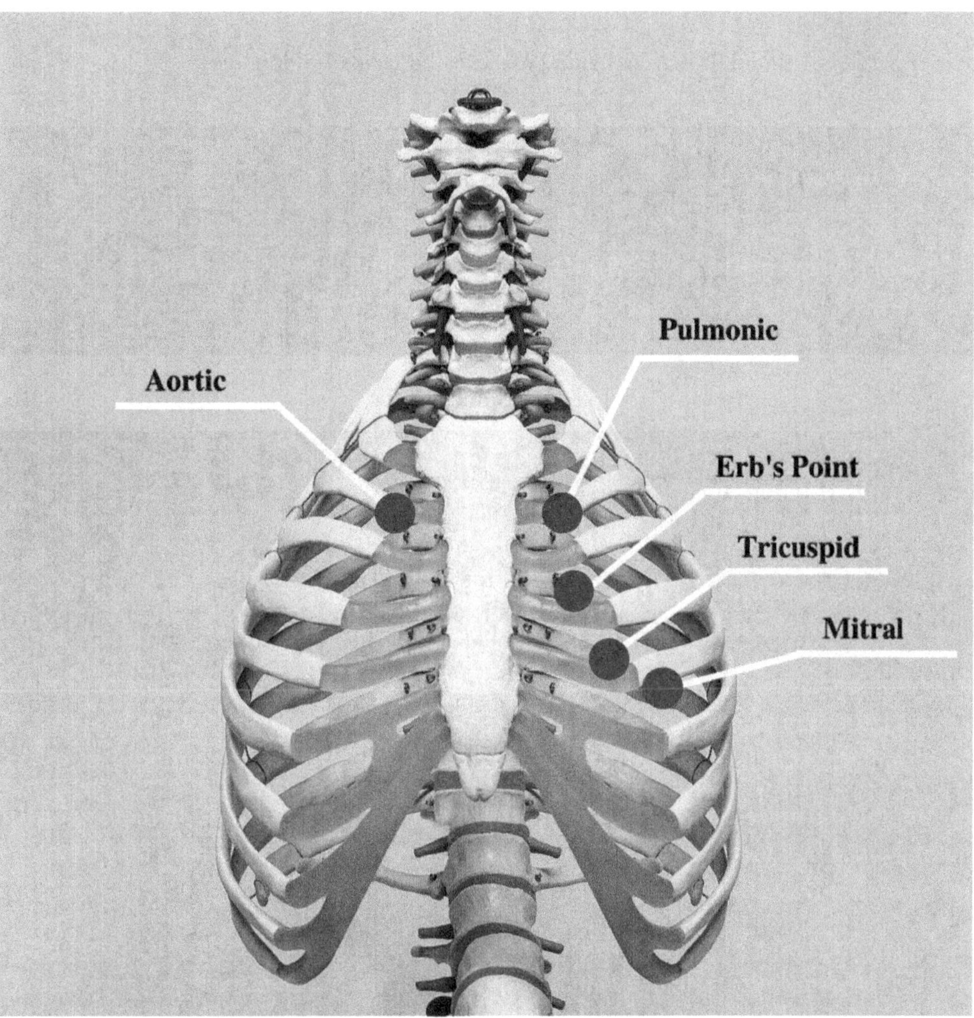

Figure 9.8 Cardiac Auscultation Areas

Auscultation usually begins at the aortic area (upper right sternal edge). Use the diaphragm of the stethoscope to carefully identify the S1 and S2 sounds. They will make a "lub-dub" sound. Note that when listening over the

17 "*Cardiac Auscultation Areas*" by Meredith Pomietlo for Chippewa Valley Technical College is licensed under CC BY 4.0. Access for free at https://drive.google.com/file/d/19LoeIQ9aEy1Rl_SnhPxYg7KlyNJu0WWM/view?usp=sharing

My Notes

area of the aortic and pulmonic valves, the "dub" (S2) will sound louder than the "lub" (S2). Move the stethoscope sequentially to the pulmonic area (upper left sternal edge), Erb's point (left third intercostal space at the sternal border), and tricuspid area (fourth intercostal space). When assessing the mitral area for female patients, it is often helpful to ask them to lift up their breast tissue so the stethoscope can be placed directly on the chest wall. Repeat this process with the bell of the stethoscope. The apical pulse should be counted over a 60-second period. For an adult, the heart rate should be between 60 and 100 with a regular rhythm to be considered within normal range. The apical pulse is an important assessment to obtain before the administration of many cardiac medications.

The first heart sound (S1) identifies the onset of systole, when the atrioventricular (AV) valves (mitral and tricuspid) close and the ventricles contract and eject the blood out of the heart. The second heart sound (S2) identifies the end of systole and the onset of diastole when the semilunar valves close, the AV valves open, and the ventricles fill with blood. When auscultating, it is important to identify the S1 ("lub") and S2 ("dub") sounds, evaluate the rate and rhythm of the heart, and listen for any extra heart sounds.

Listen to a normal S1/S2 sound. It may be helpful to use earbuds or a headphone:

Interactive Activity

An interactive or media element has been excluded from this version of the text. You can view it online here: https://wtcs.pressbooks.pub/nursingskills/?p=71

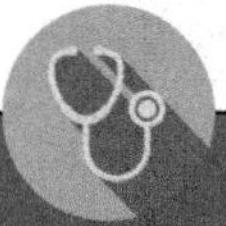

Auscultating Heart Sounds

- To effectively auscultate heart sounds, patient repositioning may be required. Ask the patient to lean forward if able, or position them to lie on their left side.
- It is common to hear lung sounds when auscultating the heart sounds. It may be helpful to ask the patient to briefly hold their breath if lung sounds impede adequate heart auscultation. Limit the holding of breath to 10 seconds or as tolerated by the patient.
- Environmental noise can cause difficulty in auscultating heart sounds. Removing environmental noise by turning down the television volume or shutting the door may be required for an accurate assessment.
- Patients may try to talk to you as you are assessing their heart sounds. It is often helpful to explain the procedure such as, "I am going to take a few minutes to listen carefully to the sounds of blood flow going through your heart. Please try not to speak while I am listening, so I can hear the sounds better."

Extra Heart Sounds

Extra heart sounds include clicks, murmurs, S3 and S4 sounds, and pleural friction rubs. These extra sounds can be difficult for a novice to distinguish, so if you notice any new or different sounds, consult an advanced practitioner

My Notes

or notify the provider. A midsystolic **click**, associated with mitral valve prolapse, may be heard with the diaphragm at the apex or left lower sternal border.

A click may be followed by a murmur. A **murmur** is a blowing or whooshing sound that signifies turbulent blood flow often caused by a valvular defect. New murmurs not previously recorded should be immediately communicated to the health care provider. In the aortic area, listen for possible murmurs of aortic stenosis and aortic regurgitation with the diaphragm of the stethoscope. In the pulmonic area, listen for potential murmurs of pulmonic stenosis and pulmonary and aortic regurgitation. In the tricuspid area, at the fourth and fifth intercostal spaces along the left sternal border, listen for the potential murmurs of tricuspid regurgitation, tricuspid stenosis, or ventricular septal defect.

Listen to a heart murmur caused by mitral valve regurgitation:

Interactive Activity

An interactive or media element has been excluded from this version of the text. You can view it online here: https://wtcs.pressbooks.pub/nursingskills/?p=71

S3 and **S4** sounds, if present, are often heard best by asking the patient to lie on their left side and listening over the apex with the bell of the stethoscope. An S3 sound, also called a **ventricular gallop**, occurs with fluid overload or heart failure when the ventricles are filling. It occurs after the S2 and sounds like "lub-dub-dah," or a sound similar to a horse galloping. The S4 sound, also called **atrial gallop**, occurs immediately before the S1 and sounds like "ta-lub-dub." An S4 sound can occur with decreased ventricular compliance or coronary artery disease.[18]

Listen to a S3 ventricular gallop:

Interactive Activity

An interactive or media element has been excluded from this version of the text. You can view it online here: https://wtcs.pressbooks.pub/nursingskills/?p=71

Listen to a S4 atrial gallop:

Interactive Activity

An interactive or media element has been excluded from this version of the text. You can view it online here: https://wtcs.pressbooks.pub/nursingskills/?p=71

18 Felner, J. M. (1990). An overview of the cardiovascular system. In Walker, H. K., Hall, W. D., & Hurst, J. W. (Eds.), *Clinical methods: The history, physical, and laboratory examinations* (3rd ed., Chapter 7). Butterworths. https://www.ncbi.nlm.nih.gov/books/NBK393/

My Notes

A **pleural friction rub** is caused by inflammation of the pericardium and sounds like sandpaper being rubbed together. It is best heard at the apex or left lower sternal border with the diaphragm as the patient sits up, leans forward, and holds their breath.

Carotid Sounds

The carotid artery may be auscultated for **bruits**. Bruits are a swishing sound due to turbulence in the blood vessel and may be heard due to atherosclerotic changes.

Palpation

Palpation is used to evaluate peripheral pulses, capillary refill, and for the presence of edema. When palpating these areas, also pay attention to the temperature and moisture of the skin.

Pulses

Compare the rate, rhythm, and quality of arterial pulses bilaterally, including the carotid, radial, brachial, posterior tibialis, and dorsalis pedis pulses. Review additional information about obtaining pulses in the "General Survey" chapter. Bilateral comparison for all pulses (except the carotid) is important for determining subtle variations in pulse strength. Carotid pulses should be palpated on one side at a time to avoid decreasing perfusion of the brain. The posterior tibial artery is located just behind the medial malleolus. It can be palpated by scooping the patient's heel in your hand and wrapping your fingers around so that the tips come to rest on the appropriate area just below the medial malleolus. The dorsalis pedis artery is located just lateral to the extensor tendon of the big toe and can be identified by asking the patient to flex their toe while you provide resistance to this movement. Gently place the tips of your second, third, and fourth fingers adjacent to the tendon, and try to feel the pulse.

The quality of the pulse is graded on a scale of 0 to 3, with 0 being absent pulses, 1 being decreased pulses, 2 is within normal range, and 3 being increased (also referred to as "bounding"). If unable to palpate a pulse, additional assessment is needed. First, determine if this is a new or chronic finding. Second, if available, use a Doppler ultrasound to determine the presence or absence of the pulse. Many agencies use Doppler ultrasound to document if a nonpalpable pulse is present. If the pulse is not found, this could be a sign of an emergent condition requiring immediate follow-up and provider notification. See Figures 9.9[19] and 9.10[20] for images of assessing pedal pulses.

19 "DSC_2277.jpg" by British Columbia Institute of Technology is licensed under CC BY 4.0. Access for free at https://opentextbc.ca/clinicalskills/chapter/2-5-focussed-respiratory-assessment/

20 "DSC_2314.jpg" by British Columbia Institute of Technology is licensed under CC BY 4.0. Access for free at https://opentextbc.ca/clinicalskills/chapter/2-5-focussed-respiratory-assessment/

My Notes

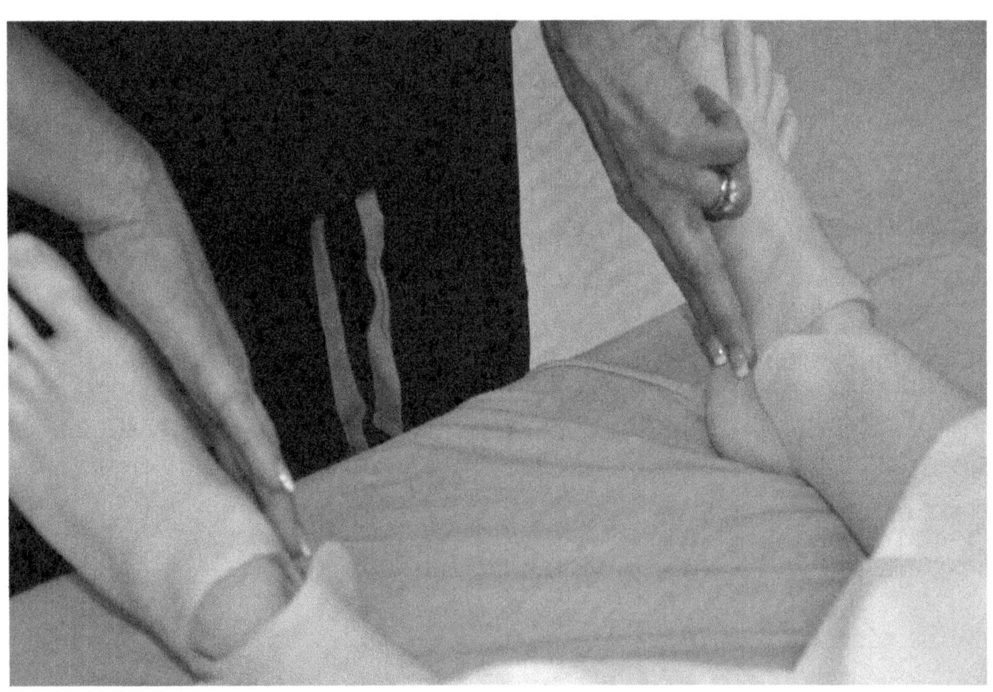

Figure 9.9 Assessing Tibial Pedal Pulses

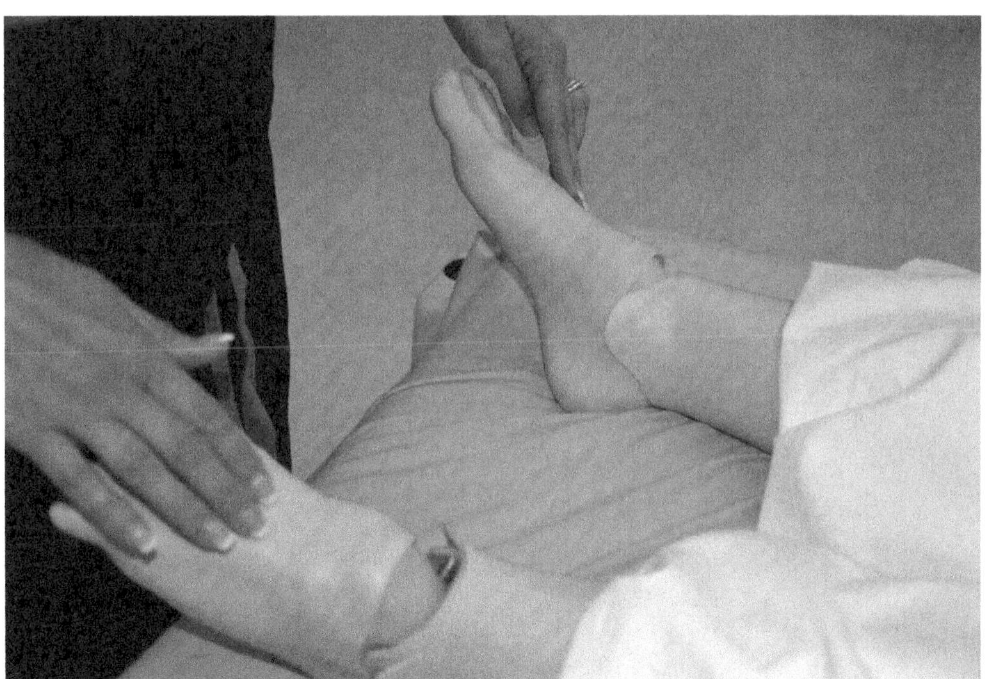

Figure 9.10 Assessing Dorsalis Pedis Pulses

My Notes

Capillary Refill

The **capillary refill** test is performed on the nail beds to monitor **perfusion**, the amount of blood flow to tissue. Pressure is applied to a fingernail or toenail until it pales, indicating that the blood has been forced from the tissue under the nail. This paleness is called **blanching**. Once the tissue has blanched, pressure is removed. Capillary refill time is defined as the time it takes for the color to return after pressure is removed. If there is sufficient blood flow to the area, a pink color should return within 2 to 3 seconds after the pressure is removed.[21]

Edema

Edema occurs when one can visualize visible swelling caused by a buildup of fluid within the tissues. If edema is present on inspection, palpate the area to determine if the edema is pitting or nonpitting. Press on the skin to assess for indentation, ideally over a bony structure, such as the tibia. If no indentation occurs, it is referred to as nonpitting edema. If indentation occurs, it is referred to as **pitting edema**. See Figure 9.11[22] for images demonstrating pitting edema.

---

21 A.D.A.M. Medical Encyclopedia [Internet]. Atlanta (GA): A.D.A.M., Inc.; c1997-2020. Capillary nail refill test; [updated 2020, Aug 9] https://medlineplus.gov/ency/article/003247.htm

22 "Combinpedal.jpg" by James Heilman, MD is licensed under CC BY-SA 3.0. Access for free at https://commons.wikimedia.org/wiki/File:Combinpedal.jpg

My Notes

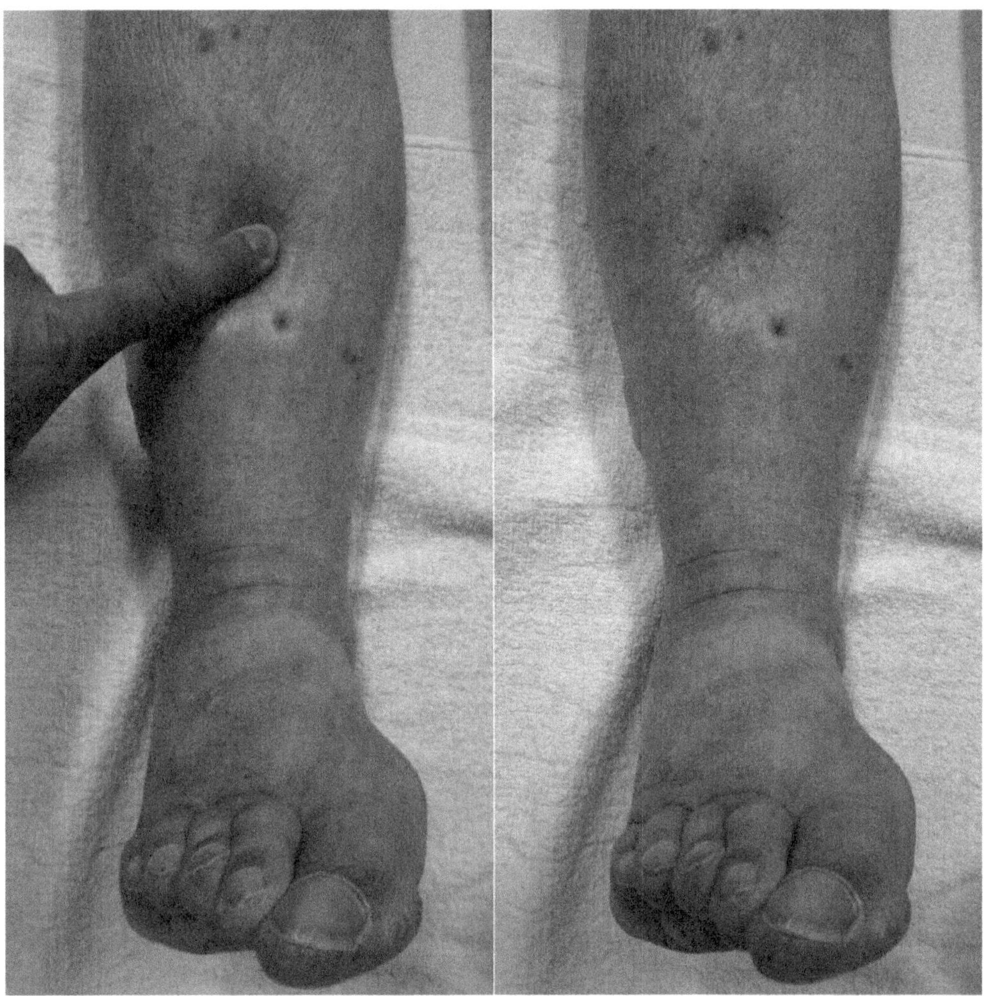

Figure 9.11 Assessing Lower Extremity Edema

Note the depth of the indention and how long it takes for the skin to rebound back to its original position. The indentation and time required to rebound to the original position are graded on a scale from 1 to 4. Edema rated at 1+ indicates a barely detectable depression with immediate rebound, and 4+ indicates a deep depression with a time lapse of over 20 seconds required to rebound. See Figure 9.12[23] for an illustration of grading edema. Additionally, it is helpful to note edema may be difficult to observe in larger patients. It is also important to monitor for sudden changes in weight, which is considered a probable sign of fluid volume overload.

23 "Grading of Edema" by Meredith Pomietlo for Chippewa Valley Technical College is licensed under CC BY 4.0. Access for free at https://drive.google.com/file/d/1dRiBmujU9KGrRgi0QpsgeJkcXL7ASWRT/view?usp=sharing

My Notes

Grade 1	**0–2 mm indentation; rebounds immediately.**
Grade 2	**3–4 mm indentation; rebounds in < 15 seconds.**
Grade 3	**5–6 mm indentation; up to 30 seconds to rebound.**
Grade 4	**8 mm indentation; > 20 seconds to rebound.**

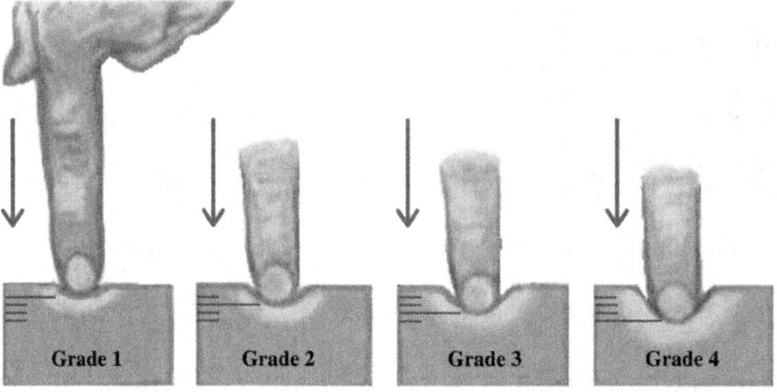

Figure 9.12 Grading of Edema

Heaves or Thrills

You may observe advanced practice nurses and other health care providers palpating the anterior chest wall to detect any abnormal pulsations the underlying cardiac chambers and great vessels may produce. Precordial movements should be evaluated at the apex (mitral area). It is best to examine the precordium with the patient supine because if the patient is turned on the left side, the apical region of the heart is displaced against the lateral chest wall, distorting the chest movements.[24] A **heave or lift** is a palpable lifting sensation under the sternum and anterior chest wall to the left of the sternum that suggests severe right ventricular hypertrophy. A **thrill** is a vibration felt on the skin of the precordium or over an area of turbulence, such as an arteriovenous fistula or graft.

Life Span Considerations

The cardiovascular assessment and expected findings should be modified according to common variations across the life span.

Infants and Children

A murmur may be heard in a newborn in the first few days of life until the **ductus arteriosus** closes.

24 Felner, J. M. (1990). An overview of the cardiovascular system. In Walker, H. K., Hall, W. D., & Hurst, J. W. (Eds.), *Clinical methods: The history, physical, and laboratory examinations* (3rd ed., Chapter 7). Butterworths. https://www.ncbi.nlm.nih.gov/books/NBK393/

My Notes

When assessing the cardiovascular system in children, it is important to assess the apical pulse. Parameters for expected findings vary according to age group. After a child reaches adolescence, a radial pulse may be assessed. Table 9.3c outlines the expected apical pulse rate by age.

Table 9.3c Expected Apical Pulse by Age

Age Group	Heart Rate
Preterm	120-180
Newborn (0 to 1 month)	100-160
Infant (1 to 12 months)	80-140
Toddler (1 to 3 years)	80-130
Preschool (3 to 5 years)	80-110
School Age (6 to 12 years)	70-100
Adolescents (13 to 18 years)	60-90

Listen to pediatric heart tones:

Interactive Activity

An interactive or media element has been excluded from this version of the text. You can view it online here: https://wtcs.pressbooks.pub/nursingskills/?p=71

Older Adults

In adults over age 65, irregular heart rhythms and extra sounds are more likely. An "irregularly irregular" rhythm suggests **atrial fibrillation**, and further investigation is required if this is a new finding.

Listen to atrial fibrillation:

Interactive Activity

An interactive or media element has been excluded from this version of the text. You can view it online here: https://wtcs.pressbooks.pub/nursingskills/?p=71

My Notes

For more information on atrial fibrillation, visit https://www.cdc.gov/heartdisease/atrial_fibrillation.htm

Expected Versus Unexpected Findings

After completing a cardiovascular assessment, it is important for the nurse to use critical thinking to determine if any findings require follow-up.

Depending on the urgency of the findings, follow-up can range from calling the health care provider to calling the rapid response team. Table 9.3d compares examples of expected findings, meaning those considered within normal limits, to unexpected findings, which require follow-up. Critical conditions are those that should be reported immediately and may require notification of a rapid response team.

Table 9.3d Expected Versus Unexpected Findings on Cardiac Assessment

Assessment	Expected Findings	Unexpected Findings (Document and notify the provider if this is a new finding*)
Inspection	Apical impulse may or may not be visible	Scars not previously documented that could indicate prior cardiac surgeries Heave or lift observed in the precordium Chest anatomy malformations
Palpation	Apical pulse felt over midclavicular fifth intercostal space	Apical pulse felt to the left of the midclavicular fifth intercostal space Additional movements over precordium such as a heave, lift, or thrill
Auscultation	S1 and S2 heart sounds in a regular rhythm	New irregular heart rhythm Extra heart sounds such as a murmur, S3, or S4
***CRITICAL CONDITIONS to report immediately**		Symptomatic tachycardia at rest (HR>100 bpm) Symptomatic bradycardia (HR<60 bpm) New systolic blood pressure (<100 mmHg) Orthostatic blood pressure changes (see "Blood Pressure" chapter for more information) New irregular heart rhythm New extra heart sounds such as a murmur, S3, or S4 New abnormal cardiac rhythm changes Reported chest pain, calf pain, or worsening shortness of breath

See Table 9.3e for a comparison of expected versus unexpected findings when assessing the peripheral vascular system.

My Notes

Table 9.3e Expected Versus Unexpected Peripheral Vascular Assessment Findings		
Assessment	**Expected Findings**	**Unexpected Findings (Document or notify provider if new finding*)**
Inspection	Skin color uniform and appropriate for race bilaterally Equal hair distribution on upper and lower extremities Absence of jugular vein distention (JVD) Absence of edema Sensation and movement of fingers and toes intact	Cyanosis or pallor, indicating decreased perfusion Decreased or unequal hair distribution Presence of jugular vein distention (JVD) in an upright position or when head of bed is 30-45 degrees New or worsening edema Rapid and unexplained weight gain Impaired movement or sensation of fingers and toes
Palpation	Skin warm and dry Pulses present and equal bilaterally Absence of edema Capillary refill less than 2 seconds	Skin cool, excessively warm, or diaphoretic Absent, weak/thready, or bounding pulses New irregular pulse New or worsening edema Capillary refill greater than 2 seconds Unilateral warmth, redness, tenderness, or edema, indicating possible deep vein thrombosis (DVT)
Auscultation	Carotid pulse	Carotid bruit
***CRITICAL CONDITIONS to report immediately**		Cyanosis Absent pulse (and not heard using Doppler device) Capillary refill time greater than 3 seconds Unilateral redness, warmth, and edema, indicating a possible deep vein thrombosis (DVT)

Interactive Activity

An interactive or media element has been excluded from this version of the text. You can view it online here: https://wtcs.pressbooks.pub/nursingskills/?p=71

Interactive Activity

An interactive or media element has been excluded from this version of the text. You can view it online here: https://wtcs.pressbooks.pub/nursingskills/?p=71

My Notes

9.4 SAMPLE DOCUMENTATION

Sample Documentation of Expected Cardiac & Peripheral Vascular Findings

Patient denies chest pain or shortness of breath. Vital signs are within normal limits. Point of maximum impulse palpable at the fifth intercostal space of the midclavicular line. No lifts, heaves, or thrills identified on inspection or palpation. JVD absent. S1 and S2 heart sounds in regular rhythm with no murmurs or extra sounds. Skin is warm, pink, and dry. Capillary refill is less than two seconds. Color, movement, and sensation are intact in upper and lower extremities. Peripheral pulses are present (+2) and equal bilaterally. No peripheral edema is noted. Hair is distributed evenly on lower extremities.

Sample Documentation of Unexpected Cardiac & Peripheral Vascular Findings

Patient reports increase in breathing difficulty and increased swelling of bilateral lower extremities over the last three days. Diminished pulses (+1) bilaterally and pitting edema (+2) in the bilateral lower extremities. Upon auscultation, an S3 heart sound is noted and the patient has bilateral crackles in the posterior bases of the lungs. Skin is pink, warm, and dry with capillary refill of < 2 seconds. All other pulses are present (+2), and no other areas of edema are noted. JVD is absent.

9.5 CHECKLIST FOR CARDIOVASCULAR ASSESSMENT

My Notes

Use the checklist below to review the steps for completion of a "Cardiovascular Assessment."[1]

Steps

Disclaimer: Always review and follow agency policy regarding this specific skill.

1. Gather supplies: stethoscope and watch with a second hand.
2. Perform safety steps:
    - Perform hand hygiene.
    - Check the room for transmission-based precautions.
    - Introduce yourself, your role, the purpose of your visit, and an estimate of the time it will take.
    - Confirm patient ID using two patient identifiers (e.g., name and date of birth).
    - Explain the process to the patient and ask if they have any questions.
    - Be organized and systematic.
    - Use appropriate listening and questioning skills.
    - Listen and attend to patient cues.
    - Ensure the patient's privacy and dignity.
    - Assess ABCs.
3. Conduct a focused interview related to cardiovascular and peripheral vascular disease.
    - Ask relevant focused questions based on patient status. See Tables 9.3a and 9.3b for example questions.
4. Inspect:
    - Face, lips, and extremities for pallor or cyanosis
    - Neck for jugular vein distension (JVD) in upright position or with head of bed at 30-45 degree angle
    - Chest for deformities and wounds/scars on chest
    - Bilateral arms/hands, noting color, warmth, movement, sensation (CWMS), edema, and color of nail beds
    - Bilateral legs, noting CWMS, edema to lower legs and feet, presence of superficial distended veins, and color of nail beds
5. Auscultate with both the bell and the diaphragm of the stethoscope over five auscultation areas of the heart. Auscultate the apical pulse at the fifth intercostal space, midclavicular line for one minute. Note the rate and

1 This work is a derivative of Clinical Procedures for Safer Patient Care by British Columbia Institute of Technology licensed under CC BY 4.0. Access for free at https://opentextbc.ca/clinicalskills/front-matter/introduction-edit-this-version/

My Notes

rhythm. Identify the S1 and S2 sounds and follow up on any unexpected findings (e.g., extra sounds or irregular rhythm).

6. Palpate the radial, brachial, dorsalis pedis, and posterior tibialis pulses bilaterally. Palpate the carotid pulse one side at a time. Note presence/amplitude of pulse and any unexpected findings requiring follow-up.
7. Palpate the nail beds for capillary refill. Document the capillary refill time as less than or greater than 2 seconds.
8. Assist the patient to a comfortable position, ask if they have any questions, and thank them for their time.
9. Ensure safety measures when leaving the room:
    - CALL LIGHT: Within reach
    - BED: Low and locked (in lowest position and brakes on)
    - SIDE RAILS: Secured
    - TABLE: Within reach
    - ROOM: Risk-free for falls (scan room and clear any obstacles)
10. Perform hand hygiene.
11. Document the assessment findings. Report any concerns according to agency policy.

9.6 SUPPLEMENTARY VIDEOS ON CARDIOVASCULAR ASSESSMENT

My Notes

Video Reviews for Assessing the Heart and Lungs and the Apical Pulse

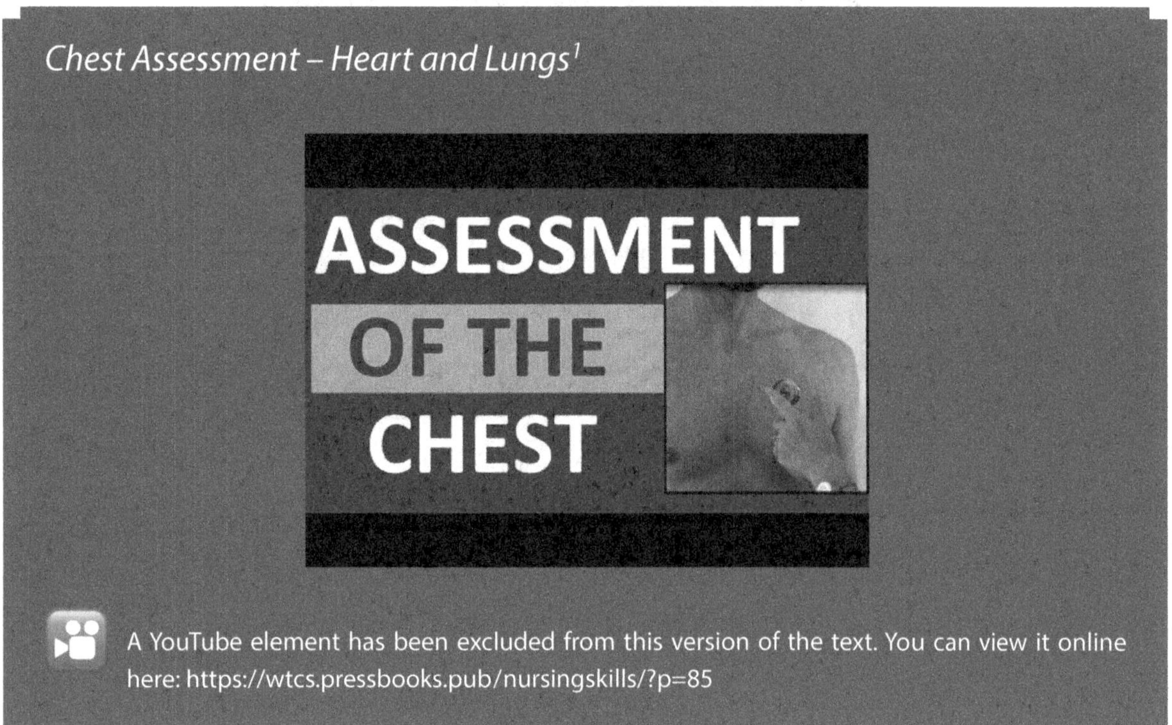

Chest Assessment – Heart and Lungs[1]

A YouTube element has been excluded from this version of the text. You can view it online here: https://wtcs.pressbooks.pub/nursingskills/?p=85

1 RegisteredNurseRN. (2017, December 13). *Chest assessment nursing | Heart & lung assessment | Head-to-toe exam.* [Video]. YouTube. All rights reserved. https://youtu.be/*kv3B81mWc1E*

My Notes

Assessing the Apical Pulse[2]

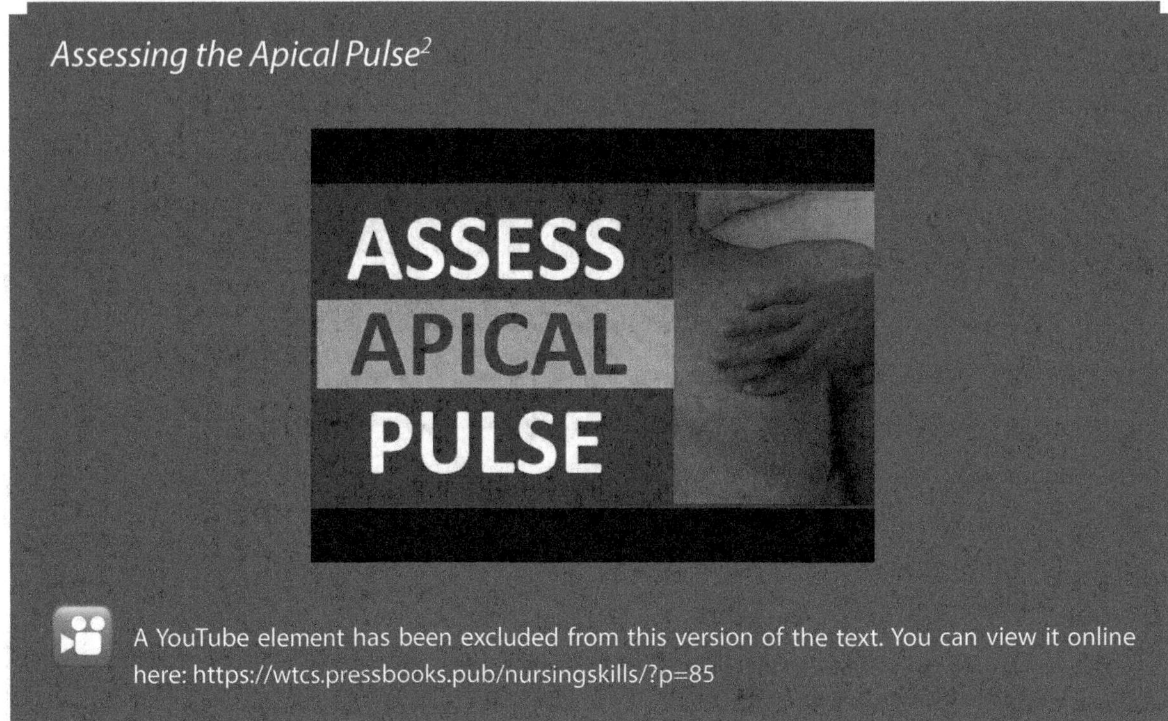

A YouTube element has been excluded from this version of the text. You can view it online here: https://wtcs.pressbooks.pub/nursingskills/?p=85

2 RegisteredNurseRN. (2017, September 5). *Apical pulse assessment location nursing | Auscultate and palpate apical pulse.* [Video]. YouTube. All rights reserved. https://youtu.be/RpaY7wM3QoM

9.7 LEARNING ACTIVITIES

My Notes

Learning Activities

(Answers to "Learning Activities" can be found in the "Answer Key" at the end of the book. Answers to interactive activity elements will be provided within the element as immediate feedback.)

1. As you walk into your patient's room, you notice the patient appears to be short of breath. Your patient states, "I have been short of breath and tired for the past week." Upon assessment of your patient, you notice JVD, labored breathing, lung sounds with crackles in the posterior bases, and +2 edema to the lower extremities bilaterally.

   From your assessment findings, determine the most likely disease state that is being described.

   a. Hypertension

   b. Pulmonary Embolism

   c. Heart Failure

   d. Stroke

2. Your patient puts on the call light. You enter the room and notice the patient appears to be in distress. The patient states, "I cannot catch my breath and my heart feels like it is going to explode." The patient's vital signs are T 98, P 148, BP 112/68, and pulse oximetry 88% on room air. You apply oxygen at 2 liters/minute via nasal cannula and notify the health care provide (HCP). The HCP orders a stat ECG. The patient's pulse oximetry increases to 94% with the oxygen, and the patient states, "I feel less short of breath but my heart is still racing." Upon assessment of heart sounds, the apical pulse is 134 and irregular. The ECG results indicate atrial fibrillation.

   What would be your next action?

   a. Leave the room and see your other patients.

   b. Stay with the patient and notify the HCP of the ECG results.

   c. Have the CNA stay with your patient as you take a break.

   d. Stay with the patient and wait for them to calm down.

Interactive Activity

An interactive or media element has been excluded from this version of the text. You can view it online here: https://wtcs.pressbooks.pub/nursingskills/?p=102

My Notes

Interactive Activity

An interactive or media element has been excluded from this version of the text. You can view it online here: https://wtcs.pressbooks.pub/nursingskills/?p=102

Interactive Activity

An interactive or media element has been excluded from this version of the text. You can view it online here: https://wtcs.pressbooks.pub/nursingskills/?p=102

Interactive Activity

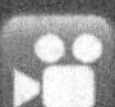

An interactive or media element has been excluded from this version of the text. You can view it online here: https://wtcs.pressbooks.pub/nursingskills/?p=102

Interactive Activity

An interactive or media element has been excluded from this version of the text. You can view it online here: https://wtcs.pressbooks.pub/nursingskills/?p=102

IX GLOSSARY

My Notes

Atrial fibrillation: An irregular heartbeat that is often fast and increases the risk of heart attack or stroke.

Blanching: The whiteness that occurs when pressure is placed on tissue or a nail bed, causing blood to leave the area.

Bruit: A swishing sound when auscultating the carotid arteries. This indicates turbulence in the blood vessel due to atherosclerotic changes.

Capillary refill: The time it takes for color to return after pressure is applied to tissue causing blanching.

Click: Clicking sound heard on auscultation of the precordium; often heard in patients with heart valve abnormalities.

Cyanosis: A bluish discoloration of the skin, lips, and nail beds. It is an indication of decreased perfusion and oxygenation.

Deep Vein Thrombosis (DVT): A blood clot that forms in a vein deep in the body.

Ductus arteriosus: Shunt that connects the pulmonary artery and aorta in the developing fetus.

Dyspnea: A feeling of shortness of breath.

Edema: Swelling in tissues caused by fluid retention.

Heave or lift: Palpable lifting sensation under the sternum and anterior chest wall to the left of the sternum; it suggests severe right ventricular hypertrophy.

Jugular Vein Distension (JVD): Occurs when the increased pressure of the superior vena cava causes the jugular vein to bulge, making it most visible on the right side of a person's neck.

Murmur: A blowing or whooshing sound heard on auscultation of the precordium that signifies turbulent blood flow in the heart often caused by a valvular defect.

Orthopnea: A feeling of shortness of breath when lying flat.

Pallor: A reduced amount of oxyhemoglobin in the skin or mucous membranes. Skin and mucous membranes present with a pale skin color.

Paroxysmal nocturnal dyspnea: An attack of severe shortness of breath that generally occurs at night.

Perfusion: The amount of blood flow to tissue.

Peripheral edema: Swelling due to an accumulation of fluid in tissues perfused by the peripheral vascular system.

Pitting edema: An accumulation of fluid in tissue and causes an indentation when the area is pressed.

Pleural friction rub: Uncommon heart sounds produced when the parietal and visceral pericardium become inflamed, generating a creaky-scratchy noise as they rub together.

Precordium: The region of the thorax in front of the heart.

Pulmonary embolism: A blood clot that lodges in one of the arteries that go from the heart to the lung.

Sphygmomanometer: An instrument for measuring blood pressure typically consisting of an inflatable rubber cuff.

Syncope: A temporary loss of consciousness usually related to insufficient blood flow to the brain.

Thrill: A vibration felt with palpation of the precordium.

Chapter 10

Respiratory Assessment

10.1 RESPIRATORY ASSESSMENT INTRODUCTION

My Notes

Learning Objectives

- Perform a respiratory assessment
- Differentiate between normal and abnormal lung sounds
- Modify assessment techniques to reflect variations across the life span
- Document actions and observations
- Recognize and report deviations from norms

The evaluation of the respiratory system includes collecting subjective and objective data through a detailed interview and physical examination of the thorax and lungs. This examination can offer significant clues related to issues associated with the body's ability to obtain adequate oxygen to perform daily functions. Inadequacy in respiratory function can have significant implications for the overall health of the patient.

My Notes

10.2 RESPIRATORY BASIC CONCEPTS

The main function of our respiratory system is to provide the body with a constant supply of oxygen and to remove carbon dioxide. To achieve these functions, muscles and structures of the thorax create the mechanical movement of air into and out of the lungs called **ventilation**. **Respiration** includes ventilation and gas exchange at the alveolar level where blood is oxygenated and carbon dioxide is removed. When completing a respiratory assessment, it is important for the nurse to understand the external and internal structures involved with respiration and ventilation. See Figure 10.1[3] for an illustration of the upper and lower respiratory system structures. Notice the lobular division of the lung structures and the bronchial tree.

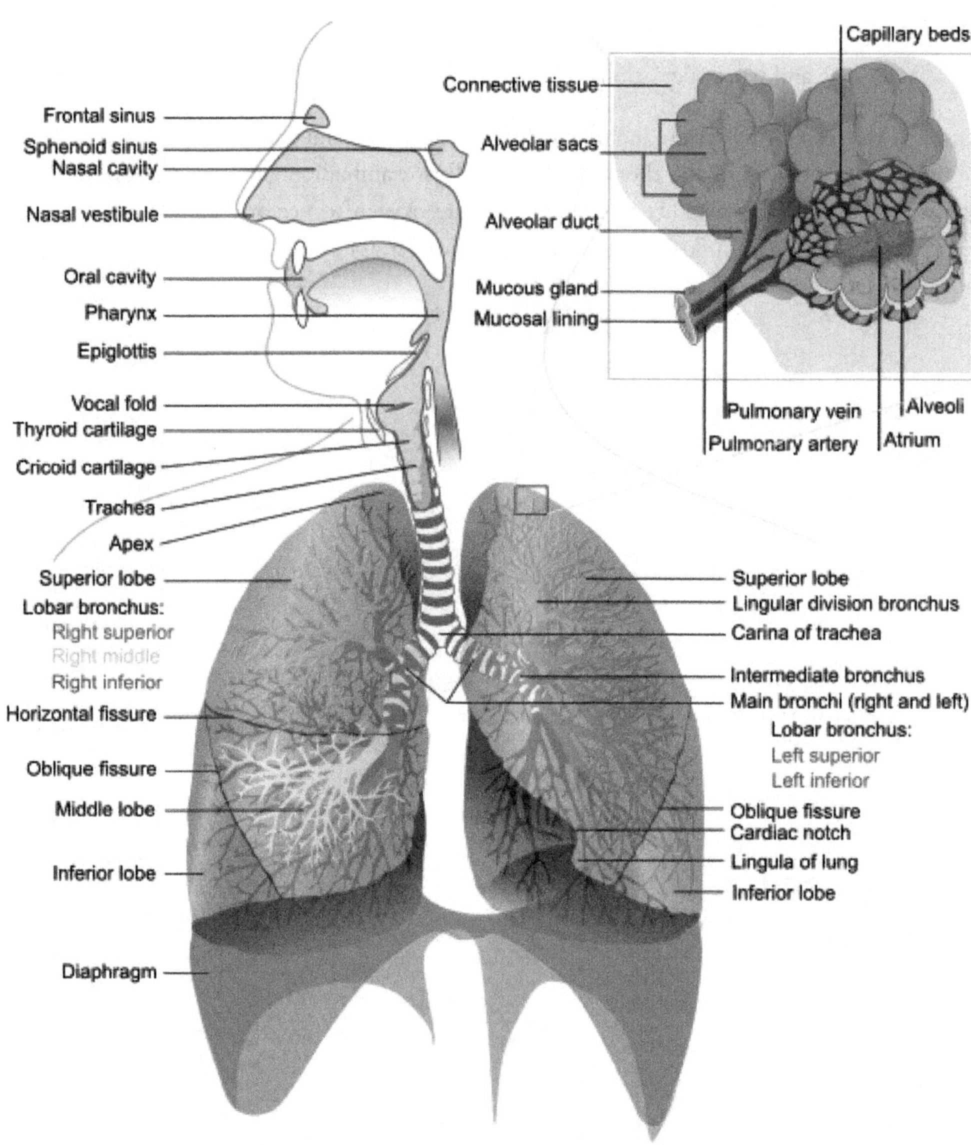

Figure 10.1 Respiratory System Structures

3 "Respiratory_system_complete_en.png" by British Columbia Institute of Technology is licensed under CC BY 4.0. Access for free at https://opentextbc.ca/clinicalskills/chapter/2-5-focussed-respiratory-assessment/

My Notes

For more information on basic oxygenation concepts, visit the "Oxygen Therapy" chapter of this book.

For more information about applying the nursing process to patients experiencing decreased oxygenation, visit the "Oxygenation" chapter in Open RN *Nursing Fundamentals*.

For a detailed review of the respiratory system, common respiratory disorders, and related medications, visit the "Respiratory" chapter of the Open RN *Nursing Pharmacology* textbook. Specific sections of this chapter include the following:

- "Overview of the Respiratory System"
- "Diseases of the Respiratory System"
- "Respiratory Medication Classes"

Video Reviews of the Anatomy of the Respiratory System and Breathing Mechanics

Respiratory System Anatomy[4]

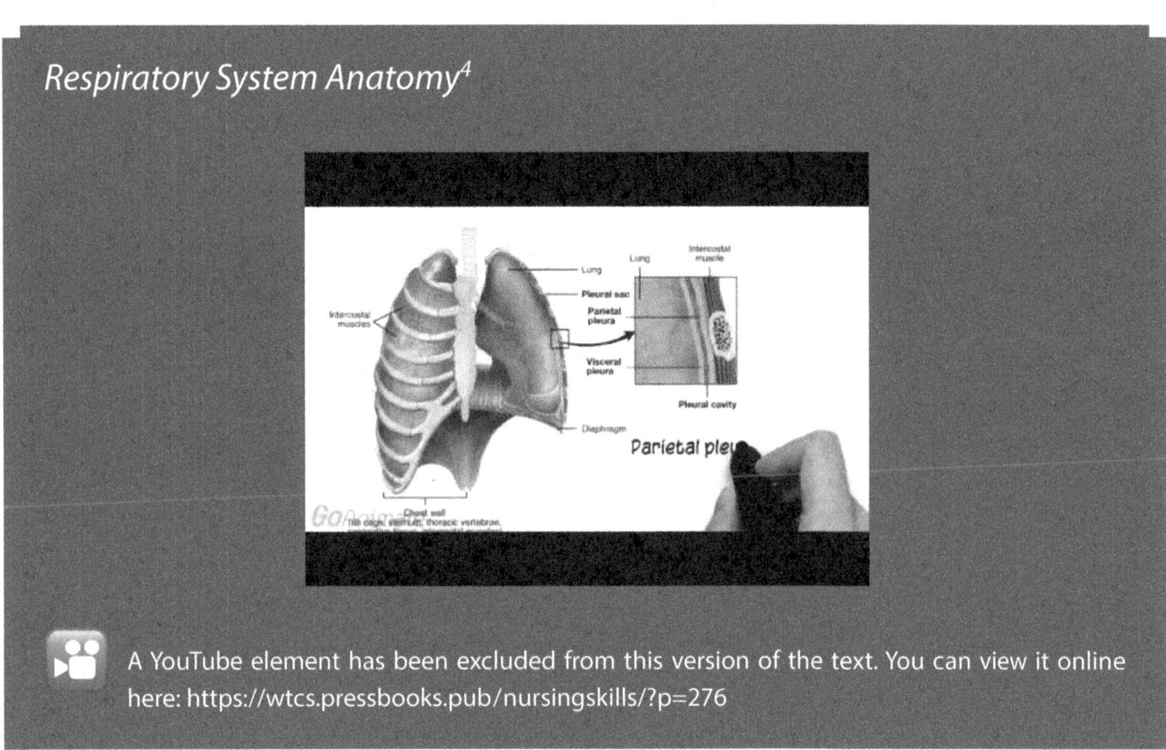

A YouTube element has been excluded from this version of the text. You can view it online here: https://wtcs.pressbooks.pub/nursingskills/?p=276

4 Forciea, B. (2015, May 13). *Respiratory system anatomy (v2.0)*. [Video]. YouTube. All rights reserved. Video used with permission. https://youtu.be/aqTwrdMS6CE

My Notes

Respiratory System: Breathing Mechanics[1]

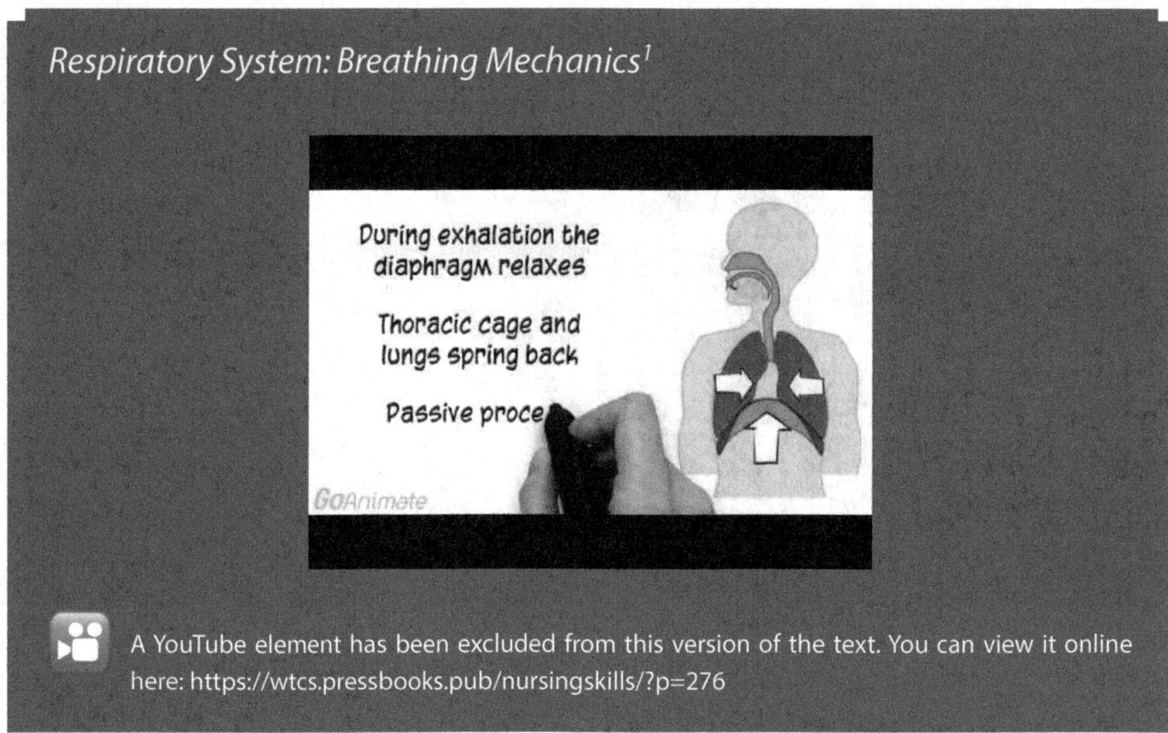

A YouTube element has been excluded from this version of the text. You can view it online here: https://wtcs.pressbooks.pub/nursingskills/?p=276

---

1 Forciea, B. (2015, May 12). *Anatomy and physiology: Respiratory system: Breathing mechanics (v2.0)*. [Video]. YouTube. All rights reserved. Video used with permission. https://youtu.be/X-J5Xgg3l6s

10.3 RESPIRATORY ASSESSMENT

My Notes

With an understanding of the basic structures and primary functions of the respiratory system, the nurse collects subjective and objective data to perform a focused respiratory assessment.

Subjective Assessment

Collect data using interview questions, paying particular attention to what the patient is reporting. The interview should include questions regarding any current and past history of respiratory health conditions or illnesses, medications, and reported symptoms. Consider the patient's age, gender, family history, race, culture, environmental factors, and current health practices when gathering subjective data. The information discovered during the interview process guides the physical exam and subsequent patient education. See Table 10.3a for sample interview questions to use during a focused respiratory assessment.[1]

1 This work is a derivative of Clinical Procedures for Safer Patient Care by British Columbia Institute of Technology and is licensed under CC BY 4.0. Access for free at https://opentextbc.ca/clinicalskills/

My Notes

Table 10.3a Interview Questions for Subjective Assessment of the Respiratory System

Interview Questions	Follow-up
Have you ever been diagnosed with a respiratory condition, such as asthma, COPD, pneumonia, or allergies? **Do you use oxygen or peak flow meter?** **Do you use home respiratory equipment like CPAP, BiPAP, or nebulizer devices?**	Please describe the conditions and treatments.
Are you currently taking any medications, herbs, or supplements for respiratory concerns?	Please identify what you are taking and the purpose of each.
Have you had any feelings of breathlessness (dyspnea)?	Note: If the shortness of breath is severe or associated with chest pain, discontinue the interview and obtain emergency assistance. Are you having any shortness of breath now? If yes, please rate the shortness of breath from 0-10 with "0" being none and "10" being severe? Does anything bring on the shortness of breath (such as activity, animals, food, or dust)? If activity causes the shortness of breath, how much exertion is required to bring on the shortness of breath? When did the shortness of breath start? Is the shortness of breath associated with chest pain or discomfort? How long does the shortness of breath last? What makes the shortness of breath go away? Is the shortness of breath related to a position, like lying down? Do you sleep in a recliner or upright in bed? Do you wake up at night feeling short of breath? How many pillows do you sleep on? How does the shortness of breath affect your daily activities?
Do you have a cough?	When you cough, do you bring up anything? What color is the phlegm? Do you cough up any blood (**hemoptysis**)? Do you have any associated symptoms with the cough such as fever, chills, or night sweats? How long have you had the cough? Does anything bring on the cough (such as activity, dust, animals, or change in position)? What have you used to treat the cough? Has it been effective?

My Notes

Interview Questions	Follow-up
Do you smoke or vape?	What products do you smoke/vape? If cigarettes are smoked, how many packs a day do you smoke? How long have you smoked/vaped? Have you ever tried to quit smoking/vaping? What strategies gave you the best success? Are you interested in quitting smoking/vaping? If the patient is ready to quit, the five successful interventions are the "5 A's": Ask, Advise, Assess, Assist, and Arrange. **Ask** – Identify and document smoking status for every patient at every visit. **Advise** – In a clear, strong, and personalized manner, urge every user to quit. **Assess** – Is the user willing to make a quitting attempt at this time? **Assist** – For the patient willing to make a quitting attempt, use counseling and pharmacotherapy to help them quit. **Arrange** – Schedule follow-up contact, in person or by telephone, preferably within the first week after the quit date.[2]

Life Span Considerations

Depending on the age and capability of the child, subjective data may also need to be retrieved from a parent and/or legal guardian.

Pediatric

- Is your child up-to-date with recommended immunizations?
- Is your child experiencing any cold symptoms (such as runny nose, cough, or nasal congestion)?
- How is your child's appetite? Is there any decrease or change recently in appetite or wet diapers?
- Does your child have any hospitalization history related to respiratory illness?
- Did your child have any history of frequent ear infections as an infant?

Older Adult

- Have you noticed a change in your breathing?
- Do you get short of breath with activities that you did not before?
- Can you describe your energy level? Is there any change from previous?

2 Massey, D., & Meredith, T. (2011). Respiratory assessment 1: Why do it and how to do it? *British Journal of Cardiac Nursing, 5(*11), 537–541. https://doi.org/10.12968/bjca.2010.5.11.79634

My Notes

Objective Assessment

A focused respiratory objective assessment includes interpretation of vital signs; inspection of the patient's breathing pattern, skin color, and respiratory status; palpation to identify abnormalities; and auscultation of lung sounds using a stethoscope. For more information regarding interpreting vital signs, see the "General Survey" chapter. The nurse must have an understanding of what is expected for the patient's age, gender, development, race, culture, environmental factors, and current health condition to determine the meaning of the data that is being collected.

Evaluate Vital Signs

The vital signs may be taken by the nurse or delegated to unlicensed assistive personnel such as a nursing assistant or medical assistant. Evaluate the respiratory rate and pulse oximetry readings to verify the patient is stable before proceeding with the physical exam. The normal range of a respiratory rate for an adult is 12-20 breaths per minute at rest, and the normal range for oxygen saturation of the blood is 94–98% (SpO_2).[3] **Bradypnea** is less than 12 breaths per minute, and **tachypnea** is greater than 20 breaths per minute.

As a general rule of thumb, respiratory rates outside the normal range or oxygen saturation levels less than 95% indicate respiration or ventilation is compromised and requires follow-up. There are disease processes, such as chronic obstructive pulmonary disease (COPD), where patients consistently exhibit below normal oxygen saturations; therefore, trends and deviations from the patient's baseline normal values should be identified. A change in respiratory rate is an early sign of deterioration in a patient, and failing to recognize such a change can result in poor outcomes. For more information on obtaining and interpreting vital signs, see the "General Survey" chapter.

Inspection

Inspection during a focused respiratory assessment includes observation of level of consciousness, breathing rate, pattern and effort, skin color, chest configuration, and symmetry of expansion.

- Assess the level of consciousness. The patient should be alert and cooperative. **Hypoxemia** (low blood levels of oxygen) or **hypercapnia** (high blood levels of carbon dioxide) can cause a decreased level of consciousness, irritability, anxiousness, restlessness, or confusion.
- Obtain the respiratory rate over a full minute. The normal range for the respiratory rate of an adult is 12-20 breaths per minute.
- Observe the breathing pattern, including the rhythm, effort, and use of **accessory muscles**. Breathing effort should be nonlabored and in a regular rhythm. Observe the depth of respiration and note if the respiration is shallow or deep. Pursed-lip breathing, nasal flaring, audible breathing, intercostal **retractions**, anxiety, and use of accessory muscles are signs of respiratory difficulty.

---

3 This work is a derivative of *Nursing Pharmacology* by Open RN licensed under CC BY 4.0. Access for free at https://wtcs.pressbooks.pub/pharmacology/

My Notes

Inspiration should last half as long as expiration unless the patient is active, in which case the inspiration-expiration ratio increases to 1:1.

- Observe pattern of expiration and patient position. Patients who experience difficulty expelling air, such as those with emphysema, may have prolonged expiration cycles. Some patients may experience difficulty with breathing specifically when lying down. This symptom is known as **orthopnea**. Additionally, patients who are experiencing significant breathing difficulty may experience most relief while in a "tripod" position. This can be achieved by having the patient sit at the side of the bed with legs dangling toward the floor. The patient can then rest their arms on an overbed table to allow for maximum lung expansion. This position mimics the same position you might take at the end of running a race when you lean over and place your hands on your knees to "catch your breath."
- Observe the patient's color in their lips, face, hands, and feet. Patients with light skin tones should be pink in color. For those with darker skin tones, assess for pallor on the palms, conjunctivae, or inner aspect of the lower lip. **Cyanosis** is a bluish discoloration of the skin, lips, and nail beds, which may indicate decreased perfusion and oxygenation. **Pallor** is the loss of color, or paleness of the skin or mucous membranes and usually the result of reduced blood flow, oxygenation, or decreased number of red blood cells.
- Inspect the chest for symmetry and configuration. The trachea should be midline, and the clavicles should be symmetrical. See Figure 10.2[4] for visual landmarks when inspecting the thorax anteriorly, posteriorly, and laterally. Note the location of the ribs, sternum, clavicle, and scapula, as well as the underlying lobes of the lungs.
  - Chest movement should be symmetrical on inspiration and expiration.
  - Observe the anterior-posterior diameter of the patient's chest and compare to the transverse diameter. The expected anteroposterior-transverse ratio should be 1:2. A patient with a 1:1 ratio is described as **barrel-chested**. This ratio is often seen in patients with chronic obstructive pulmonary disease due to hyperinflation of the lungs. See Figure 10.3[5] for an image of a patient with a barrel chest.
  - Older patients may have changes in their anatomy, such as **kyphosis**, an outward curvature of the spine.
- Inspect the fingers for clubbing if the patient has a history of chronic respiratory disease. **Clubbing** is a bulbous enlargement of the tips of the fingers due to chronic hypoxia. See Figure 10.4[6] for an image of clubbing.

---

4 "Anterior_Chest_Lines.png," "Posterior_Chest_Lines.png," and "Lateral_Chest_Lines.png" by Meredith Pomietlo for Chippewa Valley Technical College are licensed under CC BY 4.0. Access for free at https://drive.google.com/file/d/1-pUwwi83dvY1Eaw08dDomLSF-UZ_qojq/view?usp=sharing

5 "Normal A-P Chest Image.jpg" and "Barrel Chest.jpg" by Meredith Pomietlo for Chippewa Valley Technical College are licensed under CC BY 4.0. Access for free at https://drive.google.com/file/d/1V-438AwaQK6eXLjvNMhhVoxg4yxz7fH0/view?usp=sharing

6 "Clubbing of fingers in IPF.jpg" by IPFeditor is licensed under CC BY-SA 3.0. Access for free at https://commons.wikimedia.org/wiki/File:Clubbing_of_fingers_in_IPF.jpg

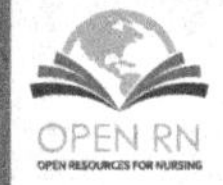

My Notes

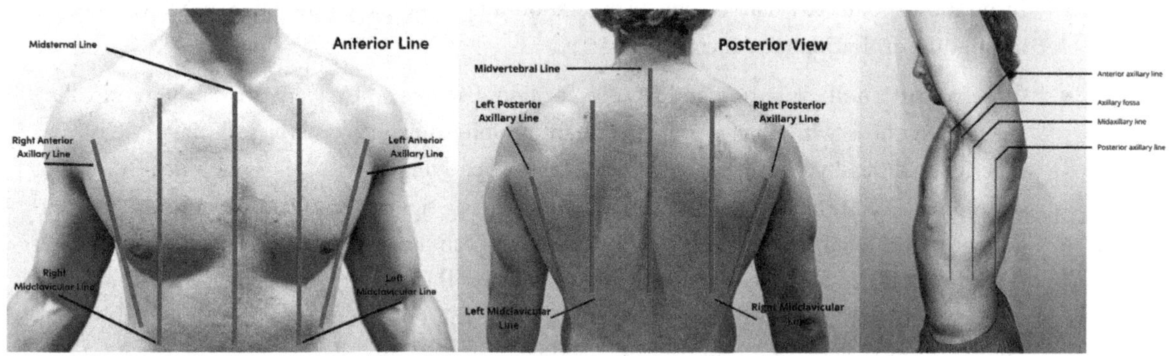

Figure 10.2 Landmarks of the Anterior, Posterior, and Lateral Thorax

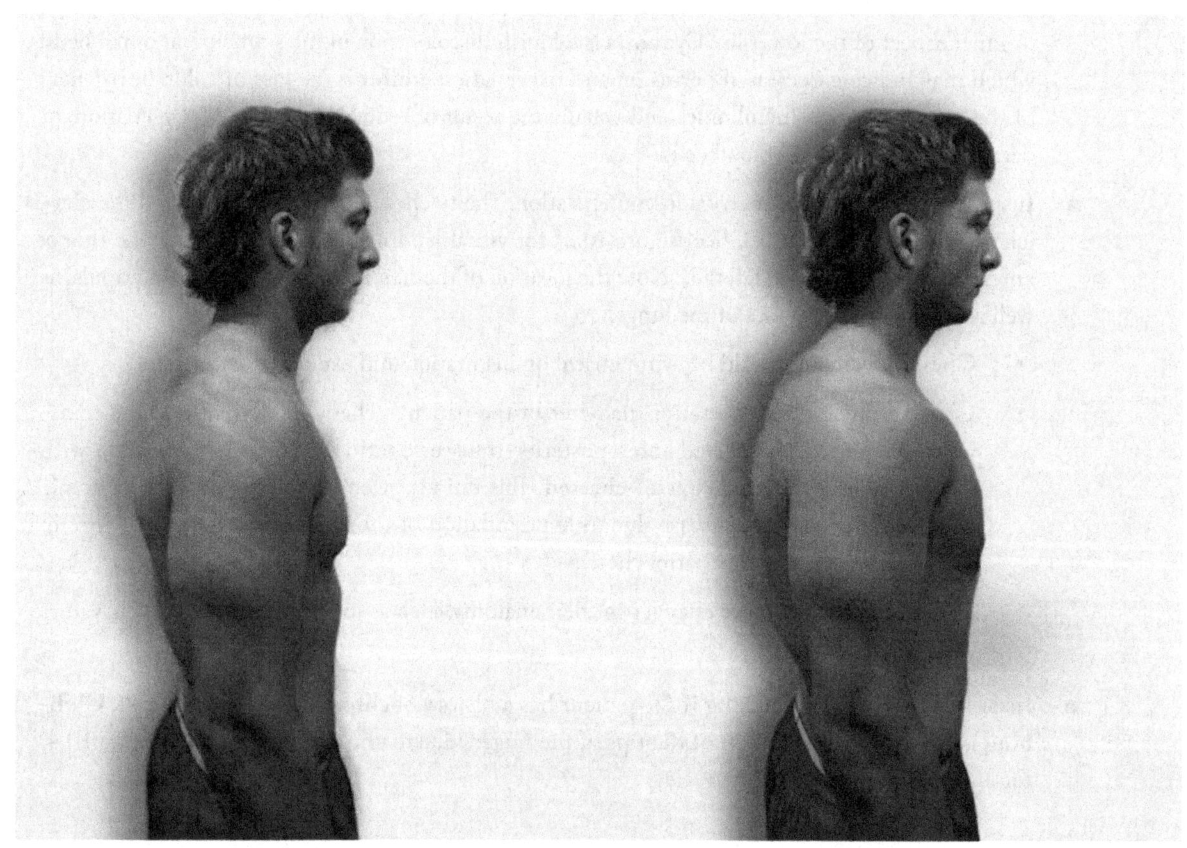

Figure 10.3 Comparison of Chest with Normal Anterior/Posterior Diameter (A) to a Barrel Chest(B)

My Notes

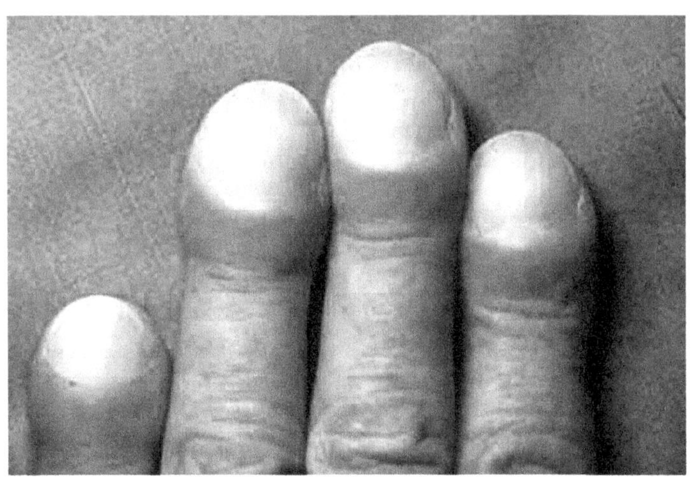

Figure 10.4 Clubbing of the Fingers

Palpation

- Palpation of the chest may be performed to investigate for areas of abnormality related to injury or procedural complications. For example, if a patient has a chest tube or has recently had one removed, the nurse may palpate near the tube insertion site to assess for areas of air leak or crepitus. **Crepitus** feels like a popping or crackling sensation when the skin is palpated and is a sign of air trapped under the subcutaneous tissues. If palpating the chest, use light pressure with the fingertips to examine the anterior and posterior chest wall. Chest palpation may be performed to assess specifically for growths, masses, crepitus, pain, or tenderness.
- Confirm symmetric chest expansion by placing your hands on the anterior or posterior chest at the same level, with thumbs over the sternum anteriorly or the spine posteriorly. As the patient inhales, your thumbs should move apart symmetrically. Unequal expansion can occur with pneumonia, thoracic trauma, such as fractured ribs, or pneumothorax.

Auscultation

Using the diaphragm of the stethoscope, listen to the movement of air through the airways during inspiration and expiration. Instruct the patient to take deep breaths through their mouth. Listen through the entire respiratory cycle because different sounds may be heard on inspiration and expiration. As you move across the different lung fields, the sounds produced by airflow vary depending on the area you are auscultating because the size of the airways change.

Listen to normal breath sounds on inspiration and expiration.

Interactive Activity

An interactive or media element has been excluded from this version of the text. You can view it online here: https://wtcs.pressbooks.pub/nursingskills/?p=279

Correct placement of the stethoscope during auscultation of lung sounds is important to obtain a quality assessment. The stethoscope should not be placed over clothes or hair because these may create inaccurate sounds from

My Notes

friction. The best position to listen to lung sounds is with the patient sitting upright; however, if the patient is acutely ill or unable to sit upright, turn them side to side in a lying position. Avoid listening over bones, such as the scapulae or clavicles or over the female breasts to ensure you are hearing adequate sound transmission. Listen to sounds from side to side rather than down one side and then down the other side. This side-to-side pattern allows you to compare sounds in symmetrical lung fields. See Figures 10.5[7] and 10.6[8] for landmarks of stethoscope placement over the anterior and posterior chest wall.

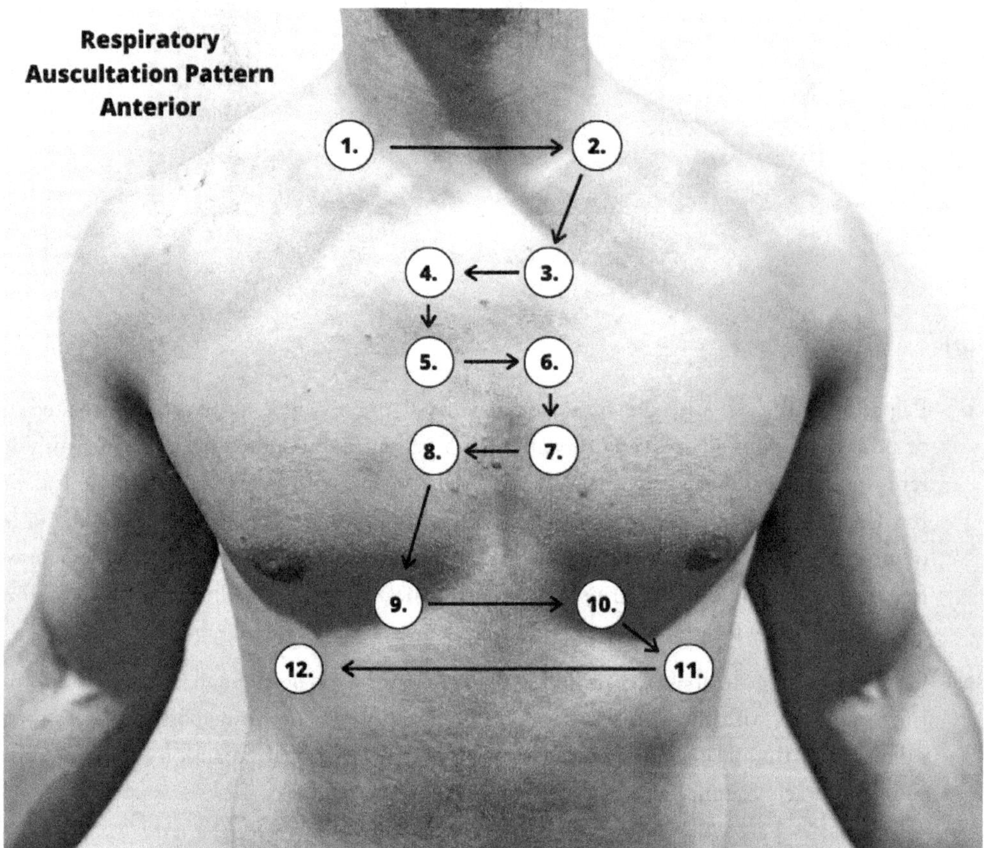

Figure 10.5 Anterior Auscultation Areas

7 "Anterior Respiratory Auscultation Pattern.png" by Meredith Pomietlo for Chippewa Valley Technical College is licensed under CC BY 4.0. Access for free at https://drive.google.com/file/d/1G1pjWedp05uMv41pnDQme_kBReWpbTpS/view?usp=sharing

8 "Posterior Respiratory Auscultation Pattern.png" by Meredith Pomietlo for Chippewa Valley Technical College is licensed under CC BY 4.0. Access for free at https://drive.google.com/file/d/1aKllXU4A0sjOMq2_pVItLi5PTYYU5njp/view?usp=sharing

My Notes

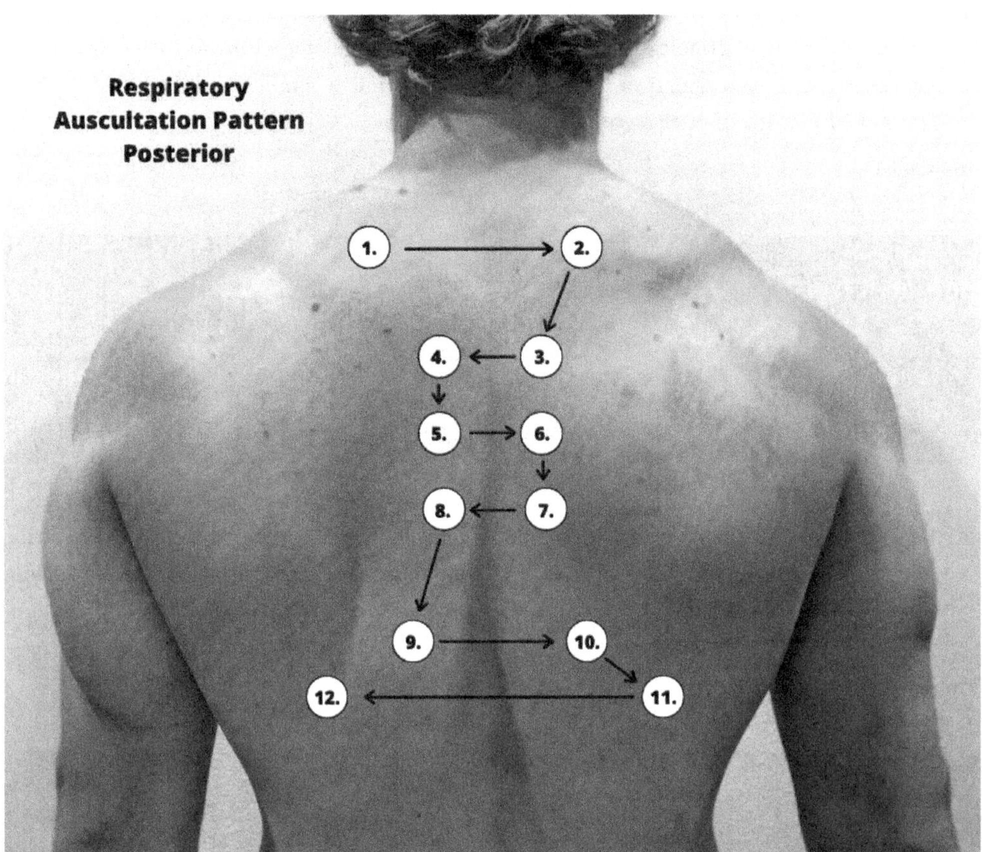

Figure 10.6 Posterior Auscultation Areas

When assessing patients who are experiencing shortness of breath (or fatigue easily), it may be helpful to begin auscultation in the bases and progress upward to other lung fields as tolerated by the patient. This ensures that assessment of the vulnerable lower lobes is achieved prior to patient fatigue.

Expected Breath Sounds

It is important upon auscultation to have awareness of expected breath sounds in various anatomical locations.

- **Bronchial breath sounds** are heard over the trachea and larynx and are high-pitched and loud.
- **Bronchovesicular sounds** are medium-pitched and heard over the major bronchi.
- **Vesicular breath sounds** are heard over the lung surfaces, are lower-pitched, and often described as soft, rustling sounds.

Adventitious Lung Sounds

Adventitious lung sounds are sounds heard in addition to normal breath sounds. They most often indicate an airway problem or disease, such as accumulation of mucus or fluids in the airways, obstruction, inflammation, or infection. These sounds include rales/crackles, rhonchi/wheezes, stridor, and pleural rub:

My Notes

- **Fine crackles**, also called **rales**, are popping or crackling sounds heard on inspiration that occur in association with conditions that cause fluid to accumulate within the alveolar and interstitial spaces, such as heart failure or pneumonia. The sound is similar to that produced by rubbing strands of hair together close to your ear.

Listen to fine crackles:

Interactive Activity

 An interactive or media element has been excluded from this version of the text. You can view it online here: https://wtcs.pressbooks.pub/nursingskills/?p=279

- **Wheezes** are whistling-type noises produced during expiration (and sometimes inspiration) when air is forced through airways narrowed by bronchoconstriction or associated mucosal edema. For example, patients with asthma commonly have wheezing.

Listen to wheezes:

Interactive Activity

 An interactive or media element has been excluded from this version of the text. You can view it online here: https://wtcs.pressbooks.pub/nursingskills/?p=279

- **Stridor** is heard only on inspiration. It is associated with mechanical obstruction at the level of the trachea/upper airway.

Listen to stridor:

Interactive Activity

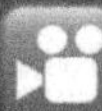 An interactive or media element has been excluded from this version of the text. You can view it online here: https://wtcs.pressbooks.pub/nursingskills/?p=279

- **Pleural rub** may be heard on either inspiration or expiration and sounds like the rubbing together of leather. A pleural rub is heard when there is inflammation of the lung pleura, resulting in friction as the surfaces rub against each other.[9]

9 This work is a derivative of Clinical Procedures for Safer Patient Care by British Columbia Institute of Technology and is licensed under CC BY 4.0. Access for free at https://opentextbc.ca/clinicalskills/

Life Span Considerations

My Notes

Children

There are various respiratory assessment considerations that should be noted with assessment of children.

- The respiratory rate in children less than 12 months of age can range from 30-60 breaths per minute, depending on whether the infant is asleep or active.
- Infants have irregular or periodic newborn breathing in the first few weeks of life; therefore, it is important to count the respirations for a full minute. During this time, you may notice periods of **apnea** lasting up to 10 seconds. This is not abnormal unless the infant is showing other signs of distress. Signs of respiratory distress in infants and children include nasal flaring and sternal or intercostal retractions.
- Up to three months of age, infants are considered "obligate" nose-breathers, meaning their breathing is primarily through the nose.
- The anteroposterior-transverse ratio is typically 1:1 until the thoracic muscles are fully developed around six years of age.

Older Adults

As the adult person ages, the cartilage and muscle support of the thorax becomes weakened and less flexible, resulting in a decrease in chest expansion. Older adults may also have weakened respiratory muscles, and breathing may become more shallow. The anteroposterior-transverse ratio may be 1:1 if there is significant curvature of the spine (kyphosis).

Percussion

Percussion is an advanced respiratory assessment technique that is used by advanced practice nurses and other health care providers to gather additional data in the underlying lung tissue. By striking the fingers of one hand over the fingers of the other hand, a sound is produced over the lung fields that helps determine if fluid is present. Dull sounds are heard with high-density areas, such as pneumonia or **atelectasis**, whereas clear, low-pitched, hollow sounds are heard in normal lung tissue.

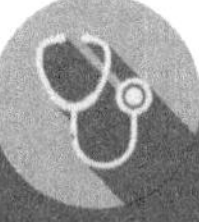

- **Because infants breathe primarily through the nose, nasal congestion can limit the amount of air getting into the lungs.**
- **Attempt to assess an infant's respiratory rate while the infant is at rest and content rather than when the infant is crying. Counting respirations by observing abdominal breathing movements may be easier for the novice nurse than counting breath sounds, as it can be difficult to differentiate lung and heart sounds when auscultating newborns.**
- **Auscultation of lungs during crying is not a problem. It will enhance breath sounds.**
- **The older patient may have a weakening of muscles that support respiration and breathing. Therefore, the patient may report tiring easily during the assessment when taking deep breaths. Break up the assessment by listening to the anterior lung sounds and then**

My Notes

the heart sounds and allowing the patient to rest before listening to the posterior lung sounds.

- Patients with end-stage COPD may have diminished lung sounds due to decreased air movement. This abnormal assessment finding may be the patient's baseline or normal and might also include wheezes and fine crackles as a result of chronic excess secretions and/or bronchoconstriction.[10, 11]

Expected Versus Unexpected Findings

See Table 10.3b for a comparison of expected versus unexpected findings when assessing the respiratory system.[12]

10 This work is a derivative of Clinical Procedures for Safer Patient Care by British Columbia Institute of Technology and is licensed under CC BY 4.0. Access for free at https://opentextbc.ca/clinicalskills/

11 Honig, E. (1990). An overview of the pulmonary system. In Walker, H. K., Hall, W. D., Hurst, J. W. (Eds.), *Clinical methods: The history, physical, and laboratory examinations* (3rd ed.). Butterworths. https://www.ncbi.nlm.nih.gov/books/NBK356/

12 This work is a derivative of Clinical Procedures for Safer Patient Care by British Columbia Institute of Technology and is licensed under CC BY 4.0. Access for free at https://opentextbc.ca/clinicalskills/

My Notes

Table 10.3b Expected Versus Unexpected Respiratory Assessment Findings		
Assessment	**Expected Findings**	**Unexpected Findings (Document and notify provider if a new finding*)**
Inspection	Work of breathing effortless Regular breathing pattern Respiratory rate within normal range for age Chest expansion symmetrical Absence of cyanosis or pallor Absence of accessory muscle use, retractions, and/or nasal flaring Anteroposterior: transverse diameter ratio 1:2	Labored breathing Irregular rhythm Increased or decreased respiratory rate Accessory muscle use, pursed-lip breathing, nasal flaring (infants), and/or retractions Presence of cyanosis or pallor Asymmetrical chest expansion Clubbing of fingernails
Palpation	No pain or tenderness with palpation. Skin warm and dry; no crepitus or masses	Pain or tenderness with palpation, crepitus, palpable masses, or lumps
Percussion	Clear, low-pitched, hollow sound in normal lung tissue	Dull sounds heard with high-density areas, such as pneumonia or atelectasis
Auscultation	Bronchovesicular and vesicular sounds heard over appropriate areas Absence of adventitious lung sounds	Diminished lung sounds Adventitious lung sounds, such as fine crackles/rales, wheezing, stridor, or pleural rub
***CRITICAL CONDITIONS to report immediately**		Decreased oxygen saturation <92%[13] Pain Worsening dyspnea Decreased level of consciousness, restlessness, anxiousness, and/or irritability

Interactive Activity

An interactive or media element has been excluded from this version of the text. You can view it online here: https://wtcs.pressbooks.pub/nursingskills/?p=279

13 Hill, B., & Annesley, S. H. (2020). Monitoring respiratory rate in adults. *British Journal of Nursing, 29*(1), 12–16. https://doi.org/10.12968/bjon.2020.29.1.12

My Notes

10.4 SAMPLE DOCUMENTATION

Sample Documentation of Expected Findings

Patient denies cough, chest pain, or shortness of breath. Denies past or current respiratory illnesses or diseases. Symmetrical anterior and posterior thorax. Anteroposterior-transverse ratio is 1:2. Respiratory rate is 16 breaths/minute, unlabored, regular, and inaudible through the nose. No retractions, accessory muscle use, or nasal flaring. Chest rise and fall are equal bilaterally. Skin is pink, warm, and dry. No crepitus, masses, or tenderness upon palpation of anterior and posterior chest. Lung sounds clear bilaterally in all lobes anteriorly and posteriorly. No adventitious sounds. SpO2 saturation 99% on room air.

Sample Documentation of Unexpected Findings

Patient reports shortness of breath for five to six hours. Patient has labored breathing at rest. Nail beds are cyanotic. Respiratory rate is tachypneic at 32/minute with neck and abdominal accessory muscle use. Lung expansion is symmetrical. Pursed-lip breathing noted with intermittent productive cough. Reports coughing up blood-tinged green sputum for two days. Anterior and posterior chest walls have no tenderness, masses, or crepitus upon palpation. On auscultation bilateral coarse crackles over lung bases. Expiratory wheezes are audible and heard with stethoscope scattered throughout lung fields. Pulse oximetry 93% on room air.

10.4 CHECKLIST FOR RESPIRATORY ASSESSMENT

My Notes

Use the checklist below to review the steps for completion of a "Respiratory Assessment."[14]

Steps

Disclaimer: Always review and follow agency policy regarding this specific skill.

1. Gather supplies: stethoscope and pulse oximeter.
2. Perform safety steps:
   - Perform hand hygiene.
   - Check the room for transmission-based precautions.
   - Introduce yourself, your role, the purpose of your visit, and an estimate of the time it will take.
   - Confirm patient ID using two patient identifiers (e.g., name and date of birth).
   - Explain the process to the patient and ask if they have any questions.
   - Be organized and systematic.
   - Use appropriate listening and questioning skills.
   - Listen and attend to patient cues.
   - Ensure the patient's privacy and dignity.
   - Assess ABCs.
3. Obtain subjective data related to history of respiratory diseases, current symptoms, medications, and history of smoking using the suggested interview questions in *Table 10.3a*.
4. Obtain and analyze vital signs including the pulse oximetry reading. Act appropriately on unexpected findings outside the normal range.
5. Assist the patient to a seated position if tolerated. Provide privacy while exposing only those areas of assessment.
   - Assess level of consciousness for signs of hypoxia/hypercapnia
   - Count respiratory rate for one minute
   - Observe respirations for rhythm pattern, depth, symmetry, and work of breathing
   - Observe configuration and symmetry of the chest. Compare anterior-posterior diameter to the transverse diameter
   - Inspect skin color of lips, face, hands, and feet

   Note that early signs of hypoxia may include anxiety, confusion, restlessness, change in mental status, and/or level of consciousness (LOC).

14 This work is a derivative of Clinical Procedures for Safer Patient Care by British Columbia Institute of Technology and is licensed under CC BY 4.0. Access for free at https://opentextbc.ca/clinicalskills/

My Notes

6. Palpate:
    - Inspect anterior/posterior chest wall for areas of tenderness, crepitus, lumps, or masses
    - Compare for bilaterally equal chest expansion
7. Auscultate: Use correct stethoscope placement directly on the skin over designated auscultation areas. Identify any adventitious sounds.
8. Assist the patient back to a comfortable position, ask if they have any questions, and thank them for their time.
9. Ensure safety measures when leaving the room:
    - CALL LIGHT: Within reach
    - BED: Low and locked (in lowest position and brakes on)
    - SIDE RAILS: Secured
    - TABLE: Within reach
    - ROOM: Risk-free for falls (scan room and clear any obstacles)
10. Perform hand hygiene.
11. Document the assessment findings. Report any concerns according to agency policy.

10.6 SUPPLEMENTARY VIDEO ON RESPIRATORY ASSESSMENT

My Notes

Video Review of Heart & Lung Assessment | Head-to-Toe Exam[15]

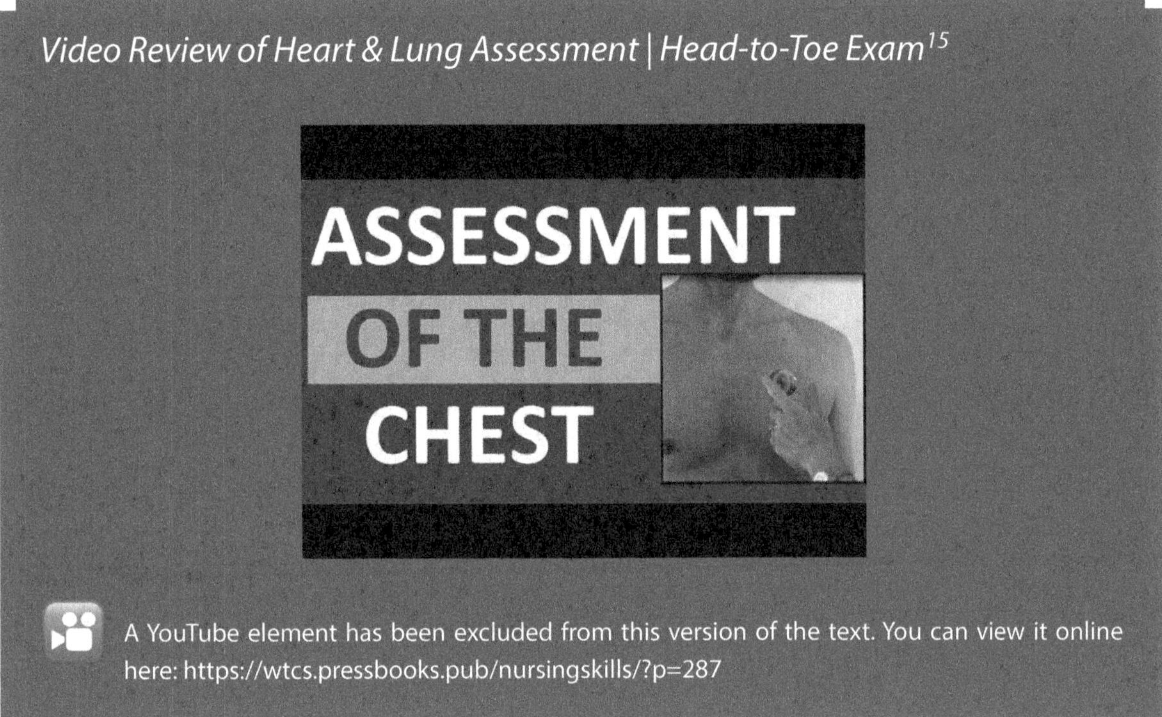

A YouTube element has been excluded from this version of the text. You can view it online here: https://wtcs.pressbooks.pub/nursingskills/?p=287

15 RegisteredNurseRN. (2017, December 17). *Chest assessment nursing | Heart & lung assessment | Head-to-toe Exam.* [Video]. YouTube. All rights reserved. Video used with permission. https://youtu.be/kv3B81mWc1E

My Notes

10.7 LEARNING ACTIVITIES

Learning Activities

(Answers to "Learning Activities" can be found in the "Answer Key" at the end of the book. Answers to interactive activity elements will be provided within the element as immediate feedback.)

1. An elderly client is admitted to the medical floor with increased shortness of breath, new productive cough, and low- grade fever. The nurse begins the physical examination of the respiratory system.

   What is the best position for the client to assume for the physical exam?

   a. Supine

   b. Sitting upright

   c. Semi-Fowlers

   d. Left-lateral

2. During the course of the preceding patient's physical exam, auscultation of the lungs reveals rhonchi in the upper airways and coarse crackles in the right lower base. The nurse knows that rhonchi and crackles may indicate ________ or ________ in the airways.

3. A client has pneumonia, which is currently being treated with antibiotics, and reports feeling better since being hospitalized. The nurse assesses the client's oxygen saturation using a pulse oximeter by placing the probe on the client's finger. The reading is 89%.

   Which of the following actions should the nurse perform first?

   a. Assess the pulse oximeter probe site to ensure an accurate reading.

   b. Administer oxygen and monitor the pulse oximetry until it reaches 95 percent.

   c. Raise the head of the bed and ask the client to take several deep breaths.

   d. Contact the provider and recommend prescribing a chest X-ray.

Interactive Activity

An interactive or media element has been excluded from this version of the text. You can view it online here: https://wtcs.pressbooks.pub/nursingskills/?p=291

My Notes

Interactive Activity

An interactive or media element has been excluded from this version of the text. You can view it online here: https://wtcs.pressbooks.pub/nursingskills/?p=291

Interactive Activity

An interactive or media element has been excluded from this version of the text. You can view it online here: https://wtcs.pressbooks.pub/nursingskills/?p=291

Interactive Activity

An interactive or media element has been excluded from this version of the text. You can view it online here: https://wtcs.pressbooks.pub/nursingskills/?p=291

My Notes

X GLOSSARY

Accessory muscles: Muscles other than the diaphragm and intercostal muscles that may be used for labored breathing.

Apnea: Absence of respirations.

Atelectasis: Alveoli or an entire lung is collapsed, allowing no air movement.

Barrel-chested: An equal AP-to-transverse diameter that often occurs in patients with COPD due to hyperinflation of the lungs.

Bradypnea: Decreased respiratory rate or slow breath less than normal range according to the patient's age.

Bronchial breath sounds: High-pitched hollow sounds heard over trachea and the larynx.

Bronchovesicular sounds: Mixture of low- and high-pitched sounds heard over major bronchi.

Clubbing: A change in the configuration where the tips of the nails curve around the fingertips, usually caused by chronic low levels of oxygen in the blood.

Crackles: Also referred to as "rales"; sound like popping or crackling noises during inspiration. Associated with inflammation and fluid accumulation in the alveoli.

Crepitus: Air trapped under a subcutaneous layer of the skin; creates a popping or crackling sensation as the area is palpated.

Cyanosis: Bluish discoloration of the skin, lips, and nail beds. It is an indication of decreased perfusion and oxygenation.

Dyspnea: A subjective feeling of breathlessness.

Hemoptysis: Blood-tinged mucus secretions from the lungs.

Hypercapnia: Increased carbon dioxide levels in the blood.

Hypoxemia: Decreased levels of oxygen in the blood.

Kyphosis: Outward curvature of the back; often described as "hunchback."

Orthopnea: Breathlessness or a feeling of shortness of breath when lying in a reclined position.

Pallor: A reduced amount of oxyhemoglobin in the skin or mucous membranes and causes skin and mucous membranes to present with a pale skin color.

Rales: Another term used for crackles.

Respiration: Includes ventilation and gas exchange at the alveolar level where blood is oxygenated and carbon dioxide is removed.

Retractions: The "pulling in" of muscles between the ribs or in the neck when breathing, indicating difficulty breathing or respiratory distress.

Stridor: High-pitched crowing sounds heard over the upper airway and larynx indicating obstruction.

Tachypnea: Rapid and often shallow breathing greater than normal range according to the patient's age.

Ventilation: The mechanical movement of air into and out of the lungs.

Vesicular sounds: Low-pitched soft sounds like "rustling leaves" heard over alveoli and small bronchial airways.

Wheeze: High-pitched sounds heard on expiration or inspiration associated with bronchoconstriction or bronchospasm.

Chapter 11

Oxygen Therapy

My Notes

11.1 OXYGEN THERAPY INTRODUCTION

My Notes

Learning Objectives

- Implement interventions to improve a patient's oxygenation status
- Correctly apply oxygen equipment
- Set flow rate using fixed and portable equipment
- Survey the environment for potential safety hazards
- Use pulse oximetry
- Assess patient response to oxygen therapy
- Adapt procedures to reflect variations across the life span
- Document actions and observations
- Recognize and report significant deviations from norms

The air we breathe contains 21% oxygen and is crucial for life. Several body systems must work collaboratively during the oxygenation process to take in oxygen from the air, carry it through the bloodstream, and adequately oxygenate tissues. First, the airway must be open and clear. The chest and lungs must mechanically move air in and out of the lungs. The bronchial airways must be open and clear so that air can reach the alveoli, where oxygen is absorbed into the bloodstream and carbon dioxide is released during exhalation. The heart must effectively pump this oxygenated blood to and from the lungs and through the systemic arteries. The hemoglobin in the blood must be in adequate amounts to sufficiently carry the oxygen to the tissues, where it is released and carbon dioxide is absorbed and carried back to the lungs.

Several medical conditions, such as asthma, chronic obstructive pulmonary disease (COPD), pneumonia, heart disease, and anemia can impair a person's ability to sufficiently complete this oxygenation process, thus requiring the administration of supplemental oxygen. This chapter will review basic concepts related to oxygenation, provide an overview of oxygenation equipment, and apply the nursing process to the administration of supplemental oxygen. Oxygen is considered a medication and, therefore, requires a prescription and continuous monitoring by the nurse to ensure its safe and effective use.

My Notes

11.2 BASIC CONCEPTS OF OXYGENATION

When assessing a patient's oxygenation status, it is important for the nurse to have an understanding of the underlying structures of the respiratory system to best understand their assessment findings. Visit the "Respiratory Assessment" chapter for more information about the structures of the respiratory system.

For more information about common respiratory conditions and medications used to treat them, visit the "Respiratory" chapter in Open RN *Nursing Pharmacology*.

Video Review for Oxygenation Basics

View the TED-Ed Oxygen's Journey Video on YouTube[1]
Breathing Mechanics[2]

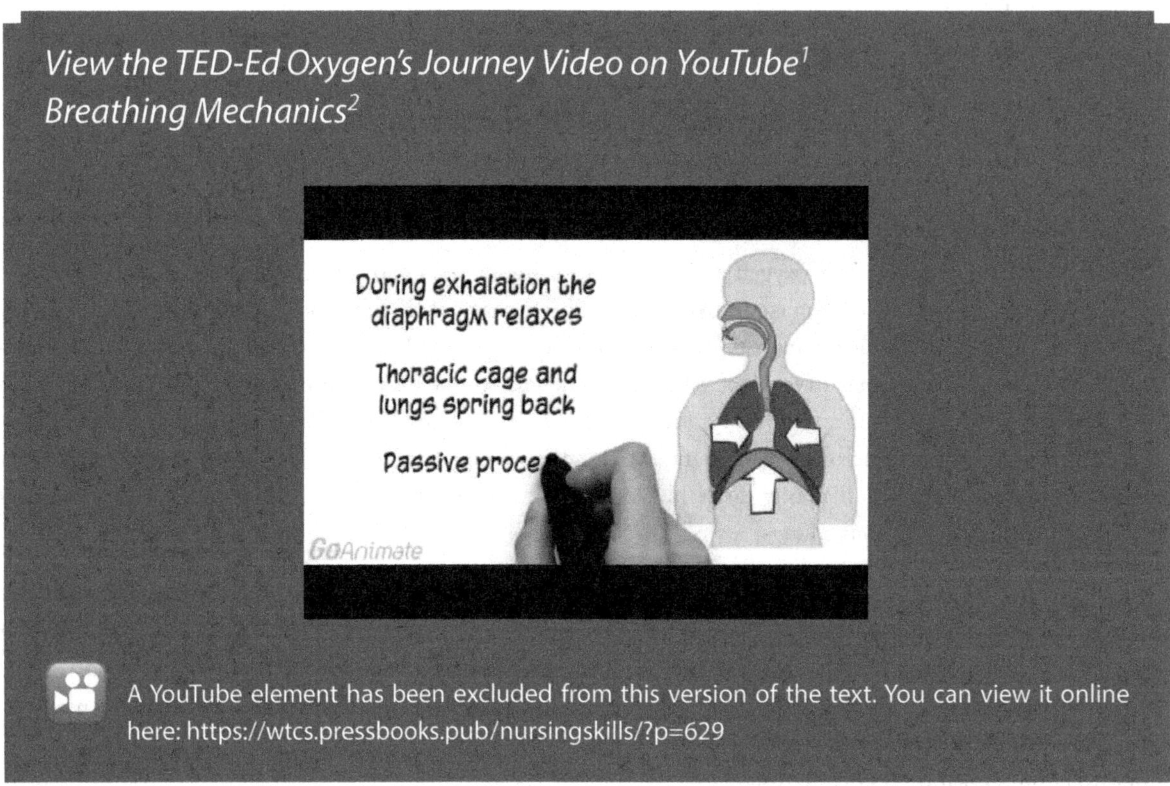

A YouTube element has been excluded from this version of the text. You can view it online here: https://wtcs.pressbooks.pub/nursingskills/?p=629

1 TED-Ed. (2017, April 13). *Oxygen's surprisingly complex journey through your body - Edna Butler.* [Video]. YouTube. All rights reserved. https://youtu.be/GVU_zANtroE

2 Forciea, B. (2015, May 12). *Anatomy and physiology: Respiratory system: Breathing mechanics (v2.0).* [Video]. YouTube. All rights reserved. Video used with permission. https://youtu.be/X-J5Xgg3l6s

My Notes

Gas Exchange[3]

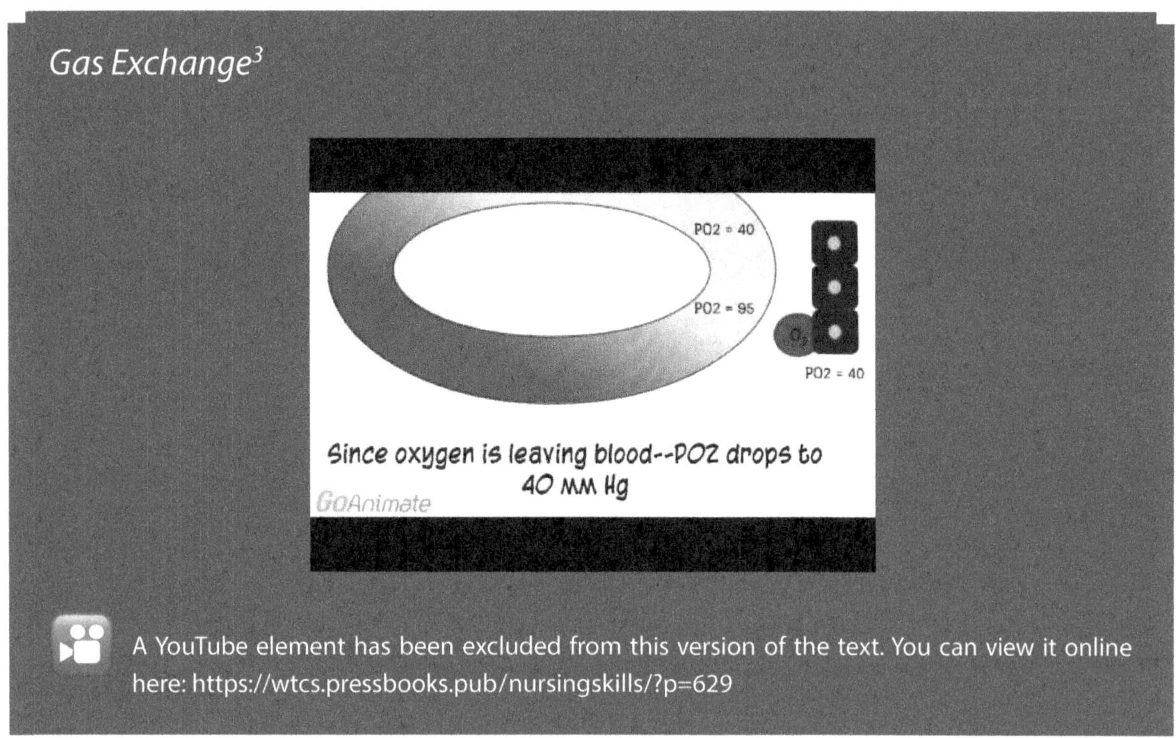

A YouTube element has been excluded from this version of the text. You can view it online here: https://wtcs.pressbooks.pub/nursingskills/?p=629

Carbon Dioxide Transport[4]

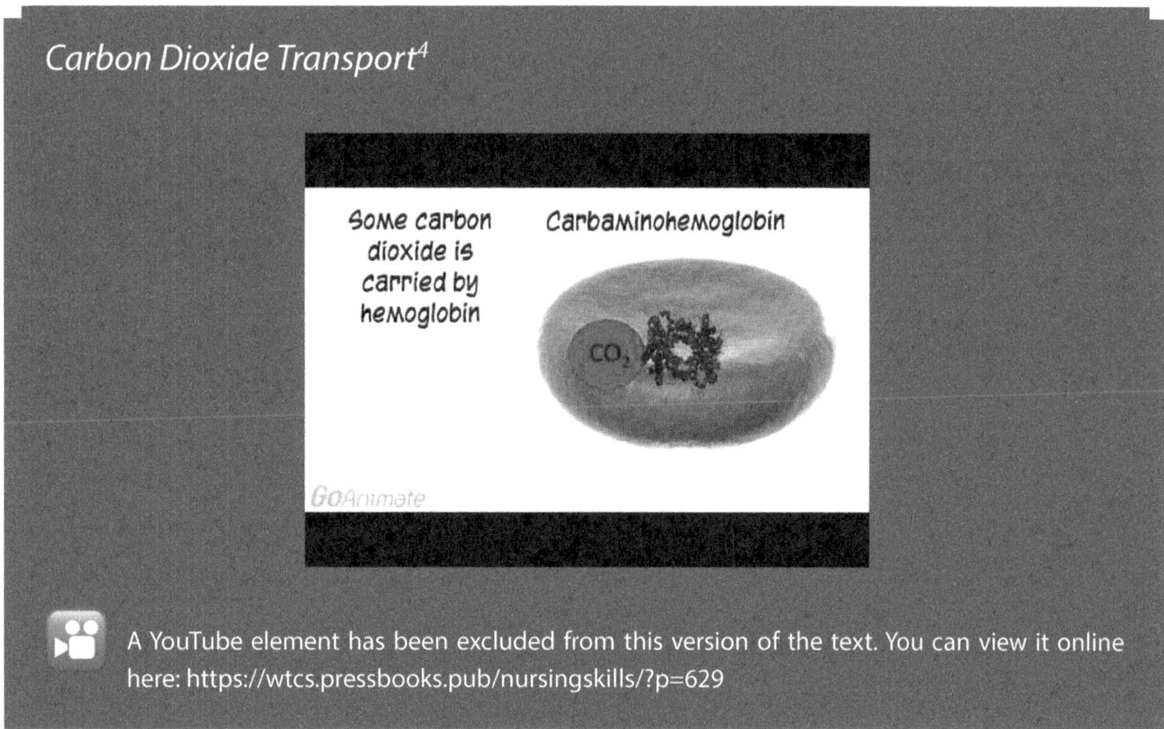

A YouTube element has been excluded from this version of the text. You can view it online here: https://wtcs.pressbooks.pub/nursingskills/?p=629

3 Forciea, B. (2015, May 12). *Respiratory system: Gas exchange (v2.0)*. [Video]. YouTube. All rights reserved. Video used with permission. https://youtu.be/uVWko7_v7MM

4 Forciea, B. (2015, May 12). *Respiratory system: C02 transport (v2.0)*. [Video]. YouTube. All rights reserved. Video used with permission. https://youtu.be/BmrvqZoxHYI

My Notes

Assessing Oxygenation Status

A patient's oxygenation status is routinely assessed using pulse oximetry, referred to as **SpO2**. SpO2 is an estimated oxygenation level based on the saturation of hemoglobin measured by a pulse oximeter. Because the majority of oxygen carried in the blood is attached to hemoglobin within the red blood cell, SpO2 estimates how much hemoglobin is "saturated" with oxygen. The target range of SpO2 for an adult is 94-98%.[5] For patients with chronic respiratory conditions, such as COPD, the target range for SpO2 is often lower at 88% to 92%. Although SpO2 is an efficient, noninvasive method to assess a patient's oxygenation status, it is an estimate and not always accurate. For example, if a patient is severely anemic and has a decreased level of hemoglobin in the blood, the SpO2 reading is affected. Decreased peripheral circulation can also cause a misleading low SpO2 level.

A more specific measurement of oxygen and carbon dioxide in the blood is obtained through an **arterial blood gas (ABG)**. ABG results are often obtained for patients who have deteriorating or unstable respiratory status requiring urgent and emergency treatment. An ABG is a blood sample that is typically drawn from the radial artery by a respiratory therapist, emergency or critical care nurse, or health care provider. ABG results evaluate oxygen, carbon dioxide, pH, and bicarbonate levels. The partial pressure of oxygen in the blood is referred to as **PaO2**. The normal PaO2 level of a healthy adult is 80 to 100 mmHg. The PaO2 reading is more accurate than a SpO2 reading because it is not affected by hemoglobin levels. The **PaCO2** level is the partial pressure of carbon dioxide in the blood. The normal PaCO2 level of a healthy adult is 35-45 mmHg. The normal range of pH level for arterial blood is 7.35-7.45, and the normal range for the bicarbonate **(HCO3)** level is 22-26. The **SaO2** level is also obtained, which is the calculated arterial oxygen saturation level. See Table 11.2a for a summary of normal ranges of ABG values.[6]

Table 11.2a Normal Ranges of ABG Values

Value	Description	Normal Range
pH	Acid-base balance of blood	7.35-7.45
PaO2	Partial pressure of oxygen	80-100 mmHg
PaCO2	Partial pressure of carbon dioxide	35-45 mmHg
HCO3	Bicarbonate level	22-26 mEq/L
SaO2	Calculated oxygen saturation	95-100%

5 Hill, B., & Annesley, S. H. (2020). Monitoring respiratory rate in adults. *British Journal of Nursing, 29*(1), 12–16. https://doi.org/10.12968/bjon.2020.29.1.12

6 This work is a derivative of Clinical Procedures for Safer Patient Care by British Columbia Institute of Technology and is licensed under CC BY 4.0. Access for free at https://opentextbc.ca/clinicalskills/

Hypoxia and Hypercapnia

My Notes

Hypoxia is defined as a reduced level of tissue oxygenation. Hypoxia has many causes, ranging from respiratory and cardiac conditions to anemia. **Hypoxemia** is a specific type of hypoxia that is defined as decreased partial pressure of oxygen in the blood (PaO2), measured by an arterial blood gas (ABG).

Early signs of hypoxia are anxiety, confusion, and restlessness. As hypoxia worsens, the patient's level of consciousness and vital signs will worsen, with increased respiratory rate and heart rate and decreased pulse oximetry readings. Late signs of hypoxia include bluish discoloration of the skin and mucous membranes called **cyanosis**. Cyanosis is most easily seen around the lips and in the oral mucosa. A sign of chronic hypoxia is clubbing, a gradual enlargement of the fingertips (see Figure 11.1[7]). See Table 11.2b for symptoms and signs of hypoxia.[8]

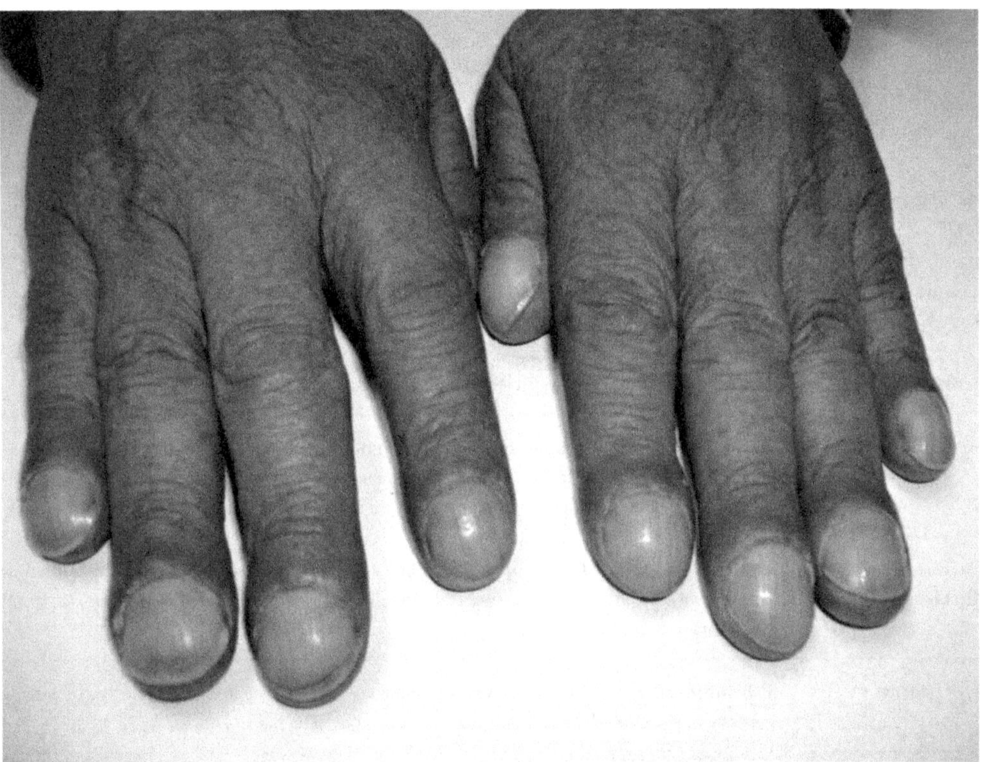

Figure 11.1 Clubbing of Fingertips

Hypercapnia is an elevated level of carbon dioxide in the blood. This level is measured by the PaCO2 level in an ABG test and is indicated when the PaCO2 level is higher than 45. Hypercapnia is typically caused by hypoventilation or areas of the alveoli that are ventilated but not perfused. In a state of hypercapnia or hypoventilation, there is an accumulation of carbon dioxide in the blood. The increased carbon dioxide causes the pH of the blood to drop, leading to a state of respiratory acidosis. You can read more about respiratory acidosis in the "Fluids and Electrolytes" chapter of the Open RN *Nursing Fundamentals* book. Patients with hypercapnia can present with

7 "Acopaquia.jpg" by Desherinka is licensed under CC BY-SA 4.0. Access for free at https://commons.wikimedia.org/wiki/File:Acopaquia.jpg

8 This work is a derivative of Clinical Procedures for Safer Patient Care by British Columbia Institute of Technology and is licensed under CC BY 4.0. Access for free at https://opentextbc.ca/clinicalskills/

My Notes

tachycardia, **dyspnea**, flushed skin, confusion, headaches, and dizziness. If the hypercapnia develops gradually over time, such as in a patient with chronic obstructive pulmonary disease (COPD), symptoms may be mild or may not be present at all. Hypercapnia is managed by addressing its underlying cause. A noninvasive positive pressure device such as a BiPAP may provide support to patients who are having trouble breathing normally, but if this is not sufficient, intubation may be required.[9]

Table 11.2b Symptoms and Signs of Hypoxia

Signs & Symptoms	Description
Restlessness	Patient may become increasingly fidgety, move about the bed, demonstrate signs of anxiety and agitation. Restlessness is an early sign of hypoxia.
Tachycardia	An elevated heart rate (above 100 beats per minute in adults) can be an early sign of hypoxia.
Tachypnea	An increased respiration rate (above 20 breaths per minute in adults) is an indication of respiratory distress.
Shortness of breath (Dyspnea)	Shortness of breath is a subjective symptom of not getting enough air. Depending on severity, dyspnea causes increased levels of anxiety.
Oxygen saturation level (SpO2)	Oxygen saturation levels should be above 94% for an adult without an underlying respiratory condition.
Use of accessory muscles	Use of neck or intercostal muscles when breathing is an indication of respiratory distress.
Noisy breathing	Audible noises with breathing are an indication of respiratory conditions. Assess lung sounds with a stethoscope for adventitious sounds such as wheezing, rales, or crackles. Secretions can plug the airway, thereby decreasing the amount of oxygen available for gas exchange in the lungs.
Flaring of nostrils or pursed lip breathing	Flaring is a sign of hypoxia, especially in infants. Pursed-lip breathing is a technique often used in patients with COPD. This breathing technique increases the amount of carbon dioxide exhaled so that more oxygen can be inhaled.
Position of patient	Patients in respiratory distress may sit up or lean over by resting arms on their legs to enhance lung expansion. Patients who are hypoxic may not be able to lie flat in bed.
Ability of patient to speak in full sentences	Patients in respiratory distress may be unable to speak in full sentences or may need to catch their breath between sentences.
Skin color (Cyanosis)	Changes in skin color to bluish or gray are a late sign of hypoxia.
Confusion or loss of consciousness (LOC)	This is a worsening sign of hypoxia.
Clubbing	Clubbing, a gradual enlargement of the fingertips, is a sign of chronic hypoxia.

9 This work is a derivative of StatPearls by Patel, Miao, Yetiskul, and Majmundar and is licensed under CC BY 4.0. Access for free at https://www.ncbi.nlm.nih.gov/books/NBK430685/

Treating Hypoxia

My Notes

Acute hypoxia is a medical emergency and should be treated promptly with oxygen therapy. Failure to initiate oxygen therapy when needed can result in serious harm or death of the patient. Although oxygen is considered a medication that requires a prescription, oxygen therapy may be initiated without a physician's order in emergency situations as part of the nurse's response to the "ABCs," a common abbreviation for airway, breathing, and circulation. Most agencies have a protocol in place that allows nurses to apply oxygen in emergency situations. After applying oxygen as needed, the nurse then contacts the provider, respiratory therapist, or rapid response team, depending on the severity of hypoxia.

Devices such high flow oxymasks, CPAP, BiPAP, or mechanical ventilation may be initiated by the respiratory therapist or provider to deliver higher amounts of inspired oxygen. Various types of oxygenation devices are further explained in the "Oxygenation Equipment" section.

Prescription orders for oxygen therapy will include two measurements of oxygen to be delivered – the oxygen flow rate and the fraction of inspired oxygen (FiO2). The oxygen flow rate is the number dialed up on the oxygen flow meter between 1 L/minute and 15 L/minute. **Fio2** is the concentration of oxygen the patient inhales. Room air contains 21% oxygen concentration, so the FiO2 for supplementary oxygen therapy will range from 21% to 100% concentration.

In addition to administering oxygen therapy, there are several other interventions the nurse should consider implementing to a hypoxic patient. Additional interventions used to treat hypoxia in conjunction with oxygen therapy are outlined in Table 11.2c.[10]

Table 11.2c Interventions to Manage Hypoxia

Interventions	Additional Information
Raise the Head of the Bed	Raising the head of the bed to high Fowler's position promotes effective chest expansion and diaphragmatic descent, maximizes inhalation, and decreases the work of breathing. Patients with COPD who are short of breath may gain relief by sitting upright or leaning over a bedside table while in bed.
Encourage Enhanced Breathing and Coughing Techniques	Enhanced breathing and coughing techniques such as using pursed-lip breathing, coughing and deep breathing, huffing technique, incentive spirometry, and flutter valves may assist patients to clear their airway while maintaining their oxygen levels. See the following "Enhanced Breathing and Coughing Techniques" section for additional information regarding these techniques.
Manage Oxygen Therapy and Equipment	If the patient is already on supplemental oxygen, ensure the equipment is turned on, set at the required flow rate, correctly positioned on the patient, and properly connected to an oxygen supply source. If a portable tank is being used, check the oxygen level in the tank. Ensure the connecting oxygen tubing is not kinked, which could obstruct the flow of oxygen. Feel for the flow of oxygen from the exit ports on the oxygen equipment. In hospitals where medical air and oxygen are used, ensure the patient is connected to the oxygen flow port. Hospitals in America follow the national standard that oxygen flow ports are green and air outlets are yellow.

10 This work is a derivative of Clinical Procedures for Safer Patient Care by British Columbia Institute of Technology and is licensed under CC BY 4.0. Access for free at https://opentextbc.ca/clinicalskills/

My Notes

Interventions	Additional Information
Assess the Need for Respiratory Medications	Pharmacological management is essential for patients with respiratory disease such as asthma, COPD, or severe allergic response. Bronchodilators effectively relax smooth muscles and open airways. Glucocorticoids relieve inflammation and also assist in opening air passages. Mucolytics decrease the thickness of pulmonary secretions so that they can be expectorated more easily.
Provide Oral Suctioning if Needed	Some patients may have a weakened cough that inhibits their ability to clear secretions from the mouth and throat. Patients with muscle disorders or those who have experienced a cerebral vascular accident (CVA) are at risk for aspiration pneumonia, which is caused by the accidental inhalation of material from the mouth or stomach. Provide oral suction if the patient is unable to clear secretions from the mouth and pharynx. See the chapter on "Tracheostomy Care and Suctioning" for additional details on suctioning.
Provide Pain Relief If Needed	Provide adequate pain relief if the patient is reporting pain. Pain increases anxiety and may inhibit the patient's ability to take in full breaths.
Consider the Side Effects of Pain Medications	A common side effect of pain medication is sedation and respiratory depression. For more information about interventions to manage respiratory depression, see the "Oxygenation" chapter in the Open RN *Nursing Fundamentals* textbook.
Consider Other Devices to Enhance Clearance of Secretions	Chest physiotherapy and specialized devices assist with secretion clearance, such as handheld flutter valves or vests that inflate and vibrate the chest wall. Consider requesting a consultation with a respiratory therapist based on the patient's situation.
Plan Frequent Rest Periods Between Activities	Patients experiencing hypoxia often feel short of breath and fatigue easily. Allow the patient to rest frequently, and space out interventions to decrease oxygen demand in patients whose reserves are likely limited.
Consider Other Potential Causes of Dyspnea	If a patient's level of dyspnea is worsening, assess for other underlying causes in addition to the primary diagnosis. Are there other respiratory, cardiovascular, or hematological conditions such as anemia occurring? Start by reviewing the patient's most recent hemoglobin and hematocrit lab results. Completing a thorough assessment may reveal abnormalities in these systems to report to the health care provider.
Consider Obstructive Sleep Apnea	Patients with obstructive sleep apnea (OSA) are often not previously diagnosed prior to hospitalization. The nurse may notice the patient snores, has pauses in breathing while snoring, or awakens not feeling rested. These signs may indicate the patient is unable to maintain an open airway while sleeping, resulting in periods of apnea and hypoxia. If these apneic periods are noticed but have not been previously documented, the nurse should report these findings to the health care provider for further testing and follow-up. Testing consists of using continuous pulse oximetry while the patient is sleeping to determine if the patient is hypoxic during these episodes and if a CPAP device should be prescribed. See the box below for additional information regarding OSA.
Anxiety	Anxiety often accompanies the feeling of dyspnea and can worsen it. Anxiety in patients with COPD is chronically undertreated. It is important for the nurse to address the feelings of anxiety and dyspnea. Anxiety can be relieved by teaching enhanced breathing and coughing techniques, encouraging relaxation techniques, or administering antianxiety medications.

My Notes

Obstructive Sleep Apnea (OSA) is the most common type of sleep apnea. See Figure 11.2[11] for an illustration of OSA. As soft tissue falls to the back of the throat, it impedes the passage of air (blue arrows) through the trachea and is characterized by repeated episodes of complete or partial obstructions of the upper airway during sleep. The episodes of breathing cessations are called "apneas," meaning "without breath." Despite the effort to breathe, apneas are associated with a reduction in blood oxygen saturation due to the obstruction of the airway. Treatment for OSA often includes the use of a CPAP device.

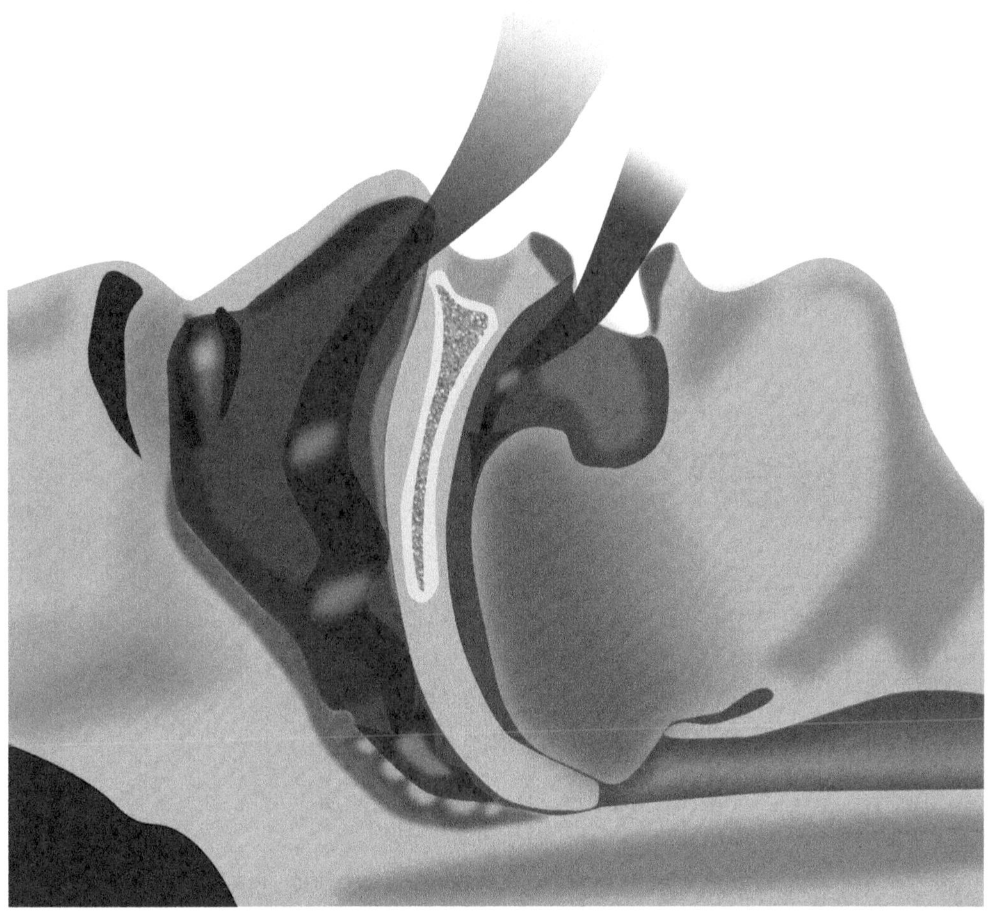

Figure 11.2 Obstructive Sleep Apnea

Enhanced Breathing and Coughing Techniques

In addition to oxygen therapy and the interventions listed in Table 11.2c to implement for a patient experiencing dyspnea and hypoxia, there are several techniques a nurse can teach a patient to use to enhance their breathing

11 "Obstruction ventilation apnée sommeil.svg" by Habib M'henni is in the Public Domain. Access for free at https://commons.wikimedia.org/wiki/File:Obstruction_ventilation_apnée_sommeil.svg

My Notes

and coughing. These techniques include pursed-lip breathing, incentive spirometry, coughing and deep breathing, and the huffing technique.

Pursed-Lip Breathing

Pursed-lip breathing is a technique that allows people to control their oxygenation and ventilation. The technique requires a person to inspire through the nose and exhale through the mouth at a slow controlled flow. See Figure 11.3[12] for an illustration of pursed-lip breathing. This type of exhalation gives the person a puckered or pursed appearance. By prolonging the expiratory phase of respiration, a small amount of positive end-expiratory pressure (PEEP) is created in the airways that helps to keep them open so that more air can be exhaled, thus reducing air trapping that occurs in some conditions such as COPD. Pursed-lip breathing often relieves the feeling of shortness of breath, decreases the work of breathing, and improves gas exchange. People also regain a sense of control over their breathing while simultaneously increasing their relaxation.[13]

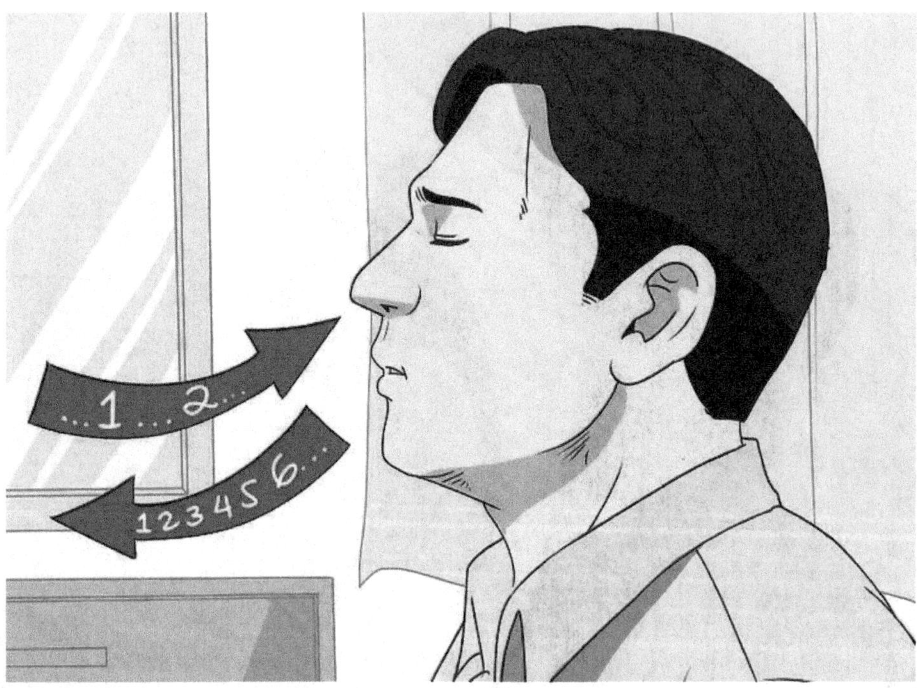

Figure 11.3 Pursed-Lip Breathing

View the COPD Foundation's YouTube video to learn more about pursed-lip breathing: Breathing Techniques.[14]

12 This work is derivative of "aid611002-v4-728px-Live-With-Chronic-Obstructive-Pulmonary-Disease-Step-8.jpg" by unknown and is licensed under CC BY-NC-SA 3.0. Access for free at https://www.wikihow.com/Live-With-Chronic-Obstructive-Pulmonary-Disease.

13 This work is a derivative of StatPearls by Nguyen and Duong and is licensed under CC BY 4.0. Access for free at https://www.ncbi.nlm.nih.gov/books/NBK430685/

14 COPD Foundation. (2020, April 17). Breathing techniques. [Video]. YouTube. All rights reserved. https://youtu.be/ZJPJjZRHmy8

Incentive Spirometry

My Notes

An incentive spirometer is a medical device often prescribed after surgery to prevent and treat atelectasis. Atelectasis occurs when alveoli become deflated or filled with fluid and can lead to pneumonia. See Figure 11.4[15] for an image of a patient using an incentive spirometer. While sitting upright, the patient should breathe in slowly and deeply through the tubing with the goal of raising the piston to a specified level. The patient should attempt to hold their breath for 5 seconds, or as long as tolerated, and then rest for a few seconds. This technique should be repeated by the patient 10 times every hour while awake.[16] The nurse may delegate this intervention to unlicensed assistive personnel, but the frequency in which it is completed and the volume achieved should be documented and monitored by the nurse.

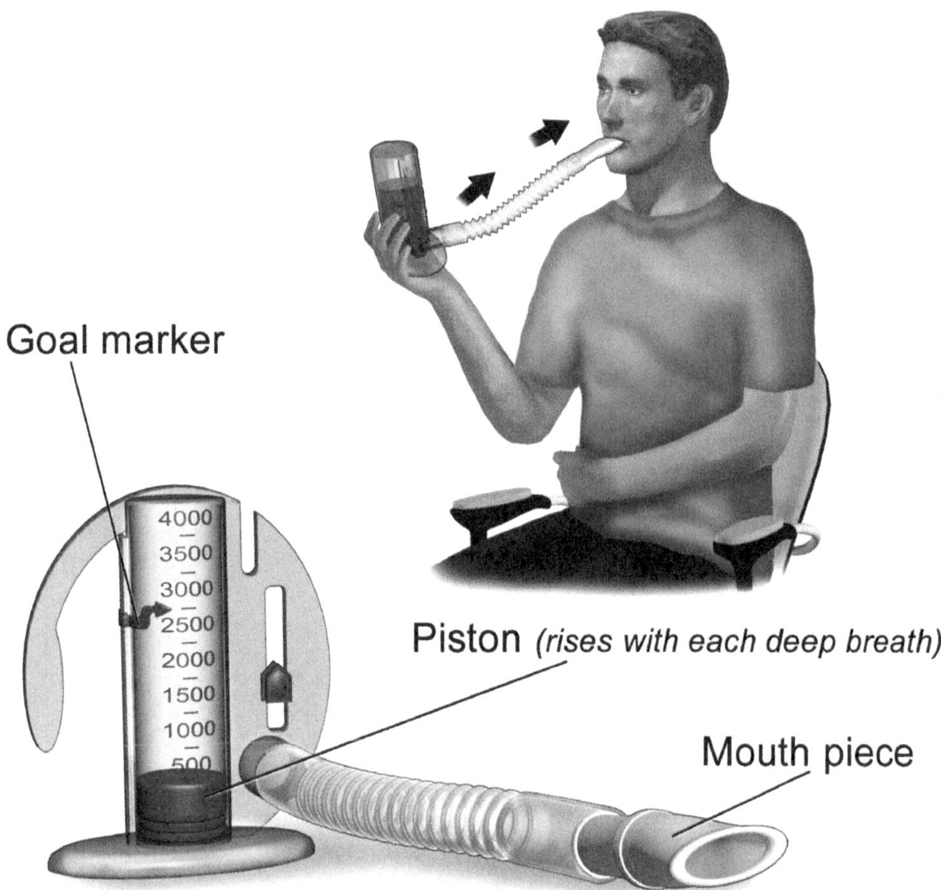

Figure 11.4 Using an Incentive Spirometer

15 "Incentive Spirometer.pngsommeil.svg" by BruceBlaus is licensed under CC BY-SA 4.0. Access for free at https://commons.wikimedia.org/wiki/File:Incentive_Spirometer.png

16 Cleveland Clinic. (2018, May 2). *Incentive spirometer.* https://my.clevelandclinic.org/health/articles/4302-incentive-spirometer

My Notes

Coughing and Deep Breathing

Teaching the coughing and deep breathing technique is similar to incentive spirometry but no device is required. The patient is encouraged to take deep, slow breaths and then exhale slowly. After each set of breaths, the patient should cough. This technique is repeated 3 to 5 times every hour.

Huffing Technique

The huffing technique is helpful for patients who have difficulty coughing. Teach the patient to inhale with a medium-sized breath and then make a sound like "Ha" to push the air out quickly with the mouth slightly open.

Vibratory PEP Therapy

Vibratory Positive Expiratory Pressure (PEP) therapy uses handheld devices such as "flutter valves" or "Acapella" devices for patients who need assistance in clearing mucus from their airways. These devices (see Figure 11.5[17]) require a prescription and are used in collaboration with a respiratory therapist or advanced health care provider. To use Vibratory PEP therapy, the patient should sit up, take a deep breath, and blow into the device. A flutter valve within the device creates vibrations that help break up the mucus so the patient can cough it up and spit it out. Additionally, a small amount of positive end-expiratory pressure (PEEP) is created in the airways that helps to keep them open so that more air can be exhaled.

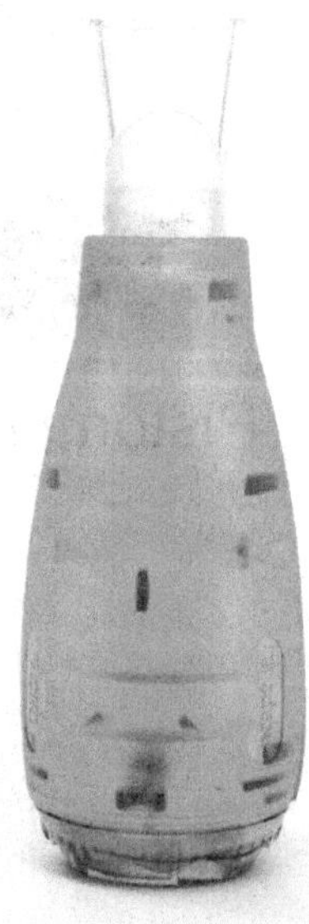

Figure 11.5 Flutter Valve Device

---

17 "Flutter Valve Breathing Device 3I3A0982.jpg" by Deanna Hoyord, Chippewa Valley Technical College is licensed under CC BY 4.0. Access for free at https://drive.google.com/file/d/1u6RY0DHrx9-pw71Mtp1DiOc1kv9w_43M/view?usp=sharing

My Notes

Visit NHS University Hospitals Plymouth Physiotherapy's "Acapella" video on YouTube to review using a flutter valve device.[18]

18 NHS University Hospitals Plymouth Physiotherapy. (2015, May 12). *Acapella.* [Video]. YouTube. https://youtu.be/XOvonQVCE6Y

My Notes

11.3 OXYGENATION EQUIPMENT

There are several types of equipment a nurse may use when providing oxygen therapy to a patient. Each device is described in detail below.

Pulse Oximeter

A pulse oximeter is a commonly used portable device used to obtain a patient's oxygen saturation level at the bedside or in a clinic. See Figure 11.6[1] for an image of a portable pulse oximeter. The pulse oximeter, commonly referred to as a "Pulse Ox," is an electronic device that measures the oxygen saturation of hemoglobin in a patient's red blood cells, referred to as SpO2. The normal range for SpO2 for an adult without an underlying respiratory condition is above 92%. The pulse oximeter analyzes light produced by the probe as it passes through the finger to determine the saturation level of the hemoglobin molecule. Pulse oximeter probes can be attached to a patient's finger, forehead, nose, foot, ear, or toe. However, pulse oximetry readings can be inaccurate if the patient is wearing nail polish, has reduced perfusion of the extremities due to a cardiovascular condition, or has other molecules attached to hemoglobin such as in the case of carbon monoxide poisoning.[2]

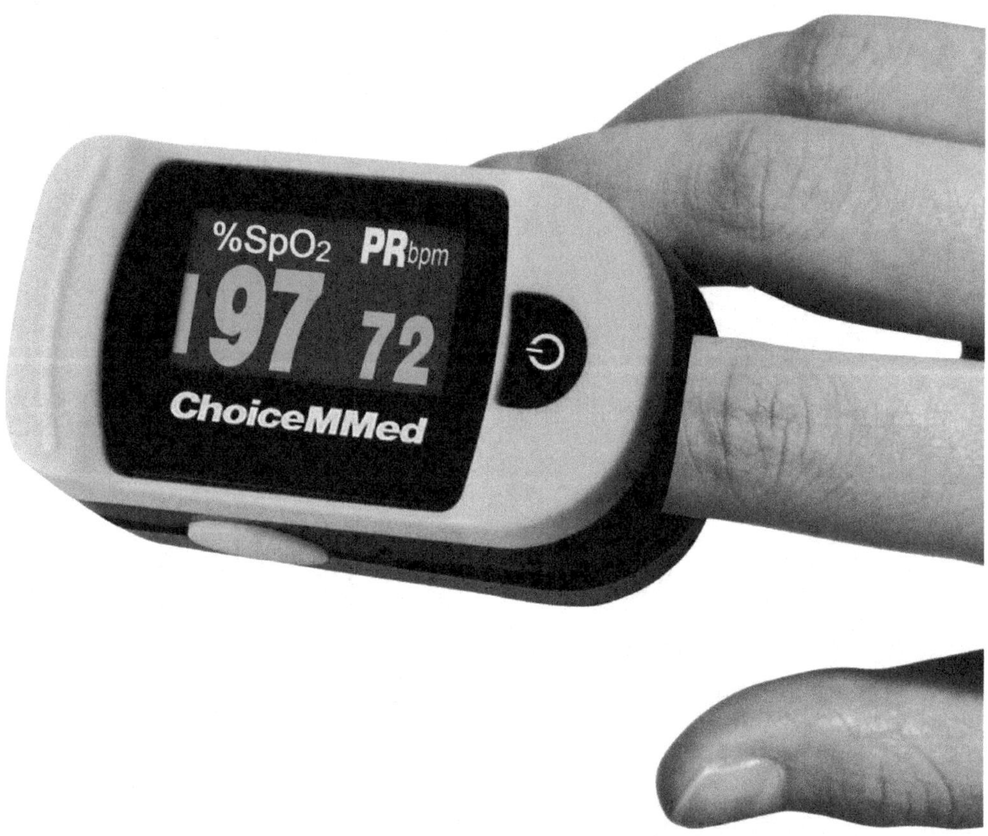

Figure 11.6 Portable Pulse Oximeter

1 "OxyWatch_C20_Pulse_Oximeter.png" by *Thinkpaul* is licensed under CC BY-SA 3.0. Access for free at https://commons.wikimedia.org/wiki/File:OxyWatch_C20_Pulse_Oximeter.png

2 American Lung Association. (2020, May 27). *Pulse oximetry*. https://www.lung.org/lung-health-diseases/lung-procedures-and-tests/pulse-oximetry

Oxygen Flow Meter

My Notes

In inpatient settings, rooms are equipped with wall-mounted oxygen supply outlets that are nationally standardized in a green color, whereas air outlets are standardized with a yellow color. Oxygen flow meters are attached to the green oxygen outlets, and then the oxygenation device is attached to the flow meter. See Figure 11.7[3] for an image of an oxygen flow meter. An oxygen flow meter consists of a glass cylinder containing a steel ball with an opening through which oxygen from the supply source is injected through an adapter. This adapter is commonly referred to as a "tree" because of its appearance. Oxygen is turned on, and the flow rate of oxygen is controlled by turning the green valve on the side of the glass cylinder. The flow rate is set according to the location of a steel ball inside the cylinder and the numbered lines on the glass cylinder. For example, in Figure 11.7, the flow rate is currently set at 2 liter per minute (L/min). It is essential to implement safety precautions whenever oxygen is used. Read more about "Safety with Oxygen Therapy" later in this section.

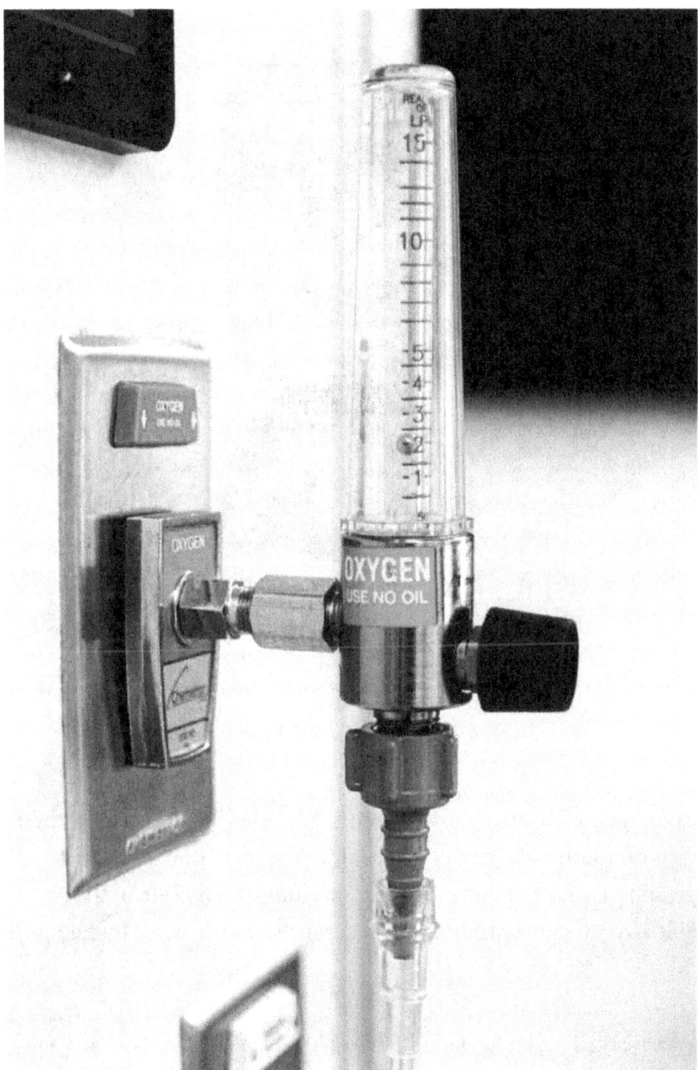

Figure 11.7 Oxygen Flow Meter

3 "Oxygen Regulator3I3A1063.jpg" by Deanna Hoyord, Chippewa Valley Technical College is licensed under CC BY 4.0. Access for free at https://drive.google.com/file/d/1SmRsl6JBNSH_DR6JCB7ZcDKzm2Kn59J1/view?usp=sharing

My Notes

Portable Oxygen Supply Devices

Portable oxygen tanks are commonly used when transporting a patient to procedures within the hospital or to other agencies. See Figure 11.8[4] for an image of a portable oxygen tank. Oxygenation devices are connected to the tank in a similar manner as the wall-mounted oxygen flow meter. It is crucial for nurses and transporters to ensure the tank has an adequate amount of oxygen for use during transport, is turned on, and the appropriate flow rate is set.

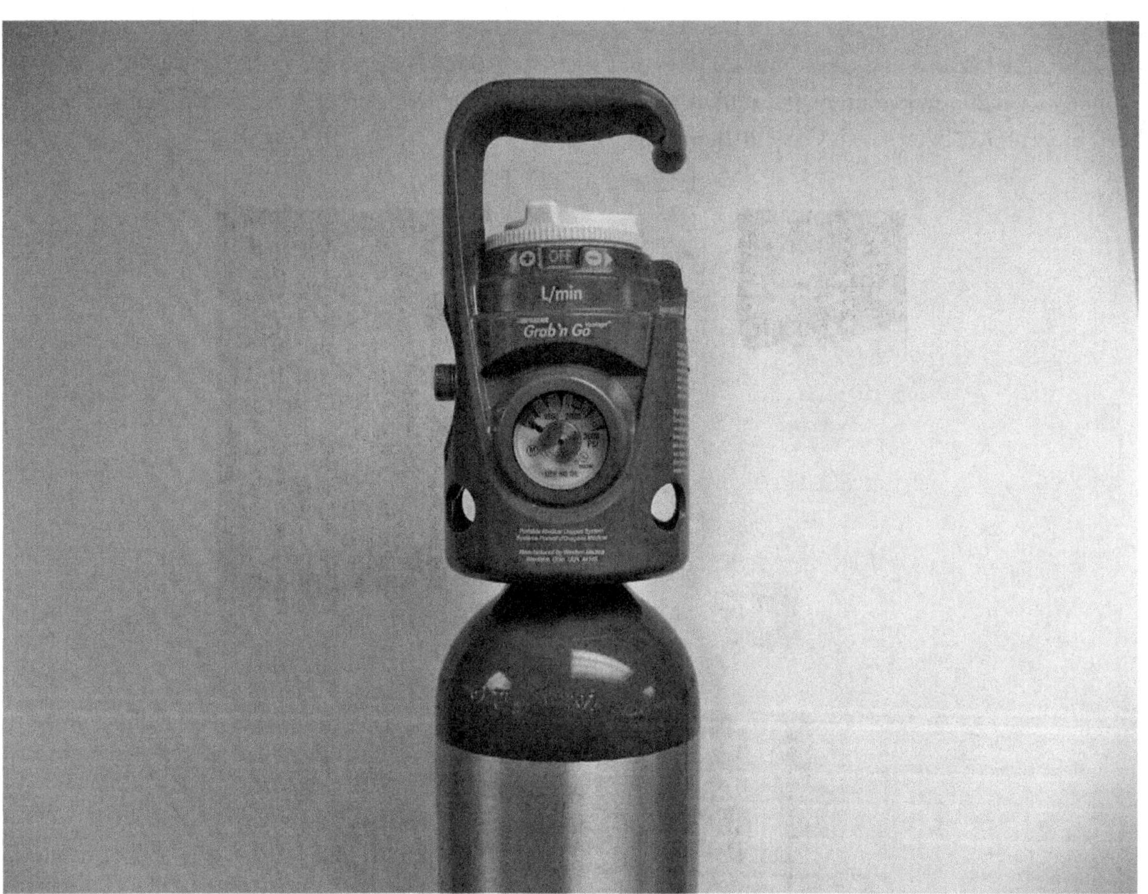

Figure 11.8 Portable Oxygen Tank

Instead of oxygen tanks, oxygen concentrators are commonly used by patients in their home environment. See Figure 11.9[5] for an image of a home oxygen concentrator. Oxygen concentrators are also produced in portable sizes that are lightweight and easy for patient use while travelling and mobile in the community. See Figure 11.10[6] for an image of a portable oxygen concentrator. Oxygen concentrators work by taking the 21% concentration of

---

4 "RECALLED_–_Portable_oxygen_cylinder_units_(8294127015).jpg" by The U.S. Food and Drug Administration is in the Public Domain. Access for free at https://commons.wikimedia.org/wiki/File:RECALLED_–_Portable_oxygen_cylinder_units_(8294127015).jpg

5 "Invacare Perfecto 2 Oxygen Concentrator.JPG" by BrokenSphere / Wikimedia Commons is licensed under CC BY-SA 3.0. Access for free at https://commons.wikimedia.org/wiki/File:Invacare_Perfecto_2_Oxygen_Concentrator.JPG

6 "Portable Oxygen Concentrator by Inogen.jpg" by Oxystore is licensed under CC BY-SA 4.0. Access for free at https://en.wikipedia.org/wiki/File:Portable_Oxygen_Concentrator_by_Inogen.jpg

oxygen in the air, running it through a molecular sleeve to remove the nitrogen and concentrating the oxygen to a 96% level, thus producing between 1 and 6 liters per minute of oxygen. Oxygen concentrators may provide pulse flow or continuous flow. Pulse flow only occurs on inhalation, whereas continuous flow delivers oxygen throughout the entire breath cycle. Pulse versions are the most lightweight because oxygen is provided only as needed by the patient.[7]

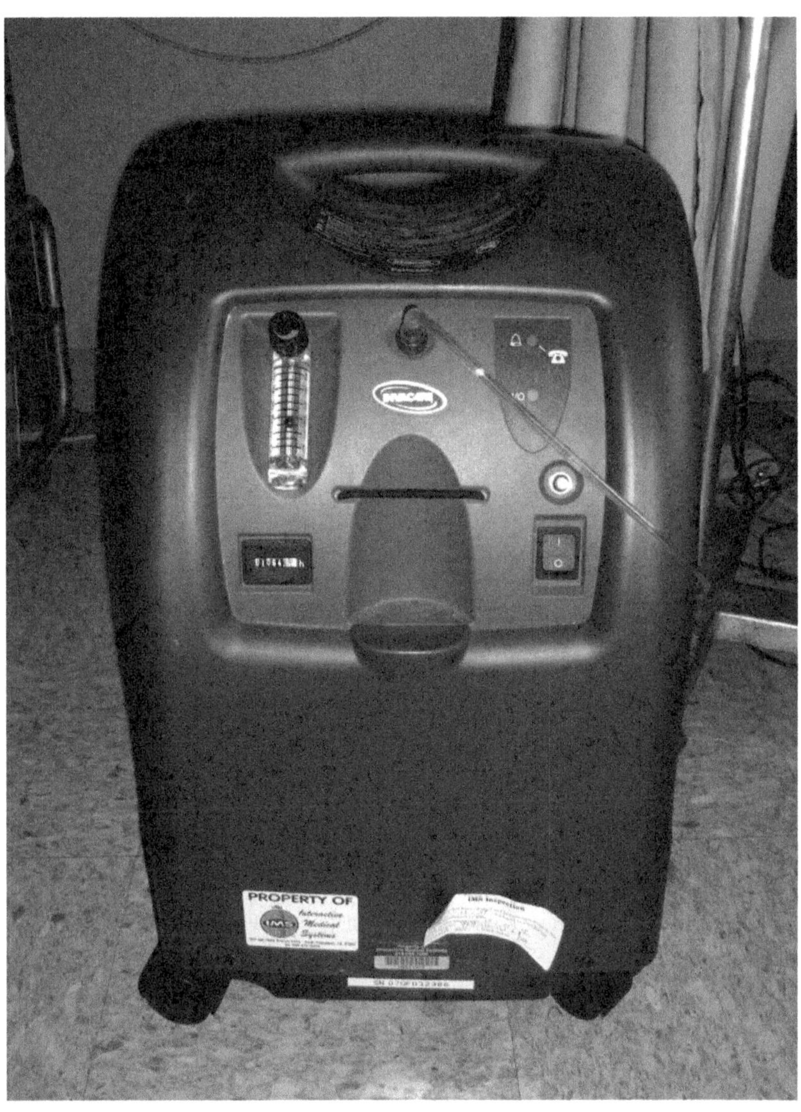

Figure 11.9 Home Oxygen Concentrator

7 Gibson, C. M. (Ed.). *Portable oxygen concentrator.* WikiDoc. https://www.wikidoc.org/index.php/Portable_oxygen_concentrator

My Notes

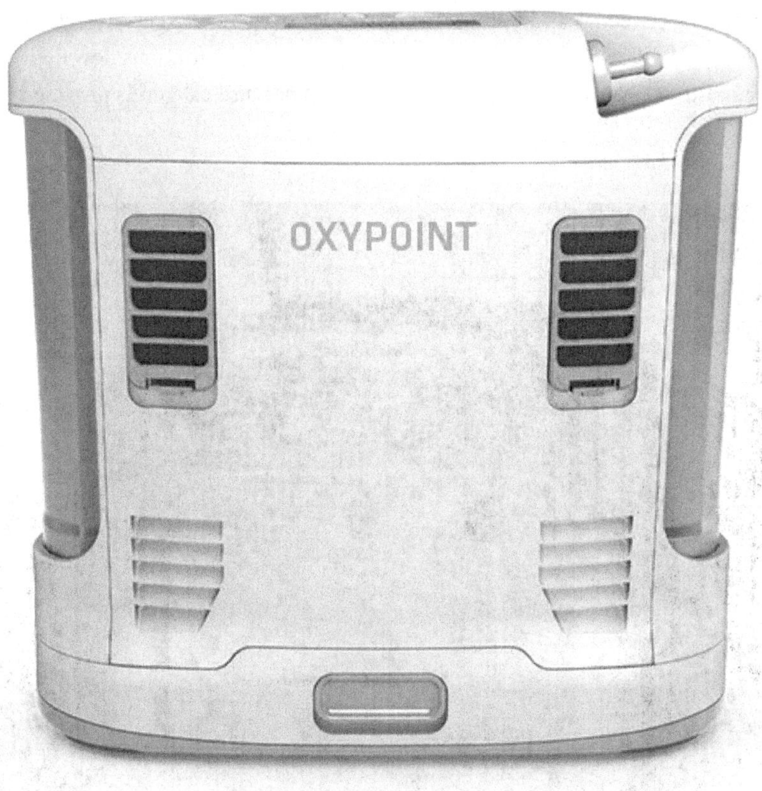

Figure 11.10 Portable Oxygen Concentrator

Nasal Cannula

A nasal cannula is the simplest oxygenation device and consists of oxygen tubing connected to two short prongs that are inserted into the patient's nares. See Figure 11.11[8] for an image of a nasal cannula. The tubing is connected to the flow meter of the oxygen supply source. To prevent drying out the patient's mucus membranes, humidification may be added for hospitalized patients receiving oxygen flow rates greater than 4 L/minute or for those receiving oxygen therapy for longer periods of time.[9]

Nasal cannulas are the most common type of oxygen equipment. They are used for short- and long-term therapy (i.e., COPD patients) and are best used with stable patients who require low amounts of oxygen.

Flow rate: Nasal cannulas can have a flow rate ranging from 1 to 5 liters per minute (L/min), with a 4% increase in FiO2 for every liter of oxygen, resulting in range of fraction of inspired oxygen (FiO2) levels of 24-44%.

---

8 "Image00011.jpg" by British Columbia Institute of Technology is licensed under CC BY 4.0. Access for free at https://opentextbc.ca/clinicalskills/chapter/5-5-oxygen-therapy-systems/

9 Duck, A. (2009, December 14). *Does oxygen need humidification?* https://www.nursingtimes.net/clinical-archive/respiratory-clinical-archive/does-oxygen-need-humidification-14-12-2009/

My Notes

Advantages: Nasal cannulas are easy to use, inexpensive, and disposable. They are convenient because the patient can talk and eat while receiving oxygen.

Limitations: The nasal prongs of nasal cannula are easily dislodged, especially when the patient is sleeping. The tubing placed on the face can cause skin breakdown in the nose and above the ears, so the nurse must vigilantly monitor these areas. Based on agency policy, the nurse should add padding to the oxygen tubing as needed to avoid skin breakdown and may apply a water-based lubricant to prevent drying. However, petroleum-based lubricant should not be used due to the risk of flammability. Nasal cannulas are not as effective if the patient is a mouth breather or has blocked nostrils, a deviated septum, or nasal polyps.[10]

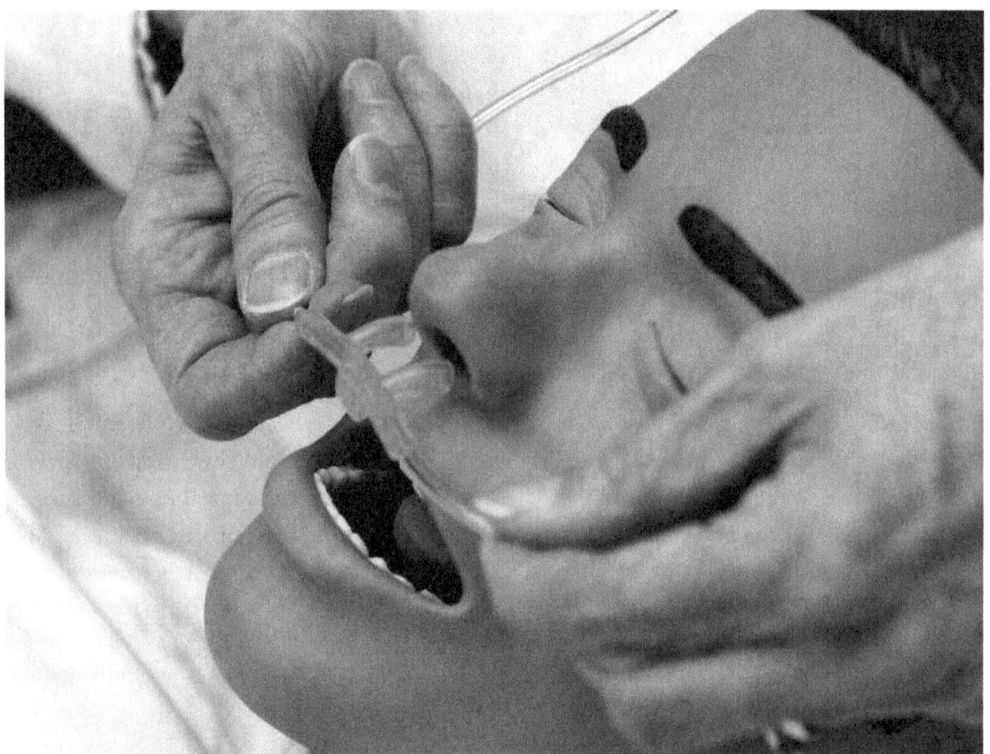

Figure 11.11 Nasal Cannula

High-Flow Nasal Cannula

High-flow nasal cannula therapy is an oxygen supply system capable of delivering up to 100% humidified and heated oxygen at a flow rate of up to 60 liters per minute.[11] Patients with high-flow nasal cannulas are generally in critical condition and require advanced monitoring. See Figure 11.12[12] for an illustration of a high-flow nasal cannula system that is initially set up by a respiratory therapist and then maintained by a nurse.

---

10 This work is a derivative of Clinical Procedures for Safer Patient Care by British Columbia Institute of Technology and is licensed under CC BY 4.0. Access for free at https://opentextbc.ca/clinicalskills/

11 This work is a derivative of StatPearls by Sharma, Danckers, Sanghavi, and Chakraborty and is licensed under CC BY 4.0. Access for free at https://www.ncbi.nlm.nih.gov/books/NBK430685/

12 "HFT diagram.png" by *Strangecow* is in the Public Domain. Access for free at https://en.wikipedia.org/wiki/File:HFT_diagram.png

My Notes

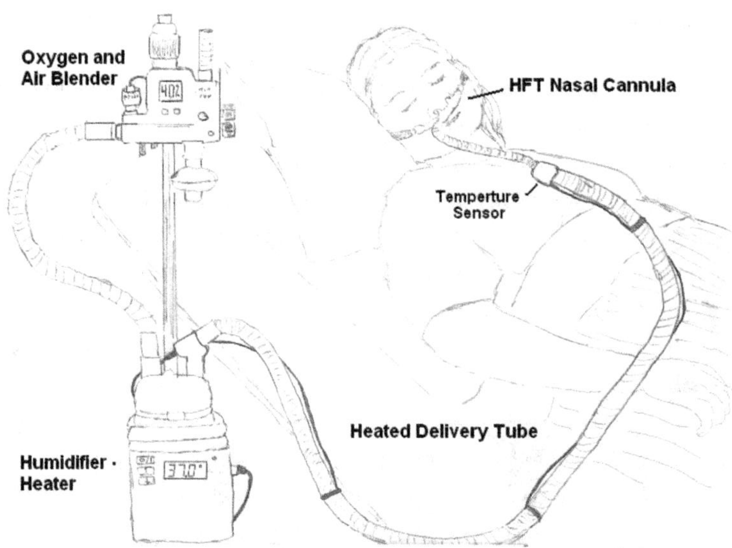

Figure 11.12 High-Flow Nasal Cannula System

Simple Mask

A simple mask fits over the mouth and nose of the patient and contains exhalation ports (i.e., holes on the side of the mask) through which the patient exhales carbon dioxide. These holes should always remain open. The mask is held in place by an elastic band placed around the back of the head. It also has a metal piece near the top that can be pinched and shaped over the patient's nose to create a better fit. Humidified air may be attached if the oxygen concentrations are drying for the patient. See Figure 11.13[13] for an image of a simple face mask.

Flow Rate: Simple masks should be set to a flow rate of 6 to 10 L/min, resulting in oxygen concentration (FiO2) levels of 35%-50%. The flow rate should never be set below 6 L/min because this can result in the patient rebreathing their exhaled carbon dioxide.

Advantages: Face masks are used to provide moderate oxygen concentrations. Their efficiency in oxygen delivery depends on how well the mask fits and the patient's respiratory demands.

Disadvantages: Face masks must be removed when eating, and they may feel confining for some patients who feel claustrophobic with the mask on.[14]

13 "DSC_2086.jpg" by British Columbia Institute of Technology is licensed under CC BY 4.0. Access for free at https://opentextbc.ca/clinicalskills/chapter/5-5-oxygen-therapy-systems/

14 This work is a derivative of Clinical Procedures for Safer Patient Care by British Columbia Institute of Technology is licensed under CC BY 4.0. Access for free at https://opentextbc.ca/clinicalskills/

My Notes

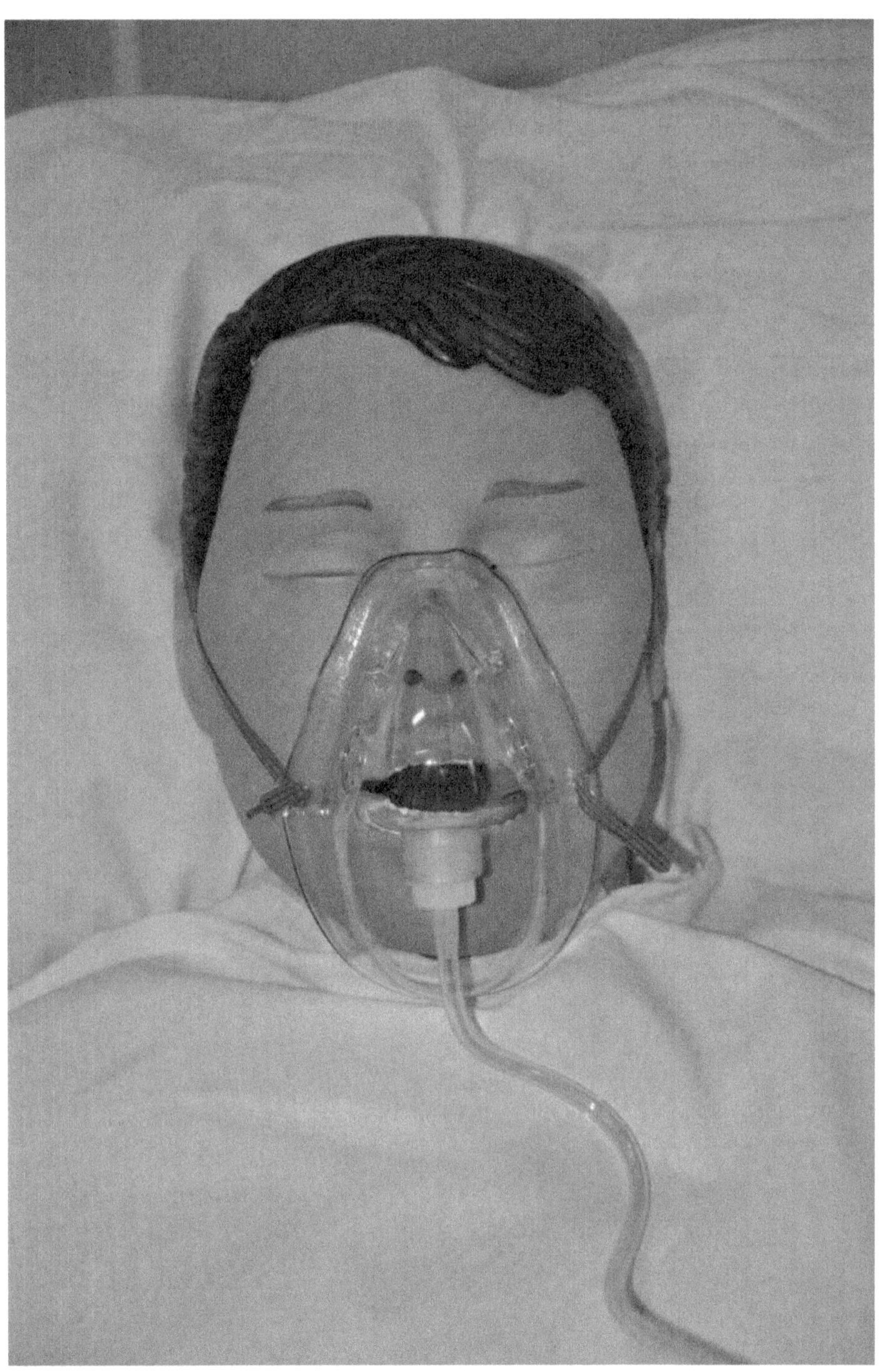

Figure 11.13 Simple Face Mask

My Notes

Non-Rebreather Mask

A non-rebreather mask consists of a mask attached to a reservoir bag that is attached with tubing to a flow meter. See Figure 11.14[15] for an image of a non-rebreather mask. It has a series of one-way valves between the mask and the bag and also on the covers on the exhalation ports. The reservoir bag should never totally deflate; if the bag deflates, there is a problem and immediate intervention is required. The one-way valves function so that on inspiration, the patient only breathes in from the reservoir bag; on exhalation, carbon dioxide is directed out through the exhalation ports. Non-rebreather masks are used for patients who can breathe on their own but require higher concentrations of oxygen to maintain satisfactory blood oxygenation levels.

Flow rate: The flow rate for a non-rebreather mask should be set to deliver a **minimum** of 10 to 15 L/minute. The reservoir bag should be inflated prior to placing the mask on the patient. With a good fit, the non-rebreather mask can deliver between 60% and 80% FiO2.

Advantages: Non-rebreather masks deliver high levels of oxygen noninvasively to patients who can otherwise breathe unassisted.

Disadvantages: Due to the one-way valves in non-rebreather masks, there is a high risk of suffocation if the gas flow is interrupted. The mask requires a tight seal and may feel hot and confining to the patient. It will interfere with talking, and the patient cannot eat with the mask on.

15 "DSC_2083.jpg" by British Columbia Institute of Technology is licensed under CC BY 4.0. Access for free at https://opentextbc.ca/clinicalskills/chapter/5-5-oxygen-therapy-systems/

My Notes

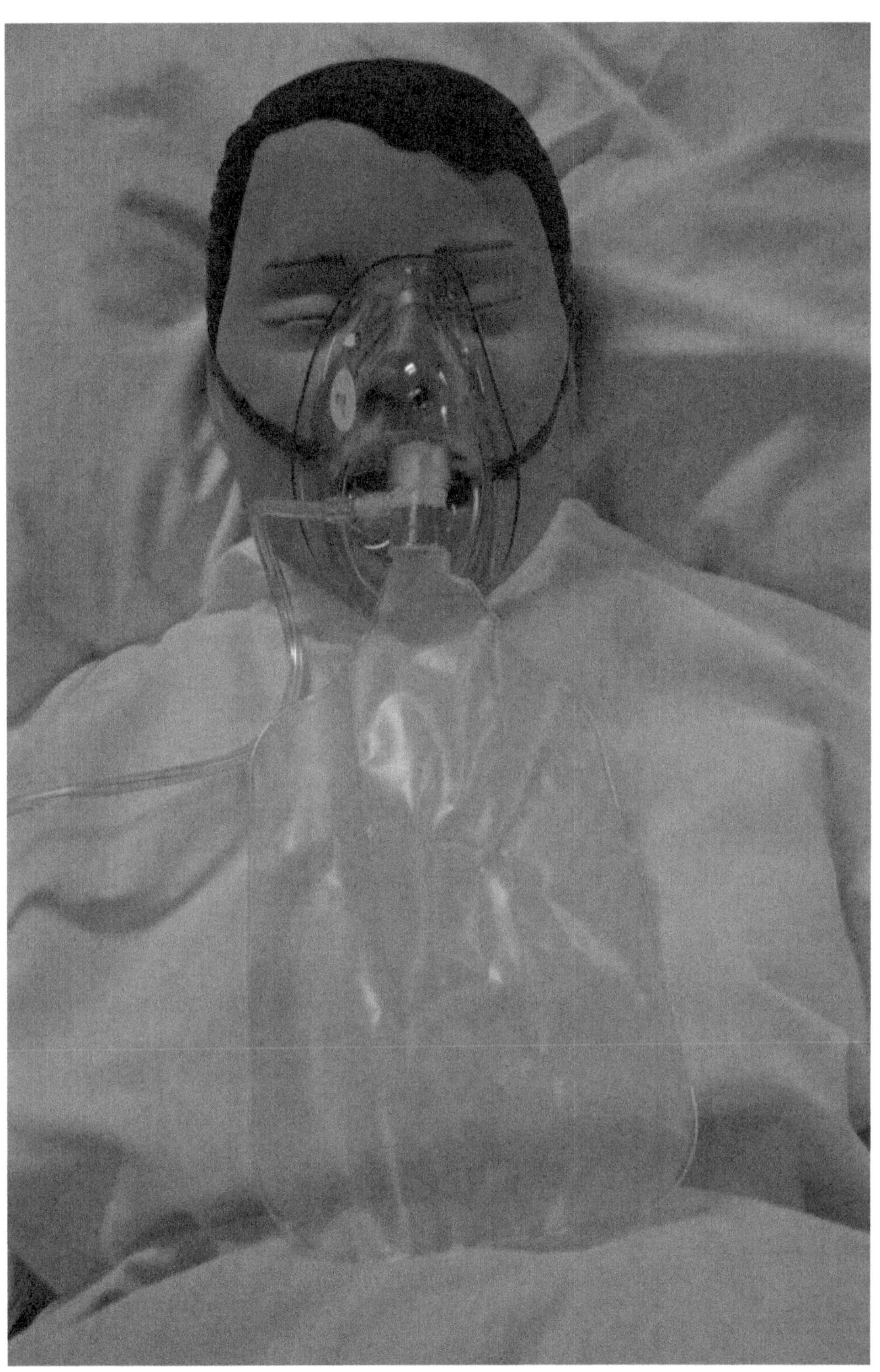

Figure 11.14 Non-Rebreather Mask

My Notes

Partial Rebreather Mask

The partial rebreather mask looks very similar to the non-rebreather mask. The difference between the masks is a partial rebreather mask does not contain one-way valves, so the patient's exhaled air mixes with their inhaled air. A partial rebreather mask requires 10-15 L/min of oxygen, but only delivers 35-50% FiO2.

Venturi Mask

Venturi masks are indicated for patients who require a specific amount of supplemental oxygen to avoid complications, such as those with chronic obstructive pulmonary disease (COPD). Different types of adaptors are attached to a face mask that set the flow rate to achieve a specific FiO2 ranging from 24% to 60%. Venturi adapters are typically set up by a respiratory therapist, but in some facilities they may be set up by a nurse according to agency policy.

Flow rate: The flow rate depends on the adaptor and does not correspond to the flow meter. Consult with a respiratory therapist before changing the flow rate.

Advantages: A specific amount of FiO2 is delivered to patients whose breathing status may be affected by high levels of oxygen.

Continuous Positive Airway Pressure (CPAP)

A continuous positive airway pressure (CPAP) device is used for people who are able to breathe spontaneously on their own but need help in keeping their airway unobstructed, such as those with obstructive sleep apnea. (See Table 11.2c in the "Basic Concepts of Oxygenation" section for more information about obstructive sleep apnea.) The CPAP device consists of a special mask that covers the patient's nose, or nose and mouth, and is attached to a machine that continuously applies mild air pressure to keep the patient's airways from collapsing.

A prescription is required for a CPAP device in the hospital or patient's home environment. In the hospital, the FiO2 is set up with the CPAP mask by the respiratory therapist. In a home setting, an adapter is added so that oxygen is attached using a flowmeter with preprogrammed settings so the patient and/or nurse are only required to turn the machine on before sleeping and off upon awakening. It is important to keep the mask and tubing clean to prevent infection, so be sure to follow agency policy for cleaning the equipment regularly. If a humidifier is attached, distilled water or sterile water should be used to fill it, but never tap water. See Figure 11.15[16] for an illustration of a patient wearing a CPAP device while sleeping.

---

16 "Depiction of a sleep apnea patient using a CPAP machine" by https://www.myupchar.com/en is licensed under CC BY 4.0. Access for free at https://commons.wikimedia.org/wiki/File:Depiction_of_a_Sleep_Apnea_patient_using_a_CPAP_machine.png

My Notes

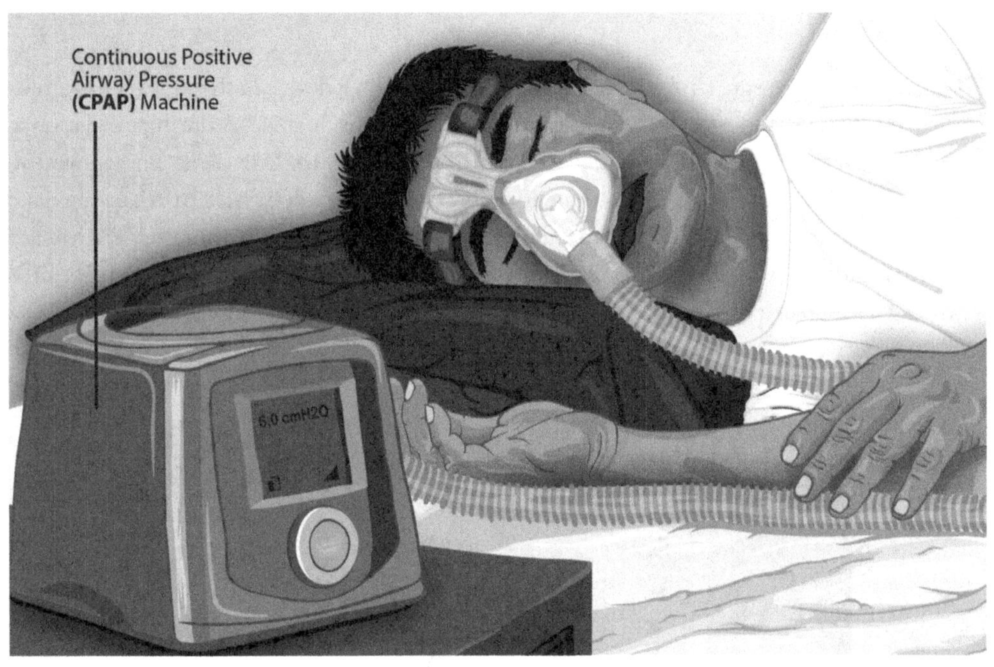

Figure 11.15 CPAP Machine

Video Review of FDA Recommendations on How to Use a CPAP Mask[17]

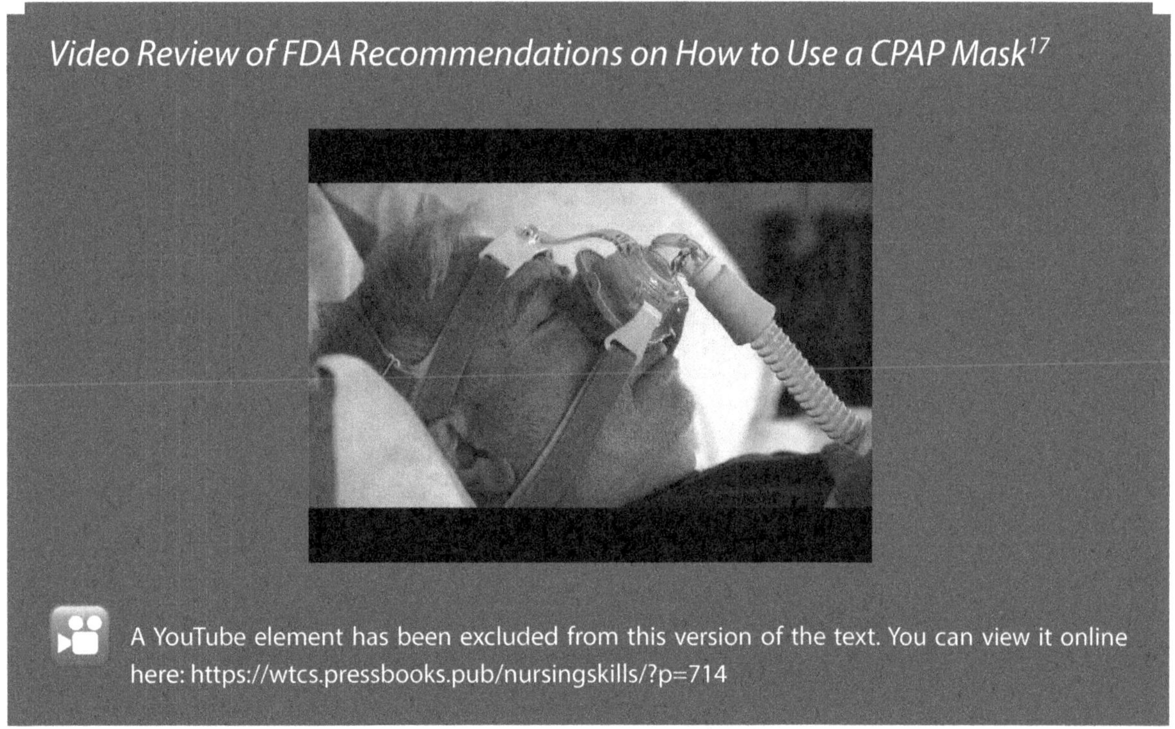

A YouTube element has been excluded from this version of the text. You can view it online here: https://wtcs.pressbooks.pub/nursingskills/?p=714

17 U.S. Food and Drug Administration. (2012, December 12). *CPAP tips from FDA.* [Video]. YouTube. https://youtu.be/B10ABypyGOo

My Notes

BiPAP

A Bilevel Positive Airway Pressure (BiPAP) device is similar to a CPAP device in that it is used to prevent airways from collapsing, but BiPAP devices have two pressure settings. One setting occurs during inhalation and a lower pressure setting is used during exhalation. Patients using BiPAP devices in their home environment for obstructive sleep apnea often find these two pressures more tolerable because they don't have to exhale against continuous pressure. In acute-care settings, BiPAP devices are also used for patients in acute respiratory distress as a noninvasive alternative to intubation and mechanical ventilation and are managed by respiratory therapists. BiPAP devices in home settings are set up in a similar manner as CPAP machines for ease of use. See Figure 11.16[18] for an image of a simulated patient wearing a BiPAP mask in a hospital setting with continuous pulse oximetry monitoring.

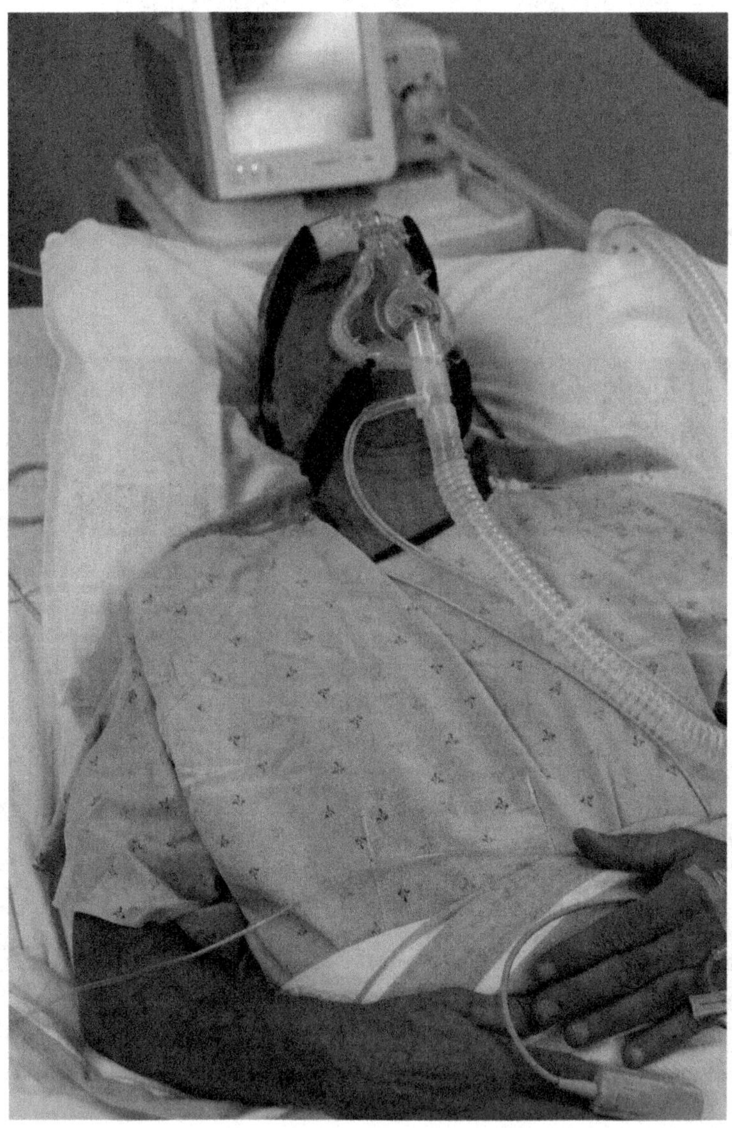

Figure 11.16 Simulated Patient Wearing a BiPAP Mask

18 "Simulated patient wearing a BiPAP mask" by Chippewa Valley Technical College is licensed under CC BY 4.0. Access for free at https://drive.google.com/file/d/1Cvn7l4-oypXIeMGV6-Qi-bvkGhzShyIs/view?usp=sharing

Bag Valve Mask (Ambu Bag)

My Notes

A bag valve mask, commonly known as an "Ambu bag," is a handheld device used in emergency situations for patients who are not breathing (respiratory arrest) or who are not breathing adequately (respiratory failure). In this manner, this device is different from the other devices because it assists with **ventilation**, the movement of air into and out of the lungs, as well as oxygenation. See Figure 11.17[19] for an image of a bag valve mask. Bag valve masks are produced in different sizes for infants, children, and adults to prevent lung injury, so it is important to use the correct size for the patient.

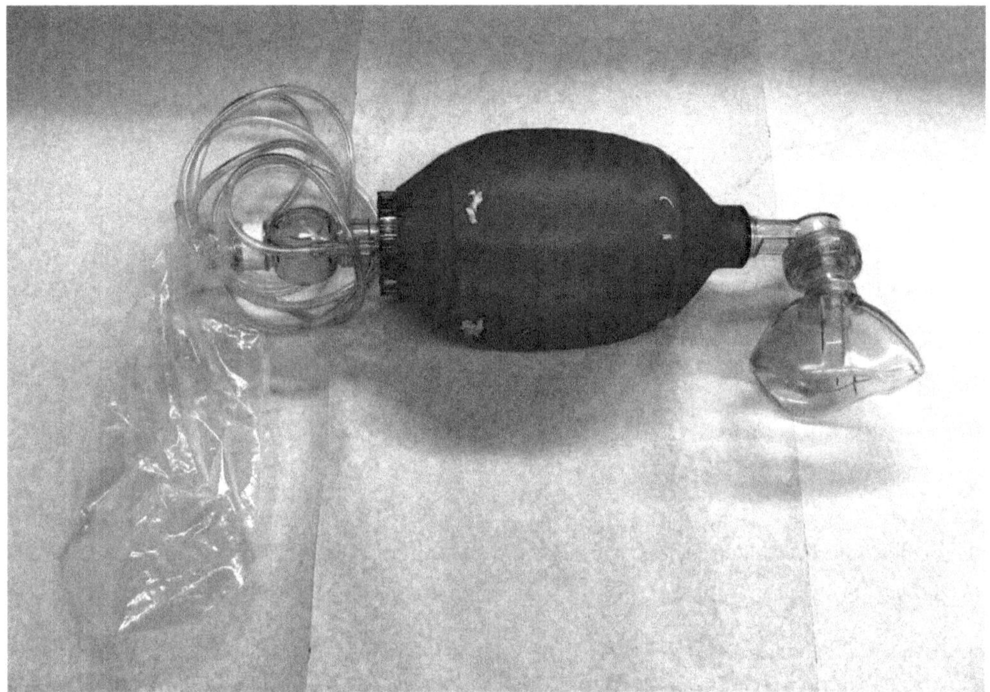

Figure 11.17 Bag Valve Mask

When using a bag mask valve, the rescuer manually compresses the bag to force air into the lungs. Squeezing the bag once every 5 to 6 seconds for an adult or once every 3 seconds for an infant or child provides an adequate respiratory rate. In inpatient settings, the bag mask valve is attached to an oxygen supply to increase the concentration of oxygenation provided with each breath. See Figure 11.18[20] for an illustration of operating a bag valve mask.

It is vital to obtain a tight seal of the mask to the patient's face, but this is difficult for a single rescuer to achieve. Therefore, two rescuers are recommended; one rescuer performs a jaw thrust maneuver, secures the mask to the patient's face with both hands, and focuses on maintaining a leak-proof mask seal, while the other rescuer squeezes the bag and focuses on the amount and the timing.

---

19 "Ballon ventilation 1.jpg" by Rama is licensed under CC BY-SA 2.0 FR. Access for free at https://commons.wikimedia.org/wiki/File:Ballon_ventilation_1.jpg

20 "Resuscitator 3 - Operation (PSF).png" by Pearson Scott Foresman is in the Public Domain. Access for free at https://commons.wikimedia.org/wiki/File:Resuscitator_3_-_Operation_(PSF).png

My Notes

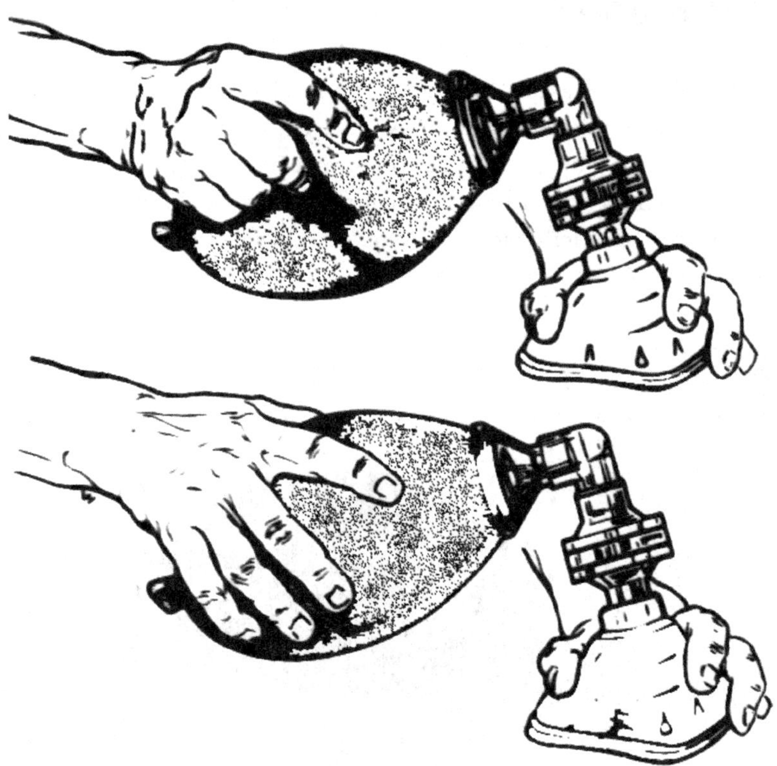

Figure 11.18 Operation of a Bag Valve Mask

Flow rate: The flow rate for a bag valve mask attached to an oxygen source should be set to 15 L/minute, resulting in FiO_2 of 100%.

Advantages: A bag valve mask is portable and provides immediate assistance to patients in respiratory failure or respiratory arrest. It also can be used to hyperoxygenate patients before procedures that can cause hypoxia, such as tracheal suctioning.

Disadvantages: The rate and depth of compression of the bag must be closely monitored to prevent injury to the patient. In the event of respiratory failure when the patient is still breathing, the bag compressions must be coordinated with the patient's inhalations to ensure that oxygen is delivered and asynchrony of breaths is prevented. Complications may also result from overinflating or overpressurizing the patient. Complications include lung injury or the inflation of the stomach that can lead to aspiration of stomach contents. Additionally, rescuers may tire after a few minutes of manually compressing the bag, resulting in less than optimal ventilation. Alternatively, an endotracheal tube (ET) can be inserted by an advanced practitioner to substitute for the mask portion of this device. See more information about endotracheal tubes below.

Endotracheal Intubation

My Notes

When a patient is receiving general anesthesia prior to a procedure or surgery or is experiencing respiratory failure or respiratory arrest, an endotracheal tube (ET) is inserted by an advanced practitioner, such as a respiratory therapist, paramedic, or anesthesiologist, to maintain a secure airway. The ET tube is sealed within the trachea with an inflatable cuff, and oxygen is supplied via a bag valve mask or via mechanical ventilation. See Figure 11.19[21] for an image of a cuffed endotracheal tube.

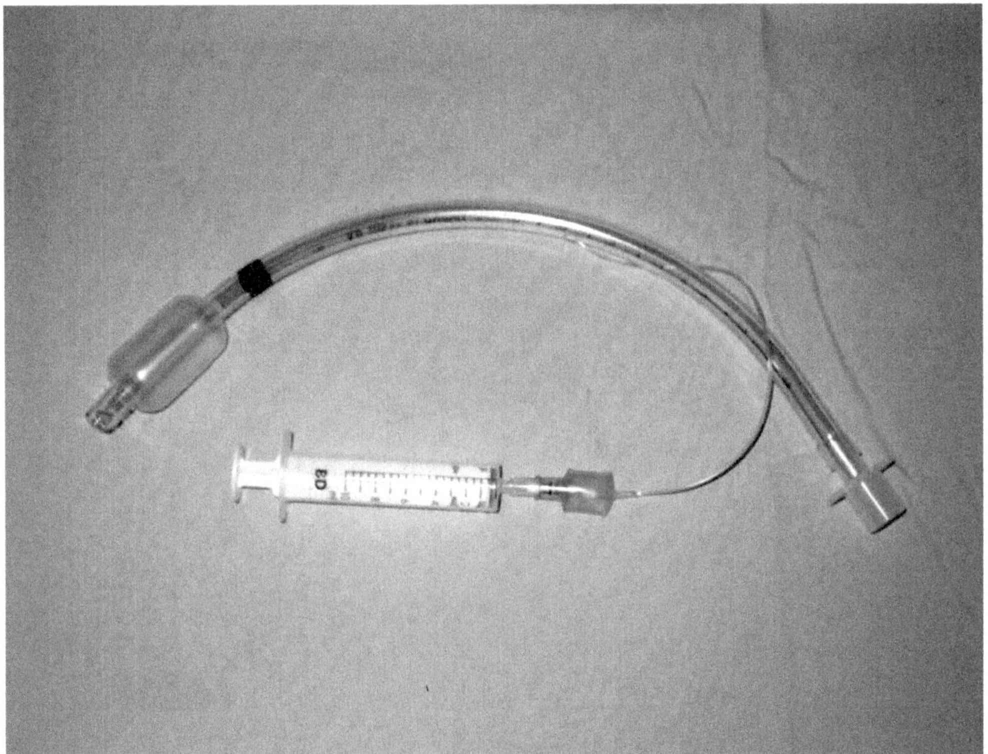

Figure 11.19 An Endotracheal Tube

21 "Sondeintubation.jpg" by bigomar2 is licensed under CC BY-SA 3.0. Access for free at https://commons.wikimedia.org/wiki/File:Sondeintubation.jpg

My Notes

Mechanical Ventilator

A mechanical ventilator is a machine attached to an endotracheal tube to assist or replace spontaneous breathing. Mechanical ventilation is termed invasive because it requires placement of a device inside the trachea through the mouth, such as an endotracheal tube. Mechanical ventilators are managed by respiratory therapists via protocol or provider order. FiO2 can be set from 21-100%. Nurses collaborate with respiratory therapists and the health care providers regarding the overall care of the patient on a mechanical ventilator. See Figure 11.20[22] for an image of a simulated patient who is intubated with an endotracheal tube and attached to a mechanical ventilator.

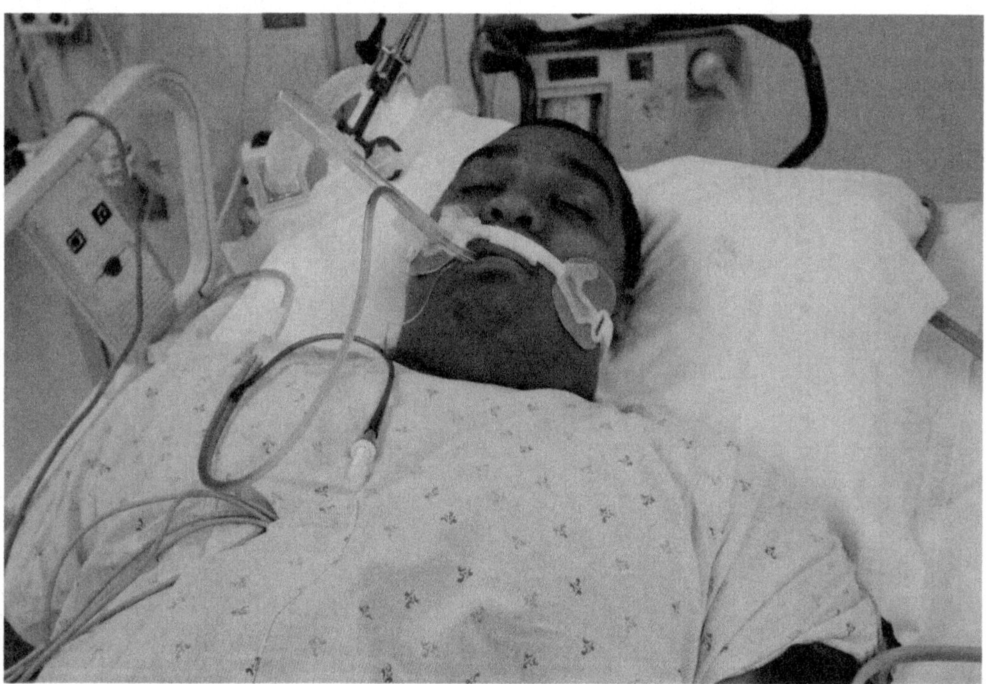

Figure 11.20 Simulated Intubated Patient on a Mechanical Ventilator

Tracheostomy

A tracheostomy is a surgically-made hole called a stoma that goes from the front of the patient's neck into the trachea. A tracheostomy tube is placed through the stoma and directly into the trachea to maintain an open (patent) airway and to administer oxygen. A tracheostomy may be performed emergently or as a planned procedure. Read more about tracheostomies in the "Tracheostomy Care and Suctioning" chapter.

Flow Rates and Oxygen Percentages

When administering oxygen to a patient, it is important to ensure that oxygen flow rates are appropriately set according to the type of administration device. Review Table 11.3a to review appropriate settings for various types of oxygenation devices.

---

22 "Simulated intubated patient on a mechanical ventilator" by ARISE project is licensed under CC BY 4.0. Access for free at https://drive.google.com/file/d/14nP861zcUCaJ8-0r44ckAuyw1NrkRo30/view?usp=sharing

My Notes

Table 11.3a Settings of Oxygenation Devices	
Device	**Flow Rates and Oxygen Percentage**
Nasal Cannula	Flow rate: 1-6 L/min FiO2: 24% to 44%
High-Flow Nasal Cannula	Flow rate: up to 60 L/min FiO2: Up to 100%
Simple Mask	Flow rate: 6-10 L/min FiO2: 28% to 50%
Non-Rebreather Mask	Flow rate: 10 to 15 L/min FiO2: 60-80% Safety Note: The reservoir bag should always be partially inflated.
CPAP, BiPAP, Venturi Mask, Mechanical Ventilator	Use the settings provided by the respiratory therapist and/or provider order.
Bag Valve Mask	Flow rate: 15 L/min FiO2: 100% Squeeze the bag once every 5 to 6 seconds for an adult or once every 3 seconds for an infant or child.

My Notes

Safety with Oxygen Therapy

Oxygen therapy supports life, but it also supports fire. While there are many benefits to oxygen therapy, there are also many hazards. Oxygen must be administered cautiously and according to the safety guidelines in Table 11.3b.[23]

Table 11.3b Oxygen Therapy Safety Guidelines

Guideline	Additional Information
Remember that oxygen is a medication.	Oxygen is a medication and should not be adjusted without consultation with a physician or respiratory therapist.
Store oxygen cylinders correctly.	When using oxygen cylinders, store them upright, chained, or in appropriate holders so that they will not fall. Full oxygen tanks should be stored separately from partially-full or empty oxygen tanks.
Use tank holders appropriately.	When transporting a patient, proper tank holders must be used per Joint Commission guidelines. Tanks should never be placed on the patient's bed.
Do not allow smoking near the oxygen devices.	Oxygen supports combustion. No smoking is permitted around any oxygen delivery devices in the hospital or home environment.
Keep oxygen cylinders away from heat sources.	Keep oxygen delivery systems at least 5 feet from any heat source.
Check for electrical hazards in the home or hospital prior to use.	Determine that electrical equipment in the room or home is in safe working condition. A small electrical spark in the presence of oxygen will result in a serious fire. The use of a gas stove, kerosene space heater, or smoker is unsafe in the presence of oxygen. Avoid items that may create a spark (e.g., electrical razor, hair dryer, synthetic fabrics that cause static electricity, or mechanical toys) with nasal cannula in use. Petroleum-based lubricants should not be used on the lips or around the nasal cannula.
Check levels of oxygen in portable tanks.	Check oxygen levels of portable tanks before transporting a patient to ensure that there is enough oxygen in the tank.

23 This work is a derivative of Clinical Procedures for Safer Patient Care by British Columbia Institute of Technology and is licensed under CC BY 4.0. Access for free at https://opentextbc.ca/clinicalskills/

11.4 NURSING PROCESS RELATED TO OXYGEN THERAPY

When administering oxygen therapy, it is important for the nurse to assess the patient before, during, and after the procedure and document the findings.

Subjective Assessment

Prior to initiating oxygen therapy, if conditions warrant, the nurse should briefly obtain a history of respiratory conditions and collect data regarding current symptoms associated with the patient's feeling of shortness of breath. The duration of this focused assessment should be modified based on the severity of the patient's dyspnea. See Table 11.4 for focused interview questions related to oxygen therapy. This information is used to customize the oxygen delivery device and flow rate for the patient. For example, supplemental oxygen is typically initiated in nonemergency situations with a nasal cannula at 1-2 liters per minute (L/min), but a patient with a history of chronic obstructive pulmonary disease (COPD) may require a different device such as a Venturi mask.

Table 11.4 Focused Interview Questions for Subjective Assessment of Dyspnea

Interview Questions	Follow-up
Please rate your current feeling of shortness of breath from 0-10, "0" being no shortness of breath and "10" being the worst shortness of breath you have ever experienced.	Note: If the shortness of breath is severe, associated with chest pain, or if there are imminent signs of respiratory failure, discontinue the subjective assessment and obtain emergency assistance.
Are you experiencing any additional symptoms such as chest pain, cough, or a feeling of swelling in your throat or tongue?	Please describe. Note: If the patient describes severe symptoms that could indicate imminent blockage of the airway, obtain emergency assistance. When did it start? Is the cough productive of phlegm? If yes, what color and what is the amount? Does the chest pain radiate elsewhere?
Have you ever been diagnosed with respiratory conditions such as asthma or COPD?	Please describe.
Are you currently taking any medications, herbs, or supplements to help you breathe?	Please identify what you are taking and the dosage. If you are using inhalers on an as-needed basis, how often are you using them and has the frequency increased lately?
Have you received oxygen therapy previously?	Please describe. Do you use oxygen therapy at home? What is your normal flow rate? Do you use CPAP or BiPAP devices at home?
Do you smoke?	Have you considered quitting?

My Notes

Objective Assessment

Prior to applying supplemental oxygen, objective data regarding patient status should quickly be obtained such as airway clearance, respiratory rate, pulse oximetry, and lung sounds. Signs of cyanosis in the skin or nail bed assessment should also be noted. Within a few minutes after initiating oxygen administration, the nurse should evaluate for improvement of these indicators, and if no improvement is noted, then additional actions should be taken. At any point, if the nurse feels that the patient's condition is deteriorating, emergency action should be taken such as calling the rapid response team or 911.

Depending upon the severity of patient condition, serial ABG results may also be monitored to determine effectiveness of oxygenation interventions.

After oxygen therapy is initiated, it is important to closely monitor for skin breakdown at pressure points. For example, nasal cannula tubing often causes skin breakdown in the nares or over the ears, so protective foam dressings may need to be applied.

Life Span Considerations

Children

Different sized oxygen equipment is used for infants and children. Additionally, oxygen tubing may need to be secured to a child's face with tape to prevent them from pulling it off. For infants, the pulse oximeter probe is usually attached to the palm or foot.

Older Adults

If a patient is oxygen-dependent, ensure that extension tubing is applied so the patient is able to reach the bathroom with the oxygen device in place. However, be aware of the increased risk for falls due to the excess tubing. Keeping the oxygen tubing coiled up at the head of the bed or on the bedside table closest to the bathroom will decrease the patient's risk of falling. Advise the patient to ask for assistance when getting up to use the restroom.

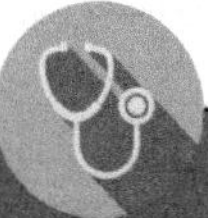

- Safety Tip: When oxygen is in use, teach the patient about safety considerations with oxygen use because it is very flammable. See the "Safety with Oxygen Therapy" section in "Oxygenation Equipment" for more details.
- After administering oxygen, instruct the patient to inhale through their nose with slow, deep breaths and to breathe out through their mouth.
- If a patient is experiencing worsening dyspnea with decreased oxygen saturation levels compared to their baseline levels, apply oxygen and stay with the patient until their oxygen saturation level increases and they report feeling less short of breath. Providing a physical presence is an important intervention for the associated anxiety that accompanies dyspnea. Consider asking a team member for assistance.
- Based on the patient's condition, it may be helpful to institute additional interventions to improve oxygenation. See Table 11.2c in the "Basic Concepts of Oxygenation" section for interventions to improve hypoxia.

11.5 SAMPLE DOCUMENTATION

My Notes

Sample Documentation of Expected Findings

Patient has a history of COPD and reported feeling short of breath after getting up to use the bathroom this morning. Respirations were 24/minute, pulse oximetry 88% on room air, and lungs sounds were diminished. Oxygen applied via nasal cannula at 2 Lpm, and the patient was encouraged to take slow deep breaths in through their nose and out of their mouth. After five minutes, the pulse oximetry was 94%, the respiratory rate decreased to 16/minute, and the patient reported the feeling of shortness of breath had subsided.

Sample Documentation of Unexpected Findings

Patient has a history of COPD and heart failure and reported feeling short of breath after getting up to use the bathroom this morning. Respirations were 30/minute, pulse oximetry was 88% on room air, and lungs had crackles in the lower posterior lobes. Oxygen was applied via nasal cannula at 2 Lpm and the patient was encouraged to cough and deep breathe. After five minutes, the respiratory rate and pulse oximetry readings did not improve. Dr. Smith was notified at 0715 and an order for a STAT chest X-ray was received, followed by an order for furosemide 40 mg IV STAT. Furosemide was administered, and 30 minutes later the pulse oximetry increased to 92%, respiratory rate decreased to 18/minute, and there was urine output of 500 mL with reduced crackles in the lower posterior lobes. Patient reported feeling less short of breath.

My Notes

11.6 CHECKLIST FOR OXYGEN THERAPY

Use the checklist below to review the steps for "Managing Oxygen Therapy."

Steps

Disclaimer: Always review and follow agency policy regarding this specific skill.

1. Verify provider order or protocol.
2. Gather supplies: pulse oximeter, oxygen delivery device, and tubing.
3. Perform safety steps:
    - Perform hand hygiene.
    - Check the room for transmission-based precautions.
    - Introduce yourself, your role, the purpose of your visit, and an estimate of the time it will take.
    - Confirm patient ID using two patient identifiers (e.g., name and date of birth).
    - Explain the process to the patient and ask if they have any questions.
    - Be organized and systematic.
    - Use appropriate listening and questioning skills.
    - Listen and attend to patient cues.
    - Ensure the patient's privacy and dignity.
    - Assess ABCs.
4. Perform a focused respiratory assessment including airway, respiratory rate, pulse oximetry rate, and lung sounds.
5. Employ safety measures for oxygen therapy.
6. Connect flow meter to oxygen supply source.
7. Apply adapter for tubing.
8. Connect nasal cannula tubing to flow meter.
9. Set oxygen flow at prescribed rate.
10. When using a nasal cannula, place the prongs into the patient's nares and fit the tubing around their ears. When using a mask, place the mask over the patient's mouth and nose, secure a firm seal, and tighten the straps around the head. If using a non-rebreather mask, partially inflate the reservoir bag before applying the mask. Place the patient in an upright position as clinically appropriate.
11. Evaluate patient's response to oxygen therapy including airway, respiratory rate, pulse oximetry reading, and reported dyspnea.
12. Institute additional interventions to improve oxygenation as needed.
13. Adapt this procedure to reflect variations across the life span.

My Notes

14. Assist the patient to a comfortable position, ask if they have any questions, and thank them for their time.

15. Ensure safety measures when leaving the room:

    - CALL LIGHT: Within reach
    - BED: Low and locked (in lowest position and brakes on)
    - SIDE RAILS: Secured
    - TABLE: Within reach
    - ROOM: Risk-free for falls (scan room and clear any obstacles)

16. Perform hand hygiene.

17. Document the assessment findings. Report any concerns according to agency policy.

My Notes

11.7 SUPPLEMENTARY VIDEOS ON OXYGEN THERAPY

Video Reviews for Oxygen

Therapy Using an Incentive Spirometer[1]

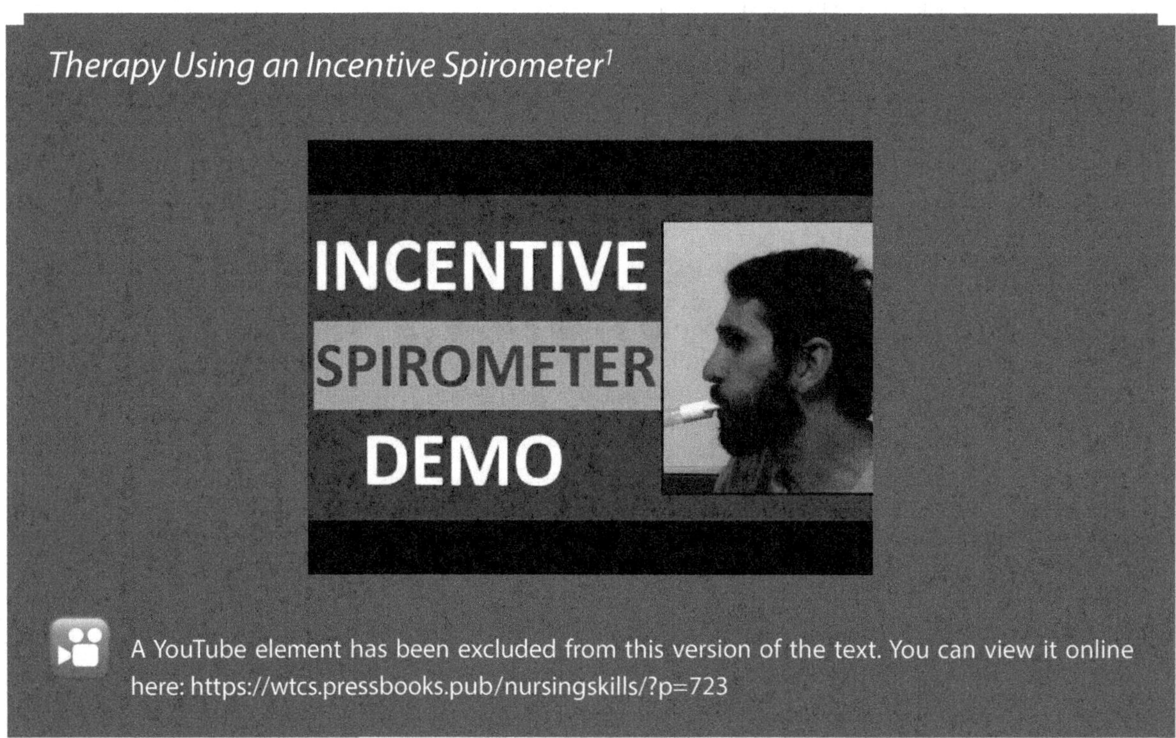

A YouTube element has been excluded from this version of the text. You can view it online here: https://wtcs.pressbooks.pub/nursingskills/?p=723

View Oxford Medical Education's "Oxygen Therapy and Delivery" video on YouTube[2]

1 RegisteredNurseRN. (2016, October 18). *Incentive spirometry (spirometer) demonstration instruction | Incentive spirometer procedure*. [Video]. YouTube. All rights reserved. Video used with permission. https://youtu.be/pZxq6oroGhk

2 Oxford Medical Education. (2012, May 13). *Oxygen therapy and delivery - How to prescribe oxygen*. [Video]. YouTube. All rights reserved. This video is included on the basis of Fair Use. https://youtu.be/Nc2zl2SeQNo

11.8 LEARNING ACTIVITIES

My Notes

Learning Activities

(Answers to "Learning Activities" can be found in the '"Answer Key'" at the end of the book. Answers to interactive activity elements will be provided within the element as immediate feedback.)

1. Your patient turns on their call light. Upon entering your patient's room, they say they are short of breath. Prioritize your actions from first to sixth.

Institute actions to improve oxygenation

Apply oxygen as ordered

Reassess pulse oximetry

Teach oxygen safety

Assess lung sounds

Assess pulse oximetry

Priority	Actions
First	
Second	
Third	
Four	
Fifth	
Sixth	

Interactive Activity

An interactive or media element has been excluded from this version of the text. You can view it online here: https://wtcs.pressbooks.pub/nursingskills/?p=726

An interactive or media element has been excluded from this version of the text. You can view it online here: https://wtcs.pressbooks.pub/nursingskills/?p=726

An interactive or media element has been excluded from this version of the text. You can view it online here: https://wtcs.pressbooks.pub/nursingskills/?p=726

My Notes

XI GLOSSARY

Clubbing: A gradual enlargement of the fingertips in patients with respiratory conditions that cause chronic hypoxia.

Cyanosis: A bluish discoloration of the skin and mucous membranes caused by lack of oxygenation to the tissues.

Dyspnea: A subjective feeling of not being able to get enough air; also called shortness of breath.

FiO2: Fraction of inspired oxygen (i.e., the concentration of oxygen inhaled). Room air contains 21% oxygen levels, and oxygenation devices can increase the inhaled concentration of oxygen up to 100%. However, FiO2 levels should be decreased as soon as feasible to do so to prevent lung injury.

Hypercapnia: Elevated carbon dioxide levels in the blood, indicated by PaCO2 level greater than 45 in an ABG test.

Hypoxemia: Decreased dissolved oxygen in the arterial blood, indicated by a PaO2 level less than 80 mmHg in an ABG test.

Hypoxia: A reduced level of tissue oxygenation.

Obstructive Sleep Apnea (OSA): Characterized by repeated occurrences of complete or partial obstructions of the upper airway during sleep, resulting in apneic episodes.

PaO2: The partial pressure of dissolved oxygen in the blood measured by arterial blood gas samples.

SpO2: An estimated oxygenation level based on the saturation level of hemoglobin measured by a pulse oximeter.

Ventilation: The mechanical movement of air into and out of the lungs.

Chapter 12

Abdominal Assessment

12.1 ABDOMINAL ASSESSMENT INTRODUCTION

My Notes

Learning Objectives

- Perform an abdominal assessment
- Differentiate normal and abnormal bowel sounds
- Modify assessment techniques to reflect variations across the life span
- Document actions and observations
- Recognize and report significant deviations from norms

A thorough assessment of the abdomen provides valuable information regarding the function of a patient's gastrointestinal (GI) and genitourinary (GU) systems. Understanding how to properly assess the abdomen and recognizing both normal and abnormal assessment findings will allow the nurse to provide high-quality care to the patient.

My Notes

12.2 GASTROINTESTINAL BASICS

It is important for the nurse to be aware of the underlying structures of the abdomen when completing a gastrointestinal or genitourinary assessment. See Figure 12.1[1] for an illustration of the gastrointestinal system and the bladder. See Figure 12.2[2] for an illustration of the male urinary system. Know the position of the organs within the abdominal cavity as you learn to auscultate, palpate, and percuss the abdomen.

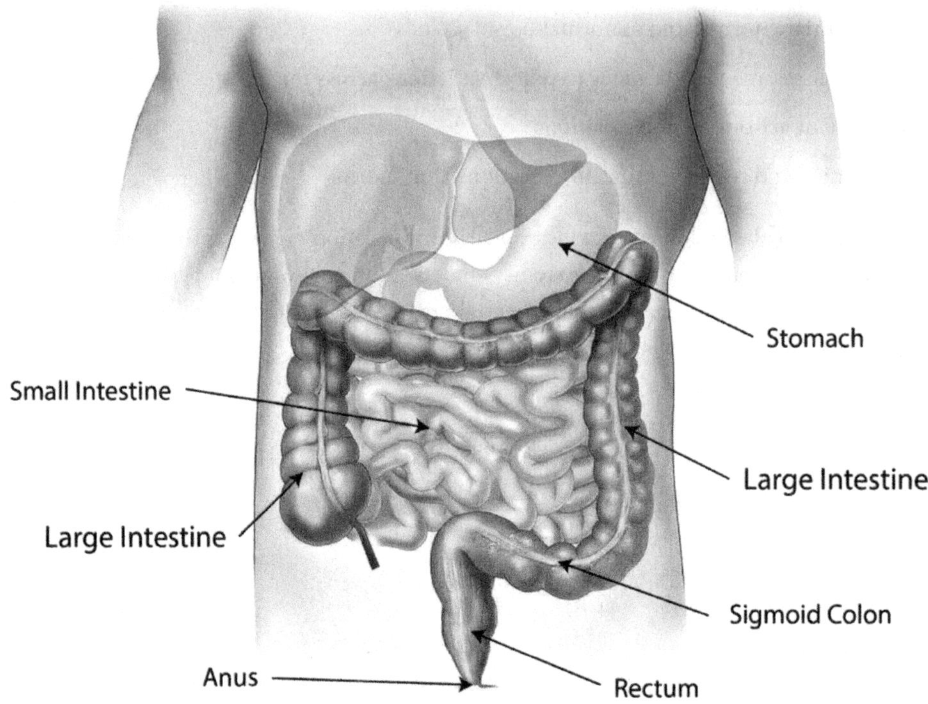

Figure 12.1 Gastrointestinal System

1 "abdomen-intestine-large-small-1698565" by bodymybody is licensed under CC0. Access for free at https://pixabay.com/illustrations/abdomen-intestine-large-small-1698565/

2 "Urinary_System_(Male).png" by BruceBlaus is licenced under CC BY-SA 4.0. Access for free at https://commons.wikimedia.org/wiki/File:Urinary_System_(Male).png

My Notes

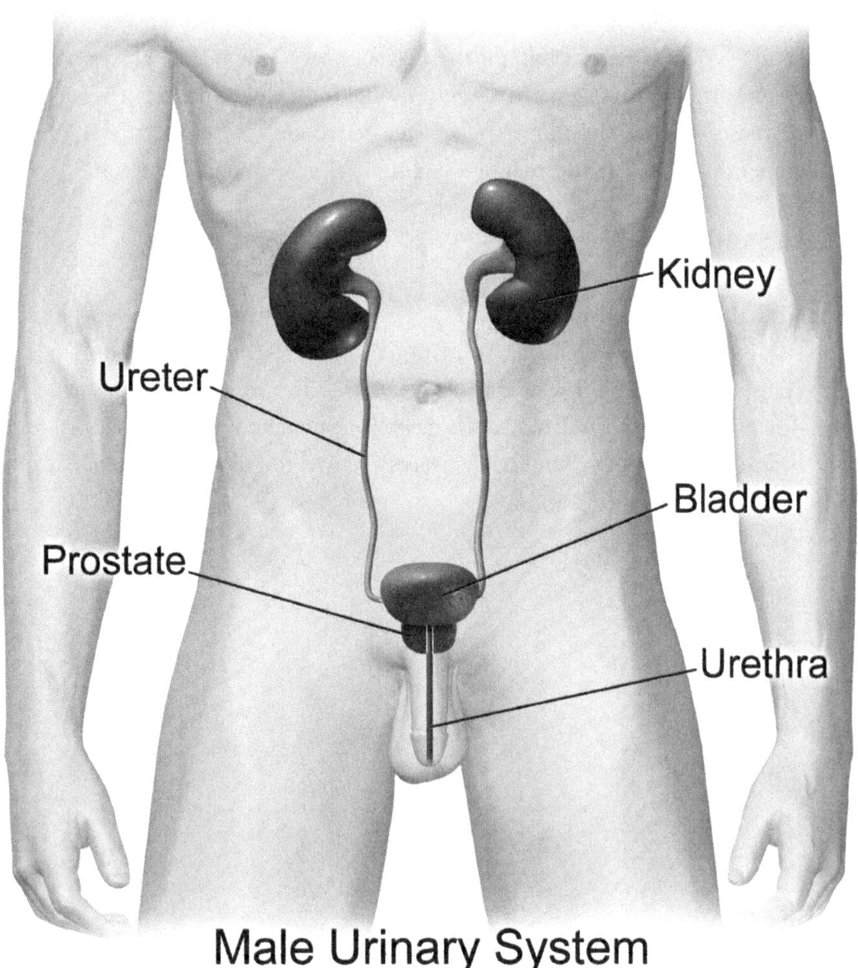

Figure 12.2 Male Urinary System

For a detailed overview of the gastrointestinal system, common GI disorders, and related GI medications, visit the "Gastrointestinal" chapter of the Open RN *Nursing Pharmacology* textbook. Specific sections of the chapter include the following:

- "GI System Review" for additional review of the anatomy of the GI system
- "Antidiarrheals and Laxatives" for more information about treating diarrhea and constipation
- "Antiemetics" for more information about treating nausea and vomiting
- "Hyperacidity and Acid Controlling Medication" for more information about treating acid reflux and gastric ulcers

My Notes

12.3 GASTROINTESTINAL AND GENITOURINARY ASSESSMENT

The gastrointestinal (GI) system is responsible for the ingestion of food and the absorption of nutrients. Additionally, the GI and genitourinary (GU) systems are responsible for the elimination of waste products.[1] Therefore, during assessment of these systems, the nurse collects subjective and objective data regarding the underlying structures of the abdomen, as well as the normal functioning of the GI and GU systems.

Subjective Assessment

A focused gastrointestinal and genitourinary subjective assessment collects data about the signs and symptoms of GI and GU diseases, including any digestive or nutritional issues, relevant medical or family history of GI and GU disease, and any current treatment for related issues.[2] Table 12.3a outlines interview questions used to explore medical and surgical history, symptoms related to the gastrointestinal and genitourinary systems, and associated medications. Information gained from the interview process is used to tailor the subsequent physical assessment and create a plan for patient care and education.[3]

1 This work is a derivative of Clinical Procedures for Safer Patient Care by British Columbia Institute of Technology and is licensed under CC BY 4.0. Access for free at https://opentextbc.ca/clinicalskills/

2 This work is a derivative of Clinical Procedures for Safer Patient Care by British Columbia Institute of Technology and is licensed under CC BY 4.0. Access for free at https://opentextbc.ca/clinicalskills/

3 This work is a derivative of Clinical Procedures for Safer Patient Care by British Columbia Institute of Technology and is licensed under CC BY 4.0. Access for free at https://opentextbc.ca/clinicalskills/

My Notes

Table 12.3a Interview Questions for Subjective Assessment of GI and GU Systems

Interview Questions	Follow-up
Have you ever been diagnosed with a gastro-intestinal (GI), kidney, or bladder condition?	Please describe the conditions and treatments.
Have you ever had abdominal surgery?	Please describe the surgery and if you experienced any complications.
Are you currently taking any medications, herbs, or supplements?	Please describe.
Do you have any abdominal pain?	Are there any associated symptoms with the pain such as fever, nausea, vomiting, or change in bowel pattern? Are you having bloody stools (**hematochezia**); dark, tarry stools (**melena**); abdominal distention; or vomiting of blood (**hematemesis**)? When did the pain start to occur? (Onset) Where is the pain? (Location) When it occurs, how long does the pain last? (Duration) Can you describe what the pain feels like? (Characteristics) What brings on the pain? (Aggravating factors) What relieves the pain? (Alleviating factors) Does the pain radiate anywhere? (Radiation) What have you used to treat the pain? (Treatment) What effect has the pain had on you? (Effects) How severe is the pain from 0-10 when it occurs? (Severity)
Have you had any issues with nausea, vomiting, food intolerance, heartburn, ulcers, change in appetite, or weight?	Please describe. What treatment did you use for these symptoms? What is your typical diet in a 24-hour period?

My Notes

Do you have any difficulty swallowing food or liquids (dysphagia)?	Please describe. Have you ever been diagnosed with a stroke or transient ischemic attack (TIA)?
When was your last bowel movement?	Have there been any changes in pattern or consistency of your stool? Are you passing any gas?
Have you had any issues with constipation or diarrhea?	Please describe. How long have you had these issues? What treatment did you use for these symptoms? If constipation: ■ Has constipation been a problem for you throughout your life? ■ How frequently do you usually have a bowel movement? If diarrhea: ■ Are your stools watery or is there some form to them? ■ How many episodes of diarrhea have you had in the past 24 hours?
Do you experience any pain or discomfort with urination (dysuria)?	Please describe. If you have discomfort while urinating, is the discomfort internal or external? Do you use any treatment for these symptoms?
Do you experience frequent urination (urinary frequency)?	Please describe. Does the frequency occur during daytime or nighttime hours?
Do you ever experience a strong urge to urinate that makes it difficult to reach the bathroom in time (urinary urgency)?	Does this strong urge ever result in a leakage of urine? Does the urge come and go or is it continuous?
Do you have any leakage of urine when you cough, sneeze, or jump (urinary incontinence)? **Do you have difficulty starting the flow of urine?**	Have you tried any treatment for this issue?

Gastrointestinal

My Notes

Pain is the most common complaint related to abdominal problems and can be attributed to multiple underlying etiologies. Because of the potential variability of contributing factors, a careful and thorough assessment of this chief complaint should occur. Additional associated questions include asking if bloody stools (**hematochezia**); dark, tarry stools (**melena**); bloating (abdominal distention); or vomiting of blood (**hematemesis**) are occurring.

Nausea, vomiting, diarrhea, and constipation are common issues experienced by hospitalized patients due to adverse effects of medications or medical procedures. Read more details about commonly occurring gastrointestinal conditions in the "Elimination" chapter in Open RN *Nursing Fundamentals.* It is important to ask a hospitalized patient daily about the date of their last bowel movement and flatus so that a bowel management program can be initiated if necessary. If a patient is experiencing diarrhea, it is important to assess and monitor for signs of dehydration or electrolyte imbalances. Dehydration can be indicated by dry skin, dry mucous membranes, or sunken eyes. These symptoms may require contacting the health care provider for further treatment. Read additional information about fluid and electrolyte imbalances in the "Fluids and Electrolytes" chapter in Open RN *Nursing Fundamentals.*

Additional specialized assessments of GI system function can include examination of the oropharynx and esophagus. For example, patients who have experienced a cerebrovascular accident (CVA), also called a "stroke," may experience difficulty swallowing (**dysphagia**). The nurse is often the first to notice these difficulties when swallowing pills, liquid, or food and can advocate for treatment to prevent complications, such as unintended weight loss or **aspiration pneumonia**.[4]

Genitourinary

The nursing assessment of the genitourinary system generally focuses on bladder function. Ask about urinary symptoms, including **dysuria**, **urinary frequency**, or **urinary urgency**. Dysuria is any discomfort associated with urination and often signifies a urinary tract infection. Patients with dysuria commonly experience burning, stinging, or itching sensation. In elderly patients, changes in mental status may be the presenting symptom of a urinary tract infection. In women with dysuria, asking whether the discomfort is internal or external is important because vaginal inflammation can also cause dysuria as urine passes by the inflamed labia.

Abnormally frequent urination (e.g., every hour or two) is termed urinary frequency. In older adults, urinary frequency often occurs at night and is termed nocturia. Frequency of normal urination varies considerably from individual to individual depending on personality traits, bladder capacity, or drinking habits. It can also be a symptom of a urinary tract infection, pregnancy in females, or prostate enlargement in males.

Urinary urgency is an abrupt, strong, and often overwhelming need to urinate. Urgency often causes **urinary incontinence**, a leakage of urine. When patients experience urinary urgency, the desire to urinate may be constant with only a few milliliters of urine eliminated with each voiding.[5] Read additional information about commonly occurring genitourinary system alterations in the "Elimination" chapter in Open RN *Nursing Fundamentals.*

---

4 Ferguson, C. M. (1990). An overview of the gastrointestinal system. In Walker, H. K., Hall, W. D., Hurst, J. W. (Eds.), *Clinical methods: The history, physical, and laboratory examinations* (3rd ed.). Butterworths. https://www.ncbi.nlm.nih.gov/books/NBK405/

5 Wrenn, K. (1990). Dysuria, frequency, and urgency. In Walker, H. K., Hall, W. D., Hurst, J. W. (Eds.), *Clinical methods: The history, physical, and laboratory examinations* (3rd ed.). Butterworths. https://www.ncbi.nlm.nih.gov/books/NBK291/

My Notes

Life Span Considerations

Infants

Eating and elimination patterns of infants require special consideration based on the stage of development.

- Ask parents about feeding habits. Is the baby being breastfed or formula fed? If formula fed, how does the child tolerate the formula?
- Note that the expected abdominal contour of an infant is called **protuberant**, which means bulging.
- Assess the umbilical cord; it should dry and fall off on its own within two weeks of life.
- Observe for respiratory movement in the abdomen of the infant.

Children

The expected abdominal contour of a child is protuberant until about the age of 4. Children often cannot provide more information than "my stomach hurts"; they may have symptoms of decreased school attendance due to abdominal discomfort.

Older Adults

Constipation may be more common in older adults due to decreased physical mobility and oral intake. Urinary urgency, urinary frequency, urinary retention, nocturia, and urinary incontinence are also common concerns for older adults.

Objective Assessment

Physical examination of the abdomen includes inspection, auscultation, palpation, and percussion. Note that the order of physical assessment differs for the abdominal system compared to other systems. Palpation should occur after the auscultation of bowel sounds so that accurate, undisturbed bowel sounds can be assessed. The abdomen is roughly divided into four quadrants: right upper, right lower, left upper, and left lower (see Figure 12.3[6]). When assessing the abdomen, consider the organs located in the quadrant you are examining.

---

6 "Blausen 0005 AbdominopelvicQuadrants.png" by BruceBlaus is licensed under CC BY 3.0. Access for free at https://commons.wikimedia.org/wiki/File:Blausen_0005_AbdominopelvicQuadrants.png

My Notes

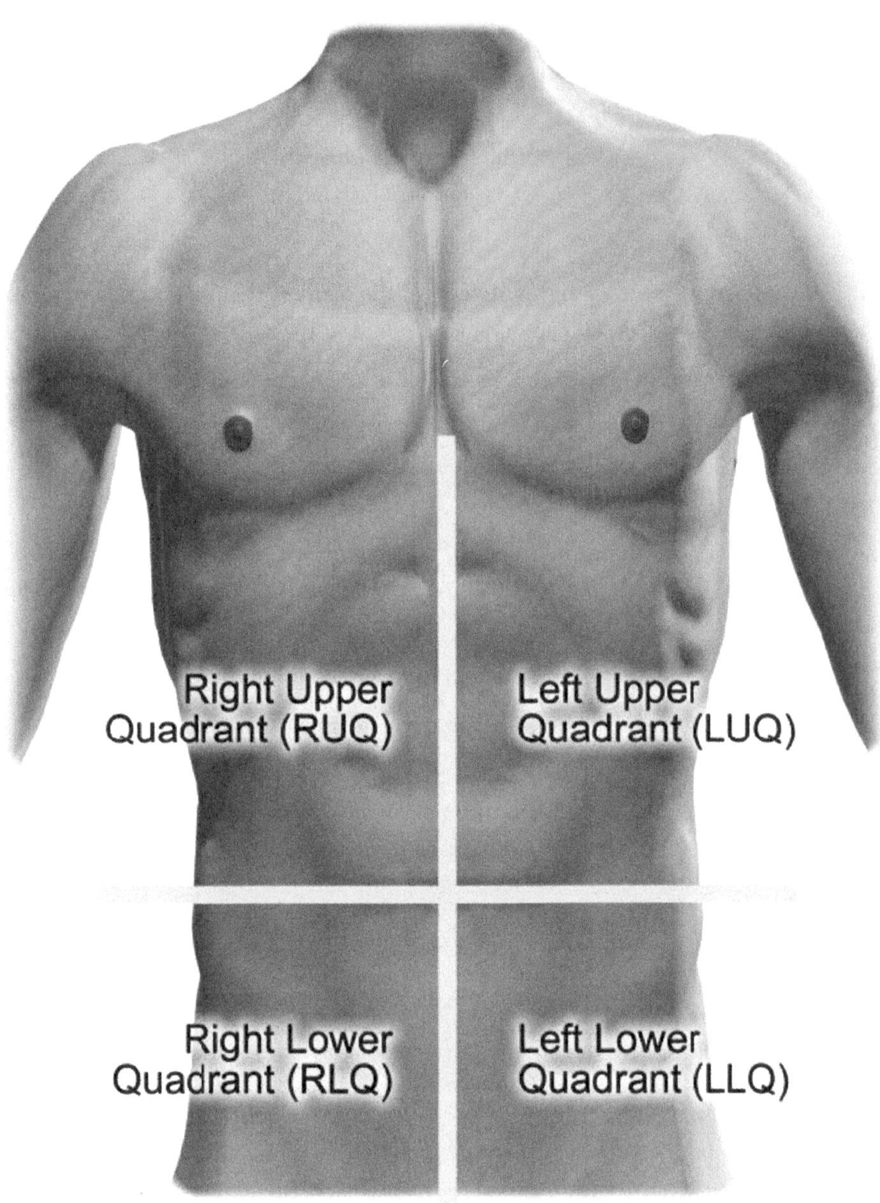

Figure 12.3 Four Quadrants of the Abdomen

In preparation for the physical assessment, the nurse should create an environment in which the patient will be comfortable. Encourage the patient to empty their bladder prior to the assessment. Warm the room and stethoscope to decrease tensing during assessment.

My Notes

Inspection

The abdomen is inspected by positioning the patient supine on an examining table or bed. The head and knees should be supported with small pillows or folded sheets for comfort and to relax the abdominal wall musculature. The patient's arms should be at their side and not folded behind the head, as this tenses the abdominal wall. Ensure the patient is covered adequately to maintain privacy, while still exposing the abdomen as needed for a thorough assessment. Visually examine the abdomen for overall shape, masses, skin abnormalities, and any abnormal movements.

- Observe the general contour and symmetry of the entire abdominal wall. The contour of the abdomen is often described as flat, rounded, **scaphoid** (sunken), or protuberant (convex or bulging).
- Assess for **distention**. Generalized distention of the abdomen can be caused by obesity, bowel distention from gas or liquid, or fluid buildup.
- Assess for masses or bulges, which may indicate structural deformities like hernias or related to disorders in abdominal organs.
- Assess the patient's skin for uniformity of color, integrity, scarring, or **striae**. Striae are white or silvery elongated marks that occur when the skin stretches, especially during pregnancy or excessive weight gain.
- Note the shape of the umbilicus; it should be inverted and midline.
- Carefully note any scars, and correlate these scars with the patient's recollection of previous surgeries or injury.
- Document any abnormal movement or pulsations. Visible intestinal peristalsis can be caused by intestinal obstruction. Pulsations may be seen in the epigastric area in patients who are especially thin, but otherwise should not be observed.[7, 8]

Auscultation

Auscultation, or the listening, of the abdomen, follows inspection for more accurate assessment of bowel sounds. Use a warmed stethoscope to assess the frequency and characteristics of the patient's bowel sounds, which are also referred to as peristaltic murmurs.

Begin your assessment by gently placing the diaphragm of your stethoscope on the skin in the right lower quadrant (RLQ), as bowel sounds are consistently heard in that area. Bowel sounds are generally high-pitched, gurgling sounds that are heard irregularly. Move your stethoscope to the next quadrant in a clockwise motion around the abdominal wall.

It is not recommended to count abdominal sounds because the activity of normal bowel sounds may cycle with peak-to-peak periods as long as 50 to 60 minutes.[9] The majority of peristaltic murmurs are produced by the stom-

---

7 This work is a derivative of Clinical Procedures for Safer Patient Care by British Columbia Institute of Technology and is licensed under CC BY 4.0. Access for free at https://opentextbc.ca/clinicalskills/

8 Ferguson, C. M. (1990). Inspection, auscultation, palpation, and percussion of the abdomen. In Walker, H. K., Hall, W. D., Hurst, J. W. (Eds.), *Clinical methods: The history, physical, and laboratory examinations* (3rd ed.). Butterworths. https://www.ncbi.nlm.nih.gov/books/NBK420/

9 McGee, S. R. (2012). *Evidence-based physical diagnosis* (3rd ed.). Elsevier Saunders. https://kimhournet.files.wordpress.com/2018/12/mcgee-evidence-based-physical-diagnosis-3rd-ed1.pdf

My Notes

ach, with the remainder from the large intestine and a small contribution from the small intestine. Because the conduction of peristaltic murmur is heard throughout all parts of the abdomen, the source of peristaltic murmur is not always at the site where it is heard. If the conduction of peristaltic sounds is good, auscultation at a single location is considered adequate.[10]

Hyperactive bowel sounds may indicate bowel obstruction or gastroenteritis. Sometimes you may be able to hear a patient's bowel sounds without a stethoscope, often described as "stomach growling" or **borborygmus**. This is a common example of hyperactive sounds. **Hypoactive bowel sounds** may be present with constipation, after abdominal surgery, peritonitis, or paralytic ileus. As you auscultate the abdomen, you should not hear vascular sounds. If heard, this finding should be reported to the health care provider.[11, 12]

Palpation

Palpation, or touching, of the abdomen involves using the flat of the hand and fingers (not the fingertips) to detect palpable organs, abnormal masses, or tenderness[13] (see Figure 12.4[14]). When palpating the abdomen of a patient reporting abdominal pain, the nurse should palpate that area last. Light palpation is primarily used by bedside nurses to assess for musculature, abnormal masses, and tenderness. Deep palpation is a technique used by advanced practice clinicians to assess for enlarged organs. Lightly palpate the abdomen by pressing into the skin about 1 centimeter beginning in the RLQ. Continue to move around the abdomen in a clockwise manner.

Palpate the bladder for distention. Note the patient response to palpation, such as pain, guarding, rigidity, or rebound tenderness. **Guarding** refers to voluntary contraction of the abdominal wall musculature, usually the result of fear, anxiety, or the touch of cold hands. **Rigidity** refers to involuntary contraction of the abdominal musculature in response to peritoneal inflammation, a reflex the patient cannot control.[15] **Rebound tenderness** is another sign of peritoneal inflammation or peritonitis. To elicit rebound tenderness, the clinician maintains

---

10 Mayumi, T., Yoshida, M., Tazuma, S., Furukawa, A., Nishii, O., Shigematsu, K., Azuhata, T., Itakura, A., Kamei, S., Kondo, H., Maeda, S., Mihara, H., Mizooka, M., Nishidate, T., Obara, H., Sato, N., Takayama, Y., Tsujikawa, T., Fujii, T., Miyata, T., Maruyama, I., Honda, H., & Hirata, K. (2015). Practice guidelines for primary care of acute abdomen. *J Hepato-biliary Pancreat Sci, 23*, 3–36. https://doi.org/10.1002/jhbp.303

11 This work is a derivative of Clinical Procedures for Safer Patient Care by British Columbia Institute of Technology and is licensed under CC BY 4.0. Access for free at https://opentextbc.ca/clinicalskills/

12 Ferguson, C. M. (1990). Inspection, auscultation, palpation, and percussion of the abdomen. In Walker, H. K., Hall W. D., Hurst J. W. (Eds.), *Clinical methods: The history, physical, and laboratory examinations* (3rd ed.). Butterworths. https://www.ncbi.nlm.nih.gov/books/NBK420/

13 Ferguson, C. M. (1990). An overview of the gastrointestinal system. In Walker, H. K., Hall W. D., Hurst J. W. (Eds.), *Clinical methods: The history, physical, and laboratory examinations* (3rd ed.). Butterworths. https://www.ncbi.nlm.nih.gov/books/NBK405/

14 "DSC_2286-1024x678.jpg" by British Columbia Institute of Technology is licensed under CC BY 4.0. Access for free at https://opentextbc.ca/clinicalskills/chapter/2-5-focussed-respiratory-assessment/

15 McGee, S. R. (2012). *Evidence-based physical diagnosis* (3rd ed.). Elsevier Saunders. https://kimhournet.files.wordpress.com/2018/12/mcgee-evidence-based-physical-diagnosis-3rd-ed1.pdf

My Notes

pressure over an area of tenderness and then withdraws the hand abruptly. If the patient winces with pain upon withdrawal of the hand, the test is positive.[16, 17, 18]

Note: If the patient has a Foley catheter in place, additional assessments are included in the "Facilitation of Elimination" chapter.

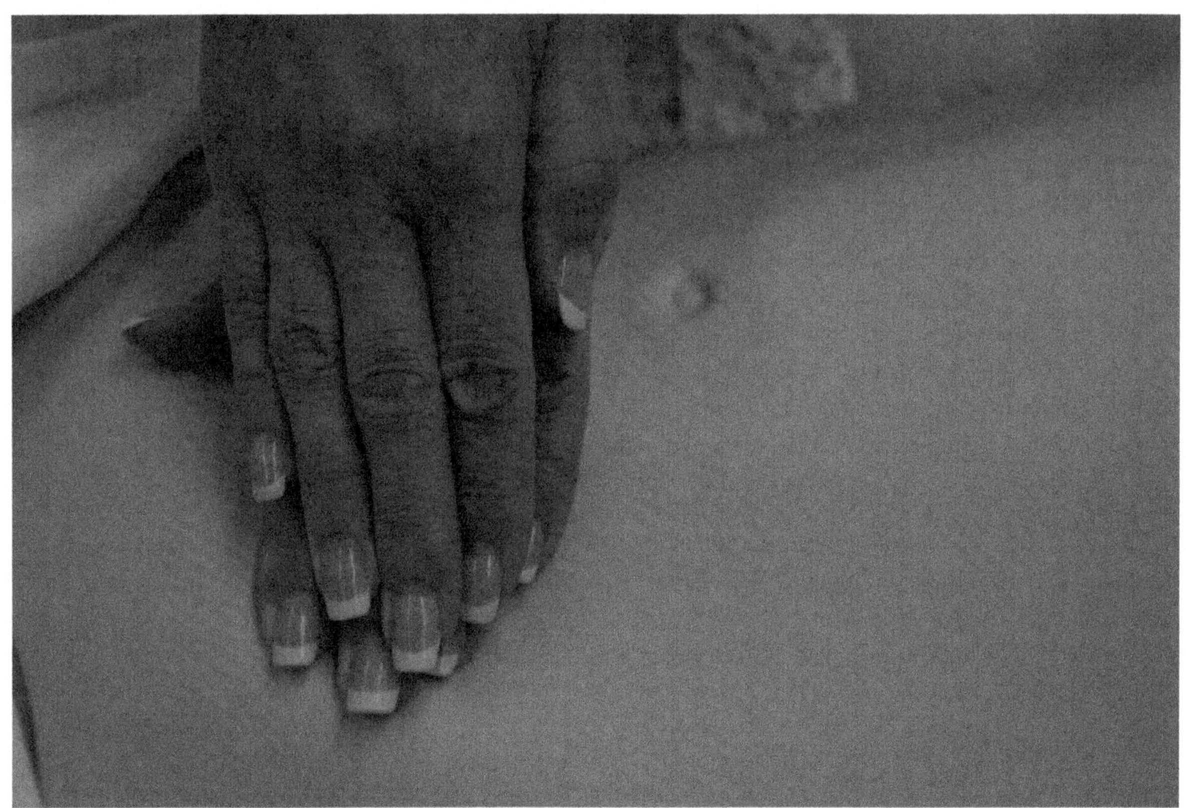

Figure 12.4 Light Palpation of the Abdomen

16 This work is a derivative of Clinical Procedures for Safer Patient Care by British Columbia Institute of Technology and is licensed under CC BY 4.0. Access for free at https://opentextbc.ca/clinicalskills/

17 Ferguson, C. M. (1990). Inspection, auscultation, palpation, and percussion of the abdomen. In Walker, H. K., Hall, W. D., Hurst, J. W. (Eds.), *Clinical methods: The history, physical, and laboratory examinations* (3rd ed.). Butterworths. https://www.ncbi.nlm.nih.gov/books/NBK420/

18 McGee, S. R. (2012). *Evidence-based physical diagnosis* (3rd ed.). Elsevier Saunders. https://kimhournet.files.wordpress.com/2018/12/mcgee-evidence-based-physical-diagnosis-3rd-ed1.pdf

Percussion

My Notes

You may observe advanced practice nurses and other health care providers percussing the abdomen to obtain additional data. Percussing can be used to assess the liver and spleen or to determine if costovertebral angle (CVA) tenderness is present, which is related to inflammation of the kidney.

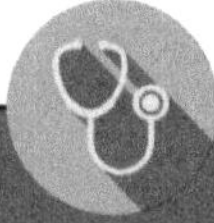

- **Encourage the patient to empty their bladder prior to palpation.**
- **When palpating the abdomen, ask the patient to bend their knees when lying in a supine position to enhance relaxation of abdominal muscles.**

See Table 12.3b for a comparison of expected versus unexpected findings when assessing the abdomen.

Table 12.3b Expected Versus Unexpected Gastrointestinal and Genitourinary Assessment Findings

Assessment	Expected Findings	Unexpected Findings (Document and notify the provider of any new findings*)
Inspection	Symmetry of shape and color Flat or rounded contour (protuberant in children until age 4) No visible lesions Intact skin Colostomy	Asymmetry Distension Scars Wounds Skin breakdown Pulsations Visible peristalsis
Auscultation	Presence of normoactive bowel sounds	Hypoactive bowel sounds Hyperactive bowel sounds Absent bowel sounds
Palpation	Absence of pain or tenderness Absence of masses	Pain on palpation Guarding Rigidity Rebound tenderness Masses noted that are not previously documented

My Notes

Assessment	Expected Findings	Unexpected Findings **(Document and notify the provider of any new findings*)**
Genitourinary	Clear, pale yellow urine Absence of pain, urgency, frequency, or retention	Dark or bloody urine, foul odor, or sediment present Dysuria Urinary frequency Urinary urgency Urinary retention
***CRITICAL CONDITIONS to report immediately**		New or worsening melena Bloody stools Hematemesis Signs of dehydration associated with diarrhea and vomiting, such as <30mL urine/hour

12.4 SAMPLE DOCUMENTATION

My Notes

Sample Documentation of Expected Findings

The patient denies abdominal pain, nausea, vomiting, bloating, constipation, diarrhea, urinary pain, urgency or frequency, change in appetite, food intolerance, dysphagia, or personal or family history. Abdominal contour is flat and symmetric. No visible lesions, pulsations, or peristalsis noted. Bowel sounds present and normoactive. Patient denies pain with palpation; no masses noted.

Sample Documentation of Unexpected Findings

The patient reports generalized abdominal pain, along with nausea and vomiting for the last two days. Abdomen is slightly distended. Bowel sounds hypoactive in all four quadrants. Pain reported at 7/10 and guarding noted with palpation of the RLQ. Dr. Smith notified at 0730.

My Notes

12.5 CHECKLIST FOR ABDOMINAL ASSESSMENT

Use this checklist below to review the steps for completion of an "Abdominal Assessment."[1]

Steps

Disclaimer: Always review and follow agency policy regarding this specific skill.

1. Gather stethoscope.
2. Perform safety steps:
    - Perform hand hygiene.
    - Check the room for transmission-based precautions.
    - Introduce yourself, your role, the purpose of your visit, and an estimate of the time it will take.
    - Confirm patient ID using two patient identifiers (e.g., name and date of birth).
    - Explain the process to the patient and ask if they have any questions.
    - Be organized and systematic.
    - Use appropriate listening and questioning skills.
    - Listen and attend to patient cues.
    - Ensure the patient's privacy and dignity.
    - Assess ABCs.
3. Conduct a focused interview related to gastrointestinal and genitourinary concerns. Ask relevant, focused questions based on patient status. See Tables 1 and 2 for sample focused questions.
4. Position the patient in the supine position and drape the patient, exposing only the areas needed for assessment.
5. Inspect the abdomen for shape/contour, symmetry, pigmentation/color, lesions/scars, pulsation, and visible peristalsis.
6. Auscultate using the diaphragm of the stethoscope to assess for bowel sounds.
7. Lightly palpate the four quadrants of the abdomen to assess for pain or masses. Palpate the suprapubic area for bladder distention. If the patient reports abdominal pain, palpate that area last.
8. Assist the patient to a comfortable position, ask if they have any questions, and thank them for their time.
9. Ensure safety measures when leaving the room:
    - CALL LIGHT: Within reach
    - BED: Low and locked (in lowest position and brakes on)
    - SIDERAILS: Secured

1 This work is a derivative of Clinical Procedures for Safer Patient Care by British Columbia Institute of Technology and is licensed under CC BY 4.0. Access for free at https://opentextbc.ca/clinicalskills/

My Notes

- TABLE: Within reach
- ROOM: Risk-free for falls (scan room and clear any obstacles)

10. Perform hand hygiene.

11. Document the assessment findings and report any concerns according to agency policy.

My Notes

12.6 SUPPLEMENTARY VIDEO ON ABDOMINAL ASSESSMENT

Video Review of Abdominal Assessment[1]

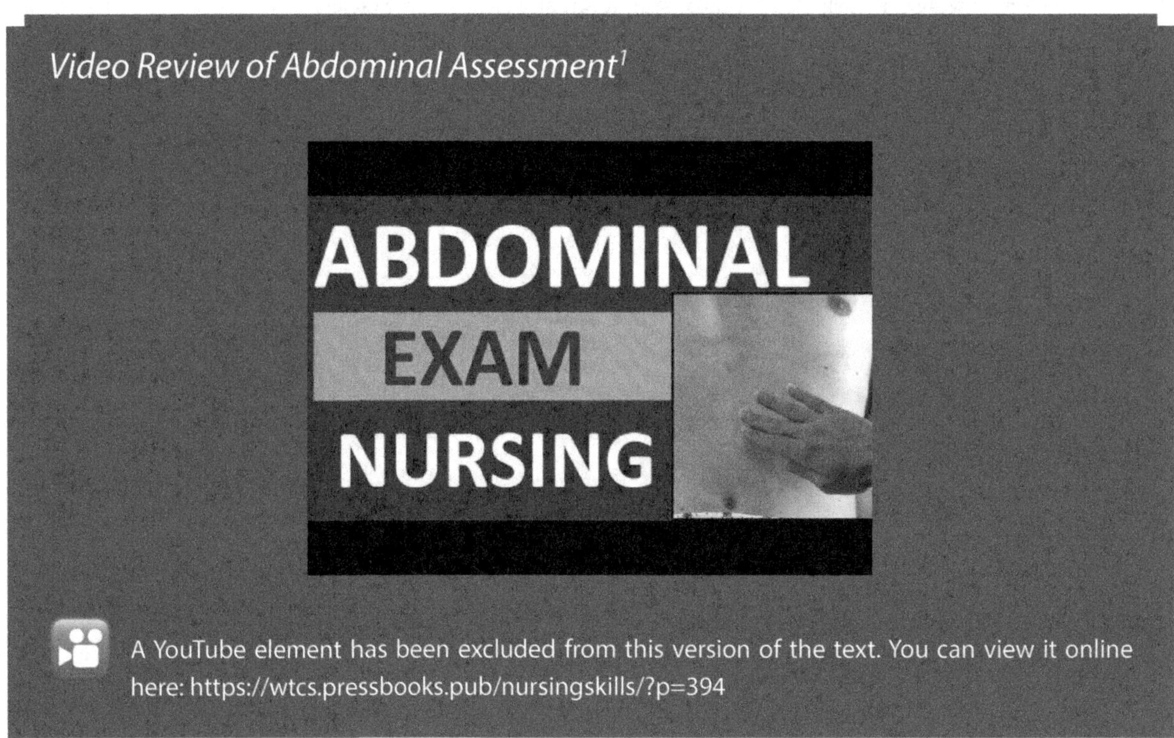

A YouTube element has been excluded from this version of the text. You can view it online here: https://wtcs.pressbooks.pub/nursingskills/?p=394

1 RegisteredNurseRN. (2017, December 29). *Abdominal examination (exam) nursing assessment | Bowel & vascular sounds, palpation, inspection*. [Video]. YouTube. All rights reserved. Video used with permission. https://youtu.be/1Xc7RYkz-CE

12.7 LEARNING ACTIVITIES

My Notes

Learning Activities

(Answers to "Learning Activities" can be found in the '"Answer Key" at the end of the book. Answers to interactive activity elements will be provided within the element as immediate feedback.)

The nurse is performing a daily assessment on a patient who had hip surgery a few days ago. The patient reports she has not had a bowel movement since prior to admission three days ago. The nurse forms a hypothesis that the patient is constipated.

1. What subjective data should the nurse plan to obtain during the assessment to investigate "cues" regarding the potential hypothesis of constipation?
   a. Nausea
   b. Vomiting
   c. Lactose intolerance
   d. Bloating
2. What objective data should the nurse plan to obtain during the assessment to investigate "cues" regarding the potential hypothesis of constipation?
   a. Bowel sounds
   b. Skin integrity
   c. Abdominal pulsations
   d. Bladder distention
3. The nurse discovers the following findings during the assessment. Which should be reported to the provider?
   a. The patient's abdomen appears flat and symmetrical.
   b. There are hypoactive bowel sounds in all quadrants.
   c. Firmness is palpated in left lower quadrant.
   d. There is a scar from a previous appendectomy.
4. The nurse calls the provider and reports the assessment findings supporting the hypothesis of constipation. A new order for Milk of Magnesia 30 mL PO is obtained and the medication is administered. A few hours later, the patient has a large bowel movement. Write a focused DAR or SOAP note documenting the patient's constipation status.

My Notes

Check your knowledge using this flashcard activity:

An interactive or media element has been excluded from this version of the text. You can view it online here: https://wtcs.pressbooks.pub/nursingskills/?p=397

Practice creating documentation in this learning activity:

An interactive or media element has been excluded from this version of the text. You can view it online here: https://wtcs.pressbooks.pub/nursingskills/?p=397

XII GLOSSARY

My Notes

Borborygmus: Hyperperistalsis, often referred to as "stomach growling."

Distention: An expansion of the abdomen caused by the accumulation of air or fluid. Patients often report "feeling bloated."

Dysphagia: Difficulty swallowing.

Dysuria: Painful urination.

Guarding: Voluntary contraction of abdominal wall musculature; may be related to fear, anxiety, or presence of cold hands.

Hematochezia: Passage of bloody stool.

Hematemesis: Blood-tinged mucus secretions from the lungs.

Hyperactive bowel sounds: Increased peristaltic activity; may be related to diarrhea, obstruction, or digestion of a meal.

Hypoactive bowel sounds: Decreased peristaltic activity; may be related to constipation following abdominal surgery or with an ileus.

Melena: Stool dark in color and tarry in consistency.

Protuberant: Convex or bulging appearance.

Rebound tenderness: Pain when hand is withdrawn during palpation.

Rigidity: Involuntary contraction of the abdominal musculature in response to peritoneal inflammation.

Scaphoid: Sunken appearance.

Stiae: White or silver markings from stretching of the skin.

Urinary frequency: Urination every hour or two.

Urinary incontinence: Involuntary leakage of urine.

Urinary urgency: An intense urge to urinate that can lead to urinary incontinence.

Chapter 13

Musculoskeletal Assessment

13.1 MUSCULOSKELETAL ASSESSMENT INTRODUCTION

My Notes

Learning Objectives

- Perform a musculoskeletal assessment
- Palpate joints for pain, swelling, change in temperature, and range of motion
- Modify assessment techniques to reflect variations across the life span
- Recognize and report significant deviations from norms
- Document actions and observations

The musculoskeletal system gives us the ability to move. It is composed of bones, muscles, joints, tendons, ligaments, and cartilage that support the body, allow movement, and protect vital organs. An assessment of the musculoskeletal system includes collecting data regarding the structure and movement of the body, as well the patient's mobility. Let's begin by reviewing the anatomy of the musculoskeletal system and common conditions a nurse may find on assessment.

My Notes

13.2 MUSCULOSKELETAL BASIC CONCEPTS

Skeleton

The skeleton is composed of 206 bones that provide the internal supporting structure of the body. See Figure 13.1[1] for an illustration of the major bones in the body. The bones of the lower limbs are adapted for weight-bearing support, stability, and walking. The upper limbs are highly mobile with large range of movements, along with the ability to easily manipulate objects with our hands and opposable thumbs.[2]

For additional information about the bones in the body, visit the OpenStax *Anatomy and Physiology* book (https://openstax.org/books/anatomy-and-physiology/pages/8-introduction).

1 "701 Axial Skeleton-01.jpg" by OpenStax is licensed under CC BY 3.0. Access for free at https://commons.wikimedia.org/wiki/File:701_Axial_Skeleton-01.jpg

2 This work is a derivative of Anatomy & Physiology by OpenStax and is licensed under CC BY 4.0. Access for free at https://openstax.org/books/anatomy-and-physiology/pages/1-introduction

My Notes

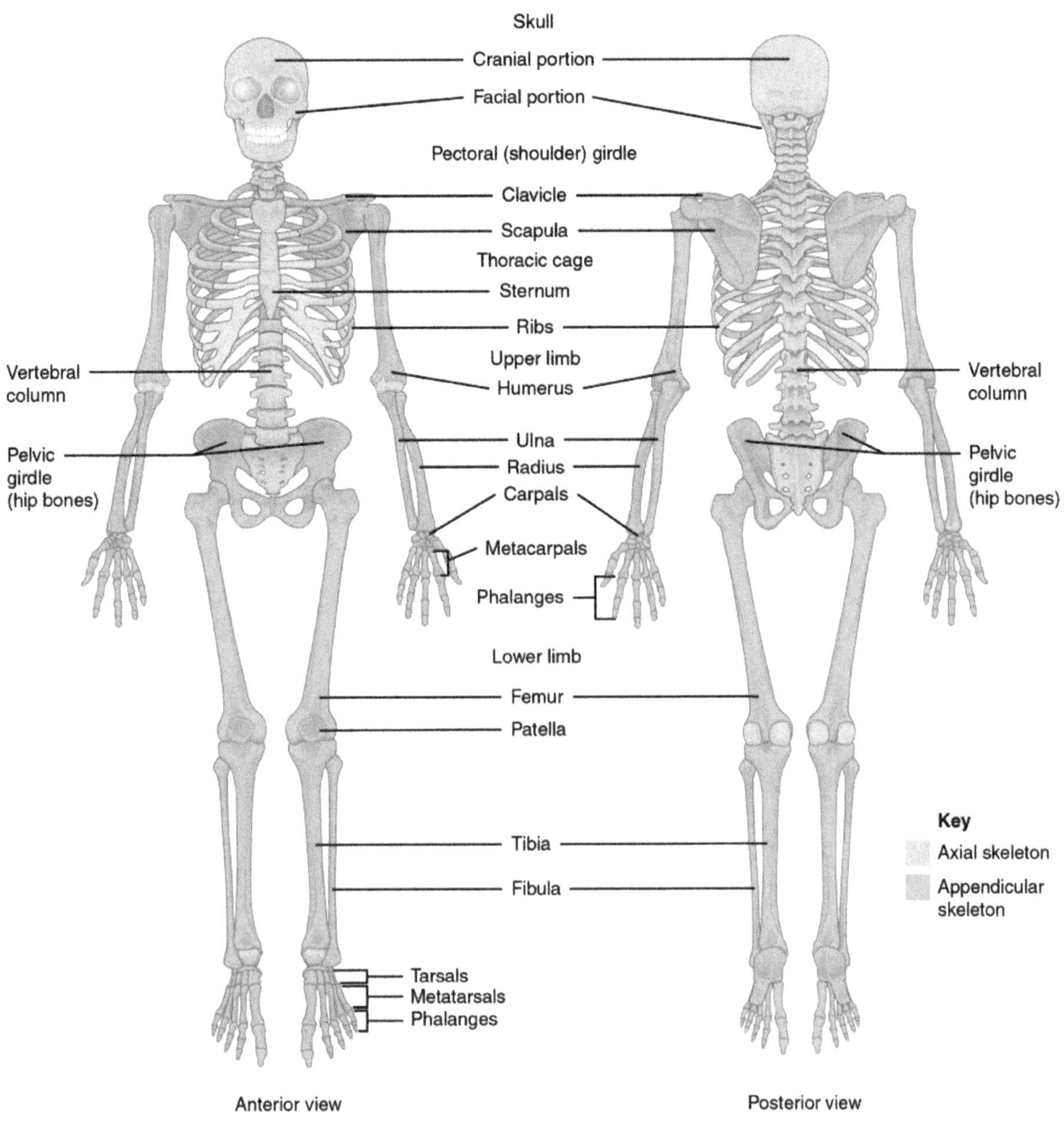

Figure 13.1 Skeletal Bones

Bones are connected together by ligaments. **Ligaments** are strong bands of fibrous connective tissue that strengthen and support the joint by anchoring the bones together and preventing their separation. Ligaments allow for normal movements of a joint while also limiting the range of these motions to prevent excessive or abnormal joint movements.[3]

---

3 This work is a derivative of Anatomy & Physiology by OpenStax and is licensed under CC BY 4.0. Access for free at https://openstax.org/books/anatomy-and-physiology/pages/preface

My Notes

Muscles

There are three types of muscle tissue: skeletal muscle, cardiac muscle, and smooth muscle. **Skeletal muscle** produces movement, assists in maintaining posture, protects internal organs, and generates body heat. Skeletal muscles are voluntary, meaning a person is able to consciously control them, but they also depend on signals from the nervous system to work properly. Other types of muscles are involuntary and are controlled by the autonomic nervous system, such as the smooth muscle within our bronchioles.[4]

See Figure 13.2[5] for an illustration of skeletal muscle.

To move the skeleton, the tension created by the contraction of the skeletal muscles is transferred to the **tendons**, strong bands of dense, regular connective tissue that connect muscles to bones.[6]

For additional information about skeletal muscles, visit the OpenStax *Anatomy and Physiology* book (https://openstax.org/books/anatomy-and-physiology/pages/8-introduction).

---

4 This work is a derivative of Anatomy & Physiology by OpenStax and is licensed under CC BY 4.0. Access for free at https://openstax.org/books/anatomy-and-physiology/pages/1-introduction

5 "1105 Anterior and Posterior Views of Muscles.jpg" by OpenStax is licensed under CC BY-SA 4.0. Access for free at https://commons.wikimedia.org/wiki/File:1105_Anterior_and_Posterior_Views_of_Muscles.jpg

6 This work is a derivative of Anatomy & Physiology by OpenStax and is licensed under CC BY 4.0. Access for free at https://openstax.org/books/anatomy-and-physiology/pages/1-introduction

My Notes

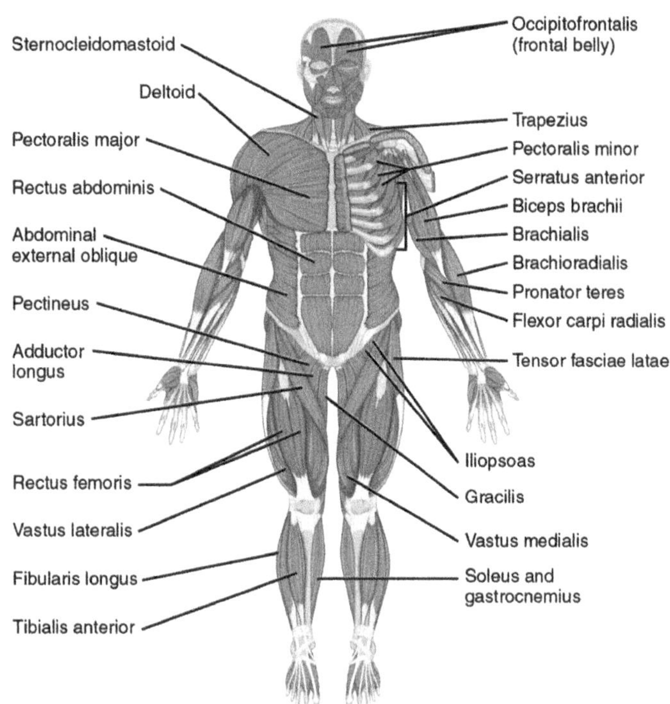

Major muscles of the body.
Right side: superficial; left side:
deep (anterior view)

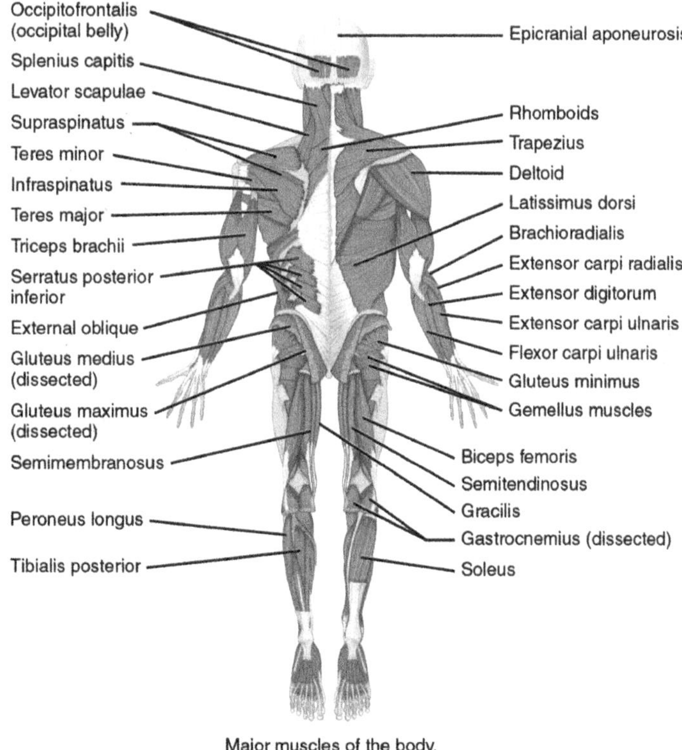

Major muscles of the body.
Right side: superficial; left side:
deep (posterior view)

Figure 13.2 Skeletal Muscle

My Notes

Muscle Atrophy

Muscle atrophy is the thinning or loss of muscle tissue. See Figure 13.3[7] for an image of muscle atrophy. There are three types of muscle atrophy: physiologic, pathologic, and neurogenic.

Physiologic atrophy is caused by not using the muscles and can often be reversed with exercise and improved nutrition. People who are most affected by physiologic atrophy are those who:

- Have seated jobs, health problems that limit movement, or decreased activity levels
- Are bedridden
- Cannot move their limbs because of stroke or other brain disease
- Are in a place that lacks gravity, such as during space flights

Pathologic atrophy is seen with aging, starvation, and adverse effects of long-term use of corticosteroids. Neurogenic atrophy is the most severe type of muscle atrophy. It can be from an injured or diseased nerve that connects to the muscle. Examples of neurogenic atrophy are spinal cord injuries and polio.[8]

Although physiologic atrophy due to disuse can often be reversed with exercise, muscle atrophy caused by age is irreversible. The effects of age-related atrophy are especially pronounced in people who are sedentary because the loss of muscle results in functional impairments such as trouble with walking, balance, and posture. These functional impairments can cause decreased quality of life and injuries due to falls.[9]

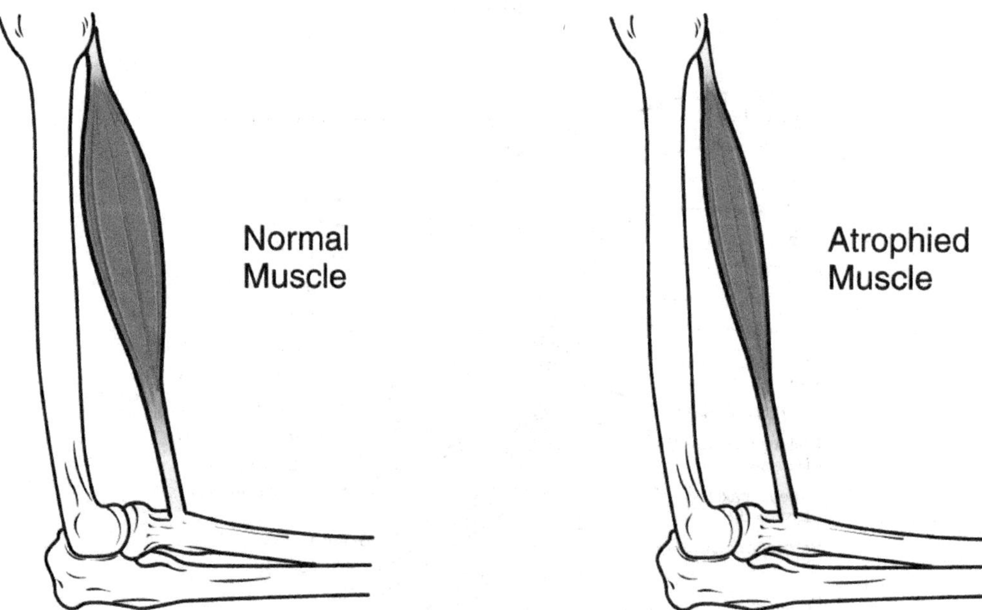

Figure 13.3 Muscle Atrophy

---

7 "1025 Atrophy.png" by OpenStax is licensed under CC BY 4.0. Access for free at https://openstax.org/books/anatomy-and-physiology/pages/10-6-exercise-and-muscle-performance.

8 A.D.A.M. Medical Encyclopedia [Internet]. Atlanta (GA): A.D.A.M., Inc.; c1997-2020. Muscle atrophy; [updated 2020, Sep 16; cited 2020, Sep 18]. https://medlineplus.gov/ency/article/003188.htm

9 This work is a derivative of Anatomy & Physiology by OpenStax and is licensed under CC BY 4.0. Access for free at https://openstax.org/books/anatomy-and-physiology/pages/1-introduction

Joints

My Notes

Joints are the location where bones come together. Many joints allow for movement between the bones. **Synovial joints** are the most common type of joint in the body. Synovial joints have a fluid-filled joint cavity where the articulating surfaces of the bones contact and move smoothly against each other. See Figure 13.4[10] for an illustration of a synovial joint.

Articular cartilage is smooth, white tissue that covers the ends of bones where they come together and allows the bones to glide over each other with very little friction. Articular cartilage can be damaged by injury or normal wear and tear. Lining the inner surface of the articular capsule is a thin synovial membrane. The cells of this membrane secrete **synovial fluid**, a thick, slimy fluid that provides lubrication to further reduce friction between the bones of the joint.[11]

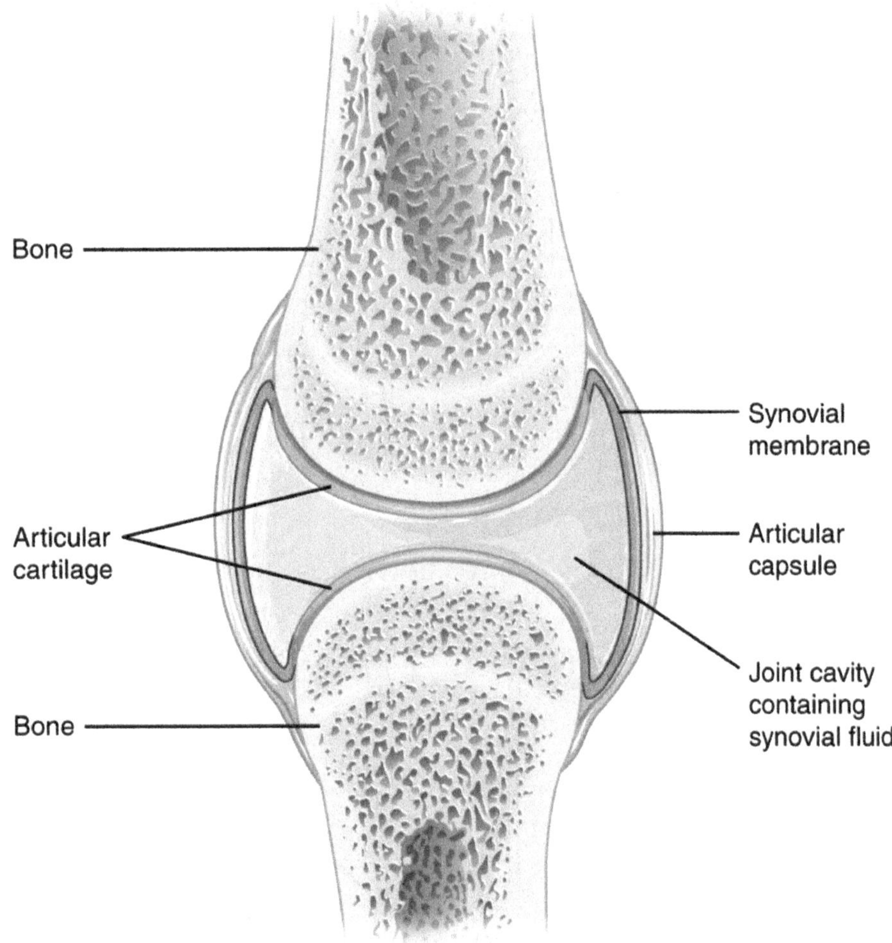

Figure 13.4 Synovial Joint

10 "907_Synovial_Joints.jpg" by OpenStax is licensed under CC BY-SA 3.0. Access for free at https://commons.wikimedia.org/wiki/File:907_Synovial_Joints.jpg

11 This work is a derivative of Anatomy & Physiology by OpenStax and is licensed under CC BY 4.0. Access for free at https://openstax.org/books/anatomy-and-physiology/pages/1-introduction

My Notes

Types of Synovial Joints

There are six types of synovial joints. See Figure 13.5[12] for an illustration of the types of synovial joints. Some joints are relatively immobile but stable. Other joints have more freedom of movement but are at greater risk of injury. For example, the hinge joint of the knee allows flexion and extension, whereas the ball and socket joint of the hip and shoulder allows flexion, extension, abduction, adduction, and rotation. The knee, hip, and shoulder joints are commonly injured and are discussed in more detail in the following subsections.

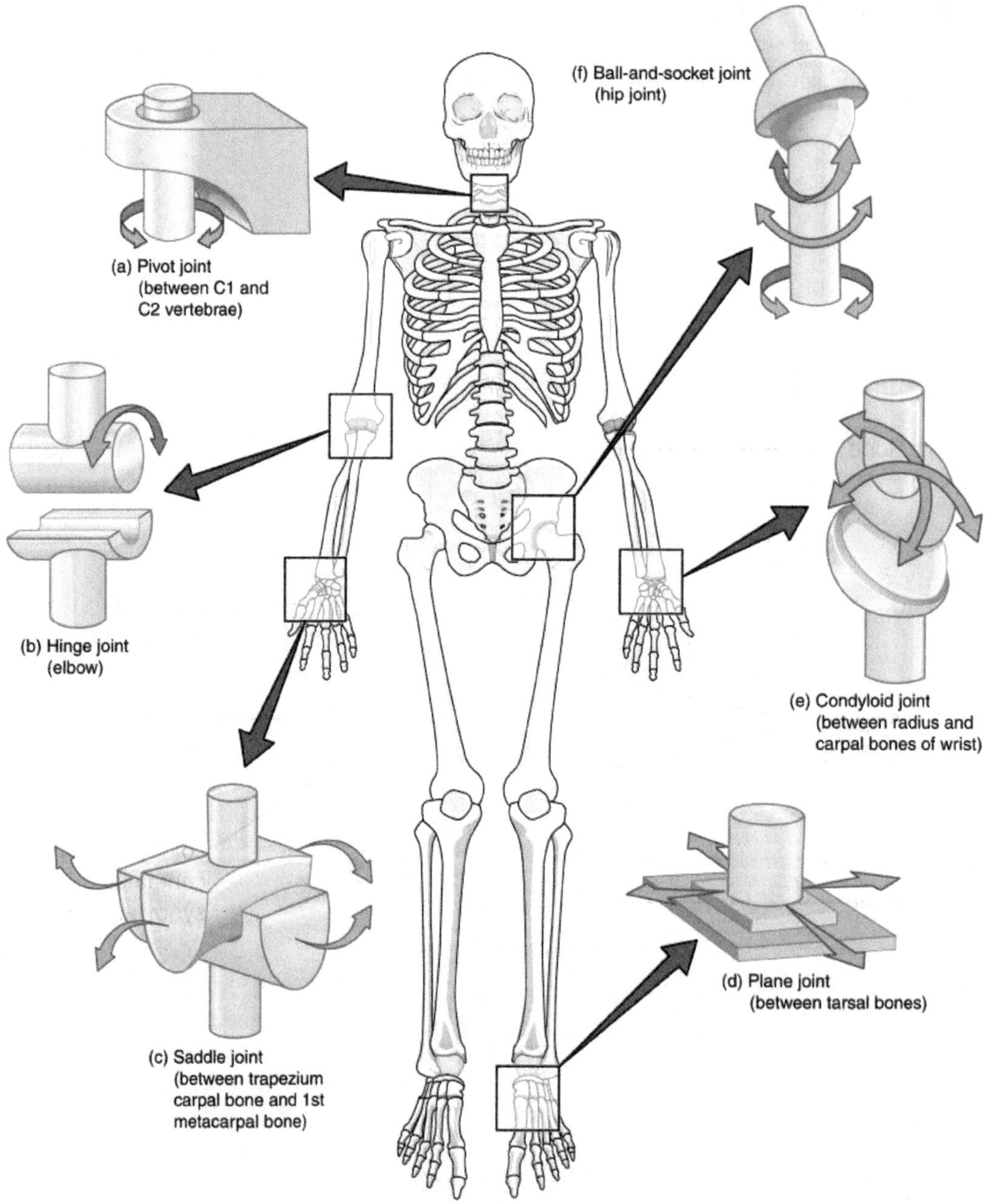

Figure 13.5 Types of Synovial Joints

---

12 "909 Types of Synovial Joints.jpg" by OpenStax is licensed under CC BY 3.0. Access for free at https://commons.wikimedia.org/wiki/File:909_Types_of_Synovial_Joints.jpg

Shoulder Joint

My Notes

The shoulder joint is a ball-and-socket joint formed by the articulation between the head of the humerus and the glenoid cavity of the scapula. This joint has the largest range of motion of any joint in the body. See Figure 13.6[13] to review the anatomy of the shoulder joint. Injuries to the shoulder joint are common, especially during repetitive abductive use of the upper limb such as during throwing, swimming, or racquet sports.[14]

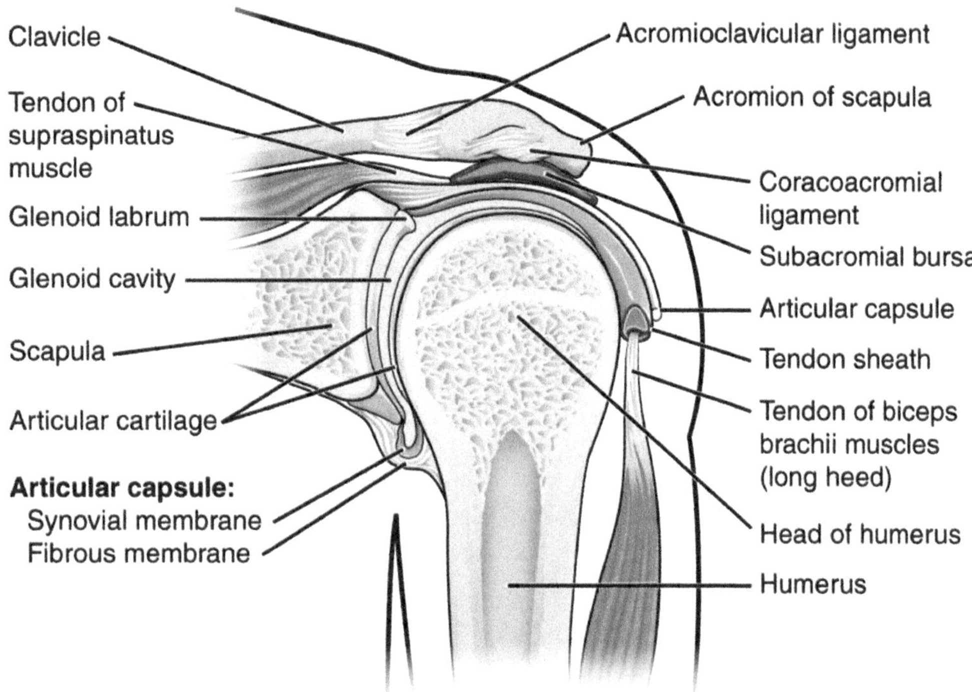

Figure 13.6 Should Joint

13 "914 Shoulder Joint.jpg" by OpenStax is licensed under CC BY 3.0. Access for free at https://commons.wikimedia.org/wiki/File:914_Shoulder_Joint.jpg

14 This work is a derivative of Anatomy & Physiology by OpenStax and is licensed under CC BY 4.0. Access for free at https://openstax.org/books/anatomy-and-physiology/pages/1-introduction

My Notes

Hip Joint

The hip joint is a ball-and-socket joint between the head of the femur and the acetabulum of the hip bone. The hip carries the weight of the body and thus requires strength and stability during standing and walking.[15]

See Figure 13.7[16] for an illustration of the hip joint.

A common hip injury in older adults, often referred to as a "broken hip," is actually a fracture of the head of the femur. Hip fractures are commonly caused by falls.[17]

See more information about hip fractures under the "Common Musculoskeletal Conditions" section.

15 This work is a derivative of Anatomy & Physiology by OpenStax and is licensed under CC BY 4.0. Access for free at https://openstax.org/books/anatomy-and-physiology/pages/1-introduction

16 "916 Hip Joint.jpg" by OpenStax is licensed under CC BY 3.0. Access for free at https://commons.wikimedia.org/wiki/File:916_Hip_Joint.jpg

17 This work is a derivative of Anatomy & Physiology by OpenStax and is licensed under CC BY 4.0. Access for free at https://openstax.org/books/anatomy-and-physiology/pages/1-introduction

My Notes

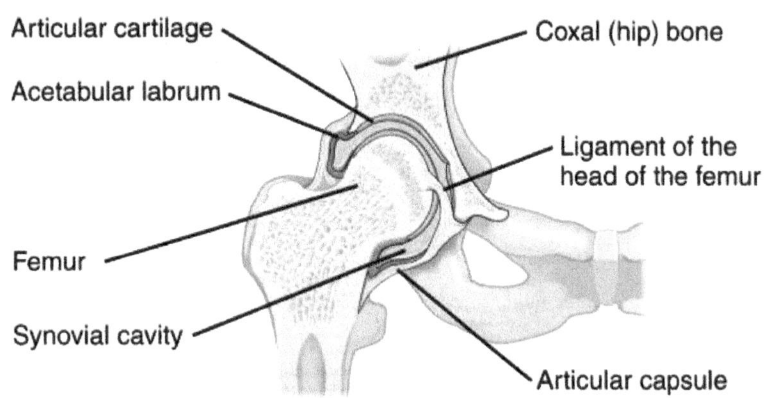

(a) Frontal section through the right hip joint

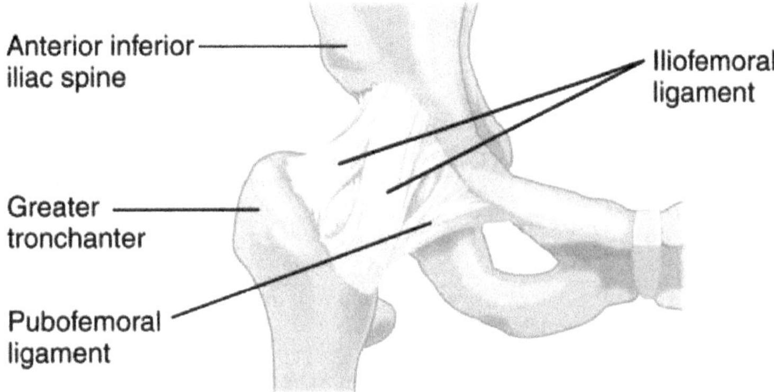

(b) Anterior view of right hip joint, capsule in place

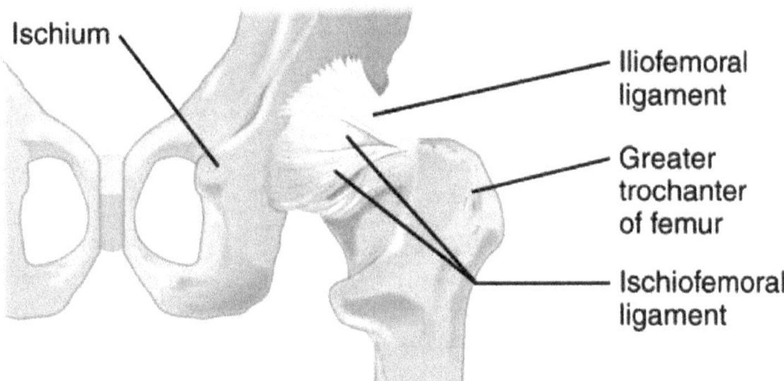

(c) Posterior view of right hip joint, capsule in place

Figure 13.7 Hip Joint

My Notes

Knee Joint

The knee functions as a hinge joint that allows flexion and extension of the leg. In addition, some rotation of the leg is available when the knee is flexed, but not when extended. See Figure 13.8[18] for an illustration of the knee joint. The knee is vulnerable to injuries associated with hyperextension, twisting, or blows to the medial or lateral side of the joint, particularly while weight-bearing.[19]

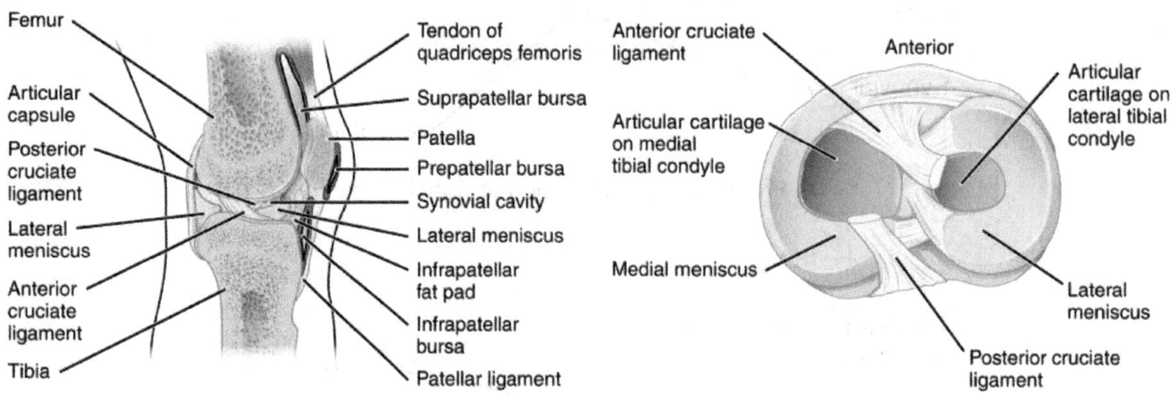

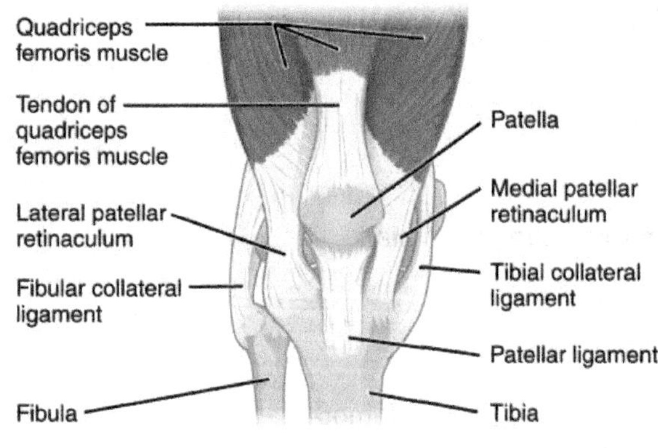

Figure 13.8 Knee Joint

18 "917 Knee Joint.jpg" by OpenStax is licensed under CC BY 3.0. Access for free at https://commons.wikimedia.org/wiki/File:917_Knee_Joint.jpg

19 This work is a derivative of Anatomy & Physiology by OpenStax and is licensed under CC BY 4.0. Access for free at https://openstax.org/books/anatomy-and-physiology/pages/1-introduction

My Notes

The knee joint has multiple ligaments that provide support, especially in the extended position. On the outside of the knee joint are the lateral collateral, medial collateral, and tibial collateral ligaments. The lateral collateral ligament is on the lateral side of the knee and spans from the lateral side of the femur to the head of the fibula. The medial collateral ligament runs from the medial side of the femur to the medial tibia. The tibial collateral ligament crosses the knee and is attached to the articular capsule and to the medial meniscus. In the fully extended knee position, both collateral ligaments are taut and stabilize the knee by preventing side-to-side or rotational motions between the femur and tibia.[20]

Inside the knee joint are the anterior cruciate ligament and posterior cruciate ligament. These ligaments are anchored inferiorly to the tibia and run diagonally upward to attach to the inner aspect of a femoral condyle. The posterior cruciate ligament supports the knee when it is flexed and weight-bearing such as when walking downhill. The anterior cruciate ligament becomes tight when the knee is extended and resists hyperextension.[21]

The patella is a bone incorporated into the tendon of the quadriceps muscle, the large muscle of the anterior thigh. The patella protects the quadriceps tendon from friction against the distal femur. Continuing from the patella to the anterior tibia just below the knee is the patellar ligament. Acting via the patella and patellar ligament, the quadriceps is a powerful muscle that extends the leg at the knee and provides support and stabilization for the knee joint.

Located between the articulating surfaces of the femur and tibia are two articular discs, the medial meniscus and lateral meniscus. Each meniscus is a C-shaped fibrocartilage that provides padding between the bones.[22]

Joint Movements

Several movements may be performed by synovial joints. **Abduction** is the movement away from the midline of the body. **Adduction** is the movement toward the middle line of the body. **Extension** is the straightening of limbs (increase in angle) at a joint. **Flexion** is bending the limbs (reduction of angle) at a joint. **Rotation** is a circular movement around a fixed point. See Figures 13.9[23] and 13.10[24] for images of the types of movements of different joints in the body.

20 This work is a derivative of Anatomy & Physiology by OpenStax and is licensed under CC BY 4.0. Access for free at https://openstax.org/books/anatomy-and-physiology/pages/1-introduction

21 This work is a derivative of Anatomy & Physiology by OpenStax and is licensed under CC BY 4.0. Access for free at https://openstax.org/books/anatomy-and-physiology/pages/1-introduction

22 This work is a derivative of Anatomy & Physiology by OpenStax and is licensed under CC BY 4.0. Access for free at https://openstax.org/books/anatomy-and-physiology/pages/1-introduction

23 "Body Movements I.jpg" by Tonye Ogele CNX is licensed under CC BY-SA 3.0. Access for free at https://commons.wikimedia.org/wiki/File:Body_Movements_I.jpg

24 "Body Movements II.jpg" by Tonye Ogele CNX is licensed under CC BY-SA 3.0. Access for free at https://commons.wikimedia.org/wiki/File:Body_Movements_II.jpg

My Notes

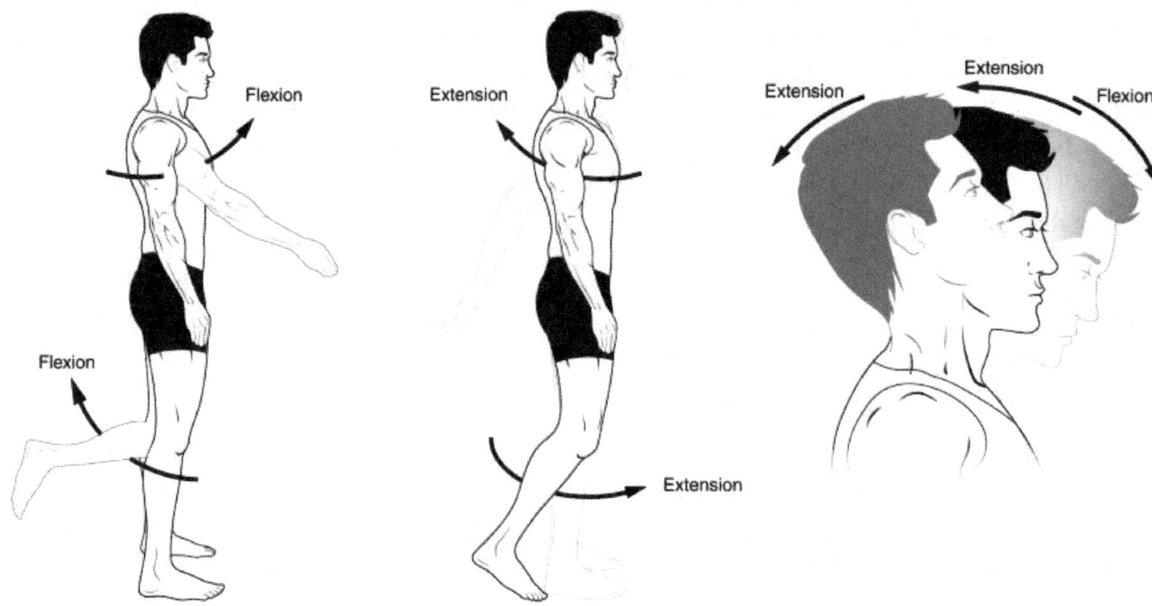

(a) and (b) Angular movements: flexion and extension at the shoulder and knees

(c) Angular movements: flexion and extension of the neck

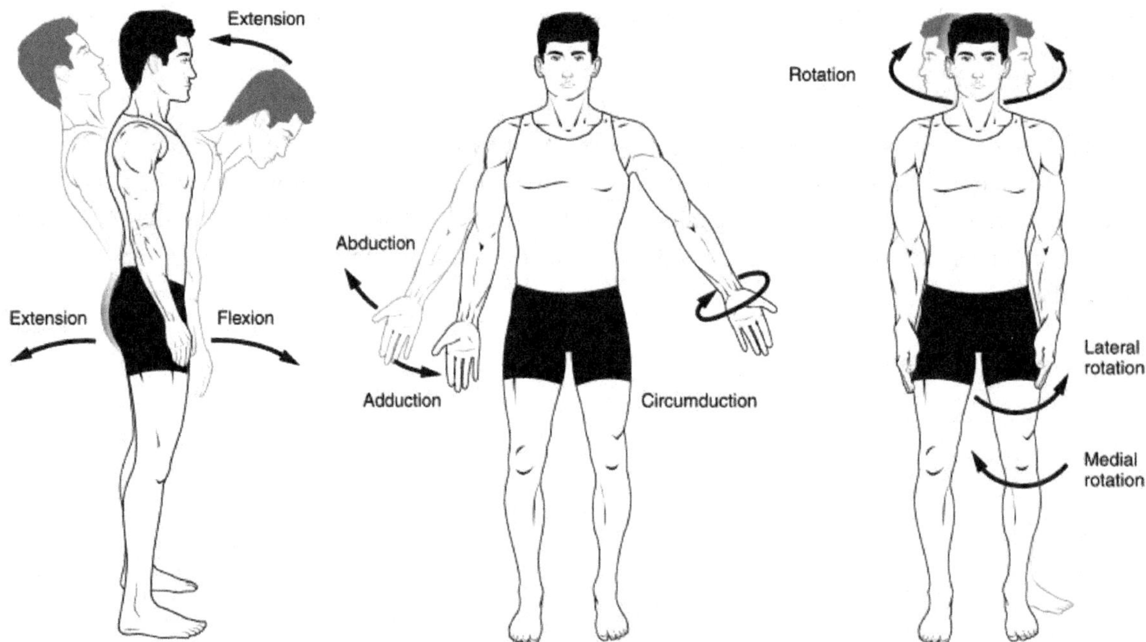

(d) Angular movements: flexion and extension of the vertebral column

(e) Angular movements: abduction, adduction, and circumduction of the upper limb at the shoulder

(f) Rotation of the head, neck, and lower limb

Figure 13.9 Joint Movements

My Notes

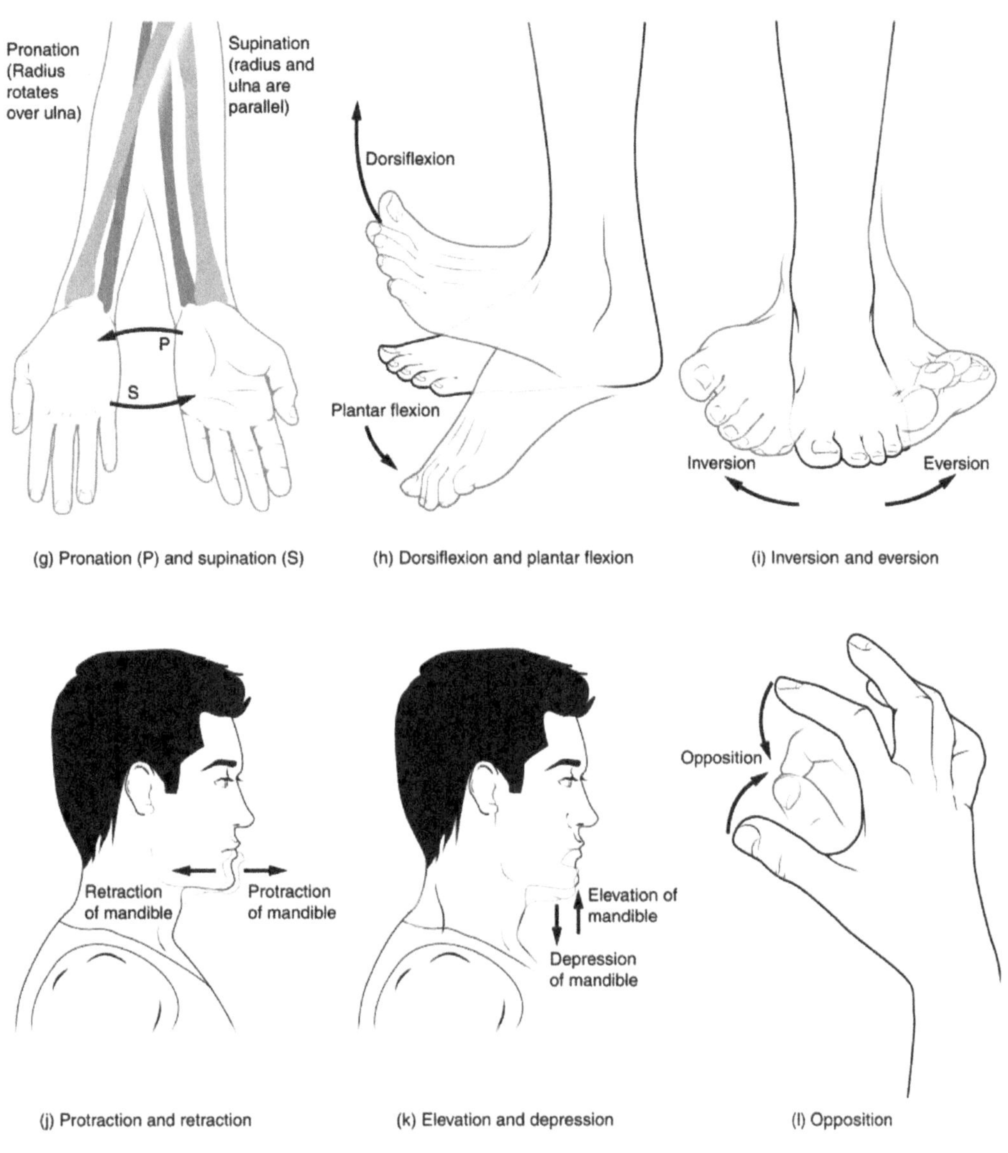

Figure 13.10 Joint Movements

My Notes

Joint Sounds

Sounds that occur as joints are moving are often referred to as **crepitus**. There are many different types of sounds that can occur as a joint moves, and patients may describe these sounds as popping, snapping, catching, clicking, crunching, cracking, crackling, creaking, grinding, grating, and clunking. There are several potential causes of these noises such as bursting of tiny bubbles in the synovial fluid, snapping of ligaments, or a disease condition. While assessing joints, be aware that joint noises are common during activity and are usually painless and harmless, but if they are associated with an injury or are accompanied by pain or swelling, they should be reported to the health care provider for follow-up.[25]

View Physitutor's YouTube video for a review of crepitus sounds: Physitutor's "Why Your Knees Crack | Joint Crepitations.[26]

---

25 Song, S. J., Park, C. H., Liang, H., & Kim, S. J. (2018). Noise around the knee. *Clinics in Orthopedic Surgery, 10*(1), 1-8. https://dx.doi.org/10.4055%2Fcios.2018.10.1.1

26 Physitutors. (2017, March 25). *Why your knees crack | Joint crepitations.* [Video]. YouTube. All rights reserved. https://youtu.be/NQOZZgh5z8I

13.3 COMMON MUSCULOSKELETAL CONDITIONS

My Notes

Now that we have reviewed the basic anatomy of the musculoskeletal system, let's review common musculoskeletal conditions that a nurse may find on assessment.

Osteoporosis

Osteoporosis is a disease that thins and weakens bones, causing them to become fragile and break easily. See Figure 13.11[1] for an illustration comparing the top right image of normal bone to the bottom right image of bone with osteoporosis. Osteoporosis is common in older women and often occurs in the hip, spine, and wrist. To keep bones strong, patients at risk are educated to eat a diet rich in calcium and vitamin D, participate in weight-bearing exercise, and avoid smoking. If needed, medications such as bisphosphonates and calcitonin are used to treat severe osteoporosis.[2]

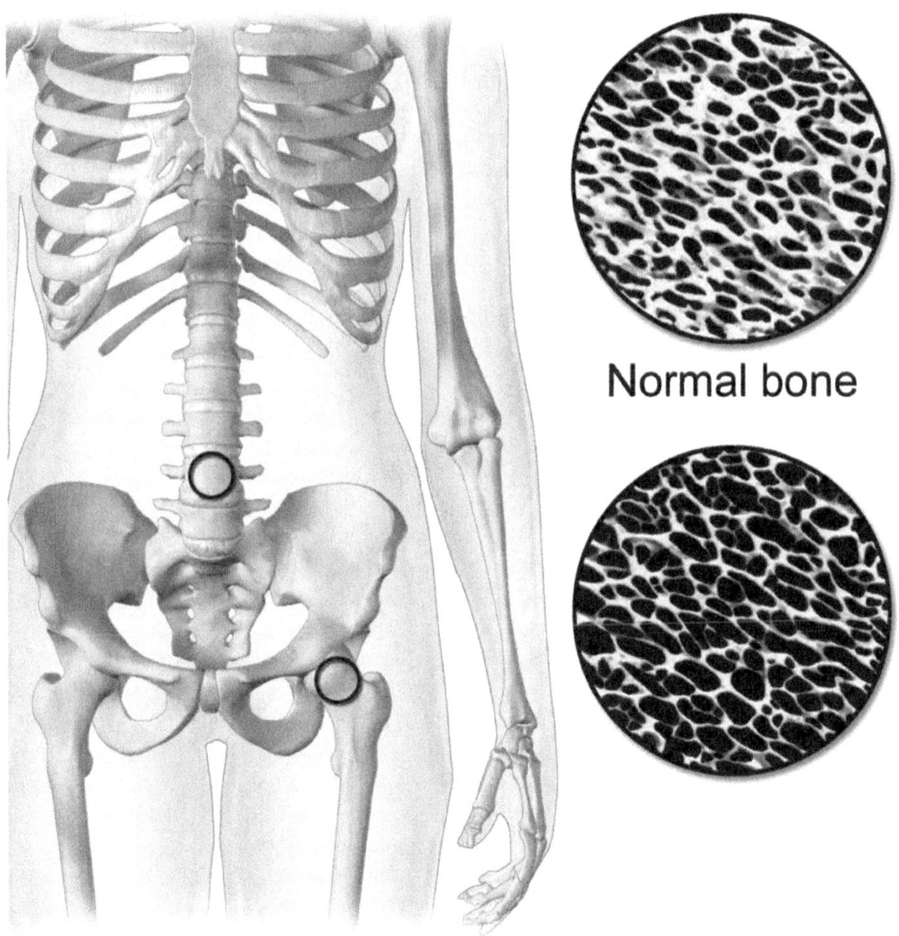

Figure 13.11 Osteoporosis

1 "Osteoporosis Effect and Locations.jpg" by *BruceBlaus* is licensed under CC BY-SA 4.0. Access for free at https://commons.wikimedia.org/wiki/File:Osteoporosis_Effect_and_Locations.jpg

2 MedlinePlus [Internet]. Bethesda (MD): National Library of Medicine (US); [updated 2020, Aug 14]. Osteoporosis; [reviewed 2017, Mar 15; cited 2020, Sep 18]. https://medlineplus.gov/osteoporosis.html

My Notes

Fracture

A **fracture** is the medical term for a broken bone. There are many different types of fractures commonly caused by sports injuries, falls, and car accidents. Additionally, people with osteoporosis are at higher risk for fractures from minor injuries due to weakening of the bones. See Figure 13.12[3] for an illustration of different types of fractures. For example, if the broken bone punctures the skin, it is called an **open fracture**. Symptoms of a fracture include the following:

- Intense pain
- Deformity (i.e., the limb looks out of place)
- Swelling, bruising, or tenderness around the injury
- Numbness and tingling of the extremity distal to the injury
- Difficulty moving a limb

A suspected fracture requires immediate medical attention and an X-ray to determine if the bone is broken. Treatment includes a cast or splint. In severe fractures, surgery is performed to place plates, pins, or screws in the bones to keep them in place as they heal.[4]

3 "612 Types of Fractures.jpg" by OpenStax is licensed under CC BY 4.0. Access for free at https://commons.wikimedia.org/wiki/File:612_Types_of_Fractures.jpg

4 MedlinePlus [Internet]. Bethesda (MD): National Library of Medicine (US); [updated 2020, Apr 20]. Fractures; [reviewed 2016, Mar 15; cited 2020, Sep 18]. https://medlineplus.gov/fractures.html

My Notes

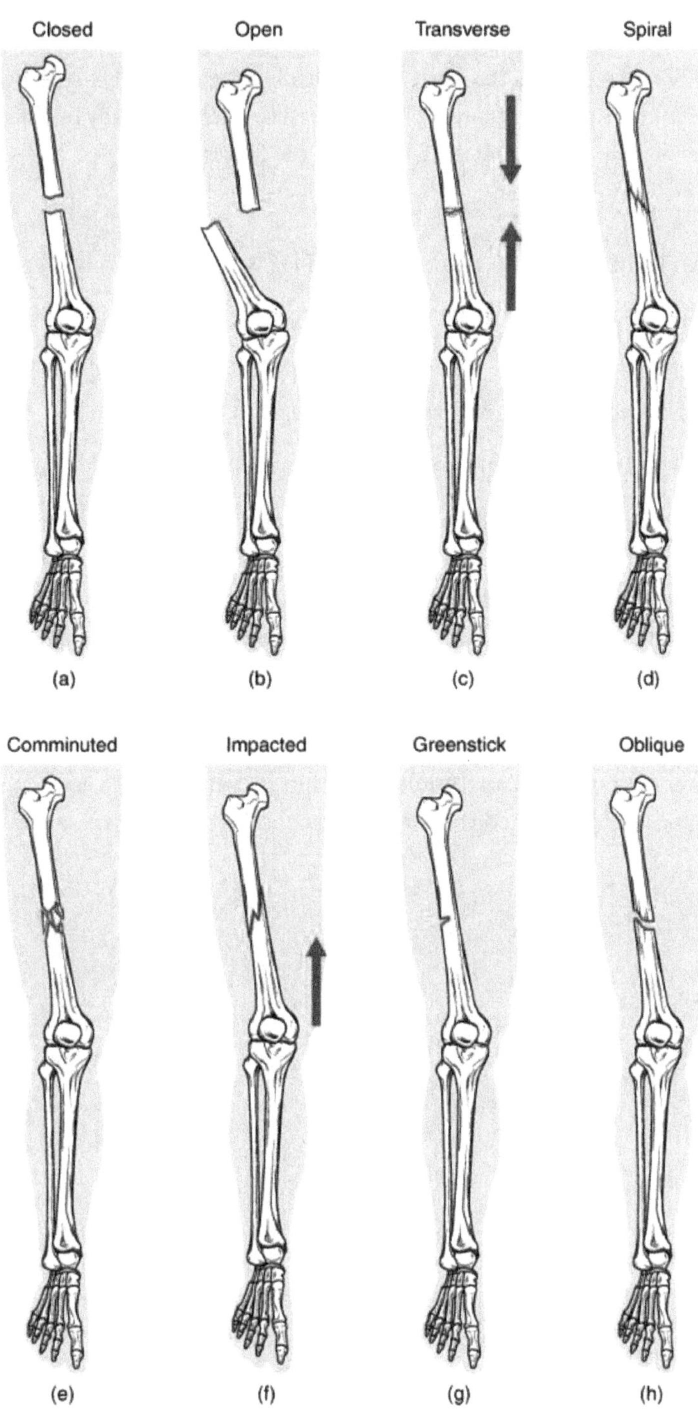

Figure 13.12 Types of Fractures

My Notes

Hip Fracture

A hip fracture, commonly referred to as a "broken hip," is actually a fracture of the femoral neck. See Figure 13.13[5] for an image of a hip fracture. Hip fractures are typically caused by a fall, especially in older adults with preexisting osteoporosis. Symptoms of a hip fracture after a fall include the following:

- Pain
- An inability to lift, move, or rotate the affected leg
- An inability to stand or put weight on the affected leg
- Bruising and swelling around the hip
- The injured leg appears shorter than the other leg
- The injured leg is rotated outwards[6]

Hip fractures typically require surgical repair within 48 hours of the injury. In approximately half of the cases of hip fractures, hip replacement is needed. See more information about hip replacement under the "Osteoarthritis" section below. In other cases, the fracture is fixed with surgery called Open Reduction Internal Fixation (ORIF) where the surgeon makes an incision to realign the bones, and then they are internally fixated (i.e., held together) with hardware like metal pins, plates, rods, or screws. After the bone heals, this hardware isn't removed unless additional symptoms occur. After surgery, the patient will need mobility assistance for a prolonged period of time from family members or in a long-term care facility, and the reduced mobility can result in additional falls if protective measures are not put into place. Additionally, hip fractures are also associated with life-threatening complications, such as pneumonia, infected pressure injuries, and blood clots that can move to the lungs causing pulmonary embolism.[7]

---

5 "Cdm hip fracture 343.jpg" by Booyabazooka is licensed under CC BY-SA 3.0. Access for free at https://commons.wikimedia.org/wiki/File:Cdm_hip_fracture_343.jpg

6 NHS (UK). (2019, October 3). Hip fracture. https://www.nhs.uk/conditions/hip-fracture/

7 This work is a derivative of Anatomy & Physiology by OpenStax and is licensed under CC BY 4.0. Access for free at https://openstax.org/books/anatomy-and-physiology/pages/1-introduction

My Notes

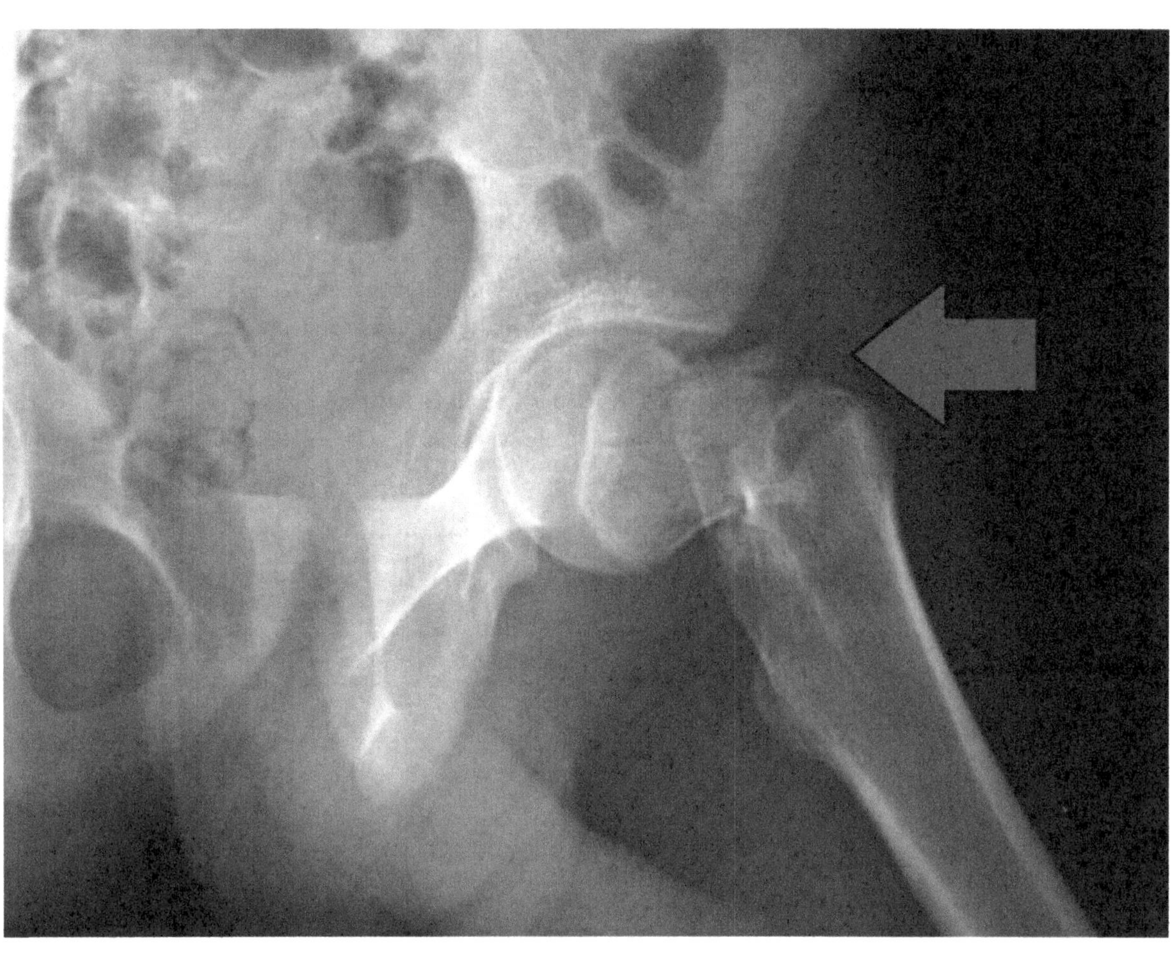

Figure 13.13 Hip Fracture

My Notes

Osteoarthritis

Osteoarthritis (OA) is the most common type of arthritis associated with aging and wear and tear of the articular cartilage that covers the surfaces of bones at a synovial joint. OA causes the cartilage to gradually become thinner, and as the cartilage layer wears down, more pressure is placed on the bones. The joint responds by increasing production of the synovial fluid for more lubrication, but this can cause swelling of the joint cavity. The bone tissue underlying the damaged articular cartilage also responds by thickening and causing the articulating surface of the bone to become rough or bumpy. As a result, joint movement results in pain and inflammation. In early stages of OA, symptoms may be resolved with mild activity that warms up the joint. However, in advanced OA, the affected joints become more painful and difficult to use, resulting in decreased mobility. There is no cure for osteoarthritis, but several treatments can help alleviate the pain. Treatments may include weight loss, low-impact exercise, and medications such as acetaminophen, nonsteroidal anti-inflammatory drugs (NSAIDs), and celecoxib. For severe cases of OA, joint replacement surgery may be required.[8]

See Figure 13.14[9] for an image comparing a normal joint to one with osteoarthritis and another type of arthritis called rheumatoid arthritis. (Rheumatoid arthritis is further explained under the "Joint Replacement" subsection.)

For more information about medications used to treat osteoarthritis, visit the "Analgesic and Musculoskeletal Medications" chapter in Open RN *Nursing Fundamentals*.

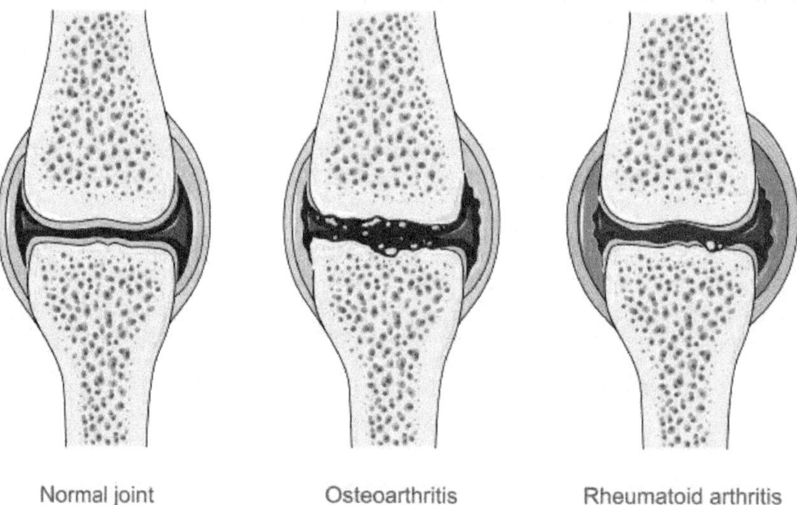

Figure 13.14 Comparison of Osteoarthritis and Rheumatoid Arthritis

8 This work is a derivative of Anatomy & Physiology by OpenStax and is licensed under CC BY 4.0. Access for free at https://openstax.org/books/anatomy-and-physiology/pages/1-introduction

9 "Osteoarthritis and rheumatoid arthritis - Normal joint Osteoarthr -- Smart-Servier.jpg" by Laboratoires Servier is licensed under CC BY-SA 3.0. Access for free at https://commons.m.wikimedia.org/wiki/File:Osteoarthritis_and_rheumatoid_arthritis_-_Normal_joint_Osteoarthr_--_Smart-Servier.jpg

Joint Replacement

My Notes

Arthroplasty, the medical term for joint replacement surgery, is an invasive procedure requiring extended recovery time, so conservative treatments such as lifestyle changes and medications are attempted before surgery is performed. See Figure 13.15[10] for an illustration of joint replacement surgery. This type of surgery involves replacing the articular surfaces of the bones with prosthesis (artificial components). For example, in hip arthroplasty, the worn or damaged parts of the hip joint, including the head and neck of the femur and the acetabulum of the pelvis, are removed and replaced with artificial joint components. The replacement head for the femur consists of a rounded ball attached to the end of a shaft that is inserted inside the femur. The acetabulum of the pelvis is reshaped and a replacement socket is fitted into its place.[11]

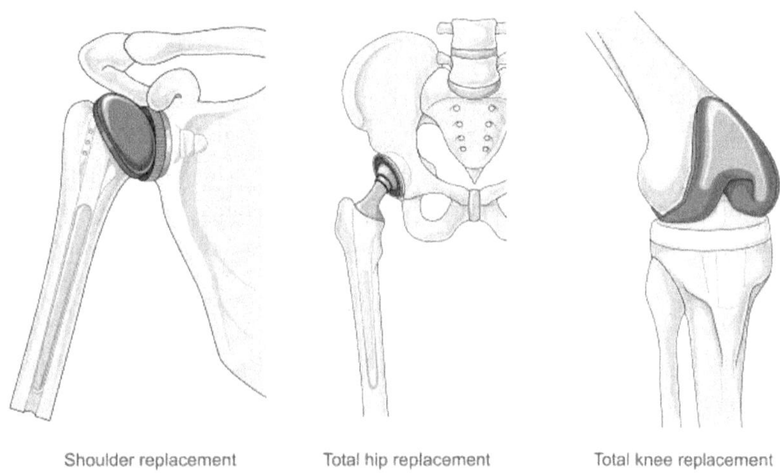

Figure 13.15 Joint Replacement

Hip Replacement

Hip replacement is surgery for people with severe hip damage often caused by osteoarthritis or a hip fracture. During a hip replacement operation, the surgeon removes damaged cartilage and bone from the hip joint and replaces them with artificial parts.[12]

The most common complication after surgery is hip dislocation. Because a man-made hip is smaller than the original joint, the ball may easily come out of its socket. Some general rules of thumb when caring for patients during the recovery period are as follows:

---

10 "Replacement surgery - Shoulder total hip and total knee replacement -- Smart-Servier.jpg" by Laboratoires Servier is licensed under CC BY-SA 3.0. Access for free at https://commons.wikimedia.org/wiki/File:Replacement_surgery_-_Shoulder_total_hip_and_total_knee_replacement_--_Smart-Servier.jpg

11 This work is a derivative of Anatomy & Physiology by OpenStax and is licensed under CC BY 4.0. Access for free at https://openstax.org/books/anatomy-and-physiology/pages/1-introduction

12 MedlinePlus [Internet]. Bethesda (MD): National Library of Medicine (US); [updated 2020, Aug 21]. Hip replacement; [reviewed 2016, Aug 31; cited 2020, Sep 18]. https://medlineplus.gov/hipreplacement.html

My Notes

- Patients should not cross their legs or ankles when they are sitting, standing, or lying down.
- Patients should not lean too far forward from their waist or pull their leg up past their waist. This bending is called hip flexion. Avoid hip flexion greater than 90 degrees.[13]

For more information about patient education after a hip replacement surgery, read the following article from *Medline Plus*: "How to Take Care of Your New Hip Joint" (https://medlineplus.gov/ency/patientinstructions/000171.htm).

Rheumatoid Arthritis

Rheumatoid arthritis (RA) is a type of arthritis that causes pain, swelling, stiffness, and loss of function in joints due to inflammation caused by an autoimmune disease. See Figure 13.16[14] for an illustration of RA in the hands causing inflammation and a common deformity of the fingers. It often starts in middle age and is more common in women. RA is different from osteoarthritis because it is an autoimmune disease, meaning it is caused by the immune system attacking the body's own tissues.[15] In rheumatoid arthritis, the joint capsule and synovial membrane become inflamed. As the disease progresses, the articular cartilage is severely damaged, resulting in joint deformation, loss of movement, and potentially severe disability. There is no known cure for RA, so treatments are aimed at alleviating symptoms. Medications such as nonsteroidal anti-inflammatory drugs (NSAIDS), corticosteroids, and antirheumatic drugs such as methotrexate are commonly used to treat rheumatoid arthritis.[16]

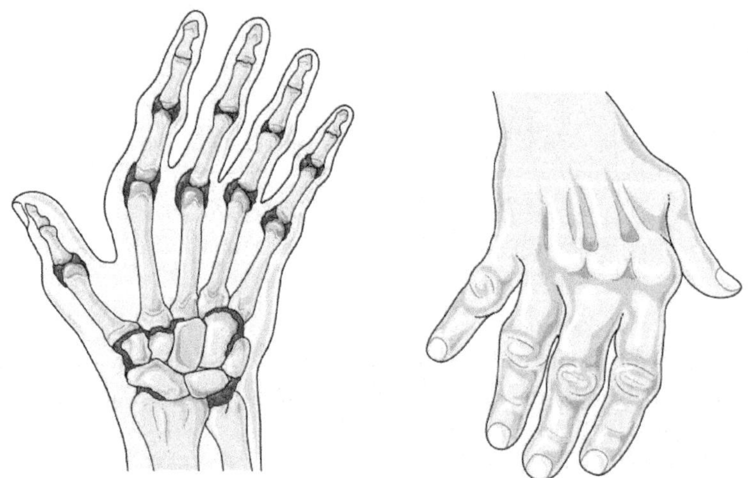

Figure 13.16 Rheumatoid Arthritis in the Hands

---

13 A.D.A.M. Medical Encyclopedia [Internet]. Atlanta (GA): A.D.A.M., Inc.; c1997-2020. Taking care of your new hip joint; [updated 2020, Sep 16; cited 2020, Sep 18]. https://medlineplus.gov/ency/patientinstructions/000171.htm

14 "Rheumatoid arthritis -- Smart- Servier (cropped).jpg" by Laboratoires Servier is licensed under *CC BY-SA 3.0*. Access for free at https://commons.wikimedia.org/wiki/File:Rheumatoid_arthritis_--_Smart-Servier_(cropped).jpg

15 MedlinePlus [Internet]. Bethesda (MD): National Library of Medicine (US); [updated 2020, Aug 14]. Rheumatoid arthritis; [reviewed 2018, May 2; cited 2020, Sep 18]. https://medlineplus.gov/rheumatoidarthritis.html

16 This work is a derivative of Anatomy & Physiology by OpenStax and is licensed under CC BY 4.0. Access for free at https://openstax.org/books/anatomy-and-physiology/pages/1-introduction

Gout

My Notes

Gout is a type of arthritis that causes swollen, red, hot, and stiff joints due to the buildup of uric acid. It typically first attacks the big toe. See Figure 13.17[17] for an illustration of gout in the joint of the big toe. Uric acid usually dissolves in the blood, passes through the kidneys, and is eliminated in urine, but gout occurs when uric acid builds up in the body and forms painful, needle-like crystals in joints. Gout is treated with lifestyle changes such avoiding alcohol and food high in purines, as well as administering antigout medications, such as allopurinol and colchicine.[18]

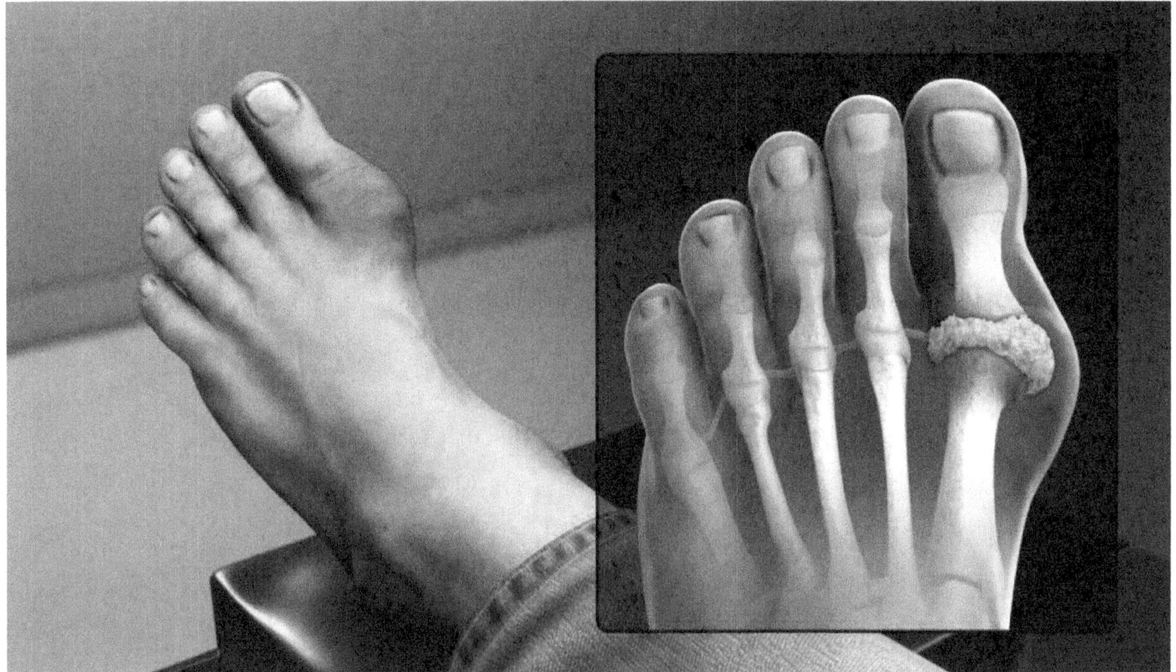

Figure 13.17 Gout

17 "Gout Signs and Symptoms.jpg" by www.scientificanimations.com/ is licensed under CC BY 4.0. Access for free at https://commons.wikimedia.org/wiki/File:Gout_Signs_and_Symptoms.jpg

18 This work is a derivative of Anatomy and Physiology by Boundless.com and is licensed under CC BY-SA 4.0. Access for free at https://courses.lumenlearning.com/boundless-ap/

Vertebral Disorders

The spine is composed of many vertebrae stacked on top of one another, forming the vertebral column. There are several disorders that can occur in the vertebral column causing curvature of the spine such as kyphosis, lordosis, and scoliosis. See Figure 13.18[19] for an illustration of kyphosis, lordosis, and scoliosis.

Kyphosis is a curving of the spine that causes a bowing or rounding of the back, often referred to as a "buffalo hump" that can lead to a hunchback or slouching posture. Kyphosis can be caused by osteoarthritis, osteoporosis, or other conditions. Pain in the middle or lower back is the most common symptom. Treatment depends upon the cause, the severity of pain, and the presence of any neurological symptoms.[20]

Lordosis is the inward curve of the lumbar spine just above the buttocks. A small degree of lordosis is normal, especially during the third trimester of pregnancy. Too much curving of the lower back is often called swayback. Most of the time, lordosis is not treated if the back is flexible because it is not likely to progress or cause problems.[21]

Scoliosis causes a sideways curve of the spine. It commonly develops in late childhood and the early teens when children grow quickly. Symptoms of scoliosis include leaning to one side and having uneven shoulders and hips. Treatment depends on the patient's age, the amount of expected additional growth, the degree of curving, and whether the curve is temporary or permanent. Patients with mild scoliosis might only need checkups to monitor if the curve is getting worse, whereas others may require a brace or have surgery.[22]

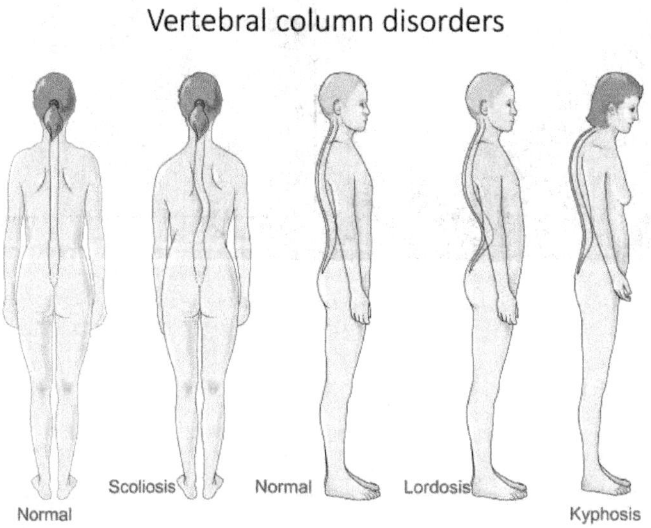

Vertebral column disorders

Figure 13.18 Vertebral Disorders

---

19 "Vertebral column disorders - Normal Scoliosis Lordosis Kyphosis -- Smart-Servier.jpg" by Laboratoires Servier is licensed under CC BY-SA 3.0. Access for free at https://commons.wikimedia.org/wiki/File:Vertebral_column_disorders_-_Normal_Scoliosis_Lordosis_Kyphosis_--_Smart-Servier.jpg

20 A.D.A.M. Medical Encyclopedia [Internet]. Atlanta (GA): A.D.A.M., Inc.; c1997-2020. Kyphosis; [updated 2020, Sep 16; cited 2020, Sep 18]. https://medlineplus.gov/ency/article/001240.htm

21 A.D.A.M. Medical Encyclopedia [Internet]. Atlanta (GA): A.D.A.M., Inc.; c1997-2020. Lordosis - lumbar; [updated 2020, Sep 16; cited 2020, Sep 18]. https://medlineplus.gov/ency/article/003278.htm

22 MedlinePlus [Internet]. Bethesda (MD): National Library of Medicine (US); [updated 2020, Apr 29]. Scoliosis; [reviewed 2016, Oct 18; cited 2020, Sep 18]. https://medlineplus.gov/scoliosis.html

Dislocation

My Notes

A **dislocation** is an injury, often caused by a fall or a blow to the joint, that forces the ends of bones out of position. Dislocated joints are typically very painful, swollen, and visibly out of place. The patient may not be able to move the affected extremity. See Figure 13.19[23] for an X-ray image of an anterior dislocation of the right shoulder where the ball (i.e., head of the humerus) has popped out of the socket (i.e., the glenoid cavity of the scapula). A dislocated joint requires immediate medical attention. Treatment depends on the joint and the severity of the injury and may include manipulation to reposition the bones, medication, a splint or sling, or rehabilitation. When properly repositioned, a joint will usually function and move normally again in a few weeks; however, once a joint is dislocated, it is more likely to become dislocated again. Instructing patients to wear protective gear during sports may help to prevent future dislocations.[24]

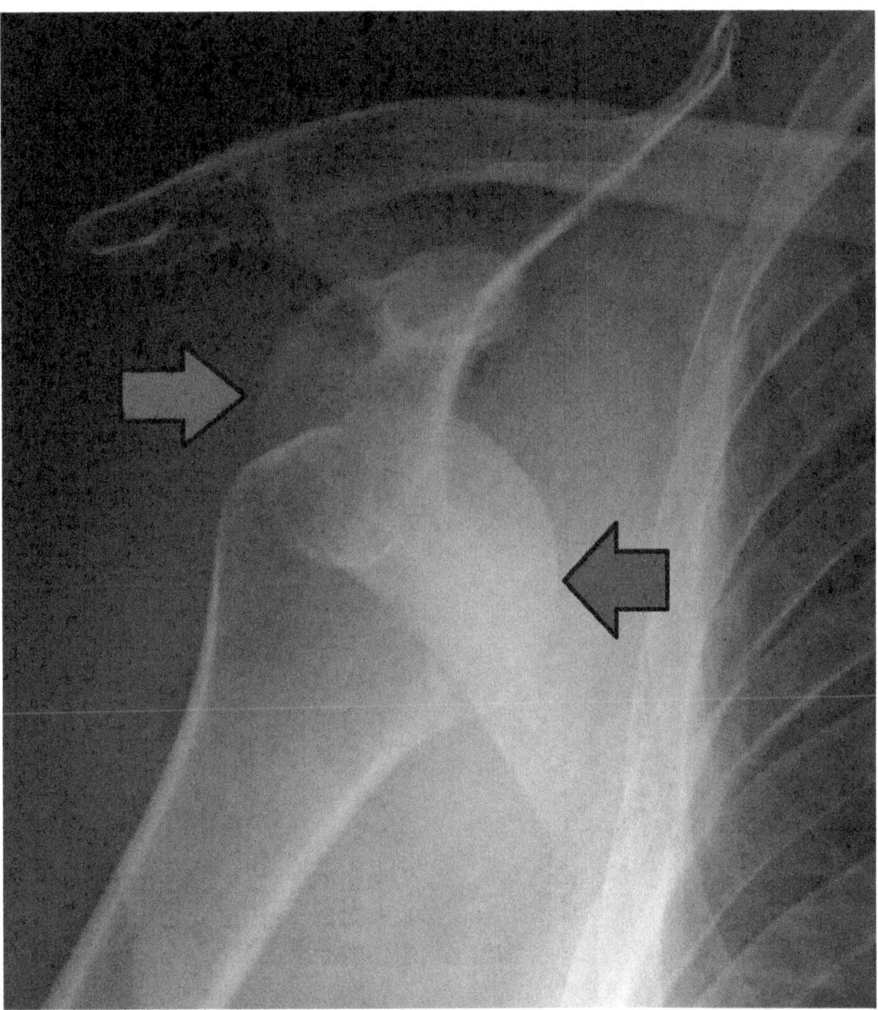

Figure 13.19 X-ray of Dislocated Shoulder

23 "AnterDisAPMark.png" by James Heilman, MD is licensed under CC BY-SA 4.0. Access for free at https://commons.wikimedia.org/wiki/File:AnterDisAPMark.png

24 MedlinePlus [Internet]. Bethesda (MD): National Library of Medicine (US); [updated 2019, Feb 7]. Dislocations; [reviewed 2016, Oct 26; cited 2020, Sep 18]. https://medlineplus.gov/dislocations.html

My Notes

Clubfoot

Clubfoot is a congenital condition that causes the foot and lower leg to turn inward and downward. A **congenital condition** means it is present at birth. See Figure 13.20[25] for an image of an infant with a clubfoot. It can range from mild and flexible to severe and rigid. Treatment by an orthopedic specialist involves using repeated applications of casts beginning soon after birth to gradually moving the foot into the correct position. Severe cases of clubfoot require surgery. After the foot is in the correct position, the child typically wears a special brace for up to three years.[26]

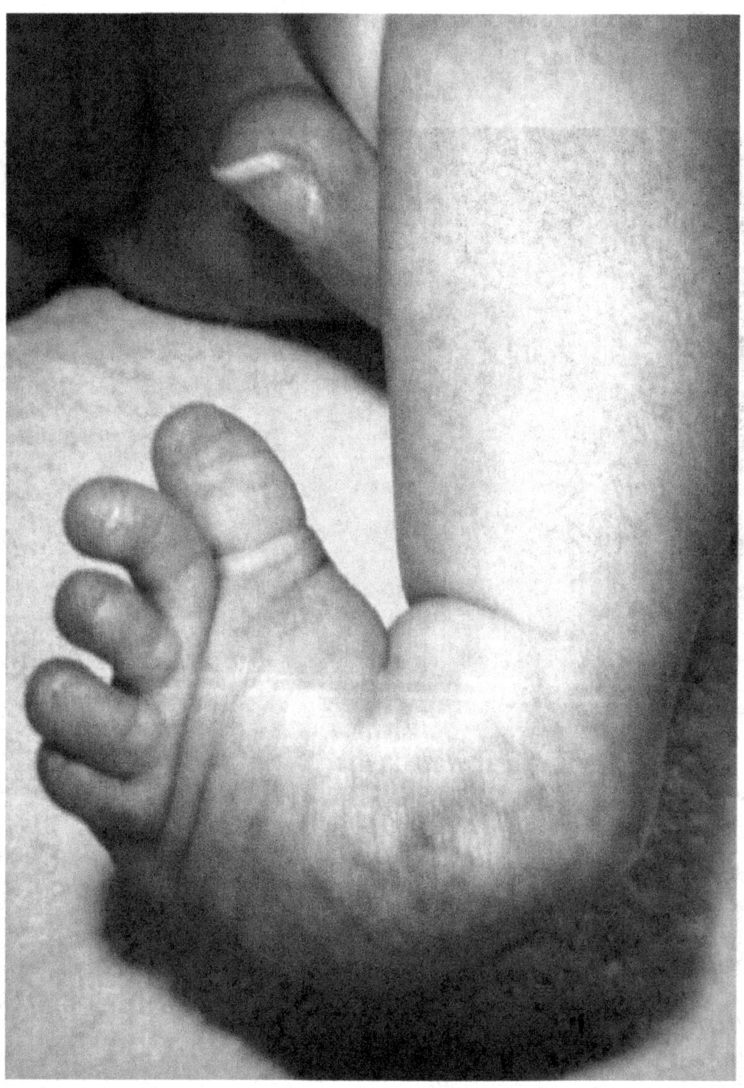

Figure 13.20 Clubfoot

25 "813 Clubfoot.jpg" by OpenStax is licensed under CC BY 3.0. Access for free at https://commons.wikimedia.org/wiki/File:813_Clubfoot.jpg

26 A.D.A.M. Medical Encyclopedia [Internet]. Atlanta (GA): A.D.A.M., Inc.; c1997-2020. Club foot; [updated 2020, Sep 16; cited 2020, Sep 18]. https://medlineplus.gov/ency/article/001228.htm

Sprains and Strains

My Notes

A **sprain** is a stretched or torn ligament caused by an injury. Ligaments are tissues that attach bones at a joint. Ankle and wrist sprains are very common, especially due to falls or participation in sports. See Figure 13.21[27] for an illustration of an ankle sprain caused by eversion or inversion of the ankle. Symptoms include pain, swelling, bruising, and the inability to move the joint. The patient may also report feeling a pop when the injury occurred.

A **strain** is a stretched or torn muscle or tendon. Tendons are tissues that connect muscle to bone. See Figure 13.22[28] for an image of a strained tendon. Strains can happen suddenly from an injury or develop over time due to chronic overuse. Symptoms include pain, muscle spasms, swelling, and trouble moving the muscle.

Treatment of sprains and strains is often referred to with the mnemonic **RICE** that stands for Resting the injured area, Icing the area, Compressing the area with an ACE bandage or other device, and Elevating the affected limb. Medications such as acetaminophen or nonsteroidal anti-inflammatory drugs (NSAIDs) may also be used.[29]

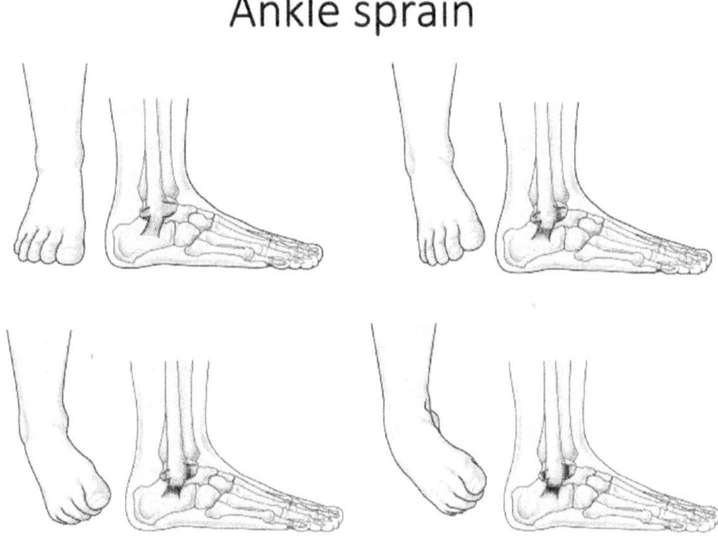

Figure 13.21 Sprained Ankle Ligaments

27 "Ankle sprain -- Smart-Servier.jpg" by Laboratoires Servier is licensed under CC BY-SA 3.0. Access for free at https://commons.wikimedia.org/wiki/File:Ankle_sprain_--_Smart-Servier.jpg

28 "3D Medical Animation Depicting Strain-Tendon.jpg" by https://www.scientificanimations.com is licensed under CC BY-SA 4.0. Access for free at https://commons.wikimedia.org/wiki/File:3D_Medical_Animation_Depicting_Strain-Tendon.jpg

29 A.D.A.M. Medical Encyclopedia [Internet]. Atlanta (GA): A.D.A.M., Inc.; c1997-2020. Sprains and strains; [updated 2020, Jun 17; reviewed 2017, Jan 3; cited 2020, Sep 18]. https://medlineplus.gov/sprainsandstrains.html

My Notes

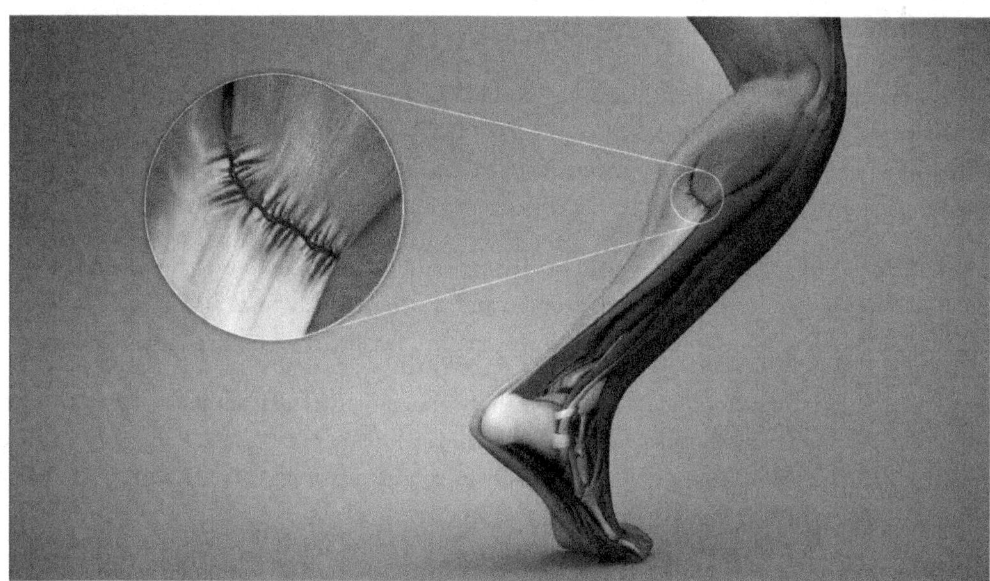

Figure 13.22 Strained Tendon

Knee Injuries and Arthroscopic Surgery

Knee injuries are common. Because the knee joint is primarily supported by muscles and ligaments, injuries to any of these structures will result in pain or knee instability. **Arthroscopic surgery** has greatly improved the surgical treatment of knee injuries and reduced subsequent recovery times. This procedure involves a small incision and the insertion of an arthroscope, a pencil-thin instrument that allows for visualization of the joint interior. Small surgical instruments are inserted via additional incisions to remove or repair ligaments and other joint structures.[30]

Contracture

A **contracture** develops when the normally elastic tissues are replaced by inelastic, fiber-like tissue. This inelastic tissue makes it difficult to stretch the area and prevents normal movement.

---

30 This work is a derivative of Anatomy & Physiology by OpenStax and is licensed under CC BY 4.0. Access for free at https://openstax.org/books/anatomy-and-physiology/pages/1-introduction

Contractures occur in the skin, the tissues underneath, and the muscles, tendons, and ligaments surrounding a joint. They affect the range of motion and function in a specific body part and can be painful. See Figure 13.23[31] for an image of severe contracture of the wrist that occurred after a burn injury.

Contracture can be caused by any of the following:

- Brain and nervous system disorders, such as cerebral palsy or stroke
- Inherited disorders, such as muscular dystrophy
- Nerve damage
- Reduced use (for example, from lack of mobility)
- Severe muscle and bone injuries
- Scarring after traumatic injury or burns

Treatments may include exercises, stretching, or applying braces and splints.[32]

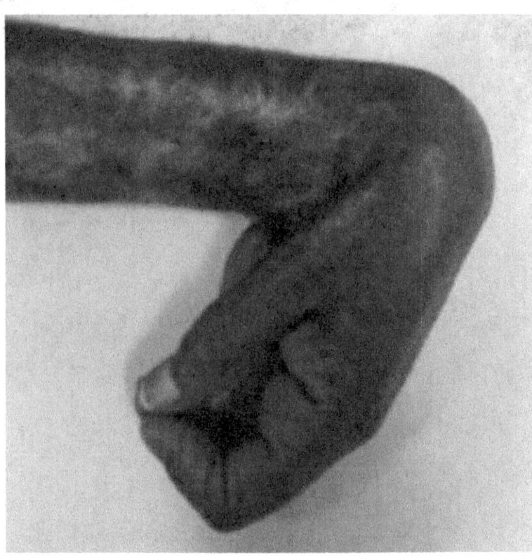

Figure 13.23 Contracture

Foot Drop

Foot drop is the inability to raise the front part of the foot due to weakness or paralysis of the muscles that lift the foot. As a result, individuals with foot drop often scuff their toes along the ground when walking or bend their knees to lift their foot higher than usual to avoid the scuffing. Foot drop is a symptom of an underlying problem and can be temporary or permanent, depending on the cause. The prognosis for foot drop depends on the cause. Foot drop caused by trauma or nerve damage usually shows partial or complete recovery, but in progressive neurological disorders, foot drop will be a symptom that is likely to continue as a lifelong disability. Treatment depends

31 "Complications of Hypertrophic Scarring.png" by Aarabi, S., Longaker, M. T., & Gurtner, G. C. is licensed under CC BY 3.0. Access for free at https://commons.wikimedia.org/wiki/File:Complications_of_Hypertrophic_Scarring.png

32 A.D.A.M. Medical Encyclopedia [Internet]. Atlanta (GA): A.D.A.M., Inc.; c1997-2020. Contracture deformity; [updated 2020, Sep 16; cited 2020, Sep 18]. https://medlineplus.gov/ency/article/003185.htm

My Notes

on the specific cause of foot drop. The most common treatment is to support the foot with lightweight leg braces. See Figure 13.24[33] for an image of a patient with foot drop treated with a leg brace. Exercise therapy to strengthen the muscles and maintain joint motion also helps to improve a patient's gait.[34]

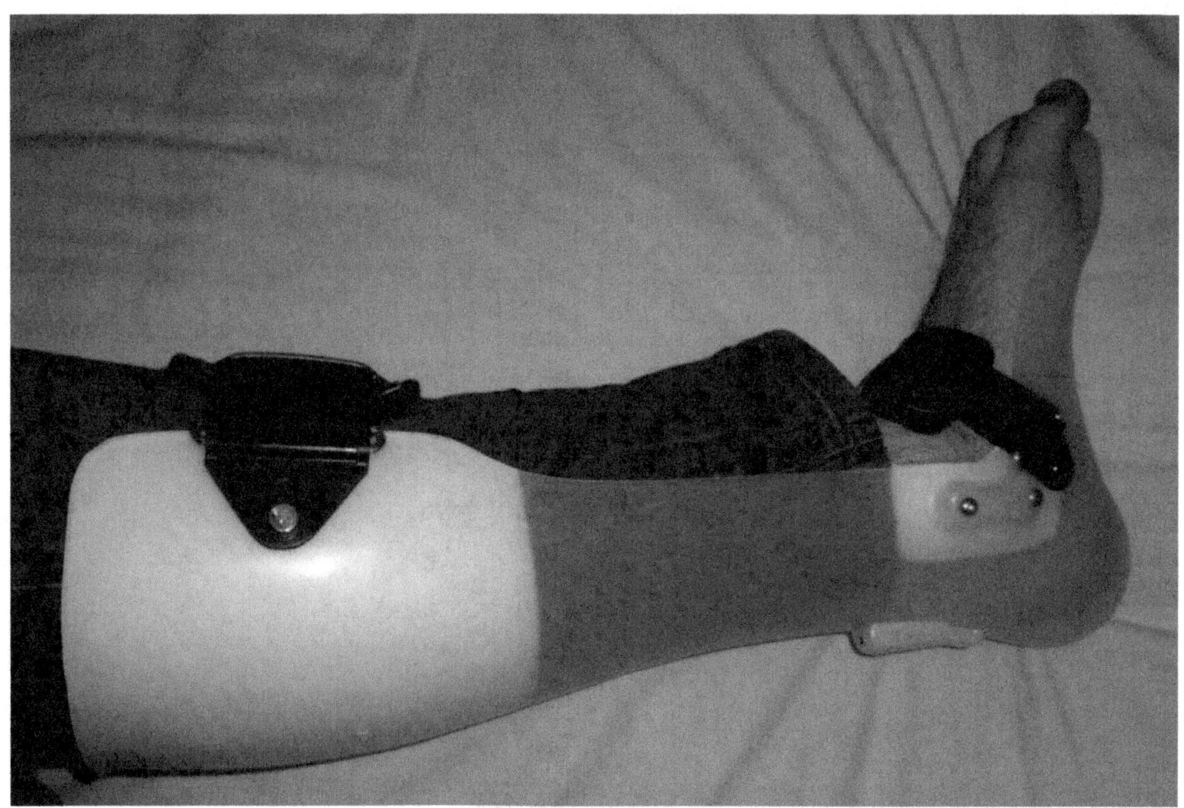

Figure 13.24 Foot Drop Treated with Leg Brace

33 "AFO brace for foot drop.JPG" by *Pagemaker787* is licensed under CC BY-SA 4.0. Access for free at https://commons.wikimedia.org/wiki/File:AFO_brace_for_foot_drop.JPG

34 National Institute of Neurological Disorders and Stroke. (2019, March 27). *Foot drop information page*. https://www.ninds.nih.gov/Disorders/All-Disorders/Foot-Drop-Information-Page

13.4 MUSCULOSKELETAL ASSESSMENT

My Notes

Now that you reviewed the anatomy of the musculoskeletal system and common musculoskeletal conditions, let's discuss the components of a routine nursing assessment.

Subjective Assessment

Collect subjective data from the patient and pay particular attention to what the patient is reporting about current symptoms, as well as past history of musculoskeletal injuries and disease. Information during the subjective assessment should be compared to expectations for the patient's age group or that patient's baseline. For example, an older client may have chronic limited range of motion in the knee due to osteoarthritis, whereas a child may have new, limited range of motion due to a knee sprain that occurred during a sports activity.

If the patient reports a current symptom, use the PQRSTU method described in the "Health History" chapter to obtain more information about this chief complaint. If the patient is experiencing acute pain or recent injury, focus on providing pain relief and/or stabilization of the injury prior to proceeding with the interview. Use information obtained during the subjective assessment to guide your physical examination. Sample focused interview questions to include during a subjective assessment of the musculoskeletal system are contained in Table 13.4a. The first question of the musculoskeletal interview is based on the six most common symptoms related to musculoskeletal disease.[1]

Table 13.4a Focused Interview Questions Related to the Musculoskeletal System

Interview Questions	Follow-up
Are you experiencing any current musculoskeletal symptoms such as muscle weakness, pain, swelling, redness, warmth, or stiffness?	Describe your concern today. How is it affecting your ability to complete daily activities? P: Does anything bring on the symptom such as activity, weight-bearing, or rest? If activity brings on the symptom, how much activity is required to bring on the symptom(s)? Does it occur at a certain time of day? Is there anything that makes it better or go away? Q: Describe the characteristics of the pain (aching, throbbing, sharp, dull). R: Is the pain localized or does it radiate to another part or area of the body? S: How severe is the pain on a scale of 0-10? T: When did the pain first start? Is it constant or does it come and go? Have you taken anything to relieve the pain?

1 Miller, S. B. (1990). An overview of the musculoskeletal system. In Walker, H. K., Hall, W. D., Hurst, J. W. (Eds.), *Clinical methods: The history, physical, and laboratory examinations* (3rd ed.). Butterworths. https://www.ncbi.nlm.nih.gov/books/NBK266/

My Notes

Interview Questions	Follow-up
Have you ever been diagnosed with a chronic musculoskeletal disease such as osteoporosis, osteoarthritis, or rheumatoid arthritis?	Please describe the conditions and treatments.
Have you ever been diagnosed with a neurological condition that affected the use of your muscles?	Please describe.
Have you had any previous surgeries on your bones or muscles, such as fracture repair or knee or hip surgery?	Please describe.
Are you currently taking any medications, herbs, or supplements for your muscles, bones, or the health of your musculoskeletal system?	Please describe.
Have you ever had a broken bone, strain, or other injury to a muscle, joint, tendon, or ligament?	Please describe.

Life Span Considerations

When conducting a subjective interview of children, additional information may be obtained from the parent or legal guardian.

Newborn

- Did your baby experience any trauma during labor and delivery?
- Did the head come first during delivery of your baby? Was the baby in breech position requiring delivery by Caesarean section?
- Were forceps used during delivery?
- Have been told your infant has a "click" within the hip(s)?
- Do you have any concern with your baby moving any joints, extremities, or neck normally? If so, describe.

Pediatric

- Has your child ever had a broken bone? If so, how was it treated?
- Has your child had any dislocation of a joint?
- Have you noticed any abnormality with your child's spine, toes, feet, or hands? If so, describe.
- Does your child have any difficulty walking, jumping, or playing? If so, describe.
- Is your child involved in sports or organized physical activities? Do you have any concerns about your child being physically able to perform these activities?

Older Adults

When assessing older adults, it is important to assess their mobility and their ability to perform activities of daily living.

My Notes

- Do you use any assistive devices such as a brace, cane, walker, or wheelchair?
- Have you fallen or had any near falls in the past few months? If so, was there any injury or did you seek medical care?
- Describe your mobility as of today. Have you noticed any changes in your ability to complete your usual daily activities such as walking, going to the bathroom, bathing, doing laundry, or preparing meals? If so, do you have any assistance available?

Objective Assessment

The purpose of a routine physical exam of the musculoskeletal system by a registered nurse is to assess function and to screen for abnormalities.

Most information about function and mobility is gathered during the patient interview, but the nurse also observes the patient's posture, walking, and movement of their extremities during the physical exam.

During a routine assessment of a patient during inpatient care, a registered nurse typically completes the following musculoskeletal assessments:

- Assess gait
- Inspect the spine
- Observe range of motion of joints
- Inspect muscles and extremities for size and symmetry
- Assess muscle strength
- Palpate extremities for tenderness[2]

While assessing an older adult, keep in mind they may have limited mobility and range of motion due to age-related degeneration of joints and muscle weakness. Be considerate of these limitations and never examine any areas to the point of pain or discomfort. Support the joints and muscles as you assess them to avoid pain or muscle spasm. Compare bilateral sides simultaneously and expect symmetry of structure and function of the corresponding body area.

Inspection

General inspection begins by observing the patient in the standing position for postural abnormalities. Observe their stance and note any abnormal curvature of the spine such as kyphosis, lordosis, or scoliosis. Ask the patient to walk away from you, turn, and walk back toward you while observing their gait and balance.

Ask the patient to sit. Inspect the size and contour of the muscles and joints and if the corresponding parts are symmetrical. Notice the skin over the joints and muscles and observe if there is tenderness, swelling, erythema, deformity, or asymmetry. Observe how the patient moves their extremities and note if there is pain with movement or any limitations in **active range of motion** (ROM). Active range of motion is the degree of movement the patient can voluntarily achieve in a joint without assistance. See Figures 13.9 and 13.10 as resources for describing joint movement.

---

2 Giddens, J. F. (2007). A survey of physical examination techniques performed by RNs: Lessons for nursing education. *Journal of Nursing Education, 46*(2), 83-87. https://doi.org/10.3928/01484834-20070201-09

My Notes

Palpation

Palpation is typically done simultaneously during inspection. As you observe, palpate each joint for warmth, swelling, or tenderness. If you observe decreased active range of motion, gently attempt passive range of motion by stabilizing the joint with one hand while using the other hand to gently move the joint to its limit of movement. **Passive range of motion** is the degree of range of motion demonstrated in a joint when the examiner is providing the movement. You may hear crepitus as the joint moves. Crepitus sounds like a crackling, popping noise that is considered normal as long as it is not associated with pain. As the joint moves, there should not be any reported pain or tenderness.

Assess muscle strength. Muscle strength should be equal bilaterally, and the patient should be able to fully resist an opposing force. Muscle strength varies among people depending on their activity level, genetic predisposition, lifestyle, and history. A common method of evaluating muscle strength is the Medical Research Council Manual Muscle Testing Scale.[3] This method involves testing key muscles from the upper and lower extremities against gravity and the examiner's resistance and grading the patient's strength on a 0 to 5 scale. See Box 13.4 for the muscle strength testing scale.

Box 13.4 Muscle Strength Scale[4]

0 – No muscle contraction

1 – Trace muscle contraction, such as a twitch

2 – Active movement only when gravity eliminated

3 – Active movement against gravity but not against resistance

4 – Active movement against gravity and some resistance

5 – Active movement against gravity and examiner's full resistance

3 This work is a derivative of StatPearls by Naqvi and Sherman and is licensed under CC BY 4.0. Access for free at https://www.ncbi.nlm.nih.gov/books/NBK430685/

4 This work is a derivative of StatPearls by Naqvi and Sherman and is licensed under CC BY 4.0. Access for free at https://www.ncbi.nlm.nih.gov/books/NBK430685/

My Notes

To assess upper extremity strength, first begin by assessing bilateral hand grip strength. Extend your index and second fingers on each hand toward the patient and ask them to squeeze them as tightly as possible. Then, ask the patient to extend their arms with their palms up. As you provide resistance on their forearms, ask the patient to pull their arms towards them. Finally, ask the patient to place their palms against yours and press while you provide resistance. See Figure 13.25[5] for images of a nurse assessing upper extremity strength.

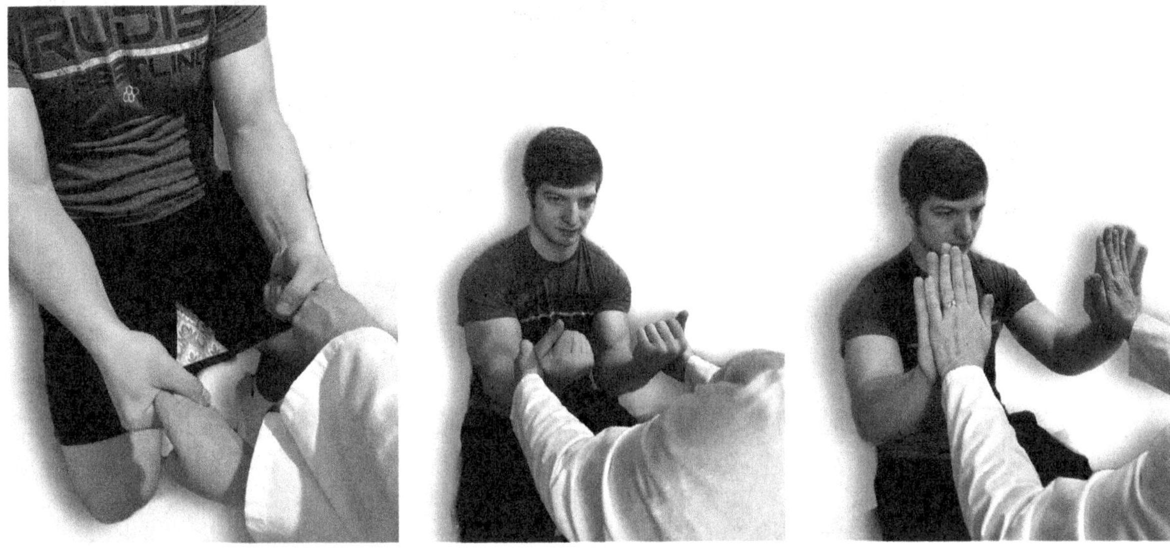

Figure 13.25 Assessing Hand Grips and Upper Extremity Strength

To assess lower extremity strength, perform the following maneuvers with a seated patient. Place your palms on the patient's thighs and ask them to lift their legs while providing resistance. Secondly, place your hands behind their calves and ask them to pull their legs backwards while you provide resistance. Place your hands on the top of their feet and ask them to pull their feet upwards against your resistance. Finally, place your hands on the soles of their feet and ask them to press downwards while you provide resistance, instructing them to "press downwards like pressing the gas pedal on a car." See Figure 13.26[6] for images of a nurse assessing lower extremity strength.

5 "Neuro Exam image 38.png," Neuro Exam image 41.png," and "Neuro Exam image 39.jpg" by Meredith Pomietlo for Chippewa Valley Technical College are licensed under CC BY 4.0. Access for free at https://drive.google.com/file/d/1D37Qu5ljGyly3xO61vqUGeQv3Zx13g9I/view?usp=sharing

6 "Musculoskeletal Exam image 2.png," "Neuro Exam image 6.png," and "Musculoskeletal Exam Image 7.png" by Meredith Pomietlo for Chippewa Valley Technical College are licensed under CC BY 4.0. Access for free at https://drive.google.com/file/d/1V-lF_5Y21OlehDMtYQi3qF2d5vGjgWlL/view?usp=sharing and https://drive.google.com/file/d/1OcXT2VxcOqr3TEacbj1XF7-BWTTki1ou/view?usp=sharing

My Notes

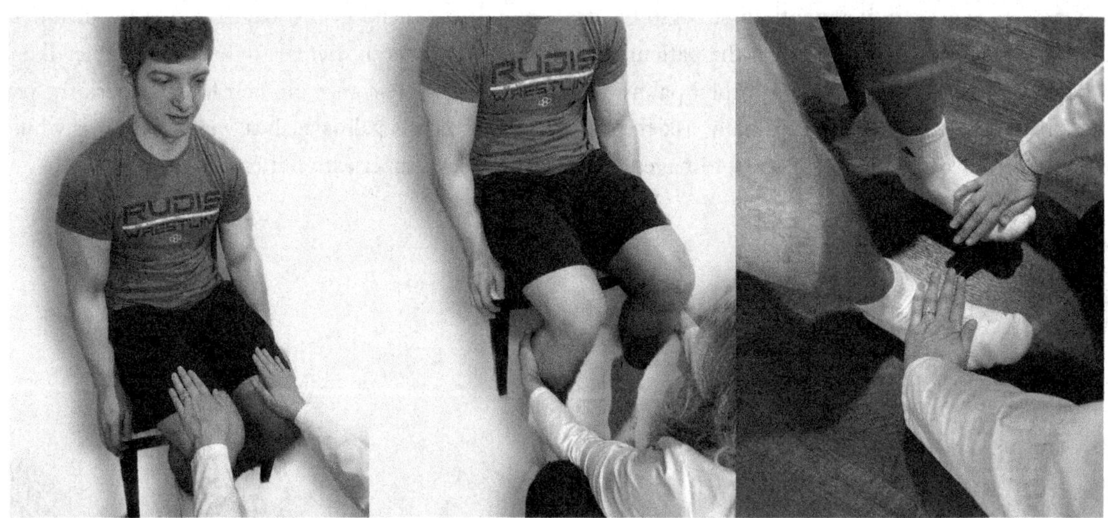

Figure 13.26 Assessing Lower Extremity Strength

To read additional details regarding a full range of motion assessment of the musculoskeletal system, visit the following chapter from *Clinical Methods: The History, Physical, and Laboratory Examinations. 3rd edition: "An Overview of the Musculoskeletal System"* (https://www.ncbi.nlm.nih.gov/books/NBK266/).

Video Review of Musculoskeletal Assessment[7]

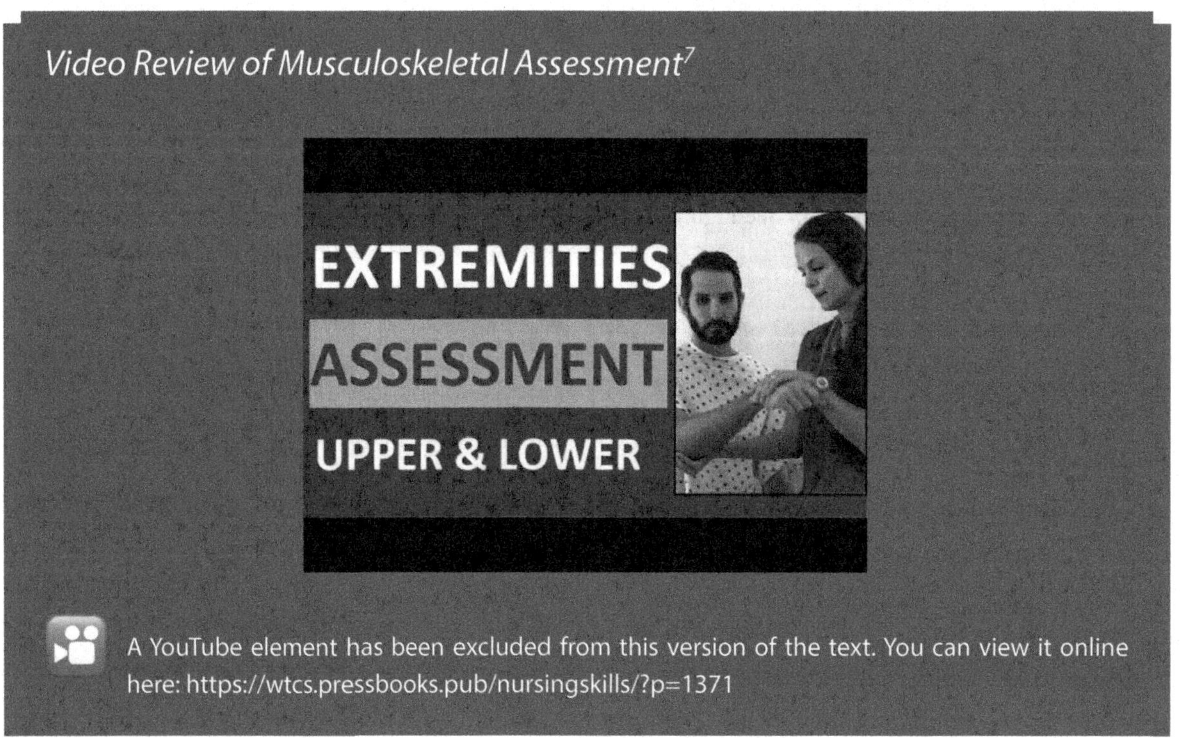

A YouTube element has been excluded from this version of the text. You can view it online here: https://wtcs.pressbooks.pub/nursingskills/?p=1371

7 RegisteredNurseRN. (2017, December 22). *Upper & lower extremities assessment nursing | Upper, lower extremity examination*. [Video]. YouTube. All rights reserved. Video used with permission. https://youtu.be/1sKnumpKT_Y

See Table 13.4b for a comparison of expected versus unexpected findings when assessing the musculoskeletal system.

My Notes

Table 13.4b Expected Versus Unexpected Findings on Musculoskeletal Assessment

Assessment	Expected Findings	Unexpected Findings (document and notify provider if a new finding*)
Inspection	Erect posture with good balance and normal gait while walking. Joints and muscles are symmetrical with no swelling, redness, or deformity. Active range of motion of all joints without difficulty. No spine curvature.	Spinal curvature is present. Poor balance or unsteady gait while walking. Swelling, bruising, erythema, or tenderness over joints or muscles. Deformity of joints. Decreased active range of motion. Contracture or foot drop present.
Auscultation	Not applicable	Crepitus associated with pain on movement.
Palpation	No palpable tenderness or warmth of joints, bones, or muscles. Muscle strength 5/5 against resistance.	Warmth or tenderness on palpation of joints, bones, or muscles. Decreased passive range of motion. Muscle strength of 3/5 or less.
***CRITICAL CONDITIONS to report immediately**		Hot, swollen, painful joint. Suspected fracture, dislocation, sprain, or strain.

My Notes

13.5 SAMPLE DOCUMENTATION

Sample Documentation of Expected Findings

Patient reports no previous history for bone trauma, disease, infection, injury, or deformity. No symptoms of joint stiffness, pain, swelling, limited function, or muscle weakness. Patient is able to perform and manage regular daily activities without limitations and reports consistent exercise consisting of walking 2 miles for 5 days a week. Joints and muscles are symmetrical bilaterally. No swelling, deformity, masses, or redness upon inspection. Nontender palpation of joints without crepitus. Full ROM of the arms and legs with smooth movement. Upper and lower extremity strength is rated at 5 out of 5. Patient is able to maintain full resistance of muscle without tenderness or discomfort.

Sample Documentation of Unexpected Findings

Patient reports, "I felt a pop in my right ankle while playing basketball this afternoon" and "My right ankle hurts when trying to walk on it." Pain is constant and worsens with weight-bearing. Patient rates pain at 4/10 at rest and 9/10 with walking and describes pain as an "aching, burning feeling." Ibuprofen and ice decrease pain. Right ankle is moderately swollen laterally and anteriorly with tenderness to palpation but no erythema, warmth, or obvious deformity. Color, motion, and sensation are intact distal to the ankle. ROM of the right ankle is limited and produces moderate pain. Minimal eversion and inversion demonstrated. Patient is unable to bear weight on the right ankle. Dr. Smith notified and an order for an ankle X-ray received. The right ankle was elevated and ice applied while the patient waits for the X-ray.

13.5 CHECKLIST FOR MUSCULOSKELETAL ASSESSMENT

My Notes

Use this checklist below to review the steps for completion of "Musculoskeletal Assessment."

Steps

Disclaimer: Always review and follow agency policy regarding this specific skill.

1. Gather supplies: assistive device (i.e., walker, cane, crutches, brace, etc.) based on patient status.
    - Check the patient chart for information prior to assessment regarding mobility status, fall risk, and use of assistive devices.
2. Perform safety steps:
    - Perform hand hygiene.
    - Check the room for transmission-based precautions.
    - Introduce yourself, your role, the purpose of your visit, and an estimate of the time it will take.
    - Confirm patient ID using two patient identifiers (e.g., name and date of birth).
    - Explain the process to the patient and ask if they have any questions.
    - Be organized and systematic.
    - Use appropriate listening and questioning skills.
    - Listen and attend to patient cues.
    - Ensure the patient's privacy and dignity.
    - Assess ABCs.
3. Perform inspection:
    - Observe the patient using their arms, legs, gait, ability to sit and stand, and posture.
    - Note symmetry; compare each side of the body.
    - Inspect overall size, bony enlargement, and alignment of muscles and joints.
    - Observe coordination and muscle function and note balance, limping, presence of deformity, or shuffling.
4. Palpate and assess range of motion (ROM) and muscle strength:
    - Gently palpate bones, joints, muscles, and surrounding tissue for heat, swelling, stiffness, tenderness, or crepitation.
    - Ask the patient to move major joints (knees, shoulders, hips, and ankles) through the expected ROM movements. Observe the quality and equality of motion bilaterally with the same body parts. Note any limitation, pain, or crepitus with movement. Use passive ROM if indicated and appropriate.
    - Assess muscle strength and tone in:
        - Hand grips

My Notes

        - Upper extremities
        - Lower extremities
    - Compare strength of symmetrical muscle groups. Upper and lower extremities on the dominant side are usually stronger. Rate muscle strength on scale of 0 to 5.

5. Assist the patient to a comfortable position, ask if they have any questions, and thank them for their time.

6. Ensure safety measures when leaving the room:

    - CALL LIGHT: Within reach
    - BED: Low and locked (in lowest position and brakes on)
    - SIDE RAILS: Secured
    - TABLE: Within reach
    - ROOM: Risk-free for falls (scan room and clear any obstacles)

7. Perform hand hygiene.

8. Document the assessment findings and report any concerns according to agency policy.

13.7 LEARNING ACTIVITIES

My Notes

Learning Activities

(Answers to "Learning Activities" can be found in the "Answer Key" at the end of the book. Answers to interactive activity elements will be provided within the element as immediate feedback.)

1. During a musculoskeletal assessment, the nurse has the patient simultaneously resist against exerted force with both upper extremities. The nurse knows this it is important to perform this assessment on both extremities simultaneously for what reason?
   a. It measures muscle strength symmetry.
   b. It provides a more accurate reading.
   c. It involves more muscle use.
   d. It decreases assessment time.
2. The nurse is testing upper body strength on an adolescent. The test indicates full ROM against gravity and full resistance. How does the nurse document these assessment findings according to the muscle strength scale?
   a. 4 out of 5
   b. 3 out of 5
   c. 5 out of 5
   d. 1 out of 5
3. A young adult presents to the urgent care with a right knee injury. The injury occurred during a basketball game. The nurse begins to perform a musculoskeletal assessment. What is the first step of the assessment?
   a. Palpation
   b. Inspection
   c. Percussion
   d. Auscultation

Check your knowledge using this flashcard activity:

An interactive or media element has been excluded from this version of the text. You can view it online here: https://wtcs.pressbooks.pub/nursingskills/?p=1377

My Notes

XIII GLOSSARY

Abduction: Joint movement away from the midline of the body.

Active range of motion: The degree of movement a patient can voluntarily achieve in a joint without assistance.

Adduction: Joint movement toward the middle line of the body.

Arthroplasty: Joint replacement surgery.

Arthroscopic surgery: A surgical procedure involving a small incision and the insertion of an arthroscope, a pencil-thin instrument that allows for visualization of the joint interior. Small surgical instruments are inserted via additional incisions to remove or repair ligaments and other joint structures.

Articular cartilage: Smooth, white tissue that covers the ends of bones where they come together at joints, allowing them to glide over each other with very little friction. Articular cartilage can be damaged by injury or normal wear and tear.

Clubfoot: A congenital condition that causes the foot and lower leg to turn inward and downward.

Congenital condition: A condition present at birth.

Contracture: A fixed or permanent tightening of muscles, tendons, ligaments, or the skin that prevents normal movement of the body part.

Crepitus: A crackling, popping noise heard on joint movement. It is considered normal when it is not associated with pain.

Dislocation: A joint injury that forces the ends of bones out of position; often caused by a fall or a blow to the joint.

Extension: Joint movement causing the straightening of limbs (increase in angle) at a joint.

Flexion: Joint movement causing the bending of the limbs (reduction of angle) at a joint.

Foot drop: The inability to raise the front part of the foot due to weakness or paralysis of the muscles that lift the foot.

Fracture: A broken bone.

Gout: A type of arthritis that causes swollen, red, hot, and stiff joints due to the buildup of uric acid, commonly starting in the big toe.

Joints: The location where bones come together.

Kyphosis: A curving of the spine that causes a bowing or rounding of the back, leading to a hunchback or slouching posture.

Ligaments: Strong bands of fibrous connective tissue that connect bones and strengthen and support joints by anchoring bones together and preventing their separation.

Lordosis: An inward curve of the lumbar spine just above the buttocks. A small degree of lordosis is normal, but too much curving is called swayback.

Muscle atrophy: The thinning or loss of muscle tissue that can be caused by disuse, aging, or neurological damage.

Open fracture: A type of fracture when the broken bone punctures the skin.

Osteoarthritis: The most common type of arthritis associated with aging and wear and tear of the articular cartilage that covers the surfaces of bones at the synovial joint.

Osteoporosis: A disease that thins and weakens bones, especially in the hip, spine, and wrist, causing them to become fragile and break easily.

Passive range of motion: The degree of range of motion a patient demonstrates in a joint when the examiner is providing the movement.

Rheumatoid arthritis: A type of arthritis that causes pain, swelling, stiffness, and loss of function in joints due to inflammation caused by an autoimmune disease.

My Notes

RICE: A mnemonic for treatment of sprains and strains that stands for: Resting the injured area, Icing the area, Compressing the area with an ACE bandage or other device, and Elevating the affected limb.

Rotation: Circular movement of a joint around a fixed point.

Scoliosis: A sideways curve of the spine that commonly develops in late childhood and the early teens.

Skeletal muscle: Voluntary muscle that produces movement, assists in maintaining posture, protects internal organs, and generates body heat.

Sprain: A stretched or torn ligament caused by an injury.

Strain: A stretched or torn muscle or tendon.

Synovial fluid: A thick fluid that provides lubrication in joints to reduce friction between the bones.

Synovial joints: A fluid-filled joint cavity where the articulating surfaces of the bones contact and move smoothly against each other. The elbow and knee are examples of synovial joints.

Tendons: Strong bands of dense, regular connective tissue that connect muscles to bones.

Chapter 14

Integumentary Assessment

14.1 INTEGUMENTARY ASSESSMENT INTRODUCTION

My Notes

Learning Objectives

- Perform an integumentary assessment including the skin, hair, and nails
- Modify assessment techniques to reflect variations across the life span and ethnic and cultural variations
- Document actions and observations
- Recognize and report significant deviations from norms

Assessing the skin, hair, and nails is part of a routine head-to-toe assessment completed by registered nurses. During inpatient care, a comprehensive skin assessment on admission establishes a baseline for the condition of a patient's skin and is essential for developing a care plan for the prevention and treatment of skin injuries.[1] Before discussing the components of a routine skin assessment, let's review the anatomy of the skin and some common skin and hair conditions.

1 Medline Industries, Inc. (n.d.). *Are you doing comprehensive skin assessments correctly? Get the whole picture.* https://www.medline.com/skin-health/comprehensive-skin-assessments-correctly-get-whole-picture/#:~:text=A%20comprehensive%20skin%20assessment%20entails,actually%20more%20than%20skin%20deep.

My Notes

14.2 BASIC INTEGUMENTARY CONCEPTS

The integumentary system includes the skin, hair, and nails. The skin is an organ that performs a variety of essential functions, such as protecting the body from invasion by microorganisms, chemicals, and other environmental factors; preventing dehydration; acting as a sensory organ; modulating body temperature and electrolyte balance; and synthesizing vitamin D.[1]

Skin

The skin is made of multiple layers of cells and tissues, which are held to underlying structures by connective tissue. See Figure 14.1[2] for an image of the layers of the skin. The skin is composed of two main layers: the uppermost thin layer called the **epidermis** made of closely packed epithelial cells, and the inner thick layer called the **dermis** that houses blood vessels, hair follicles, sweat glands, and nerve fibers. Beneath the dermis lies the **hypodermis** that contains connective tissue and adipose tissue (stored fat) to connect the skin to the underlying bones and muscles. The skin acts as a sense organ because the epidermis, dermis, and hypodermis contain specialized sensory nerve structures that detect touch, surface temperature, and pain.[3]

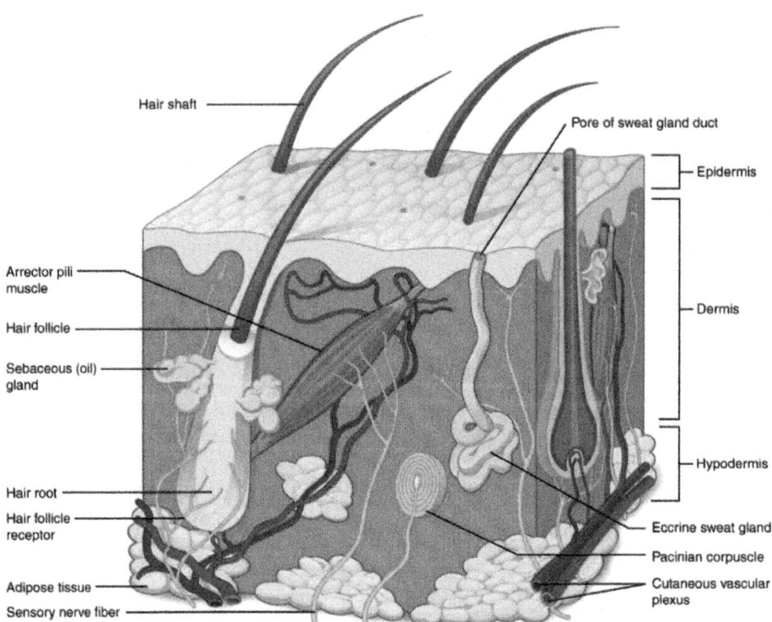

Figure 14.1 Layers of the Skin

1 This work is a derivative of Anatomy & Physiology by OpenStax and is licensed under CC BY 4.0. Access for free at https://openstax.org/books/anatomy-and-physiology/pages/1-introduction

2 "501 Structure of the skin.jpg" by OpenStax is licensed under CC BY 3.0. Access for free at https://openstax.org/books/anatomy-and-physiology/pages/5-1-layers-of-the-skin

3 This work is a derivative of Anatomy & Physiology by OpenStax and is licensed under CC BY 4.0. Access for free at https://openstax.org/books/anatomy-and-physiology/pages/1-introduction

My Notes

The color of skin is created by pigments, including melanin, carotene, and hemoglobin. **Melanin** is produced by cells called melanocytes that are scattered throughout the epidermis. See Figure 14.2[4] for an illustration of melanin and melanocytes. When there is an irregular accumulation of melanocytes in the skin, freckles appear. Dark-skinned individuals produce more melanin than those with pale skin. Exposure to the UV rays of the sun or a tanning bed causes additional melanin to be manufactured and built up, resulting in the darkening of the skin referred to as a tan. Increased melanin accumulation protects the DNA of epidermal cells from UV ray damage, but it requires about ten days after initial sun exposure for melanin synthesis to peak. This is why pale-skinned individuals often suffer sunburns during initial exposure to the sun. Darker-skinned individuals can also get sunburns, but they are more protected from their existing melanin than pale-skinned individuals.[5]

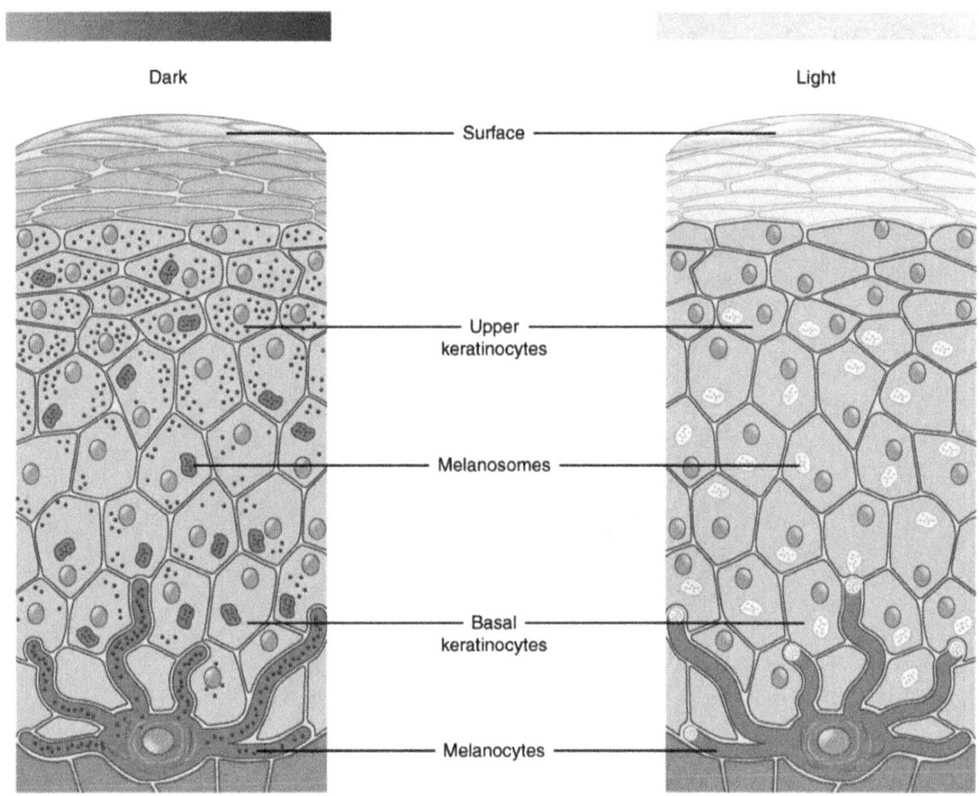

Figure 14.2 Pigmentation of the Skin

4 "504 Melanocytes.jpg" by OpenStax is licensed under CC BY 3.0. Access for free at https://openstax.org/books/anatomy-and-physiology/pages/5-1-layers-of-the-skin

5 A.D.A.M. Medical Encyclopedia [Internet]. Atlanta (GA): A.D.A.M., Inc.; c1997-2020. Skin turgor; [updated 2020, Sep 16; cited 2020, Sep 18]. https://medlineplus.gov/ency/article/003281.htm#:~:text=To%20check%20for%20skin%20turgor,back%20to%20its%20normal%20position.

My Notes

Too much sun exposure can eventually lead to wrinkling due to the destruction of the cellular structure of the skin, and in severe cases, can cause DNA damage resulting in skin cancer. Moles are larger masses of melanocytes, and although most are benign, they should be monitored for changes that indicate the presence of skin cancer. See Figure 14.3[6] for an image of moles.

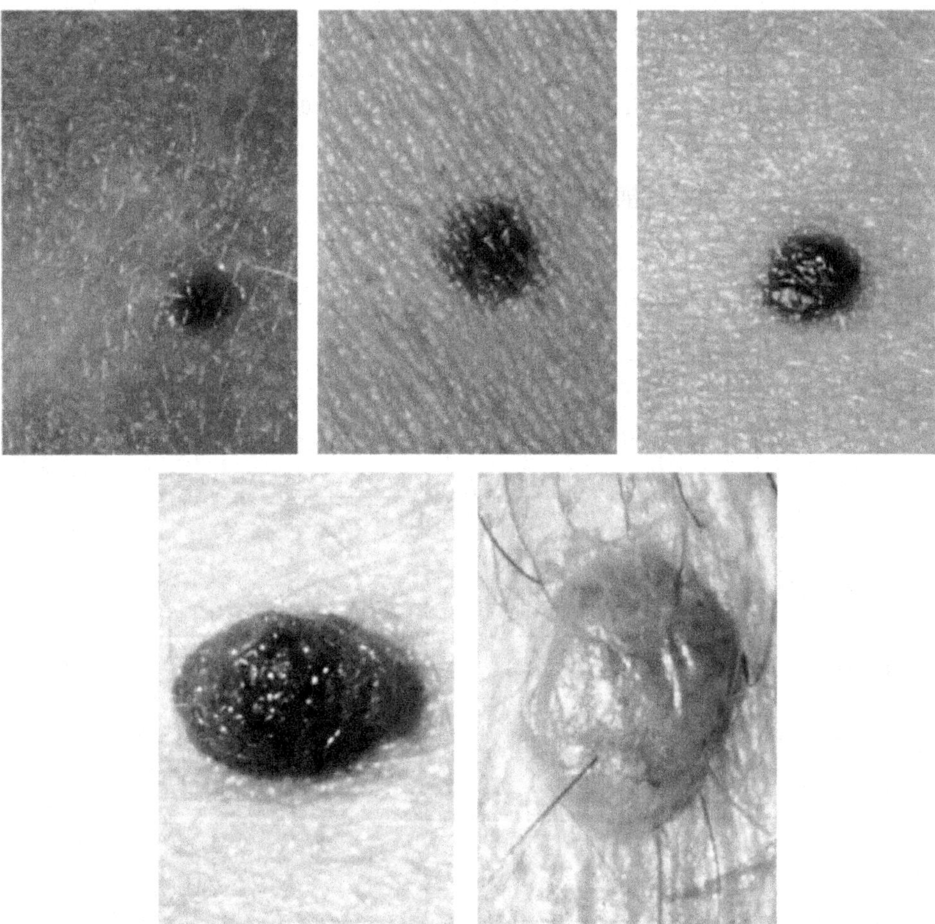

Figure 14.3 Moles

Patients are encouraged to use the **ABCDE** mnemonic to watch for signs of early-stage melanoma developing in moles. Consult a health care provider if you find these signs of melanoma when assessing a patient's skin:

- **A**symmetrical: The sides of the moles are not symmetrical
- **B**orders: The edges of the mole are irregular in shape
- **C**olor: The color of the mole has various shades of brown or black
- **D**iameter: The mole is larger than 6 mm. (0.24 in.)
- **E**volving: The shape of the mole has changed

---

6 "508 Moles.jpg" by OpenStax is licensed under CC BY 3.0. Access for free at https://openstax.org/books/anatomy-and-physiology/pages/5-1-layers-of-the-skin.

Hair

My Notes

Hair is made of dead, keratinized cells that originate in the hair follicle in the dermis. For these reasons, there is no sensation in hair. See Figure 14.4[7] for an image of a hair follicle. Hair serves a variety of functions, including protection, sensory input, thermoregulation, and communication. For example, hair on the head protects the skull from the sun. Hair in the nose, ears, and around the eyes (eyelashes) defends the body by trapping any dust particles that may contain allergens and microbes. Hair of the eyebrows prevents sweat and other particles from dripping into the eyes.

Hair also has a sensory function due to sensory innervation by a hair root plexus surrounding the base of each hair follicle. Hair is extremely sensitive to air movement or other disturbances in the environment, even more so than the skin surface. This feature is also useful for the detection of the presence of insects or other potentially damaging substances on the skin surface. Each hair root is also connected to a smooth muscle called the arrector pili that contracts in response to nerve signals from the sympathetic nervous system, making the external hair shaft "stand up." This movement is commonly referred to as goose bumps. The primary purpose for this movement is to trap a layer of air to add insulation.[8]

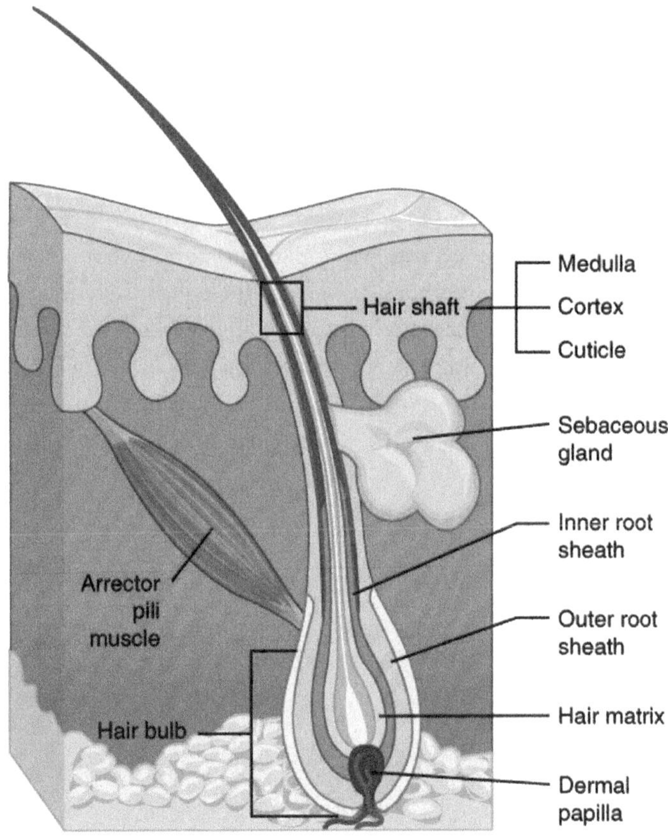

Figure 14.4 Hair Follicle

---

7 "506 Hair.jpg" by OpenStax is licensed under CC BY 3.0. Access for free at https://openstax.org/books/anatomy-and-physiology/pages/5-2-accessory-structures-of-the-skin

8 This work is a derivative of Anatomy & Physiology by OpenStax and is licensed under CC BY 4.0. Access for free at https://openstax.org/books/anatomy-and-physiology/pages/1-introduction

My Notes

Nails

The nail bed is a specialized structure of the epidermis that is found at the tips of our fingers and toes. See Figure 14.5[9] for an illustration of a fingernail. The nail body is formed on the nail bed and protects the tips of our fingers and toes as they experience mechanical stress while being used. In addition, the nail body forms a back-support for picking up small objects with the fingers.[10]

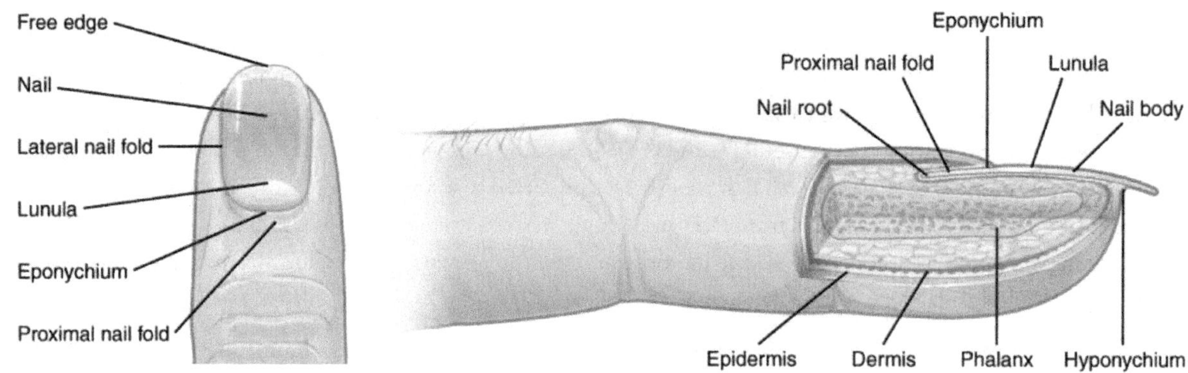

Figure 14.5 Nails

Sweat Glands

When the body becomes warm, sweat glands produce sweat to cool the body. There are two types of sweat glands that secrete slightly different products. An **eccrine sweat gland** produces hypotonic sweat for thermoregulation. See Figure 14.6[11] for an illustration of an eccrine sweat gland. These glands are found all over the skin's surface, but are especially abundant on the palms of the hand, the soles of the feet, and the forehead. They are coiled glands lying deep in the dermis, with the duct rising up to a pore on the skin surface where the sweat is released. This type of sweat is composed mostly of water and some salt, antibodies, traces of metabolic waste, and dermicidin, an antimicrobial peptide. Eccrine glands are a primary component of thermoregulation and help to maintain homeostasis.[12]

---

9 "507 Nails.jpg" by OpenStax is licensed under CC BY 3.0. Access for free at https://openstax.org/books/anatomy-and-physiology/pages/5-2-accessory-structures-of-the-skin

10 This work is a derivative of Anatomy & Physiology by OpenStax and is licensed under CC BY 4.0. Access for free at https://openstax.org/books/anatomy-and-physiology/pages/1-introduction

11 "508 Eccrine gland.jpg" by OpenStax is licensed under CC BY 3.0. Access for free at https://openstax.org/books/anatomy-and-physiology/pages/5-2-accessory-structures-of-the-skin

12 This work is a derivative of Anatomy & Physiology by OpenStax and is licensed under CC BY 4.0. Access for free at https://openstax.org/books/anatomy-and-physiology/pages/1-introduction

My Notes

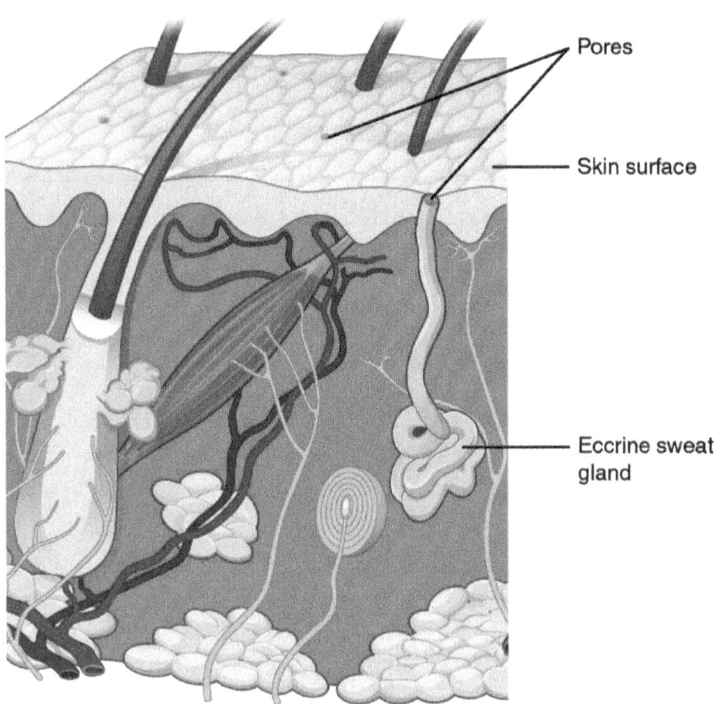

Figure 14.6 Eccrine Sweat Gland

Apocrine sweat glands are mostly found in hair follicles in densely hairy areas, such as the armpits and genital regions. In addition to secreting water and salt, apocrine sweat includes organic compounds that make the sweat thicker and subject to bacterial decomposition and subsequent odor. The release of this sweat is controlled by the nervous system and hormones and plays a role in the human pheromone response. Most commercial antiperspirants use an aluminum-based compound as their primary active ingredient to stop sweat. When the antiperspirant enters the sweat gland duct, the aluminum-based compounds form a physical block in the duct, which prevents sweat from coming out of the pore.[13]

13 This work is a derivative of Anatomy & Physiology by OpenStax and is licensed under CC BY 4.0. Access for free at https://openstax.org/books/anatomy-and-physiology/pages/1-introduction

My Notes

Skin Lesions

A **lesion** is an area of abnormal tissue. There are many terms for common skin lesions that may be described in a patient's chart. These terms are defined in Table 14.2. See Figure 14.7[14] for illustrations of common skin lesions.

Table 14.2 Medical Terms Associated with Skin Lesions and Rashes[15]

Medical Term	Definition
abscess	localized collection of pus
bulla (pl., bullae)	fluid-filled blister no more than 5 mm in diameter
carbuncle	deep, pus-filled abscess generally formed from multiple furuncles
crust	dried fluids from a lesion on the surface of the skin
cyst	encapsulated sac filled with fluid, semi-solid matter, or gas, typically located just below the upper layers of skin
folliculitis	a localized rash due to inflammation of hair follicles
furuncle (boil)	pus-filled abscess due to infection of a hair follicle
macules	smooth spots of discoloration on the skin
papules	small raised bumps on the skin, such as a mosquito bite
pseudocyst	lesion that resembles a cyst but with a less-defined boundary
purulent	pus-producing; also called suppurative
pustules	fluid- or pus-filled bumps on the skin, such as acne
pyoderma	any suppurative (pus-producing) infection of the skin
suppurative	producing pus; purulent
ulcer	break in the skin or open sore such as a venous ulcer
vesicle	small, fluid-filled lesion, such as a herpes blister
wheal	swollen, inflamed skin that itches or burns, often from an allergic reaction

14 "OSC Microbio 21 01 LesionLine.jpg" by OpenStax is licensed under CC BY 4.0. Access for free at https://commons.wikimedia.org/wiki/File:OSC_Microbio_21_01_LesionLine.jpg

15 This work is derivative of *Microbiology* by OpenStax and is licensed under CC BY 4.0. Access for free at https://openstax.org/books/microbiology/pages/1-introduction

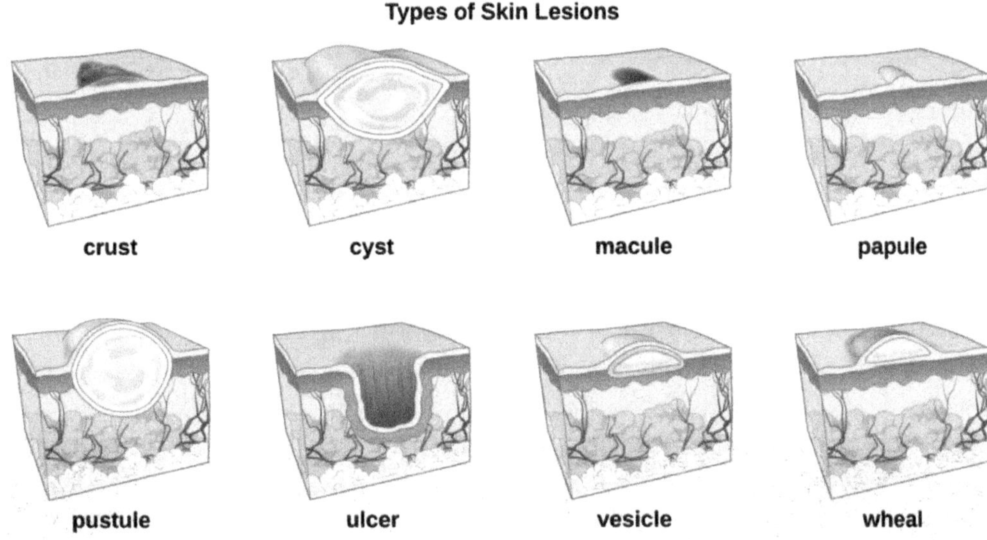

Figure 14.7 Common Types of Skin Lesions

My Notes

14.3 COMMON INTEGUMENTARY CONDITIONS

Now that we have reviewed the anatomy of the integumentary system, let's review common conditions that you may find during a routine integumentary assessment.

Acne

Acne is a skin disturbance that typically occurs on areas of the skin that are rich in sebaceous glands, such as the face and back. It is most common during puberty due to associated hormonal changes that stimulate the release of sebum. An overproduction and accumulation of sebum, along with keratin, can block hair follicles. Acne results from infection by acne-causing bacteria and can lead to potential scarring.[1] See Figure 14.8[2] for an image of acne.

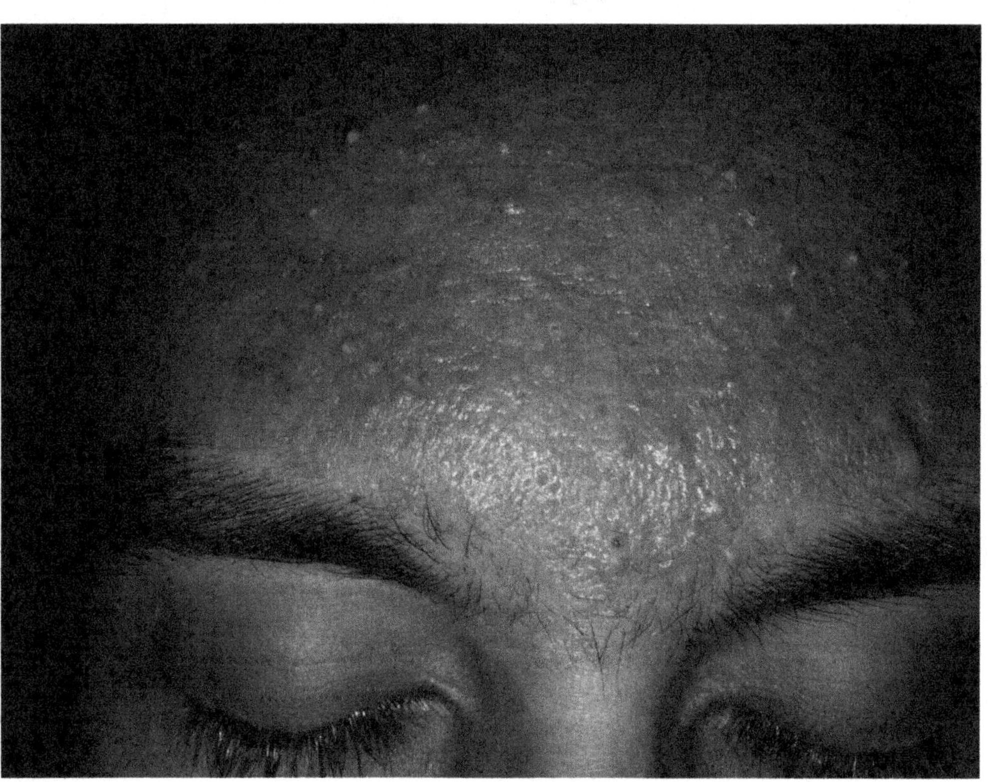

Figure 14.8 Acne

Lice and Nits

Head lice are tiny insects that live on a person's head. Adult lice are about the size of a sesame seed, but the eggs, called nits, are smaller and can appear like a dandruff flake. See Figure 14.9[3] for an image of very small white nits in a person's hair. Children ages 3-11 often get head lice at school and day care because they have head-to-head

---

1 This work is a derivative of Anatomy & Physiology by OpenStax and is licensed under CC BY 4.0. Access for free at https://openstax.org/books/anatomy-and-physiology/pages/1-introduction

2 "Acne vulgaris on a very oily skin.jpg" by Roshu Bangal is licensed under CC BY-SA 4.0. Access for free at https://commons.wikimedia.org/wiki/File:Acne_vulgaris_on_a_very_oily_skin.jpg

3 "Fig.5. Louse nites.jpg" by KostaMumcuoglu at English Wikipedia is licensed under CC BY-SA 3.0. Access for free at

My Notes

contact while playing together. Lice move by crawling and spread by close person-to-person contact. Rarely, they can spread by sharing personal belongings such as hats or hair brushes. Contrary to popular belief, personal hygiene and cleanliness have nothing to do with getting head lice. Symptoms of head lice include the following:

- Tickling feeling in the hair
- Frequent itching, which is caused by an allergic reaction to the bites
- Sores from scratching, which can become infected with bacteria
- Trouble sleeping due to head lice being most active in the dark

A diagnosis of head lice usually comes from observing a louse or nit on a person's head. Because they are very small and move quickly, a magnifying lens and a fine-toothed comb may be needed to find lice or nits. Treatments for head lice include over-the-counter and prescription shampoos, creams, and lotions such as permethrin lotion.[4]

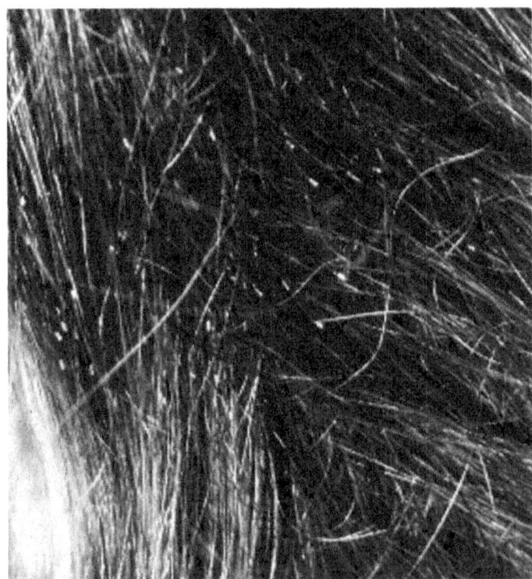

Figure 14.9 Nits

Burns

A burn results when the skin is damaged by intense heat, radiation, electricity, or chemicals. The damage results in the death of skin cells, which can lead to a massive loss of fluid due to loss of the skin's protection. Burned skin is also extremely susceptible to infection due to the loss of protection by intact layers of skin.

Burns are classified by the degree of their severity. A **first-degree burn**, also referred to as a superficial burn, only affects the epidermis. Although the skin may be painful and swollen, these burns typically heal on their own within a few days. Mild sunburn fits into the category of a first-degree burn. A **second-degree burn**, also referred to as a partial thickness burn, affects both the epidermis and a portion of the dermis. These burns result in swelling and a painful blistering of the skin. It is important to keep the burn site clean to prevent infection. With good care, a second-degree burn will heal within several weeks. A **third-degree** burn, also referred to as a full thickness burn, extends fully into the epidermis and dermis, destroying the tissue and affecting the nerve endings and

---

4 MedlinePlus [Internet]. Bethesda (MD): National Library of Medicine (US); [updated 2020, Aug 17]. Head lice; [reviewed 2016, Sep 9; cited 2020, Sep 18]. https://medlineplus.gov/headlice.html

My Notes

sensory function. These are serious burns that require immediate medical attention. A **fourth-degree burn**, also referred to as a deep full thickness burn, is even more severe, affecting the underlying muscle and bone. Third- and fourth-degree burns are usually not as painful as second-degree burns because the nerve endings are damaged. Full thickness burns require debridement (removal of dead skin) followed by grafting of the skin from an unaffected part of the body or from skin grown in tissue culture.[5] See Figure 14.10[6] for an image of a patient recovering from a second-degree burn on the hand.

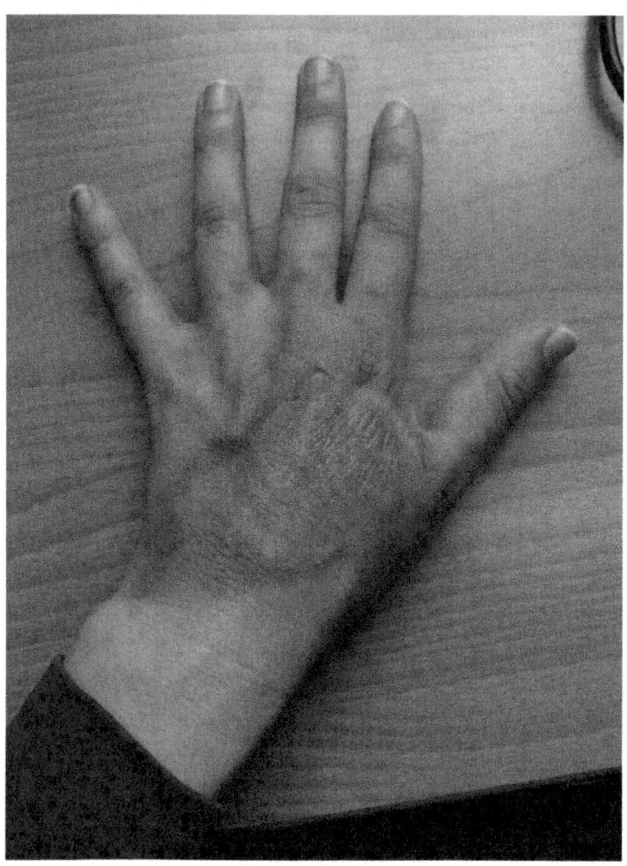

Figure 14.10 Recovering Second-Degree Burn

Severe burns are quickly measured in emergency departments using a tool called the "**rule of nines**," which associates specific anatomical locations with a percentage that is a factor of nine. Rapid estimate of the burned surface area is used to estimate intravenous fluid replacement because patients will have massive fluid losses due to the removal of the skin barrier.[7] See Figure 14.11[8] for an illustration of the rule of nines. The head is 9% (4.5% on

5 This work is a derivative of Anatomy & Physiology by OpenStax and is licensed under CC BY 4.0. Access for free at https://openstax.org/books/anatomy-and-physiology/pages/1-introduction

6 "1Veertje hand-burn-do8.jpg" by 1Veertje is licensed under CC BY-SA 3.0. Access for free at https://commons.wikimedia.org/wiki/File:1Veertje_hand-burn-d08.jpg

7 This work is a derivative of StatPearls by Moore, Waheed, and Burns and is licensed under CC BY 4.0. Access for free at https://www.ncbi.nlm.nih.gov/books/NBK430685/

8 "513 Degree of burns.jpg" by OpenStax is licensed under CC BY 3.0. Access for free at https://commons.wikimedia.org/wiki/File:513_Degree_of_burns.jpg

each side), the upper limbs are 9% each (4.5% on each side), the lower limbs are 18% each (9% on each side), and the trunk is 36% (18% on each side).

My Notes

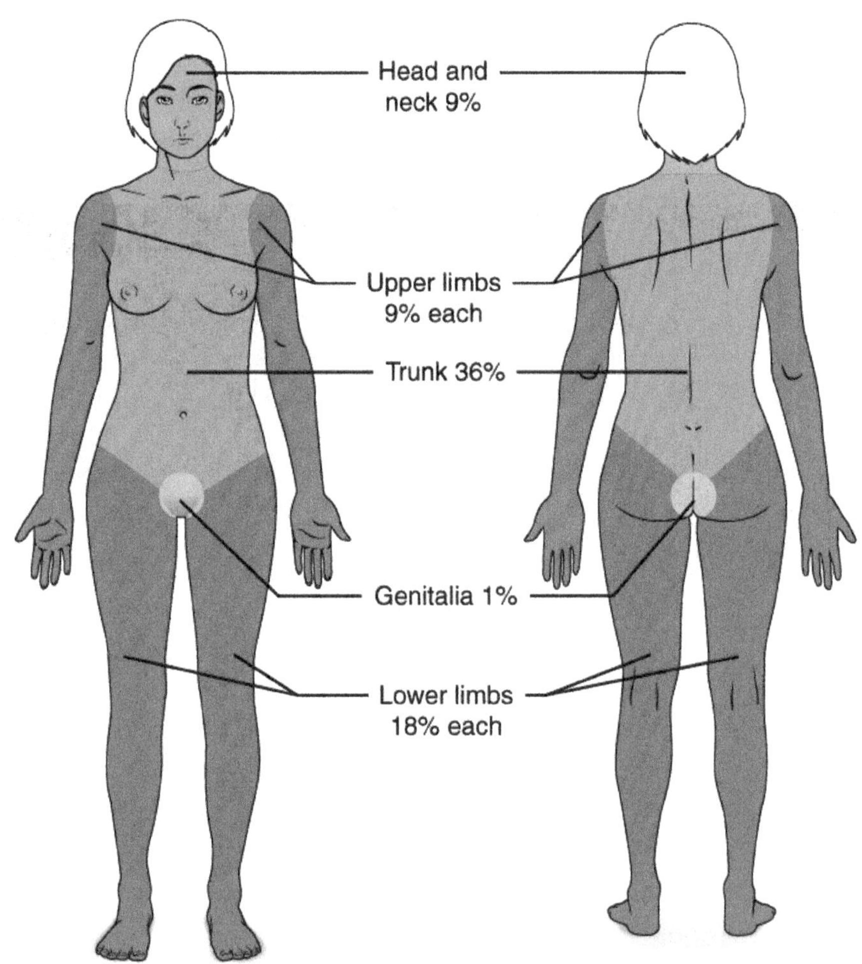

Figure 14.11 Rule of Nines

My Notes

Scars

Most cuts and wounds cause scar formation. A scar is collagen-rich skin formed after the process of wound healing. Sometimes there is an overproduction of scar tissue because the process of collagen formation does not stop when the wound is healed, resulting in the formation of a raised scar called a **keloid**.[9] Keloids are more common in patients with darker skin color. See Figure 14.12[10] for an image of a keloid that has developed from a scar on a patient's chest wall.

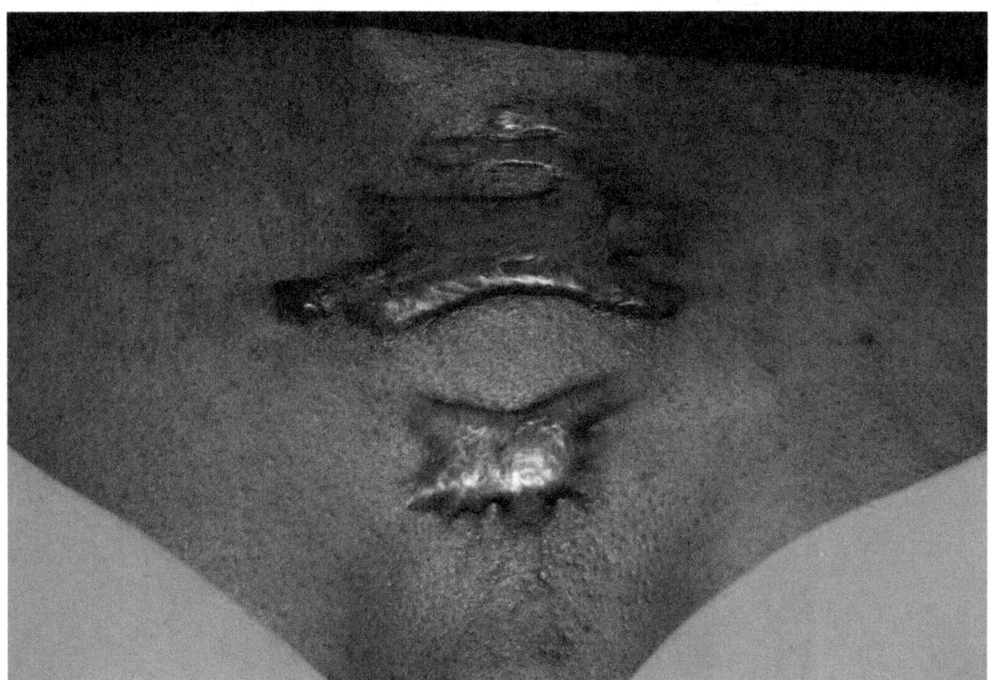

Figure 14.12 Keloid

9 This work is a derivative of Anatomy & Physiology by OpenStax and is licensed under CC BY 4.0. Access for free at https://openstax.org/books/anatomy-and-physiology/pages/1-introduction

10 "Keloid-Butterfly, Chest Wall.JPG" by Htirgan is licensed under CC BY-SA 3.0. Access for free at https://commons.wikimedia.org/wiki/File:Keloid-Butterfly,_Chest_Wall.JPG

Skin Cancer

My Notes

Skin cancer is common, with one in five Americans experiencing some type of skin cancer in their lifetime. Basal cell carcinoma is the most common of all cancers that occur in the United States and is frequently found on areas most susceptible to long-term sun exposure such as the head, neck, arms, and back. Basal cell carcinomas start in the epidermis and become an uneven patch, bump, growth, or scar on the skin surface. Treatment options include surgery, freezing (cryosurgery), and topical ointments.[11]

Squamous cell carcinoma presents as lesions commonly found on the scalp, ears, and hands. If not removed, squamous cell carcinomas can metastasize to other parts of the body. Surgery and radiation are used to cure squamous cell carcinoma. See Figure 14.13[12] for an image of squamous cell carcinoma.[13]

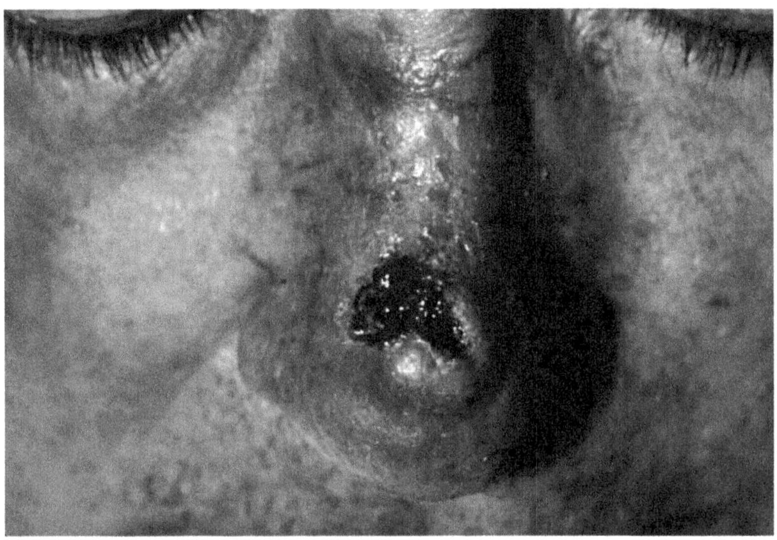

Figure 14.13 Squamous Cell Carcinoma

Melanoma is a cancer characterized by the uncontrolled growth of melanocytes, the pigment-producing cells in the epidermis. A melanoma commonly develops from an existing mole. See Figure 14.14[14] for an image of a melanoma. Melanoma is the most fatal of all skin cancers because it is highly metastatic and can be difficult to

11 This work is a derivative of Anatomy & Physiology by OpenStax and is licensed under CC BY 4.0. Access for free at https://openstax.org/books/anatomy-and-physiology/pages/1-introduction

12 "Squamous cell carcinoma (3).jpg" by unknown photographer, provided by National Cancer Institute is licensed under *CC0*. Access for free at https://openstax.org/books/anatomy-and-physiology/pages/5-4-diseases-disorders-and-injuries-of-the-integumentary-system

13 This work is a derivative of Anatomy & Physiology by OpenStax and is licensed under CC BY 4.0. Access for free at https://openstax.org/books/anatomy-and-physiology/pages/1-introduction

14 "Melanoma (2).jpg" by unknown photographer, provided by National Cancer Institute is in the Public Domain. Access for free at https://openstax.org/books/anatomy-and-physiology/pages/5-4-diseases-disorders-and-injuries-of-the-integumentary-system

My Notes

detect before it has spread to other organs. Melanomas usually appear as asymmetrical brown and black patches with uneven borders and a raised surface. Treatment includes surgical excision and immunotherapy.[15]

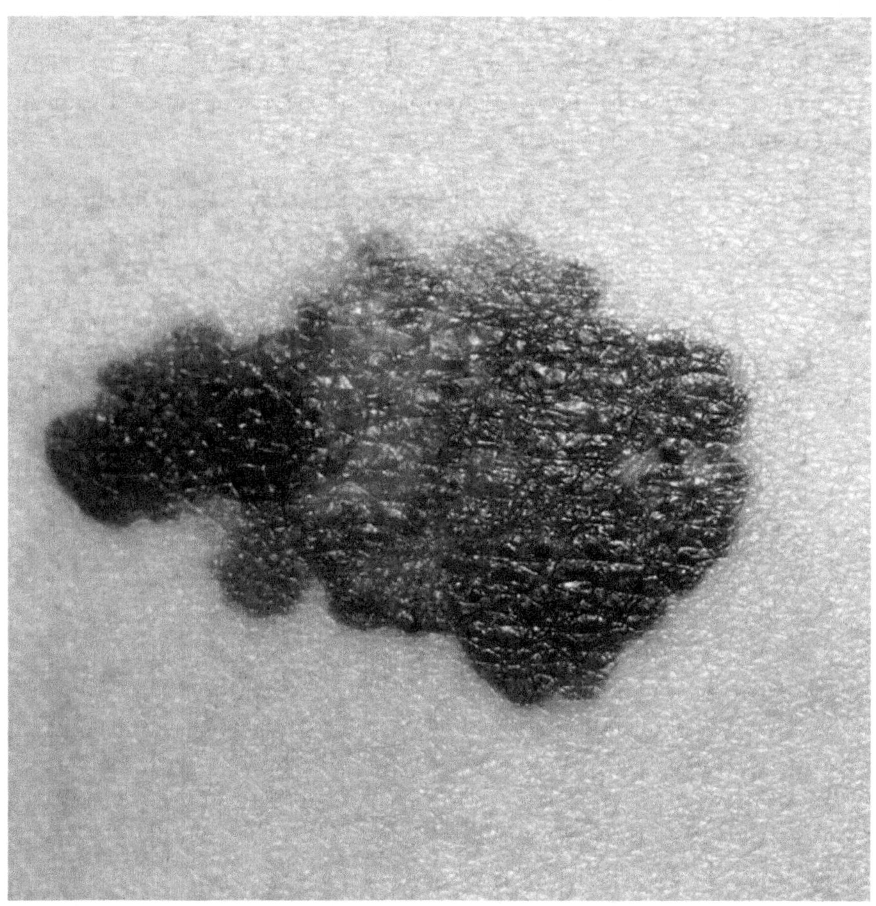

Figure 14.14 Melanoma

15 This work is a derivative of Anatomy & Physiology by OpenStax and is licensed under CC BY 4.0. Access for free at https://openstax.org/books/anatomy-and-physiology/pages/1-introduction

Fungal (Tinea) Infections

My Notes

Tinea is the name of a group of skin diseases caused by a fungus. Types of tinea include ringworm, athlete's foot, and jock itch. These infections are usually not serious, but they can be uncomfortable because of the symptoms of itching and burning. They can be transmitted by touching infected people, damp surfaces such as shower floors, or even from pets.[16] Ringworm (tinea corporis) is a type of rash that forms on the body that typically looks like a red ring with a clear center, although a worm doesn't cause it. Scalp ringworm (tinea capitals) causes itchy, red patches on the head that can leave bald spots. Athlete's foot (tinea pedis) causes itching, burning, and cracked skin between the toes. Jock itch (tinea cruris) causes an itchy, burning rash in the groin area. Fungal infections are often treated successfully with over-the-counter creams and powders, but some require prescription medicine such as nystatin. See Figure 14.15[17] for an image of a tinea in a patient's groin.[18]

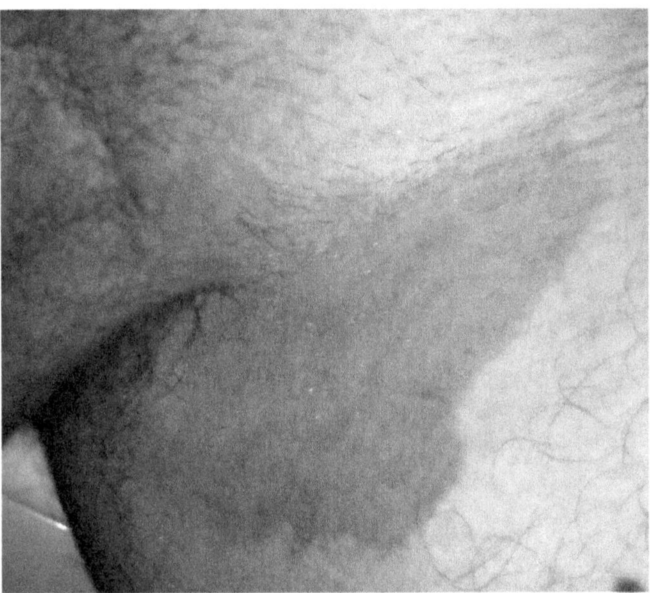

Figure 14.15 Fungal Infection in the Groin

16 MedlinePlus [Internet]. Bethesda (MD): National Library of Medicine (US); [updated 2020, Aug 17]. Tinea infections; [reviewed 2016, Apr 4; cited 2020, Sep 18]. https://medlineplus.gov/tineainfections.html#:~:text=Tinea%20is%20the%20name%20of,or%20even%20from%20a%20pet

17 "Tinea cruris.jpg" by *Robertgascoin* is licensed under CC BY-SA 3.0. Access for free at https://commons.wikimedia.org/wiki/File:Tinea_cruris.jpg

18 MedlinePlus [Internet]. Bethesda (MD): National Library of Medicine (US); [updated 2020, Aug 17]. Tinea infections; [reviewed 2016, Apr 4; cited 2020, Sep 18]. https://medlineplus.gov/tineainfections.html#:~:text=Tinea%20is%20the%20name%20of,or%20even%20from%20a%20pet

My Notes

Impetigo

Impetigo is a common skin infection caused by bacteria in children between the ages two and six. It is commonly caused by *Staphylococcus* (staph) or *Streptococcus* (strep) bacteria. See Figure 14.16[19] for an image of impetigo. Impetigo often starts when bacteria enter a break in the skin, such as a cut, scratch, or insect bite. Symptoms start with red or pimple-like sores surrounded by red skin. The sores fill with pus and then break open after a few days and form a thick crust. They are often itchy, but scratching them can spread the sores. Impetigo can spread by contact with sores or nasal discharge from an infected person and is treated with antibiotics.

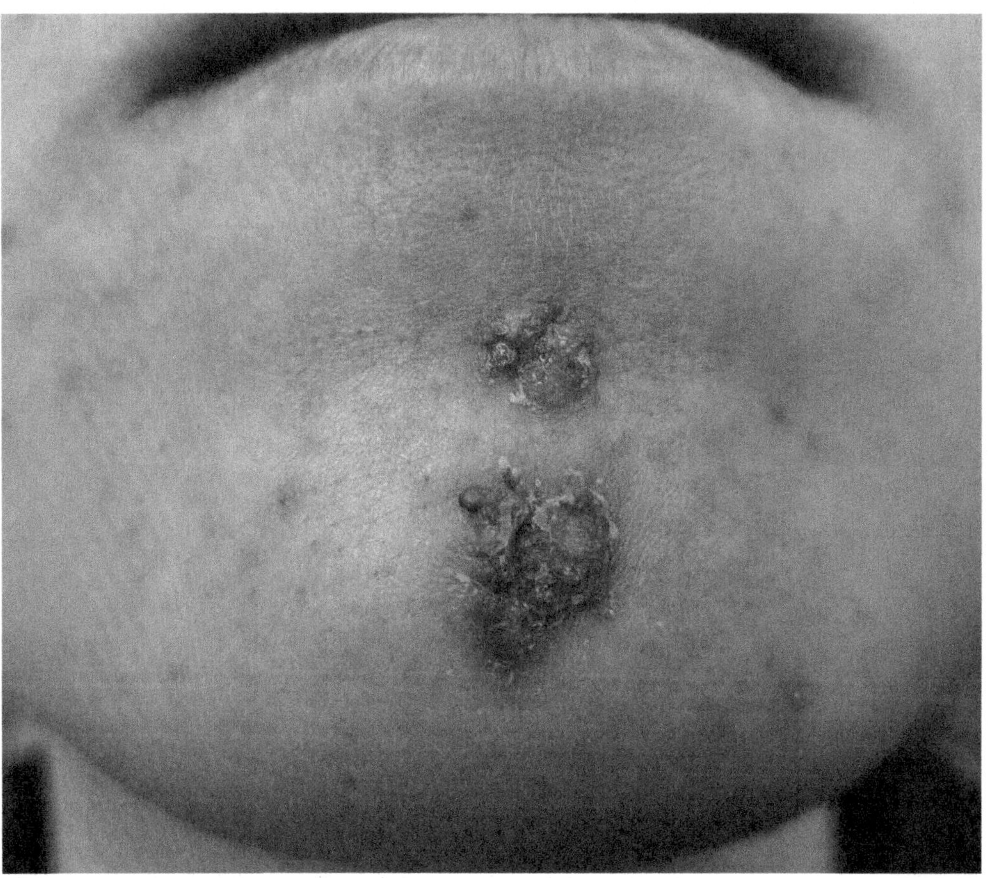

Figure 14.16 Impetigo

Edema

Edema is caused by fluid accumulation within the tissues often caused by underlying cardiovascular or renal disease. Read more about edema in the "Basic Concepts" section of the "Cardiovascular Assessment" chapter.

19 "Impetigo2020.jpg" by *James Heilman, MD* is licensed under CC BY-SA 4.0. Access for free at https://commons.wikimedia.org/wiki/File:Impetigo2020.jpg

Lymphedema

My Notes

Lymphedema is the medical term for a type of swelling that occurs when lymph fluid builds up in the body's soft tissues due to damage to the lymph system. It often occurs unilaterally in the arms or legs after surgery has been performed that injured the regional lymph nodes. See Figure 14.17[20] for an image of lower extremity edema. Causes of lymphedema include infection, cancer, scar tissue from radiation therapy, surgical removal of lymph nodes, or inherited conditions. There is no cure for lymphedema, but elevation of the affected extremity is vital. Compression devices and massage can help to manage the symptoms. See Figure 14.18[21] for an image of a specialized compression dressing used for lymphedema. It is also important to remember to avoid taking blood pressure on a patient's extremity with lymphedema.[22]

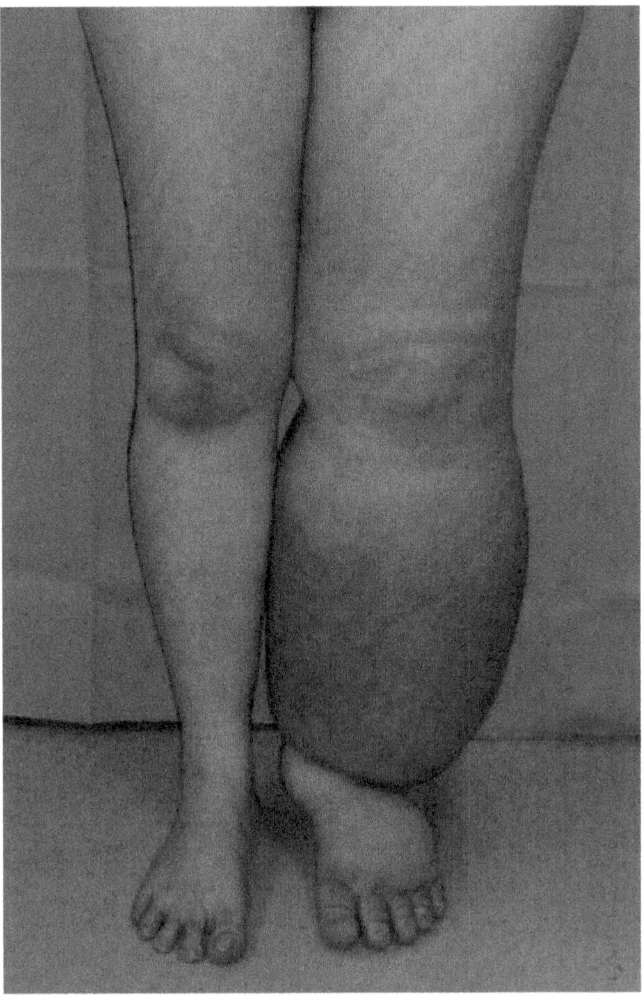

Figure 14.17 Lymphedema

---

20 "Lymphedema_limbs.JPG" by medical doctors is licensed under CC BY-SA 4.0. Access for free at https://commons.wikimedia.org/wiki/File:Lymphedema_limbs.JPG

21 "Adaptive_Kompressionsbandage_mit_Fußteil.jpg" by *Enter* is in the Public Domain. Access for free at https://commons.wikimedia.org/wiki/File:Adaptive_Kompressionsbandage_mit_Fußteil.jpg

22 MedlinePlus [Internet]. Bethesda (MD): National Library of Medicine (US); [updated 2020, Aug 27]. Lymphedema; [reviewed 2019, Jan 22; cited 2020, Sep 18]. https://medlineplus.gov/lymphedema.html

My Notes

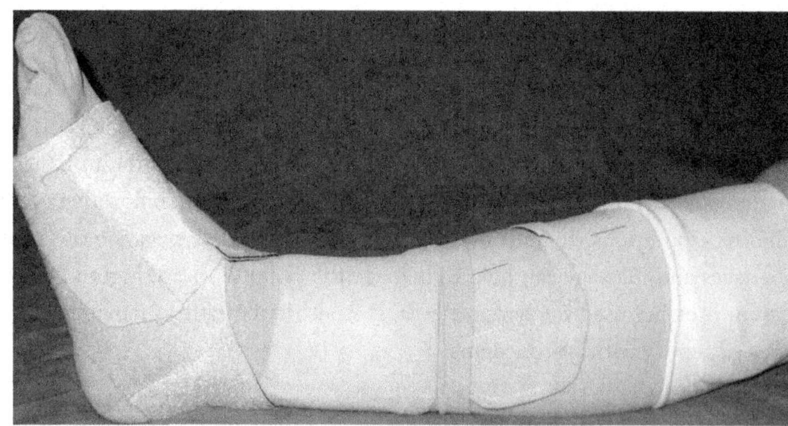

Figure 14.18 Compression Dressing for Lymphedema

Jaundice

Jaundice causes skin and sclera (whites of the eyes) to turn yellow. See Figure 14.19[23] for an image of a patient with jaundice visible in the sclera and the skin. Jaundice is caused by too much bilirubin in the body. Bilirubin is a yellow chemical in hemoglobin, the substance that carries oxygen in red blood cells. As red blood cells break down, the old ones are processed by the liver. If the liver can't keep up due to large amounts of red blood cell breakdown or liver damage, bilirubin builds up and causes the skin and sclera to appear yellow. New onset of jaundice should always be reported to the health care provider.

Many healthy babies experience mild jaundice during the first week of life that usually resolves on its own, but some babies require additional treatment such as light therapy. Jaundice can happen at any age for many reasons, such as liver disease, blood disease, infections, or side effects of some medications.[24]

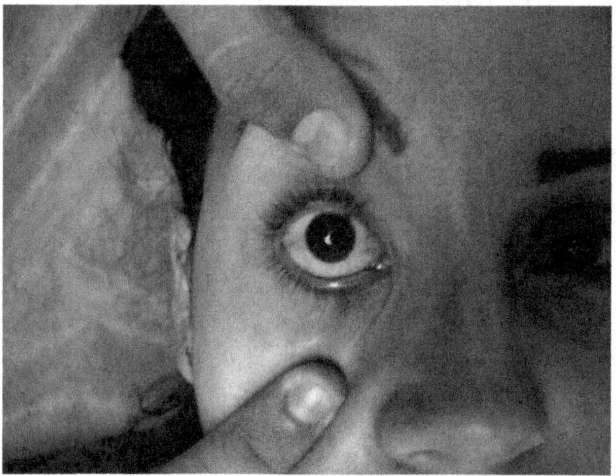

Figure 14.19 Jaundice

23 "Cholangitis Jaundice.jpg" by Bobjgalindo is licensed under CC BY-SA 4.0. Access for free at https://commons.wikimedia.org/wiki/File:Cholangitis_Jaundice.jpg

24 MedlinePlus [Internet]. Bethesda (MD): National Library of Medicine (US); [updated 2019, Oct 22]. Jaundice; [reviewed 2016, Aug 31; cited 2020, Sep 18]. https://medlineplus.gov/jaundice.html

Pressure Injuries

My Notes

Pressure injuries also called bedsores, form when a patient's skin and soft tissue press against a hard surface, such as a chair or bed, for a prolonged period of time. The pressure against a hard surface reduces blood supply to that area, causing the skin tissue to become damaged and become an ulcer. Patients are at high risk of developing a pressure injury if they spend a lot of time in one position, have decreased sensation, or have bladder or bowel leakage.[25] See Figure 14.20[26] for an image of a pressure ulcer injury on a bed-bound patient's back. Read more information about assessing and caring for pressure injury in the "Wound Care" chapter.

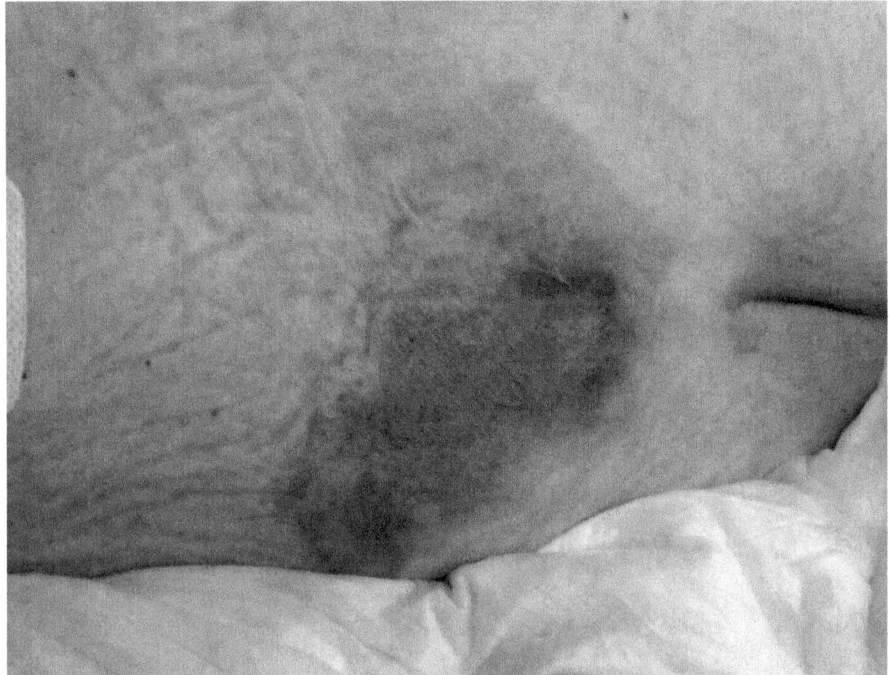

Figure 14.20 Pressure Ulcer Injury

25 A.D.A.M. Medical Encyclopedia [Internet]. Atlanta (GA): A.D.A.M., Inc.; c1997-2020. Preventing pressure ulcers; [updated 2020, Sep 16; cited 2020, Sep 18]. https://medlineplus.gov/ency/patientinstructions/000147.htm

26 "Decubitus 01.jpg" by AfroBrazilian is licensed under CC BY-SA 3.0. Access for free at https://commons.wikimedia .org/wiki/File:Decubitus_01.JPG

My Notes

Petechiae

Petechiae are tiny red dots caused by bleeding under the skin that may appear like a rash. Large petechiae are called purpura. An easy method used to assess for petechiae is to apply pressure to the rash with a gloved finger. A rash will blanch (i.e., whiten with pressure) but petechiae and purpura do not blanch. See Figure 14.21[27] for an image of petechiae and purpura. New onset of petechiae should be immediately reported to the health care provider because it can indicate a serious underlying medical condition.[28]

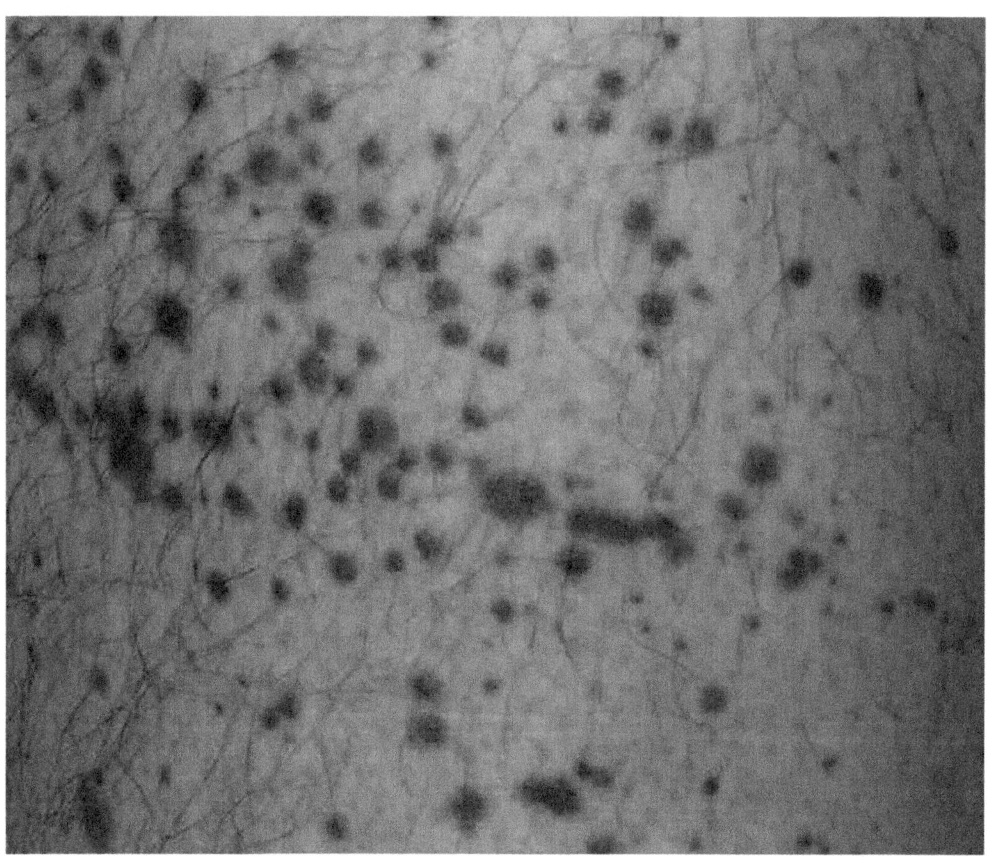

Figure 14.21 Petechiae and Purpura

27 "Purpura.jpg" by User:Hektor is licensed under CC BY-SA 3.0. Access for free at https://commons.wikimedia.org/wiki/File:Purpura.jpg

28 A.D.A.M. Medical Encyclopedia [Internet]. Atlanta (GA): A.D.A.M., Inc.; c1997-2020. Bleeding into the skin; [updated 2020, Sep 16; cited 2020, Sep 18]. https://medlineplus.gov/ency/article/003235.htm

14.4 INTEGUMENTARY ASSESSMENT

My Notes

Now that we have reviewed the anatomy of the integumentary system and common integumentary conditions, let's review the components of an integumentary assessment. The standard for documentation of skin assessment is within 24 hours of admission to inpatient care. Skin assessment should also be ongoing in inpatient and long-term care.[1]

A routine integumentary assessment by a registered nurse in an inpatient care setting typically includes inspecting overall skin color, inspecting for skin lesions and wounds, and palpating extremities for edema, temperature, and capillary refill.[2]

Subjective Assessment

Begin the assessment by asking focused interview questions regarding the integumentary system. Itching is the most frequent complaint related to the integumentary system. See Table 14.4a for sample interview questions.

Table 14.4a Focused Interview Questions for the Integumentary System

Questions	Follow-up
Are you currently experiencing any skin symptoms such as itching, rashes, or an unusual mole, lump, bump, or nodule?[3]	Use the PQRSTU method to gain additional information about current symptoms. Read more about the PQRSTU method in the "Health History" chapter.
Have you ever been diagnosed with a condition such as acne, eczema, skin cancer, pressure injuries, jaundice, edema, or lymphedema?	Please describe.
Are you currently using any prescription or over-the-counter medications, creams, vitamins, or supplements to treat a skin, hair, or nail condition?	Please describe.

1 Medline Industries, Inc. (n.d.). *Are you doing comprehensive skin assessments correctly? Get the whole picture.* https://www.medline.com/skin-health/comprehensive-skin-assessments-correctly-get-whole-picture/#:~:text=A%20comprehensive%20skin%20assessment%20entails,actually%20more%20than%20skin%20deep.

2 Giddens, J. F. (2007). A survey of physical examination techniques performed by RNs: Lessons for nursing education. *Journal of Nursing Education, 46*(2), 83-87. https://doi.org/10.3928/01484834-20070201-09

3 McKay, M. (1990). The dermatologic history. In Walker, H. K., Hall, W. D., Hurst, J. W. (Eds.), *Clinical methods: The history, physical, and laboratory* examinations (3rd ed.). https://www.ncbi.nlm.nih.gov/books/NBK207/

My Notes

Objective Assessment

There are five key areas to note during a focused integumentary assessment: color, skin temperature, moisture level, skin turgor, and any lesions or skin breakdown. Certain body areas require particular observation because they are more prone to pressure injuries, such as bony prominences, skin folds, perineum, between digits of the hands and feet, and under any medical device that can be removed during routine daily care.[4]

Inspection

Color

Inspect the color of the patient's skin and compare findings to what is expected for their skin tone. Note a change in color such as **pallor** (paleness), **cyanosis** (blueness), **jaundice** (yellowness), or **erythema** (redness). Note if there is any bruising (**ecchymosis**) present.

Scalp

If the patient reports itching of the scalp, inspect the scalp for lice and/or nits.

Lesions and Skin Breakdown

Note any lesions, skin breakdown, or unusual findings, such as rashes, petechiae, unusual moles, or burns. Be aware that unusual patterns of bruising or burns can be signs of abuse that warrant further investigation and reporting according to agency policy and state regulations.

Auscultation

Auscultation does not occur during a focused integumentary exam.

Palpation

Palpation of the skin includes assessing temperature, moisture, texture, skin turgor, capillary refill, and edema. If erythema or rashes are present, it is helpful to apply pressure with a gloved finger to further assess for **blanching** (whitening with pressure).

Temperature, Moisture, and Texture

Fever, decreased perfusion of the extremities, and local inflammation in tissues can cause changes in skin temperature. For example, a fever can cause a patient's skin to feel warm and sweaty (diaphoretic). Decreased perfusion of the extremities can cause the patient's hands and feet to feel cool, whereas local tissue infection or inflammation can make the localized area feel warmer than the surrounding skin. Research has shown that experienced practitioners can palpate skin temperature accurately and detect differences as small as 1 to 2 degrees Celsius. For accurate palpation of skin temperature, do not hold anything warm or cold in your hands for several minutes

4 Medline Industries, Inc. (n.d.). *Are you doing comprehensive skin assessments correctly? Get the whole picture.* https://www.medline.com/skin-health/comprehensive-skin-assessments-correctly-get-whole-picture/#:~:text=A%20comprehensive%20skin%20assessment%20entails,actually%20more%20than%20skin%20deep

prior to palpation. Use the palmar surface of your dominant hand to assess temperature.[5] While assessing skin temperature, also assess if the skin feels dry or moist and the texture of the skin. Skin that appears or feels sweaty is referred to as being **diaphoretic.**

My Notes

Capillary Refill

The capillary refill test is a test done on the nail beds to monitor perfusion, the amount of blood flow to tissue. Pressure is applied to a fingernail or toenail until it turns white, indicating that the blood has been forced from the tissue under the nail. This whiteness is called blanching. Once the tissue has blanched, remove pressure. Capillary refill is defined as the time it takes for color to return to the tissue after pressure has been removed that caused blanching. If there is sufficient blood flow to the area, a pink color should return within 2 seconds after the pressure is removed.[6]

View the following video demonstrating capillary refill[7]: "Cardiovascular Assessment Part Two | Capillary Refill Test."

Skin Turgor

Skin turgor may be included when assessing a patient's hydration status, but research has shown it is not a good indicator. **Skin turgor** is the skin's elasticity. Its ability to change shape and return to normal may be decreased when the patient is dehydrated. To check for skin turgor, gently grasp skin on the patient's lower arm between two fingers so that it is tented upwards, and then release. Skin with normal turgor snaps rapidly back to its normal position, but skin with poor turgor takes additional time to return to its normal position.[8] Skin turgor is not a reliable method to assess for dehydration in older adults because they have decreased skin elasticity, so other assessments for dehydration should be included.[9]

Edema

If edema is present on inspection, palpate the area to determine if the edema is pitting or nonpitting. Press on the skin to assess for indentation, ideally over a bony structure, such as the tibia. If no indentation occurs, it is referred to as nonpitting edema. If indentation occurs, it is referred to as pitting edema. See Figure 14.22[10] for an image demonstrating pitting edema. If pitting edema is present, document the depth of the indention and how

---

5 Levine, D., Walker, J. R., Marcellin-Little, D. J., Goulet, R., & Ru, H. (2018). Detection of skin temperature differences using palpation by manual physical therapists and lay individuals. *The Journal of Manual & Manipulative Therapy, 26*(2), 97-101. https://dx.doi.org/10.1080%2F10669817.2018.1427908

6 Johannsen, L.L. (2005). Skin assessment. *Dermatology Nursing, 17*(2), 165-66.

7 Nurse Saria. (2018, September 18). *Cardiovascular assessment part two | Capillary refill test.* [Video]. YouTube. All rights reserved. https://youtu.be/A6htMxo4Cks

8 A.D.A.M. Medical Encyclopedia [Internet]. Atlanta (GA): A.D.A.M., Inc.; c1997-2020. Skin turgor; [updated 2020, Sep 16; cited 2020, Sep 18]. https://medlineplus.gov/ency/article/003281.htm#:~:text=To%20check%20for%20skin%20turgor,back%20to%20its%20normal%20position

9 Nursing Times. (2015, August 3). *Detecting dehydration in older people.* https://www.nursingtimes.net/roles/older-people-nurses-roles/detecting-dehydration-in-older-people-useful-tests-03-08-2015/

10 "Combinpedal.jpg" by James Heilman, MD is licensed under CC BY-SA 3.0. Access for free at https://commons.wikimedia.org/wiki/File:Combinpedal.jpg

My Notes

long it takes for the skin to rebound back to its original position. The indentation and time required to rebound to the original position are graded on a scale from 1 to 4, where 1+ indicates a barely detectable depression with immediate rebound, and 4+ indicates a deep depression with a time lapse of over 20 seconds required to rebound. See Figure 14.23[11] for an illustration of grading edema.

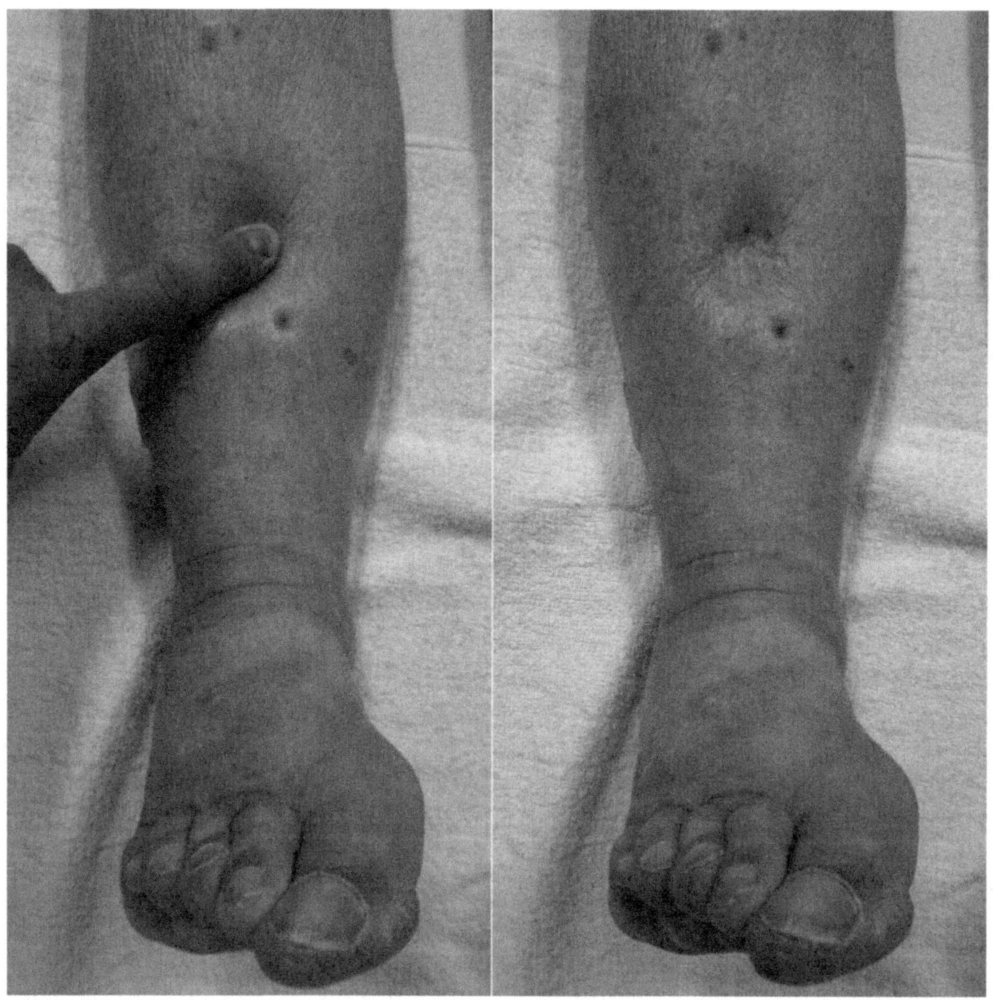

Figure 14.22 Assessing Lower Extremity Edema

11 "Grading of Edema" by Meredith Pomietlo for Chippewa Valley Technical College is licensed under CC BY 4.0. Access for free at https://drive.google.com/file/d/1dRiBmujU9KGrRgi0QpsgeJkcXL7ASWRT/view?usp=sharing

My Notes

Grade 1	0–2 mm indentation; rebounds immediately.
Grade 2	3–4 mm indentation; rebounds in < 15 seconds.
Grade 3	5–6 mm indentation; up to 30 seconds to rebound.
Grade 4	8 mm indentation; > 20 seconds to rebound.

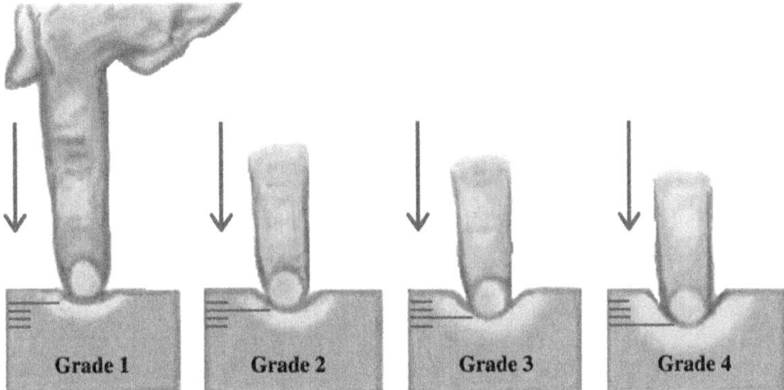

Figure 14.23 Grading of Edema

Life Span Considerations

Older Adults

Older adults have several changes associated with aging that are apparent during assessment of the integumentary system. They often have cardiac and circulatory system conditions that cause decreased perfusion, resulting in cool hands and feet. They have decreased elasticity and fragile skin that often tears more easily. The blood vessels of the dermis become more fragile, leading to bruising and bleeding under the skin. The subcutaneous fat layer thins, so it has less insulation and padding and reduced ability to maintain body temperature. Growths such as skin tags, rough patches (keratoses), skin cancers, and other lesions are more common. Older adults may also be less able to sense touch, pressure, vibration, heat, and cold.[12]

12 A.D.A.M. Medical Encyclopedia [Internet]. Atlanta (GA): A.D.A.M., Inc.; c1997-2020. Aging changes in skin; [updated 2020, Sep 16; cited 2020, Sep 18]. https://medlineplus.gov/ency/article/004014.htm#:~:text=The%20remaining%20melanocytes%20increase%20in,the%20skin's%20strength%20and%20elasticity

My Notes

When completing an integumentary assessment it is important to distinguish between expected and unexpected assessment findings. Please review Table 14.4b to review common expected and unexpected integumentary findings.

Table 14.4b Expected Versus Unexpected Findings on integumentary Assessment

Assessment	**Expected Findings**	**Unexpected Findings (Document and notify provider if it is a new finding*)**
Inspection	Skin is expected color for ethnicity without lesions or rashes.	Jaundice Erythema Pallor Cyanosis Irregular-looking mole Bruising (ecchymosis) Rashes Petechiae Skin breakdown Burns
Auscultation	Not applicable	
Palpation	Skin is warm and dry with no edema. Capillary refill is less than 3 seconds. Skin has normal turgor with no tenting.	Diaphoretic or clammy Cool extremity Edema Lymphedema Capillary refill greater than 3 seconds Tenting
***CRITICAL CONDITIONS to report immediately**		Cool and clammy Diaphoretic Petechiae Jaundice Cyanosis Redness, warmth, and tenderness indicating a possible infection

14.5 SAMPLE DOCUMENTATION

My Notes

Sample Documentation of Expected Findings

Skin is expected color for ethnicity without lesions or rashes. Skin is warm and dry with no edema. Capillary refill is less than 3 seconds. Normal skin turgor with no tenting.

Sample Documentation of Unexpected Findings

Mother brought the child into the clinic for evaluation of an "itchy rash around the mouth" that started about three days ago. Crusted pustules are present around the patient's mouth. Dr. Smith evaluated the patient and a prescription for antibiotics was provided. Mother and child were educated to use good hand hygiene practices to prevent the spread of infection.

My Notes

14.6 CHECKLIST FOR INTEGUMENTARY ASSESSMENT

Use this checklist to review the steps for completion of an "Integumentary Assessment."

Steps

Disclaimer: Always review and follow agency policy regarding this specific skill.

1. Gather supplies: penlight, nonsterile gloves, magnifying glass (optional), and wound measuring tool (optional).
2. Perform safety steps:
    - Perform hand hygiene.
    - Check the room for transmission-based precautions.
    - Introduce yourself, your role, the purpose of your visit, and an estimate of the time it will take.
    - Confirm patient ID using two patient identifiers (e.g., name and date of birth).
    - Explain the process to the patient and ask if they have any questions.
    - Be organized and systematic.
    - Use appropriate listening and questioning skills.
    - Listen and attend to patient cues.
    - Ensure the patient's privacy and dignity.
    - Assess ABCs.
3. Ask the patient if they have any known skin conditions or concerns.
4. Inspect the general color of the skin and look for any discolorations. Inspect the skin for lesions, bruising, edema, or rashes.
5. Verbalize the ABCE format for evaluating skin lesions.
6. Inspect the scalp for lesions and hair for lice or nits.
7. Inspect the nail beds for color and palpate for capillary refill.
8. Palpate the skin to assess for temperature, moisture, and turgor. Apply gloves prior to palpation as indicated.
9. Assess pressure points for skin breakdown: back of head, ears, elbows, sacrum, and heels.
10. Palpate for edema on lower extremities bilaterally. If edema is present, determine the grade of edema.
11. Assist the patient to a comfortable position, ask if they have any questions, and thank them for their time.
12. Ensure safety measures when leaving the room:
    - CALL LIGHT: Within reach
    - BED: Low and locked (in lowest position and brakes on)
    - SIDE RAILS: Secured
    - TABLE: Within reach

My Notes

- ROOM: Risk-free for falls (scan room and clear any obstacles)

13. Perform hand hygiene.
14. Document the assessment findings. Report any concerns according to agency policy.

My Notes

14.7 LEARNING ACTIVITIES

Learning Activities

(Answers to "Learning Activities" can be found in the "Answer Key" at the end of the book. Answers to interactive activity elements will be provided within the element as immediate feedback.)

Mr. Curtis is a 47-year-old patient admitted with a one-week history of progressive fatigue and ongoing diarrhea. You are completing his admission assessment. Based upon his presenting condition, what integumentary assessments might be important?

Check your knowledge about integumentary assessment using this flashcard activity:

An interactive or media element has been excluded from this version of the text. You can view it online here: https://wtcs.pressbooks.pub/nursingskills/?p=1447

Check your knowledge about integumentary conditions using this flashcard activity:

An interactive or media element has been excluded from this version of the text. You can view it online here: https://wtcs.pressbooks.pub/nursingskills/?p=1447

XIV GLOSSARY

My Notes

ABCDE: A mnemonic for assessing for melanoma developing in moles: Asymmetrical, Borders are irregular in shape, Color is various shades of brown or black, Diameter is larger than 6 mm., and the shape of the mole is Evolving.

Apocrine sweat gland: Sweat glands associated with hair follicles in densely hairy areas that release organic compounds subject to bacterial decomposition causing odor.

Blanching: To make white or pale by applying pressure.

Cyanosis: A bluish discoloration caused by lack of oxygenation of the tissue.

Dermis: The inner layer of skin with connective tissue, blood vessels, sweat glands, nerves, hair follicles, and other structures.

Diaphoretic: Excessive, abnormal sweating.

Ecchymosis: Bruising.

Eccrine sweat gland: Sweat gland that produces hypotonic sweat for thermoregulation.

Epidermis: The thin, uppermost layer of skin.

Erythema: A red color of the skin.

First-degree burn: A superficial burn that affects only the epidermis.

Fourth-degree burn: Severe burn damaging the dermis and the underlying muscle and bone.

Hypodermis: The layer of skin beneath the dermis composed of connective tissue and used for fat storage.

Jaundice: A yellowing of the skin or sclera caused by underlying medical conditions.

Keloid: A raised scar caused by overproduction of scar tissue.

Lesion: An area of abnormal tissue.

Lymphedema: A type of swelling that occurs when lymph fluid builds up in the body's soft tissues due to damage to the lymph system.

Melanin: Skin pigment produced by melanocytes scattered throughout the epidermis.

Melanoma: Skin cancer characterized by the uncontrolled growth of melanocytes that commonly develops from a mole. Melanoma is the most fatal of all skin cancers because it is highly metastatic. Melanomas usually appear as asymmetrical brown and black patches with uneven borders and a raised surface.

Petechiae: Tiny red dots caused by bleeding under the skin.

Pressure injury: Skin breakdown caused when a patient's skin and soft tissue press against a hard surface for a prolonged period of time, causing reduced blood supply and resulting in damaged tissue.

Rule of Nines: A tool used in the emergency department to assess the total body surface area burned to quickly estimate intravenous fluid requirements.

Second-degree burn: Burn affecting both the epidermis and a portion of the dermis, resulting in swelling and a painful blistering of the skin.

Skin turgor: The skin's elasticity and its ability to change shape and return to normal when gently grasped between two fingers.

Third-degree burn: Severe burn that fully extends into the epidermis and dermis, destroying the tissue and affecting the nerve endings and sensory function.

Chapter 15

Administration of Enteral Medications

15.1 ADMINISTRATION OF ENTERAL MEDICATIONS INTRODUCTION

My Notes

Learning Objectives

- Safely administer medication orally, rectally, and via enteral tubes
- Accurately check medication administration rights three times
- Calculate correct amount of medication to administer
- Explain medication information to patient
- Collect appropriate assessment data prior to and after medication administration
- Modify procedure to reflect variations across the life span
- Document actions and observations

"Enteral" means related to the intestines. The term **enteral medication** describes medications that are administered into the gastrointestinal tract including orally (PO), rectally (PR), or through a tube such as a nasogastric (NG) tube, nasointestinal (NI) tube, or percutaneous endoscopic gastrostomy (PEG) tube.

This chapter will review overall concepts related to safe medication administration, as well as specific information regarding the administration of oral medication, rectal medication, and medication via a gastric tube. Information regarding administering injections and intravenous medications can be found in "Administration of Parenteral Medications" and additional information about administering medications via other routes can be found in "Administration of Medications via Other Routes."

My Notes

15.2 BASIC CONCEPTS OF ADMINISTERING MEDICATIONS

The scope of practice regarding a nurse's ability to legally dispense and administer medication is based on each state's Nurse Practice Act.

Registered Nurses (RNs) and Licensed Practical Nurses (LPNs/LVNs) may legally administer medications that are prescribed by a health care provider, such as a physician, nurse practitioner, or physician's assistant. Prescriptions are "orders, interventions, remedies, or treatments ordered or directed by an authorized primary health care provider."[1]

For more information about the state Nurse Practice Act, visit the "Legal/Ethical" chapter in Open RN *Nursing Pharmacology*.

Types of Orders

Prescriptions are often referred to as orders in clinical practice. There are several types of orders, such as routine orders, PRN orders, standing orders, one-time orders, STAT orders, and titration orders.

- A **routine order** is a prescription that is followed until another order cancels it. An example of a routine order is "Lisinopril 10 mg PO daily."
- A **PRN** (or as-needed) order is a prescription for medication to be administered when it is requested by, or as needed by, the patient. PRN orders are typically administered based on patient symptoms, such as pain, nausea, or itching. An example of a PRN order for pain medication is "Acetaminophen 500 mg PO every 4-6 hours as needed for pain."
- A **standing order** is also referred to in practice as an "order set" or a "protocol." Standing orders are standardized prescriptions for nurses to implement to any patient in clearly defined circumstances without the need to initially notify a provider. An example of a standing order set/protocol for patients visiting an urgent care clinic reporting chest pain is to immediately administer four chewable aspirin, establish intravenous (IV) access, and obtain an electrocardiogram (ECG).
- A **one-time order** is a prescription for a medication to be administered only once. An example of a one-time order is a prescription for an IV dose of antibiotics to be administered immediately prior to surgery.
- A **STAT order** is a one-time order that is administered without delay due to the urgency of the circumstances. An example of a STAT order is "Benadryl 50 mg PO stat" for a patient having an allergic reaction.
- A **titration** order is an order in which the medication dose is either progressively increased or decreased by the nurse in response to the patient's status. Titration orders are typically used for patients in critical care as defined by agency policy. The Joint Commission requires titration orders to include the medication name, medication route, initial rate of infusion (dose/unit of time), incremental units to which the rate or dose can be increased or decreased, how often the rate or dose can be changed, the maximum rate or dose of infusion, and the objective clinical measure to be used to guide changes. An example of a titration order is "Norepinephrine 2-12

1 NCSBN.(2018). *2019 NCLEX-RN test plan*. https://www.ncsbn.org/2019_RN_TestPlan-English.pdf

micrograms/min, start at 2 mcg/min and titrate upward by 1 mcg/min every 5 minutes with continual blood pressure monitoring until systolic blood pressure >90 mm Hg."

My Notes

Components of a Medication Order

According to the Centers for Medicare & Medicaid Services, all orders for the administration of drugs and biologicals must contain the following information:[2]

- Name of the patient
- Age or date of birth
- Date and time of the order
- Drug name
- Dose, frequency, and route
- Name/Signature of the prescriber
- Weight of the patient to facilitate dose calculation when applicable. (Note that dose calculations are based on metric weight: kilograms for children/adults or grams for newborns)
- Dose calculation requirements, when applicable
- Exact strength or concentration, when applicable
- Quantity and/or duration of the prescription, when applicable
- Specific instructions for use, when applicable

When reviewing a medication order, the nurse must ensure these components are included in the prescription before administering the medication. If a pertinent piece of information is not included, the nurse must contact the prescribing provider to clarify and correct the order.

Drug Name

The name of the drug may be ordered by the generic name or brand name. The generic name is considered the safest method to use and allows for substitution of various brand medications by the pharmacist.

Dose

The dosage of a drug is prescribed using either the metric or the household system. The metric system is the most commonly accepted system internationally. Examples of standard dosage are 5 mL (milliliters) or 1 teaspoon. Standard abbreviations of metric measurement are frequently used regarding the dosage, such as mg (milligram), kg (kilogram), mL (milliliter), mcg (microgram), or L (liter). However, it is considered safe practice to avoid other abbreviations and include the full words in prescriptions to avoid errors. In fact, several abbreviations have been deemed unsafe by the Joint Commission and have been put on a "do not use" list. See the hyperlinks below to view the Joint Commission "Do Not Use List" and the Institute of Safe Medication Practices (ISMP) list of abbreviations to avoid. If a dosage is unclear or written in a confusing manner in a prescription, it is always best to clarify the order with the prescribing provider before administering the medication.

---

2 Centers for Medicare & Medicaid Services. (2014, March 14). *Memo: Requirements for hospital medication administration, particularly intravenous (IV) medications and post-operative care of patients receiving IV opioids.* https://www.cms.gov/Medicare/Provider-Enrollment-and-Certification/SurveyCertificationGenInfo/Downloads/Survey-and-Cert-Letter-14-15.pdf

My Notes

View the Joint Commission's "Do Not Use List of Abbreviations" (https://www.jointcommission.org/-/media/tjc/documents/resources/patient-safety-topics/do_not_use_list_6_28_19.pdf).

View the ISMP "List of Error-Prone Abbreviations to Avoid" (https://www.ismp.org/recommendations/error-prone-abbreviations-list).

Frequency

Frequency in prescriptions is indicated by how many times a day the medication is to be administered or how often it is to be administered in hours or minutes. Examples of frequency include verbiage such as once daily, twice daily, three times daily, four times daily, every 30 minutes, every hour, every four hours, or every eight hours. Medication times are typically indicated using military time (i.e., using a 24-hour clock). For example, 11 p.m. is indicated as "2300." Read more about military time in the "Math Calculations" chapter.

Some types of medications may be ordered "**around the clock (ATC)**." An around-the-clock frequency order indicates they should be administered at regular time intervals, such as every six hours, to maintain consistent levels of the drug in the patient's bloodstream. For example, pain medications administered at end of life are often prescribed ATC instead of PRN (as needed) to maintain optimal pain relief.

Route of Administration

Common routes of administration and standard abbreviations include the following:

- **Oral (PO)** – the patient swallows a tablet or capsule
- **Sublingual (SL)** – applied under the tongue
- **Enteral (NG or PEG)** – administered via a tube directly into the GI tract
- **Rectal (PR)** – administered via rectal suppository
- **Inhalation (INH)** – the patient breathes in medication from an inhaler
- **Intramuscular (IM)** – administered via an injection into a muscle
- **Subcutaneous** – administered via injection into the fat tissue beneath the skin (Note that "subcutaneous" is on ISMP's recommended list of abbreviations to avoid due to common errors.)
- **Transdermal (TD)** – administered by applying a patch on the skin

For more information about routes of administration and considerations regarding absorption, visit the "Kinetics and Dynamics" chapter in Open RN *Nursing Pharmacology*.

Provider Name/Signature

Signature of the prescribing provider is required on the order and can be electronic or handwritten. Verbal orders from a prescriber are not recommended, but may be permitted in some agencies for urgent situations. Verbal orders require the nurse to "repeat back" the order to the prescriber for confirmation.

Rights of Medication Administration

My Notes

Each year in the United States, 7,000 to 9,000 people die as a result of a medication error. Hundreds of thousands of other patients experience adverse reactions or other complications related to a medication. The total cost of caring for patients with medication-associated errors exceeds $40 billion each year. In addition to the monetary cost, patients experience psychological and physical pain and suffering as a result of medication errors.[3] Nurses play a vital role in reducing the number of medication errors that occur by verifying several rights of medication.

The Centers for Medicare & Medicaid Services requires nurses to verify specific information prior to the administration of medication to avoid errors, referred to as verifying the rights of medication administration.[4] These rights of medication administration are the vital last safety check by nurses to prevent errors in the chain of medication administration that includes the prescribing provider, the pharmacist, the nurse, and the patient.

It is important to remember that if a medication error occurs resulting in harm to a patient, a nurse can be held liable even if "just following orders." It is absolutely vital for nurses to use critical thinking and clinical judgment to ensure each medication is safe for each specific patient before administering it. The consequences of liability resulting from a medication error can range from being charged with negligence in a court of law, to losing one's job, to losing one's nursing license.

The six rights of medication administration must be verified by the nurse at least three times before administering a medication to a patient. These six rights include the following:

1. Right Patient
2. Right Drug
3. Right Dose
4. Right Time
5. Right Route[5]
6. Right Documentation

---

3 This work is a derivative of StatPearls by Tariq, Vashisht, Sinha, and Scherbak and is licensed under CC BY 4.0. Access for free at https://www.ncbi.nlm.nih.gov/books/NBK519065/

4 Centers for Medicare & Medicaid Services. (2014, March 14). *Memo: Requirements for hospital medication administration, particularly intravenous (IV) medications and post-operative care of patients receiving IV opioids.* https://www.cms.gov/Medicare/Provider-Enrollment-and-Certification/SurveyCertificationGenInfo/Downloads/Survey-and-Cert-Letter-14-15.pdf

5 Centers for Medicare & Medicaid Services. (2014, March 14). *Memo: Requirements for hospital medication administration, particularly intravenous (IV) medications and post-operative care of patients receiving IV opioids.* https://www.cms.gov/Medicare/Provider-Enrollment-and-Certification/SurveyCertificationGenInfo/Downloads/Survey-and-Cert-Letter-14-15.pdf

My Notes

Recent literature indicates that up to ten rights should be completed as part of a safe medication administration process. These additional rights include Right History and Assessment, Right Drug Interactions, Right to Refuse, and Right Education and Information. Information for each of these rights is further described below.[6,7]

Right Patient

Acceptable patient identifiers include, but are not limited to, the patient's full name, an identification number assigned by the hospital, or date of birth. A patient's room number must never be used as an identifier because a patient may change rooms. Identifiers must be confirmed by the patient wristband, patient identification card, patient statement (when possible), or other means outlined in the agency policy such as a patient picture included on the MAR. The nurse must confirm the patient's identification matches the **medication administration record** (MAR) and medication label prior to administration to ensure that the medication is being given to the correct patient.[8] See Figure 15.1[9] for an illustration of the nurse verifying the patient's identify by scanning their identification band and asking for their date of birth. See Figure 15.2[10] for a close-up image of a patient identification wristband.

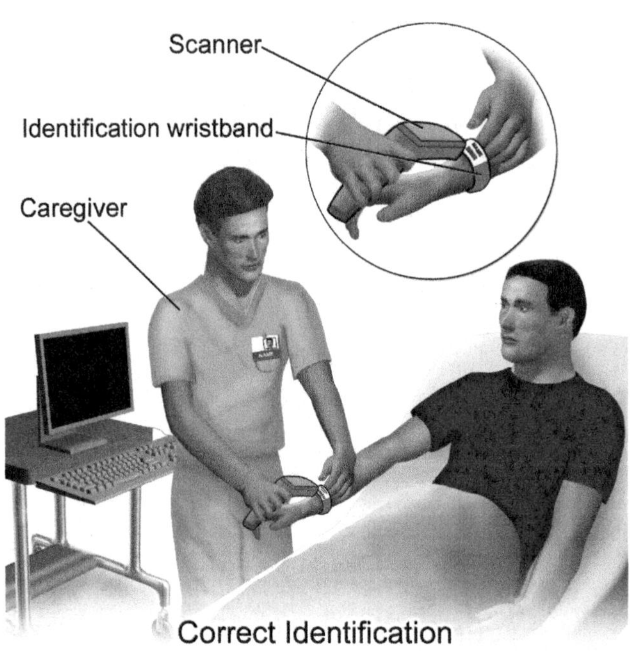

Figure 15.1 Patient Identification by Scanning Armband

---

6 Vera, M. (2020, June 30). *The 10 rights of drug administration.* Nurselabs. https://nurseslabs.com/10-rs-*rights-of-drug-administration/*

7 Butcher, H., Bulechek, G., Dochterman, J., & Wagner, C. (2018). *Nursing interventions classification (NIC).* Elsevier, pp. 250-251, 257-258.

8 Centers for Medicare & Medicaid Services. (2014, March 14). *Memo: Requirements for hospital medication administration, particularly intravenous (IV) medications and post-operative care of patients receiving IV opioids.* https://www.cms.gov/Medicare/Provider-Enrollment-and-Certification/SurveyCertificationGenInfo/Downloads/Survey-and-Cert-Letter-14-15.pdf

9 "Patient Identification.png" by BruceBlaus is licensed under CC BY-SA 4.0. Access for free at https://commons.wikimedia.org/wiki/File:Patient_Identification.png

10 "Wrist Identification Band.jpg" by Whoisjohngalt is licensed under CC BY-SA 4.0. Access for free at https://commons.wikimedia.org/wiki/File:Wrist_Identification_Band.jpg

My Notes

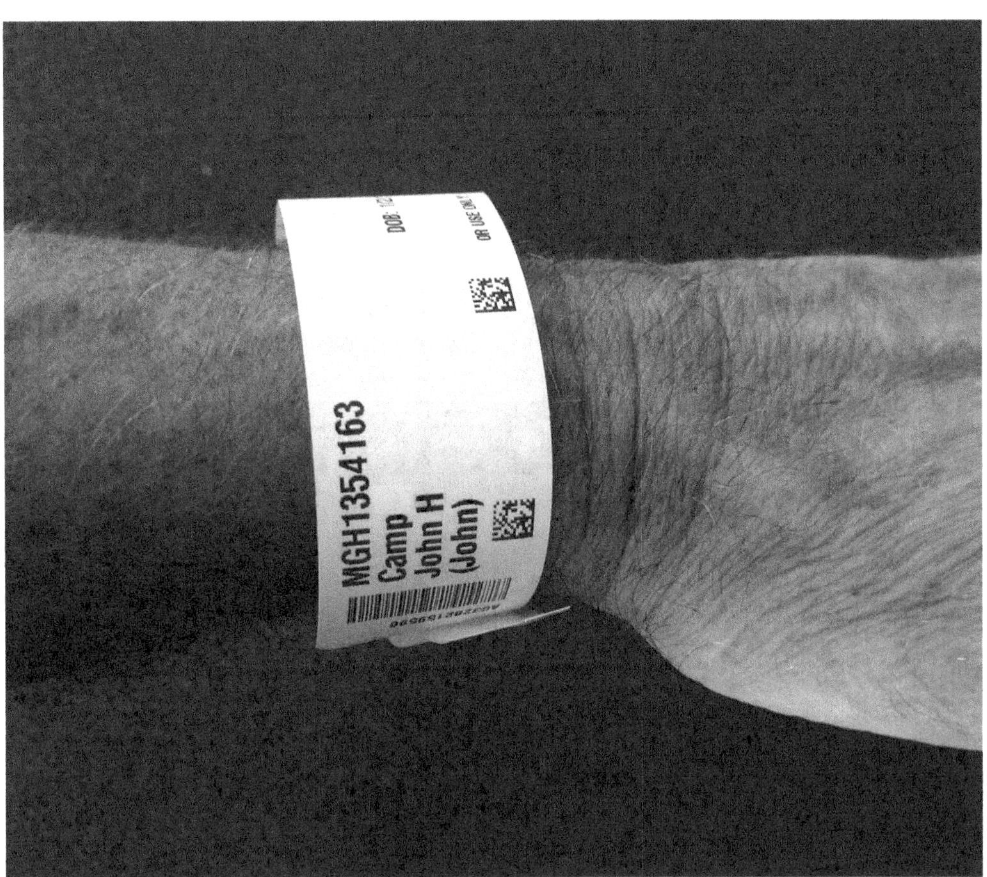

Figure 15.2 Patient Identification Band

If barcode scanning is used in an agency, this scanning is not intended to take the place of confirming two patient identifiers, but is intended to add another layer of safety to the medication administration process. The National Patient Safety Goals established by the Joint Commission state that whenever administering patient medications, at least two patient identifiers should be used.[11]

Right Drug

During this step, the nurse ensures the medication to be administered to the patient matches the order or Medication Administration Record (MAR) and that the patient does not have a documented allergy to it.[12] The Medication Administration Record (MAR), or **eMAR**, an electronic medical record, is a specific type of documentation found in a patient's chart. See Figure 15.3[13] for an image of a MAR and its components. Beware of look-alike and sound-alike medication names, as well as high-alert medications that bear a heightened risk of

---

11 The Joint Commission. (n.d.). *National patient safety goals.* https://www.jointcommission.org/standards/national-patient-safety-goals/

12 Centers for Medicare & Medicaid Services. (2014, March 14). *Memo: Requirements for hospital medication administration, particularly intravenous (IV) medications and post-operative care of patients receiving IV opioids.* https://www.cms.gov/Medicare/Provider-Enrollment-and-Certification/SurveyCertificationGenInfo/Downloads/Survey-and-Cert-Letter-14-15.pdf

13 "MAR.png" by Meredith Pomietlo for Chippewa Valley Technical College is licensed under CC BY 4.0. Access for free at https://drive.google.com/file/d/1hlq2d08NiA_njagAh0AkpNy-iWD8d9em/view?usp=sharing

My Notes

causing significant patient harm if they are used in error. The nurse should also be aware of what medication can be crushed and those that cannot be crushed. Read more information about these concerns using the hyperlinks below.

View the ISMP "Frequently Confused Medication List" (https://www.ismp.org/recommendations/confused-drug-names-list).

View the ISMP "High-Alert Medications List" (https://www.ismp.org/sites/default/files/attachments/2018-08/highAlert2018-Acute-Final.pdf).

View the ISMP "Do Not Crush List" (https://www.ismp.org/recommendations/do-not-crush).

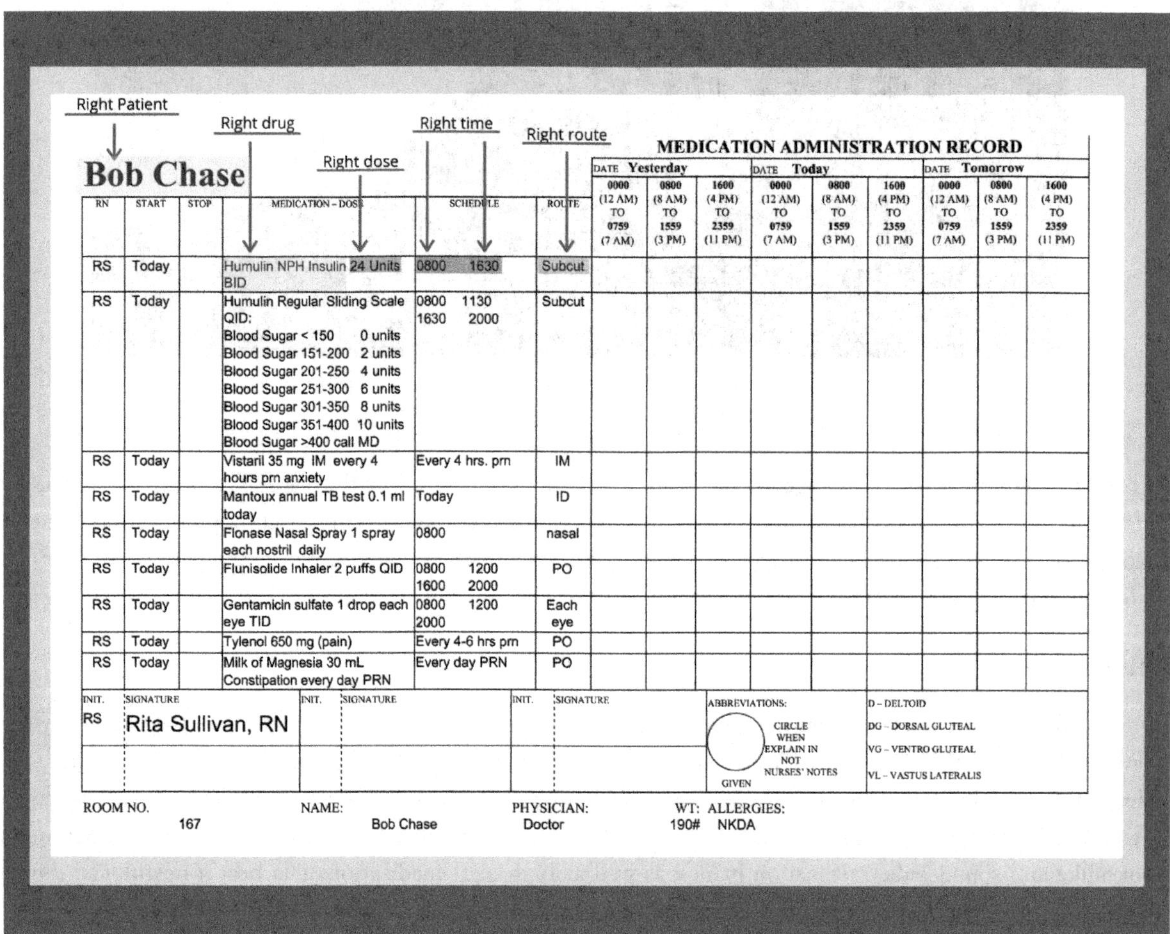

MEDICATION ADMINISTRATION RECORD

Bob Chase

RN	START	STOP	MEDICATION – DOSE	SCHEDULE	ROUTE	DATE Yesterday 0000 (12 AM) TO 0759 (7 AM)	0800 (8 AM) TO 1559 (3 PM)	1600 (4 PM) TO 2359 (11 PM)	DATE Today 0000 (12 AM) TO 0759 (7 AM)	0800 (8 AM) TO 1559 (3 PM)	1600 (4 PM) TO 2359 (11 PM)	DATE Tomorrow 0000 (12 AM) TO 0759 (7 AM)	0800 (8 AM) TO 1559 (3 PM)	1600 (4 PM) TO 2359 (11 PM)
RS	Today		Humulin NPH Insulin 24 Units BID	0800 1630	Subcut									
RS	Today		Humulin Regular Sliding Scale QID: Blood Sugar < 150 0 units Blood Sugar 151-200 2 units Blood Sugar 201-250 4 units Blood Sugar 251-300 6 units Blood Sugar 301-350 8 units Blood Sugar 351-400 10 units Blood Sugar >400 call MD	0800 1130 1630 2000	Subcut									
RS	Today		Vistaril 35 mg IM every 4 hours prn anxiety	Every 4 hrs. prn	IM									
RS	Today		Mantoux annual TB test 0.1 ml today	Today	ID									
RS	Today		Flonase Nasal Spray 1 spray each nostril daily	0800	nasal									
RS	Today		Flunisolide Inhaler 2 puffs QID	0800 1200 1600 2000	PO									
RS	Today		Gentamicin sulfate 1 drop each eye TID	0800 1200 2000	Each eye									
RS	Today		Tylenol 650 mg (pain)	Every 4-6 hrs prn	PO									
RS	Today		Milk of Magnesia 30 mL Constipation every day PRN	Every day PRN	PO									

INIT.	SIGNATURE	INIT.	SIGNATURE	INIT.	SIGNATURE
RS	Rita Sullivan, RN				

ABBREVIATIONS: CIRCLE WHEN GIVEN; EXPLAIN IN NURSES' NOTES; NOT GIVEN

D – DELTOID
DG – DORSAL GLUTEAL
VG – VENTRO GLUTEAL
VL – VASTUS LATERALIS

ROOM NO. 167 NAME: Bob Chase PHYSICIAN: Doctor WT: 190# ALLERGIES: NKDA

Figure 15.3 Medication Administration Record

Right Dose

During this step, the nurse ensures the dosage of the medication matches the prescribed dose, verifies the correct dosage range for the age and medical status of the patient, and also confirms that the prescription itself does not

My Notes

reflect an unsafe dosage level (i.e., a dose that is too high or too low).[14] For example, medication errors commonly occur in children, who typically receive a lower dose of medication than an adult. Medication errors also commonly occur in older patients who have existing kidney or liver disease and are unable to metabolize or excrete typical doses of medications.

Right Time and Frequency

During this step, the nurse verifies adherence to the prescribed frequency and scheduled time of administration of the medication.[15] This step is especially important when PRN medications are administered because it is up to the nurse to verify the time of the previous dose and compare it to the ordered frequency.

Medications should be administered on time whenever possible. However, when multiple patients are scheduled to receive multiple medications at the same time, this goal of timeliness can be challenging. Most facilities have a policy that medications can be given within a range of 30 minutes before or 30 minutes after the medication is scheduled. For example, a medication ordered for 0800 could be administered anytime between 0730 and 0830. However, some medications must be given at their specific ordered time due to pharmacokinetics of the drug. For example, if an antibiotic is scheduled every eight hours, this time frame must be upheld to maintain effective bioavailability of the drug, but a medication scheduled daily has more flexibility with time of actual administration.

Right Route

During this step, the nurse ensures the route of administration is appropriate for the specific medication and also for the patient.[16] Many medications can potentially be administered via multiple routes, whereas other medications can only be given safely via one route. Nurses must administer medications via the route indicated in the order. If a nurse discovers an error in the order or believes the route is unsafe for a particular patient, the route must be clarified with the prescribing provider before administration. For example, a patient may have a PEG tube in place, but the nurse notices the medication order indicates the route of administration as PO. If the nurse believes this medication should be administered via the PEG tube and the route indicated in the order is an error, the prescribing provider must be notified and the order must be revised indicating via PEG tube before the medication is administered.

Right Documentation

After administering medication, it is important to immediately document the administration to avoid potential errors from an unintended repeat dose.

---

14 Centers for Medicare & Medicaid Services. (2014, March 14). *Memo: Requirements for hospital medication administration, particularly intravenous (IV) medications and post-operative care of patients receiving IV opioids.* https://www.cms.gov/Medicare/Provider-Enrollment-and-Certification/SurveyCertificationGenInfo/Downloads/Survey-and-Cert-Letter-14-15.pdf

15 Centers for Medicare & Medicaid Services. (2014, March 14). *Memo: Requirements for hospital medication administration, particularly intravenous (IV) medications and post-operative care of patients receiving IV opioids.* https://www.cms.gov/Medicare/Provider-Enrollment-and-Certification/SurveyCertificationGenInfo/Downloads/Survey-and-Cert-Letter-14-15.pdf

16 Centers for Medicare & Medicaid Services. (2014, March 14). *Memo: Requirements for hospital medication administration, particularly intravenous (IV) medications and post-operative care of patients receiving IV opioids.* https://www.cms.gov/Medicare/Provider-Enrollment-and-Certification/SurveyCertificationGenInfo/Downloads/Survey-and-Cert-Letter-14-15.pdf

My Notes

In addition to checking the basic rights of medication administration and documenting the administration, it is also important for nurses to verify the following information to prevent medication errors.

Right History and Assessment

The nurse should be aware of the patient's allergies, as well as any history of any drug interactions. Additionally, nurses collect appropriate assessment data regarding the patient's history, current status, and recent lab results to identify any contraindications for the patients to receive the prescribed medication.[17]

Right Drug Interactions

The patient's history should be reviewed for any potential interactions with medications previously given or with the patient's diet. It is also important to verify the medication's expiration date before administration.

Right Education and Information

Information should be provided to the patient about the medication, including the expected therapeutic effects, as well as the potential adverse effects. The patient should be encouraged to report suspected side effects to the nurse and/or prescribing provider. If the patient is a minor, the parent may also have a right to know about the medication in many states, depending upon the circumstances.

Right of Refusal

After providing education about the medication, the patient has the right to refuse to take medication in accordance with the Nurses Code of Ethics and respect for individual patient autonomy. If a patient refuses to take the medication after proper education has been performed, the event should be documented in the patient chart and the prescribing provider notified.

Medication Dispensing

Medications are dispensed for patients in a variety of methods. During inpatient care, unit dose packaging is a common method for dispensing medications. See Figure 15.4[18] for an image of unit dose packaging.

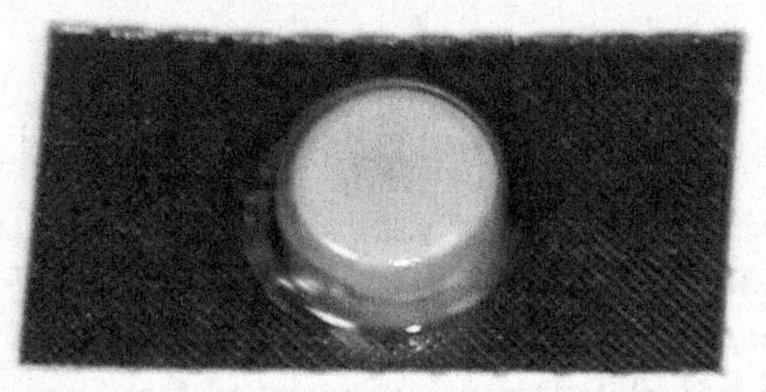

Figure 15.4 Unit Dose Packaging

17 NCSBN. (2018). *2019 NCLEX-RN test plan*. https://www.ncsbn.org/2019_RN_TestPlan-English.pdf

18 "Unit Dose Packaging.jpg" and "Unit Dose Label.jpg" by Deanna Hoyord, Chippewa Valley Technical College are licensed under CC BY 4.0. Access for free at https://drive.google.com/file/d/1llFhST_M7YSmf7lKAlHL1qRTgHe13z2V/view?usp=sharing

My Notes

Unit dose dispensing is typically used in association with a medication dispensing system, sometimes referred to in practice with brand names such as "Pyxis" or "Omnicell." Medication dispensing systems help keep medications secure by requiring a user sign-in and password. They also reduce medication errors by only allowing medications prescribed for a specific patient to be removed unless additional actions are taken. However, it is important to remember that medication errors can still occur when using a medication dispensing system if the incorrect medication is erroneously stocked in a compartment. See Figure 15.5[19] for an image of a medication dispensing system.

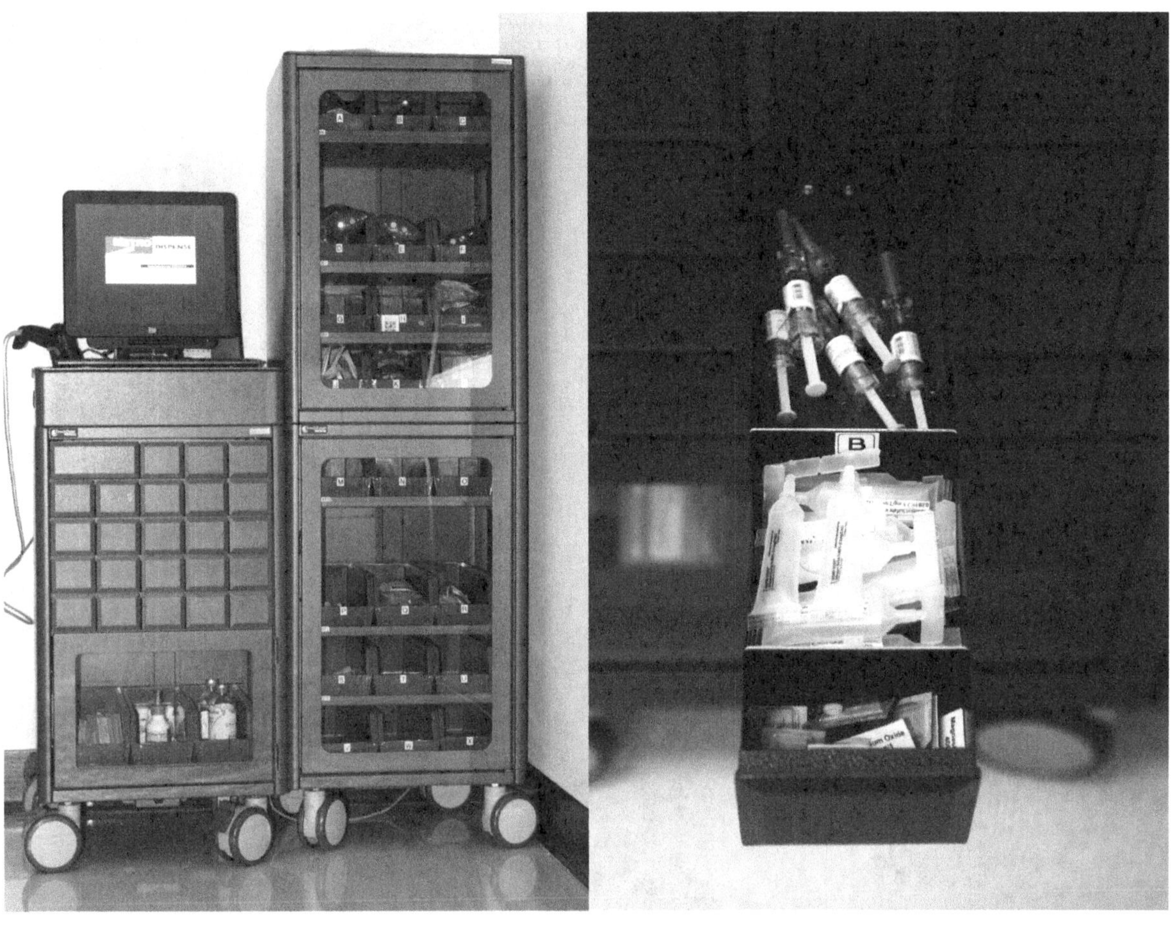

Figure 15.5 Medication Dispensing System

Bar codes are often incorporated with unit dose medication dispensing as an additional layer of safety to prevent medication errors. Each patient and medication is identified with a unique bar code. The nurse scans the patient's identification wristband with a bedside portable device and then scans each medication to be administered. The portable device will display error messages if an incorrect medication is scanned or if medication is scanned at an incorrect time. It is vital for nurses to stop and investigate the medication administration process when an error is received. The scanning device is typically linked to an electronic MAR and the medication administered is documented immediately in the patient's chart.

19 "Med Cart 1_313A0209.jpg" and "Med Cart Drawer._313A0224.jpg" by Deanna Hoyord, Chippewa Valley Technical College are licensed under CC BY 4.0. Access for free at https://drive.google.com/file/d/197qI1knbsUu-Ls9ZrNfxO3MCc9VTzsf_/view?usp=sharing

My Notes

In long-term care agencies, weekly blister cards may be used that contain a specific patient's medications for each day of the week. See Figure 15.6[20] for an image of a blister pack.

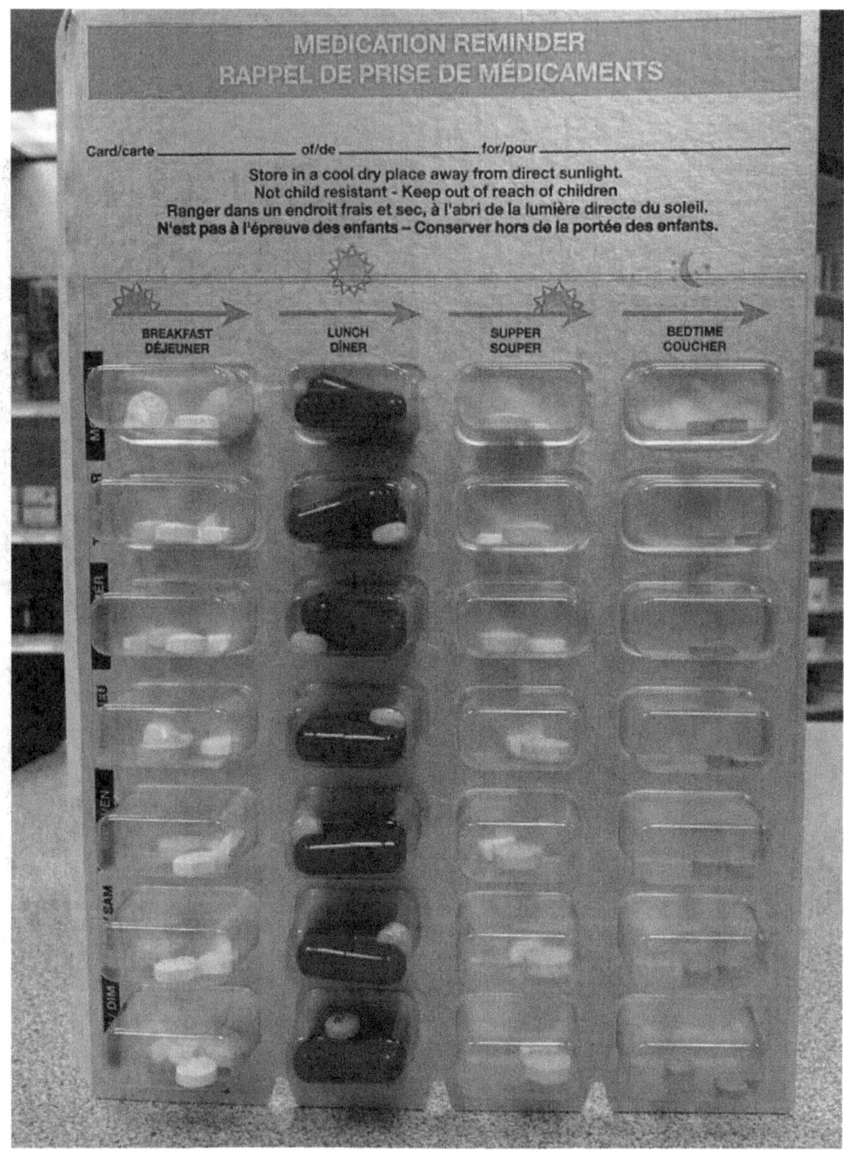

Figure 15.6 Blister Pack of Medications

Agencies using blister cards or pill bags typically store medications in a locked medication cart to keep them secure. Supplies used to administer medications are also stored on the cart. The MAR is available in printed format or electronically with a laptop computer. See Figure 15.7[21] for an image of a medication cart.

20 "Medication_blister_pack_2.jpg" by Sprinno is licensed under CC BY-SA 3.0. Access for free at https://commons.wikimedia.org/wiki/File:Medication_blister_pack_2.jpg

21 "MMI medication cart.JPG" by BrokenSphere is licensed under CC BY-SA 3.0. Access for free at https://commons.wikimedia.org/wiki/File:MMI_medication_cart.JPG

My Notes

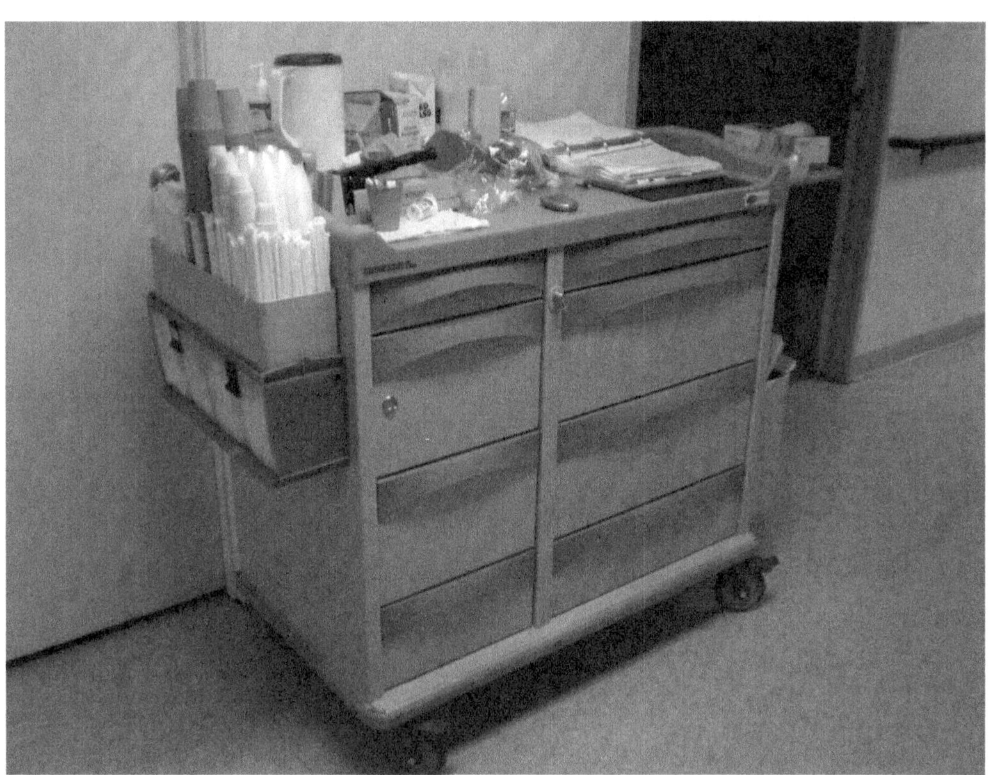

Figure 15.7 Medication Cart

Process of Medication Administration

No matter what method of medication storage and dispensing is used in a facility, the nurse must continue to verify the rights of medication administration to perform an accurate and safe medication pass. Using a medication dispensing system or bar coding does not substitute for verifying the rights, but are used to add an additional layer of safety to medication administration. Nurses can also avoid medication errors by creating a habitual process of performing medication checks when administering medication. The rights of medication administration should be done in the following order:

1. Perform the first check as the unit dose package, blister pack, or pill bag is removed from the dispensing machine or medication cart. Also, check the expiration date of the medication.

2. A second check should be performed after the medication is removed from the dispensing machine or medication cart. This step should be performed prior to pouring or removing from a multidose container. Note: Some high-alert medications, such as insulin, require a second nurse to perform a medication check at this step due to potentially life-threatening adverse effects that can occur if an error is made.

3. The third check should be performed immediately before administering the medication to the patient at the bedside or when replacing the multidose container back into the drawer.

My Notes

See Figure 15.8[22] for an image of a nurse comparing medication information on the medication packet to information on the patient's MAR.

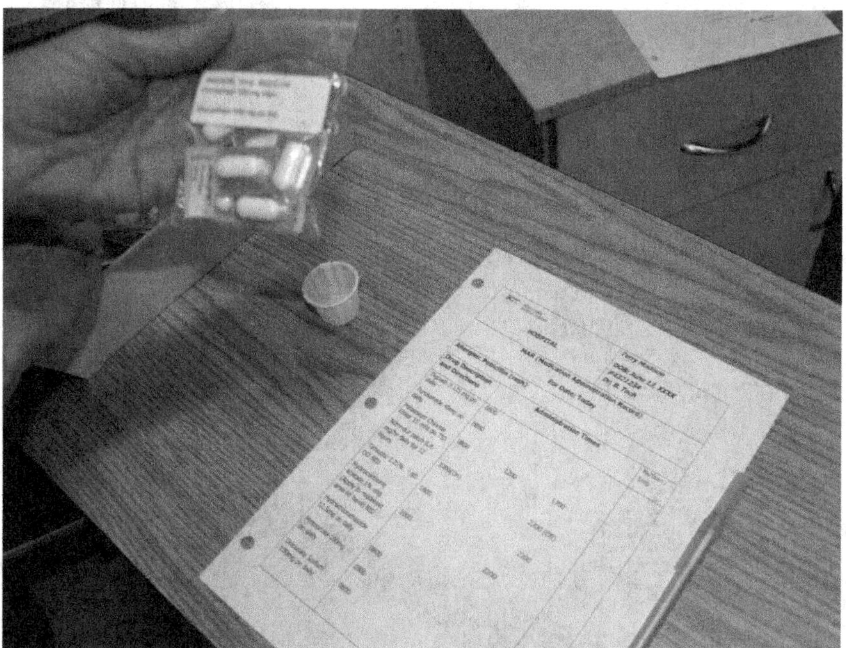

Figure 15.8 Comparing Medication Information to the MAR

When performing these three checks, the nurse should ensure this is the right medication, right patient, right dosage, right route, and right time. See Figure 15.9[23] for an image of the nurse performing patient identification prior to administering the medication. The sixth right, correct documentation, should be done immediately after the medication is administered to the patient to avoid an error from another nurse inadvertently administering the dose a second time. These six rights completed three times have greatly reduced medication errors.

As discussed earlier, other rights to consider during this process are as follows:

- Is the patient receiving this medication for the right reason?
- Have the right assessments been performed prior to giving the medication?
- Has the patient also received the right education regarding the medications?
- Is the patient exhibiting the right response to the medication?
- Is the patient refusing to take the medication? Patients have the right to refuse medication. The patient's refusal and any education or explanation provided related to the attempt to administer the medication should be documented by the nurse and the prescribing provider should be notified.

---

22 "DSC_17601-150x150.jpg" by British Columbia Institute of Technology is licensed under CC BY 4.0. Access for free at https://opentextbc.ca/clinicalskills/chapter/6-1-safe-medication-adminstration/

23 "Book-pictures-2015-430-150x150.jpg" by British Columbia Institute of Technology is licensed under CC BY 4.0. Access for free at https://opentextbc.ca/clinicalskills/chapter/6-1-safe-medication-adminstration/

My Notes

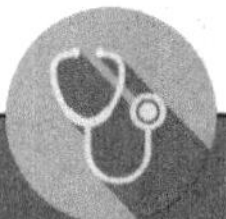

- Listen to the patient if they verbalize any concerns about medications. Explore their concerns, verify the order, and/or discuss their concerns with the prescribing provider before administering the medication to avoid a potential medication error.
- If a pill falls on the floor, it is contaminated and should not be administered. Dispose the medication according to agency policy.
- Be aware of absorption considerations of the medications you are administering. For example, certain medications such as levothyroxine should be administered on an empty stomach because food and other medications will affect its absorption.
- Nurses are often the first to notice when a patient has difficulty swallowing. If you notice a patient coughs immediately after swallowing water or has a "gurgling" sound to their voice, do not administer any medications, food, or fluid until you have reported your concerns to the heath care provider. A swallow evaluation may be needed and the route of medication may need to be changed from oral to another route to avoid aspiration.
- If your patient has a nothing by mouth (NPO) order, verify if this includes all medications. This information may be included on the MAR or the orders, and if not, verify this information with the provider. Some medications, such as diabetes medication, may be given with a sip of water in some situations where the patient has NPO status.
- If the route of administration is not accurately listed on the MAR, contact the prescribing provider before administering the medication. For example, a patient may have a PEG tube but the medication is erroneously listed as "PO" on the order.

My Notes

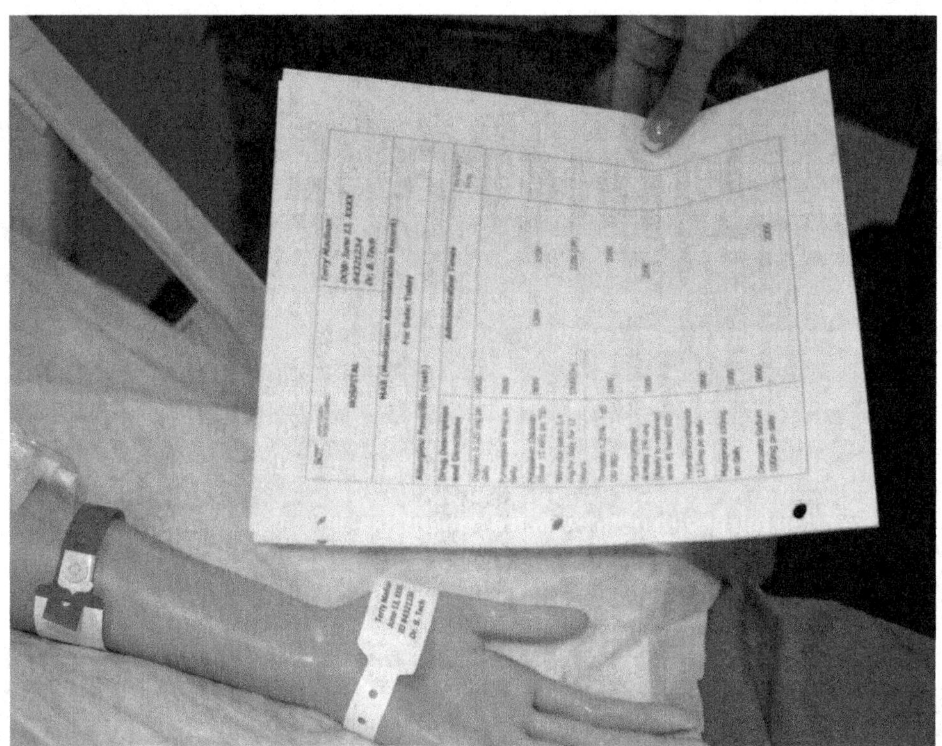

Figure 15.9 Identifying the Patient Prior to Medication Administration

For more information regarding classes of medications, administration considerations, and adverse effects to monitor, visit Open RN *Nursing Pharmacology*.

For information about specific medications, visit *DailyMed*, a current, evidence-based medication reference (https://dailymed.nlm.nih.gov/dailymed/).

Special Considerations for Administering Controlled Substances

Controlled substances, also called Scheduled Medications, are kept in a locked system and accounted for using a checks and balance system. Removal of a controlled substance from a medication dispensing system must be verified and documented by a second nurse witness. Removal of a controlled substance from a medication cart needs to be documented on an additional controlled substance record with the patient's name, the actual amount of substance given, the time it was given, associated pre-assessment data, and the name of the nurse administering the controlled substance.

Controlled substances stored in locked areas of medication carts must also be counted at every shift change by two nurses and then compared to the controlled substance administration record. If the count does not match the documentation record, the discrepancy must be reported immediately according to agency policy.

Additionally, if a partial dose of a controlled substance is administered, the remainder of the substance must be discarded in front of another nurse witness to document the event. This process is called "wasting." Follow agency policy regarding wasting of controlled substances.

My Notes

These additional safety measures help to prevent drug diversion, the use of a prescription medication for other than its intended purpose.

For more information about scheduled medications, drug diversion, and substance abuse in health care personnel, visit the "Legal/Ethical" chapter in Open RN *Nursing Pharmacology*.

Oral Medication Administration

Most medications are administered orally because it is the most convenient and least invasive route for the patient. Medication given orally has a slower onset, typically about 30-60 minutes. Prior to oral administration of medications, ensure the patient has no contraindications to receiving oral medication, is able to swallow, and is not on gastric suction. If the patient has difficulty swallowing (**dysphagia**), tablets are typically crushed and placed in a substance like applesauce or pudding for easier swallowing (based on the patient's prescribed diet). However, it is important to verify that a tablet may be crushed by consulting a drug reference or a pharmacist. For example, medications such as enteric-coated tablets, capsules, and sustained-release or long-acting drugs should never be crushed because doing so will affect the intended action of the medication. In this event, the provider must be contacted for a change in route.[24]

View the ISMP Do Not Crush List.

Position the patient receiving oral medication in an upright position to decrease the risk of aspiration. Patients should remain in this position for 30 minutes after medication administration, if possible. If a patient is unable to sit, assist them into a side-lying position. See Figure 15.10[25] for an image of a nurse positioning the patient in an upright position prior to medication administration. Offer a glass of water or other oral fluid (that is not contraindicated with the medication) to ease swallowing and improve absorption and dissolution of the medication, taking any fluid restrictions into account.[26]

Remain with the patient until all medication has been swallowed before documenting to verify the medication has been administered.[27]

If any post-assessments are required, follow up in the appropriate time frame. For example, when administering oral pain medication, follow up approximately 30 minutes to an hour after medication is given to ensure effective pain relief.

If medication is given sublingual (under the tongue) or buccal (between the cheek and gum), the mouth should be moist. Offering the patient a drink of water prior to giving the medication can help with absorption. Instruct

24 This work is a derivative of Clinical Procedures for Safer Patient Care by British Columbia Institute of Technology and is licensed under CC BY 4.0. Access for free at https://opentextbc.ca/clinicalskills/

25 "DSC_17631-150x150.jpg" by British Columbia Institute of Technology is licensed under CC BY 4.0. Access for free at https://opentextbc.ca/clinicalskills/chapter/6-1-safe-medication-adminstration/

26 This work is a derivative of Clinical Procedures for Safer Patient Care by British Columbia Institute of Technology and is licensed under CC BY 4.0. Access for free at https://opentextbc.ca/clinicalskills/

27 This work is a derivative of Clinical Procedures for Safer Patient Care by British Columbia Institute of Technology and is licensed under CC BY 4.0. Access for free at https://opentextbc.ca/clinicalskills/

My Notes

the patient to allow the medication to completely dissolve, and reinforce the importance of not swallowing or chewing the medication.

Liquid medications are available in multidose vials or single-dose containers. It may be necessary to shake liquid medications if they are suspensions prior to pouring. Make sure the label is clearly written and easy to read. When pouring a liquid medication, it is ideal to place the label in the palm of your hand so if any liquid medication runs down the outside of the bottle it does not blur the writing and make the label unidentifiable. When pouring liquid medication, read the dose at eye level measuring at the meniscus of the poured fluid. Always follow specific agency policy and procedure when administering oral medications.

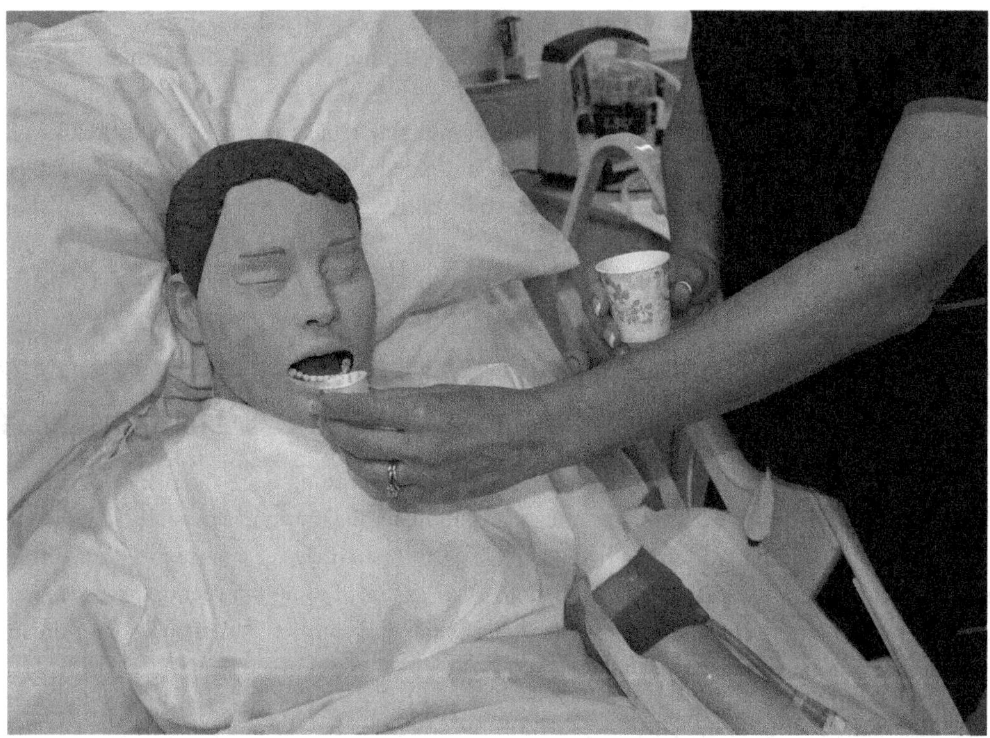

Figure 15.10 Placing the Patient in an Upright Position Prior to Medication Administration

Rectal Medication Administration

Drugs administered rectally have a faster action than the oral route and a higher bioavailability, meaning a higher amount of effective drug in the bloodstream because it has not been influenced by upper gastrointestinal tract digestive processes. Rectal administration also reduces side effects of some drugs, such as gastric irritation, nausea, and vomiting. Rectal medications may also be prescribed for their local effects in the gastrointestinal system (e.g., laxatives) or their systemic effects (e.g., analgesics when oral route is contraindicated). Rectal medications are contraindicated after rectal or bowel surgery, with rectal bleeding or prolapse, and with low platelet counts.[28]

Rectal medications are often formulated as suppositories. Suppositories are small, cone-shaped objects that melt inside the body and release medication. When administering rectal suppositories, the patient should be placed on

28 This work is a derivative of Clinical Procedures for Safer Patient Care by British Columbia Institute of Technology and is licensed under CC BY 4.0. Access for free at https://opentextbc.ca/clinicalskills/

My Notes

their left side in the Sims position. See Figure 15.11[29] for an image of patient positioning during rectal medication administration. The suppository and gloved index finger placing the suppository should be lubricated for ease of placement. Suppositories are conical and should be placed into the rectum rounded side first. The suppository should be inserted past the sphincter along the wall of the rectum. After placement, the patient should remain on their side while the medication takes effect. This time period is specific to each medication, but typically is at least 5 minutes. Make sure to avoid placing the suppository into stool. It is also important to monitor for a vasovagal response when placing medications rectally. A vasovagal response can occur when the vagus nerve is stimulated, causing the patient's blood pressure and heart rate to drop, and creating symptoms of dizziness and perspiration. Sometimes the patient can faint or even have a seizure. Patients with a history of cardiac arrhythmias should not be administered rectal suppositories due to the potential for a vasovagal response. Always follow agency policy and procedure when administering rectal medications.[30, 31]

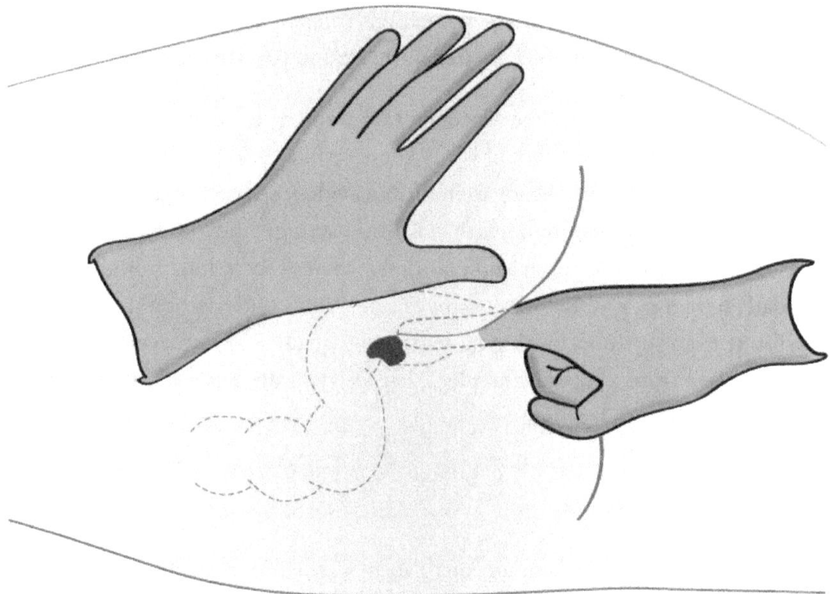

Figure 15.11 Administering a Rectal Suppository

Another type of rectal medication is an enema. An enema is the administration of a substance in liquid form into the rectum. Many enemas are formulated in disposable plastic containers. Warming the solution to body temperature prior to administration may be beneficial because cold solution can cause cramping. It is also helpful to encourage the patient to empty their bladder prior to administration to reduce feelings of discomfort. Place an incontinence pad under the patient and position them on their left side in the Sims position. Lubricate the nozzle of the container and expel air. Insert the lubricated nozzle into the rectum slowly and gently expel the contents into the rectum. Ask the patient to retain the enema based on manufacturer's recommendations.

29 "Administering-med-rectally-2.png" by British Columbia Institute of Technology is licensed under CC BY 4.0. Access for free at https://en.wikipedia.org/wiki/File:Administering-med-rectally-2.png

30 This work is a derivative of Clinical Procedures for Safer Patient Care by British Columbia Institute of Technology and is licensed under CC BY 4.0. Access for free at https://opentextbc.ca/clinicalskills/

31 Butcher, H., Bulechek, G., Dochterman, J., & Wagner, C. (2018). *Nursing interventions classification (NIC)*. Elsevier, pp. 250-251, 257-258.

My Notes

Enteral Tube Medication Administration

Medication is administered via an enteral tube when the patient is unable to orally swallow medication. Medications given through an enteral feeding tube (nasogastric, nasointestinal, percutaneous endoscopic gastrostomy {PEG}, or jejunostomy {J} tube) should be in liquid form whenever possible to avoid clogging the tube. If a liquid form is not available, medications that are safe to crush should be crushed finely and dissolved in water to keep the tube from becoming clogged. If a medication is not safe to crush, the prescribing provider should be notified and a prescription for alternative medication obtained. Capsules should be opened and emptied into liquid as indicated prior to administration, and liquids should be administered at room temperature. Keep in mind that some capsules are time-released and should not be opened. In this case, contact the provider for a change in order.[32, 33]

As always, follow agency policy for this medication administration procedure. Position the patient to at least 30 degrees and in high Fowler's position when feasible. If gastric suctioning is in place, turn off the suctioning. See Figure 15.12[34] for an image of a nurse positioning the patient prior to administration of medications via a PEG tube. Follow the tube to the point of entry into the patient to ensure you are accessing the correct tube.[35, 36]

Prior to medication administration, verify tube placement. Placement is initially verified immediately after the tube is placed with an X-ray, and the nurse should verify these results. Additionally, bedside placement is verified by the nurse before every medication pass. There are multiple evidence-based methods used to check placement. One method includes aspirating tube contents with a 60-mL syringe and observing the fluid. Fasting gastric secretions appear grassy-green, brown, or clear and colorless, whereas secretions from a tube that has perforated the pleural space typically have a pale yellow serous appearance. A second method used to verify placement is to measure the pH of aspirate from the tube. Fasting gastric pH is usually 5 or less, even in patients receiving gastric acid inhibitors. Fluid aspirated from a tube in the pleural space typically has a pH of 7 or higher.[37, 38] Note that

---

32 This work is a derivative of Clinical Procedures for Safer Patient Care by British Columbia Institute of Technology and is licensed under CC BY 4.0. Access for free at https://opentextbc.ca/clinicalskills/

33 Boullata, J.I., Carrera, A.L., Harvey, L., Escuro, A.A., Hudson, L., Mays, A., McGinnis, C., Wessel, J.J., Bajpai, S., Beebe, M.L., Kinn, T.J., Klang, M.G., Lord, L., Martin, K., Pompeii-Wolfe, C., Sullivan, J., Wood, A., Malone, A., & Guenter, P. (2017). ASPEN safe practices for enteral nutrition therapy. *Journal of Parenteral and Enteral Nutrition, 41*(1), 15-103. https://doi.org/10.1177/0148607116673053

34 "degreeLow.jpg" by British Columbia Institute of Technology is licensed under CC BY 4.0. Access for free at https://opentextbc.ca/clinicalskills/chapter/3-4-positioning-a-patient-in-bed/

35 This work is a derivative of Clinical Procedures for Safer Patient Care by British Columbia Institute of Technology and is licensed under CC BY 4.0. Access for free at https://opentextbc.ca/clinicalskills/

36 Boullata, J.I., Carrera, A.L., Harvey, L., Escuro, A.A., Hudson, L., Mays, A., McGinnis, C., Wessel, J.J., Bajpai, S., Beebe, M.L., Kinn, T.J., Klang, M.G., Lord, L., Martin, K., Pompeii-Wolfe, C., Sullivan, J., Wood, A., Malone, A., & Guenter, P. (2017). ASPEN safe practices for enteral nutrition therapy. *Journal of Parenteral and Enteral Nutrition, 41*(1), 15-103. https://doi.org/10.1177/0148607116673053

37 This work is a derivative of Clinical Procedures for Safer Patient Care by British Columbia Institute of Technology and is licensed under CC BY 4.0. Access for free at https://opentextbc.ca/clinicalskills/

38 Boullata, J.I., Carrera, A.L., Harvey, L., Escuro, A.A., Hudson, L., Mays, A., McGinnis, C., Wessel, J.J., Bajpai, S., Beebe, M.L., Kinn, T.J., Klang, M.G., Lord, L., Martin, K., Pompeii-Wolfe, C., Sullivan, J., Wood, A., Malone, A., & Guenter, P. (2017). ASPEN safe practices for enteral nutrition therapy. *Journal of Parenteral and Enteral Nutrition, 41*(1), 15-103. https://doi.org/10.1177/0148607116673053

installation of air into the tube while listening over the stomach with a stethoscope is no longer considered a safe method to check tube placement according to evidence-based practices.[39]

My Notes

After tube placement is checked, a clean 60-mL syringe is used to flush the tube with a minimum of 15 mL of water (5-10 mL for children) before administering the medication. Follow agency policy regarding flushing amount. Liquid medication, or appropriately crushed medication dissolved in water, is administered one medication at a time. Medication should not be mixed because of the risks of physical and chemical incompatibilities, tube obstruction, and altered therapeutic drug responses. Between each medication, the tube is flushed with 15 mL of water, keeping in mind the patient's fluid volume status. After the final medication is administered, the tube is flushed with 15 mL of water. The tube is then clamped, or if the patient is receiving tube feeding, it can be restarted. If the patient is receiving gastric suctioning, it can be restarted 30 minutes after medication administration.[40, 41, 42] See Figure 15.13[43] for an image of a nurse administering medication via an enteral tube.

Special considerations during this procedure include the following:

- If the patient has fluid restrictions, the amount of fluid used to flush the tube between each medication may need to be modified to avoid excess fluid intake.
- If the tube is attached to suctioning, the suctioning should be left off for 20 to 30 minutes after the medication is given to promote absorption of the medication.
- If the patient is receiving tube feedings, review information about the drugs that are being administered. If they cannot be taken with food or need to be taken on an empty stomach, the tube feeding running time will need to be adjusted.
- Be sure to document the amount of water used to flush the tube during the medication pass on the fluid intake record.
- If the patient has a chronic illness or is immunosuppressed, sterile water is suggested for use of mixing and flushing instead of tap water.
- Enteric-coated medications and other medications on the "Do Not Crush List" should not be crushed for this procedure. Instead, the prescribing provider must be notified and an order for a different form of the medication must be obtained.

---

39 ABoullata, J.I., Carrera, A.L., Harvey, L., Escuro, A.A., Hudson, L., Mays, A., McGinnis, C., Wessel, J.J., Bajpai, S., Beebe, M.L., Kinn, T.J., Klang, M.G., Lord, L., Martin, K., Pompeii-Wolfe, C., Sullivan, J., Wood, A., Malone, A., & Guenter, P. (2017). ASPEN safe practices for enteral nutrition therapy. *Journal of Parenteral and Enteral Nutrition, 41*(1), 15-103. https://doi.org/10.1177/0148607116673053

40 This work is a derivative of Clinical Procedures for Safer Patient Care by British Columbia Institute of Technology and is licensed under CC BY 4.0. Access for free at https://opentextbc.ca/clinicalskills/

41 Boullata, J.I., Carrera, A.L., Harvey, L., Escuro, A.A., Hudson, L., Mays, A., McGinnis, C., Wessel, J.J., Bajpai, S., Beebe, M.L., Kinn, T.J., Klang, M.G., Lord, L., Martin, K., Pompeii-Wolfe, C., Sullivan, J., Wood, A., Malone, A., & Guenter, P. (2017). ASPEN safe practices for enteral nutrition therapy. *Journal of Parenteral and Enteral Nutrition, 41*(1), 15-103. https://doi.org/10.1177/0148607116673053

42 Butcher, H., Bulechek, G., Dochterman, J., & Wagner, C. (2018). *Nursing interventions classification (NIC)*. Elsevier, pp. 250-251, 257-258.

43 "Administering medication into a gastric tube.jpg" by British Columbia Institute of Technology is licensed under CC BY 4.0. Access for free at https://commons.wikimedia.org/wiki/File:Administering_medication_into_a_gastric_tube.jpg

My Notes

- If the tube becomes clogged, attempt to flush it with water. If unsuccessful, notify the provider and a pancreatic enzyme solution or kit may be ordered before a new tube is placed.[44]

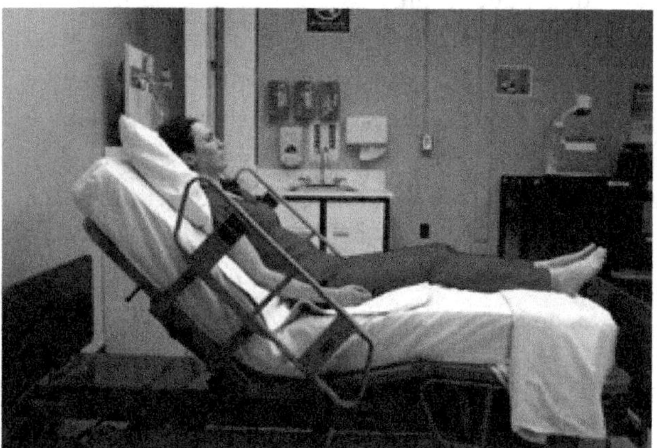

Figure 15.12 Position Patient at 30 Degrees Prior to Administering Medications via a Tube

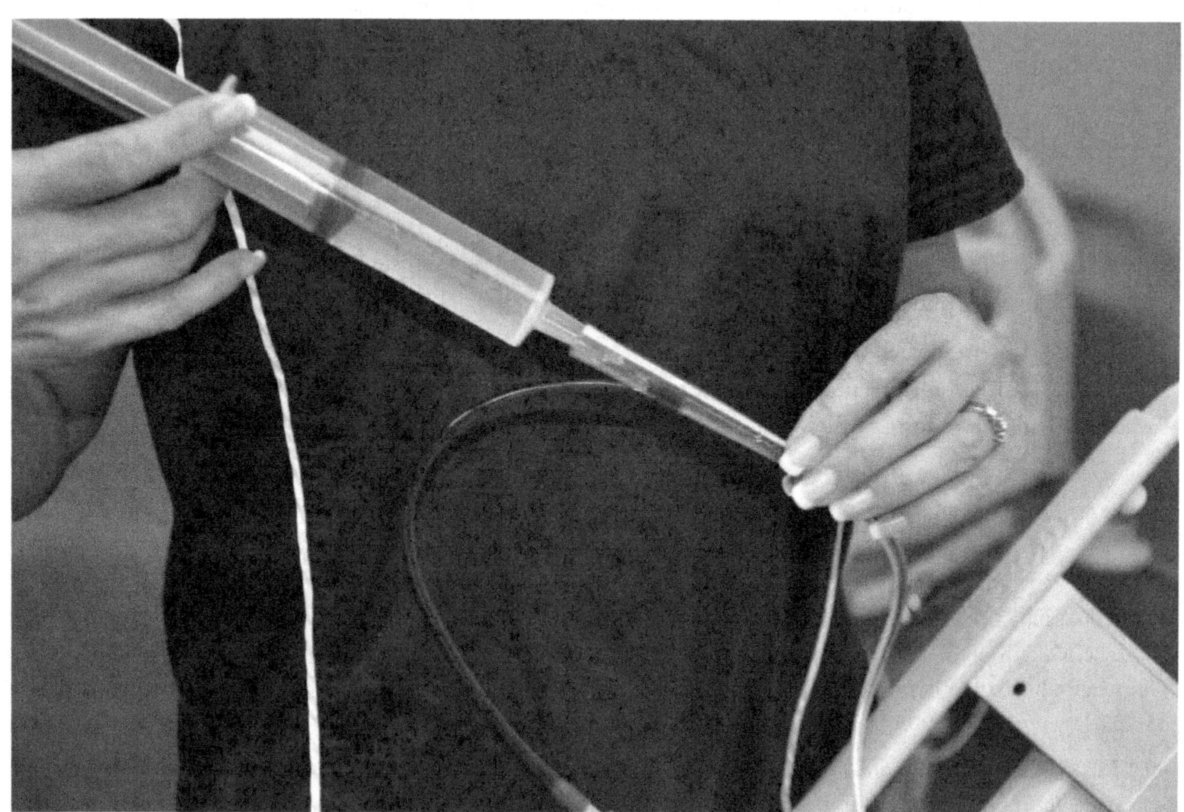

Figure 15.13 Administering Medication via a Gastric Tube

---

44 Boullata, J.I., Carrera, A.L., Harvey, L., Escuro, A.A., Hudson, L., Mays, A., McGinnis, C., Wessel, J.J., Bajpai, S., Beebe, M.L., Kinn, T.J., Klang, M.G., Lord, L., Martin, K., Pompeii-Wolfe, C., Sullivan, J., Wood, A., Malone, A., & Guenter, P. (2017). ASPEN safe practices for enteral nutrition therapy. *Journal of Parenteral and Enteral Nutrition, 41*(1), 15-103. https://doi.org/10.1177/0148607116673053

My Notes

Video Review for Crushing Medications[45]

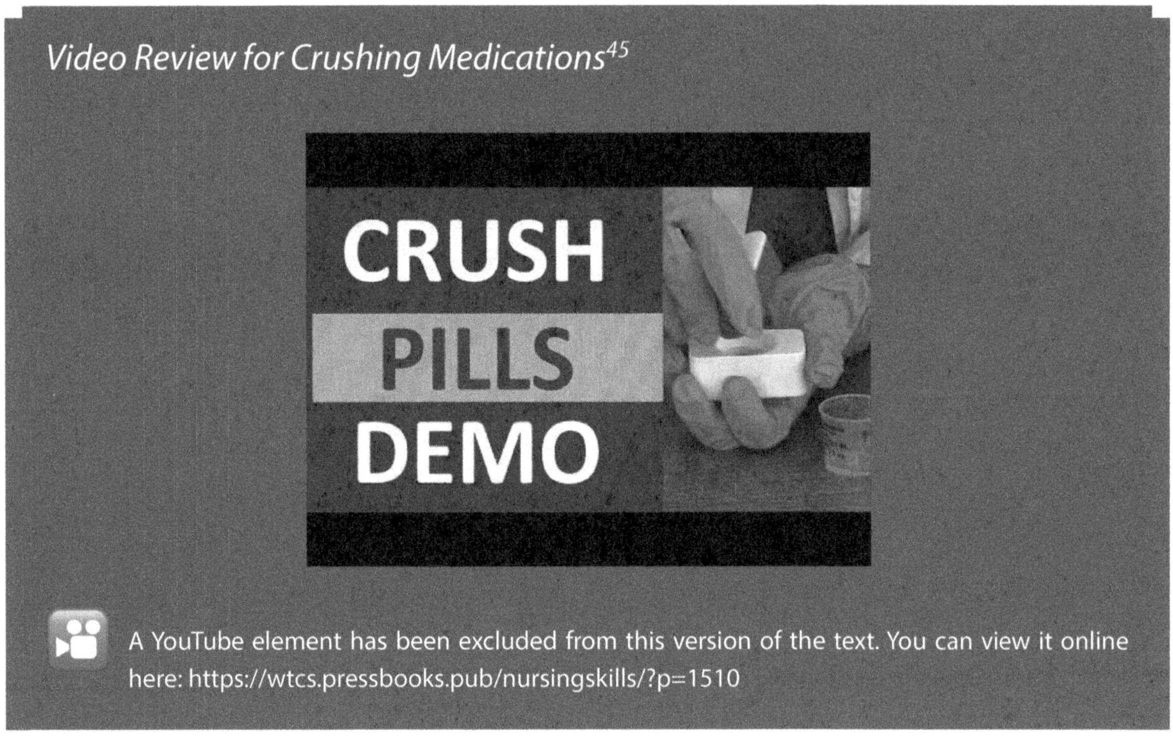

A YouTube element has been excluded from this version of the text. You can view it online here: https://wtcs.pressbooks.pub/nursingskills/?p=1510

Preventing Medication Errors

Medication errors can occur at various stages of the medication administration process, beginning with the prescribing provider, to the pharmacist preparing the medication, to the pharmacy technician stocking the medication, to the nurse administering the medication. Medication errors are most common at the ordering or prescribing stage. Typical errors include the prescribing provider writing the wrong medication, wrong route or dose, or the wrong frequency. These ordering errors account for almost 50% of medication errors. Data shows that nurses and pharmacists identify anywhere from 30% to 70% of medication-ordering errors.[46]

One of the major causes for medication errors is a distraction. Nearly 75% of medication errors have been attributed to this cause.[47] To minimize distractions, hospitals have introduced measures to reduce medication errors. For example, some hospitals set a "no-interruption zone policy" during medication dispensing and preparation and ask health care team members to only disrupt the medication administration process for emergencies. To reduce medication errors, agencies are also adopting many initiatives developed by the World Health Organization (WHO),[48] Institute for Safe Medication Practices (ISMP), the Institute of Medicine The (IOM),[49] and several

45 RegisteredNurseRN. (2017, March 22). *Crushing medications for tube feeding and oral administration.* [Video]. YouTube. All rights reserved. Video used with permission. https://youtu.be/86RzAgHu75U

46 This work is a derivative of StatPearls by Tariq, Vashisht, Sinha, and Scherbak and is licensed under CC BY 4.0. Access for free at https://www.ncbi.nlm.nih.gov/books/NBK519065/

47 This work is a derivative of StatPearls by Tariq, Vashisht, Sinha, and Scherbak and is licensed under CC BY 4.0. Access for free at https://www.ncbi.nlm.nih.gov/books/NBK519065/

48 World Health Organization (n.d.). *Patient safety.* https://www.who.int/patientsafety/medication-safety/technical-reports/en/

49 IOM. Institute of Medicine. (2007). *Preventing medication errors.* The National Academies Press. https://doi.org/10.17226/11623

My Notes

other organizations. Initiatives include measures such as avoiding error-prone abbreviations, being aware of commonly confused medication names, and instituting additional safeguards for high-alert medications. Student nurses must also be aware of conditions that may contribute to making a medication error during their clinical courses. Read more about initiatives to prevent medication errors in the hyperlinks and videos provided below.

For more information about preventing medication errors as a student nurse, visit "IMSP's Error-Prone Conditions that Lead to Student Nurse-Related Errors." When you prepare to administer medications to your patients during clinical, your instructor will ask you questions to ensure safe medication administration (https://www.ismp.org/resources/error-prone-conditions-lead-student-nurse-related-errors).

Watch a video of an instructor asking a student typical medication questions (https://youtu.be/MUn4Ec2X93g).

Video Review of Administering Medications Without Harm[50]

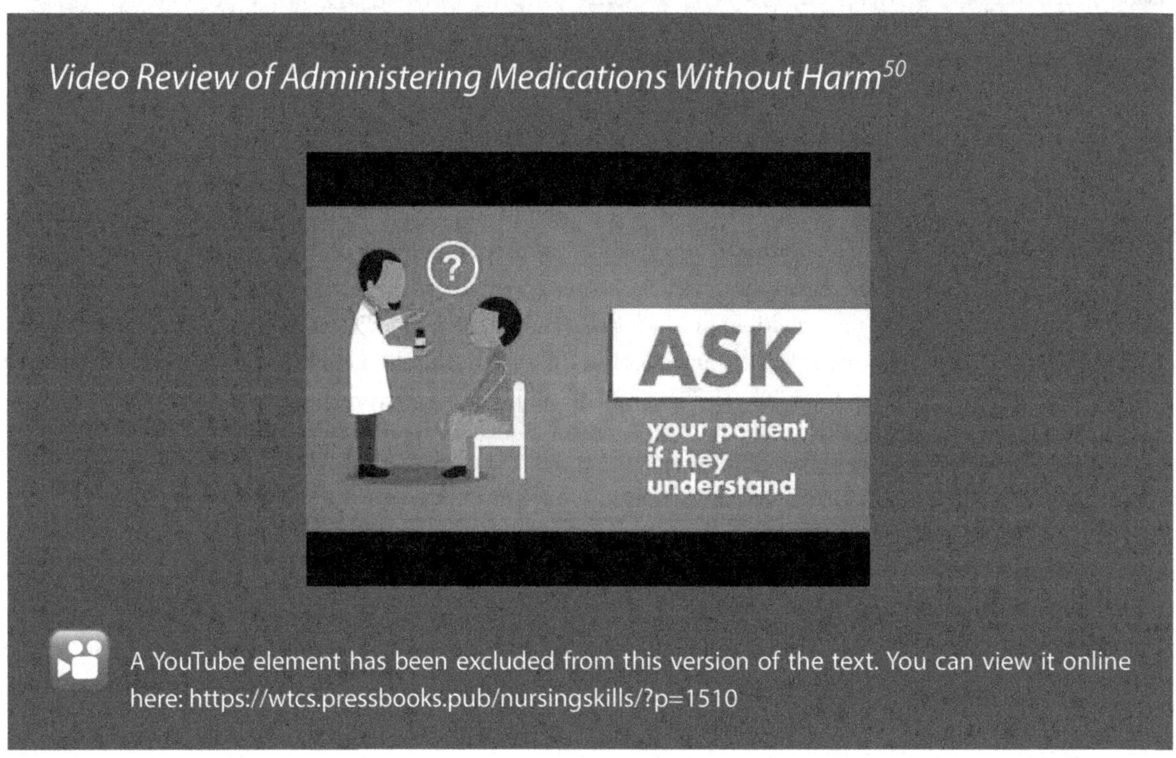

A YouTube element has been excluded from this version of the text. You can view it online here: https://wtcs.pressbooks.pub/nursingskills/?p=1510

Reporting Medication Errors

Despite multiple initiatives that have been instituted to prevent medication errors, including properly checking the rights of medication administration, medication errors happen. Examples of common errors include administering the wrong dose or an unsafe dose, giving medication to the wrong patient, administering medication by

50 World Health Organization (WHO). (2017, October 6). *WHO: Medication without harm.* [Video]. YouTube. All rights reserved. https://youtu.be/MWUM7LIXDeA

My Notes

the wrong route or at the incorrect rate, and giving a drug that is expired. If a medication error occurs, the nurse must follow specific steps of reporting according to agency policy. In the past when medication errors occurred, the individual who caused it was usually blamed for the mishap and disciplinary action resulted. However, this culture of blame has shifted, and many medication errors by well-trained and careful nurses and other health care professions are viewed as potential symptoms of a system-wide problem. This philosophy is referred to as an institution's **safety culture**. Thus, rather than focusing on disciplinary action, agencies are now trying to understand how the system failed causing the error to occur. This approach is designed to introduce safeguards at every level so that a mistake can be caught before the drug is given to the patient, which is often referred to as a "near miss." For an agency to effectively institute a safety culture, all medication errors and near misses must be reported.

When a medication error occurs, the nurse's first response should be to immediately monitor the patient's condition and watch for any side effects from the medication. Secondly, the nurse must notify the nurse manager and prescribing provider of the error. The provider may provide additional orders to counteract the medication's effects or to monitor for potential adverse reactions. In some situations, family members of the patient who are legal guardians or powers of attorney should also be notified. Lastly, a written report should be submitted documenting the incident, often referred to as an **incident report**. Incident reports are intended to identify if patterns of errors are occurring due to system-wide processes that can be modified to prevent future errors.

For more information about safety culture, visit the "Legal/Ethical" chapter in Open RN *Nursing Pharmacology*.

Life Span Considerations

Children

It can be difficult to persuade children to take medications. It is often helpful for medications to be prescribed in liquid or chewable form. For example, droppers are used for infants or very young children; the medication should be placed between the gum and cheek to prevent aspiration. Mixing medication with soft foods can also be helpful to encourage the child to swallow medications, but it is best to avoid mixing the medication with a staple food in the child's diet because of potential later refusal of the food associated with medication administration. It can be helpful to offer the child a cool item, such as a popsicle or frozen fruit bar, prior to medication administration to numb the child's tongue and decrease the taste of the medication. Other clinical tips for medication administration include asking the caregiver how the child takes medications at home and mimicking this method or asking the caregiver to administer the medication if the child trusts them more than the nurse. Oral syringes (without needles attached) may be used to administer precise dosages of medication to children. See Figure 15.14[51] of a nurse administering oral medication to a child with an oral syringe. When administering medication with an oral syringe, remember to remove the cap prior to administration because this could be a choking hazard. It is also important to educate the caregiver of the child how to properly administer the medication at the correct dosage at home.

51 "USMC-080623-M-9467O-024.jpg" by Lance Cpl. Regina A. Ochoa for the United States Marine Corps is in the Public Domain. Access for free at https://commons.wikimedia.org/wiki/File:USMC-080623-M-9467O-024.jpg

My Notes

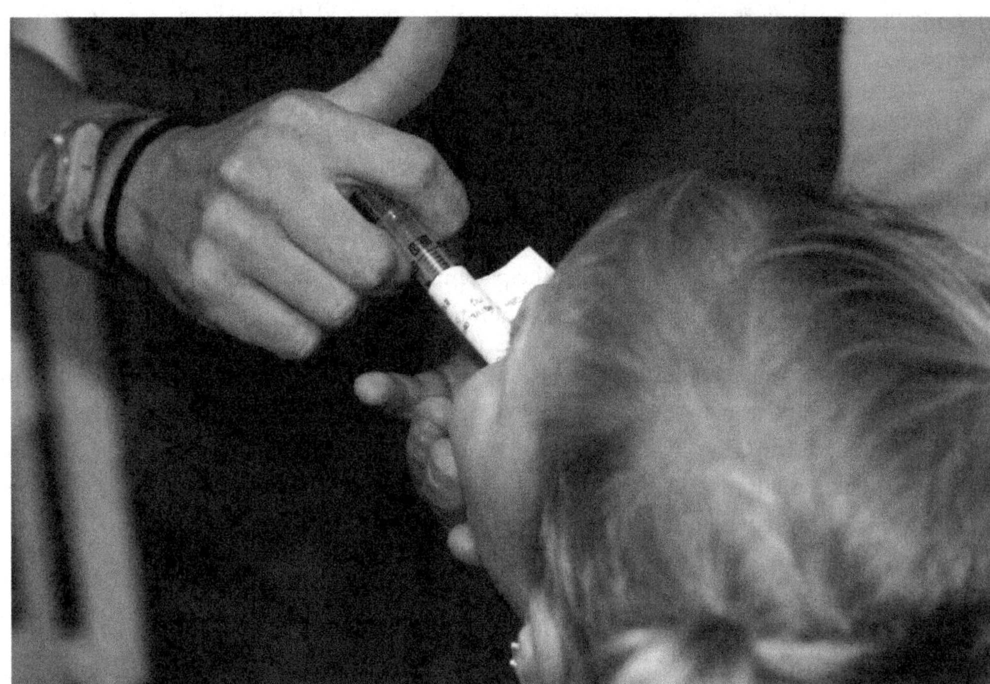

Figure 15.14 Administering Oral Medication Using an Oral Syringe to a Child

Older Adults

Many older adults have a "polypharmacy," meaning many medications to keep track of and multiple times these medications need to be taken per day. Nurses should help patients set up a schedule to remember when to take the medications. Organizing medications in medication boxes by day and time is a very helpful strategy. See Figure 15.15[52] of a medication box. Nurses can suggest to patients to have all medications filled at the same pharmacy to avoid drug-drug interactions that can occur when multiple providers are prescribing medications.

Older adults often have difficulty swallowing, so obtaining a prescription for liquid medication or crushing the medication when applicable and placing it in applesauce or pudding is helpful. Allow extra time when administering medication to an older adult to give them time to ask questions and to swallow multiple pills. Monitor for adverse effects and drug interactions in older adults, who are often taking multiple medications and may have preexisting kidney or liver dysfunction.

Be sure to address the economic needs of an older adult as it relates to their medications. Medications can be expensive and many older adults live on a strict budget. Nurses often advocate for less expensive alternatives for patients, such as using a generic brand instead of a name brand or a less expensive class of medication. Be aware that an older adult with financial concerns may try to save money by not taking medications as frequently as prescribed. Also, the older adult may "feel good" on their medications and think they don't need to monitor or take medications because they are "cured." Reinforce that "feeling good" usually means the medication is working as prescribed and should continue to be taken. Finally, empower patients to take control of managing their health by providing education and ongoing support.

---

52 "pills-4005382_960_720.jpg" by Nemo73 is licensed under CC0. Access for free at https://pixabay.com/ko/photos/%EC%95%BD-%EC%9A%94%EB%B2%95-%EA%B1%B4%EA%B0%95-%EC%9D%98%ED%95%99-%EC%A3%BC%EC%9D%98-4005382/

My Notes

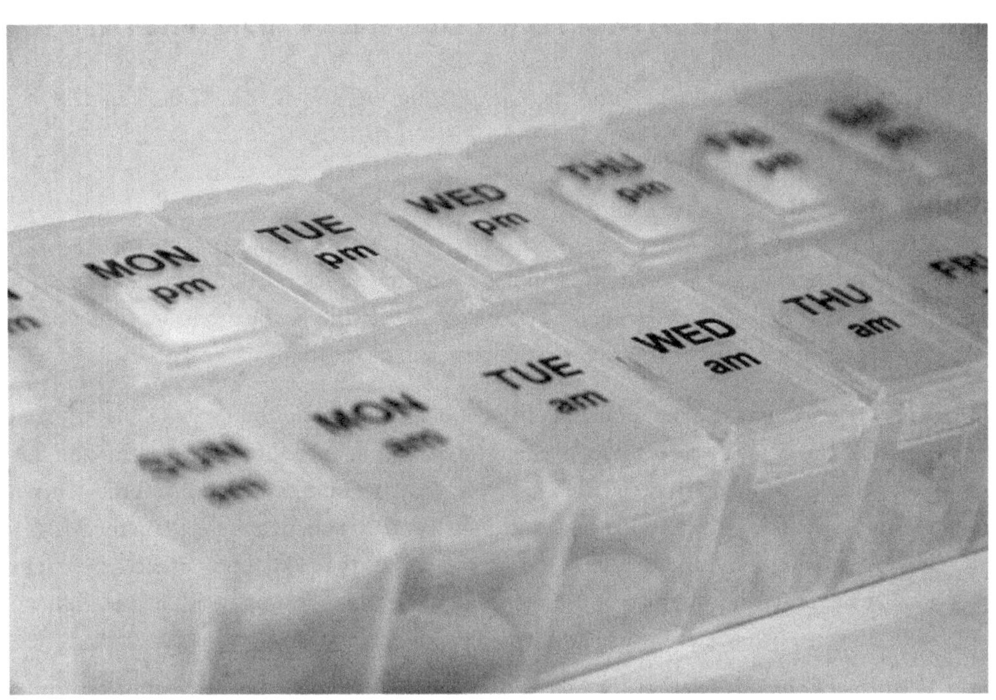

Figure 15.15 Medication Box

My Notes

15.3 ASSESSMENTS RELATED TO MEDICATION ADMINISTRATION

This section will review assessments to be performed prior to, during, and after a medication pass to ensure safe medication administration.

Pre-Administration

In addition to verifying the rights of medication administration three times, the nurse should also perform focused assessments of the patient's current status and anticipate actions of the medications and potential side effects. Here are some examples of pre-assessments before administering medication:

- **Check Vital Signs.** Before administering cardiac medication, the patient's blood pressure and heart rate are typically assessed to ensure they are within range of parameters for administration. For example, a patient is scheduled to receive a blood pressure medication, but their current blood pressure is 90/50, so the medication is withheld based on parameters stated on the MAR to withhold the medication if the systolic blood pressure is less than 100. If parameters are not provided, it is the nurse's responsibility to use clinical judgment and follow up with the prescribing provider with concerns before administering the medication.
- **Perform a Focused Respiratory Assessment.** Before administering inhaled respiratory medications such as albuterol for asthma or chronic pulmonary disease, the O2 saturation, heart rate, respiratory rate, and lungs sounds are typically assessed. The patient's response to the medication is then compared to pre-assessment data to determine effectiveness.
- **Review Lab Results.** Before administering a diuretic such as furosemide, the nurse assesses the patient's potassium level in recent lab work results. If the potassium level is lower than normal range, the nurse withholds the medication and notifies the prescribing provider.
- **Perform a Pain Assessment.** Before administering pain medication, the nurse performs a thorough pain assessment based on the mnemonic PQRSTU. (See more information about the PQRSTU mnemonic in the "Health History" chapter.) The patient's response to the medication after it is received is then compared to pre-assessment data to determine effectiveness.

During Administration

The nurse continues to assess safety during administration of medication, such as sudden changes in condition or difficulty swallowing. For example, if a patient suddenly becomes dizzy, the administration of cardiac medication is postponed until further assessments are performed. If a patient starts to cough, choke, or speak in a gurgly voice during oral or tube administration of medication, the procedure should be stopped and further assessments performed.

My Notes

Table 15.1 Summary of Safe Medication Administration Guidelines	
Guidelines	**Additional Information**
Be cautious and focused when preparing medications.	Avoid distractions. Some agencies have a no-interruption zone (NIZ) where health care providers can prepare medications without interruptions.[1]
Check and verify allergies.	Always ask the patient about their medication allergies, types of reactions, and severity of reactions. Verify the patient's medical record for documented allergies.
Use two patient identifiers and follow agency policy for patient identification.	Use at least two patient identifiers before administration and compare information against the medication administration record (MAR).[2]
Perform appropriate patient assessments before medication administration.	Assess the patient prior to administering medications to ensure the patient is receiving the correct medication, for the correct reason, and at the correct time. For example, a nurse reviews lab values and performs a cardiac assessment prior to administering cardiac medication. See more information regarding specific patient assessments during parenteral medication administration in the "Applying the Nursing Process" section.
Be diligent and perform medication calculations accurately.	Double-check and verify medication calculations. Incorrect calculation of medication dosages causes medication errors that can compromise patient safety.
Use standard procedures and evidence-based references.	Follow a standardized procedure when administering medication for every patient. Look up current medication information in evidence-based sources because information changes frequently.
Communicate with the patient before and after administration.	Provide information to the patient about the medication before administering it. Answer their questions regarding usage, dose, and special considerations. Give the patient an opportunity to ask questions and include family members if appropriate.
Follow agency policies and procedures regarding medication administration.	Avoid work-arounds. A work-around is a process that bypasses a procedure or policy in a system. For example, a nurse may "borrow" medication from one patient's drawer to give to another patient while waiting for an order to be filled by the pharmacy. Although performed with a good intention to prevent delay, these work-arounds fail to follow policies in place that ensure safe medication administration and often result in medication errors.

1 Institute for Safe Medication Practices. (2012, November 29). *Side tracks on the safety express. Interruptions lead to errors and unfinished... Wait, what was I doing?* https://www.ismp.org/resources/side-tracks-safety-express-interruptions-lead-errors-and-unfinished-wait-what-was-i-doing?id=37

2 The Joint Commission. (n.d.). *2020 hospital national patient safety goals.* https://www.jointcommission.org/standards/national-patient-safety-goals/

My Notes

Guidelines	Additional Information
Ensure medication has not expired.	Check all medications' expiration dates before administering them. Medications can become inactive after their expiration date.
Always clarify an order or procedure that is unclear.	Always verify information whenever you are uncertain or unclear about an order. Consult with the pharmacist, charge nurse, or health care provider, and be sure to resolve all questions before proceeding with medication administration.
Use available technology to administer medications.	Use available technology, such as bar code scanning, when administering medications. Bar code scanning is linked to the patient's eMAR and provides an extra level of patient safety to prevent wrong medications, incorrect doses, or wrong timing of administration. If error messages occur, it is important to follow up appropriately according to agency policy and not override them. Additionally, it is important to remember that this technology provides an additional layer of safety and should not be substituted for the checking the five rights of medication administration.
Be a part of the safety culture.	Report all errors, near misses, and adverse reactions according to agency policy. Incident reports improve patient care through quality improvement identification, analysis, and problem-solving.
Be alert.	Be alert to error-prone situations and high-alert medications. High-alert medications are those that can cause significant harm. The most common high-alert medications are anticoagulants, opiates, insulins, and sedatives. Read more about high-alert medications in the "Basic Concepts of Administering Medications" section.
Address patient concerns.	If a patient questions or expresses concern regarding a medication, stop the procedure and do not administer it. Explore the patient's concerns, review the provider's order, and, if necessary, notify the provider.

Post-Administration: Right Response

In addition to documenting the medication administration, the nurse evaluates the patient after medications have been administered to monitor the efficacy of the drug. For example, if a patient reported a pain level of "8" before PRN pain medication was administered, the nurse evaluates the patient's pain level after administration to ensure the pain level is decreasing and the pain medication was effective. This evaluation data is documented in the patient's chart.

Additionally, the nurse continually monitors for adverse effects from all of a patient's medications. For example, the first dose of an antibiotic was administered to a patient during a previous shift, but the nurse notices the patient has developed a rash. The nurse notifies the prescribing provider of the change in condition and anticipates new orders or changes in the existing orders.

15.4 CHECKLIST FOR ORAL MEDICATION ADMINISTRATION

My Notes

Use the checklist below to review the steps for completion of "Oral Medication Administration."[1]

Steps

Disclaimer: Always review and follow agency policy regarding this specific skill.

Special Considerations:

- **Plan medication administration to avoid disruption.**
- **Dispense medication in a quiet area.**
- **Avoid conversation with others.**
- **Follow agency's no-interruption zone policy.**
- **Perform hand hygiene prior to medication preparation.**
- **Prepare medications for ONE patient at a time.**

1. Gather supplies: MAR/eMAR.
2. Know the actions, special nursing considerations, safe dose ranges, purpose of administration, and potential adverse effects of the medications to be administered. Consider the appropriateness of the medication for this patient at this time.
3. Read the eMAR/MAR and select the proper medication from the medication supply system or the patient's medication drawer. Perform the first of three checks of the six rights of medication administration plus two (allergies and expiration dates). Perform necessary calculations to verify correct dosage.
    - **The right patient:** Check that you have the correct patient using two patient identifiers (e.g., name and date of birth).
    - **The right medication (drug):** Check that you have the correct medication and that it is appropriate for the patient in the current context.
    - **The right dose:** Check that the dose is safe for the age, size, and condition of the patient. Different dosages may be indicated for different conditions.
    - **The right route:** Check that the route is appropriate for the patient's current condition.
    - **The right time:** Adhere to the prescribed dose and schedule.
    - **The right documentation:** Always verify any unclear or inaccurate documentation prior to administering medications.
4. The medication label must be checked for name, dose, and route, and compared with the MAR at least three different times:
    - When the medication is taken out of the drawer.
    - When the medication is being prepared.

---

1 This work is a derivative of Clinical Procedures for Safer Patient Care by British Columbia Institute of Technology and is licensed under CC BY 4.0. Access for free at https://opentextbc.ca/clinicalskills/

My Notes

- At the bedside, prior to medication administration to the patient.

5. Prepare the required medications:

   - **Unit dose packages:** Do not open the wrapper until you are at the patient's bedside. Keep opioids and medications that require special nursing assessments separate from other medication packages.
   - **Multi-dose containers:** When removing tablets or capsules from a multi-dose bottle, pour the necessary number into the bottle cap and then place the tablets or capsules in a medication cup. Cut scored tablets, if necessary, to obtain the proper dosage. If it is necessary to touch the tablets, wear gloves.
   - **Liquid medication in a multi-dose bottle:** When pouring liquid medications out of a multi-dose bottle, hold the bottle so the label is against the palm to avoid dripping on the label. Use an appropriate measuring device when pouring liquids, and read the amount of medication at the bottom of the meniscus at eye level. Wipe the lip of the bottle with a paper towel.

6. Depending on agency policy, the third check of the label may occur at this point. If so, after all medications for one patient have been prepared, recheck the medication labels against the eMAR/MAR before taking the medications to the patient. However, many agencies require the third check to be performed at the bedside after obtaining two patient identifiers and scanning the barcode of the patient.

7. Replace any multi-dose containers in the patient's drawer or medication supply system. Lock the medication supply system before leaving it.

8. Transport the medications to the patient's bedside carefully, and keep the medications in sight at all times.

9. Perform safety steps:

   - Perform hand hygiene.
   - Check the room for transmission-based precautions.
   - Introduce yourself, your role, the purpose of your visit, and an estimate of the time it will take.
   - Confirm patient ID using two patient identifiers (e.g., name and date of birth).
   - Explain the process to the patient and ask if they have any questions.
   - Be organized and systematic.
   - Use appropriate listening and questioning skills.
   - Listen and attend to patient cues.
   - Ensure the patient's privacy and dignity.
   - Assess ABCs.

10. When identifying the patient, compare the information with the eMAR/MAR. The patient should be identified using at least two of the following methods:

    - Check the name on the patient's identification band.
    - Check the identification number on the patient's identification band.

My Notes

- Check the birth date on the patient's identification band.
- Ask the patient to state his or her name and birth date, based on facility policy.
- If a patient is unable to verbalize their name and date of birth and patient identification bands are not used, use alternative methods of identification such as a second staff member and/or a patient picture in the MAR.

11. Complete all necessary assessments before administering the medications. Check the patient's allergy bracelet or ask the patient about allergies. Explain the purpose and action of each medication to the patient.
12. Based on facility policy, the third check of the medication label typically occurs at this point. If so, recheck the label with the eMAR/ MAR before administering the medications to the patient. Scan the patient's bar code on the identification band, if bar scanning is used. If an error occurs during bar code scanning, obtain assistance before administering the medication. Most error messages are intended to warn the nurse of a potential medication error.
13. Assist the patient to an upright (or a side-lying) position if they are unable to be positioned upright:
    - Offer water or other permitted fluids with pills, capsules, tablets, and some liquid medications.
    - Ask if the patient prefers to take the medications by hand or in a cup and if they prefer all medications at once or individually.
14. Remain with the patient until each medication is swallowed. Never leave medication at the patient's bedside.
    - Note: If the patient is confused or has been known to hoard pills, have the patient open their mouth and check under the tongue.
15. Assist the patient to a comfortable position, ask if they have any questions, and thank them for their time.
16. Ensure safety measures when leaving the room:
    - CALL LIGHT: Within reach
    - BED: Low and locked (in lowest position and brakes on)
    - SIDE RAILS: Secured
    - TABLE: Within reach
    - ROOM: Risk-free for falls (scan room and clear any obstacles)
17. Perform hand hygiene.
18. Document medication administration and related assessment findings. Report any concerns according to agency policy.
19. Evaluate the patient's response to the medication within the appropriate time frame. Note: Most sublingual medications act in 15 minutes, and most oral medications act in 30 minutes. If patient presents with any adverse effects:
    - Withhold further doses.
    - Assess vital signs.

My Notes

- Notify prescriber.
- Notify pharmacy.
- Document as per agency policy.

15.5 CHECKLIST FOR RECTAL MEDICATION ADMINISTRATION

My Notes

Use the checklist below to review the steps for completion of "Rectal Medication Administration" using a rectal suppository.[1]

Steps

Disclaimer: Always review and follow agency policy regarding this specific skill.

Follow Steps 1 through 12 in the "Checklist for Oral Medication Administration."

13. If possible, have the patient defecate prior to rectal medication administration.
14. Ensure that you have water-soluble lubricant available for medication administration.
15. Explain the procedure to the patient. If a patient prefers to self-administer the suppository/enema, give specific instructions to the patient on correct procedure.
16. Raise the bed to working height:
    - Position the patient on left side with the upper leg flexed over the lower leg toward the waist (Sims position).
    - Provide privacy and drape the patient with only the buttocks and anal area exposed.
    - Place a drape underneath the patient's buttocks.
17. Apply clean, nonsterile gloves.
18. Assess the patient for diarrhea or active rectal bleeding.
19. Remove the wrapper from the suppository/tip of enema and lubricate the rounded tip of the suppository and index finger of the dominant hand with lubricant. If administering an enema, lubricate the tip of the enema.
20. Separate the buttocks with the nondominant hand and, using the gloved index finger of dominant hand, insert the suppository (rounded tip toward patient) into the rectum toward the umbilicus while having the patient take a deep breath, exhale through the mouth, and relax the anal sphincter. Insert the suppository against the rectal mucosa for optimal absorption, about 3 to 4 inches for an adult and 1 to 2 inches for a child. Do not insert the suppository into feces. If administering an enema, expel the air from the enema and then insert the tip of the enema into the rectum toward the umbilicus while having the patient take a deep breath, exhale through the mouth, and relax the anal sphincter. Roll the plastic bottle from bottom to tip until all solution has entered the rectum and colon. Remove the bottle.
21. Monitor the patient for signs of dizziness. Unintended vagal stimulation may occur, resulting in bradycardia in some patients. Be aware that the rectal route may not be suitable for certain cardiac conditions.
22. When administering a suppository, ask the patient to remain on side for 5 to 10 minutes.

---

1 This work is a derivative of Clinical Procedures for Safer Patient Care by British Columbia Institute of Technology and is licensed under CC BY 4.0. Access for free at https://opentextbc.ca/clinicalskills/

My Notes

- When administering an enema, ask the patient to retain the enema until the urge to defecate is strong, usually about 5 to 15 minutes.

23. Discard gloves by turning them inside out before disposing them. Discard used supplies as per agency policy and perform hand hygiene.
24. Assist the patient to a comfortable position, ask if they have any questions, and thank them for their time.
25. Ensure safety measures when leaving the room:
    - CALL LIGHT: Within reach
    - BED: Low and locked (in lowest position and brakes on)
    - SIDE RAILS: Secured
    - TABLE: Within reach
    - ROOM: Risk-free for falls (scan room and clear any obstacles)
26. Perform hand hygiene.
27. Document medication administration and the related assessment findings. Report any unexpected findings according to agency policy.
28. Evaluate the patient's response to the medication within the appropriate time frame.

15.6 CHECKLIST FOR ENTERAL TUBE MEDICATION ADMINISTRATION

My Notes

Use the checklist below to review the steps for completion of "Enteral Tube Medication Administration."[1]

Steps

Disclaimer: Always review and follow agency policy regarding this specific skill.

Follow Steps 1 through 12 in the "Checklist for Oral Medication Administration."

13. Prepare each medication individually in its own cup. Crush pills, open capsules, and pour liquid medication into a medication cup. Dilute the medication in 5 to 10 mL of water.
14. If administering medication to a patient who is receiving intermittent or continuous tube feeding, stop the feeding based on the following guidelines:
    - 1-2 hours prior to medication administration if medication is incompatible with feeding
    - 1 hour prior to medication administration if placement is to be assessed via the pH method
    - 30 minutes prior to medication administration if the medication should be given on an empty stomach
    - Immediately before medication administration if medication can be given with food
15. If the enteral tube is attached to suction for gastric decompression, disconnect.
16. Perform an abdominal assessment.
17. Elevate the head of the bed at least 30-45 degrees, preferably to high Fowler's position, to prevent aspiration.
18. Verify tube placement according to agency policy. (For more information on verifying tube placement, review the "Enteral Tube Management" chapter.)
19. Using a 60-mL syringe, flush the tube with at least 15 mL of water to verify patency.
20. Administer diluted medication. When administering multiple medications, each medication should be administered separately to prevent tube clogging. Flush between each medication with 15 mL of room-temperature water (unless contraindicated for the patient). For more information about preventing tube clogging, see the "Enteral Tube Management" chapter.
21. After all medications are administered, flush the tube with at least 15 mL of tepid water. If there is a risk of fluid overload, the amount of fluid used to flush between medications may be modified according to agency policy. However, it is essential to flush the tube when beginning and ending medication administration to prevent tube clogging.
22. If the tube is to be reattached to suction, clamp the enteral tube for 20-30 minutes (or the amount of time specified in the order) to permit medication absorption. If the enteral tube is attached to a continuous tube feeding, the feeding should be resumed when appropriate.

1 This work is a derivative of Clinical Procedures for Safer Patient Care by British Columbia Institute of Technology and is licensed under CC BY 4.0. Access for free at https://opentextbc.ca/clinicalskills/

My Notes

23. Elevate the head of the bed for 60 minutes after medication administration or at all times if continuous feeding is being given.

24. Record the total amount of water used to flush the tube on the client's intake and output record.

25. Document medication administered on the MAR/eMAR.

26. Assist the patient to a comfortable position, ask if they have any questions, and thank them for their time.

27. Ensure safety measures when leaving the room:

    - CALL LIGHT: Within reach
    - BED: Low and locked (in lowest position and brakes on)
    - SIDE RAILS: Secured
    - TABLE: Within reach
    - ROOM: Risk-free for falls (scan room and clear any obstacles)

28. Perform hand hygiene.

29. Document the medication administration and related assessment findings. Report any concerns according to agency policy.

30. Evaluate the patient's response to the medication within the appropriate time frame.

15.7 SUPPLEMENTARY VIDEOS

My Notes

Video Reviews of Crushing Medications, Pill Splitting, and Administering Rectal Suppositories

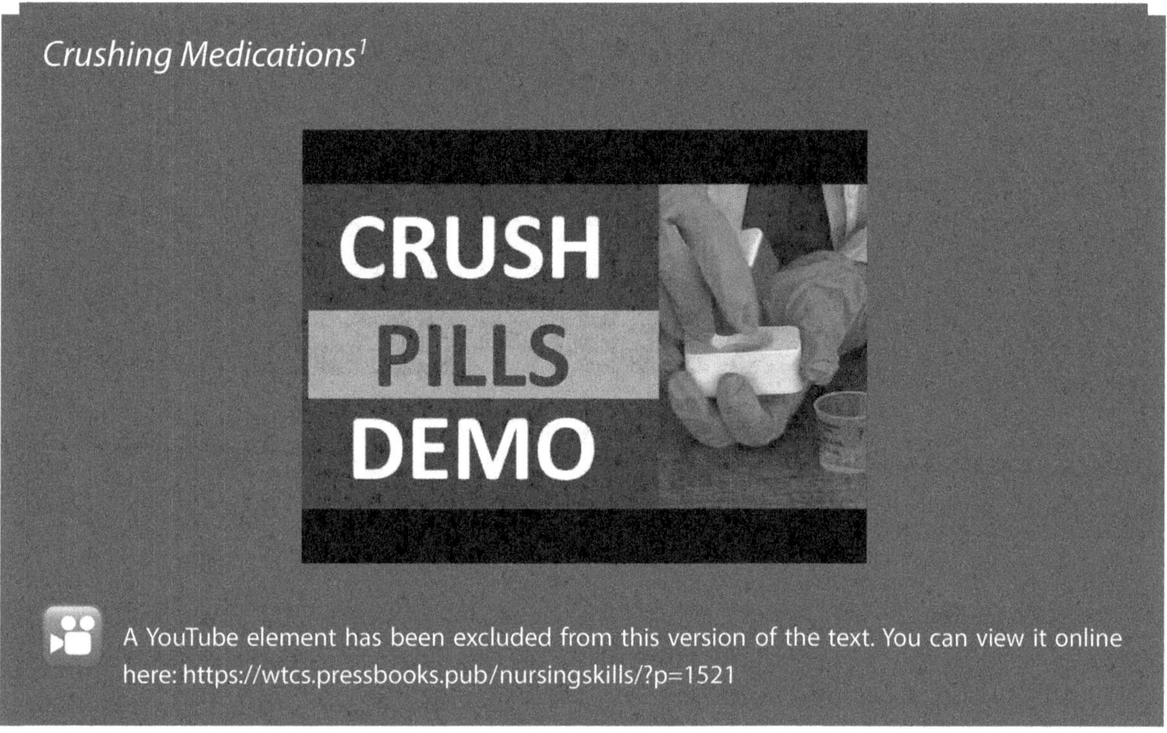
Crushing Medications[1]
CRUSH
PILLS
DEMO
A YouTube element has been excluded from this version of the text. You can view it online here: https://wtcs.pressbooks.pub/nursingskills/?p=1521

1 RegisteredNurseRN. (2017, March 22). *Crushing medications for tube feeding and oral administration | How to crush pills for nurses.* [Video]. YouTube. All rights reserved. Video used with permission. https://youtu.be/86RzAgHu75U

My Notes

Splitting Pill in Half[2]

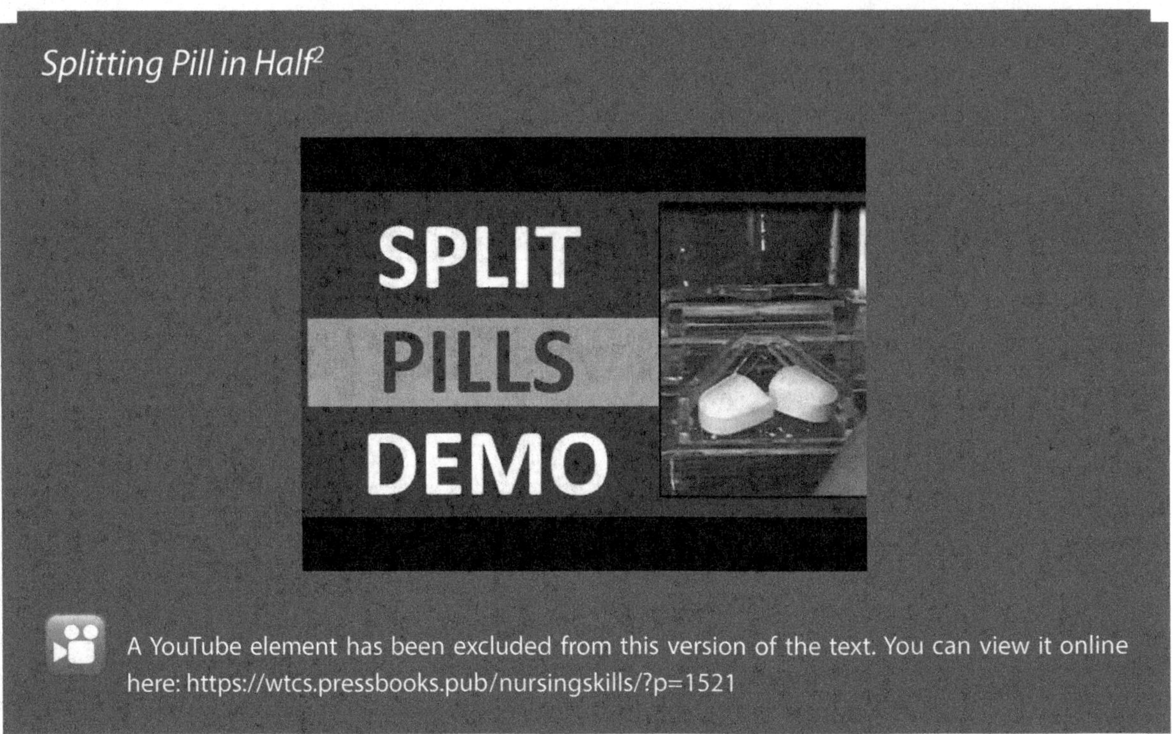

A YouTube element has been excluded from this version of the text. You can view it online here: https://wtcs.pressbooks.pub/nursingskills/?p=1521

View Agrace Hospice Care's "Giving Meds by Suppository" video on YouTube[3]

2 RegisteredNurseRN. (2017, March 18). *How to split in half | Cut a pill in half | Nursing medication administration.* [Video]. YouTube. All rights reserved. Video used with permission. https://youtu.be/uuC4jWcbamE

3 Agrace HospiceCare. (2017, August 23). *Giving meds by suppository.* [Video]. YouTube. All rights reserved. https://youtu.be/hLDyZ4QW9Fo

15.8 LEARNING ACTIVITIES

My Notes

Learning Activities

(Answers to "Learning Activities'" can be found in the '"Answer Key'" at the end of the book. Answers to interactive activity elements will be provided within the element as immediate feedback.)

1. A physician has ordered nafcillin 750 mg IM q 6 h. On hand is a 2 gram vial that states: "Add 6.8 mL of sterile water to provide a total solution of 8 mL." How many milliliters should the nurse draw up to give the patient the ordered dose?
2. What are the steps the nurse should follow if the medication is given to the wrong patient?

Check your knowledge using this flashcard activity:

An interactive or media element has been excluded from this version of the text. You can view it online here: https://wtcs.pressbooks.pub/nursingskills/?p=1523

Use this drag and drop activity to check your knowledge about different types of medication orders.

An interactive or media element has been excluded from this version of the text. You can view it online here: https://wtcs.pressbooks.pub/nursingskills/?p=1523

An interactive or media element has been excluded from this version of the text. You can view it online here: https://wtcs.pressbooks.pub/nursingskills/?p=1523

My Notes

XV GLOSSARY

Around the Clock (ATC) order: An order that reflects that medication should be administered at regular time intervals, such as every six hours, to maintain consistent levels of the drug in the patient's bloodstream

Dysphagia: Difficulty swallowing.

eMAR: Electronic medication administration record contained in a patient's electronic chart.

Enteral medications: Medications that are administered directly into the gastrointestinal tract orally, rectally, or through a tube such as a nasogastric (NG) tube, nasointestinal (NI) tube, or percutaneous endoscopic gastrostomy (PEG) tube.

Incident report: A report submitted per agency policy used to document the events surrounding a medication error.

MAR: Medication administration record contained in a patient's chart.

One-time order: A prescription for a medication to be administered only once. An example of a one-time order is a prescription for an IV dose of antibiotics to be administered immediately prior to surgery.

Prescriptions: Orders, interventions, remedies, or treatments ordered or directed by an authorized primary health care provider.

PRN (as needed) order: A prescription for medication to be administered when it is requested by, or as needed by, the patient. PRN orders are usually administered based on patient symptoms such as pain medications. An example of a PRN order is a prescription for pain medication, such as "Acetaminophen 500 mg PO every 4-6 hours as needed for pain."

Routine order: A written prescription that is followed until another order cancels it. An example of a routine order is a prescription for daily medication such as "Lisinopril 10 mg PO daily."

Safety culture: A culture established in health care agencies to empower staff to speak up about risks to patients and to report errors and near misses, all of which drive improvement in patient care and reduce the incident of patient harm.

Standing order: Standing orders are standard prescriptions for nurses to implement for patients in clearly defined circumstances without the need to notify a provider. They may also be referred to as an "order set" or a "protocol." An example of a standing order/protocol is a standard prescription for all patients coming into an urgent care reporting chest pain to immediately receive four chewable aspirin, the placement of an IV, and an electrocardiogram (ECG).

STAT order: A one-time prescription that is administered without delay. An example of a STAT order is the prescription for a dose of Benadryl to be administered to a patient having an allergic reaction.

Titration order: An order in which the medication dose is either progressively increased or decreased by the nurse in response to the patient's status.

Chapter 16

Administration of Medications Via Other Routes

16.1 ADMINISTRATION OF MEDICATIONS VIA OTHER ROUTES INTRODUCTION

My Notes

Learning Objectives

- Safely administer medications and irrigations for the eye, ear, inhalation, and vaginal routes
- Select the appropriate equipment
- Calculate correct amount to administer
- Select appropriate site
- Modify the procedure to reflect variations across the life span
- Document actions and observations
- Recognize and report significant deviations from norms

This chapter will review specific information related to administering medications via the topical, transdermal, eye, ear, inhalation, and vaginal routes. Read additional information about administering medications in the "Administration of Enteral Medications" and "Administration of Parenteral Medications" chapters.

My Notes

16.2 BASIC CONCEPTS

Topical and Transdermal Medications

Topical medications are medications that are administered via the skin or mucous membranes for direct local action, as well as for systemic effects. An **innunction** is a medication that is massaged or rubbed into the skin and includes topical creams such as nystatin antifungal cream. The **transdermal route** of medication administration includes patches or disks applied to the skin that deliver medication over an extended period of time. Common types of transdermal medications are analgesics (such as fentanyl), cardiac medications (such as nitroglycerin), hormones (such as estrogen), and nicotine patches (for smoking cessation). See Figure 16.1[1] for an image of typical packaging of a topical patch. Medications delivered transdermally provide a consistent level of the drug in the bloodstream for distribution. The transdermal route is also helpful for patients who are nauseated or having difficulty swallowing.

Heat may be applied with the administration of some inunctions. Heat causes vasodilation that enhances blood flow and improves absorption of some medication. However, heat should never be applied over patches, such as the fentanyl or nitroglycerin patches, because it increases the release of the drug and can cause overdose and death. Be sure to reference manufacturer recommendations regarding the application of heat.[2]

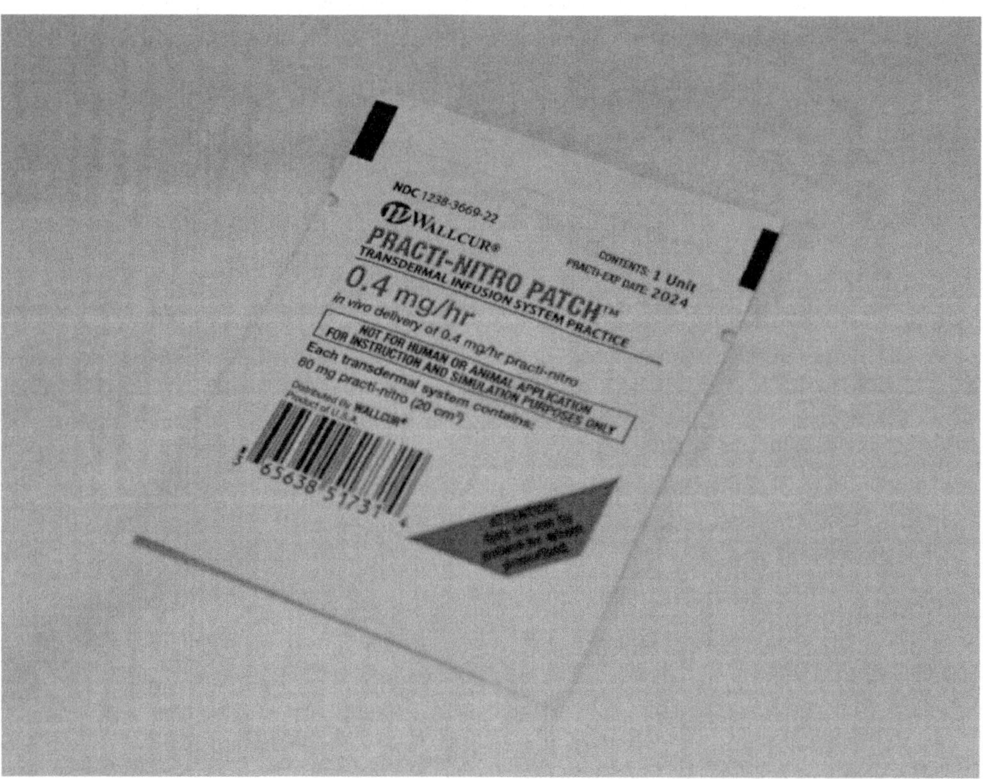

Figure 16.1 Topical Patch

1 "DSC_17661.jpg" by British Columbia Institute of Technology is licensed under CC BY 4.0. Access for free at https://opentextbc.ca/clinicalskills/chapter/administering-topical-medication/

2 Institute for Safe Medication Practices. (2015). Transdermal patches and heat sources. *NurseAdviseERR, 13*(4). https://www.ismp.org/sites/default/files/attachments/2018-04/NurseAdviseERR201504.pdf

When applying transdermal patches, the nurse should always wear gloves and check the rights of medication administration as is done with other types of medication. Before applying a new patch, the old patch should be removed, the skin around the old patch should be assessed, and the site for the patch cleansed and dried thoroughly. The skin around the patch should be monitored for any irritation or reaction to the medication or patch adhesive. Patches should not be applied to broken or irritated skin.

When applying a new patch, the nurse should remove the clear plastic backing and take care to not touch the medication surface of the patch while placing it on the patient's skin. Patches should be placed on an appropriate skin area per manufacturer guidelines, such as the upper arms or on the chest. The patch should be pressed firmly to the skin for ten seconds to ensure adhesion to the skin. For documentation purposes, the nurse should initial, date, and time a piece of tape that is applied close to the patch. The patch should not be written on directly because this may puncture the patch and cause it to become ineffective. Based on the onset of the medication, the patient should be evaluated to ensure they are responding appropriately to the therapeutic effects of the medication and not experiencing any adverse effects.

Patch placement should be routinely assessed for dislodgement per agency policy. For example, for some opioid patches like fentanyl, the nurse is required to assess and document that the patch is present during every shift. The nurse should also be aware that patches with aluminum backing can cause issues with defibrillation and MRI scans, so this type of patch should be removed prior to either of these actions.

To remove a patch, the nurse should wear gloves and remove the patch carefully so as not to tear the skin. The patch should be disposed of in the proper waste receptacle per agency policy. For example, some agencies have specific receptacles for nitroglycerin patches. Additionally, agencies have specific policies for disposal of fentanyl patches to prevent drug diversion of used patches. Patch removal should be documented in the patient's record.

Eye Instillations and Irrigations

Eye Drops

Eye drops are administered for a local effect on the eye. Examples of eye drop medications include antibiotic drops for conjunctivitis, glaucoma medication to reduce intraocular pressure, and saline drops to relieve dry eyes. The amount of drops to administer per eye is indicated on the provider order. When instilling eye drops, the nurse should perform hand hygiene, apply gloves, and check the same rights of medication administration as done with other types of medication. Prior to administration of eye medication, the patient's eyes should be assessed for new or unusual redness or drainage. If discharge is present, the eyelids should be cleansed with gauze saturated with warm water or normal saline to remove any dirt or debris that could be carried into the eye during instillation. When cleaning the eyelids, the nurse should clean from the inner canthus toward the outer canthus so as not to introduce debris or dirt into the lacrimal ducts that could cause an infection. A new gauze pad is used for each stroke. The nurse should remove gloves after cleansing, perform hand hygiene, and apply new gloves prior to medication administration.

When administering the drops, the patient should be instructed to tilt their head backwards or be positioned in a supine position with their head on a pillow looking up. When the cap of the medication is removed, it should be placed on a clean surface with care taken to keep the inside of the cap sterile and to not contaminate the dropper tip. The patient should look up and away while the nurse gently uses pressure to pull the lower lid down and expose the lower conjunctival sac. By holding the dropper close to the sac without touching it, the nurse should squeeze the bottle and allow the drop to fall into the sac, taking care to not touch the dropper to the eye. After the eye drop has been instilled, the patient should close their eye. The nurse should apply gentle pressure to the inner canthus, when appropriate, to prevent the medication from entering the lacrimal duct and causing a possible systemic

My Notes

reaction to the medication. This procedure should be repeated in the other eye as ordered. The patient should be instructed to not to rub their eye(s). During the procedure, the nurse evaluates the patient's tolerance of the medication and the procedure and documents it. See Figure 16.2[3] for an image of a nurse administering eye drops.

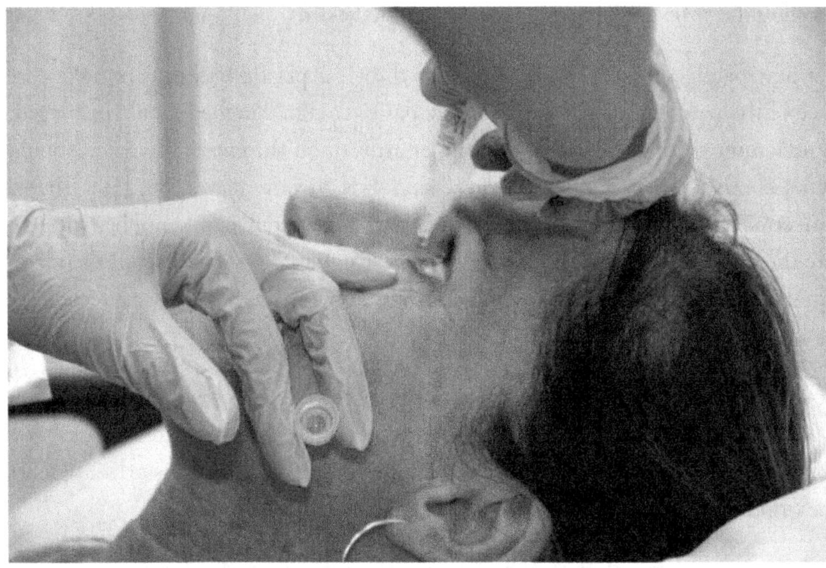

Figure 16.2 Administering Eye Drops

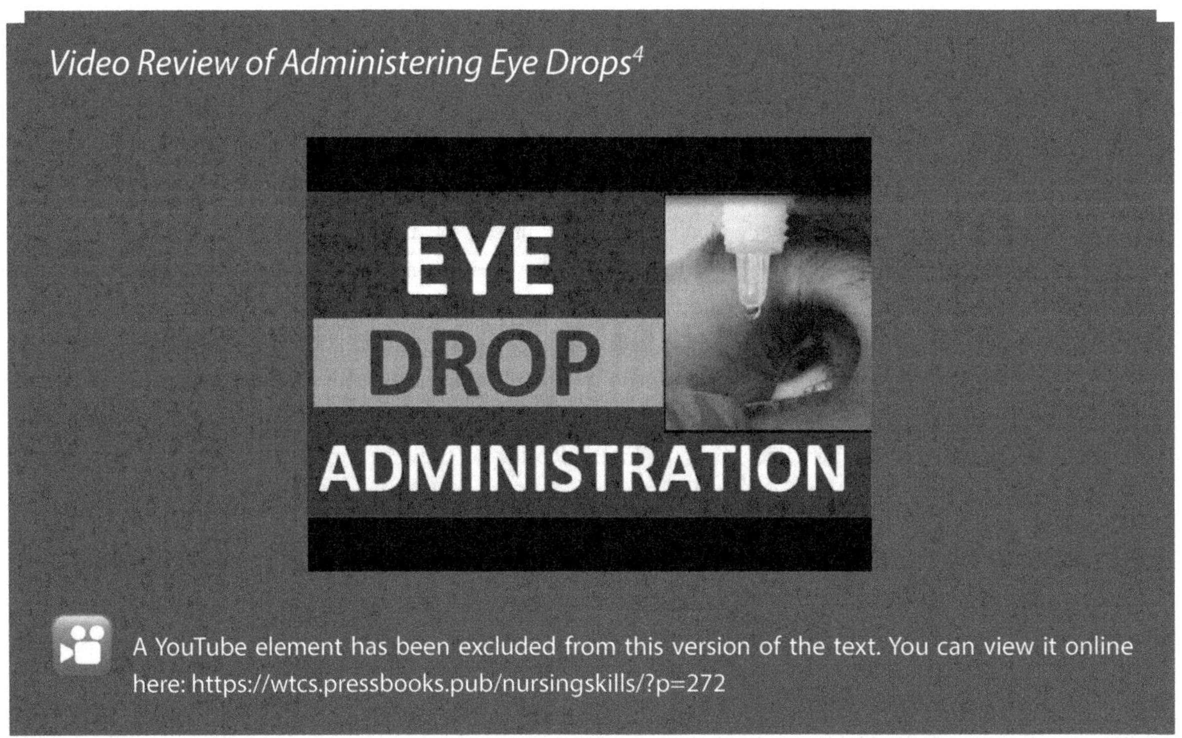

Video Review of Administering Eye Drops[4]
EYE
DROP
ADMINISTRATION

A YouTube element has been excluded from this version of the text. You can view it online here: https://wtcs.pressbooks.pub/nursingskills/?p=272

---

3 "*Instilling eye medication*" by British Columbia Institute of Technology is licensed under CC BY 4.0. Access for free at https://opentextbc.ca/clinicalskills/chapter/6-5-installing-eye-ear-and-nose-medications/

4 RegisteredNurseRN. (2017, March 24). *Eye drop administration nursing | Instill eye drops punctal occlusion for glaucoma.* [Video.] YouTube. All rights reserved. Video used with permission. https://youtu.be/TLhnsABDtco

Eye Ointment

Administering eye ointment follows the same procedure as administering eye drops, except that instead of drops, ½ inch of ointment is placed in the lower conjunctival sac. When applying the ointment, the nurse should start at the inner canthus and move outward. After application, the patient should be instructed to close their eyelid and move the eye to spread the ointment so it is absorbed. They should be advised they may experience blurry vision for a few minutes until the medication is absorbed.

Eye Irrigations

Eye irrigations are used to flush foreign bodies from the eye, such as debris or chemicals, using large amounts of saline. The amount of solution and length of time used to irrigate the eye depends on the contaminant. Follow agency policy when performing eye irrigation. For example, some emergency eye flush stations provide a 15-minute flush to the eye. Care should be taken to not contaminate the other eye while removing the debris unless it is necessary to flush both eyes.

Ear Instillations and Irrigations

Medications and fluids may be instilled into the ear for local effect, including antibiotics, analgesics, wax softeners, and irrigation fluid to remove foreign objects or wax buildup. Medications and fluids are instilled into the outer ear canal, with the tympanic membrane forming a thin barrier to the middle and inner ear. However, if the tympanic membrane is ruptured, instillation of ear drops is generally contraindicated unless a sterile, no-touch technique is used. However, if a patient has a surgical opening in the tympanic membrane (i.e., tympanostomy tubes have been placed), ear drops may be prescribed but caution must be taken not to introduce debris into the middle or inner air.

Ear Drops

When administering ear drops, the nurse should carefully follow the dosage and amount of drops per ear according to the provider order. The nurse should perform hand hygiene, apply gloves, and check the same rights of medication administration as is completed with other types of medication. The external ear should be cleaned of debris prior to drops being instilled. The patient should be positioned so the affected ear is tilted in the uppermost position. If the patient is lying in bed, position the patient so they are lying with the unaffected ear against the pillow and the affected ear upward. When removing the cap of the medication, caution should be used to not touch the dropper or the inside of the cap to avoid contamination. The pinna of the ear should be grasped and pulled backwards and upwards for an adult. For children, the pinna should be pulled straight back, and for infants, it should be pulled down and back. This movement straightens the auditory canal and prepares it for instillation. The nurse should squeeze the bottle so that the drops of medication fall onto the side of the auditory canal and not directly onto the tympanic membrane. The medication should run towards the tympanic membrane after it is instilled. The tragus can be massaged to help move the medication into place. The patient should remain in this lying position for five minutes. After five minutes, this procedure can be repeated on the other ear, if ordered. Evaluation of the patient should be performed post administration to assess if the patient tolerated the procedure and if anticipated therapeutic effects occurred. When instilling medication or fluids into the ear, monitor for side effects such as dizziness or nausea. See Figure 16.3[5] for an image of a nurse administering ear drops.

---

5 "DSC_2273.jpg" by British Columbia Institute of Technology is licensed under CC BY 4.0. Access for free at https://opentextbc.ca/clinicalskills/chapter/6-5-installing-eye-ear-and-nose-medications/

My Notes

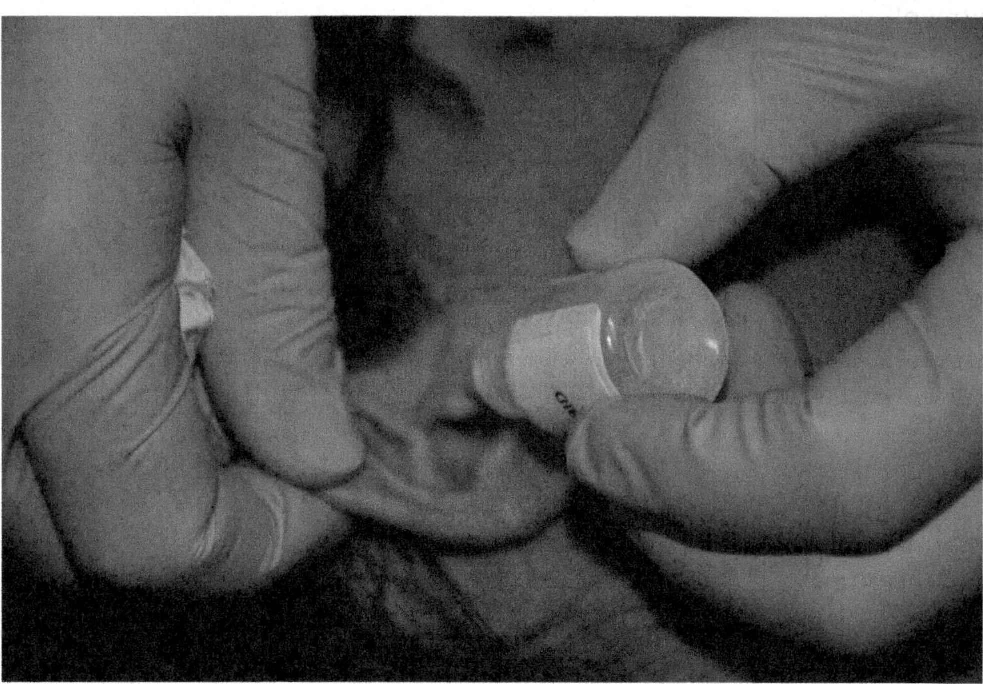

Figure 16.3 Administering Ear Drops

Ear Irrigations

Ear irrigations are typically performed to remove wax buildup or foreign bodies from the external ear canal. Normal saline at room temperature is typically used, although a mixture of saline and hydrogen peroxide can also be used. A 60-cc needleless syringe is typically used to irrigate the ear, or a spray bottle with a soft angio catheter can also be used. Ask the patient to hold an emesis basin under the ear to catch the expelled irrigant. During and after the irrigation, the patient should be evaluated for side effects such as dizziness, nausea, or pain.

Nasal Instillation

Medications administered via the nasal passage are typically used to treat allergies, sinus infections, and nasal congestion. Nasal spray or drops should be administered via the nasal passage using a clean technique. The nurse should perform hand hygiene, apply gloves, and perform the same rights of medication administration as is completed with other types of medications. The patient should be given tissues and asked to blow their nose. Position the patient with their head tilted backwards while sitting or lying supine looking upwards. The nurse should insert the tip of the spray bottle or the nasal dropper into one nare while occluding the other nare and then activate the spray as the patient inhales. The bottle should remain compressed as it is removed from the nose to prevent contamination. The patient should be instructed to hold their breath for a few seconds and then breathe through their mouth. Repeat this procedure in the other nare if ordered. Wipe the outside of the bottle with clean tissue before storing it, and advise the patient to avoid blowing their nose for 5-10 minutes after nasal instillation. Note any unexpected situations such as nosebleeds or increased congestion.[6]

---

6 Djupesland, P. G. (2012). Nasal drug delivery devices: Characteristics and performance in a clinical perspective - a review. *Drug Delivery and Translational Research, 3,* 42-62. https://doi.org/10.1007/s13346-012-0108-9

Vaginal Instillations

My Notes

Vaginal instillations are typically used to administer hormone therapy and antifungal treatment. Vaginal applications can be supplied in foams, suppositories that melt with body heat, creams, and tablets. The patient should be asked to void prior to placement. The nurse should perform hand hygiene, apply gloves, perform the same rights of medication administration as is completed with other types of medications, and provide privacy. Position the patient on their back with knees flexed. Perineal care should be performed by the nurse prior to administration of the medication. After perineal care, remove gloves, perform hand hygiene, and apply new gloves. Fill a vaginal applicator with cream or foam or open the suppository to be placed. Lubricate the applicator or your gloved finger with water-based lubricant. With the nondominant hand, spread the labia and place the applicator into the full length of the vagina, push the plunger, and then remove the applicator. If a suppository is being placed, insert the rounded end of the suppository with your index finger, placing it along the posterior wall of the vagina. Ask the patient to remain in the supine position for 5-10 minutes for optimal absorption. If possible, administer the medication at bedtime so the patient can remain in the supine position for an extended period of time to enhance absorption. Assess the patient for any unexpected situations, such as the suppository coming out. See Figure 16.4[7] for an illustration of vaginal administration of cream medication.

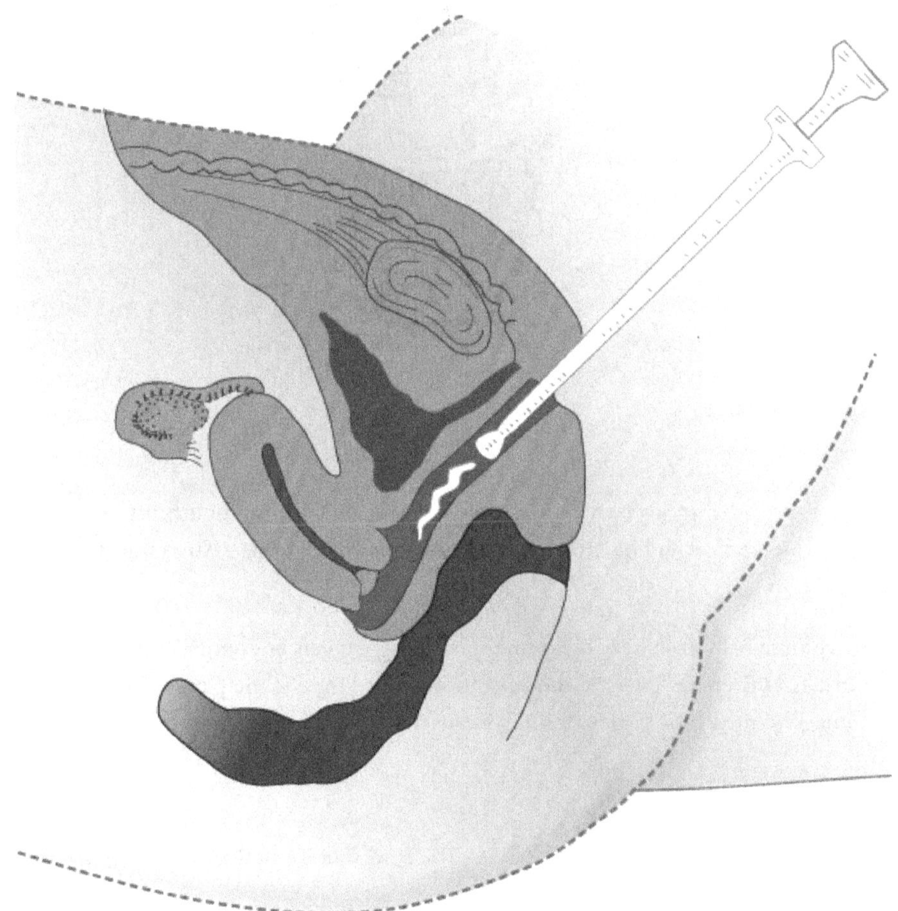

Figure 16.4 Administering Vaginal Medication

7 "Administering-med-vaginally-appliator.png" by British Columbia Institute of Technology is licensed under CC BY 4.0. Access for free at https://opentextbc.ca/clinicalskills/chapter/6-4-rectal-and-vaginal-medications/

My Notes

Inhaled Medications

The lungs have a large surface area with an increased amount of blood flow, so medications are easily absorbed. Medications inhaled from the mouth into the lungs can be administered using a **Metered Dose Inhaler** (MDI), a **Dry Powder Inhaler** (DPI), or a **small-volume nebulizer**. A metered dose inhaler (MDI) provides a mist of medication that is inhaled through the mouth into the lungs. See Figure 16.5[8] for an image of an albuterol MDI. However, during inhalation from an MDI, small medication particles can get trapped on the tongue or aerosolize into the air and not make it into the lungs, so a spacer is optimally used for full absorption of medication.

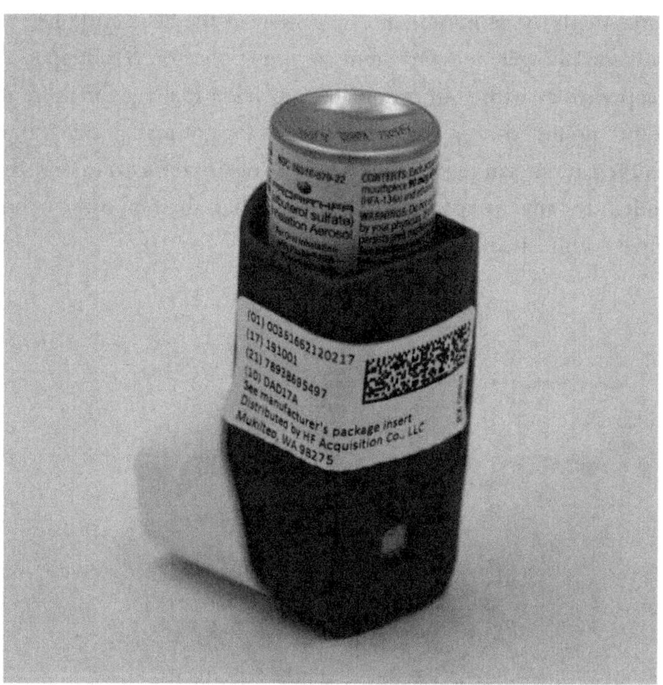

Figure 16.5 Albuterol Metered Dose Inhaler (MDI)

A DPI is medication provided in a powder form that is inhaled from the mouth into the lungs using a quick breath to activate the medication and move it into the lungs from the inhaler. An example of Advair Diskus DPI is illustrated in Figure 16.6.[9]

Hand-held, small-volume nebulizers provide a fine mist using oxygen or compressed air to transport the liquid medication from the nebulizer cup into the mouth and into the lungs as the patient breathes normally. See Figure 16.7[10] for an image of medication packaged for use with nebulizers.[11]

---

8 This work is derivative of "RESIZED+SERIALIZED+1202-1.jpg" courtesy of the *U.S.National Library of Medicine*. This image is included on the basis of Fair Use.

9 This work is a derivative of "advair-diskus-spl-graphic-16.jpg" courtesy of the *U.S.National Library of Medicine*. This image is included on the basis of Fair Use.

10 "Ipratropium_Bromide_(1).JPG" by *Intropin* is licensed under CC BY-SA 3.0. Access for free at https://commons.wikimedia.org/wiki/File:Ipratropium_Bromide_(1).JPG

11 Ari, A. & Restrepo, R. D. (2012). Aerosol delivery device selection for spontaneously breathing patients: 2012. *Respiratory Care, 57*(4), 613-626. http://rc.rcjournal.com/content/respcare/57/4/613.full.pdf

My Notes

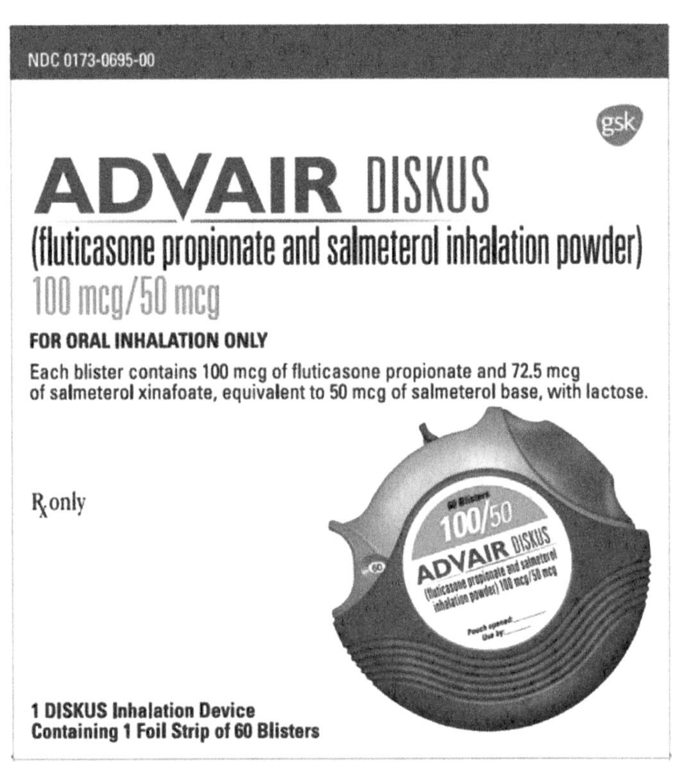

Figure 16.6 Advair Dry Powder Inhaler (DPI)

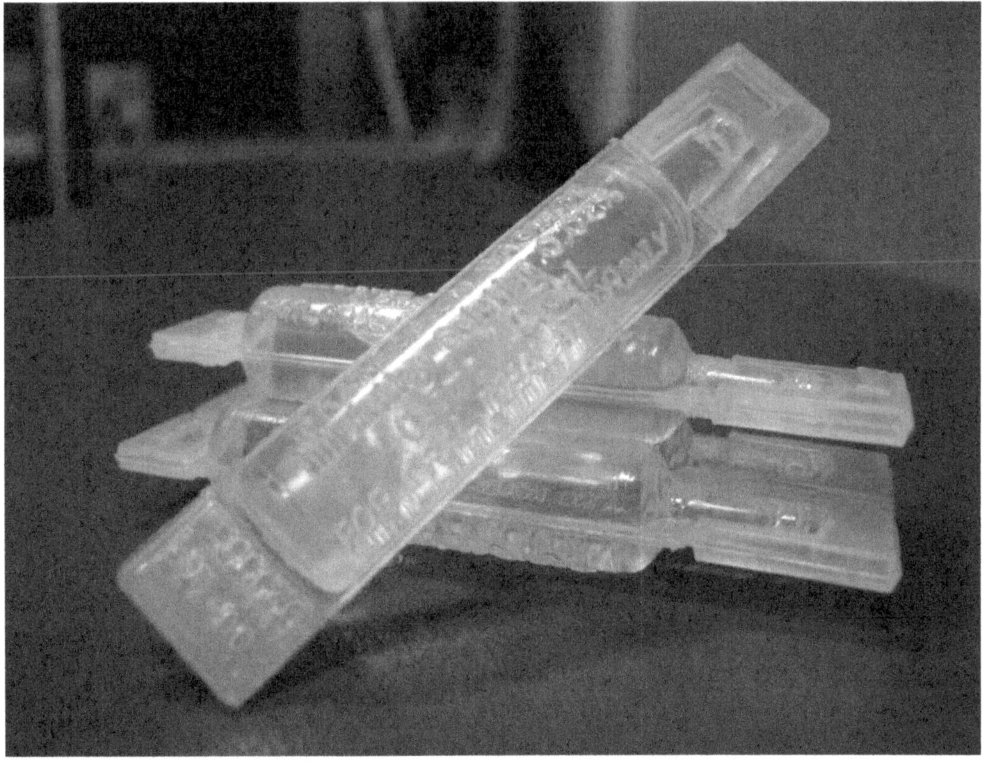

Figure 16.7 Medication for Nebulizer Inhalation

My Notes

Before administering an inhaler, the nurse should perform hand hygiene and check medication rights as with all medication. If the patient is self-administering the medication, advise them to wash their hands. The patient's respiratory system should be assessed and documented before and after the administration of inhaled medications, including assessment of respiratory rate, pulse oximetry, heart rate, and lung sounds.

When administering an MDI, the nurse should shake the inhaler and add a spacer onto the mouthpiece. The use of spacers with MDIs is considered best practice because they help ensure the medication is inhaled rather than inadvertently placed in the mouth. They also reduce waste by ensuring the patient receives the full amount of medication. The patient should be instructed to exhale while placing the spacer's mouthpiece into their mouth. The inhaler is depressed to move the aerosolized medication into the spacer, and the patient should breathe in normally through the spacer to receive the medication. If a spacer is not available, the patient should exhale and hold the inhaler mouthpiece about 1 to 2 inches away from their mouth to help ensure the medication is inhaled via the larynx and not sprayed onto the posterior pharynx. As the inhaler is depressed, the patient should inhale the medication deeply through their mouth and into their lungs. The patient should be advised to hold their breath for 5 to 10 seconds after inhaling the medication and then exhale through pursed lips. The patient should wait for 1 to 5 minutes between each puff of medication. When administering inhaled corticosteroids via MDI, the patient should rinse their mouth with water afterwards to prevent fungal infection.[12]

When using a DPI, the nurse should load the medication into the devices as required and then activate the inhaler per the manufacturer's guidelines. The patient should be instructed to exhale and then place their lips around the mouthpiece and inhale strongly and deeply. After they have inhaled, they should hold their breath for 10 seconds or as long as comfortable and then exhale through pursed lips. The patient should wait 1 to 5 minutes between puffs of medication. If the DPI contains a corticosteroid medication, the patient should gargle and rinse with tap water to decrease the risk of developing a fungal infection.

When using a small-volume nebulizer, the nurse pours the liquid medication into the medication cup of the nebulizer. When possible, the patient should be sitting or positioned in high Fowler's position to enhance deep breaths and absorption of medication. The bottom end of the tubing is attached to the oxygen flowmeter, and the flow rate should be set between 6-10 L/minute, based on the manufacturer's recommendations. The top end of the tubing is connected to either a nebulizer mask or mouthpiece. The patient should be instructed to inhale slowly through the device into their mouth and hold each breath for a slight pause before exhaling. Remain with the patient during the nebulizer treatment, which usually takes about 15 minutes. After treatment, the patient should be encouraged to cough and perform oral care. The patient's respiratory system should be reevaluated after the administration of inhaled medications to document therapeutic effects, as well as to monitor for adverse effects.[13]

Inhalers should be cleaned after use per the manufacturer's directions. Most MDI and DPI inhalers track how much medication is left in the canister. Patients should be advised to obtain refills of these medications before the inhaler runs out of doses.

---

12 Ari, A. & Restrepo, R. D. (2012). Aerosol delivery device selection for spontaneously breathing patients: 2012. *Respiratory Care, 57*(4), 613-626. http://rc.rcjournal.com/content/respcare/57/4/613.full.pdf

13 Gregory, K. L., Wilken, L., & Hart, M. K. (2017). *Pulmonary disease aerosol delivery devices: A guide for physicians, nurses, pharmacists, and other health care professionals* (3rd ed.). American Association for Respiratory Care. https://www.aarc.org/wp-content/uploads/2018/03/aersol-guides-for-hcp.pdf

My Notes

Video Review of Administering Inhaled Medication with a Spacer[14]

A video element has been excluded from this version of the text. You can watch it online here: https://wtcs.pressbooks.pub/nursingskills/?p=2727

14 ARISE. (2016). *Inhaler with spacer MVI_7500-ARISE.mp4*. [Video]. Licensed under CC BY 3.0. Access for free at https://www.youtube.com/watch?v=-qNySzIGHWQ&list=PLyzTdm5SU2AQNw4X2tOW8Nli-4hPv_u8c&index=5

My Notes

16.3 CHECKLIST FOR TRANSDERMAL, EYE, EAR, INHALATION, AND VAGINAL ROUTES MEDICATION ADMINISTRATION

Use the checklist below to review the steps for completion of "Transdermal, Eye, Ear, Inhalation, and Vaginal Routes for Medication Administration."

Steps

Disclaimer: Always review and follow agency policy regarding this specific skill.

Follow Steps 1 through 12 in 15.4 "Checklist for Oral Medication Administration."

13. A. Transdermal Patch:

- Perform hand hygiene and apply clean gloves
- Remove the old patch (if present).
- Clean the skin with mild soap and water. Dry the area completely.
- Assess the skin for any breaks or rashes. Do not use these areas.
- Apply a new patch wearing gloves. Rotate application site based on manufacturer recommendations. Be careful not to touch the medication surface.
- Press firmly to the patient's skin for about ten seconds.
- Date, time, and initial a piece of tape and place this next to the patch.
- Perform hand hygiene.

B. Eye Drops:

- Perform hand hygiene.
- Clean the eyes from the inner canthus to the outer canthus using water or normal saline.
- Tilt the patient's head back or have them lying supine with their head on a pillow.
- Remove the cap and keep inside sterile. Do not touch the dropper.
- Pull the lower conjunctival sac open.
- Squeeze the ordered drops into the conjunctival sac.
- Apply gentle pressure over the inner canthus.
- Repeat in the other eye if ordered.
- Perform hand hygiene.

C. Ear Drops:

- Perform hand hygiene.
- Clean the external ear of debris.
- Tilt the patient's head so the affected ear is uppermost.
- Remove the cap and keep inside sterile. Do not touch the dropper.
- Straighten the auditory canal properly for the age of the patient:
    - Adult: Pinna pulled up and back

My Notes

    - Child: Pinna pulled straight back
    - Infant and child under three: Pinna pulled back and down
- Squeeze the bottle and allow drop(s) to fall on the side of the auditory canal.
- Release the pinna and massage the tragus to help with movement of the drop into the canal.
- Keep the patient in a lying position with the affected ear up for 5 minutes.
- Repeat in the other ear if ordered.
- Perform hand hygiene.

D. Nose Spray:

- Perform hand hygiene.
- Have the patient blow their nose.
- Have the patient tilt their head back.
- Instruct the patient to inhale with administration if necessary.
- Close the opposite nare.
- Place a bottle or dropper in the affected nare.
- Squeeze the bottle or dropper and have the patient inhale.
- Keep the bottle or dropper compressed and remove from the nare.
- Instruct the patient to hold their breath for a few seconds and then breath out through the mouth.
- Repeat in other nare if ordered.
- Clean tip of bottle with tissue or cloth.
- Perform hand hygiene.

E. Vaginal Cream or Suppository:

- Have the patient void prior to medication administration.
- Position the patient on their back with their knees flexed.
- Perform perineal care. Dispose gloves and perform hand hygiene.
- Put on new gloves.
- Fill the vaginal applicator with the correct dose and lubricate the applicator, OR open the suppository and lubricate dominant index finger and suppository.
- With the nondominant hand spread the labia.
- Insert the applicator completely OR insert the suppository along the posterior vaginal wall.
- Instruct the patient to remain in supine position for 5-10 minutes.
- Perform hand hygiene.

F. Metered-Dose Inhaler (MDI):

- Perform hand hygiene.
- Shake the inhaler.

My Notes

- IF SPACER IS USED: Attach the inhaler opposite to the mouthpiece.
- Have the patient place the mouthpiece of the spacer into their mouth and grasp with teeth and seal lips around the mouthpiece.
- Push down on inhaler to release medication.
- Instruct the patient to inhale slowly and deeply through the mouthpiece of the spacer.
- IF NO SPACER USED: Patient should exhale out breath and hold the inhaler one to two inches from their mouth and inhale slowly and deeply as they push down on the inhaler to release the medication. The patient will then hold their breath for 5 to 10 seconds and release their breath through pursed lips. This can be repeated for a second puff after 1-5 minutes.
- Instruct the patient to rinse mouth after finishing with the inhaler.

G. Dry Powder Inhaler (DPI):

- Perform hand hygiene.
- Remove the mouthpiece cover and load the medication if necessary.
- Activate the inhaler per manufacturer directions.
- Have the patient exhale out slowly and completely.
- Instruct the patient to place the mouthpiece of the inhaler in their mouth and inhale deeply and forcefully for at least 2-3 seconds.
- Remind the patient to hold their breath for 10 seconds and then breath out through pursed lips.
- Instruct the patient to rinse mouth after finishing with the inhaler.

14. Assist the patient to a comfortable position, ask if they have any questions, and thank them for their time.
15. Ensure safety measures when leaving the room:
    - CALL LIGHT: Within reach
    - BED: Low and locked (in lowest position and brakes on)
    - SIDE RAILS: Secured
    - TABLE: Within reach
    - ROOM: Risk-free for falls (scan room and clear any obstacles)
16. Perform hand hygiene.
17. Document medication administration and related assessment findings. Report any concerns according to agency policy.

16.4 LEARNING ACTIVITIES

My Notes

Learning Activities

(Answers to "Learning Activities" can be found in the "Answer Key" at the end of the book. Answers to interactive activity elements will be provided within the elements as immediate feedback.)

1. You are caring for an elderly patient who is complaining of pain, severe nausea, and who has difficulty swallowing. In addition to intravenous medication administration, what route of medication delivery might be beneficial for this patient? Please provide rationale for your selection.
2. Which of the following transdermal medication administration actions are correct? (Select all that apply).
   a. The nurse may apply heat to all medication patches to help aid absorption of the medication.
   b. When placing a patch, the nurse should press the patch firmly to the skin to ensure adequate adherence.
   c. Gloves are required for patch application and removal.
   d. Transdermal patches may be placed directly into the trash.
   e. Date and location of patch application should be promptly documented in the medication administration record (MAR).

Check your knowledge with this flashcard learning activity:

An interactive or media element has been excluded from this version of the text. You can view it online here: https://wtcs.pressbooks.pub/nursingskills/?p=2739

Check your knowledge with these quiz questions:

An interactive or media element has been excluded from this version of the text. You can view it online here: https://wtcs.pressbooks.pub/nursingskills/?p=2739

My Notes

XVI GLOSSARY

Dry Powder Inhaler (DPI): An inhaler with medication provided in a powder form that is inhaled from the mouth into the lungs using a quick breath to activate the medication and move it into the lungs. An example of a DPI is tiotropium (Spiriva).

Innunction: A medication that is massaged or rubbed into the skin.

Metered Dose Inhaler (MDI): An inhaler that provides a mist of medication that is inhaled through the mouth into the lungs. An example of an MDI is albuterol. Optimal administration is achieved with a spacer attached to the inhaler.

Small-volume nebulizers: Devices that provide a fine mist using oxygen or compressed air to transport the medication from a nebulizer cup into the mouth and into the lungs as the patient breathes normally through a mask or pipe device.

Topical medications: Medications administered via the skin or mucous membranes for direct local action, as well as for systemic effects.

Transdermal route: Patches or disks applied to the skin that deliver medication over an extended period of time.

Chapter 17

Enteral Tube Management

17.1 ENTERAL TUBE MANAGEMENT INTRODUCTION

My Notes

Learning Objectives

- Administer enteral nutrition
- Perform irrigation and suctioning of enteral tubes
- Select appropriate equipment
- Explain the procedure to the patient
- Assess tube placement
- Implement measures to prevent displacement of tube
- Modify procedures to reflect variations across the life span
- Document actions and observations
- Recognize and report significant deviations from norms

Enteral tubes are tubes placed in the gastrointestinal tract. Enteral tubes are used as an alternate route for feeding and medication administration, as well as for stomach decompression. **Stomach decompression** is a medical term that refers to removing stomach contents by using suctioning. Stomach decompression is commonly used after surgery or trauma to reduce pressure from fluids and gas that cause pain, nausea, vomiting, and potential aspiration of stomach contents into the lungs.

The nurse's responsibilities when caring for a patient with an enteral tube include the following:

- assessing tube placement and patency
- assessing and cleansing the insertion site
- administering tube feeding
- administering medication
- irrigating/flushing the tube
- suctioning the tube
- monitoring for complications

Administering enteral medication is discussed in "Administration of Enteral Medications." The remaining responsibilities related to maintaining enteral tubes will be discussed in this chapter.

My Notes

17.2 BASIC CONCEPTS OF ENTERAL TUBES

Gastrointestinal Function

It is important to understand the anatomy and functioning of the gastrointestinal system before administering feedings or medications through an enteral tube. See Figure 17.1[1] for an illustration of the anatomy of the gastrointestinal system.

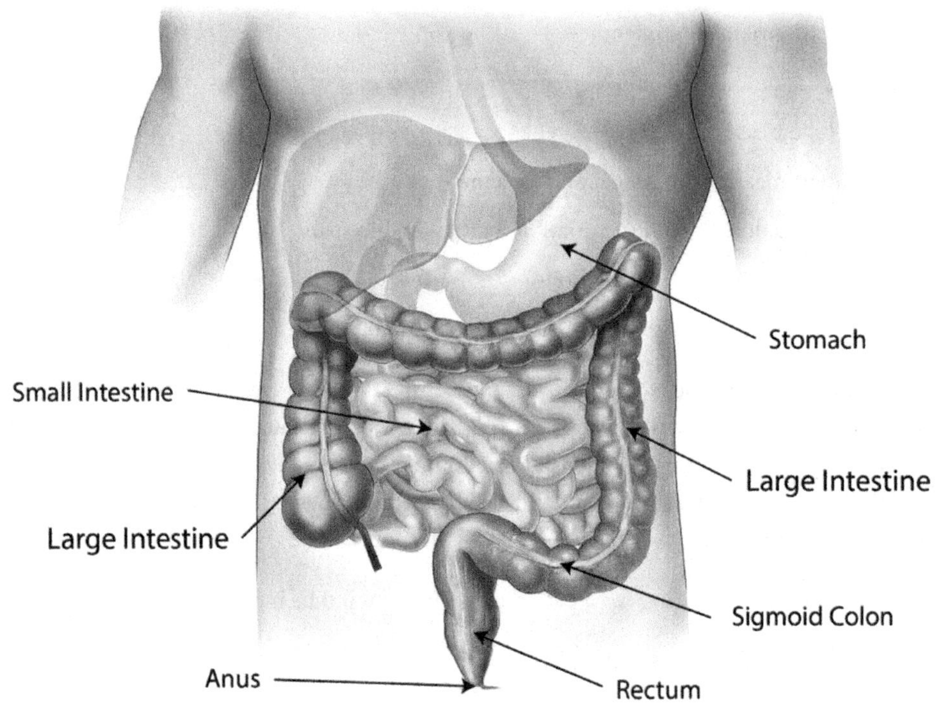

Figure 17.1 Anatomy of the Gastrointestinal System

For more information about the digestive function of the gastrointestinal system, visit the "Gastrointestinal System" chapter in Open RN *Nursing Pharmacology*.

Enteral Nutrition

Enteral nutrition is indicated for patients who need nutritional supplementation and have a functioning gastrointestinal tract, but cannot swallow food safely. Feedings can be administered via enteral tubes placed into the stomach or into the small intestine (usually the jejunum). For example, enteral feeding is commonly used for patients with the following conditions:

- Impaired swallowing (such as from a stroke or Parkinson's disease)

1 "abdomen-intestine-large-small-1698565" by bodymybody is licenced under CCO. Access for free at https://pixabay.com/illustrations/abdomen-intestine-large-small-1698565/

My Notes

- Decreased level of consciousness
- Respiratory distress requiring mechanical ventilation
- Oropharyngeal or esophageal obstruction (such as in head or neck cancer)
- Hypercatabolic states (such as in severe burns)[2]

For short-term feeding, NG tubes are used. If the duration of feeding is longer than four weeks or if access through the nose is contraindicated, a surgery is performed to place the tube directly through the gastrointestinal wall (for example, PEG or PEJ tubes).

Patients who are not candidates for enteral nutrition are prescribed parenteral nutrition. Parenteral nutrition is a concentrated intravenous solution containing glucose, amino acids, minerals, electrolytes, and vitamins. A lipid solution is typically administered as a separate infusion. This combination of solutions is called total parenteral nutrition because it supplies complete nutritional support. Parenteral nutrition is administered via a large central intravenous line, typically the subclavian or internal jugular vein, because it is irritating to the blood vessels.

Types of Enteral Tubes

There are several different types of enteral tubes based on their location in the gastrointestinal system, as well as their function. Three commonly used enteral tubes are the nasogastric tube, the percutaneous endoscopic gastrostomy (PEG) tube, and the percutaneous endoscopic jejunostomy (PEJ) tube. See Figure 17.2[3] for an illustration of common enteral tubes. NG tubes are typically used for a short period of time (less than four weeks), whereas PEG and PEJ tubes are inserted for long-term enteral nutrition. Some institutions also place nasoduodenal (ND) tubes to provide long-term enteral nutrition.[4]

---

2 Wireko, B. M., & Bowling, T. (2010). Enteral tube feeding. *Clinical Medicine, 10*(6), 616–619. https://doi.org/10.7861/clinmedicine.10-6-616

3 "Types and Placement of Enteral Tubes.png" by Meredith Pomietlo for Chippewa Valley Technical College is licensed under CC BY 4.0. Access for free at https://drive.google.com/file/d/1UC7HMzQXFR00MRM6h2Q_Ec96EadcV_o2/view?usp=sharing

4 Best, C. (2019). Selection and management of commonly used enteral feeding tubes. *Nursing Times, 15*(3), 43-47. https://www.nursingtimes.net/clinical-archive/nutrition/selection-and-management-of-commonly-used-enteral-feeding-tubes-18-02-2019/

My Notes

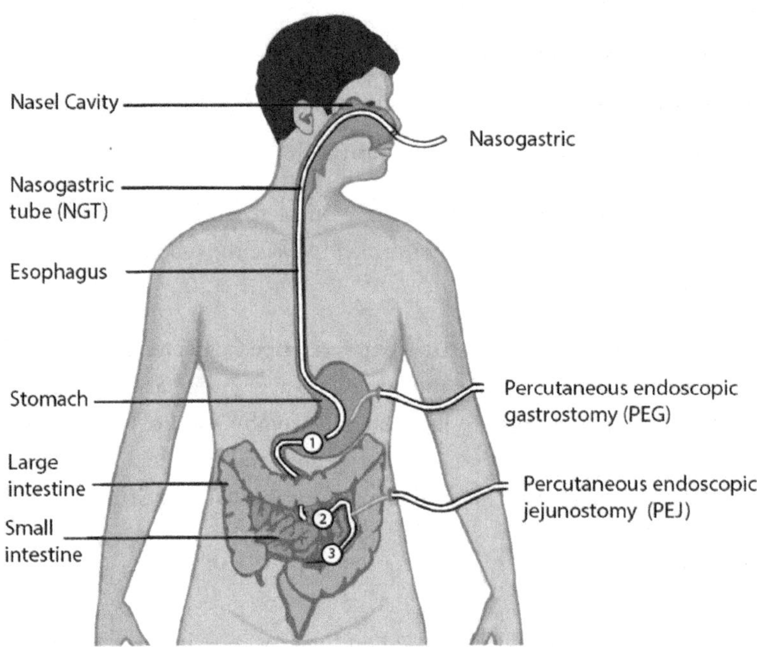

Figure 17.2 Types and Placement of Enteral Tubes

A nasogastric (NG) tube is a single- or double-lumen tube that is inserted into the nasopharynx through the esophagus and into the stomach. NG tubes can be used for feeding, medication administration, and suctioning. NG tubes used for feeding and medication administration are small and flexible, whereas NG tubes used for suctioning are larger and more rigid. NG tubes are secured externally on the patient's nose or cheek by adhesive tape or a fixation device, so this area should be assessed daily for signs of pressure damage. See Figure 17.3[5] for an image of a small bore feeding tube.

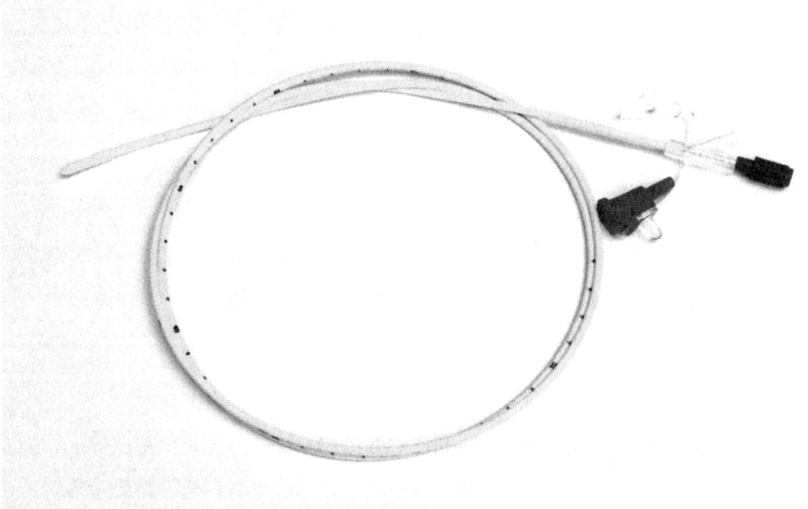

Figure 17.3 Small Bore NG Tube

5 "Enteral_feeding_tube_stylet_retracted.png" by *Tenbergen* is licensed under CC BY-SA 4.0. Access for free at https://commons.wikimedia.org/wiki/File:Enteral_feeding_tube_stylet_retracted.png

My Notes

An example of a large bore nasogastric tube is the Salem Sump. Large bore nasogastric tubes, such as the Salem Sump, are used for gastric decompression. The Salem Sump has a double lumen that includes a venting system. One lumen is used to empty the stomach, and the other lumen is used to provide a continuous flow of air. The continuous flow of air reduces negative pressure and prevents gastric mucosa from being drawn into the catheter, which causes mucosal damage. This terminal end also has an anti-reflux valve to prevent gastric secretions from traveling through the wrong lumen. See Figure 17.4[6] for an example of a double-lumen enteral tube.

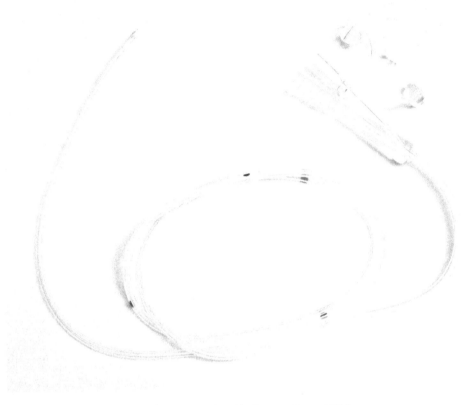

Figure 17.4 Double-Lumen Enteral Tube

Other types of tubes are placed through the patient's abdominal wall and are used for long-term enteral feeding. A percutaneous endoscopic gastrostomy (PEG) tube is placed via an endoscopic procedure into the stomach. Alternatively, a percutaneous endoscopic jejunostomy (PEJ) tube is placed in the jejunum of the small intestine for patients who cannot tolerate the administration of enteral formula or medications into the stomach due to medical conditions such as delayed gastric emptying. See Figure 17.5[7] for an image of a PEG tube insertion kit and the appearance of an enteral tube as it exits from a patient's abdomen.

6 "Silicone_dual_lumen_stomach_tube_with_plug_removed.png" by Tenbergen is licensed under CC BY-SA 4.0. Access for free at https://commons.wikimedia.org/wiki/File:Silicone_dual_lumen_stomach_tube_with_plug_removed.png

7 "PEG_tube_kit.jpg" by Gilo1969 and "Percutaneous_endoscopic_gastrostomy-tube.jpg" by Pflegewiki-User HoRaMi are licensed under CC BY-SA 3.0. Access for free at https://commons.wikimedia.org/wiki/File:PEG_tube_kit.jpg

My Notes

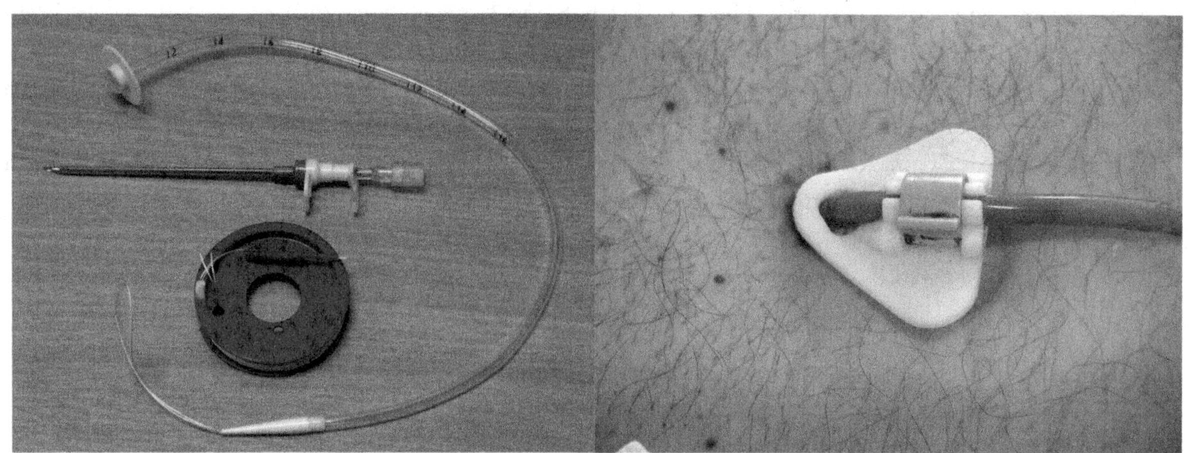

Figure 17.5 PEG Tube

Assessing Tube Placement

Feedings or medications administered into an incorrectly placed enteral tube result in life-threatening aspiration pneumonia. The placement of an enteral tube is immediately verified after insertion by an X-ray to ensure it has not been inadvertently placed into the trachea and down into the bronchi. See Figure 17.6[8] for an image of an X-ray demonstrating correct placement of an enteral tube in the stomach as indicated by the lower red arrow. (This X-ray also demonstrates an endotracheal tube correctly placed in the trachea as indicated by the top arrow.) After X-ray verification, the tube should be marked with adhesive tape and/or a permanent marker to indicate the point on the tube where the feeding tube enters the nares or penetrates the abdominal wall. This number on the tube at the entry point should be documented in the medical record and communicated during handoff reports. At the start of every shift, nurses evaluate if the incremental marking or external tube length has changed. If a change is observed, bedside tests such as visualization or pH testing of tube aspirate can help determine if the tube has become dislocated. If in doubt, a radiograph should be obtained to determine tube location.[9]

8 "ETTubeandNGtubeMarked.png" by James Heilman, MD is licensed under CC BY-SA 4.0. Access for free at https://commons.wikimedia.org/wiki/File:ETTubeandNGtubeMarked.png

9 Boullata, J. I., Carrera, A. L., Harvey, L., Escuro, A. A., Hudson, L., Mays, A., McGinnis, C., Wessel, J. J., Bajpai, S., Beebe, M. L., Kinn, T. J., Klang, M. G., Lord, L., Martin, K., Pompeii-Wolfe, C., Sullivan, J., Wood, A., Malone, A., & Guenter, P. (2017). ASPEN safe practices for enteral nutrition therapy. *Journal of Parenteral and Enteral Nutrition, 41*(1), 15-103. https://doi.org/10.1177/0148607116673053

My Notes

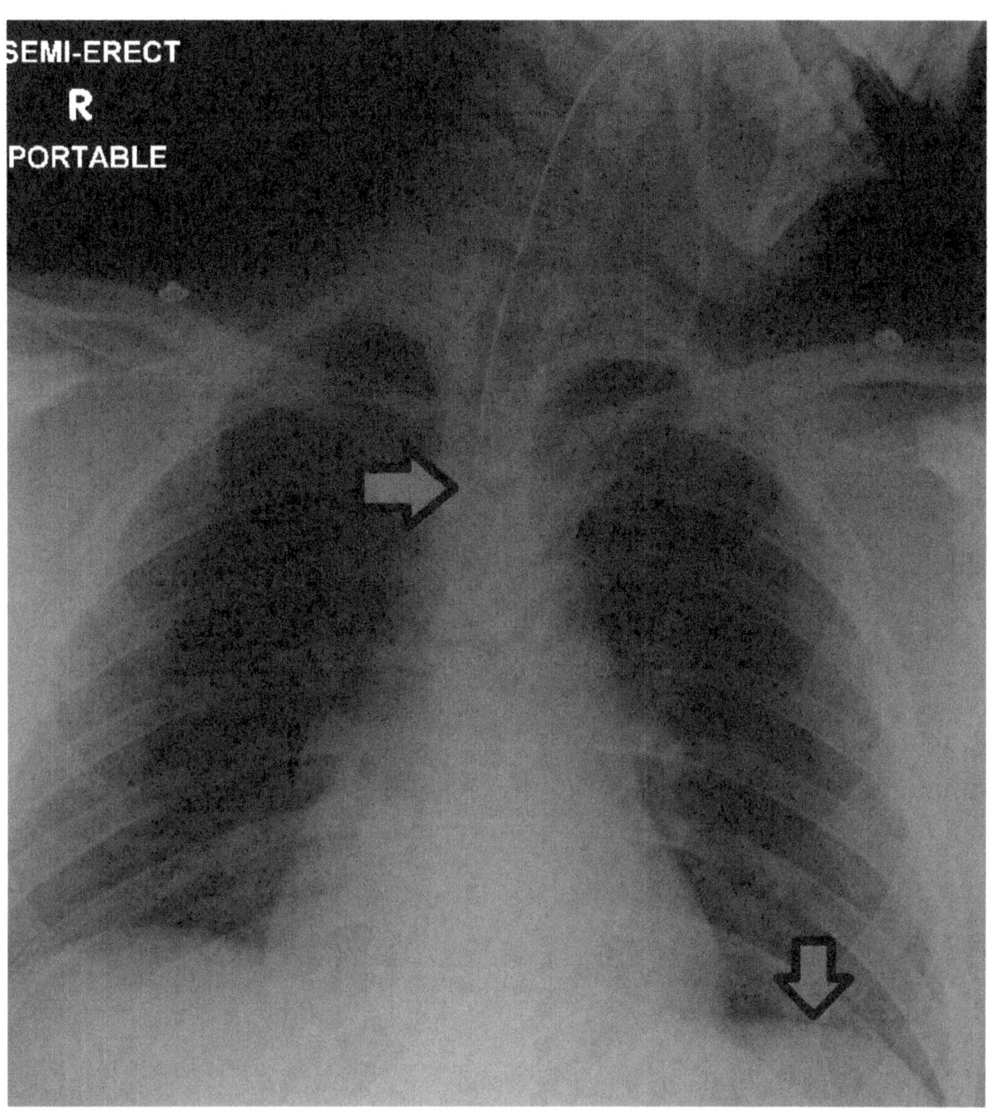

Figure 17.6 Placement Verification by X-Ray

After the initial verification of tube placement by X-ray, it is possible for the tube to migrate out of position due to the patient coughing, vomiting, and moving. For this reason, the nurse must routinely check tube placement before every use. The American Association of Critical-Care Nursing recommends that the position of a feeding tube should be checked and documented every four hours and prior to the administration of enteral feedings

My Notes

and medications by measuring the visible tube length and comparing it to the length documented during X-ray verification.[10, 11, 12]

Older methods of checking tube placement included observing aspirated GI contents or the administration of air with a syringe while auscultating (commonly referred to as the "whoosh test"). However, research has determined these methods are unreliable and should no longer be used to verify placement.[13, 14]

Checking the pH of aspirated gastric contents is an alternative method to verify placement that may be used in some agencies. Gastric aspirate should have a pH of less than or equal to 5.5 using pH indicator paper that is marked for use with human aspirate. However, caution should be used with this method because enteral formula and some medications alter the gastric pH.[15]

Follow agency policy for assessing and documenting tube placement. Additionally, if the patient develops respiratory symptoms that indicate potential aspiration, immediately notify the provider and withhold enteral feedings and medications until the placement is verified.

Assessing and Cleaning the Tube Insertion Site

The area of tube insertion should be assessed daily for signs of pressure damage. For NG tubes, the adhesive used to secure the tube can be irritating and cause skin breakdown. PEG and PEJ tubes may have fluid seepage around the insertion point that can cause skin breakdown if not cleaned regularly. Follow agency policy for cleansing the external insertion site for PEG and PEJ tubes. Cleansing is typically performed using gauze moistened with water or saline and then allowed to air dry before the fixation plate is repositioned. Because skin surrounding the insertion site is prone to breakdown, barrier cream or dressings may be prescribed to prevent breakdown.[16, 17]

---

10 Lemyze, M. (2010). The placement of nasogastric tubes. *CMAJ : Canadian Medical Association Journal*, *182*(8), 802. https://doi.org/10.1503/cmaj.091099

11 Simons, S. R., & Abdallah, L. M. (2012). Bedside assessment of enteral tube placement: Aligning practice with evidence. *American Journal of Nursing, 112*(2), 40-46. https://doi.org/10.1097/01.naj.0000411178.07179.68

12 Boullata, J. I., Carrera, A. L., Harvey, L., Escuro, A. A., Hudson, L., Mays, A., McGinnis, C., Wessel, J. J., Bajpai, S., Beebe, M. L., Kinn, T. J., Klang, M. G., Lord, L., Martin, K., Pompeii-Wolfe, C., Sullivan, J., Wood, A., Malone, A., & Guenter, P. (2017). ASPEN safe practices for enteral nutrition therapy. *Journal of Parenteral and Enteral Nutrition, 41*(1), 15-103. https://doi.org/10.1177/0148607116673053

13 Simons, S. R., & Abdallah, L. M. (2012). Bedside assessment of enteral tube placement: Aligning practice with evidence. *American Journal of Nursing, 112*(2), 40-46. https://doi.org/10.1097/01.naj.0000411178.07179.68

14 Boullata, J. I., Carrera, A. L., Harvey, L., Escuro, A. A., Hudson, L., Mays, A., McGinnis, C., Wessel, J. J., Bajpai, S., Beebe, M. L., Kinn, T. J., Klang, M. G., Lord, L., Martin, K., Pompeii-Wolfe, C., Sullivan, J., Wood, A., Malone, A., & Guenter, P. (2017). ASPEN safe practices for enteral nutrition therapy. *Journal of Parenteral and Enteral Nutrition, 41*(1), 15-103. https://doi.org/10.1177/0148607116673053

15 Best, C. (2019). Selection and management of commonly used enteral feeding tubes. *Nursing Times, 15*(3), 43-47. https://www.nursingtimes.net/clinical-archive/nutrition/selection-and-management-of-commonly-used-enteral-feeding-tubes-18-02-2019/

16 Blumenstein, I., Shastri, Y. M., & Stein, J. (2014). Gastroenteric tube feeding: Techniques, problems and solutions. *World Journal of Gastroenterology, 20*(26), 8505–8524. https://doi.org/10.3748/wjg.v20.i26.8505

17 Best, C.(2019). Selection and management of commonly used enteral feeding tubes. *Nursing Times, 15*(3), 43-47. https://www.nursingtimes.net/clinical-archive/nutrition/selection-and-management-of-commonly-used-enteral-feeding-tubes-18-02-2019/

Tube Feeding

My Notes

Enteral Nutrition (EN) refers to nutrition provided directly into the gastrointestinal (GI) tract through an enteral tube that bypasses the oral cavity. Each year in the United States, over 250,000 hospitalized patients from infants to older adults receive EN. It is also used widely in rehabilitation, long-term care, and home settings. EN requires a multidisciplinary team approach, including a registered dietician, health care provider, pharmacist, and bedside nurses. The registered dietician performs a nutrition assessment and determines what type of enteral nutrition is appropriate to promote improved patient outcomes. The health care provider writes the order for the enteral nutrition. Prescriptions for enteral nutrition should be reviewed by the nurse for the following components: type of enteral nutrition formula, amount and frequency of free water flushes, route of administration, administration method, and rate. Any concerns about the components of the prescription should be verified with the provider before tube feeding is administered.[18]

Tube feeding can be administered using gravity to provide a bolus feeding or via a pump to provide continuous or intermittent feeding. Feedings via a pump are set up in mL/hr, with the rate prescribed by the health care provider. See Figure 17.7[19] for an image of an enteral tube feeding pump and the associated tubing. Note that tubing used for enteral feeding is indicated by specific colors (such as purple in Figure 17.7). A global safety initiative, referred to as "EnFit," is in progress to ensure all devices used with enteral feeding, such as extension sets, syringes, PEG tubes, and NG tubes have specific EnFit ends that can only be used with tube feeding sets. This new safety design will avoid inadvertent administration of enteral feeding into intravenous tubing that can cause life-threatening adverse effects.

Review the "Checklist for NG Tube Enteral Feeding by Gravity with Irrigation" section for additional information regarding administering bolus feedings by gravity.

18 Boullata, J. I., Carrera, A. L., Harvey, L., Escuro, A. A., Hudson, L., Mays, A., McGinnis, C., Wessel, J. J., Bajpai, S., Beebe, M. L., Kinn, T. J., Klang, M. G., Lord, L., Martin, K., Pompeii-Wolfe, C., Sullivan, J., Wood, A., Malone, A., & Guenter, P. (2017). ASPEN safe practices for enteral nutrition therapy. *Journal of Parenteral and Enteral Nutrition, 41*(1), 15-103. https://doi.org/10.1177/0148607116673053

19 "Open_system_enteral_feeding.jpg" by *Ashashyou* is licensed under CC BY-SA 3.0. Access for free at https://commons.wikimedia.org/wiki/File:Open_system_enteral_feeding.jpg

My Notes

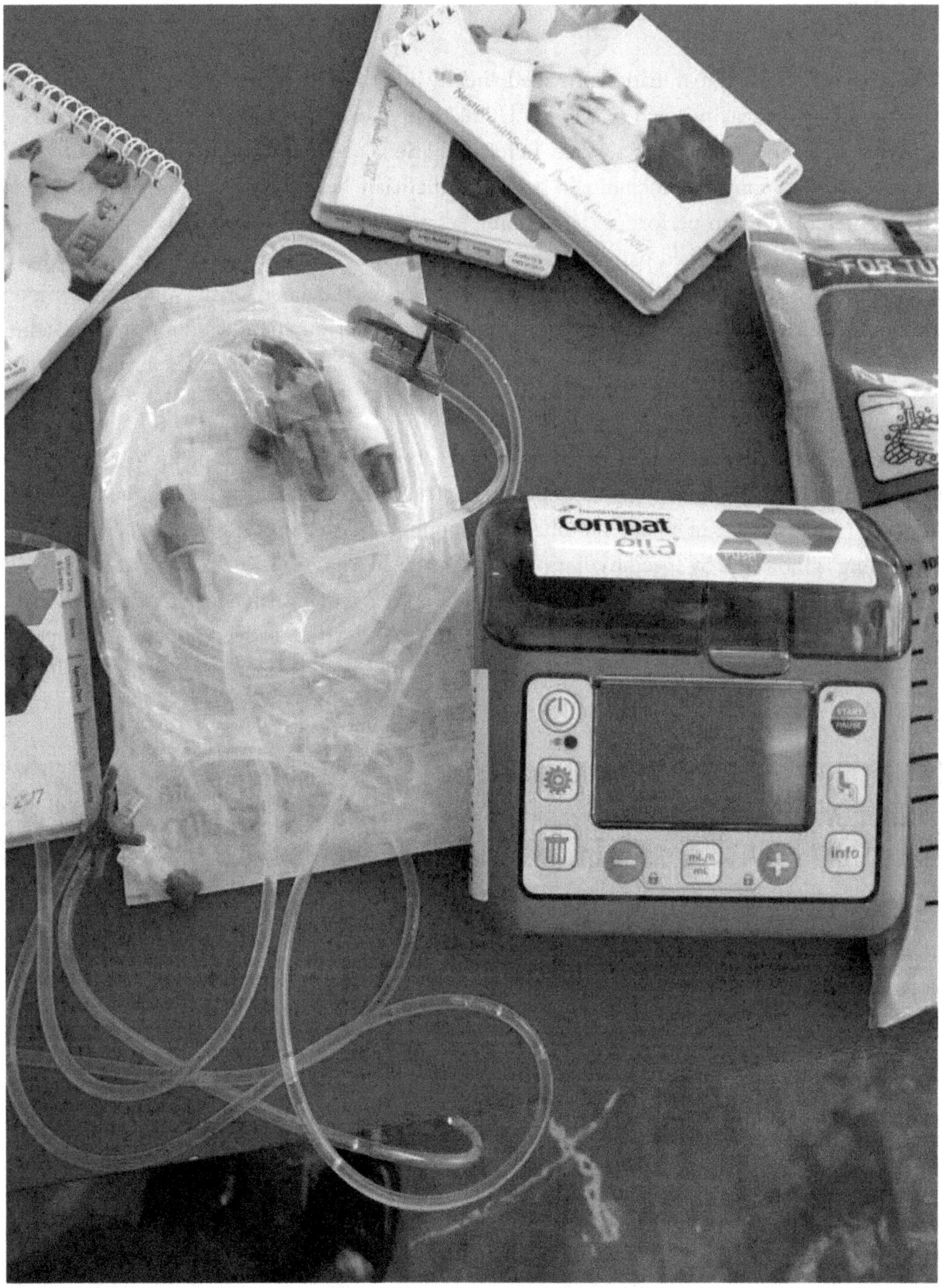

Figure 17.7 Enteral Feeding Pump and Tubing

Life Span Considerations

Enteral feeding is administered to infants and children via a syringe, gravity feeding set, or feeding pump. The method selected is dependent on the nature of the feeding and clinical status of the child.[20]

---

20 The Royal Children's Hospital Melbourne. (2017, December). *Enteral feeding and medication administration*. https://www.rch.org.au/rchcpg/hospital_clinical_guideline_index/Enteral_feeding_and_medication_administration/

Complications of Enteral Feeding

My Notes

The most serious complication of enteral feeding is inadvertent respiratory aspiration of gastric contents, causing life-threatening aspiration pneumonia. Other complications include tube clogging, tubing misconnections, and patient intolerance of enteral feeding.[21]

Reducing Risk of Aspiration

In addition to verifying tube placement as discussed in an earlier section, nurses perform additional interventions to prevent aspiration. The American Association of Critical-Care Nurses recommends the following guidelines to reduce the risk for aspiration:

- Maintain the head of the bed at 30°-45° unless contraindicated
- Use sedatives as sparingly as possible
- Assess feeding tube placement at four-hour intervals
- Observe for change in the amount of external length of the tube
- Assess for gastrointestinal intolerance at four-hour intervals[22]

Measurement of **gastric residual volume (GRV)** is performed by using a 60-mL syringe to aspirate stomach contents through the tube. It has traditionally been used to assess aspiration risk with associated interventions such as slowing or stopping the enteral feeding. GRVs in the range of 200–500 mL cause interventions such as slowing or stopping the feeding to reduce risk of aspiration. However, according to recent research, it is not appropriate to stop enteral nutrition for GRVs less than 500 mL in the absence of other signs of intolerance because of the impact on the patient's overall nutritional status. Additionally, the aspiration of gastric residual volumes can contribute to tube clogging.[23] Follow agency policy regarding measuring gastric residual volume and implementing interventions to prevent aspiration.

Managing Tube Clogging

Feeding tubes are prone to clogging for a variety of reasons. The risk of clogging may result from tube properties (such as narrow tube diameter), the tube tip location (stomach vs. small intestine), insufficient water flushes, aspiration for gastric residual volume (GRV), contaminated formula, and incorrect medication preparation and

---

21 Blumenstein, I., Shastri, Y. M., & Stein, J. (2014). Gastroenteric tube feeding: Techniques, problems and solutions. *World Journal of Gastroenterology, 20*(26), 8505–8524. https://doi.org/10.3748/wjg.v20.i26.8505

22 Boullata, J. I., Carrera, A. L., Harvey, L., Escuro, A. A., Hudson, L., Mays, A., McGinnis, C., Wessel, J. J., Bajpai, S., Beebe, M. L., Kinn, T. J., Klang, M. G., Lord, L., Martin, K., Pompeii-Wolfe, C., Sullivan, J., Wood, A., Malone, A., & Guenter, P. (2017). ASPEN safe practices for enteral nutrition therapy. *Journal of Parenteral and Enteral Nutrition, 41*(1), 15-103. https://doi.org/10.1177/0148607116673053

23 Boullata, J. I., Carrera, A. L., Harvey, L., Escuro, A. A., Hudson, L., Mays, A., McGinnis, C., Wessel, J. J., Bajpai, S., Beebe, M. L., Kinn, T. J., Klang, M. G., Lord, L., Martin, K., Pompeii-Wolfe, C., Sullivan, J., Wood, A., Malone, A., & Guenter, P. (2017). ASPEN safe practices for enteral nutrition therapy. *Journal of Parenteral and Enteral Nutrition, 41*(1), 15-103. https://doi.org/10.1177/0148607116673053

My Notes

administration. A clogged feeding tube can result in decreased nutrient delivery or delayed administration of medication, and, if not corrected, the patient may require additional surgical intervention to replace the tube.[24]

Research supports using water as the best choice for initial declogging efforts. Instill warm water into the tube using a 60-mL syringe, and apply a gentle back-and-forth motion with the plunger of the syringe. Research shows that the use of cranberry juice and carbonated beverages to flush the tube can worsen tube occlusions because the acidic pH of these fluids can cause proteins in the enteral formula to precipitate within the tube. If water does not work, a pancreatic enzyme solution, an enzymatic declogging kit, or mechanical devices for clearing feeding tubes are the best second-line options.[25]

To prevent enteral tubes from clogging, it is important to follow these guidelines:

- Flush feeding tubes at a minimum of once a shift.
- Flush feeding tubes immediately before and after intermittent feedings. During continuous feedings, flush at standardized, scheduled intervals.
- Flush feeding tubes before and after medication administration and follow appropriate medication administration practices.
- Limit gastric residual volume checks because the acidic gastric contents may cause protein in enteral formulas to precipitate within the lumen of the tube.[26]

Preventing Tubing Misconnections

In April 2006, The Joint Commission issued a Sentinel Event Alert on tubing misconnections due to enteral feedings being inadvertently infused into intravenous lines with life-threatening results. A color-coded enteral tubing connection design was developed to visually communicate the difference between enteral tubing and intravenous tubing. In addition to tubing design, follow these guidelines to prevent tubing misconnection errors:

- Make tubing connections under proper lighting.
- Do not modify or adapt IV or feeding devices because doing so may compromise the safety features incorporated into their design.

---

24 Boullata, J. I., Carrera, A. L., Harvey, L., Escuro, A. A., Hudson, L., Mays, A., McGinnis, C., Wessel, J. J., Bajpai, S., Beebe, M. L., Kinn, T. J., Klang, M. G., Lord, L., Martin, K., Pompeii-Wolfe, C., Sullivan, J., Wood, A., Malone, A., & Guenter, P. (2017). ASPEN safe practices for enteral nutrition therapy. *Journal of Parenteral and Enteral Nutrition, 41*(1), 15-103. https://doi.org/10.1177/0148607116673053

25 Boullata, J. I., Carrera, A. L., Harvey, L., Escuro, A. A., Hudson, L., Mays, A., McGinnis, C., Wessel, J. J., Bajpai, S., Beebe, M. L., Kinn, T. J., Klang, M. G., Lord, L., Martin, K., Pompeii-Wolfe, C., Sullivan, J., Wood, A., Malone, A., & Guenter, P. (2017). ASPEN safe practices for enteral nutrition therapy. *Journal of Parenteral and Enteral Nutrition, 41*(1), 15-103. https://doi.org/10.1177/0148607116673053

26 Boullata, J. I., Carrera, A. L., Harvey, L., Escuro, A. A., Hudson, L., Mays, A., McGinnis, C., Wessel, J. J., Bajpai, S., Beebe, M. L., Kinn, T. J., Klang, M. G., Lord, L., Martin, K., Pompeii-Wolfe, C., Sullivan, J., Wood, A., Malone, A., & Guenter, P. (2017). ASPEN safe practices for enteral nutrition therapy. *Journal of Parenteral and Enteral Nutrition, 41*(1), 15-103. https://doi.org/10.1177/0148607116673053

- When making a reconnection, routinely trace lines back to their origins and then ensure that they are secure.
- As part of a hand-off process, recheck connections and trace all tubes back to their origins.[27]

Managing Intolerances and Imbalances

Patients should be monitored daily for signs of tube feeding intolerance, such as abdominal bloating, nausea, vomiting, diarrhea, cramping, and constipation. If cramping occurs during bolus feedings, it can be helpful to administer the enteral nutritional formula at room temperature to prevent symptoms.[28] Notify the provider of signs of intolerance with anticipated changes in the prescription regarding the type of formula or the rate of administration. Electrolytes and blood glucose levels should also be monitored, as ordered, for signs of imbalances.[29, 30]

Tube Irrigation

Enteral tubes are routinely flushed to maintain patency. Follow agency policy when flushing a tube. Typically, tap water and a 60-mL syringe are used to flush enteral tubes.[31] See Figure 17.8[32] for an image of a nurse irrigating an NG tube.

The steps for irrigating enteral tubes are typically the following:

- Draw the required amount of water into the 60-mL syringe and dispel excess air.
- If the tube has a clamp, close it.
- Open the distal end of the tube and connect the syringe.
- Open the clamp.
- Administer the water.
- Close the clamp.

---

27 Boullata, J. I., Carrera, A. L., Harvey, L., Escuro, A. A., Hudson, L., Mays, A., McGinnis, C., Wessel, J. J., Bajpai, S., Beebe, M. L., Kinn, T. J., Klang, M. G., Lord, L., Martin, K., Pompeii-Wolfe, C., Sullivan, J., Wood, A., Malone, A., & Guenter, P. (2017). ASPEN safe practices for enteral nutrition therapy. *Journal of Parenteral and Enteral Nutrition, 41*(1), 15-103. https://doi.org/10.1177/0148607116673053

28 The Royal Children's Hospital Melbourne. (2017, December). Enteral feeding and medication administration. https://www.rch.org.au/rchcpg/hospital_clinical_guideline_index/Enteral_feeding_and_medication_administration/

29 Blumenstein, I., Shastri, Y. M., & Stein, J. (2014). Gastroenteric tube feeding: Techniques, problems and solutions. *World Journal of Gastroenterology, 20*(26), 8505–8524. https://doi.org/10.3748/wjg.v20.i26.8505

30 Boullata, J. I., Carrera, A. L., Harvey, L., Escuro, A. A., Hudson, L., Mays, A., McGinnis, C., Wessel, J. J., Bajpai, S., Beebe, M. L., Kinn, T. J., Klang, M. G., Lord, L., Martin, K., Pompeii-Wolfe, C., Sullivan, J., Wood, A., Malone, A., & Guenter, P. (2017). ASPEN safe practices for enteral nutrition therapy. *Journal of Parenteral and Enteral Nutrition, 41*(1), 15-103. https://doi.org/10.1177/0148607116673053

31 Best, C. (2019). Selection and management of commonly used enteral feeding tubes. *Nursing Times, 15(*3), 43-47. https://www.nursingtimes.net/clinical-archive/nutrition/selection-and-management-of-commonly-used-enteral-feeding-tubes-18-02-2019/

32 "DSC_1667.jpg" by British Columbia Institute of Technology is licensed under CC BY 4.0. Access for free at https://opentextbc.ca/clinicalskills/chapter/10-2-nasogastric-tubes

My Notes

- Remove the syringe and refill it with water if indicated.
- Repeat as needed to obtain the desired flushing volume.
- Once completed, remove the syringe, close the tube cap, and reopen the clamp.[33]

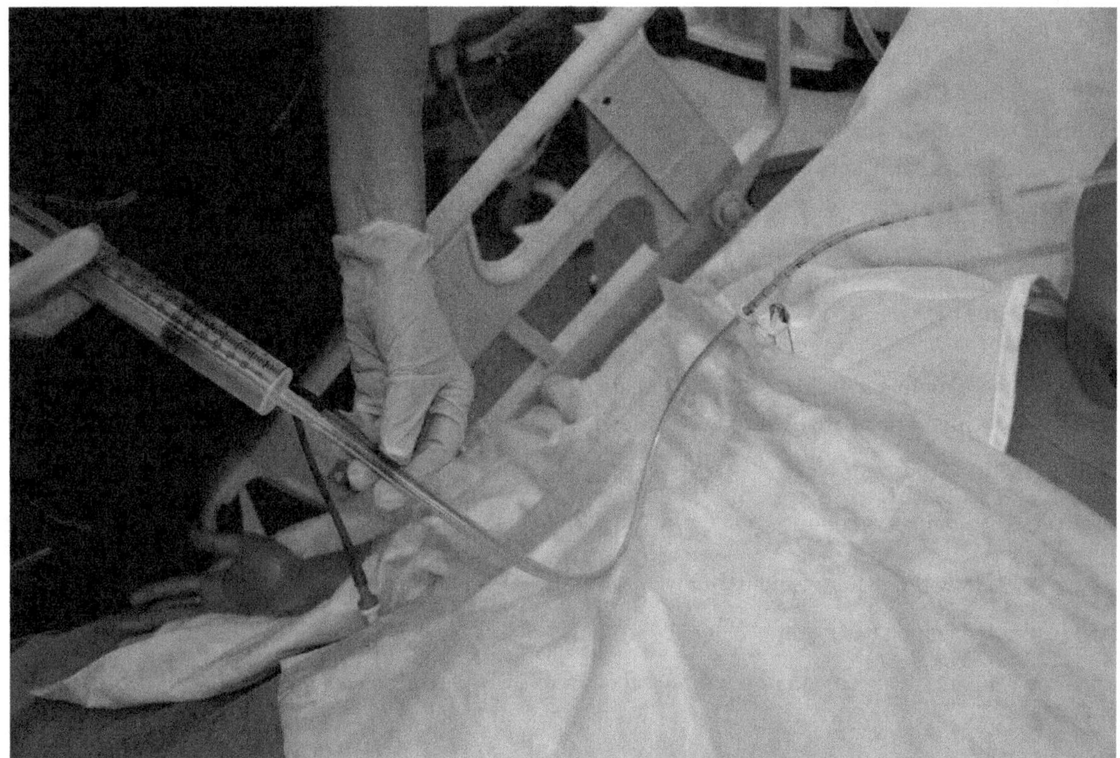

Figure 17.8 Irrigating an NG Tube

Tube Suctioning

NG tubes may be used to remove gastric content, referred to as gastric decompression. In these situations, the stomach is drained by gravity or by connection to a suction pump to prevent nausea, vomiting, gastric distension, or to wash the stomach of toxins. This procedure is commonly used for post-operative patients who have not yet regained peristalsis or for patients with a small bowel obstruction to remove the accumulation of stomach bile. It is also used in the emergency department for patients with some types of poisonings or overdoses and is commonly referred to as "pumping out the stomach."

For patients receiving suctioning via enteral tubes, the drainage amount and color should be documented every shift.

33 Best, C. (2019). Selection and management of commonly used enteral feeding tubes. *Nursing Times, 15*(3), 43-47. https://www.nursingtimes.net/clinical-archive/nutrition/selection-and-management-of-commonly-used-enteral-feeding-tubes-18-02-2019/

17.3 ASSESSMENTS RELATED TO ENTERAL TUBES

My Notes

When caring for patients with enteral tubes, it is important for the nurse to routinely assess and document the patient's condition.

Subjective Assessment

When a patient is receiving enteral feeding, the nurse should assess the patient's tolerance of tube feeding.

Table 17.3 Focused Interview Questions for Tube Feeding

Interview Questions	Follow-up
How long have you been receiving tube feeding?	Tell me more about why you are receiving tube feeding and how you feel about the tube feeding. (Patients may experience psychosocial reactions to receiving tube feeding that can be addressed with therapeutic communication.)
Are you experiencing symptoms of stomach cramping, nausea, vomiting, excess gas, diarrhea, or constipation?	Please describe.
Are you experiencing any discomfort where the tube is inserted?	Please describe.
Have you noticed any coughing or respiratory symptoms after receiving tube feeding?	Please describe.

Objective Assessment

Objective assessments for patients with enteral tubes include assessing skin integrity, tube placement, gastrointestinal function, and for signs of complications:

- Assess the tube insertion site daily for signs of pressure injury and skin breakdown. Cleanse and protect the area as indicated.
- Assess tube placement every four hours and prior to administration of feedings or medications according agency policy. Verify the visible tube length and compare it to the length documented after X-ray verification.
- Trace the tubing from the insertion site to prevent tubing misconnections.
- Assess the abdomen. If tube suctioning is in place, the suction should be turned off prior to auscultation. Bowel sounds should be present in all four quadrants, and the abdomen should be soft and nondistended.
- Monitor the patient's weight and overall nutritional status in collaboration with the multidisciplinary team.
- Monitor serum electrolytes and blood glucose as indicated.

My Notes

17.4 SAMPLE DOCUMENTATION

Sample Documentation of Expected Findings

Tube Feeding

Patient's abdomen is soft, nondistended, and bowel sounds are present in all four quadrants. Head of the bed elevated to 45 degrees. Placement of tube verified with measurement of the tube at the nares at 55 cm and gastric aspirate had a pH 4. Patient tolerated 240 mL of tube feeding by gravity followed by a 30-mL water flush.

Tube Irrigation

Irrigated NG tube with 30 mL of water with no resistance. Patient tolerated flush without symptoms.

Tube Suctioning

NG tube connected to low-intermittent suction (LIS) at 60 mmHg. Output from the NGT is green with a volume of 100 mLs in eight hours.

Sample Documentation of Unexpected Findings

Tube Feeding

Patient's abdomen is soft, nondistended, and bowel sounds are present in all four quadrants. Head of the bed elevated to 45 degrees. Placement of tube verified with measurements of tube at nares at 55 cm and gastric aspirate with a pH of 4. After 100 mLs of tube feeding was infused, the patient complained of feeling full and nauseated. Tube feeding infusion stopped and the head of the bed maintained at a 45-degree angle. Will reassess gastric volume residual in one hour and determine if tube feeding will be resumed.

Tube Irrigation

Attempted to irrigate NG tube with 30 mLs of water, but resistance was felt with procedure. Unable to inject water flush into the NGT. Dr. Smith notified of findings at 1320.

Tube Suctioning

Patient's abdomen is slightly distended and bowel sounds are hypoactive in all four quadrants. Patient reports increased nausea over the last two hours. NGT connected to low-intermittent suction (LIS) at 60 mmHg. Output from the NGT is mahogany colored with a volume of 800 mLs in eight hours. Dr. Smith notified of findings at 1640.

17.5 CHECKLIST FOR NG TUBE ENTERAL FEEDING BY GRAVITY WITH IRRIGATION

My Notes

Use the checklist below to review the steps for completion of the "NG Tube Enteral Feeding by Gravity with Irrigation."

Steps

Disclaimer: Always review and follow agency policy regarding this specific skill.

1. Verify the provider's order.
2. Gather supplies: stethoscope, gloves, towel, irrigating solution (usually water), and irrigation set with irrigating syringe, pH tape, and prescribed tube feeding.
3. Perform safety steps:
   - Perform hand hygiene.
   - Check the room for transmission-based precautions.
   - Introduce yourself, your role, the purpose of your visit, and an estimate of the time it will take.
   - Confirm patient ID using two patient identifiers (e.g., name and date of birth).
   - Explain the process to the patient and ask if they have any questions.
   - Be organized and systematic.
   - Use appropriate listening and questioning skills.
   - Listen and attend to patient cues.
   - Ensure the patient's privacy and dignity.
   - Assess ABCs.
4. Don the appropriate PPE as indicated.
5. Perform abdominal and nasogastric tube assessment:
   - Assess skin integrity on the nose and ensure the tube is securely attached.
   - Use a flashlight to look in the nares to assess swelling, redness, or bleeding.
   - Ask the patient to open their mouth and look for curling of the tube in the patient's mouth. The tube should go straight down into the esophagus.
   - Lower the blankets and move the gown up to expose the abdomen. Inspect from two locations.
   - Auscultate bowel sounds and then palpate the abdomen. If the patient is receiving NG suctioning, turn off the suction prior to auscultation.
6. Check for tube placement:
   - Verify tube measurement at insertion site based on documentation.

My Notes

- If agency policy dictates, test the pH of the aspirate. The pH should be equal or less than 5.5.
- If agency policy dictates, measure and document residual amount. Instill residual back into gastric tube if placement was confirmed.

7. Draw up 30 mL of water in a 60-mL syringe. (If applicable, use sterile water according to agency policy.)
8. Connect the syringe to the tubing port (not the blue pigtail).
9. Instill 30 mL water.
10. Reconnect the plug tube or clamp tube.
11. Remove the plunger from the syringe and attach the syringe to the NG tube.
12. Complete tube feeding administration:
    - Verify the order for the type of formula, amount, method of administration, and rate.
    - Check the expiration date on the formula.
    - Verify if the tops of the containers need cleaning or if feeding needs mixing/shaking.
    - Add the formula to the syringe until the ordered amount is administered. Hold the syringe above the insertion site and allow it to enter via gravity.
    - Assess the patient for tolerance of the feeding. Slow infusion as necessary. Do not allow air to enter the tube when refilling the syringe.
    - After formula is administered, flush the NG tube with 30 mL of water.
    - If a patient is unable to tolerate the feeding, slow or stop the infusion. Document and report the intolerance.
13. Disconnect the syringe and plug the NG tube.
14. Maintain the patient at or above a 30-degree angle for a minimum of one hour to prevent aspiration. Ask the patient if they have any questions and thank them for their time.
15. Perform hand hygiene.
16. Ensure safety measures when leaving the room:
    - CALL LIGHT: Within reach
    - BED: Low and locked (in lowest position and brakes on)
    - SIDE RAILS: Secured
    - TABLE: Within reach
    - ROOM: Risk-free for falls (scan room and clear any obstacles)
17. Document assessment findings and report any concerns according to agency policy. When documenting the procedure, include the following:
    - Time performed
    - Irrigation solution used
    - Quantity instilled

My Notes

- Residual amount, color, odor, and consistency
- Method for checking the placement (including pH of gastric contents, if performed)
- Related assessments
- Amount of tube feeding
- Patient tolerance for the procedure

My Notes

17.6 CHECKLIST FOR NG SUCTION

Use the checklist below to review the steps for completion of the "NG Suction."

Steps

Disclaimer: Always review and follow agency policy regarding this specific skill.

1. Verify the provider's order.
2. Gather supplies: nonsterile gloves.
3. Perform safety steps:
    - Perform hand hygiene.
    - Check the room for transmission-based precautions.
    - Introduce yourself, your role, the purpose of your visit, and an estimate of the time it will take.
    - Confirm patient ID using two patient identifiers (e.g., name and date of birth).
    - Explain the process to the patient and ask if they have any questions.
    - Be organized and systematic.
    - Use appropriate listening and questioning skills.
    - Listen and attend to patient cues.
    - Ensure the patient's privacy and dignity.
    - Assess ABCs.
4. Don the appropriate PPE as indicated.
5. Perform abdominal and nasogastric tube assessment:
    - Assess skin integrity on the nose and ensure the tube is securely attached.
    - Use a flashlight to look in the nares to assess swelling, redness, or bleeding.
    - Ask the patient to open their mouth and look for curling of the tube in the patient's mouth. The tube should go straight down into the esophagus.
    - Lower the blankets and move the gown up to expose the abdomen. Inspect from two locations.
    - Auscultate bowel sounds and then palpate the abdomen.

    Rationale: Performing a nasogastric and abdominal assessment is important for determining signs of complications such as skin breakdown and necessity for suction.
6. Don gloves.
7. Attach the NG tube to the suction canister.
8. Set the rate of suction according to provider order:

My Notes

- Low intermittent suction is usually ordered. Low range on the suction device is from 0 to 80 mmHg. Starting between 40-60 mmHg is recommended. The suction level should not exceed 80 mmHg.
- Observe for the gastric content to flow into the tubing and then the canister.

9. Monitor canister output and document color, odor, consistency, and amount.
10. Perform hand hygiene.
11. Ensure safety measures when leaving the room:
    - CALL LIGHT: Within reach
    - BED: Low and locked (in lowest position and brakes on)
    - SIDE RAILS: Secured
    - TABLE: Within reach
    - ROOM: Risk-free for falls (scan room and clear any obstacles)
12. Document the procedure and related assessment findings. Report any concerns according to agency policy.

My Notes

17.7 LEARNING ACTIVITIES

Learning Activities

(Answers to "Learning Activities" can be found in the "Answer Key" at the end of the book. Answers to interactive activity elements will be provided within the element as immediate feedback.)

1. As you are administering tube feeding to your patient, they complain of feeling full. What is the next step to take?
    a. Continue with administering the tube feeding.
    b. Stop the tube feeding and check the gastric residual.
    c. Stop the tube feeding and waste the remaining feeding.
    d. Slow or stop the infusion based on the patient's response.

Video Review of Tube Feeding Calculations[1]

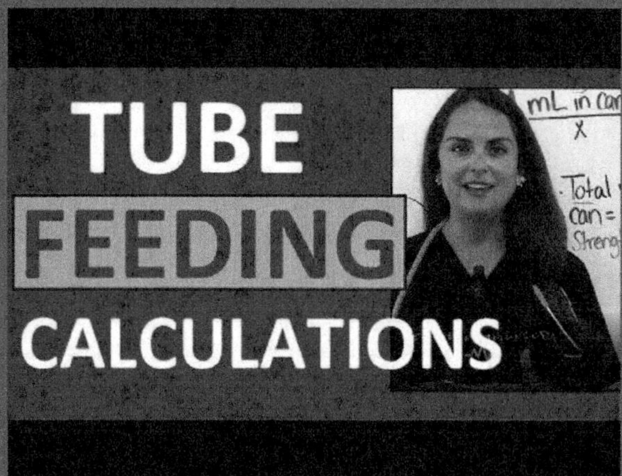

 A YouTube element has been excluded from this version of the text. You can view it online here: https://wtcs.pressbooks.pub/nursingskills/?p=3031

Interactive Activity

 An interactive or media element has been excluded from this version of the text. You can view it online here: https://wtcs.pressbooks.pub/nursingskills/?p=3031

1 RegisteredNurseRN. (2020, May 18). *Tube feeding nursing calculations problems dilution enteral.* [Video]. YouTube. All rights reserved. Video used with permission. https://youtu.be/CwfJ-sQ-xOQ

My Notes

Interactive Activity

An interactive or media element has been excluded from this version of the text. You can view it online here: https://wtcs.pressbooks.pub/nursingskills/?p=3031

Interactive Activity

An interactive or media element has been excluded from this version of the text. You can view it online here: https://wtcs.pressbooks.pub/nursingskills/?p=3031

My Notes

XVII GLOSSARY

Enteral Nutrition (EN): Nutrition provided directly into the gastrointestinal (GI) tract through an enteral tube that bypasses the oral cavity.

Gastric Residual Volume (GRV): Stomach contents aspirated with a 60-mL syringe, typically performed for patients receiving enteral feeding to assess aspiration risk with associated interventions such as slowing or stopping tube feeding. GRVs in the range of 200–500 mL should raise concern and lead to the implementation of measures to reduce risk of aspiration.

Stomach Decompression: Using suctioning through a nasogastric tube to remove the contents of the stomach.

Chapter 18

Administration of Parenteral Medications

18.1 ADMINISTRATION OF PARENTERAL MEDICATIONS INTRODUCTION

My Notes

Learning Objectives

- Safely administer medication via the intradermal, subcutaneous, and intramuscular routes
- Maintain aseptic technique
- Select appropriate equipment
- Calculate correct amount of medication to administer
- Correctly select site using anatomical landmarks
- Modify procedure to reflect variations across the life span
- Document actions and observations
- Recognize and report significant deviations from norms

Administering medication by the parenteral route is defined as medications placed into the tissues and the circulatory system by injection. There are several reasons why medications may be prescribed via the parenteral route. Medications administered parenterally are absorbed more quickly compared to oral ingestion, meaning they have a faster onset of action. Because they do not undergo digestive processes in the gastrointestinal tract, they are metabolized differently, resulting in a stronger effect than oral medications. The parenteral route may also be prescribed when patients are nauseated or unable to swallow.

Although an injectable medication has many benefits, there are additional safety precautions the nurse must take during administration because an injection is considered an invasive procedure. Injections cause a break in the protective barrier of the skin, and some are administered directly into the bloodstream so there is increased risk of infection and rapid development of life-threatening adverse reactions.

There are four potential routes of parenteral injections, including intradermal (IM), subcutaneous (SQ), intramuscular (IM), and intravenous (IV). An **intradermal** injection is administered in the dermis just below the epidermis. A **subcutaneous** injection is administered into adipose tissue under the dermis. An **intramuscular** injection is administered into a muscle. **Intravenous** medications are injected directly into the bloodstream. Administering medication via the intravenous (IV) route is discussed in the "IV Therapy Management" chapter. This chapter will describe several evidence-based guidelines for safe administration of parenteral medications.

My Notes

18.2 BASIC CONCEPTS

Syringes

Syringes are used to administer parenteral medications. A disposable syringe is a sterile device that is available in various sizes ranging from 0.5 mL to 60 mL. A syringe consists of a plunger, a barrel, and a needle hub. Syringes may be supplied individually or with a needle and protective cover attached. See Figure 18.1[1] for an illustration of the parts of a syringe.

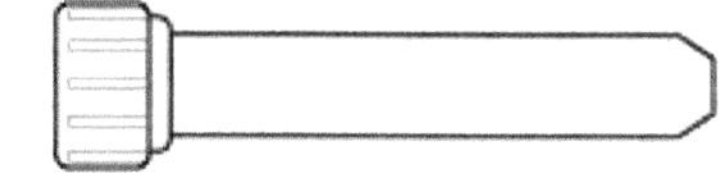

Disposable syringe and needle (parts labelled)

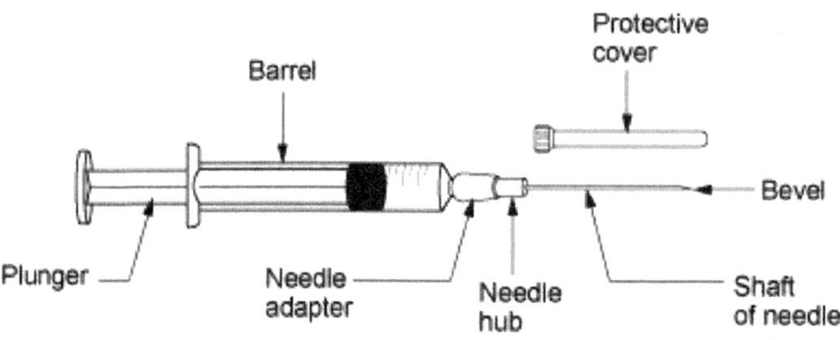

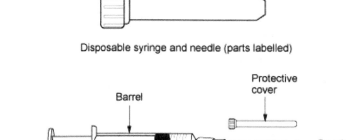

Figure 18.1 Parts of a Syringe

Luer lock syringes have threads in the needle hub that provide a secure connection of needles, tubing, or other devices. See Figure 18.2[2] for an image of a Luer lock syringe with a barrel and a readable scale. This image shows a syringe that holds 12 cc, also referred to as 12 mL. When withdrawing medication, match up the top of the plunger and the line on the barrel scale with the amount of medication you need to administer. In this image, 3 mL of medication is contained in the syringe.

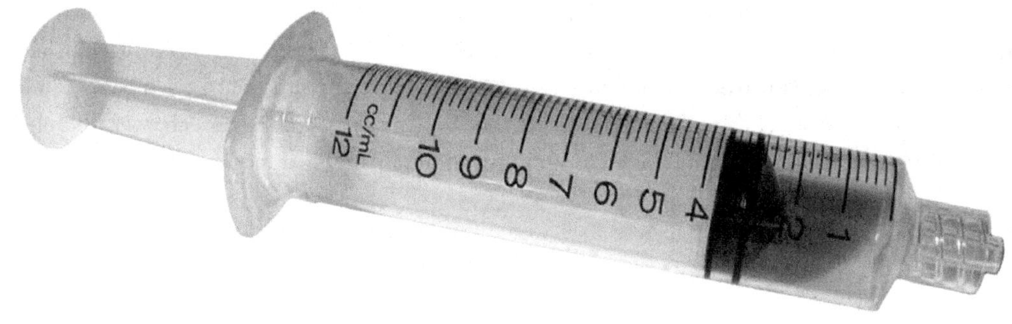

Figure 18.2 Luer Lock Syringe

1 "Labeled syringe.png" by British Columbia Institute of Technology is licensed under CC BY 4.0. https://opentextbc.ca/clinicalskills/chapter/safe-injection-administration-and-preparing-medication-from-ampules-and-vials/

2 "Syringe.jpg" by Erich Schulz, Brisbane is in the Public Domain. Access for free at https://commons.wikimedia.org/wiki/File:Syringe.jpg

My Notes

Video Review of How to Read a Syringe[3]

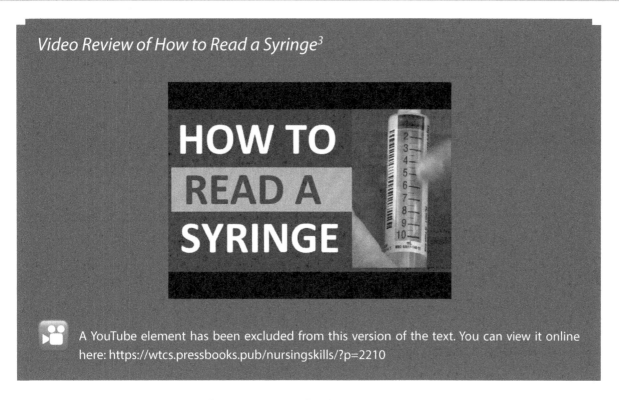

A YouTube element has been excluded from this version of the text. You can view it online here: https://wtcs.pressbooks.pub/nursingskills/?p=2210

Insulin is administered using a specific insulin syringe. Insulin syringes are marked in units, not milliliters (mL), because insulin is prescribed by providers in units, not mLs. A regular syringe marked in milliliters should never be used to administer insulin. All insulin syringes have orange caps for quick identification, but verify the markings are in units to prevent a medication error. See Figure 18.3[4] for an image of a 50-unit insulin syringe with a white safety shield attached.

3 RegisteredNurseRN. (2017, June 12). *How to read a syringe 3 ml, 1 ml, insulin, & 5 ml/cc | Reading a syringe plunger.* [Video]. YouTube. All rights reserved. Video used with permission. https://youtu.be/_TnDr8cKums

4 "Insulin Syringe 3I3A0783.jpg" by Deanna Hoyord, for Chippewa Valley Technical College is licensed under CC BY 4.0. Access for free at https://drive.google.com/file/d/1aL5h5h4J1E7BKP5gJz_103536Jtxest_/view?usp=sharing

My Notes

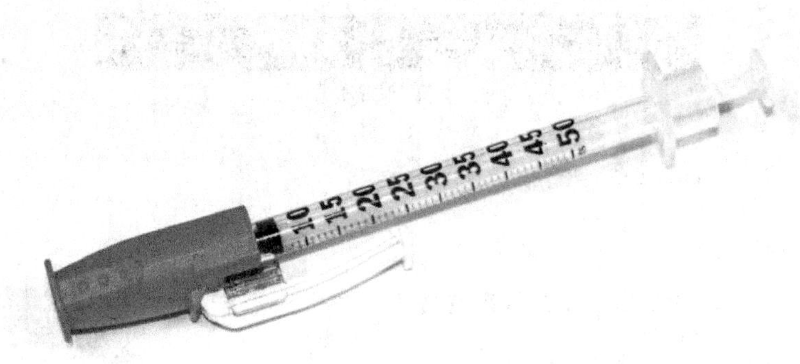

Figure 18.3 Insulin Syringe

Needles

Needles are made out of stainless steel. They are sterile and disposable and are available in various lengths and sizes. A needle is made up of the hub, shaft, and bevel. The hub fits onto the tip of the syringe. All three parts must remain sterile at all times. The bevel is the tip of the needle that is slanted to create a slit into the skin. See Figure 18.4[5] for an image of a bevel.

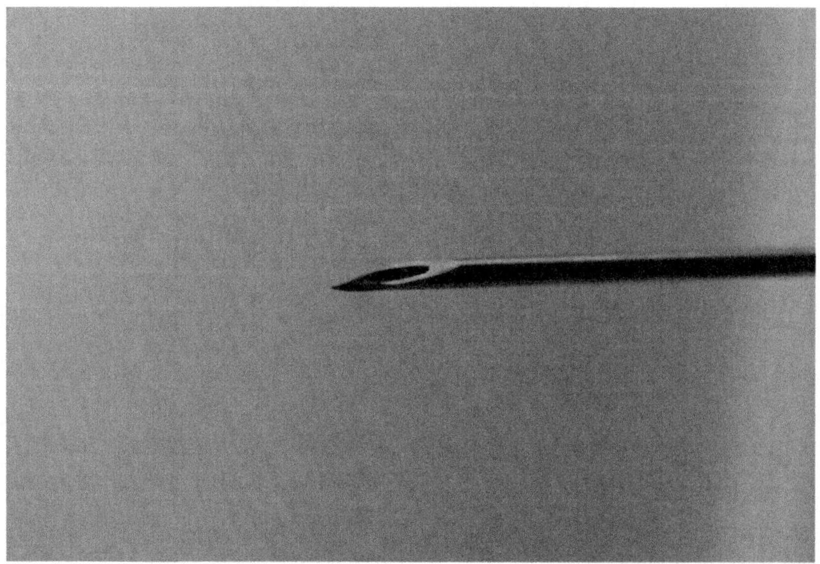

Figure 18.4 Bevel of a Needle

5 "Beveled tip of a hypodermic needle 20090714 005.JPG" by Politikaner is licensed under CC BY-SA 3.0. Access for free at https://commons.wikimedia.org/wiki/File:Beveled_tip_of_a_hypodermic_needle_20090714_005.JPG

Gauge and Length

My Notes

The **gauge** of a needle refers to its diameter. Needles range in various sized gauges from small diameter (25 to 29 gauge) to large diameter (18 to 22 gauge). Note that the larger the diameter of a needle, the smaller the gauge number. Larger diameter needles (18-22 gauge) are typically used to administer thicker medications or blood products. See Figure 18.5[6] for an image comparing various needle lengths and gauges. Read more about needle gauges according to type of injection in Table 18.2 in the "Anatomic Location" subsection.

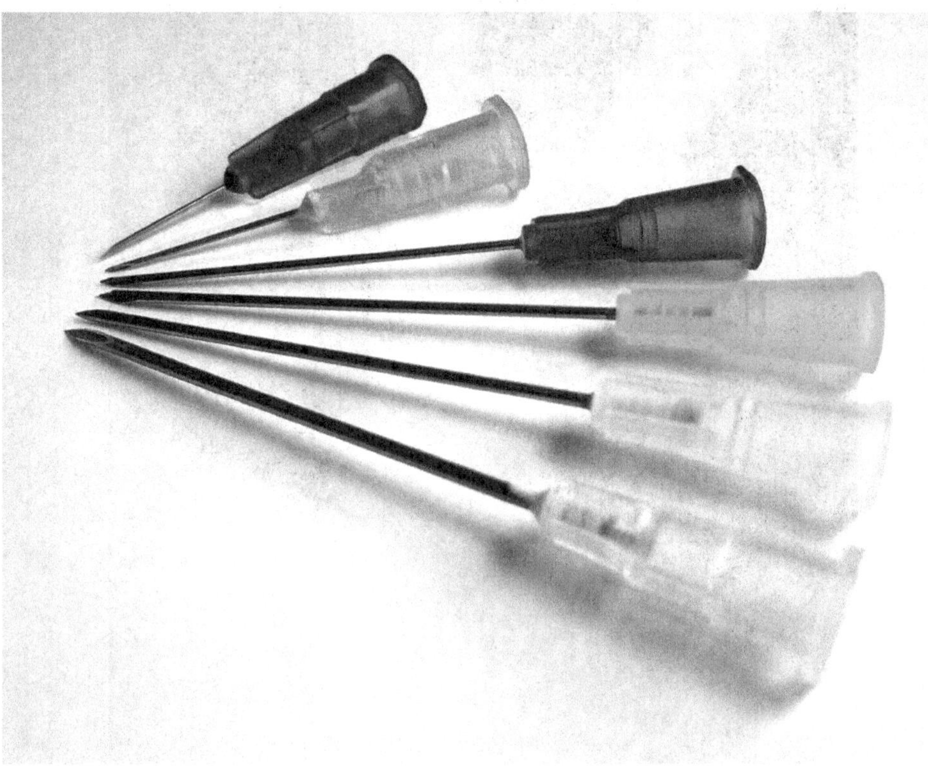

Figure 18.5 Needle Lengths and Gauges

Gauge and length are marked on the outer packaging of needles. Needle length varies from 1/8 inches to 3 inches and is selected based on the type of injection. Nurses select the appropriate gauge and length according to the medication ordered, the anatomical location selected, and the patient's body mass and age. For example, an intramuscular injection requires a longer needle to reach muscle tissue than an intradermal injection that is inserted just under the epidermis. Read more about needle length according to type of injection in Table 18.2 in the "Anatomic Location" section.

Many needles have safety shields attached to prevent needlestick injuries. See Figure 18.6[7] for an image of a syringe inserted into a vial of medication with a needle and a type of safety shield attached.

---

6 "HypodermicNeedles.jpg" by Zephyris is licensed under CC BY-SA 3.0. Access for free at https://commons.wikimedia.org/wiki/File:HypodermicNeedles.jpg

7 "Book-pictures-2015-527.jpg" by British Columbia Institute of Technology is licensed under CC BY 4.0. Access for free at https://opentextbc.ca/clinicalskills/chapter/safe-injection-administration-and-preparing-medication-from-ampules-and-vials/

My Notes

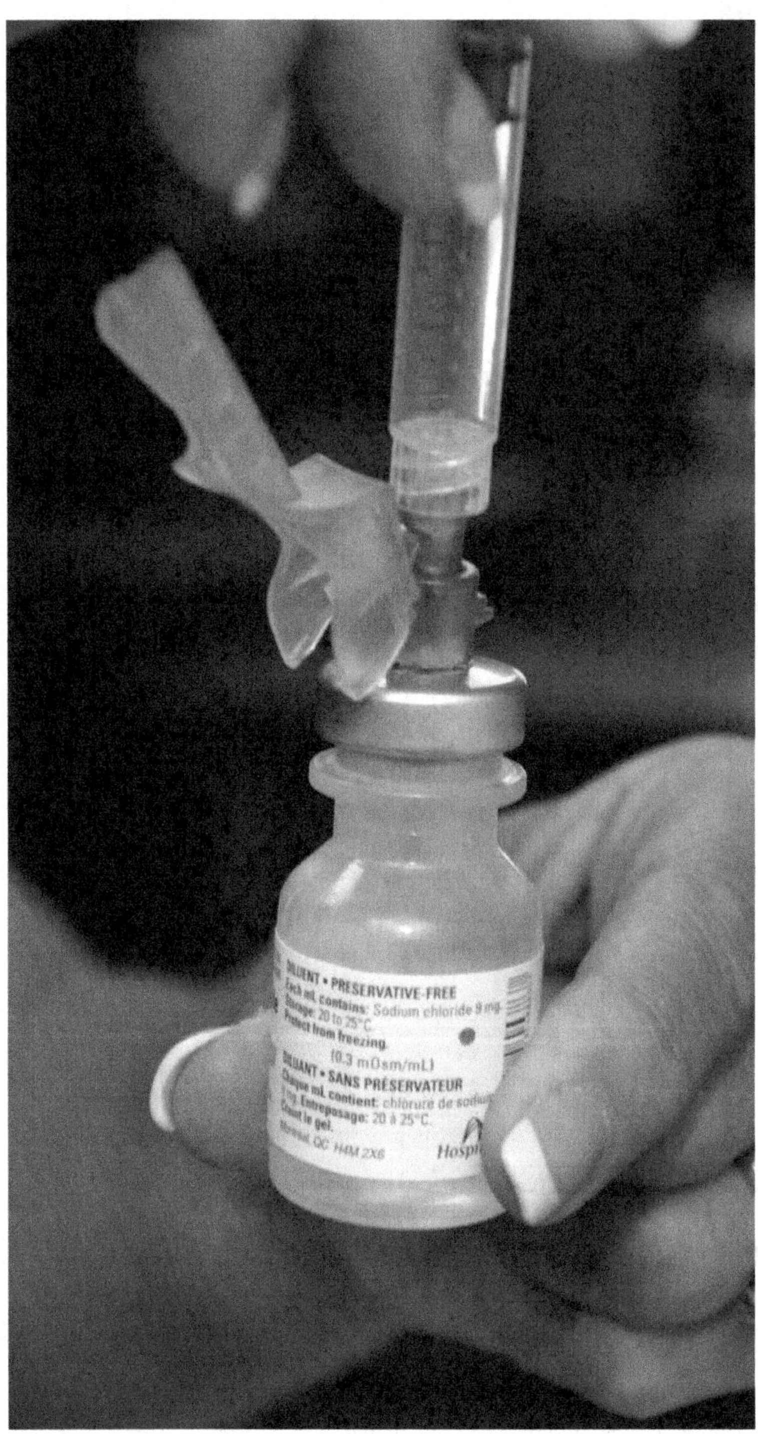

Figure 18.6 Safety Shield on Needle

Needle Insertion Angle and Removal

When administering an injection, the syringe should be held like a dart to prevent inadvertent release of medication as the needle is inserted. The needle should be inserted at the proper angle depending on the type of injection. See Table 18.2 for additional details regarding angles of insertion for each type of injection. The needle should be

My Notes

inserted all the way to the hub smoothly and quickly to reduce discomfort of the injection. See Figure 18.7[8] for an illustration of angles of insertion for each type of injection. After the needle is inserted, it is important to hold the syringe steady to prevent tissue damage. The needle should be removed at the same angle used for insertion.[9]

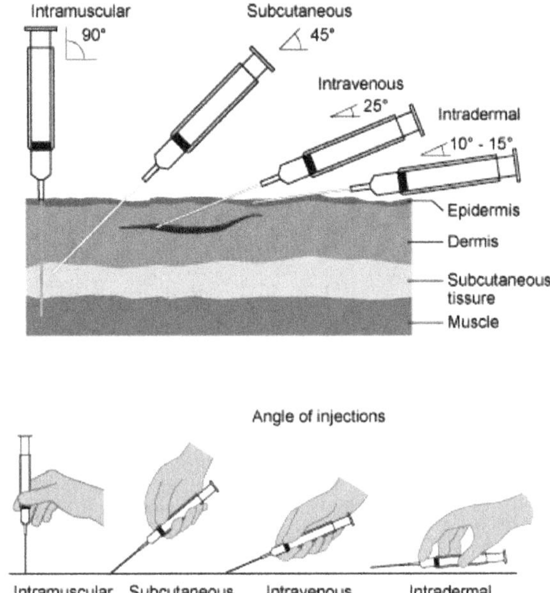

Figure 18.7 Angles of Insertion

Anatomical Location

It is important for the nurse to select the correct anatomical location for parenteral medication administration according to the type of injection prescribed and for optimal absorption of the medications. Injection of medication into the correct location also prevents injury to the tissues, nerves, blood vessels, and bones. Table 18.2 summarizes anatomical locations, needle sizes, amount of fluid, and the degree of angle of the needle insertion for each type of parenteral injection with life span and other considerations provided. Additional details regarding each type of injection are discussed later in this chapter.

---

8 "Needle-insertion-angles-1.png" by British Columbia Institute of Technology is licensed under CC BY 4.0. Access for free at https://opentextbc.ca/clinicalskills/chapter/safe-injection-administration-and-preparing-medication-from-ampules-and-vials/

9 This work is a derivative of Clinical Procedures for Safer Patient Care by British Columbia Institute of Technology and is licensed under CC BY 4.0. Access for free at https://opentextbc.ca/clinicalskills/

My Notes

Table 18.2 Summarized Injection Information

Injection Types	Anatomic Locations	Needle Gauge and Length	Total Amount of Injectable Fluid	Degree of Angle When Injecting	Considerations
Intradermal	■ Upper third of the forearm ■ Outer aspects upper arms ■ Between scapula	■ 25-27G ■ 3/8" to 5/8"	0.1 mL	5-15 degree	The forearm is the recommended site for tuberculosis (TB) testing for all ages. Allergy testing may be performed between the scapulae. Older adults have decreased skin elasticity, so the skin should be held taut to ensure the medication is administered properly.
Subcutaneous	■ Outer upper arms ■ Anterior thighs ■ Upper outer gluteal area ■ Upper back ■ Abdomen	■ 25-31G ■ 1/2" to 5/8"	Up to 1 mL Up to 0.5 mL in infants and small children	45-90 degree	The older patient's skin is less elastic, and subcutaneous tissue may be reduced in the skinfolds. The upper abdomen should be used for patients with less subcutaneous tissue.

My Notes

Injection Types	Anatomic Locations	Needle Gauge and Length	Total Amount of Injectable Fluid	Degree of Angle When Injecting	Considerations
Intramus-cular	■ Ventrogluteal ■ Vastus lateralis ■ Deltoid	■ 18 to 25G ■ 1/2" to 1 1/2" (based on age/ size of patient and site used)	0.5-1 mL (infants and children) 2-5 mL (adults)	90 degree	The vastus lateralis site is preferred for infants because that muscle is most developed. The ventrogluteal site is recom-mended in adults. The deltoid site is recommended for vaccinations in adults.

Preparing Medications

Ampules

Parenteral medications are supplied in sterile vials, ampules, and prefilled syringes. **Ampules** are small glass containers containing liquid medication ranging from 1 mL to 10 mL sizes. They have a scored neck to indicate where to break the ampule. See Figure 18.8[10] for an image of an ampule of epinephrine.

---

10 "Epinephrine 1-1000 (1).JPG" by *Intropin* is licensed under CC BY 3.0. Access for free at https://commons.wikimedia.org/wiki/File:Epinephrine_1-1000_(1).JPG

My Notes

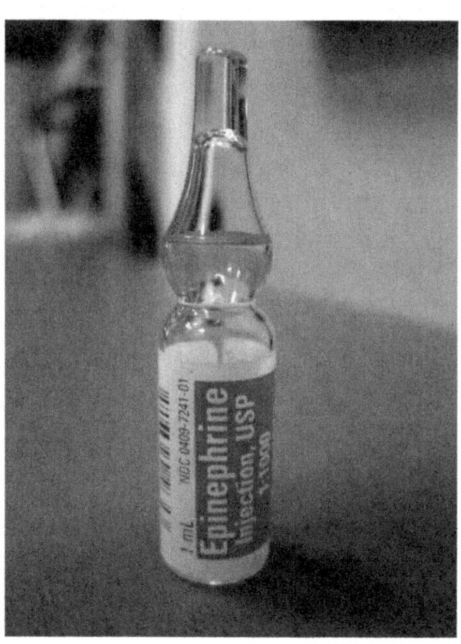

Figure 18.8 Ampule of Epinephrine

Medication is withdrawn from an ampule using a syringe with a special needle called a blunt fill filter needle. These needles have a blunt end to prevent needlestick injuries and a filter to prevent glass particles from being drawn up into the syringe. See Figure 18.9[11] for an image of a blunt fill filter needle. Filter needles should never be used to inject medication into a patient. The filter needle should be removed and replaced with a needle appropriate in size and gauge for the type of injection and the anatomical location of the patient.

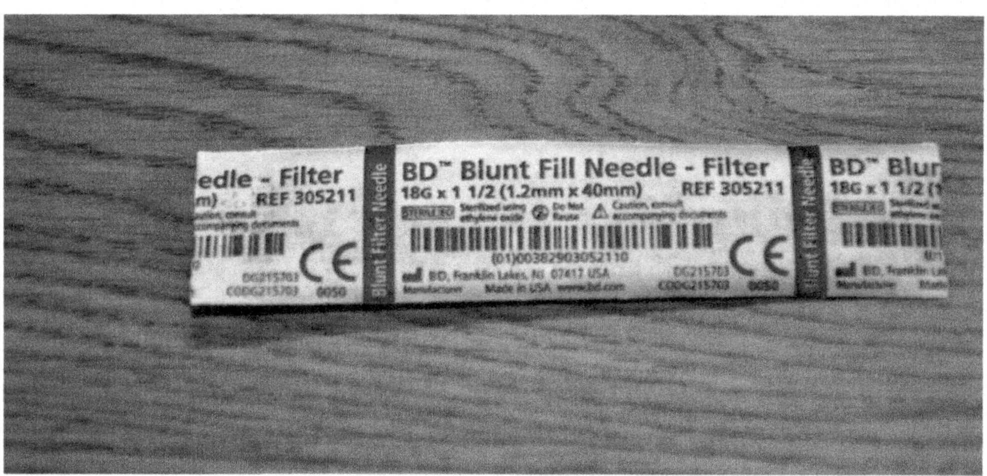

Figure 18.9 Blunt Fill Filter Needle

11 "Oct-2-2015-009.jpg" by British Columbia Institute of Technology is licensed under CC BY 4.0. Access for free at https://opentextbc.ca/clinicalskills/chapter/safe-injection-administration-and-preparing-medication-from-ampules-and-vials/

My Notes

When breaking open an ampule, it is important to use appropriate steps to avoid injury. First, tap the ampule while holding it upright to move fluid down out of the neck. Place a piece of gauze around the neck, and then snap the neck away from your hands. See Figure 18.10[12] for an illustration of how to safely open an ampule.

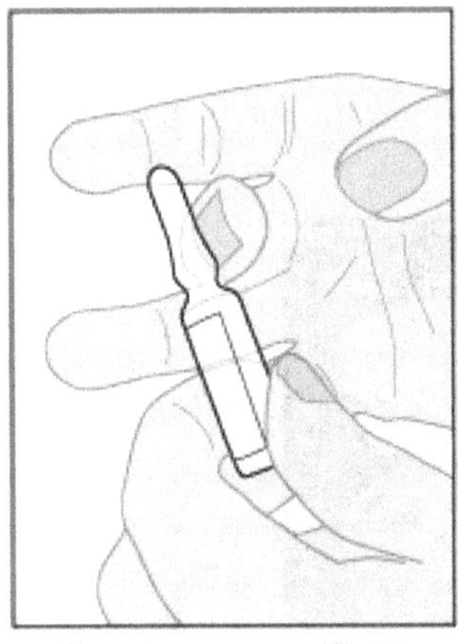

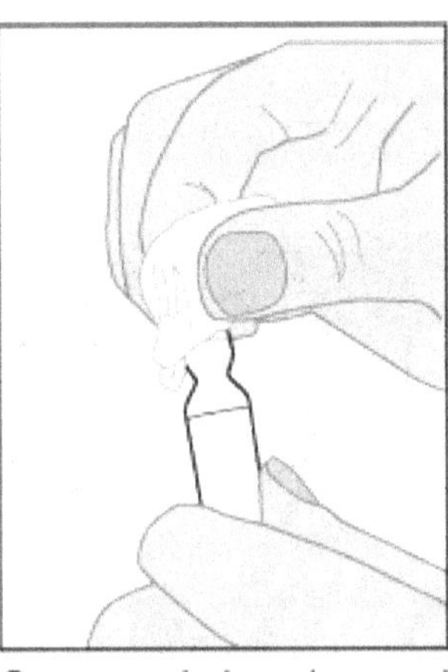

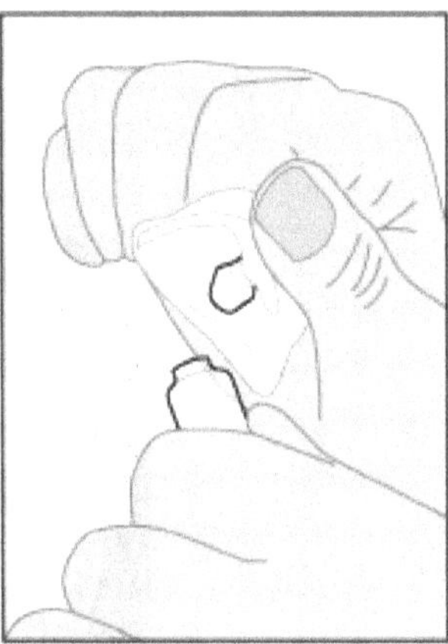

Figure 18.10 Opening an Ampule

Video Review of Withdrawing Medication from an Ampule[1]

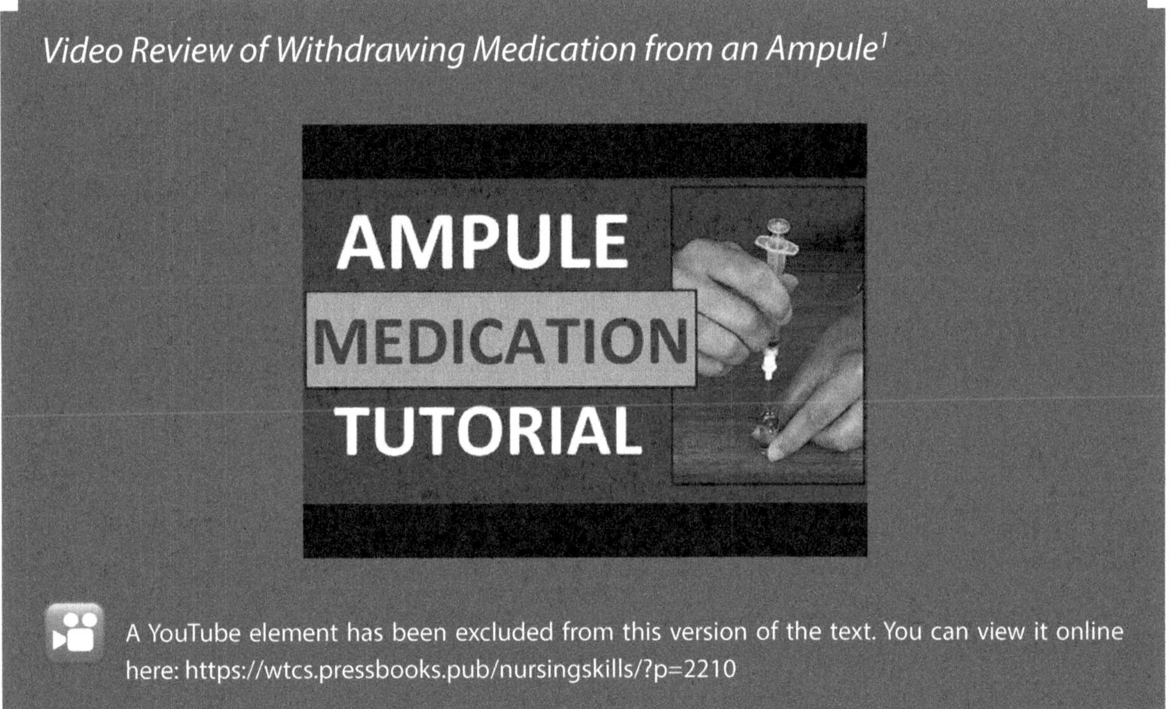

A YouTube element has been excluded from this version of the text. You can view it online here: https://wtcs.pressbooks.pub/nursingskills/?p=2210

12 "Preparing-an-ampule-1.png" by British Columbia Institute of Technology is licensed under CC BY 4.0. Access for free at https://opentextbc.ca/clinicalskills/chapter/safe-injection-administration-and-preparing-medication-from-ampules-and-vials/

1 RegisteredNurseRN. (2019, September 5). *Ampule medication administration nursing clinical skills.* [Video]. YouTube. All rights reserved. Video used with permission. https://youtu.be/mFKj3_Wk8m8

My Notes

Vials

A vial is a single- or multi-dose plastic container with a rubber seal top. Most rubber seals are covered by a plastic cap. See Figure 18.11[2] for an image of a medication dispensed in a vial. A single-use vial must be discarded after one use. Multi-dose vials are used for medications like insulin and must be labelled with the date it was opened. Refer to agency policy regarding how long an open vial may be used and how it should be stored. For example, insulin is typically refrigerated until the vial is opened, and then it can be stored at room temperature for 28 days.

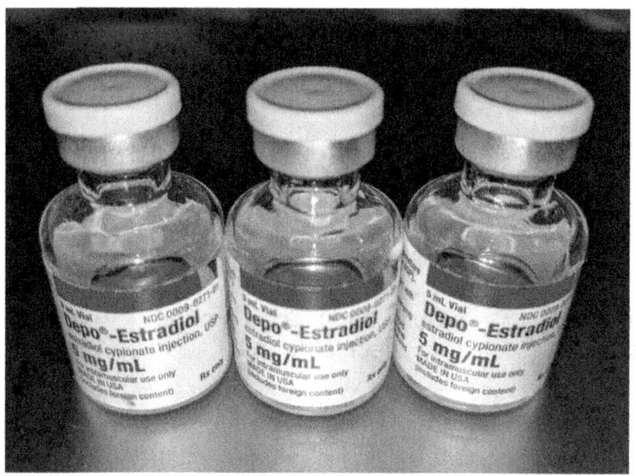

Figure 18.11 Vial

A vial is a closed system. Air must be injected prior to medication withdrawal to maintain a pressure gradient so that solution can be removed from the vial. It is also important to closely observe and maintain the tip of the needle within the level of medication inside the vial as it is removed. See Figure 18.12[3] for an image of removing medication from a vial.

To remove medication from a vial, pull air into the syringe to match the amount of medication you plan to remove. Hold the syringe like a pencil and insert the needle into the rubber stopper on the top of the vial. Push the plunger down until all of the air is in the bottle. This helps to keep the right amount of pressure in the bottle and makes it easier to draw up the medication. With the needle still in the vial, turn the bottle and syringe upside down (vial above syringe). Pull the plunger to fill the syringe to the desired amount. Check the syringe for air bubbles. If you see any large bubbles, push the plunger until the air is purged out of the syringe. Pull the plunger back down to the desired dose. Remove the needle from the bottle. Be careful to not let the needle touch anything until you are ready to inject.[4]

---

2 "Depo-Estradiol (estradiol cypionate) vials.jpg" by Medgirl131 is licensed under CC BY-SA 4.0. Access for free at https://commons.wikimedia.org/wiki/File:Depo-Estradiol_(estradiol_cypionate)_vials.jpg

3 " Syringe-1973129 340.jpg" by Myriams Zilles from Pixabay is licensed under CC0. Access for free at https://pixabay.com/sv/photos/sprutan-nål-engångsspruta-1973129/

4 American Association of Diabetes Educators. (n.d.). *Insulin injection know-how.* https://www.diabeteseducator.org/docs/default-source/legacy-docs/_resources/pdf/general/Insulin_Injection_How_To_AADE.pdf

My Notes

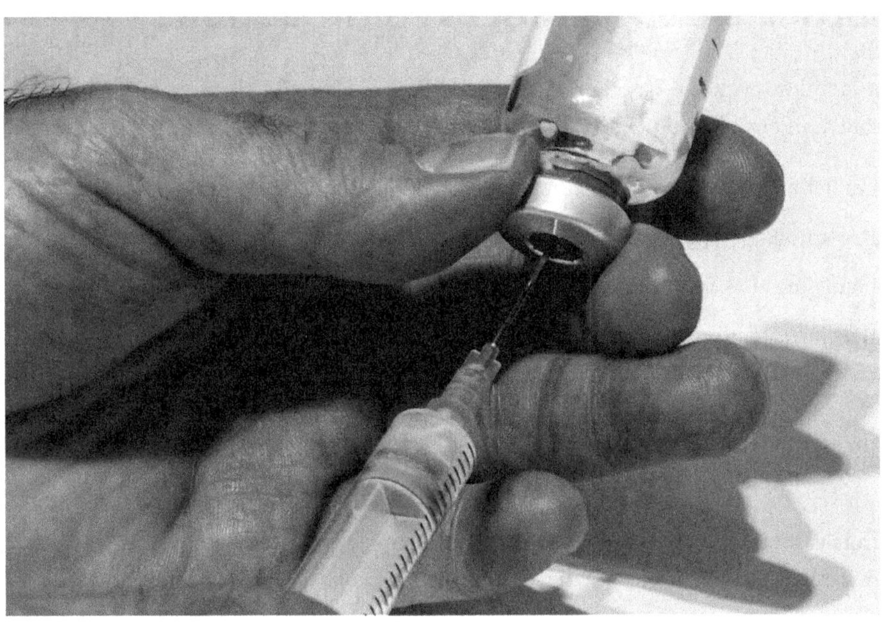

Figure 18.12 Removing Medication From a Vial

Prefilled Syringes

Prefilled syringes can provide greater patient safety by reducing the potential for inadvertent needlesticks and exposure to toxic products that can occur while withdrawing medication from vials. Prefilled syringes, with premeasured dosage, can reduce dosing errors and waste. They are especially useful during emergent situations that require rapid administration of medication. See Figure 18.13[5] for an image of a prefilled syringe.

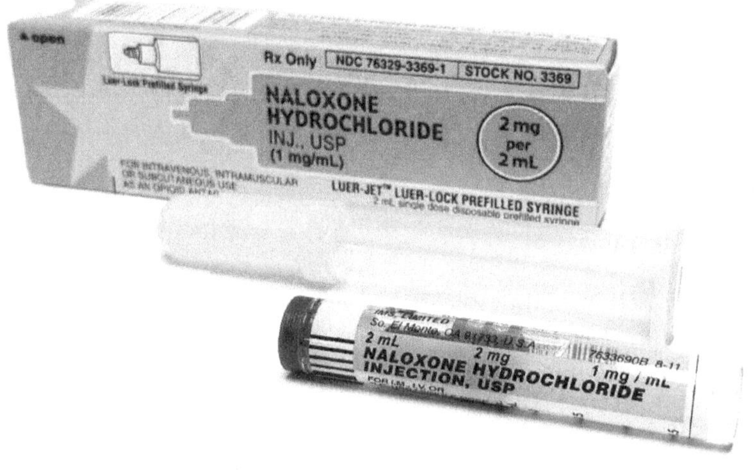

Figure 18.13 Prefilled Syringe

5 "Naloxone_5.jpg" by Intropin (Mark Oniffrey) is licensed under CC BY-SA 4.0. Access for free at https://commons.wikimedia.org/wiki/File:Naloxone_5.jpg

My Notes

18.3 EVIDENCE-BASED PRACTICES FOR INJECTIONS

It is important to follow evidence-based practices regarding parenteral medication administration to provide safe and effective care. Evidence-based practices include the following:

- Guidelines for preventing medication errors
- Recommendations to prevent infection from injections
- Guidelines for patient safety and comfort
- Recommendations to prevent needlestick injuries

Each of these practices is further described in the following sections.

Guidelines for Preventing Medication Errors

Medication errors can occur at various steps of the medication administration process. It is important to follow a standardized method for parenteral medication administration. Agency policies on medication preparation, administration, and documentation may vary, so it is important to receive agency training on using their medication system to avoid errors. See Table 18.3a for a summary of guidelines for safe medication administration.[1]

Additional details about preventing medication errors can be found in the "Administration of Enteral Medications" chapter.

Table 18.3a Summary of Safe Medication Administration Guidelines

Guidelines	Additional Information
Be cautious and focused when preparing medications.	Avoid distractions. Some agencies have a no-interruption zone (NIZ) where health care providers can prepare medications without interruptions.[2]
Check and verify allergies.	Always ask the patient about their medication allergies, types of reactions, and severity of reactions. Verify the patient's medical record for documented allergies.
Use two patient identifiers and follow agency policy for patient identification.	Use at least two patient identifiers before administration and compare information against the medication administration record (MAR).[3]

1 This work is a derivative of Clinical Procedures for Safer Patient Care by British Columbia Institute of Technology (BCIT) and is licensed under CC BY 4.0. Access for free at https://opentextbc.ca/clinicalskills/

2 Institute for Safe Medication Practices. (2012, November 29). *Side tracks on the safety express. Interruptions lead to errors and unfinished... Wait, what* was I doing? https://www.ismp.org/resources/side-tracks-safety-express-interruptions-lead-errors-and-unfinished-wait-what-was-i-doing?id=37

3 The Joint Commission. (n.d.). *2020 Hospital national patient saf*ety goals. https://www.jointcommission.org/standards/national-patient-safety-goals/

My Notes

Guidelines	Additional Information
Perform appropriate patient assessments before medication administration.	Assess the patient prior to administering medications to ensure the patient is receiving the correct medication, for the correct reason, and at the correct time. For example, a nurse reviews lab values and performs a cardiac assessment prior to administering cardiac medication. See more information regarding specific patient assessments during parenteral medication administration in the "Applying the Nursing Process" section.
Be diligent and perform medication calculations accurately.	Double-check and verify medication calculations. Incorrect calculation of medication dosages causes medication errors that can compromise patient safety.
Use standard procedures and evidence-based references.	Follow a standardized procedure when administering medication for every patient. Look up current medication information in evidence-based sources because information changes frequently.
Communicate with the patient before and after administration.	Provide information to the patient about the medication before administering it. Answer their questions regarding usage, dose, and special considerations. Give the patient an opportunity to ask questions and include family members if appropriate.
Follow agency policies and procedures regarding medication administration.	Avoid work-arounds. A work-around is a process that bypasses a procedure or policy in a system. For example, a nurse may "borrow" medication from one patient's drawer to give to another patient while waiting for an order to be filled by the pharmacy. Although performed with a good intention to prevent delay, these work-arounds fail to follow policies in place that ensure safe medication administration and often result in medication errors.
Ensure medication has not expired.	Check all medications' expiration dates before administering them. Medications can become inactive after their expiration date.
Always clarify an order or procedure that is unclear.	Always verify information whenever you are uncertain or unclear about an order. Consult with the pharmacist, charge nurse, or health care provider, and be sure to resolve all questions before proceeding with medication administration.
Use available technology to administer medications.	Use available technology, such as bar code scanning, when administering medications. Bar code scanning is linked to the patient's eMAR and provides an extra level of patient safety to prevent wrong medications, incorrect doses, or wrong timing of administration. If error messages occur, it is important to follow up appropriately according to agency policy and not override them. Additionally, it is important to remember that this technology provides an additional layer of safety and should not be substituted for the checking the five rights of medication administration.
Be a part of the safety culture.	Report all errors, near misses, and adverse reactions according to agency policy. Incident reports improve patient care through quality improvement identification, analysis, and problem-solving.

My Notes

Guidelines	Additional Information
Be alert.	Be alert to error-prone situations and high-alert medications. High-alert medications are those that can cause significant harm. The most common high-alert medications are anticoagulants, opiates, insulins, and sedatives. Read more about high-alert medications in the "Administration of Enteral Medications" chapter.
Address patient concerns.	If a patient questions or expresses concern regarding a medication, stop the procedure and do not administer it. Explore the patient's concerns, review the provider's order, and, if necessary, notify the provider.

Preventing Infection

Administering parenteral medications is considered an invasive procedure. It is imperative to take additional measures when administering parenteral medications to prevent health care associated infections. The Centers for Disease Control and Prevention provides several recommendations for safe injection practices to prevent contamination and spread of pathogens. These recommendations include hand hygiene, prevention of needle/syringe contamination, preparation of the patient's skin, prevention of contamination of the solution, and use of new, sterile equipment for each injection.[4,5,6] Each of these recommendations is discussed below.

Perform Hand Hygiene

Always perform hand hygiene before preparing and after administering the injection with facility-approved, alcohol-based hand sanitizer. See more information about performing effective hand hygiene in the "Aseptic Technique" chapter.

Prevent Needle/Syringe Contamination

Keep the parts of the needle and syringe sterile. Keep the tip of the syringe sterile and keep it covered with a cap or needle. Avoid letting the needle touch unsterile surfaces, such as the outer edges of the ampule or vial, the surface of the needle cap, or the counter. Always keep the needle covered with a cap when not in use and avoid touching the length of the plunger.

After administration, use the scoop-cap method to recap the needle to avoid needlestick injuries and place the used syringe/needle immediately in the sharps container.

---

4 This work is a derivative of Clinical Procedures for Safer Patient Care by British Columbia Institute of Technology and is licensed under CC BY 4.0. Access for free at https://opentextbc.ca/clinicalskills/

5 Centers for Disease Control and Prevention. (2019, June 20). *Injection safety.* https://www.cdc.gov/injectionsafety/providers/provider_faqs.html

6 Centers for Disease Control and Prevention. (2011, April 1). *Safe injection practices to prevent transmission of infections to patients.* https://www.cdc.gov/injectionsafety/ip07_standardprecaution.html

My Notes

Video Review of Scoop-Cap Technique[7]

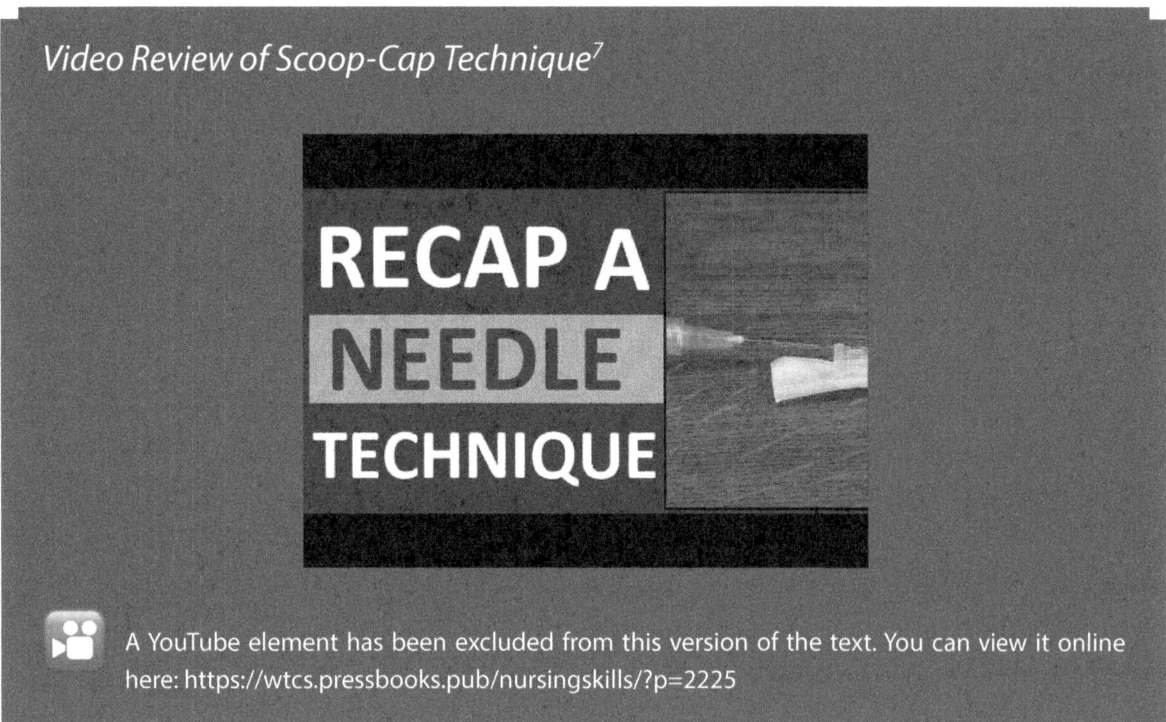

A YouTube element has been excluded from this version of the text. You can view it online here: https://wtcs.pressbooks.pub/nursingskills/?p=2225

Prepare Patient's Skin

Wash the patient's skin with soap and water if it is soiled. Follow agency policy for skin preparation. When using an alcohol swab, use a circular motion to rub the area for 15 seconds, and then let the area dry for 30 seconds. If cleaning a site, move from the center of the site outward in a 5-cm (2 in.) radius.

Prevent Contamination of Solution

Use single-dose vials or ampules whenever possible. Do not keep multi-dose vials in patient treatment areas. Discard a container if sterility is compromised or questionable. Medications from ampules should be used immediately and then discarded appropriately. Additional information about ampules is provided in the "Basic Concepts" section.

Use New Sterile Equipment

Use a new, sterile syringe and needle with each patient. Inspect packaging for intactness and discard if there are rips or torn corners. If single-use equipment is not available, use syringes and needles designed for steam sterilization.

Guidelines for Patient Safety and Comfort During Injections

With proper preparation and technique, injections can be given safely and effectively to patients to prevent harm. It is essential to use correct needle sizes and angles of insertion and select appropriate anatomical locations based on patient age, size, and type of injection to avoid complications.[8]

---

7 RegisteredNurseRN. (2021, February 25). *Recap a needle using the one-hand scoop technique nursing skill | Medication administration.* [Video]. YouTube. All rights reserved. Video used with permission. https://youtu.be/bEeAo2jCJjw

8 This work is a derivative of Clinical Procedures for Safer Patient Care by British Columbia Institute of Technology and is licensed under CC BY 4.0. Access for free at https://opentextbc.ca/clinicalskills/

My Notes

For example, for intramuscular injections the ventrogluteal site is preferred in adults because it has the greatest muscle thickness, is free of nerves and blood vessels, and has a small layer of fat, resulting in less painful administration and optimal absorption of the medication.

Use the correct needle length according to the type of injection to ensure delivery of medication into the correct layer of tissue and to reduce complications such as abscesses, pain, and bruising. Needle selection should be based on the patient's size, gender, and injection site. Be aware that women tend to have more adipose tissue around the buttocks and deltoid fat pad, which means a longer needle is required. Larger diameter (smaller gauge) needles have been found to reduce pain, swelling, and redness after an injection because less pressure is required to depress the plunger.

Removing medication residue on the tip of the needle has been shown to reduce pain and discomfort of the injection. To remove residue from the needle, change needles after medication is removed from a vial and before it is administered to the patient. Additionally, place the bevel side of the needle up on the patient's skin for quick and smooth injection of the needle into the tissue.

Proper positioning of the patient will facilitate proper landmarking of the site and may reduce perception of pain from the injection. Position the patient's limbs in a relaxed, comfortable position to reduce muscle tension. For example, when giving an intramuscular injection in the deltoid, have the patient relax their arm by placing their hand in their lap.

The nurse can also encourage relaxation techniques to help decrease the patient's anxiety-heightened pain. For example, divert the patient's attention away from the injection procedure by chatting about other topics.[9]

Recommendations for Preventing Needlestick Injuries

Nurses are at high risk for needlestick injuries when administering injections. Needlestick injuries can result in the transmission of blood-borne pathogens and should always be reported according to agency policy for appropriate follow-up. Table 18.3b outlines guidelines for preventing needlestick injuries.[10]

9 This work is a derivative of Clinical Procedures for Safer Patient Care by British Columbia Institute of Technology and is licensed under CC BY 4.0. Access for free at https://opentextbc.ca/clinicalskills/

10 This work is a derivative of Clinical Procedures for Safer Patient Care by British Columbia Institute of Technology and is licensed under CC BY 4.0. Access for free at https://opentextbc.ca/clinicalskills/

My Notes

Table 18.3b Guidelines for Preventing Needlestick Injuries

Practice Guidelines	Additional Information
Do not recap needles with both hands.	Recapping needles with two hands creates high risk for needlestick injuries. Use the scoop-cap method by laying the cap on a hard surface and using one hand to hold the syringe and scoop up the cap from the surface. Whenever possible, use devices with safety features such as a safety shield on needles so that recapping is not necessary.
Dispose of the needle immediately after injection.	Immediately dispose of used needles in an approved sharps disposal container that is puncture-proof and leakproof.
Reduce or eliminate all hazards related to needles.	Use a needleless system and engineered safety devices for prevention of needlestick injuries when preparing injectable medications whenever possible.
Plan disposal of sharps before injection.	Plan for the safe handling and disposal of needles and other sharp objects before beginning the procedure. Locate the sharps container before administration, so that you can quickly dispose of the sharps after injection.
Follow all standard policies related to prevention or treatment of injury.	Follow all agency policies regarding infection control, hand hygiene, standard precautions, and blood and body fluid exposure management.
Report all injuries.	Report all needlestick injuries and sharp-related injuries immediately. Know how to manage needlestick injuries and follow agency policy regarding exposure to blood-borne pathogens. These policies help decrease the risk of contracting a blood-borne illness.
Participate in required training and education.	Attend training on injury-prevention strategies related to needles and safety devices per agency policy.

My Notes

18.4 ADMINISTERING INTRADERMAL MEDICATIONS

Intradermal injections (ID) are administered into the dermis just below the epidermis. See Figure 18.14[1] for an image of the layers of the skin. Intradermal (ID) injections have the longest absorption time of all parenteral routes because there are fewer blood vessels and no muscle tissue. These types of injections are used for sensitivity testing because the patient's reaction is easy to visualize and the degree of reaction can be assessed. Examples of intradermal injections include tuberculosis (TB) and allergy testing.[2]

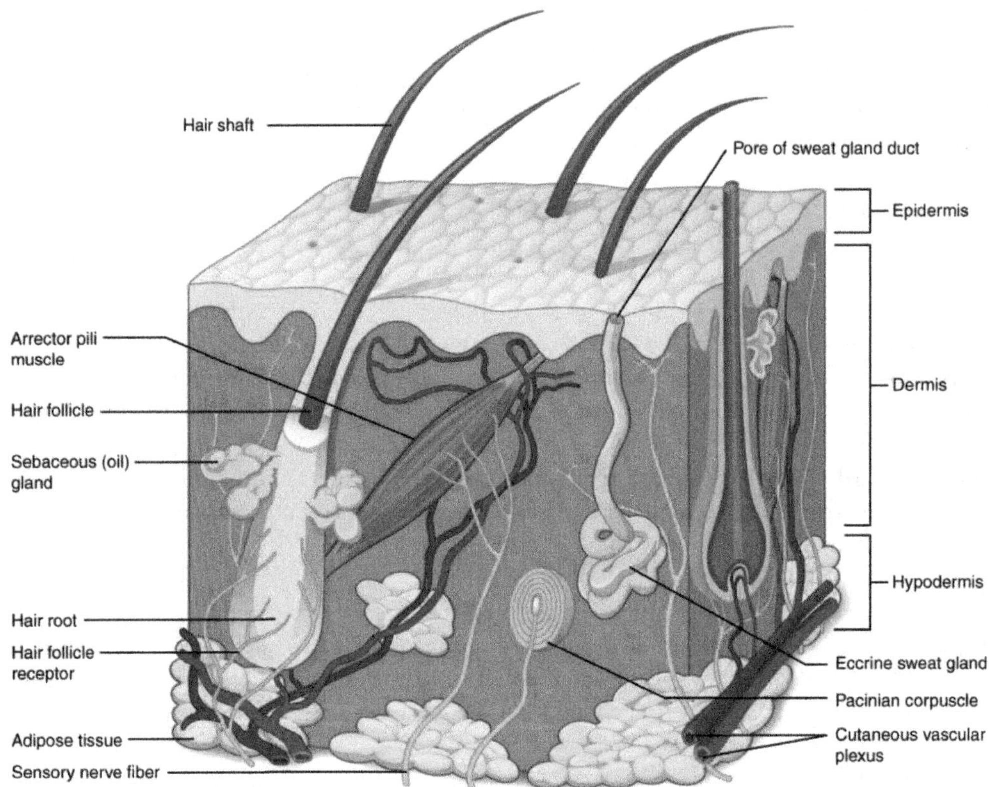

Figure 18.14 Layers of Skin

1 "501 Structure of the skin.jpg" by OpenStax is licensed under CC BY 3.0. Access for free at https://openstax.org/books/anatomy-and-physiology/pages/5-1-layers-of-the-skin

2 This work is a derivative of Clinical Procedures for Safer Patient Care by British Columbia Institute of Technology and is licensed under CC BY 4.0. Access for free at https://opentextbc.ca/clinicalskills/

Anatomic Sites

My Notes

The most common anatomical sites used for intradermal injections are the inner surface of the forearm and the upper back below the scapula. The nurse should select an injection site that is free from lesions, rashes, moles, or scars that may alter the visual inspection of the test results. See Figure 18.15[3] for an image of the nurse inspecting a patient's forearm site prior to injection.

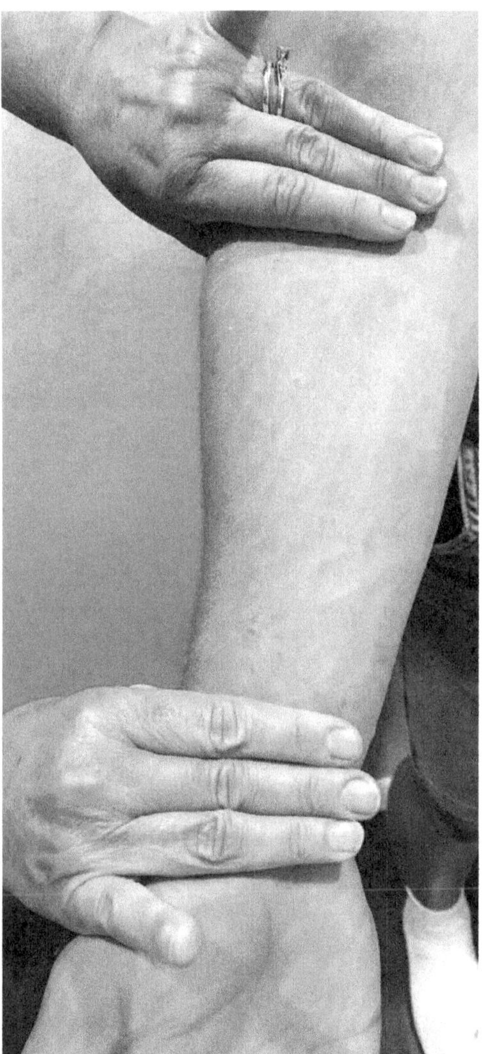

Figure 18.15 Inspecting the Forearm Site Prior to Injection

3 "*Inspecting Forearm*" by Meredith Pomietlo for Chippewa Valley Technical College is licensed under CC BY 4.0. Access for free at https://drive.google.com/file/d/1yuhbt30LS2BYA98vb4Re0lCdhvmcyoi2/view?usp=sharing

My Notes

Description of Procedure

Clean the site with an alcohol swab or antiseptic swab for 30 seconds using a firm, circular motion. Allow the site to dry. Allowing the skin to dry prevents introducing alcohol into the tissue, which can be irritating and uncomfortable.[4]

Use a tuberculin syringe, calibrated in tenths and hundredths of a milliliter, with a needle length of 1/4 inches o1/2 inches and a gauge of 26 or 27.[5] See Figure 18.16[6] for an image of a tuberculin syringe. Remove the cap from the needle by pulling it off in a straight motion. A straight motion helps prevent needlestick injury.

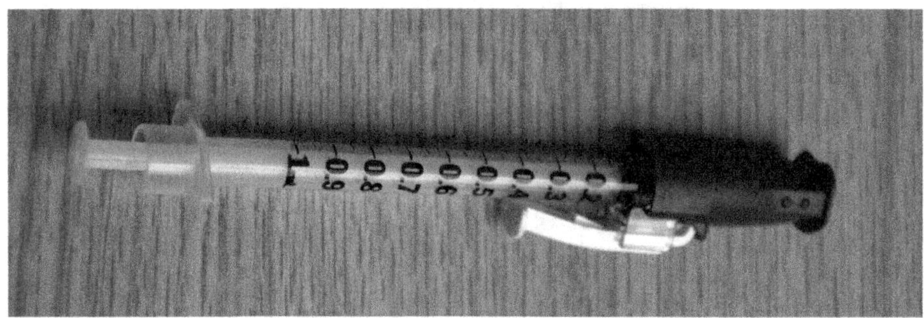

Figure 18.16 Tuberculin Syringe

The dosage of an intradermal injection is usually under 0.5 mL, and the angle of administration for an ID injection is 5 to 15 degrees. Using your nondominant hand, spread the skin taut over the injection site. Taut skin provides easy entrance for the needle and is also important to do for older adults, whose skin is less elastic. See Figure 18.17[7] holding the skin taut prior to injection.[8]

4 This work is a derivative of Clinical Procedures for Safer Patient Care by British Columbia Institute of Technology and is licensed under CC BY 4.0. Access for free at https://opentextbc.ca/clinicalskills/

5 This work is a derivative of Clinical Procedures for Safer Patient Care by British Columbia Institute of Technology and is licensed under CC BY 4.0. Access for free at https://opentextbc.ca/clinicalskills/

6 "Book-pictures-2015-544.jpg" by British Columbia Institute of Technologyis licensed under CC BY 4.0. Access for free at https://opentextbc.ca/clinicalskills/chapter/6-7-intradermal-subcutaneous-and-intramuscular-injections/

7 "Book-pictures-2015-623.jpg" by British Columbia Institute of Technologyis licensed under CC BY 4.0. Access for free at https://opentextbc.ca/clinicalskills/chapter/6-7-intradermal-subcutaneous-and- intramuscular-injections/

8 This work is a derivative of Clinical Procedures for Safer Patient Care by British Columbia Institute of Technology and is licensed under CC BY 4.0. Access for free at https://opentextbc.ca/clinicalskills/

My Notes

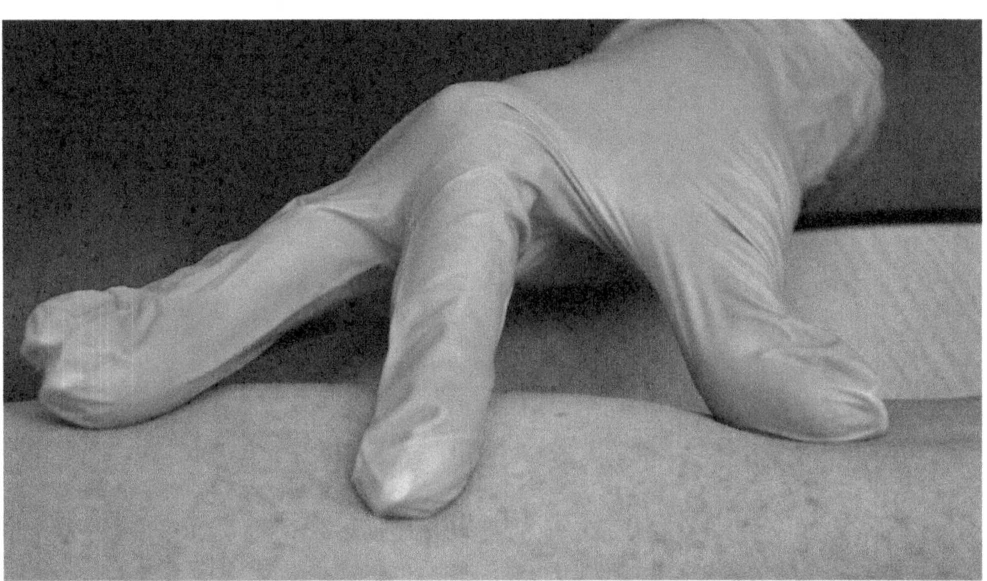

Figure 18.17 Holding Skin Taut

Hold the syringe in the dominant hand between the thumb and forefinger, with the bevel of the needle up at a 5- to 15-degree angle at the selected site. Place the needle almost flat against the patient's skin, bevel side up, and insert the needle into the skin. Keeping the bevel side up allows for smooth piercing of the skin and induction of the medication into the dermis. Advance the needle no more than an eighth of an inch to cover the bevel. Once the syringe is in place, use the thumb of the nondominant hand to push on the plunger to slowly inject the medication.[9] See Figure 18.18[10] for an image of a nurse administering an intradermal injection.

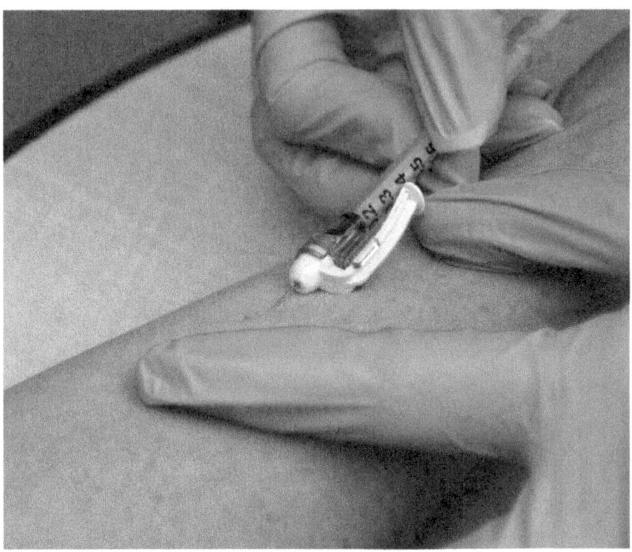

Figure 18.18 Intradermal Injection

9 This work is a derivative of Clinical Procedures for Safer Patient Care by British Columbia Institute of Technology and is licensed under CC BY 4.0. Access for free at https://opentextbc.ca/clinicalskills/

10 "Intradermal_injection.jpg" by British Columbia Institute of Technologyis licensed under CC BY 4.0. Access for free at https://opentextbc.ca/clinicalskills/chapter/6-7-intradermal-subcutaneous-and-intramuscular-injections/

My Notes

After the ID injection is completed, a **bleb** (small blister) should appear under the skin. The presence of the bleb indicates that the medication has been correctly placed in the dermis. See Figure 18.19[11] for an image of a bleb.

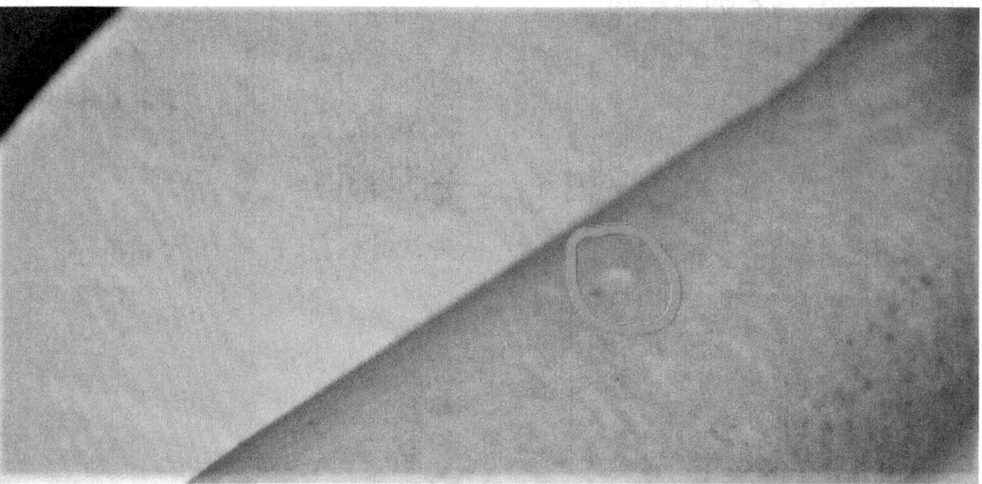

Figure 18.19 Bleb

Carefully withdraw the needle out of the insertion site using the same angle it was placed so as not to disturb the bleb. Withdrawing at the same angle as insertion also minimizes discomfort to the patient and damage to the tissue. Do not massage or cover the site. Massaging the area may spread the solution to the underlying subcutaneous tissue. Discard the syringe in the sharps container. If administering a TB test, advise the patient to return for a reading in 48-72 hours. Discard used supplies, remove gloves, perform hand hygiene, and document.[12]

11 This work is derivative of "Book-pictures-2015-636.jpg" by British Columbia Institute of Technologyand is licensed under CC BY 4.0. Access for free at https://opentextbc.ca/clinicalskills/chapter/6-7-intradermal-subcutaneous-and-intramuscular-injections/

12 This work is a derivative of Clinical Procedures for Safer Patient Care by British Columbia Institute of Technology and is licensed under CC BY 4.0. Access for free at https://opentextbc.ca/clinicalskills/

18.5 ADMINISTERING SUBCUTANEOUS MEDICATIONS

My Notes

Subcutaneous injections are administered into the adipose tissue layer called "subcutis" below the dermis. See an image of the subcutis (hypodermis) layer in Figure 18.20.[1] Medications injected into the subcutaneous layer are absorbed at a slow and steady rate.

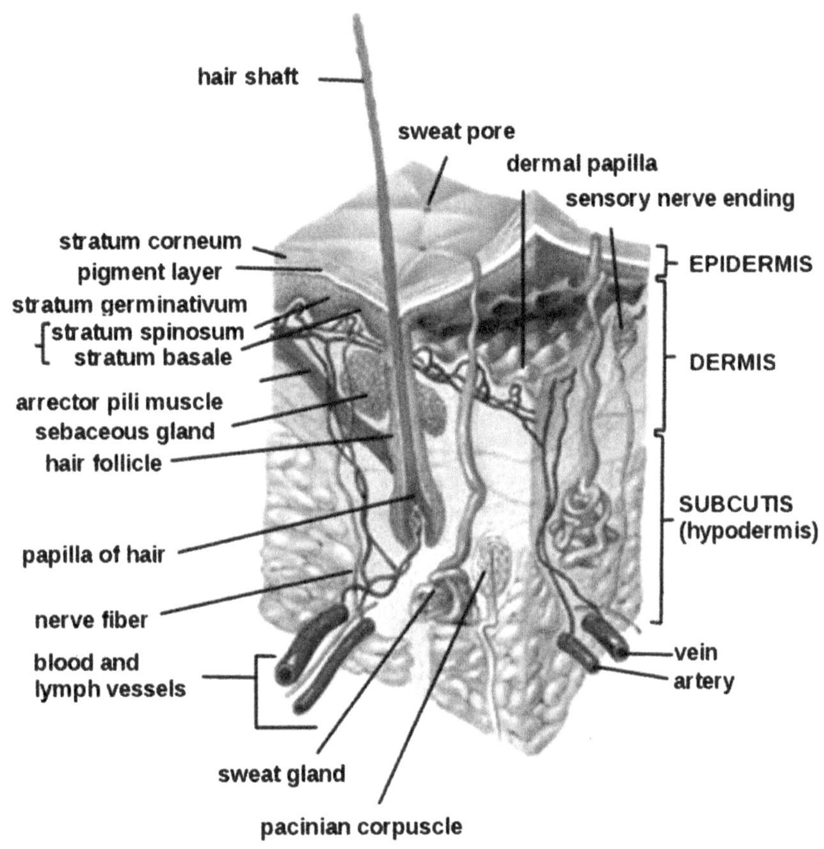

Figure 18.20 Subcutis Layer of Skin

Anatomic Sites

Sites for subcutaneous injections include the outer lateral aspect of the upper arm, the abdomen (from below the costal margin to the iliac crest and more than two inches from the umbilicus), the anterior upper thighs, the upper back, and the upper ventral gluteal area.[2] See Figure 18.21[3] for an illustration of commonly used subcutaneous

1 "HumanSkinDiagram.jpg" by Daniel de Souza Telles is licensed under CC BY-SA 3.0. Access for free at https://commons.wikimedia.org/wiki/File:HumanSkinDiagram.jpg

2 This work is a derivative of Clinical Procedures for Safer Patient Care by British Columbia Institute of Technology and is licensed under CC BY 4.0. Access for free at https://opentextbc.ca/clinicalskills/

3 "Subcutaneous-injection-sites-274x300.png" by British Columbia Institute of Technology is licensed under CC BY 4.0. Access for free at https://opentextbc.ca/clinicalskills/chapter/6-7-intradermal-subcutaneous-and-intramuscular-injections/

My Notes

injection sites. These areas have large surface areas that allow for rotation of subcutaneous injections within the same site when applicable.

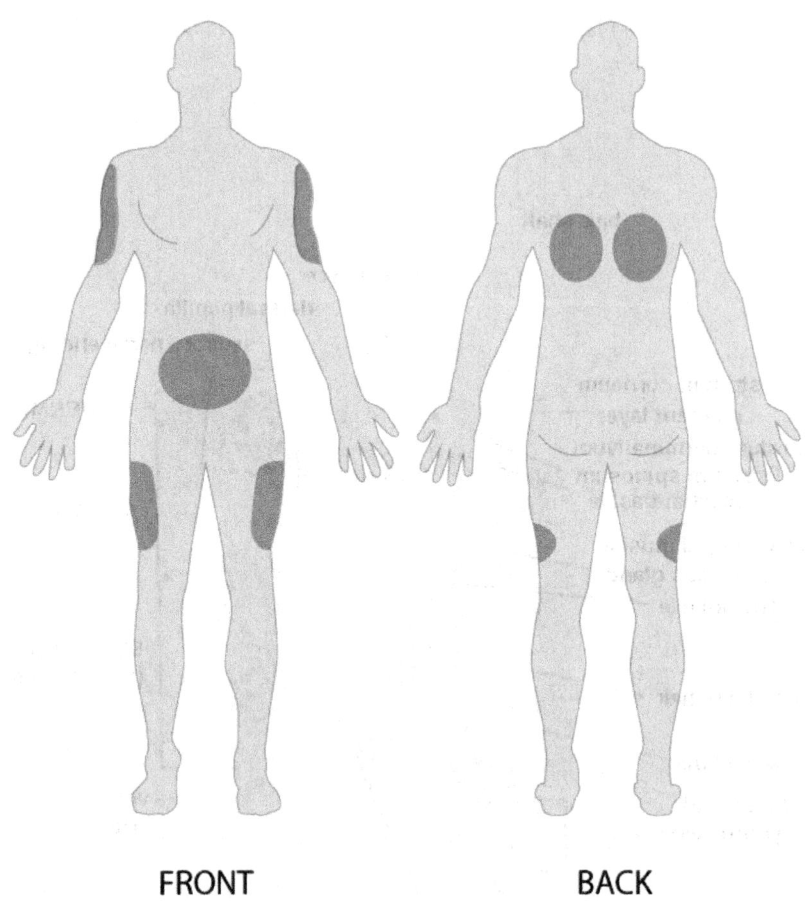

Figure 18.21 Common Subcutaneous Injection Sites

Prior to injecting the medication, inspect the skin area. Avoid skin areas that are bruised, open, scarred, or over bony prominences. Medical conditions that impair the blood flow to a tissue area contraindicate the use of subcutaneous injections in that area. For example, if a patient has an infection in an area of their skin called "cellulitis," then subcutaneous injections should not be given in that area.

Description of Procedure

Nurses select the appropriate needle size for subcutaneous injection based on patient size. Subcutaneous needles range in gauge from 25-31 and in length from ½ inch to ⅝ inch. Prior to administering the injection, determine the amount of subcutaneous tissue present and use this information to select the needle length. A 45- or 90-degree angle is used for a subcutaneous injection. A 90-degree angle is used for normal-sized adult patients or obese patients, and a 45-degree angle is used for patients who are thin or have with less adipose tissue at the injection site. The volume of solution in a subcutaneous injection should be no more than 1 mL for adults and 0.5 mL for children. Larger amounts may not be absorbed appropriately and may cause increased discomfort for the patient.[4]

---

4 This work is a derivative of Clinical Procedures for Safer Patient Care by British Columbia Institute of Technology and is licensed under CC BY 4.0. Access for free at https://opentextbc.ca/clinicalskills/

My Notes

When administering a subcutaneous injection, assess the patient for any contraindications for receiving the medication. Apply nonsterile gloves after performing hand hygiene to reduce your risk of exposure to blood. Position the patient in a comfortable position and select an appropriate site for injection. Cleanse the site with an alcohol swab or antiseptic swab for 30 seconds using a firm, circular motion, and then allow the site to dry. Allowing the skin to dry prevents introducing alcohol into the tissue, which can be irritating and uncomfortable. Remove the needle cap with the nondominant hand, pulling it straight off to avoid needlestick injury.

Grasp and pinch the area selected as an injection site.[5] See Figure 18.22[6] for an image of a nurse grasping the back of a patient's upper arm with the nondominant hand in preparation of a subcutaneous injection at the anatomical site indicted with an "X."

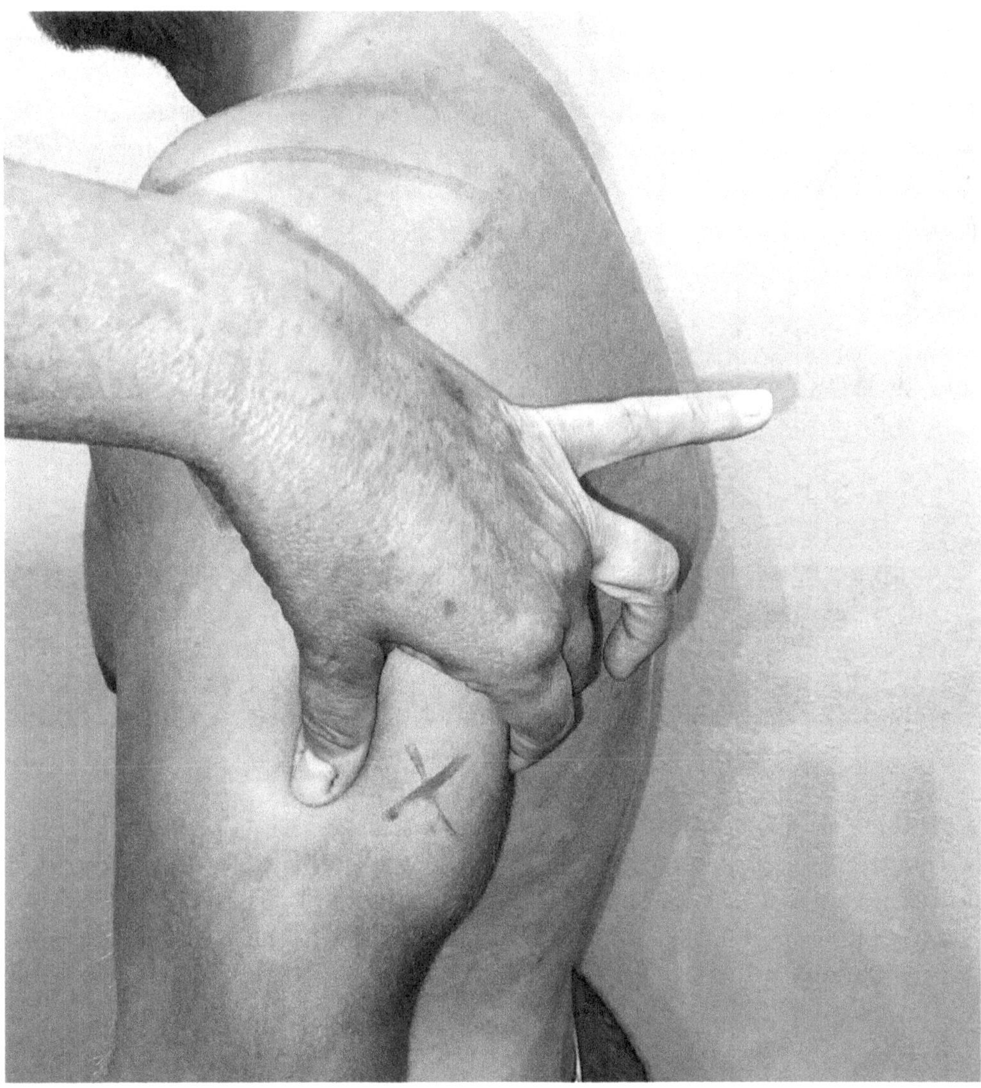

Figure 18.22 Grasping and Pinching Area

5 This work is a derivative of Clinical Procedures for Safer Patient Care by British Columbia Institute of Technology and is licensed under CC BY 4.0. Access for free at https://opentextbc.ca/clinicalskills/

6 "Upper Posterior Arm" by Meredith Pomietlo for Chippewa Valley Technical College is licensed under CC BY 4.0. Access for free at https://drive.google.com/file/d/10Zc5ayZ1s3CAgv-xRKp23sv3TA4Gm3--/view?usp=sharing

My Notes

Hold the syringe in the dominant hand between the thumb and forefinger like a dart. Insert the needle quickly at a 45- to 90-degree angle, depending on the size of the patient and the amount of adipose tissue. After the needle is in place, release the tissue with your nondominant hand. With your dominant hand, inject the medication at a rate of 10 seconds per mL. Avoid moving the syringe.[7] See Figure 18.23[8] for an image of a subcutaneous injection.

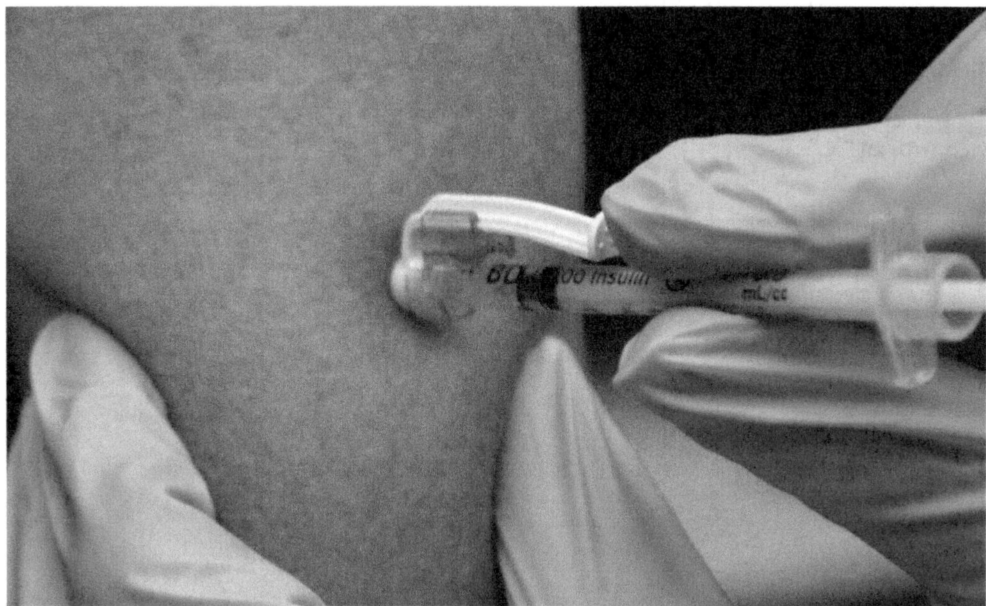

Figure 18.23 Subcutaneous Injection

When injecting heparin or when using an insulin pen, continue pinching the skin during the injection and release the skinfold immediately before withdrawing the needle.

Withdraw the needle quickly at the same angle at which it was inserted. Using a sterile gauze, apply gentle pressure at the site after the needle is withdrawn. Do not massage the site. Massaging after a heparin injection can contribute to the formation of a hematoma. Do not recap the needle to avoid puncturing oneself. Apply the safety shield and dispose of the syringe/needle in a sharps container. See Figure 18.24[9] for an image of a needle after the safety shield has been applied. Remove gloves and perform hand hygiene.[10]

7 This work is a derivative of Clinical Procedures for Safer Patient Care by British Columbia Institute of Technology and is licensed under CC BY 4.0. Access for free at https://opentextbc.ca/clinicalskills/

8 "Book-pictures-2015-650.jpg" by British Columbia Institute of Technology is licensed under CC BY 4.0. Access for free at https://opentextbc.ca/clinicalskills/chapter/6-7-intradermal-subcutaneous-and-intramuscular-injections/

9 "Sept-22-2015-040.jpg" by British Columbia Institute of Technology is licensed under CC BY 4.0. Access for free at https://opentextbc.ca/clinicalskills/chapter/6-7-intradermal-subcutaneous-and-intramuscular-injections/

10 This work is a derivative of Clinical Procedures for Safer Patient Care by British Columbia Institute of Technology and is licensed under CC BY 4.0. Access for free at https://opentextbc.ca/clinicalskills/

My Notes

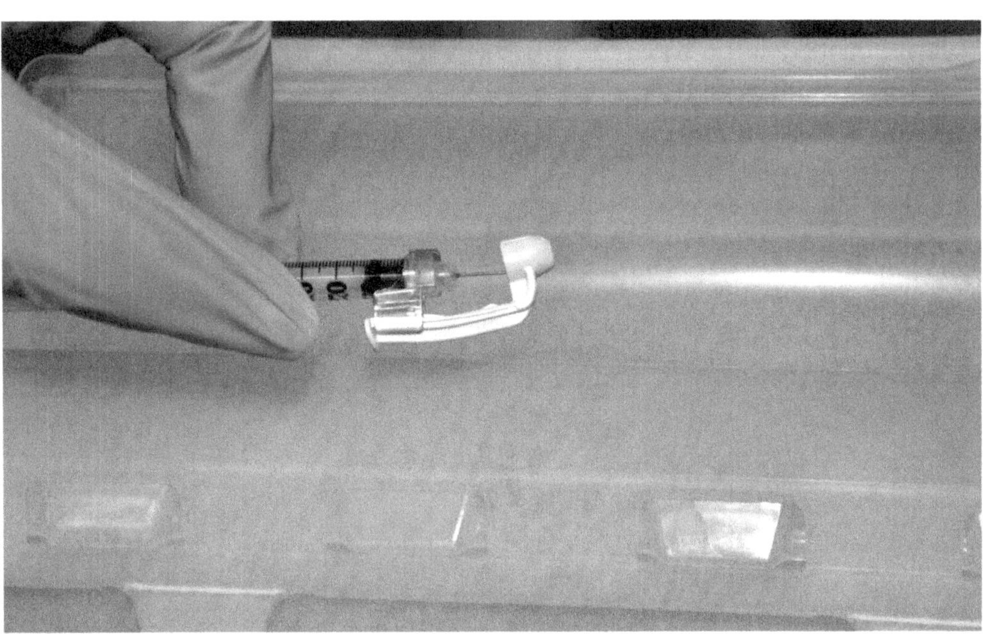

Figure 18.24 Needle with Safety Shield Applied

Examples of common medications administered via subcutaneous injection include insulin and heparin. Special considerations for each of these medications are discussed below.

Insulin Injections

Insulin is considered a high-alert medication requiring special care to prevent medication errors. Care must be taken to ensure the correct type and amount of insulin are administered at the correct time. It is highly recommended to have insulin dosages double-checked by another nurse before administration because of the potential for life-threatening adverse effects that can occur due to medication errors. Some agencies require this second safety check.

Only insulin syringes should be used to administer insulin injection. Insulin syringes are supplied in 30-, 50-, or 100-unit measurements, so read the barrel increments (calibration) carefully. Insulin is always ordered and administered in unit dosage. Insulin dosage may be based on the patient's pre-meal blood sugar reading and a sliding scale protocol that indicates the number of units administered based on the blood sugar reading.[11,12]

There are rapid-, short-, intermediate-, and long-acting insulins. For each type of insulin, it is important to know the onset, peak, and duration of the insulin so that it can be timed appropriately with the patient's food intake. It is essential to time the administration of insulin with food intake to avoid hypoglycemia. When administering insulin before a meal, always ensure the patient is not nauseated and is able to eat. Short- or rapid-acting insulin may be administered up to 15-30 minutes before meals. Intermediate insulin is typically administered twice daily,

---

11 This work is a derivative of Clinical Procedures for Safer Patient Care by British Columbia Institute of Technology and is licensed under CC BY 4.0. Access for free at https://opentextbc.ca/clinicalskills/

12 American Diabetes Association. (n.d.). *Insulin basics.* https://www.diabetes.org/diabetes/medication-management/insulin-other-injectables/insulin-basics

My Notes

at breakfast and dinner, and long-acting insulin is typically administered in the evening.[13, 14] When administering cloudy insulin preparations such as NPH insulin (Humulin-N), gently roll the vial between the palms of your hands to resuspend the medication before withdrawing it from the vial.[15, 16] See Figure 18.25[17] for an image of insulin NPH that is cloudy in color.

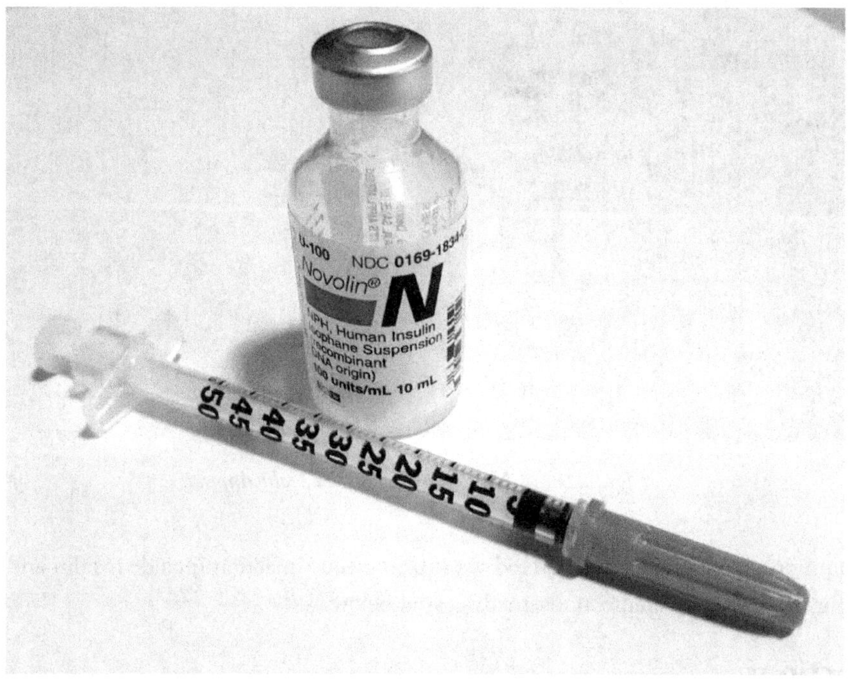

Figure 18.25 NPH Insulin

Preparing Insulin in a Syringe

When withdrawing insulin from a vial, check the insulin vial to make sure it is the right kind of insulin and that there are no clumps or particles in it. Also, make sure the insulin is not past its expiration date. Pull air into the syringe to match the amount of insulin you plan to remove. Hold the syringe like a pencil and insert the needle into the rubber stopper on the top of the vial. Push the plunger down until all of the air is in the bottle.

This helps to keep the right amount of pressure in the bottle and makes it easier to draw up the insulin. With the needle still in the vial, turn the bottle and syringe upside down (vial above syringe). Pull the plunger to fill the

---

13 This work is a derivative of Clinical Procedures for Safer Patient Care by British Columbia Institute of Technology and is licensed under CC BY 4.0. Access for free at https://opentextbc.ca/clinicalskills/

14 American Diabetes Association. (n.d.). *Insulin basics.* https://www.diabetes.org/diabetes/medication-management/insulin-other-injectables/insulin-basics

15 This work is a derivative of Clinical Procedures for Safer Patient Care by British Columbia Institute of Technology and is licensed under CC BY 4.0. Access for free at

16 American Diabetes Association. (n.d.). *Insulin basics.* https://www.diabetes.org/diabetes/medication-management/insulin-other-injectables/insulin-basics

17 "insulin-syringe" by biologycorner is licensed under CC BY-NC 2.0. Access for free at https://www.flickr.com/photos/biologycorner/31950868730

syringe to the desired amount. Check the syringe for air bubbles. If you see any large bubbles, push the plunger until the air is purged out of the syringe. Pull the plunger back down to the desired dose. Remove the needle from the bottle. Be careful to not let the needle touch anything until you are ready to inject.[18]

Mixing Two Types of Insulin

If a patient is ordered two types of insulin, some insulins may be mixed together in one syringe. For example, insulin NPH (Novolin-N) can be mixed with insulin regular (Humulin-R), insulin aspart (Novolog), or insulin lispro (Humalog). However, some types of insulin cannot be mixed with other insulin, such as insulin glargine (Lantus) or insulin detemir (Levemir).[19, 20]

When mixing insulin, gather your insulin supplies. Check the insulin vials to make sure they are the right kinds of insulin, there are no clumps or particles in them, and the expiration dates have not passed. Gently mix intermediate or premixed insulin by turning the vial on its side and rolling it between the palms of your hands. Prepare the insulin vials by injecting air into the intermediate insulin vial. Remove the cap from the needle. With the vial of insulin below the syringe, inject an amount of air equal to the dose of intermediate insulin that you will be taking. Do not draw out the insulin into the syringe yet. Remove the needle from the vial. Inject air into the rapid-acting insulin vial equal to the rapid-acting insulin dose. With the needle still in the vial, turn the vial upside down (vial above the syringe) and pull the plunger to fill the syringe with the desired dose. Check the syringe for air bubbles. If you see any large bubbles, push the plunger until the air is purged out of the syringe. Pull the plunger back down to the desired dose. Remove the needle from the vial and recheck your dose. Insert the needle into the vial of cloudy insulin. Turn the vial upside down (vial above syringe) and pull the plunger to draw the dose of intermediate-acting insulin. Because the short-acting insulin is already in the syringe, pull the plunger to the total number of units you need. Do not inject any of the insulin back into the vial because the syringe now contains a mixture of intermediate- and rapid-acting insulin. Remove the needle from the vial and be careful to not let the needle touch anything until you are ready to inject.[21]

When mixing insulin, it is important to always draw up the short-acting insulin first to prevent it from being contaminated with the long-acting insulin. See Figure 18.26[22] for an illustration of the order to follow when mixing insulin.

---

18 American Association of Diabetes Educators. (n.d.). *Insulin injection know-how.* https://www.diabeteseducator.org/docs/default-source/legacy-docs/_resources/pdf/general/Insulin_Injection_How_To_AADE.pdf

19 This work is a derivative of Clinical Procedures for Safer Patient Care by British Columbia Institute of Technology and is licensed under CC BY 4.0. Access for free at https://opentextbc.ca/clinicalskills/

20 American Diabetes Association. (n.d.). *Insulin basics.* https://www.diabetes.org/diabetes/medication-management/insulin-other-injectables/insulin-basics

21 American Association of Diabetes Educators. (n.d.). *Insulin injection know-how.* https://www.diabeteseducator.org/docs/default-source/legacy-docs/_resources/pdf/general/Insulin_Injection_How_To_AADE.pdf

22 "Mixing Insulin" by Meredith Pomietlo for Chippewa Valley Technical College is licensed under CC BY 4.0. Access for free at https://drive.google.com/file/d/1AwJlZ87zhUBVIYkdwP4qvYG_5mjsTtWv/view?usp=sharing

My Notes

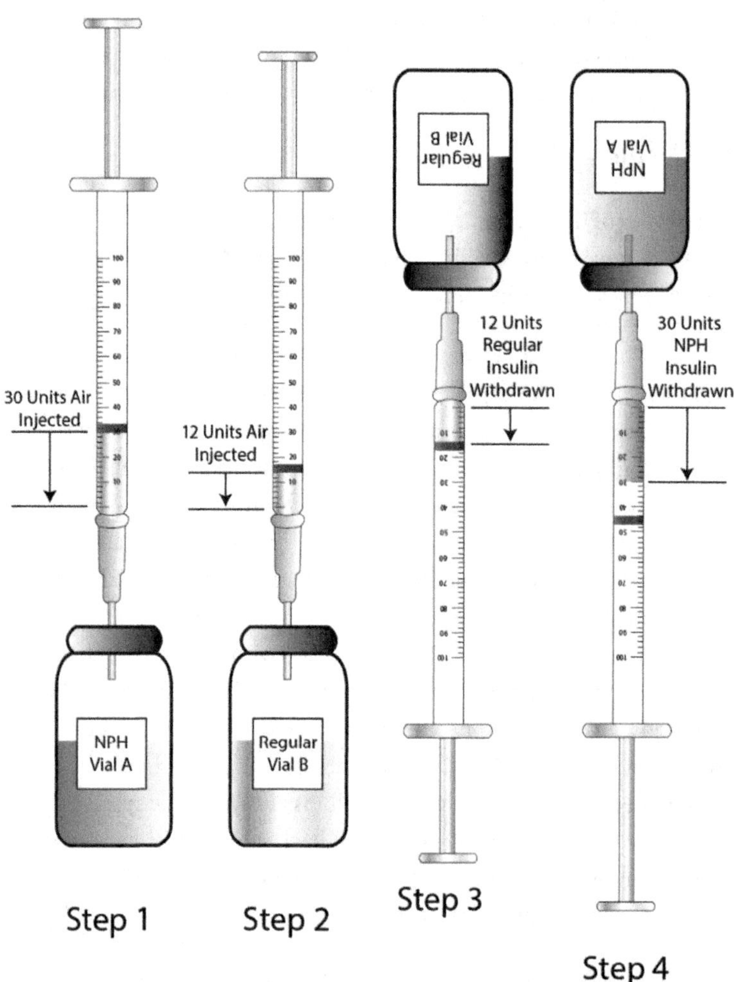

Figure 18.26 Mixing Insulin

One anatomic region should be selected for a patient's insulin injections to maintain consistent absorption, and then sites should be rotated within that region. The abdomen absorbs insulin the fastest, followed by the arms, thighs, and buttocks. It is no longer necessary to rotate anatomic regions, as was once done, because newer insulins have a lower risk for causing hypertrophy of the skin.[23, 24]

Insulin Pens

Insulin pens are a newer technology designed to be used multiple times for a single person, using a new needle for each injection. See Figure 18.27[25] for an image of an insulin pen. Insulin pens must never be used for more than one person. Regurgitation of blood into the insulin cartridge can occur after injection, creating a risk of blood-borne

23 This work is a derivative of Clinical Procedures for Safer Patient Care by British Columbia Institute of Technology and is licensed under CC BY 4.0. Access for free at https://opentextbc.ca/clinicalskills/

24 American Diabetes Association. (n.d.). *Insulin basics.* https://www.diabetes.org/diabetes/medication-management/insulin-other-injectables/insulin-basics

25 "Insulin_pen_(labeled).jpg" by User:Wesalius is licensed under CC BY 4.0. Access for free at https://commons.wikimedia.org/wiki/File:Insulin_pen_(labeled).jpg

My Notes

pathogen transmission if the pen is used for more than one person, even when the needle is changed.[26] Prefilled insulin pens consist of a prefilled cartridge of insulin to which a special, single-use needle is attached. When using an insulin pen for subcutaneous insulin administration, a few additional steps must be taken according to manufacturer guidelines. The needle should be primed with two units of insulin, and then the dosage should be dialed in the dose window. The pen should be held with the hand using four fingers so that the thumb can be used to fully depress the plunger button. The pen should be left in place for ten seconds after the insulin is injected to aid in absorption.[27]

Insulin pens are often prescribed for home use because of their ease of use. Patients and family members must be educated on how to correctly use an insulin pen before discharge. To evaluate a patient's knowledge of how to correctly administer insulin, ask them to "return demonstrate" the procedure to you.[28, 29]

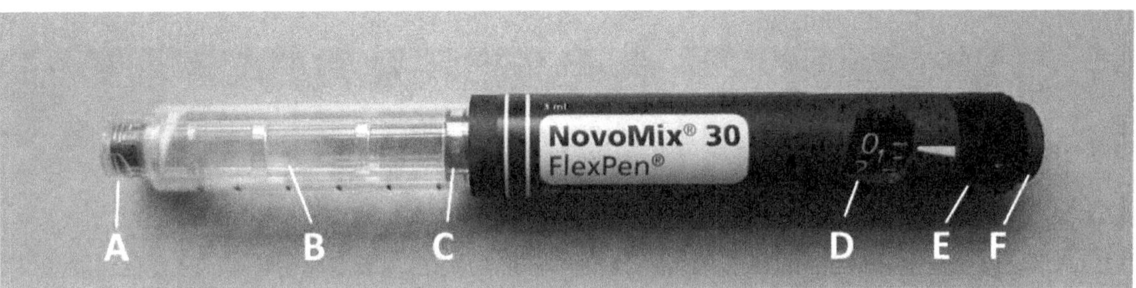

Figure 18.27 Insulin Pen A) tip, B) medication chamber, C) plunger, D) dose window, E) dose selection dial, F) plunger button

Special Considerations for Insulin

- Insulin vials are stored in the refrigerator until they are opened. When removed, it should be labelled with an open date and expiration date according to agency policy. When a vial is in use, it should be at room temperature. Do not inject cold insulin because this can cause discomfort.
- Patients who take insulin should monitor their blood sugar (glucose) levels as prescribed by their health care provider.
- Vials of insulin should be inspected prior to use. Any change in appearance may indicate a change in potency. Check the expiration date and do not use it if it has expired.
- All health care workers should be aware of the signs and symptoms of hypoglycemia. Signs and symptoms of hypoglycemia include fruity breath, restlessness, agitation, confusion, slurring of

26 Centers for Disease Control and Prevention. (2012, January 4). *CDC clinical reminder: Insulin pens must never be used for more than one person.* https://www.cdc.gov/injectionsafety/clinical-reminders/insulin-pens.html

27 American Association of Diabetes Educators. (n.d.). *Insulin injection know-how.* https://www.diabeteseducator.org/docs/default-source/legacy-docs/_resources/pdf/general/Insulin_Injection_How_To_AADE.pdf

28 This work is a derivative of Clinical Procedures for Safer Patient Care by British Columbia Institute of Technology and is licensed under CC BY 4.0. Access for free at https://opentextbc.ca/clinicalskills/

29 American Diabetes Association. (n.d.). *Insulin basics.* https://www.diabetes.org/diabetes/medication-management/insulin-other-injectables/insulin-basics

My Notes

words, clammy skin, inability to concentrate or follow commands, hunger, and nausea. Follow agency policy regarding hypoglycemic reactions.[30]

For more information about injecting insulin, read the following American Association of Diabetes Educators PDF:
"Insulin Injection Know-How"

For additional details about different types of insulin, hypoglycemia, and safety considerations when administering insulin, visit the "Antidiabetics" section of the "Endocrine" chapter in Open RN *Nursing Pharmacology*.

Video Review of Mixing Insulin[31]

A YouTube element has been excluded from this version of the text. You can view it online here: https://wtcs.pressbooks.pub/nursingskills/?p=2577

Heparin Injections

Heparin is an anticoagulant medication used to treat or prevent blood clots. It comes in various strengths and can be administered subcutaneously or intravenously. Heparin is also considered a high-alert medication because of the potential life-threatening harm that can result from a medication error. See Figure 18.28[32] for an image of a prefilled syringe of enoxaparin (Lovenox), a low-molecular weight heparin, that is typically dispensed in prefilled syringes. Review specific guidelines regarding heparin administration in Table 18.5.[33]

30 American Diabetes Association. (n.d.). *Insulin basics.* https://www.diabetes.org/diabetes/medication-management/insulin-other-injectables/insulin-basics

31 RegisteredNurseRN. (2016, July 15). *How to mix insulin NPH and regular insulin nursing | Mixing insulin clear to cloudy.* [Video]. YouTube. All rights reserved. Video used with permission. https://youtu.be/O_kXOnrYYRA

32 "syringe-103060_1920.jpg" by Stux from Pixabay is licensed under CC0. Access for free at https://pixabay.com/photos/syringe-disposable-syringe-blister-103059/

33 This work is a derivative of Clinical Procedures for Safer Patient Care by British Columbia Institute of Technology and is licensed under CC BY 4.0. Access for free at https://opentextbc.ca/clinicalskills/

My Notes

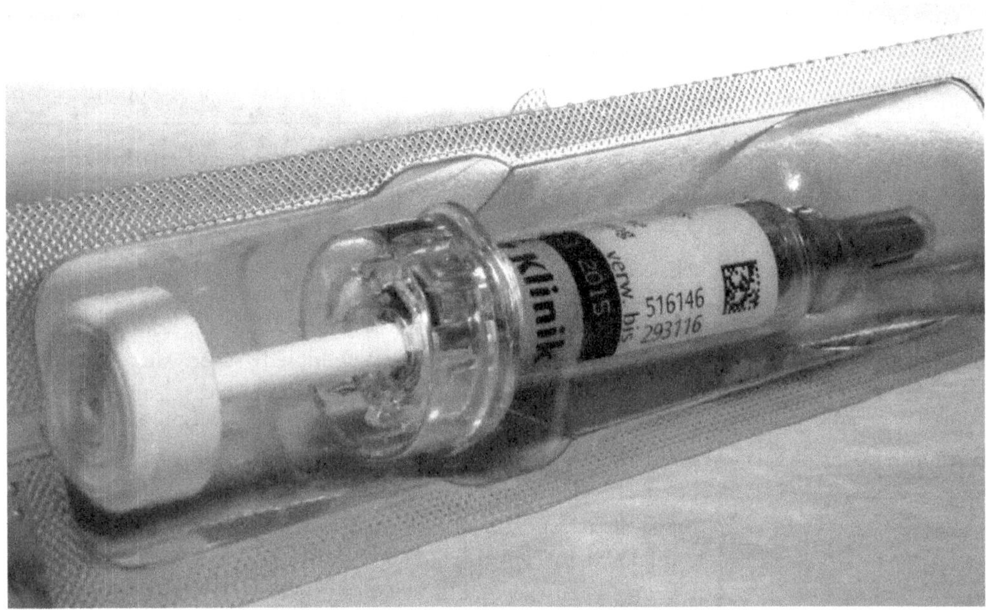

Figure 18.28 Low-Molecular Weight Heparin

For more information about heparin, visit the "Blood Coagulation Modifiers" section of the "Cardiovascular and Renal System" chapter in Open RN *Nursing Pharmacology*.

Table 18.5 Specific Guidelines for Administering Heparin[34]

Guidelines	Additional Information
Remember that heparin is considered a high-alert medication.	Heparin is available in vials and prefilled syringes in a variety of concentrations. Because of the dangerous adverse effects of the medication, it is considered a high-alert medication. Always follow agency policy regarding the preparation and administration of heparin.
Rotate heparin injection sites.	It is important to rotate heparin sites to avoid bruising in one location. Heparin is absorbed best in the abdominal area, at least 2 inches (5 cm.) away from the umbilicus.
Know the risks associated with heparin.	There are many risks associated with the administration of heparin, including bleeding, hematuria, hematemesis, bleeding gums, and melena. Monitor, document, and report these side effects when a patient is receiving heparin.

34 This work is a derivative of Clinical Procedures for Safer Patient Care by British Columbia Institute of Technology and is licensed under CC BY 4.0. Access for free at https://opentextbc.ca/clinicalskills/

My Notes

Guidelines	Additional Information
Review lab values.	Review lab values (PTT and aPTT) before and after heparin administration. If injecting low-molecular weight heparin (enoxaparin), review platelet count because heparin can cause thrombocytopenia.
Follow administration standards for prepackaged heparin and enoxaparin syringes.	Many agencies use prepackaged heparin and enoxaparin syringes. Always follow the standards for safe medication administration when using prefilled syringes.
Assess patient conditions prior to administration.	Some medical conditions increase the patient's risk for hemorrhage (severe bleeding), such as recent childbirth, severe kidney and liver disease, cerebral or aortic aneurysm, and cerebral vascular accidents (CVA).
Assess other medications and diet.	Over-the-counter (OTC) herbal medications, such as garlic, ginger, and horse chestnut, may interact with heparin. Additional medications that may interact or cause increased risk of bleeding include aspirin, NSAIDs, cephalosporins, antithyroid agents, thrombolytics, and probenecids. Foods like green leafy vegetables can alter the therapeutic effect of heparin.

Device Technology

A jet injector is a medical device used for vaccinations and other subcutaneous injections that uses a high-pressure, narrow stream of fluid to penetrate the skin instead of a hypodermic needle. An example of a flu vaccine approved for administration to adults aged 18-64 is AFLURIA © Quadrivalent. The most common injection-site adverse reactions of the jet injector flu vaccine up to seven days post-vaccination were tenderness, swelling, pain, redness, itching, and bruising.[35] Insulin can also be successfully administered via a jet injector, with research demonstrating improved glucose control because the insulin is spread out over a larger area of tissue and enters the bloodstream faster than when administered by an insulin pen or needle. Patients have indicated preference for insulin delivered by the jet injector compared to the insulin pen or syringe because it is needle-free with less tissue injury and pain as compared to the needle injection.[36] See Figure 18.29[37] for an image comparing insulin delivery devices.

35 Centers for Disease Control and Prevention. (2020, August 20). *Flu vaccination by jet injector*. https://www.cdc.gov/flu/prevent/jet-injector.htm

36 Guo, L., Xiao, X., Sun, X., & Qi, C. (2017). Comparison of jet injector and insulin pen in controlling plasma glucose and insulin concentrations in type 2 diabetic patients. *Medicine, 96*(1), e5482. https://doi.org/10.1097/MD.0000000000005482

37 "Insulin_Delivery_Devices.png" by BruceBlaus is licensed under CC BY-SA 4.0. Access for free at https://commons.wikimedia.org/wiki/File:Insulin_Delivery_Devices.png

My Notes

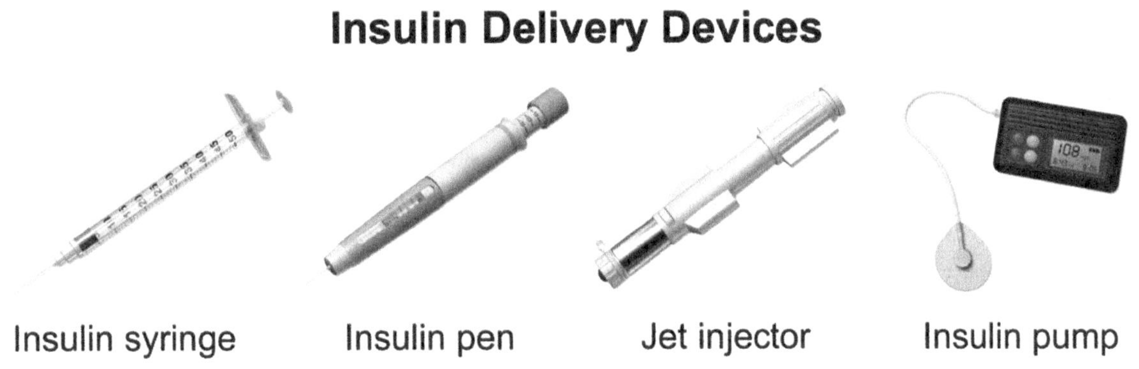

Insulin Delivery Devices

Insulin syringe Insulin pen Jet injector Insulin pump

Figure 18.29 Insulin Delivery Devices

Another type of new technology used to continuously deliver subcutaneous insulin is the insulin pump. Pumps are a computerized device attached to the body, either with tubing or attached to the skin. They are programmed to release small doses of insulin (continuously or as a surge bolus dose) close to mealtime to control the rise in blood sugar after a meal. They work by closely mimicking the body's normal release of insulin. Insulin doses are delivered through a flexible plastic tube called a catheter. With the aid of a small needle, the catheter is inserted through the skin into the fatty tissue and is taped in place.[38] See Figure 18.30[39] for an image of an insulin pump infusion set attached to a patient.

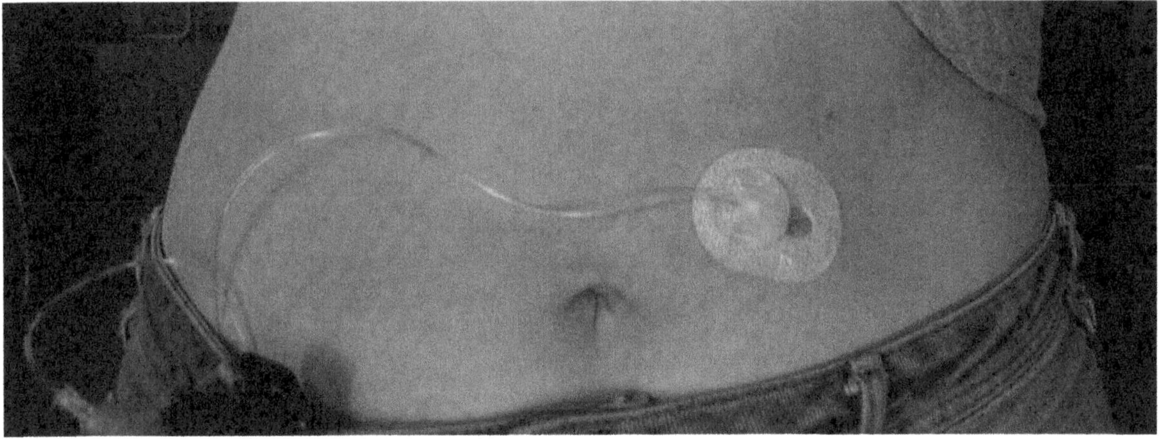

Figure 18.30 Insulin Pump

38 American Diabetes Association. (n.d.). *Device technology*. https://www.diabetes.org/diabetes/device-technology

39 "insulin pump day 1" by Erin Stevenson O'Connor is licensed under CC BY-SA 2.0. Access for free at https://www.flickr.com/photos/kirinqueen/159638798/

My Notes

18.6 ADMINISTERING INTRAMUSCULAR MEDICATIONS

The intramuscular (IM) injection route is used to place medication in muscle tissue. Muscle has an abundant blood supply that allows medications to be absorbed faster than the subcutaneous route.

Factors that influence the choice of muscle to use for an intramuscular injection include the patient's size, as well as the amount, viscosity, and type of medication. The length of the needle must be long enough to pass through the subcutaneous tissue to reach the muscle, so needles up to 1.5 inches long may be selected. However, if a patient is thin, a shorter needle length is used because there is less fat tissue to advance through to reach the muscle. Additionally, the muscle mass of infants and young children cannot tolerate large amounts of medication volume. Medication fluid amounts up to 0.5-1 mL can be injected in one site in infants and children, whereas adults can tolerate 2-5 mL. Intramuscular injections are administered at a 90-degree angle. Research has found administering medications at 10 seconds per mL is an effective rate for IM injections, but always review the drug administration rate per pharmacy or manufacturer's recommendations.[1]

Anatomic Sites

Anatomic sites must be selected carefully for intramuscular injections and include the ventrogluteal, vastus lateralis, and the deltoid. The vastus lateralis site is preferred for infants because that muscle is most developed. The ventrogluteal site is generally recommended for IM medication administration in adults, but IM vaccines may be administered in the deltoid site. Additional information regarding injections in each of these sites is provided in the following subsections.

Ventrogluteal

This site involves the gluteus medius and minimus muscle and is the safest injection site for adults and children because it provides the greatest thickness of gluteal muscles, is free from penetrating nerves and blood vessels, and has a thin layer of fat. To locate the ventrogluteal site, place the patient in a supine or lateral position. Use your right hand for the left hip or your left hand for the right hip. Place the heel or palm of your hand on the greater trochanter, with the thumb pointed toward the belly button. Extend your index finger to the anterior superior iliac spine and spread your middle finger pointing towards the iliac crest. Insert the needle into the "V" formed between your index and middle fingers. This is the preferred site for all oily and irritating solutions for patients of any age.[2] See Figure 18.31[3] for an image demonstrating how to accurately locate the ventrogluteal site using your hand.

1 This work is a derivative of Clinical Procedures for Safer Patient Care by British Columbia Institute of Technology and is licensed under CC BY 4.0. Access for free at https://opentextbc.ca/clinicalskills/

2 This work is a derivative of Clinical Procedures for Safer Patient Care by British Columbia Institute of Technology and is licensed under CC BY 4.0. Access for free at https://opentextbc.ca/clinicalskills/

3 "Im-ventrogluteal-300x244.png" by British Columbia Institute of Technology is licensed under CC BY 4.0. Access for free at https://opentextbc.ca/clinicalskills/chapter/6-8-iv-push-medications-and-saline-lock-flush/

My Notes

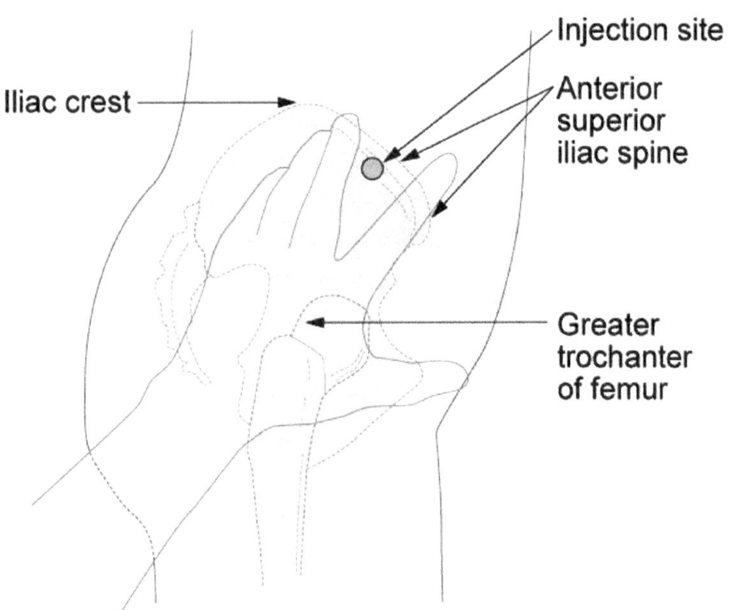

Figure 18.31 Locating the Ventrogluteal Site

The needle gauge used at the **ventrogluteal** site is determined by the solution of the medication ordered. An aqueous solution can be given with a 20- to 25-gauge needle, whereas viscous or oil-based solutions are given with 18- to 21-gauge needles. The needle length is based on patient weight and body mass index. A thin adult may require a 5/8-inch to 1-inch (16 mm to 25 mm) needle, while an average adult may require a 1-inch (25 mm) needle, and a larger adult (over 70 kg) may require a 1-inch to 1½-inch (25 mm to 38 mm) needle. Children and infants require shorter needles. Refer to agency policies regarding needle length for infants, children, and adolescents. Up to 3 mL of medication may be administered in the ventrogluteal muscle of an average adult and up to 1 mL in children. See Figure 18.32[4] for an image of locating the ventrogluteal site on a patient.

4 "Injection Site Image1.heic" by Meredith Pomietlo for Chippewa Valley Technical College is licensed under CC BY 4.0. Access for free at https://drive.google.com/file/d/13jkVZwlkbAlsLtJhRR6-XismNIAg3MDb/view?usp=sharing

My Notes

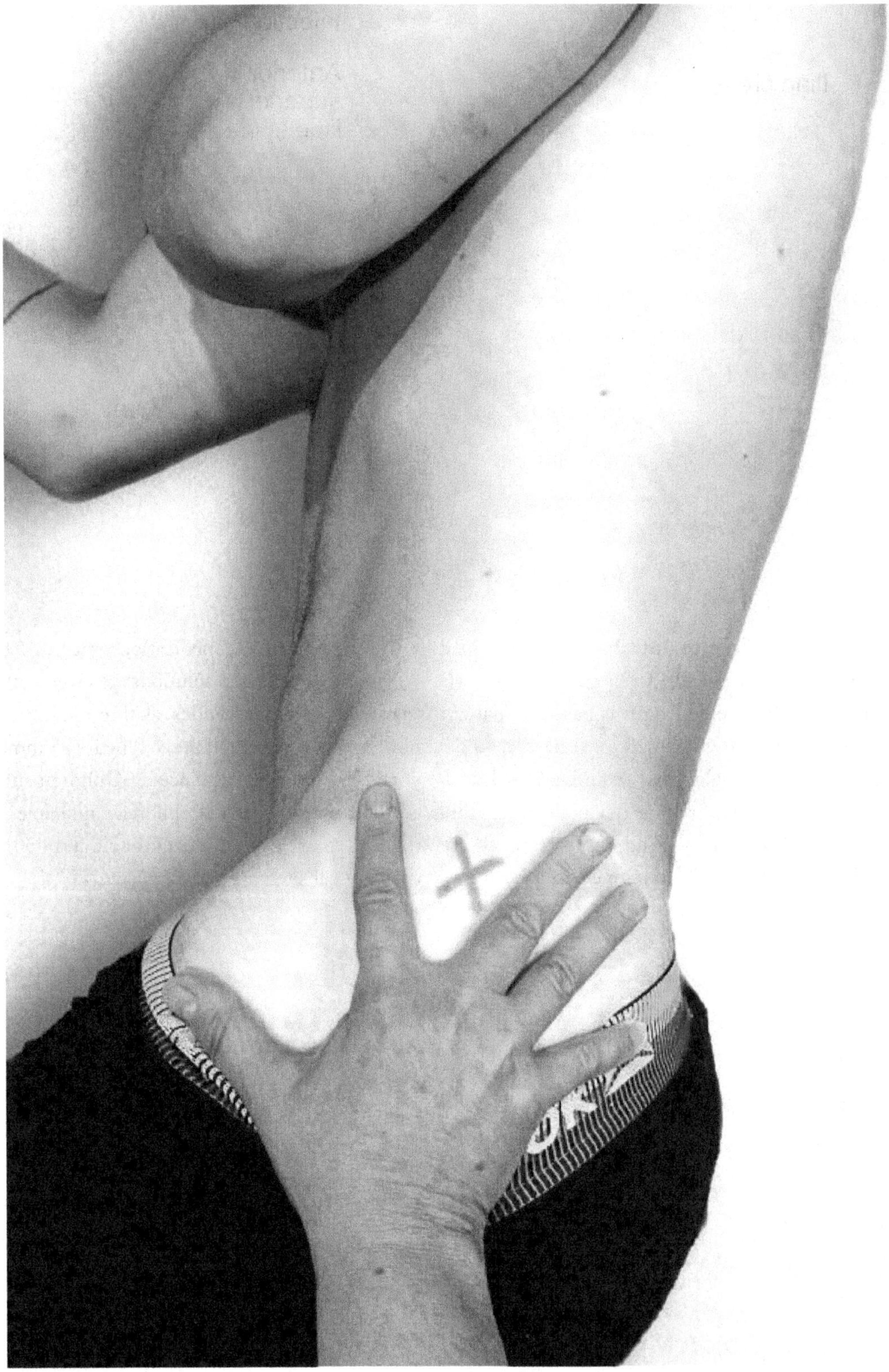

Figure 18.32 Ventrogluteal Site

My Notes

Vastus Lateralis

The **vastus lateralis** site is commonly used for immunizations in infants and toddlers because the muscle is thick and well-developed. This muscle is located on the anterior lateral aspect of the thigh and extends from one hand's breadth above the knee to one hand's breadth below the greater trochanter. The outer middle third of the muscle is used for injections. To help relax the patient, ask the patient to lie flat with knees slightly bent or have the patient in a sitting position. See Figure 18.33[5] for an image of the vastus lateralis injection site.

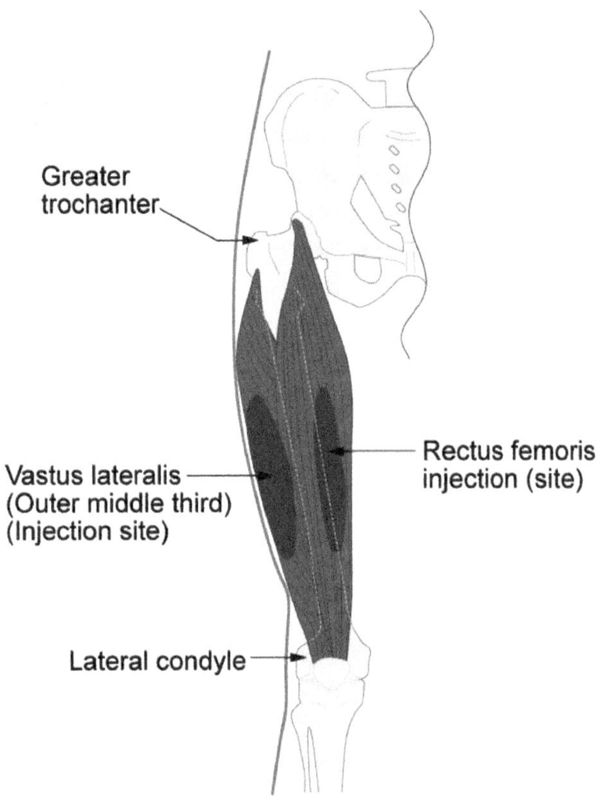

Figure 18.33 Vastus Lateralis Site

The length of the needle used at the vastus lateralis site is based on the patient's age, weight, and body mass index. In general, the recommended needle length for an adult is 1 inch to 1 ½ inches (25 mm to 38 mm), but the needle length is shorter for children. Refer to agency policy for pediatric needle lengths. The gauge of the needle is determined by the type of medication administered. Aqueous solutions can be given with a 20- to 25-gauge needle; oily or viscous medications should be administered with 18- to 21-gauge needles. A smaller gauge needle (22 to 25 gauge) should be used with children. The maximum amount of medication for a single injection in an adult is 3 mL. See Figure 18.34[6] for an image of an intramuscular injection being administered at the vastus lateralis site.

---

5 "Im-vastus-lateralis.png" by British Columbia Institute of Technology is licensed under CC BY 4.0. Access for free at https://opentextbc.ca/clinicalskills/chapter/6-7-intradermal-subcutaneous-and-intramuscular-injections/

6 "Vastus Lateralis Site" by Meredith Pomietlo for Chippewa Valley Technical College is licensed under CC BY 4.0. Access for free at https://drive.google.com/file/d/1ltTpqnI2iLgsbc6UyZn0vG1EG2Ju2mdL/view?usp=sharing

My Notes

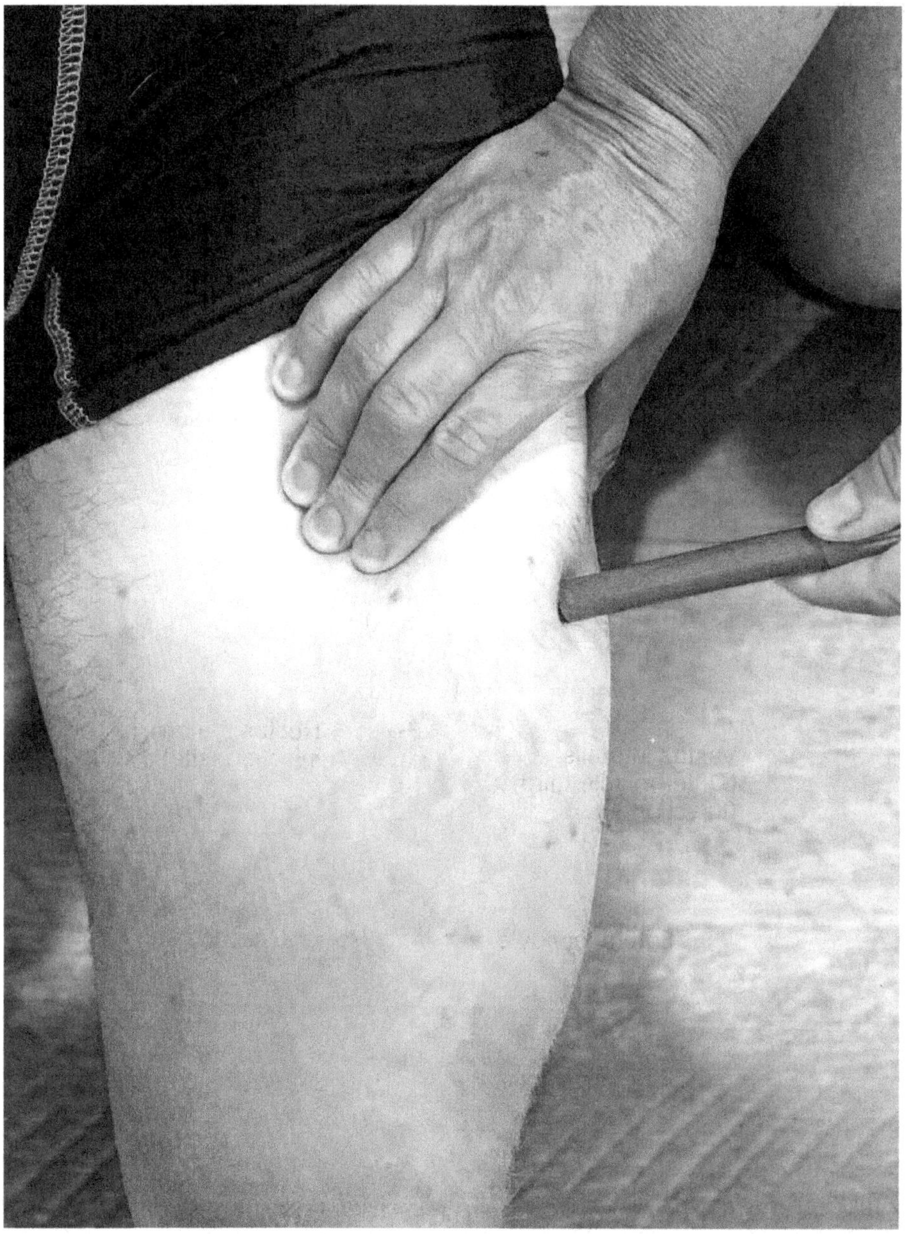

Figure 18.34 Intramuscular Injection at Vastus Lateralis Site

Deltoid

My Notes

The **deltoid** muscle has a triangular shape and is easy to locate and access. To locate the injection site, begin by having the patient relax their arm. The patient can be standing, sitting, or lying down. To locate the landmark for the deltoid muscle, expose the upper arm and find the acromion process by palpating the bony prominence. The injection site is in the middle of the deltoid muscle, about 1 inch to 2 inches (2.5 cm to 5 cm) below the acromion process. To locate this area, lay three fingers across the deltoid muscle and below the acromion process. The injection site is generally three finger widths below in the middle of the muscle. See Figure 18.35[7] for an illustration for locating the deltoid injection site.

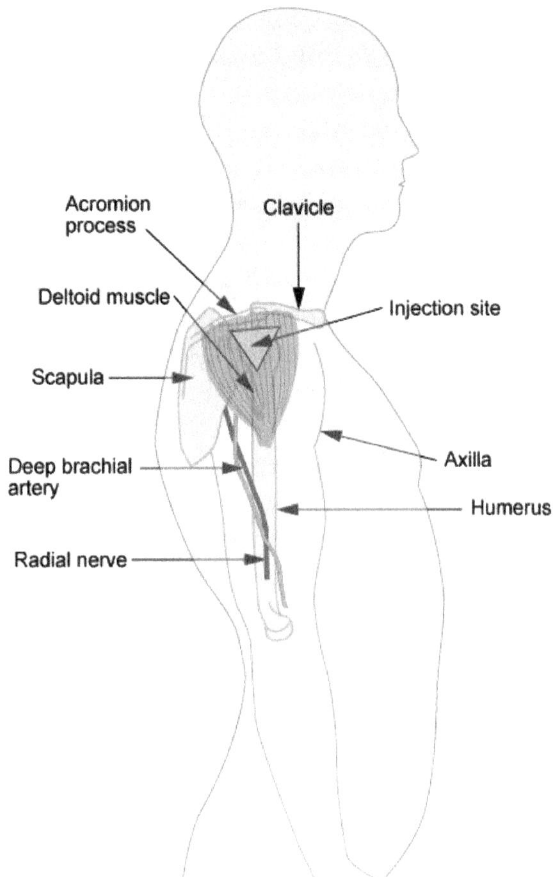

Figure 18.35 Locating the Deltoid Injection Site

Select the needle length based on the patient's age, weight, and body mass. In general, for an adult male weighing 60 kg to 118 kg (130 to 260 lbs), a 1-inch (25 mm) needle is sufficient. For women under 60 kg (130 lbs), a ⅝-inch (16 mm) needle is sufficient, while for women between 60 kg and 90 kg (130 to 200 lbs) a 1-inch (25 mm) needle is required. A 1 ½-inch (38 mm) length needle may be required for women over 90 kg (200 lbs) for a deltoid IM injection. For immunizations, a 22- to 25-gauge needle should be used. Refer to agency policy regarding

7 "Im-deltoid.png" by British Columbia Institute of Technology is licensed under CC BY 4.0. Access for free at https://opentextbc.ca/clinicalskills/chapter/6-7-intradermal-subcutaneous-and-intramuscular-injections/

My Notes

specifications for infants, children, adolescents, and immunizations. The maximum amount of medication for a single injection is generally 1 mL. See Figure 18.36[8] for an image of locating the deltoid injection site on a patient.

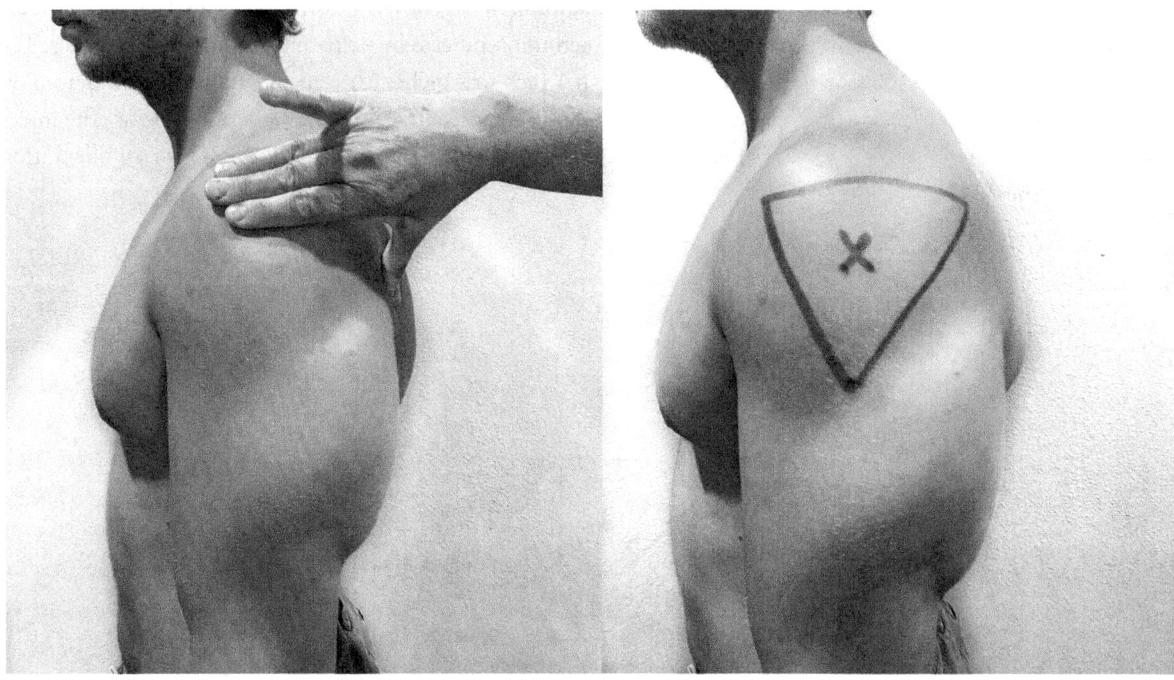

Figure 18.36 The Deltoid Injection Site

Description of Procedure

When administering an intramuscular injection, the procedure is similar to a subcutaneous injection, but instead of pinching the skin, stabilize the skin around the injection site with your nondominant hand. With your dominant hand, hold the syringe like a dart and inject the needle quickly into the muscle at a 90-degree angle using a steady and smooth motion. After the needle pierces the skin, use the thumb and forefinger of the nondominant hand to hold the syringe. If aspiration is indicated according to agency policy and manufacturer recommendations, pull the plunger back to aspirate for blood. If no blood appears, inject the medication slowly and steadily. If blood appears, discard the syringe and needle and prepare the medication again. See Figure 18.37[9] for an image of aspirating for blood. After the medication is completely injected, remove the needle using a smooth, steady motion. Remove the needle at the same angle at which it was inserted. Cover the injection site with sterile gauze using gentle pressure and apply a Band-Aid if needed.[10]

---

8 "Injection Site Image 3.jpg" and "Injection Site Image 2.jpg" by Meredith Pomietlo for Chippewa Valley Technical College are licensed under CC BY 4.0. Access for free at https://drive.google.com/file/d/1Lly6r7cYT3LjpecCktoMY4cLU5c91NDY/view?usp=sharing

9 "Sept-22-2015-111.jpg" by British Columbia Institute of Technology is licensed under CC BY 4.0. Access for free at https://opentextbc.ca/clinicalskills/chapter/6-8-iv-push-medications-and-saline-lock-flush/

10 This work is a derivative of Clinical Procedures for Safer Patient Care by British Columbia Institute of Technology and is licensed under CC BY 4.0. Access for free at https://opentextbc.ca/clinicalskills/

My Notes

Because the injection sites recommended for immunizations do not contain large blood vessels, the CDC recommends there is no longer the need to aspirate when administering vaccines.[11]

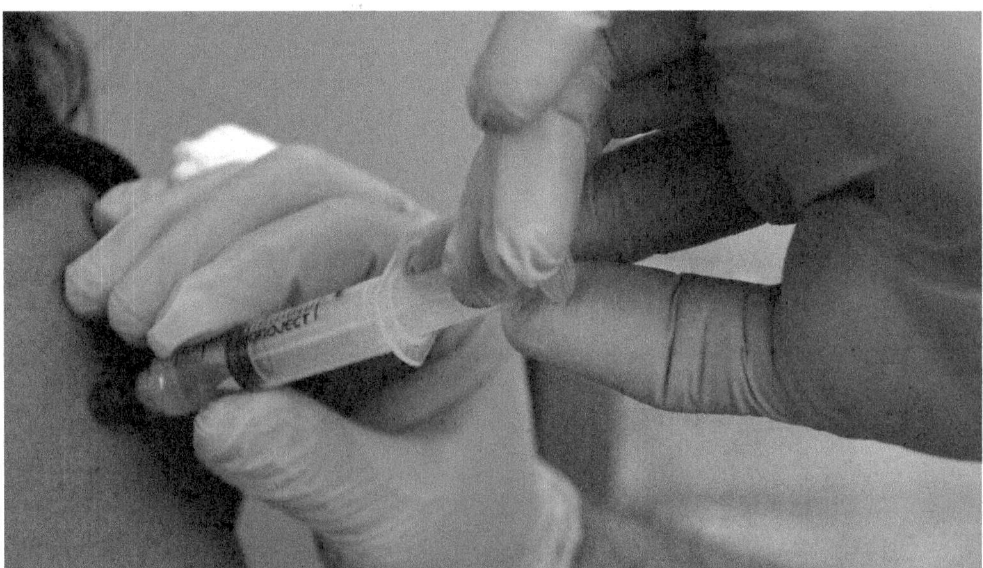

Figure 18.37 Aspirating for Blood

Z-track Method for IM injections

Evidence-based practice supports using the **Z-track method** for administration of intramuscular injections. This method prevents the medication from leaking into the subcutaneous tissue, allows the medication to stay in the muscles, and can minimize irritation.[12]

The Z-track method creates a zigzag path to prevent medication from leaking into the subcutaneous tissue. This method may be used for all injections or may be specified by the medication.

Displace the patient's skin in a Z-track manner by pulling the skin down or to one side about 1 inch (2 cm) with your nondominant hand before administering the injection. With the skin held to one side, quickly insert the needle at a 90-degree angle. After the needle pierces the skin, continue pulling on the skin with the nondominant hand, and at the same time, grasp the lower end of the syringe barrel with the fingers of the nondominant hand to stabilize it. Move your dominant hand and pull the end of the plunger to aspirate for blood, if indicated. If no blood appears, inject the medication slowly. Once the medication is given, leave the needle in place for ten seconds.

---

11 Centers for Disease Control and Prevention. (2019, April 15). *Vaccine administration*. https://www.cdc.gov/vaccines/pubs/pinkbook/vac-admin.html

12 Yilmaz, D., Khorshid, L., & Dedeoğlu, Y. (2016). The effect of the z-track technique on pain and drug leakage in intramuscular injections. *Clinical Nurse Specialist, 30*(6), E7-E12. https://doi.org/10.1097/nur.0000000000000245

My Notes

After the medication is completely injected, remove the needle using a smooth, steady motion, and then release the skin. See Figure 18.38[13] for an illustration of the Z-track method.

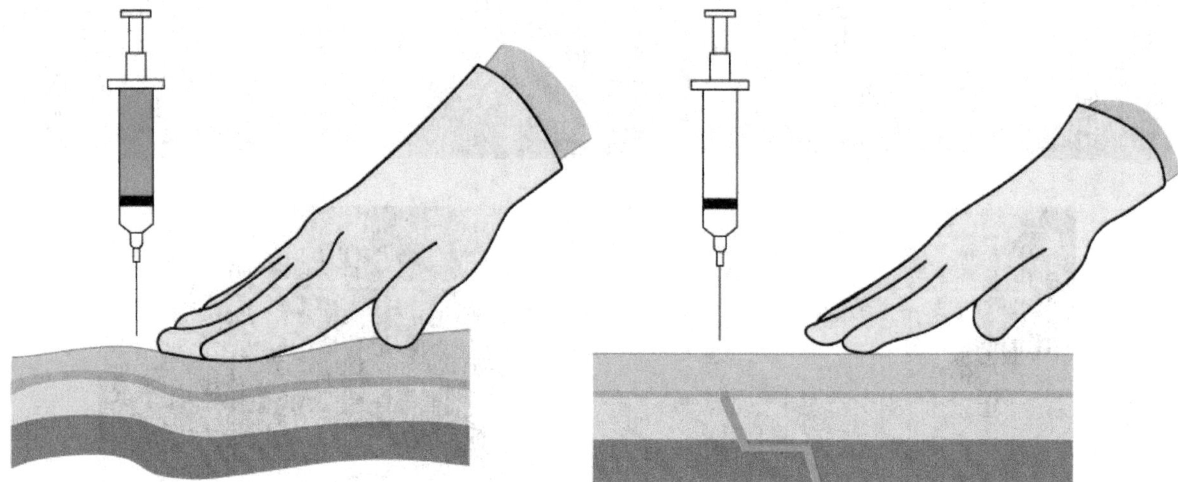

Figure 18.38 Z-track Method

Special Considerations for IM Injections

- Avoid using sites with atrophied muscle because they will poorly absorb medications.
- If repeated IM injections are given, sites should be rotated to decrease the risk of hypertrophy.
- Older adults and thin patients may only tolerate up to 2 milliliters in a single injection.
- Choose a site that is free from pain, infection, abrasions, or necrosis.
- The dorsogluteal site should be avoided for intramuscular injections because of the risk for injury. If the needle inadvertently hits the sciatic nerve, the patient may experience partial or permanent paralysis of the leg.

13 "Z-track-process-1.png" and "Z-track-process-3.png" by British Columbia Institute of Technology are licensed under CC BY 4.0. Access for free at https://opentextbc.ca/clinicalskills/chapter/6-8-iv-push-medications-and-saline-lock-flush/

Video Reviews of Administering Intramuscular Injections

My Notes

Z-Track Method[14]

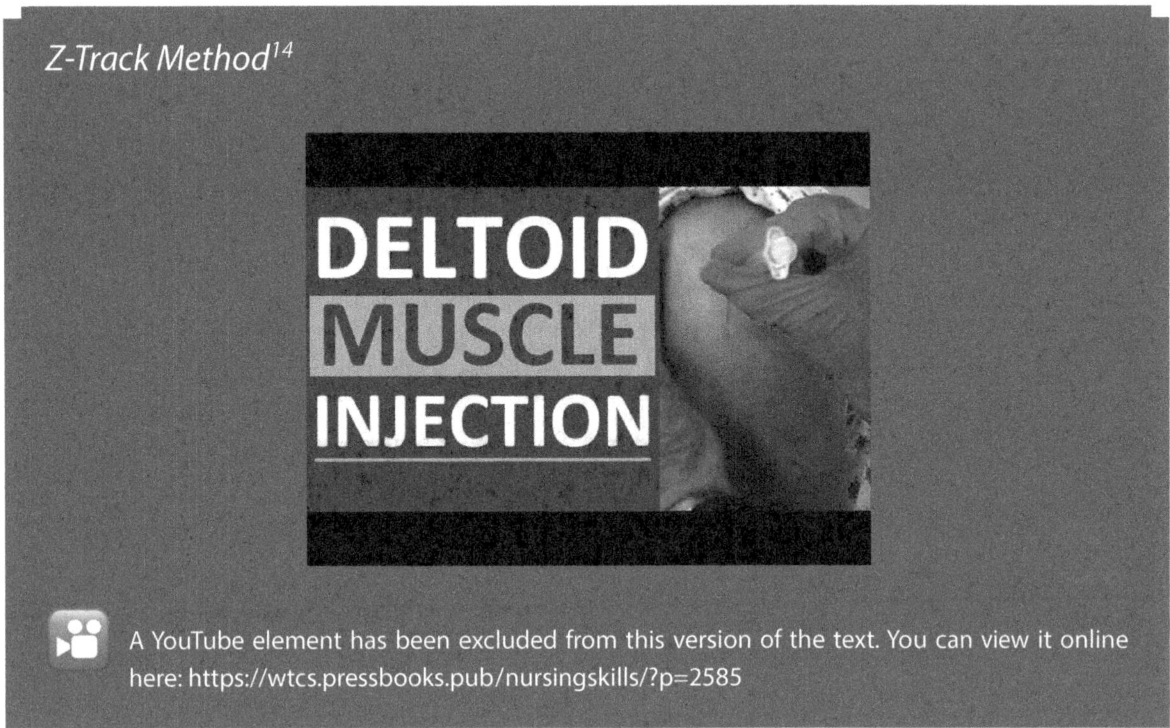

A YouTube element has been excluded from this version of the text. You can view it online here: https://wtcs.pressbooks.pub/nursingskills/?p=2585

IM injection Ventrogluteal Site

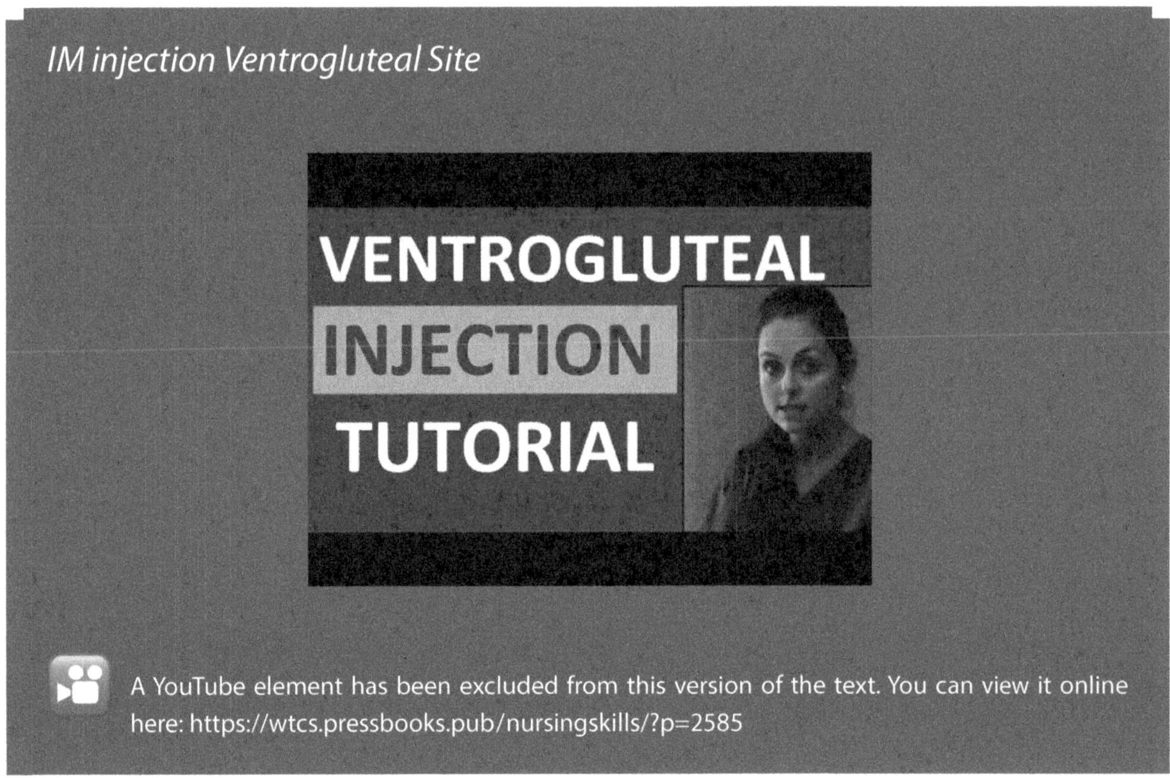

A YouTube element has been excluded from this version of the text. You can view it online here: https://wtcs.pressbooks.pub/nursingskills/?p=2585

14 RegisteredNurseRN. (2018, November 19). *Intramuscular injection in deltoid muscle with Z-Track Technique.* [Video]. YouTube. All rights reserved. Video used with permission. https://youtu.be/DBHnd3N-5Ns

My Notes

IM injection Dorsogluteal Site[15]

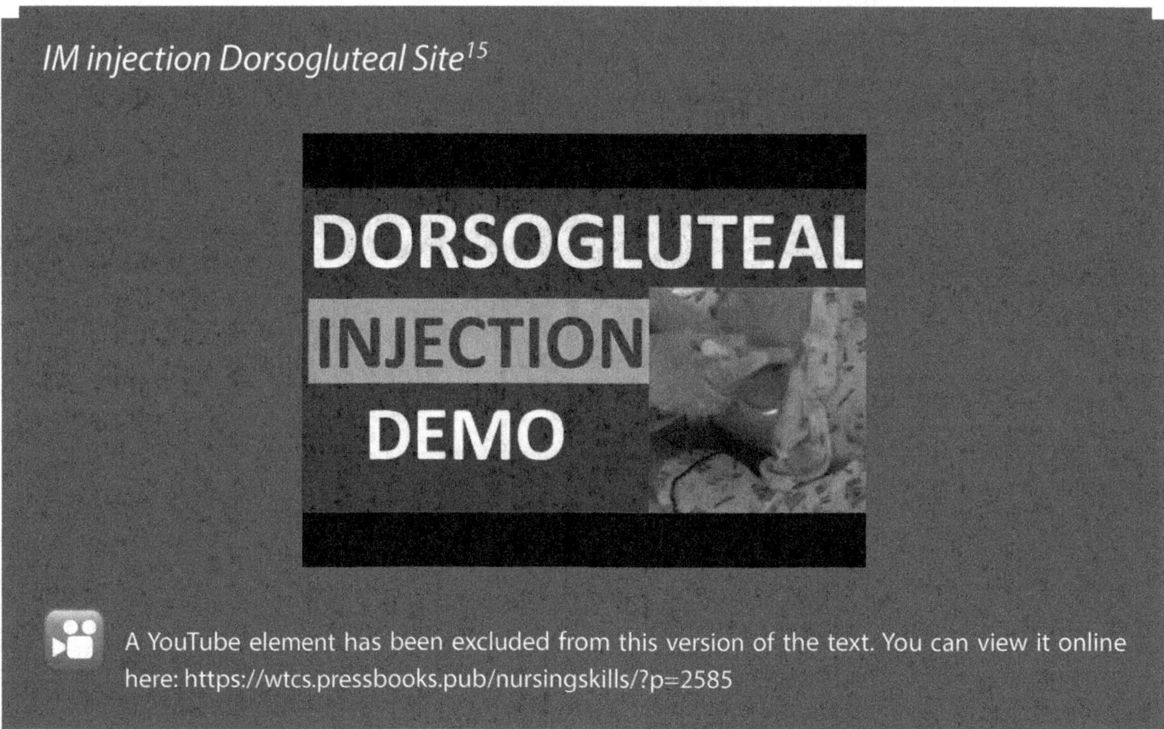

A YouTube element has been excluded from this version of the text. You can view it online here: https://wtcs.pressbooks.pub/nursingskills/?p=2585

15 RegisteredNurseRN. (2014, August 8). *How to give an IM intramuscular injection in the buttocks | Dorsogluteal hip injection technique*. [Video]. YouTube. All rights reserved. Video used with permission. https://youtu.be/v_pRjbM2sV8

18.7 APPLYING THE NURSING PROCESS

My Notes

Assessments Prior to Injection Administration

When administering any parenteral injection, the nurse assesses the patient prior to administration for safe medication administration. See Table 18.7 to review assessments prior to medication administration.

Table 18.7 Assessments Prior to Injection Administration

Assessment	Rationale/Considerations
Check the MAR with the written medication prescription for accuracy and completeness.	Prevent medication errors.
Perform the rights of medication administration, including patient's name, medication name and dose, route, time of administration, and verify the expiration date. Label syringes with medication names as you prepare them.	Prevent medication errors. Discard medication if expired. Label syringes during the procedure to administer medications safely according to the Joint Commission.[1]
Assess and review a patient's current medical condition, past medical history, and medication history.	Identify the need for the medication, as well as any possible contraindications for the administration of prescribed medication to the specific patient.
Assess the patient's history of medication allergies or nondrug allergies that may interfere with the medication. If there is a history of allergic reactions, document the type of reaction if possible (e.g., hives, rash, swelling, difficulty breathing). If there is an allergy to prescriber medication, do not prepare it and notify the prescribing provider.	Safely administer medication.
Review a current, evidence-based drug reference to determine medication action, indication for medication, normal dosage range, and potential side effects. Identify peak and onset times, as well as any nursing considerations.	Safely administer medication and plan to monitor the patient's response. For example, by knowing the peak onset of fast-acting insulin, the nurse anticipates when the patient may be most at risk for a hypoglycemic reaction.

1 The Joint Commission. (n.d.). 2020 Hospital national patient safety goals. https://www.jointcommission.org/standards/national-patient-safety-goals/

My Notes

Assessment	Rationale/Considerations
Review and assess pertinent laboratory results (i.e., blood glucose, prothrombin times). Be aware of abnormal kidney and liver function results because they may affect metabolism of medication. Notify the prescriber of any concerns.	Collect data to determine if the medication should be withheld to ensure proper dosage and to establish a baseline for measuring the patient's response to the drug.
Observe the patient's verbal and nonverbal reactions to the injection.	Be aware of the patient's level of anxiety and use distractions and other therapeutic techniques to reduce pain and anxiety.
Perform patient assessments, such as vital signs, lung sounds, or pain level, as indicated, prior to medication administration.	Obtain baseline data to ensure medication administration is appropriate at this time and to establish a baseline for measuring the patient's response to the medication.
Assess for contraindications to subcutaneous or intramuscular injections such as muscle atrophy or decreased blood flow to the tissue.	Assess for contraindications because reduced muscle and blood flow interfere with the drug absorption and distribution.
Assess the patient's knowledge of the medication.	Perform patient education about the medication as needed.
Assess the skin and tissue quality around the area of the intended injection site. Note any bruising, nonintact skin, abrasions, masses, or scar tissue. Avoid these areas and choose another recommended location.	Assess skin and tissue quality to avoid unnecessary or further injury to the already compromised skin integrity. Areas that are scarred or atrophied can affect the absorption and distribution of the medication.

Evaluation

Nurses evaluate for possible complications of parenteral medication administration that may occur as a result of a medication error or as an adverse reaction. Complications may occur if a medication is prepared incorrectly, if the medication is injected incorrectly, or if an adverse effect occurs after the medication is injected. Unexpected outcomes can occur such as nerve or tissue damage, ineffective absorption of the medication, pain, bleeding, or infection.

An adverse reaction may develop as a result of an injected medication. An adverse reaction may also occur despite appropriate administration of medication and can happen for various reasons. A reaction may be evident within minutes or days after the exposure to the injectable medication. An unexpected outcome may range from a minor reaction, like a skin rash, to serious and life-threatening events such as anaphylaxis, hemorrhaging, and even death.

If a suspected complication occurs during administration, immediately stop the injection. Assess and monitor vital signs, notify the health care provider, and document an incident report.

18.8 CHECKLISTS FOR PARENTERAL MEDICATION ADMINISTRATION

My Notes

Checklist for Parenteral Site Identification

Use the checklist below to review the steps for completion of "Parenteral Site Identification."

Directions: Identify parenteral injection sites, needle size/gauge, injection angle, and the appropriate amount that can be administered in each of the parenteral routes: intradermal, subcutaneous, and intramuscular.

1. Describe the appropriate needle gauge, length, number of cc's, and angle for an intradermal injection:
    - 25-27G
    - 3/8" to 5/8"
    - 0.1 mL (for TB testing)
    - 5 to 15 degree angle
2. Demonstrate locating the intradermal injection sites on a peer:
    - Upper third of the forearm
    - Outer aspects upper arms
    - Between scapula
3. Describe the appropriate needle gauge, length, number of mL, and angle for a subcutaneous injection:
    - 25-31G
    - to 5/8"
    - Up to 1 mL
    - 45 to 90 degree angle
4. Demonstrate locating the subcutaneous injection sites on a peer:
    - Anterior thighs
    - Abdomen
5. Describe the appropriate needle gauge, length, number of mL, and angle for an adult intramuscular:
    - 18-25G
    - – 1 ½" (based on age/size of patient and site used)
    - <0.5 – 1 mL (infants and children), 2-5 mL (adults)
    - 90-degree angle
6. Demonstrate locating the intramuscular injection sites on a peer:
    - Ventrogluteal
    - Vastus laterus
    - Deltoid
7. Explain how you would modify assessment techniques to reflect variations across the life span and body size variations.

My Notes

Checklist for Parenteral Medication Injections

Use the checklist below to review the steps for completion of "Parenteral Medication Injections."

Steps

Disclaimer: Always review and follow agency policy regarding this specific skill.

Special Considerations:

- Plan medication administration to avoid disruption.
- Dispense medication in a quiet area.
- Avoid conversation with others.
- Follow agency's no-interruption zone policy.
- Prepare medications for ONE patient at a time.
- Plan for disposal of sharps in an appropriate sharps disposal container.

1. Check the orders and MAR for accuracy and completeness; clarify any unclear orders.
2. Review pertinent information related to the medications: labs, last time medication was given, and medication information: generic name, brand name, dose, route, time, class, action, purpose, side effects, contraindications, and nursing considerations.
3. Gather available supplies: correctly sized syringes and needles appropriate for medication, patient's size, and site of injection; diluent (if required); tape or patient label for each syringe; nonsterile gloves; sharps container; and alcohol wipes.
4. Perform hand hygiene.
5. While withdrawing medication from the medication dispensing system, perform the first check of the six rights of medication administration. Check expiration date and perform any necessary calculations.
6. Select the correct type of syringe and needle size appropriate for the medication, patient size, and site of injection.

Preparing the Medication for Administration

7. Scrub the top of the vial of the correct medication. State the correct dose to be drawn.
8. Remove the cap from the needle. Pull back on the plunger to draw air into the syringe equal to the dose.
9. With the vial on a flat surface, insert the needle. Invert the vial and withdraw the correct amount of the medication. Expel any air bubbles. Remove the needle from the vial.
10. Using the scoop method, recap the needle.
11. Perform the second check of the six rights of medication administration, looking at the vial, syringe, and MAR.
12. Label the syringe with the name of the drug and dose.

Additional Preparation Steps When Mixing Two Types of Insulin in One Syringe

My Notes

Intermediate-Acting (NPH) and Short-Acting (Regular) insulins

a. Place the vials side by side on a flat surface: NPH on left and regular insulin on the right.

b. With an alcohol pad, scrub off the vial top of the NPH insulin. Using a new alcohol pad, scrub the vial top of the regular insulin. Discard any prep pads.

c. Select the correct insulin syringe that will exactly measure the TOTAL dose of the amount of NPH and regular doses (30- and 50-unit syringes measure single units; 100-unit syringes only measure even numbered doses).

d. Pull back on the plunger to draw air into the syringe equal to the dose of NPH insulin.

e. With the NPH vial on a flat surface, remove the cap from the syringe, insert the needle into the NPH vial, and inject air. Do not let the tip of the needle touch the insulin solution. Withdraw the needle.

f. Pull back on the plunger to draw air into the syringe equal to the dose of the regular insulin.

g. With the regular vial on a flat surface, remove the cap from the syringe, insert the needle into the regular vial, and inject air.

h. With the needle still in the vial, invert the regular insulin vial and withdraw the correct dose. Remove the needle from the vial. Cap the needle using the scoop method.

i. Roll the NPH insulin vial between your hands to mix the solution. Uncap the needle and insert the needle into the NPH insulin vial. Withdraw the correct amount of NPH insulin. Withdraw the needle and recap using the scoop method.

j. Perform the second medication check of the combined dose looking at the vial, syringe, and MAR, verifying all the rights.

k. Label the syringe with the name of the combined medications and doses.

Alternative Preparation Using an Insulin Pen

a. Select the correct insulin pen to be used for the injection. Identify the dose to be given.

b. Remove the cap from the insulin pen and clean the top (hub) with an alcohol prep pad. Attach the insulin pen needle without contaminating the needle or pen hub.

c. Turn the dial to two units and push the injection button to prime the pen.

d. Turn the dial to the correct dose.

e. Perform the second medication check looking at the insulin pen and MAR, verifying all the rights.

Administration of Parenteral Medication

13. Knock, enter the room, greet the patient, and provide for privacy.

14. Perform safety steps:

My Notes

- Perform hand hygiene.
- Check the room for transmission-based precautions.
- Introduce yourself, your role, the purpose of your visit, and an estimate of the time it will take.
- Confirm patient ID using two patient identifiers (e.g., name and date of birth).
- Explain the process to the patient and ask if they have any questions.
- Be organized and systematic.
- Use appropriate listening and questioning skills.
- Listen and attend to patient cues.
- Ensure the patient's privacy and dignity.
- Assess ABCs.

15. Perform the third check of the six rights of medication administration at the patient's bedside after performing patient identification.

16. Perform the following steps according to the type of parenteral medication.

Intradermal – Administration of a Tb Test

a. Correctly identify the sites and verbalize the landmarks used for intradermal injections.

b. Select the correct site for the TB test, verbalizing the anatomical landmarks and skin considerations.

c. Put on nonsterile gloves if contact with blood or body fluids is likely or if your skin or the patient's skin isn't intact.

d. Use an alcohol swab in a circular motion to clean the skin at the site; place the pad above the site to mark the site, if desired.

e. Using the nondominant hand, gently pull the skin away from the site.

f. Insert the needle with the bevel facing upward, slowly at a 5- to 15-degree angle, and then advance no more than an eighth of an inch to cover the bevel.

g. Use the thumb of the nondominant hand to push on the plunger to slowly inject the medication. Inspect the site, noting if a small bleb forms under the skin surface.

h. Carefully withdraw the needle straight back out of the insertion site so not to disturb the bleb (do not massage or cover the site).

i. Activate the safety feature of the needle and place the syringe in the sharps container.

j. Teach the patient to return for a TB skin test reading in 48-72 hours and not to press on the site or apply a Band-Aid.

Subcutaneous – Administration of Insulin in a Syringe

a. Correctly identify the sites and verbalize the landmarks used for subcutaneous injections. Ask the patient regarding a preferred site of medication administration.

My Notes

b. Put on nonsterile gloves if contact with blood or body fluids is likely or if your skin or the patient's skin isn't intact.

c. Select an appropriate site and clean with an alcohol prep in a circular motion. Place the pad above the site to mark the location, if desired. Remove the cap from the needle without contaminating the needle.

d. Pinch approximately an inch of subcutaneous tissue, creating a skinfold.

e. Inject the needle at 90-degree angle, release the patient's skin, and inject the medication. Withdraw the needle.

f. Activate the safety feature of the needle and place the syringe in a sharps container.

Subcutaneous – Administration With an Insulin Pen

a. Select the site and clean with an alcohol prep in a circular motion. Place the pad above the site to mark the location, if desired. Remove the cap from the needle without contaminating the needle.

b. Put on nonsterile gloves if contact with blood or body fluids is likely or if your skin or the patient's skin isn't intact.

c. Pinch approximately an inch of subcutaneous tissue, creating a skinfold.

d. Inject the needle quickly at a 90-degree angle, continue to hold the skinfold, and inject the medication. After the medication is injected, count to 10, remove the needle, and release the skinfold.

e. Dispose of the needle in a sharps container. Replace the top cap to the insulin pen.

Intramuscular – Deltoid

a. Correctly identify the site and verbalize the landmarks used for a deltoid injection.

b. Put on nonsterile gloves if contact with blood or body fluids is likely or if your skin or the patient's skin isn't intact.

c. Use an alcohol swab in a circular motion to clean the skin at the site. Place a pad above the site to mark the location. Remove the cap from the needle without contaminating the needle.

d. Depending on the muscle mass of the deltoid, either grasp the body of the muscle between the thumb and forefingers of the nondominant hand or spread the skin taut.

e. Inject the needle at a 90-degree angle.

f. Follow agency policy and manufacturer recommendations regarding aspiration.

g. Continue to hold the muscle fold and inject the medication. After the medication is injected, count to 10, remove the needle, and release the muscle fold.

h. Activate the safety on the syringe. Place the syringe in a sharps container.

Intramuscular – Vastus Lateralis

a. Correctly identify the site and verbalize the landmarks to locate the vastus lateralis site.

My Notes

b. Put on nonsterile gloves if contact with blood or body fluids is likely or if your skin or the patient's skin isn't intact.

c. Use an alcohol swab in a circular motion to clean the skin at the site. Place the pad above the site to mark the location. Remove the cap from the needle without contaminating the needle.

d. Depending on the muscle mass of the vastus lateralis, either grasp the body of the muscle between the thumb and forefingers of the nondominant hand or spread the skin taut.

e. Inject the needle at a 90-degree angle.

f. Follow agency policy and manufacturer recommendations regarding aspiration.

g. Continue to hold the muscle fold and inject the medication. After the medication is injected, count to 10, remove the needle, and release the muscle fold.

h. Activate the safety on the syringe. Put the needle in a sharps container.

Intramuscular – Ventrogluteal (Using the Z-Track Technique)

a. Correctly identify and verbalize the landmarks used to locate the ventrogluteal site.

b. Put on nonsterile gloves if contact with blood or body fluids is likely or if your skin or the patient's skin isn't intact.

c. Use an alcohol swab in a circular motion to clean the skin at the site and place a pad above the site to mark the location. Remove the cap from the needle without contaminating the needle.

d. Place the ulnar surface of the hand approximately 1 – 3 inches from the selected site; press down and pull the skin and subcutaneous tissue to the side or downward.

e. Maintaining tissue traction, hold the syringe like a dart and insert the needle into the skin at 90 degrees.

f. Maintaining tissue traction, use the available thumb and index finger to help stabilize the syringe.

g. Follow agency policy and manufacturer recommendations regarding aspiration. If aspiration is required, pull back the plunger and observe for blood return. If there is no blood return, inject the medication. If blood return is observed, remove the needle, and prepare a new medication.

h. Maintaining tissue traction, wait 10 seconds with the needle still in the skin to allow the muscle to absorb the medication. Withdraw the needle from the site and then release traction. Do not rub/massage the site.

i. Activate the safety feature of the needle; place in a sharps container.

Following Conclusion of All Injections

17. Assess site; apply Band-Aid if necessary and appropriate.

18. Remove gloves. Perform hand hygiene.

19. Ensure safety measures before leaving the room:

    - CALL LIGHT: Within reach
    - BED: Low and locked (in lowest position and brakes on)

My Notes

- SIDE RAILS: Secured
- TABLE: Within reach
- ROOM: Risk-free for falls (scan room and clear any obstacles)

20. Document medication administered, including the site used for the injection.

My Notes

18.9 SAMPLE DOCUMENTATION

Patient reports post-surgical pain at a level of 8/10. Patient is grimacing when moving in the bed and describes pain as a dull constant ache located in the right lower abdomen surgical incision area that is aggravated by moving or repositioning. Blood pressure 146/80, heart rate 94 bpm, respirations 22 per minute, temperature (tympanic) 98.8°F, pulse oximetry 98%. Last pain medication Ketorolac 30 mg (IM) given 8 hours ago. Incision site is dry and intact. Ketorolac 30mg IM administered per health provider's prescription in the left ventrogluteal area with 22-gauge needle, length 1 ½ inches. Patient tolerated the procedure without difficulty or increased pain. Injection site post-procedure without bleeding or hematoma.

18.10 LEARNING ACTIVITIES

My Notes

Learning Activities

(Answers to "Learning Activities" can be found in the "Answer Key" at the end of the book. Answers to interactive activity elements will be provided within the element as immediate feedback.)

1. An older, frail patient is prescribed a flu vaccine that is an aqueous or water-based solution. The patient's deltoid muscle is not very prominent, and the patient has very little fat over the deltoid. The needles available are 23 G 5⁄8 inch, 22 G 1 inch, and 20 G 1 1⁄2 inch.
   a. What needle size/length would work best for this particular medication and patient? ***Give the reason for your selection.***
2. A patient is hospitalized on the surgical floor. Pain medication is prescribed to be given by intramuscular route. After calculating, the volume to be administered is 2 mL. The patient has a large amount of adipose tissue around her hips and buttocks region and weighs 253 pounds. The needle sizes available include 27 G 3⁄8 inch, 25 G 5⁄8 inch, 22 G 1 inch, 21 G 1 1⁄2 inch, and 20 G 2 inches.
   a. What needle size/length and injection site would work best for this particular medication and patient? ***Give the reason for your selection.***
3. The nurse is teaching a patient how to mix 5 units of regular insulin and 15 units of NPH insulin in the same syringe. The nurse determines further instruction is needed if the patient does which of the following?
   a. Injects 5 units of air into the regular insulin vial first and withdraws 5 units of regular insulin
   b. Injects 15 units of air into the NPH insulin vial but does not withdraw the medication
   c. Withdraws 5 units of regular insulin before withdrawing 15 units of NPH insulin
   d. Calculates the combined total insulin dose as 20 units after withdrawing the regular insulin from the vial

Interactive Activity

An interactive or media element has been excluded from this version of the text. You can view it online here: https://wtcs.pressbooks.pub/nursingskills/?p=2607

Interactive Activity

An interactive or media element has been excluded from this version of the text. You can view it online here: https://wtcs.pressbooks.pub/nursingskills/?p=2607

My Notes

XVIII GLOSSARY

Ampules: Small glass containers of liquid medication ranging from 1 mL to 10 mL sizes.

Bleb: A small, raised circle that appears after administration of an intradermal medication indicating correct placement into the dermis.

Deltoid: Commonly used for intramuscular vaccinations in adults because it has a triangular shape and is easy to locate and access. The injection site is in the middle of the deltoid muscle, about 1 to 2 inches below the acromion process.

Gauge: Refers to the diameter of a needle. Gauges can vary from very small diameter (25 to 29 gauge) to large diameter (18 to 22 gauge).

Intradermal injection: Medication administered in the dermis just below the epidermis.

Intramuscular injection: Medication administered into a muscle.

Intravenous injection: Medication administered directly into the bloodstream.

Subcutaneous injection: Medication administered into the subcutaneous tissue just under the dermis.

Vastus lateralis: A muscle located on the anterior lateral aspect of the thigh and extends from one hand's breadth above the knee to one hand's breadth below the greater trochanter. It is commonly used for immunizations in infants and toddlers because the muscle is thick and well-developed.

Ventrogluteal: The safest intramuscular injection site for adults and children because it provides the greatest thickness of gluteal muscles, is free from penetrating nerves and blood vessels, and has a thin layer of fat.

Z-track method: A method for administering intramuscular injections that prevents the medication from leaking into the subcutaneous tissue, allows the medication to stay in the muscles, and minimizes irritation.

Chapter 19

Specimen Collection

19.1 SPECIMEN COLLECTION INTRODUCTION

My Notes

Learning Objectives

- Accurately collect specimens for blood glucose monitoring, nasal swabs, and oropharyngeal swabs
- Modify procedure to reflect variations across the life span
- Maintain standard and transmission-based precautions
- Select appropriate equipment
- Explain procedure to patient
- Document actions and observations
- Recognize and report significant deviations from norms

This chapter will describe specimen collection for blood glucose monitoring, nasal swabs, oropharyngeal swabs, sputum, and stool.

Additional information regarding obtaining wound cultures can be found in "Wound Care," and information about obtaining urine cultures can be found in the "Facilitation of Elimination."

My Notes

19.2 BLOOD GLUCOSE MONITORING

Blood glucose monitoring is performed on patients with diabetes mellitus and other conditions that cause elevated blood sugar levels. Diabetes mellitus is a common medical condition that affects the body's ability to produce insulin in the pancreas and use insulin at the cellular level. There are two types of diabetes mellitus, type 1 and type 2. Type 1 diabetes mellitus is an autoimmune disease that damages the beta cells of the pancreas so they do not produce insulin; thus, synthetic insulin must be administered by injection or infusion. It typically begins in childhood or adolescence. Type 2 diabetes mellitus accounts for approximately 95 percent of all cases and is highly correlated with obesity and inactivity. During type 2 diabetes, the cells of the body become resistant to the effects of insulin, and the pancreas increases its production of insulin. However, over time, the pancreas may no longer be able to produce insulin. In many cases, type 2 diabetes can be managed by moderate weight loss, regular physical activity, and a healthy diet. However, if blood glucose levels cannot be controlled with healthy lifestyle choices, oral diabetic medication is prescribed and eventually, the administration of insulin may be required.[1] Prediabetes is a medical condition where blood sugar levels are higher than normal, but not high enough yet to be diagnosed as type 2 diabetes. Approximately one in three American adults have prediabetes. Gestational diabetes is a type of diabetes that occurs during pregnancy in women who did not have diabetes before they were pregnant.

Diabetic patients require frequent blood glucose monitoring to administer customized medication therapy to prevent long-term complications from occurring. Hospitalized patients who do not have diabetes may also require frequent blood glucose monitoring due to elevations that can occur as a result of the stress of hospitalization, surgical procedures, and side effects of medications. Additionally, patients receiving enteral feedings typically have their blood glucose monitored every six hours. Health care providers prescribe the frequency of blood glucose monitoring; testing is typically performed before meals and at bedtime. For some patients, a **standardized sliding-scale insulin** protocol may be prescribed with instructions on the medication administration record (MAR) for administration of insulin based on their blood glucose results.[2,3] See Table 19.2 for an example of a sliding-scale insulin protocol.

---

1 This work is a derivative of *Nursing Pharmacology* by Open RN licensed under CC BY 4.0. Access for free at https://wtcs.pressbooks.pub/pharmacology/

2 This work is a derivative of Clinical Procedures for Safer Patient Care by British Columbia Institute of Technology and is licensed under CC BY 4.0. Access for free at https://opentextbc.ca/clinicalskills/

3 Donihi, A. C., DiNardo, M. M., DeVita, M. A., & Korytkowski, M. T. (2006). Use of a standardized protocol to decrease medication errors and adverse events related to sliding scale insulin. *Quality & Safety in Health Care, 15*(2), 89–91. https://doi.org/10.1136/qshc.2005.014381

Table 19.2 Sample Sliding-Scale Insulin Protocol	
Instructions: Check patient's blood sugar before meals, at bedtime, and as needed for symptoms of hypoglycemia or hyperglycemia. Use the following table to administer insulin lispro PRN.	
Blood Sugar Range	**Lispro Insulin Instructions**
Less than 70	Hold all insulin and initiate hypoglycemia protocol.
70-150	0 units
151-174	2 units
175-199	4 units
200-224	6 units
225-249	8 units
250-274	10 units
275-299	12 units
Greater than 300	Administer 14 units and call the provider.

Hypoglycemia

When caring for patients with diabetes mellitus and monitoring their blood glucose readings, it is important to continually monitor for signs of hypoglycemia. **Hypoglycemia** is defined as blood sugar readings less than 70 and signs and symptoms such as the following:

- Shakiness
- Feeling nervous or anxious
- Sweating, chills, and clamminess
- Irritability or impatience
- Confusion
- Fast heartbeat
- Feeling light-headed or dizzy
- Hunger
- Nausea
- Color draining from the skin (pallor)
- Feeling sleepy
- Feeling weak or having no energy

My Notes

- Blurred/impaired vision
- Tingling or numbness in the lips, tongue, or cheeks
- Headaches
- Coordination problems or clumsiness
- Nightmares or crying out during sleep
- Seizures[4]

A low blood sugar level triggers the release of epinephrine (adrenaline), the "fight-or-flight" hormone. Epinephrine causes the symptoms of hypoglycemia such as a rapid heartbeat, sweating, and anxiety. If a patient's blood sugar level continues to drop, the brain has impaired functioning. This may lead to seizures and a coma.[5]

If a nurse suspects hypoglycemia is occuring, a blood sugar reading should be obtained and appropriate actions taken. Most agencies have a hypoglycemia protocol based on the "15-15 Rule." The **15-15 rule** is to provide 15 grams of carbohydrate and recheck the blood glucose after 15 minutes. If the reading is still below 70 mg/dL, another serving of 15 grams of carbohydrate should be provided and the process continued until the blood sugar is above 70 mg/dL. Fifteen grams of carbohydrate includes options like 4 ounces of juice or regular soda, hard candy, or glucose tablets. If a patient is experiencing severe hypoglycemia and cannot swallow, a glucagon injection or intravenous administration of dextrose may be required.[6]

Hyperglycemia

Hyperglycemia is defined as elevated blood glucose and often causes signs and symptoms such as frequent urination and increased thirst. Hyperglycemia occurs when the patient's body does not produce enough insulin or cannot use the insulin properly at the cellular level. There are many potential causes of hyperglycemia, such as not receiving enough medication to effectively control blood glucose, eating more than planned, exercising less than planned, or increased stress from an illness, surgery, hospitalization, or other life events.

If a patient's blood glucose is greater than 240 mg/dL, their urine is typically checked for ketones. Ketones indicate a condition called ketoacidosis may be occurring. Ketoacidosis occurs in patients whose pancreas is no longer creating insulin, so fats are broken down for energy and waste products called ketones are produced. If the kidneys cannot effectively eliminate ketones in the urine, they build up in the blood and cause ketoacidosis. **Ketoacidosis** is a life-threatening condition that requires immediate notification of the provider for treatment. Symptoms of ketoacidosis include fruity-smelling breath, nausea, vomiting, very dry mouth, and shortness of breath. Treatment of ketoacidosis often requires the administration of intravenous insulin while the patient is closely monitored in a critical care inpatient unit.[7]

---

4 American Diabetes Association. (n.d.). *Hypoglycemia (Low blood sugar).* https://www.diabetes.org/diabetes/medication-management/blood-glucose-testing-and-control/hypoglycemia

5 American Diabetes Association. (n.d.). *Hypoglycemia (Low blood sugar).* https://www.diabetes.org/diabetes/medication-management/blood-glucose-testing-and-control/hypoglycemia

6 American Diabetes Association. (n.d.). *Hypoglycemia (Low blood sugar).* https://www.diabetes.org/diabetes/medication-management/blood-glucose-testing-and-control/hypoglycemia

7 American Diabetes Association. (n.d.). *Hyperglycemia (High blood glucose).* https://www.diabetes.org/diabetes/medication-management/blood-glucose-testing-and-control/hyperglycemia

My Notes

For more information about diabetes mellitus, measuring blood sugar levels, and diabetic medications, visit the "Endocrine" chapter in Open RN *Nursing Pharmacology*.

Glucometer Use

It is typically the responsibility of a nurse to perform bedside blood glucose readings, but in some agencies, this procedure may be delegated to trained nursing assistants or medical assistants. See Figure 19.1[8] for an image of a standard bedside glucometer kit that contains a glucometer, lancets, reagent strips, and calibration drops. Prior to performing a blood glucose test, read the manufacturer's instructions and agency policy because they may vary across devices and sites. Ensure the glucometer has been calibrated per agency policy.[9]

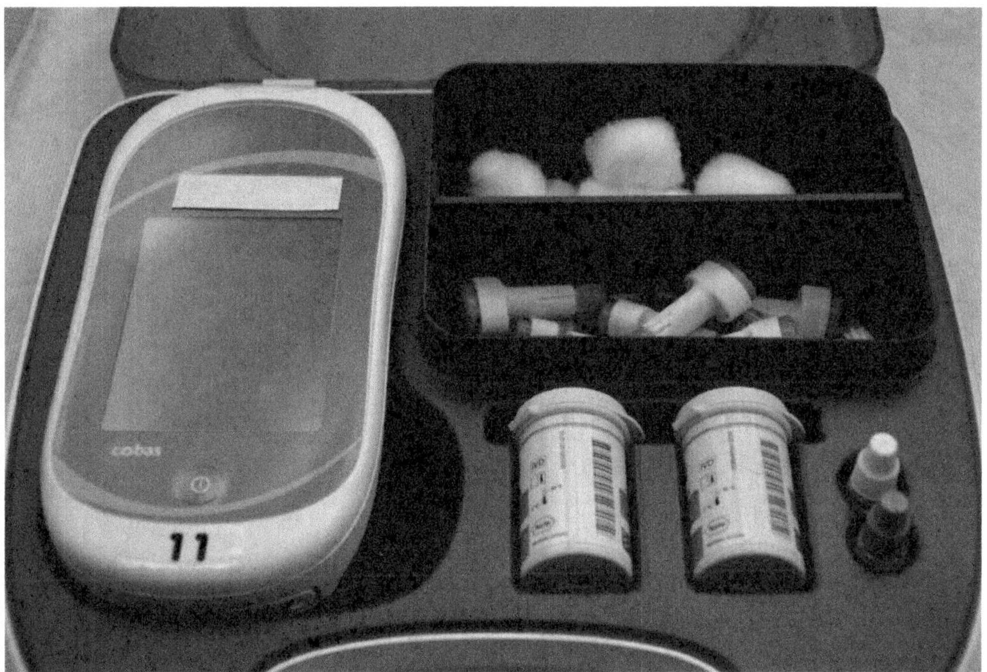

Figure 19.1 Bedside Glucometer

Before beginning the procedure, determine if there are any conditions present that could affect the reading. For example, is the patient fasting? Has the patient already begun eating? Is the patient demonstrating any symptoms of hypoglycemia or hyperglycemia? Keep your patient safe by applying your knowledge of diabetes, the medication being administered, and the uniqueness of the patient to make appropriate clinical judgments regarding the procedure and associated medication administration.[10]

---

8 "DSC_0718.jpg" by British Columbia Institute of Technology is licensed under CC BY 4.0. Access for free at https://opentextbc.ca/clinicalskills/chapter/8-2-glucometer-use/

9 This work is a derivative of Clinical Procedures for Safer Patient Care by British Columbia Institute of Technology and is licensed under CC BY 4.0. Access for free at https://opentextbc.ca/clinicalskills/

10 This work is a derivative of Clinical Procedures for Safer Patient Care by British Columbia Institute of Technology and is licensed under CC BY 4.0. Access for free at https://opentextbc.ca/clinicalskills/

My Notes

See the "Checklist for Blood Glucose Monitoring" for details regarding the procedure. It is often important to keep the patient's hand warm and in a dependent position to promote vasodilation and obtain a good blood sample. If necessary, warm compresses can be applied for 10 minutes prior to the procedure to promote vasodilation. Follow the manufacturer's instructions to prepare the glucometer for measurement. After applying clean gloves, clean the patient's skin with an alcohol wipe for 30 seconds, allow the site to dry, and then puncture the skin using the lancet. See Figure 19.2[11] for an image of performing a skin puncture using a lancet.

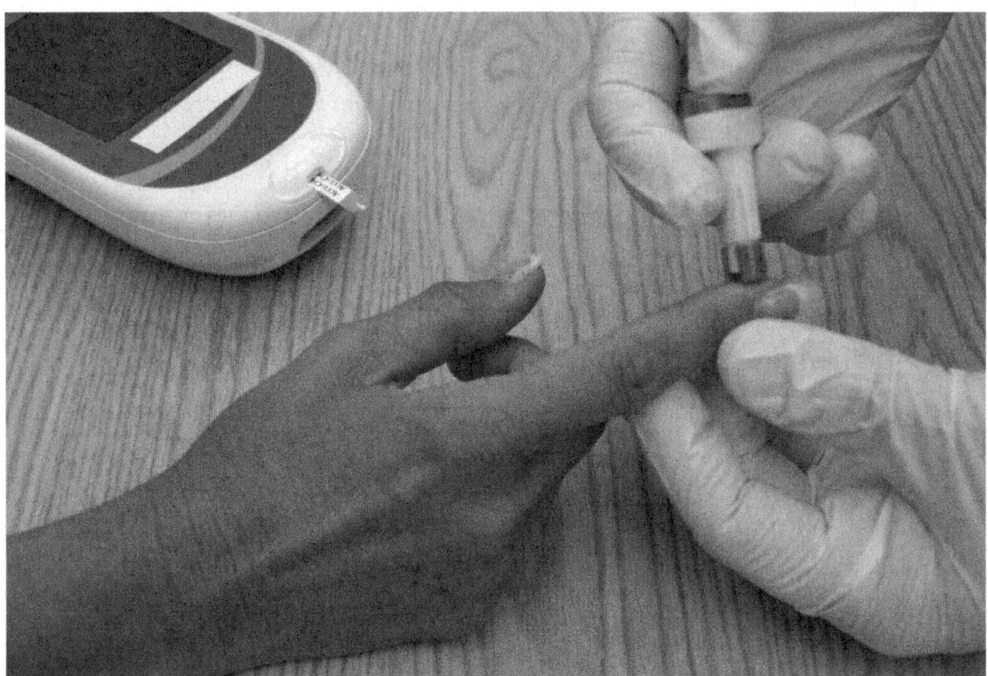

Figure 19.2 Using a Lancet to Perform a Skin Puncture

If needed, gently squeeze above the site to obtain a large drop of blood. Do not milk or massage the finger because it may introduce excess tissue fluid and hemolyze the specimen. Wipe away the first drop of blood and use the second drop for the blood sample. Follow agency policy and manufacturer instructions regarding placement of the drop of blood for absorption on the reagent strip. See Figure 19.3[12] for an image of a nurse absorbing the patient's drop of blood on the reagent strip. Timeliness is essential in gathering an appropriate specimen before clotting occurs or the glucometer times out.

11 "DSC_1130.jpg" by British Columbia Institute of Technology is licensed under CC BY 4.0. Access for free at https://opentextbc.ca/clinicalskills/chapter/8-2-glucometer-use/

12 "DSC_1141.jpg" by British Columbia Institute of Technology is licensed under CC BY 4.0. Access for free at https://opentextbc.ca/clinicalskills/chapter/8-2-glucometer-use/

My Notes

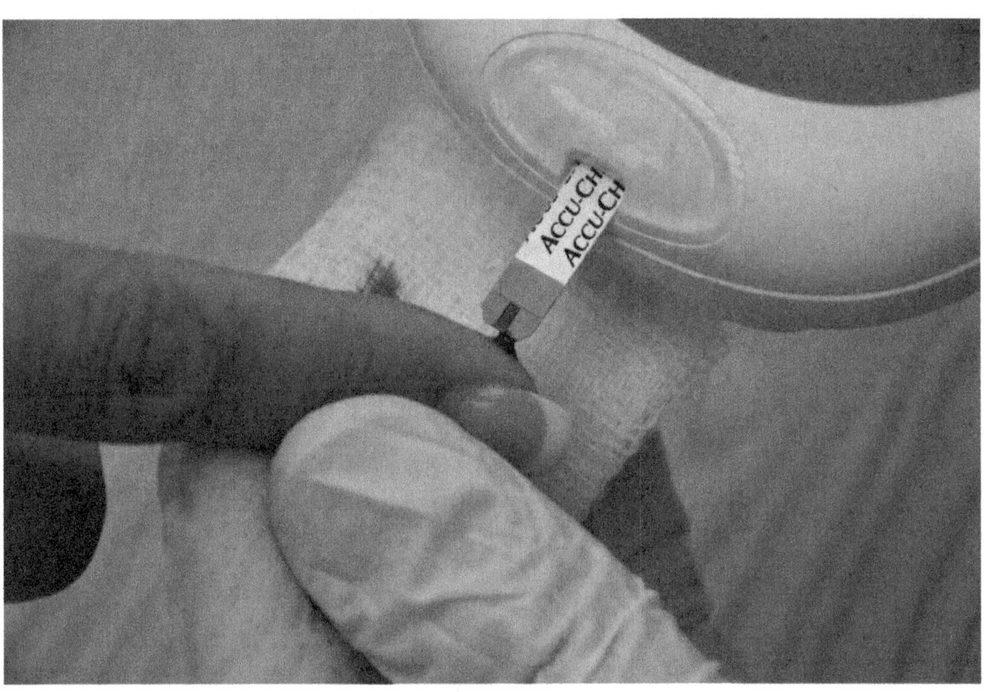

Figure 19.3 Obtaining Drop of Blood

Cleanse the glucometer and document the blood glucose results according to agency policy. Report any concerns about patient symptoms or blood sugar results according to agency policy.

Life Span Considerations

Blood glucose samples should be taken from the heel of newborns and infants up to the age of six months. When obtaining a sample from the heel, the sample is taken from the medial or lateral plantar surface.

My Notes

Video Review of Obtaining a Bedside Blood Sugar[13]

A YouTube element has been excluded from this version of the text. You can view it online here: https://wtcs.pressbooks.pub/nursingskills/?p=2957

13 RegisteredNurseRN. (2015, August 12). *How to prick finger tips with a lancet device for checking a blood sugar | Nursing skills.* [Video]. YouTube. All rights reserved. Video used with permission. https://youtu.be/JPJ4l7QZ9eM

19.3 NASAL SPECIMEN COLLECTION

My Notes

Specimen collections from a patient's anterior nasal cavity and nasopharynx are used to test for multiple viral illnesses such as influenza and COVID-19. Nasal swabs can be performed by the nurse or the patient with proper education. It is vital to understand the anatomy of these areas to obtain an accurate sample so that patients receive the appropriate care they need. See Figure 19.4[1] for an image of the anatomy of the head and neck.

Review the "Checklist for Obtaining a Nasal Swab" for details about performing a nasal swab procedure.

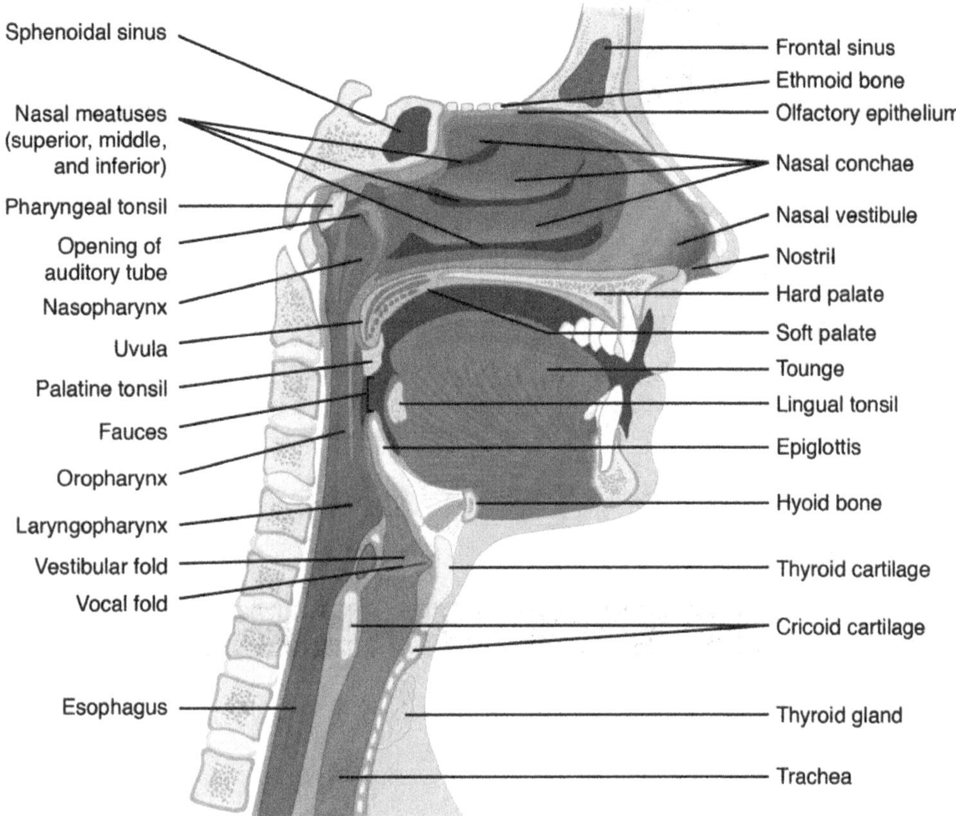

Figure 19.4 Anatomy of the Head and Neck

1 2303 Anatomy of Nose-Pharynx-Mouth-Larynx.jpg" by OpenStax is licensed under CC BY 3.0. Access for free at https://commons.wikimedia.org/wiki/File:2303_Anatomy_of_Nose-Pharynx-Mouth-Larynx.jpg

My Notes

Video Reviews of Nasopharyngeal Specimens and COVID-19 Testing

Collection of Nasopharyngeal Specimens with the Swab Technique[2]

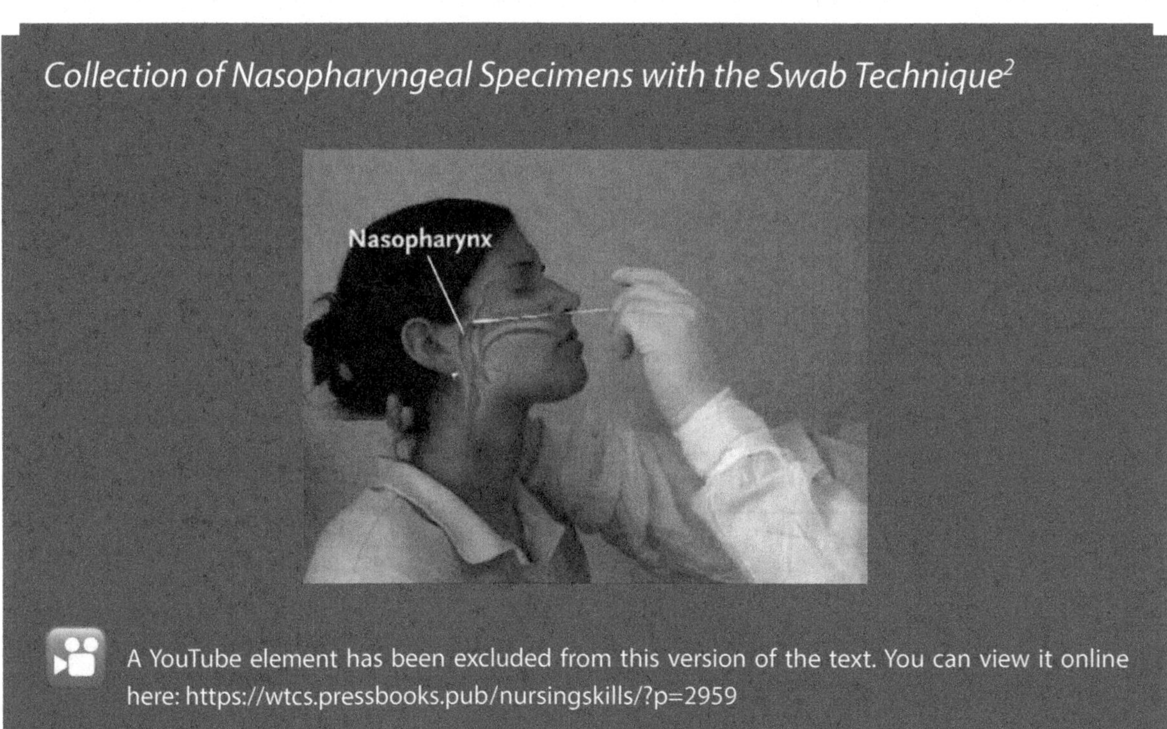

A YouTube element has been excluded from this version of the text. You can view it online here: https://wtcs.pressbooks.pub/nursingskills/?p=2959

Introduction to COVID-19 Tests[3]

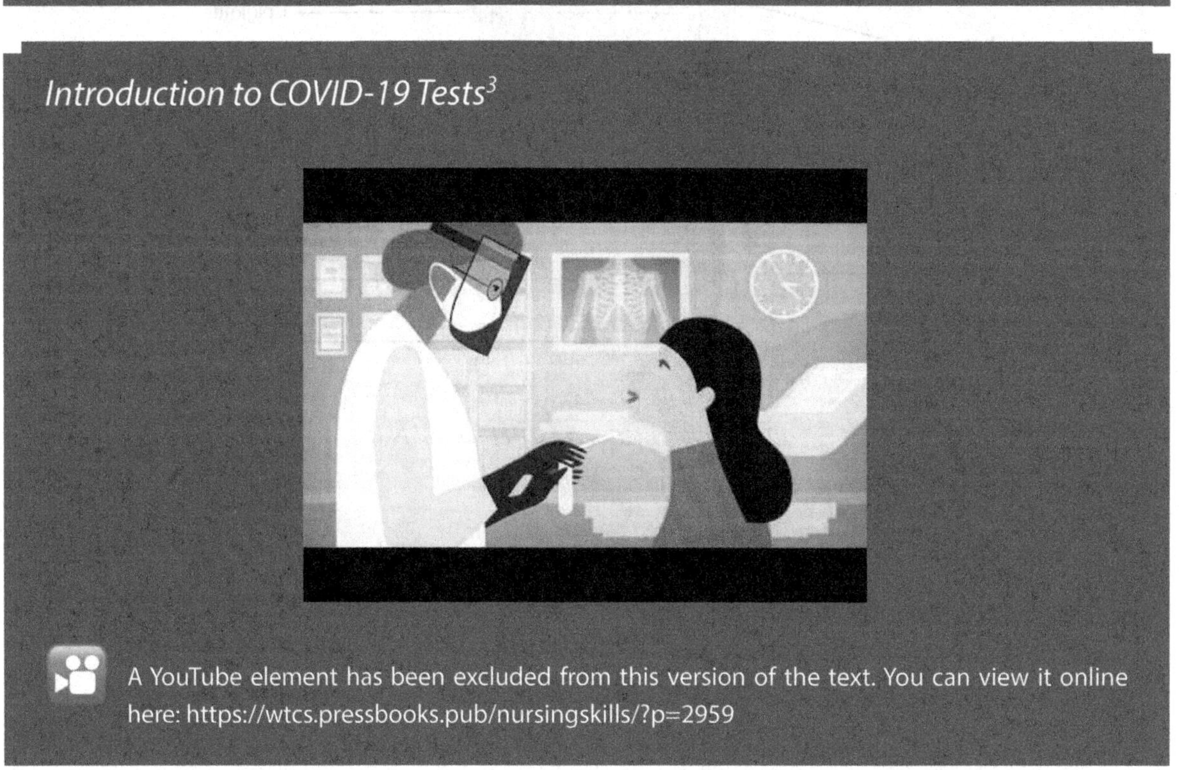

A YouTube element has been excluded from this version of the text. You can view it online here: https://wtcs.pressbooks.pub/nursingskills/?p=2959

2 NEJMVideo. (2009, November 23). *NEJM procedure: Collection of nasopharyngeal specimens with the swab technique.* [Video]. YouTube. All rights reserved. This video is included on the basis of Fair Use. https://youtu.be/DVJNWefmHjE

3 U.S. Food and Drug Administration. (2020, June 4). *An introduction to COVID-19 tests.* [Video]. YouTube. All rights reserved. https://youtu.be/5hu7_xIsCRgt

19.4 OROPHARYNGEAL SPECIMEN COLLECTION

My Notes

The **oropharynx** is the part of the throat at the back of the mouth behind the oral cavity. It includes the back third of the tongue, the soft palate, the side and back walls of the throat, and the tonsils.[1] When obtaining a specimen from this area, it is important to avoid the tongue and teeth. Depending on the test ordered, the nurse may obtain the specimen from the tonsils alone or the posterior pharynx (throat) and the tonsils. Keep in mind that if you are ever unsure about how to accurately obtain a specimen, lab technicians are a great resource.

See the "Checklist for Oropharyngeal Testing" for additional details about performing the procedure.

Life Span Considerations

Infants and Children

Specimen collection on infants and children may require the support of another health care provider or a parent. Educate the patient and the parent about the procedure and the expectations if the parent decides to assist with the specimen collection. During specimen collection, it's important that the patient is immobile to prevent injury to the nasal cavity, nasopharyngeal, or oropharynx.

View Medscape's YouTube video to review oropharyngeal testing: "How to Perform a Throat Swab"[2]

1 National Cancer Institute. (n.d.). *Oropharynx.* https://www.cancer.gov/publications/dictionaries/cancer-terms/def/oropharynx

2 Medscape. (2018, August 23). *How to perform a throat swab on a patient.* [Video]. YouTube. All rights reserved. https://youtu.be/-uyBJ0nv4oI

My Notes

19.5 SPUTUM SPECIMEN COLLECTION

Sputum specimens collected by expectoration are commonly used for cytology, culture and sensitivity, and acid-fast bacilli (AFB) testing.

Cytologic examination identifies abnormal cells such as cancer. Culture and sensitivity testing identifies specific infectious microorganisms and their sensitivity to antibiotics. Optimally, sputum samples used for culture and sensitivity testing should be collected before initiating antibiotic therapy because antibiotics affect the results. AFB testing, along with culture and sensitivity testing, is used to diagnose tuberculosis (TB). When testing for TB, at least three consecutive samples are collected, with at least one being an early morning sample.

Prior to implementing the procedure, it is helpful to ensure the patient is well-hydrated. Hydration helps thin and loosen sputum and increases the likelihood of obtaining an adequate sample. If the patient is prescribed nebulizer treatments, it is helpful to administer this treatment prior to the procedure to help mobilize secretions. It is also important to assess if the patient is experiencing pain related to coughing. For example, pain following chest or abdominal surgery can inhibit the patient from taking deep breaths and expectorating. In this case, pain medication should be provided prior to performing the procedure. Patients can also be encouraged to support surgical wounds with a pillow while coughing to provide additional support and comfort.

It is best to obtain sputum samples in the early morning because secretions accumulate overnight. The patient can rinse their mouth with water prior to the procedure, but avoid mouthwash or toothpaste because these products can affect the microorganisms in the sample. Remove dentures if they are present.

Be aware that droplets and aerosols may be generated when collecting sputum specimens, so use appropriate personal protective equipment when entering the room and during the procedure based on the patient's condition. Explain the procedure to the patient, the type of specimen required, and the difference between oral secretions and sputum. Position the patient in a seated position in a chair or at the side of the bed, or place them in high Fowler's position.

Instruct the patient to take three slow, deep breaths and then cough deeply. Repeat this process until the patient has produced sputum, with rest periods between each maneuver.

When the patient has mobilized sputum, instruct them to expectorate directly into a sterile specimen container without touching the inside or rim of the container. The specimen should be at least 5 mL (one teaspoon); ask the patient to continue producing and expectorating sputum until this amount is achieved. Assess the sputum specimen to ensure it is sputum and not saliva. Sputum appears thick and opaque, whereas saliva appears thin, clear, and watery.

Cap the specimen container tightly and ensure it is labeled with the patient's name. Place the specimen in a transport bag and send it to the laboratory for analysis. Document the time and date the sputum specimen was collected and the characteristics of the sputum, including amount and color.

If a patient is unable to expectorate a sputum sample, other interventions may be required to mobilize secretions. It is often helpful to collaborate with a respiratory therapist for assistance in this situation. Interventions may include nebulizers, hydration, deep-breathing exercises, chest percussion, and postural drainage. If these interventions are not successful, a sputum sample may be obtained via oropharyngeal or endotracheal suctioning; these methods are used to obtain sputum samples for patients who are intubated.[1,2,3]

My Notes

Read South Dakota Department of Health's PDF with instructions for collecting a sputum sample: "Sputum Collection Instructions" (https://doh.sd.gov/documents/diseases/infectious/SputumCollection.pdf)

1 Shepherd, E. (2017). Specimen collection 4: Procedure for obtaining a sputum specimen. *Nursing Times, 113*(10), 49-51. https://www.nursingtimes.net/clinical-archive/assessment-skills/specimen-collection-4-procedure-for-obtaining-a-sputum-specimen-11-09-2017/

2 Sputum collection by expectoration. (2020). Lippincott procedures. http://procedures.lww.com

3 South Dakota Department of Health (2018, February). *Sputum collection instructions.* https://doh.sd.gov/documents/diseases/infectious/SputumCollection.pdf

My Notes

19.6 STOOL SPECIMEN COLLECTION

Stool samples are collected from patients to test for cancer, parasites, or for occult blood (i.e., hidden blood). Follow specific instructions from the laboratory for collecting the sample.

The Guaiac-Based Fecal Occult Blood Test (gFOBT) is a commonly used test to find hidden blood in the stool that is not visibly apparent. As a screening test for colon cancer, it is typically obtained by the patient in their home using samples from three different bowel movements. Nurses may assist in gFOBT specimen collection during inpatient care.

Before the test, the patient should avoid red meat for three days and should not take aspirin or nonsteroidal anti-inflammatory drugs (NSAIDs), such as ibuprofen, for seven days prior to the test. (Blood from the meat can cause a false positive test, and aspirin and NSAIDS can cause bleeding, leading to a false positive result.) Vitamin C (more than 250 mg a day) from supplements, citrus fruits, or citrus juices should be avoided for 3 to 7 days before testing because it can affect the chemicals in the test and make the result negative, even if blood is present.

To perform a gFOBT in an inpatient setting, perform the following steps.

- Verify the patient has not consumed red meat for three days, has not taken aspirin or NSAIDs for seven days prior to the test, and has not had vitamin C greater than 250 mg daily for the past 3-7 days because these substances can affect the results.
- Explain the procedure to the patient. Instruct them to flush the toilet before defecating to remove any potential chemicals and to not place toilet paper in the toilet after defecating. Request they notify you when they have had a bowel movement.
- Review the manufacturer's instructions because different test kits may have different instructions. Contact the laboratory with any questions.
- Label the card with the patient's name and medical information per agency policy. Open the flap of the guaiac test card.
- Apply nonsterile gloves. Use the applicator stick to apply a thin smear of the stool specimen to one of the squares of filter paper on the card. Obtain a second specimen from a different part of the stool and apply it to the second square of filter paper on the card. (Occult blood isn't typically equally dispersed throughout the stool.)
- Place the labeled test card in a transport bag and send it to the laboratory for analysis.
- If you are working in an agency where nurses apply the guaiac developer solution to the card, allow the specimen to dry for 3 to 5 minutes. Open the reverse side of the card and apply two drops of guaiac developer solution to each square. A blue reaction will occur within 60 seconds if the test is positive. The absence of a blue color after 60 seconds is considered a negative test.
- Document the date and time of the test and any unusual characteristics of the stool sample.[1,2]

---

1 American Cancer Society (2020, June 29). *Colorectal cancer screening tests.* https://www.cancer.org/cancer/colon-rectal-cancer/detection-diagnosis-staging/screening-tests-used.htm

2 A.D.A.M. Medical Encyclopedia [Internet]. Atlanta (GA): A.D.A.M., Inc.; c1997-2021. Stool guaiac test; [updated 2021, February 26]. https://medlineplus.gov/ency/article/003393.htm

19.7 SAMPLE DOCUMENTATION

My Notes

Sample Documentation of Expected Findings

Patient alert and oriented x 3, sitting in a wheelchair and awaiting breakfast. Patient denies symptoms of hypoglycemia or hyperglycemia. Bedside blood glucose obtained with results of 135 mg/dL. 2 units of regular insulin given per sliding scale. Breakfast delivered to the patient.

Sample Documentation of Unexpected Findings

0730: Patient alert and oriented x 3, sitting in a wheelchair and awaiting breakfast. Denies symptoms of hypoglycemia and hyperglycemia. Bedside blood glucose obtained with results of 185 mg/dL. 6 units of regular insulin given per sliding scale along with 34 units of scheduled NPH insulin as breakfast tray was delivered to patient.

0900: Patient only ate 25% of breakfast and complains of headache, fatigue, and dizziness. Patient is shaking and irritable but alert and oriented x 3. Blood glucose was rechecked and results were 65 mg/dL. 4 ounces of orange juice was provided.

0915: Blood glucose rechecked and results were 95 mg/dL. Patient states, "I'm feeling much better and not dizzy anymore." Shakiness has resolved. Provided a peanut butter sandwich per patient request. Will continue to monitor the patient for signs of hypoglycemia. Call light within reach.

My Notes

19.8 CHECKLIST FOR BLOOD GLUCOSE MONITORING

Use the checklist below to review the steps for completion of "Blood Glucose Monitoring."

Steps

Disclaimer: Always review and follow agency policy regarding this specific skill.

1. Prepare before completing the procedure:
   - Review the patient's medical history and current medications.
     - Note if the patient is receiving anticoagulant therapy. Anticoagulant therapy may result in prolonged bleeding at the puncture site and require pressure to the site.
   - Assess the patient for signs and symptoms of hyperglycemia or hypoglycemia to correlate data to pursue acute action due to an onset of symptoms.
   - Determine if the test requires special timing, for example, before or after meals.
     - Blood glucose monitoring is typically performed prior to meals and the administration of antidiabetic medications.
2. Gather supplies: nonsterile gloves, alcohol swab, lancet, 2" x 2" gauze or cotton ball, reagent strips, and blood glucose meter.
   - Determine if the blood glucose meter needs to be calibrated according to agency policy to ensure accuracy of readings.
   - Read and understood the manufacturer's instructions and agency policy for the blood glucose meters.
3. Perform safety steps:
   - Perform hand hygiene.
   - Check the room for transmission-based precautions.
   - Introduce yourself, your role, the purpose of your visit, and an estimate of the time it will take.
   - Confirm patient ID using two patient identifiers (e.g., name and date of birth).
   - Explain the process to the patient and ask if they have any questions.
   - Be organized and systematic.
   - Use appropriate listening and questioning skills.
   - Listen and attend to patient cues.
   - Ensure the patient's privacy and dignity.
   - Assess ABCs.
4. Have the patient wash their hands with soap and warm water, and position the patient comfortably in a semi-upright position in a bed or upright in a chair. Encourage the patient to keep their hands warm. Washing reduces transmission of microorganisms and increases blood flow to the puncture site.
   - Agency policy may require use of an alcohol swab to clean the puncture site.

- Ensure that the puncture site is completely dry prior to skin puncture.

5. Remove a reagent strip from the container and reseal the container cap to keep the strips free from damage from environmental factors. Do not touch the test pad portion of the reagent strip.
6. Follow the manufacturer's instructions to prepare the meter for measurement.
7. Place the unused reagent strip in the glucometer or on a clean, dry surface (e.g., paper towel) with the test pad facing up, based on manufacturer recommendations.
8. Apply nonsterile gloves.
9. Keep the area to be punctured in a dependent position. Do not milk or massage the finger site:
    - Dependent position will increase blood flow to the area.
    - Do not milk or massage the finger because it may introduce excess tissue fluid and hemolyze the specimen.
    - Warm water, dangling the hand for 15 seconds, and a warm towel stimulate the blood flow to the fingers.
    - Avoid having the patient stand during the procedure to reduce the risk of fainting.
10. Select the appropriate puncture site. Cleanse the site with an alcohol swab for 30 seconds and allow it to dry. Perform the skin puncture with the lancet, using a quick, deliberate motion against the patient's skin:
    - The patient may have a preference for the site used. For example, the patient may prefer not to use a specific finger for the skin puncture. However, keep in mind their preferred site may be contraindicated. For example, do not use the hand on the same side as a mastectomy.
    - Avoid fingertip pads; use the sides of fingers.
    - Avoid fingers that are calloused, have broken skin, or are bruised.
11. Gently squeeze above the site to produce a large droplet of blood.
    - Do not contaminate the site by touching it.
    - The droplet of blood needs to be large enough to cover the test pad on the reagent strip.
    - Wipe away the first drop of blood with gauze.
12. Transfer the second drop of blood to the reagent strip per manufacturer's instructions:
    - The test pad must absorb the droplet of blood for accurate results. Smearing the blood will alter results.
    - The timing and specific instructions for measurement will vary between blood glucose meters. Be sure to read the instructions carefully to ensure accurate readings.
13. Apply pressure, or ask the patient to apply pressure, to the puncture site using a 2" x 2" gauze pad or clean tissue to stop the bleeding at the site.
14. Read the results on the unit display.
15. Turn off the meter and dispose of the test strip, 2" x 2" gauze, and lancet according to agency policy. Use caution with the lancet to prevent an unintentional sharps injury.

My Notes

16. Remove gloves.
17. Perform hand hygiene.
18. Assist the patient to a comfortable position, review test results with the patient, ask if they have any questions, and thank them for their time.
19. Ensure safety measures when leaving the room:
    - CALL LIGHT: Within reach
    - BED: Low and locked (in lowest position and brakes on)
    - SIDE RAILS: Secured
    - TABLE: Within reach
    - ROOM: Risk-free for falls (scan room and clear any obstacles)
20. Document the results and related assessment findings. Report critical values according to agency policy, such as values below 70 or greater than 300, and any associated symptoms. Read more about hypoglycemia and hyperglycemia in the "Blood Glucose Monitoring" section of this chapter.

19.9 CHECKLIST FOR OBTAINING A NASAL SWAB

My Notes

Use the checklist below to review the steps for completion of "Obtaining a Nasal Swab."

Steps

Disclaimer: Always review and follow agency policy regarding this specific skill.

1. Gather supplies: N95 respirator (or face mask if respirators are not available), gloves, gown, eye protection (goggles or disposable face shields that cover the front and sides of the face), and physical barriers (e.g., plexiglass) if needed.

2. Apply appropriate PPE: gown, N95 respirator (or face mask if a respirator is not available), gloves, and eye protection are needed for staff collecting specimens or working within 6 feet of the person being tested.

3. Perform safety steps:

    - Perform hand hygiene.
    - Check the room for transmission-based precautions.
    - Introduce yourself, your role, the purpose of your visit, and an estimate of the time it will take.
    - Confirm patient ID using two patient identifiers (e.g., name and date of birth).
    - Explain the process to the patient and ask if they have any questions.
    - Be organized and systematic.
    - Use appropriate listening and questioning skills.
    - Listen and attend to patient cues.
    - Ensure the patient's privacy and dignity.
    - Assess ABCs.

4. Open the sampling kit using clean technique on a clean surface. The kit should contain a biohazard bag, specimen container, and a nasal swab.

5. Remove the swab from the container being careful not to touch the soft end with your gloved hand or any other surface, which could contaminate the swab and either obscure the results or infect the patient.

6. Insert the swab into the nostril:

    - Anterior Nasal Swab: Have the patient tilt their head back at a 70-degree angle. Do not insert the swab more than a half an inch into the nostril.
    - Nasopharyngeal Swab: Insert until resistance is encountered or the distance is equivalent to that from the ear to the nostril of the patient, indicating contact with the nasopharynx.

7. Leave the swab in place as directed:

    - Anterior Nasal Swab: Leave in place for 10 to 15 seconds.
    - Nasopharyngeal Swab: Leave the swab in place for several seconds to absorb secretions.

My Notes

8. Gently remove the swab:
    - Anterior Nasal Swab: Gently remove the swab after repeating Steps 6 & 7 in the other nostril.
    - Nasopharyngeal Swab: Slowly remove the swab while rotating it.
9. Place the swab in the sterile tube and snap the end off the swab at the break line. Place the cap on the tube.
10. Label the tube with the patient's name, date of birth, medical record number, today's date, your initials, time, and specimen type.
11. Place the specimen into the biohazard bag.
12. Remove the nonsterile gloves and place them in the appropriate receptacle.
13. Perform hand hygiene.
14. Assist the patient to a comfortable position, ask if they have any questions, and thank them for their time.
15. Ensure safety measures when leaving the room:
    - CALL LIGHT: Within reach
    - BED: Low and locked (in lowest position and brakes on)
    - SIDE RAILS: Secured
    - TABLE: Within reach
    - ROOM: Risk-free for falls (scan room and clear any obstacles)
16. Follow agency policy regarding transportation of the specimen to the lab. Report results appropriately when they are received.

19.10 CHECKLIST FOR OROPHARYNGEAL TESTING

My Notes

Use the checklist below to review the steps for completion of "Oropharyngeal Testing."

Steps

Disclaimer: Always review and follow agency policy regarding this specific skill.

1. Gather supplies: testing kit or swab, gloves, tongue depressor, and mask. Other PPE such as a face shield, respirator, or gown may be required based on the patient condition.
2. Perform safety steps:
    - Perform hand hygiene.
    - Check the room for transmission-based precautions.
    - Introduce yourself, your role, the purpose of your visit, and an estimate of the time it will take.
    - Confirm patient ID using two patient identifiers (e.g., name and date of birth).
    - Explain the process to the patient and ask if they have any questions.
    - Be organized and systematic.
    - Use appropriate listening and questioning skills.
    - Listen and attend to patient cues.
    - Ensure the patient's privacy and dignity.
    - Assess ABCs.
3. Apply nonsterile gloves. Inform the patient the procedure may be uncomfortable and cause gagging.
4. Open the supplies.
5. Ask the patient to open their mouth wide and tilt their head back.
6. Insert the tongue blade to depress the tongue. If the patient can depress their tongue so that it is out of the way of the swab, the tongue blade may not be needed.
7. Insert the swab into the posterior pharynx and tonsillar areas. Rub the swab over both tonsillar pillars and posterior oropharynx and avoid touching the tongue, teeth, and gums.
8. Place the swab in the sterile tube and snap the end off the swab at the break line. Place the cap on the tube.
9. Label the tube with the patient's name, date of birth, medical record number, today's date, your initials, time, and specimen type.
10. Place the specimen into the biohazard bag.
11. Remove nonsterile gloves and place them in the appropriate receptacle.
12. Perform hand hygiene.
13. Assist the patient to a comfortable position, ask if they have any questions, and thank them for their time.

My Notes

14. Ensure safety measures when leaving the room:
    - CALL LIGHT: Within reach
    - BED: Low and locked (in lowest position and brakes on)
    - SIDE RAILS: Secured
    - TABLE: Within reach
    - ROOM: Risk-free for falls (scan room and clear any obstacles)
15. Follow agency policy regarding transportation of the specimen to the lab. Report results appropriately when they are received.

19.11 LEARNING ACTIVITIES

My Notes

Learning Activities

(Answers to "Learning Activities" can be found in the "Answer Key" at the end of the book. Answers to interactive activity elements will be provided within the element as immediate feedback.)

You are caring for an elderly diabetic patient who requires a morning glucose check. You gather the calibrated glucometer and lancet, but have difficulty obtaining a capillary blood glucose from the patient's fingerstick. What strategies might you use to facilitate blood flow?

Check your knowledge using this flash card activity:

An interactive or media element has been excluded from this version of the text. You can view it online here: https://wtcs.pressbooks.pub/nursingskills/?p=2967

Check your understanding of hypoglycemia with this activity:

An interactive or media element has been excluded from this version of the text. You can view it online here: https://wtcs.pressbooks.pub/nursingskills/?p=2967

My Notes

XIX GLOSSARY

15-15 Rule: A rule in an agency's hypoglycemia protocols that includes providing 15 grams of carbohydrate, then repeating the blood glucose reading in 15 minutes, and then repeating as needed until the patient's blood glucose reading is above 70.

Hyperglycemia: Elevated blood glucose reading with associated signs and symptoms such as frequent urination and increased thirst.

Hypoglycemia: A blood glucose reading less than 70 associated with symptoms such as irritability, shakiness, hunger, weakness, or confusion. If not rapidly treated, hypoglycemia can cause seizures and a coma.

Ketoacidosis: A life-threatening complication of hyperglycemia that can occur in patients with type 1 diabetes mellitus that is associated with symptoms such as fruity-smelling breath, nausea, vomiting, severe thirst, and shortness of breath.

Oropharynx: The part of the throat at the back of the mouth behind the oral cavity. It includes the back third of the tongue, the soft palate, the side and back walls of the throat, and the tonsils.

Standardized sliding-scale insulin protocol: Standardized instructions for administration of adjustable insulin dosages based on a patient's premeal blood glucose readings.

Chapter 20

Wound Care

20.1 WOUND CARE INTRODUCTION

My Notes

Learning Objectives

- Assess tissue condition, wounds, drainage, and pressure injuries
- Cleanse and irrigate wounds
- Apply a variety of wound dressings
- Obtain a wound culture specimen
- Use appropriate aseptic or sterile technique
- Explain procedure to patient
- Adapt procedures to reflect variations across the life span
- Recognize and report significant deviations in wounds
- Document actions and observations

Wound healing is a complex physiological process that restores function to skin and tissue that have been injured. The healing process is affected by several external and internal factors that either promote or inhibit healing. When providing wound care to patients, nurses, in collaboration with other members of the health care team, assess and manage external and internal factors to provide an optimal healing environment.[1]

Complex wounds often require care by specialists. Certified wound care nurses assess, treat, and create care plans for patients with complex wounds, ostomies, and incontinence conditions. They act as educators and consultants to staff nurses and other health care professionals. This chapter will discuss wound care basics for entry-level nurses. Request a consultation by a certified wound care nurse when caring for patients with complex or nonhealing wounds.

1 Cox, J. (2019). Wound care 101. *Nursing*, *49*(10). https://doi.org/10.1097/01.nurse.0000580632.58318.08

My Notes

20.2 BASIC CONCEPTS RELATED TO WOUNDS

PHASES OF WOUND HEALING

When skin is injured, there are four phases of wound healing that take place: hemostasis, inflammatory, proliferative, and maturation.[1] See Figure 20.1[2] for an illustration of the phases of wound healing.

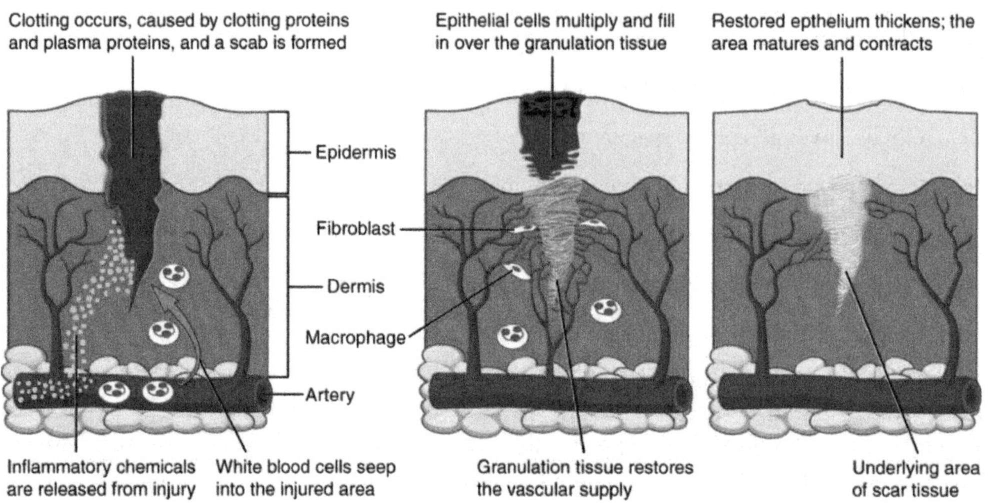

Figure 20.1 Phases of Wound Healing

To illustrate the phases of wound healing, imagine that you accidentally cut your finger with a knife as you were slicing an apple. Immediately after the injury occurs, blood vessels constrict and clotting factors are activated. This is referred to as the hemostasis phase. Clotting factors form clots that stop the bleeding and act as a barrier to prevent bacterial contamination. Platelets release growth factors that alert various cells to start the repair process at the wound location. The **hemostasis phase** lasts up to 60 minutes, depending on the severity of the injury.[3,4]

After the hemostasis phase, the **inflammatory phase** begins. Vasodilation occurs so that white blood cells in the bloodstream can move into the wound to start cleaning the wound bed. The inflammatory process appears to the observer as **edema** (swelling), **erythema** (redness), and exudate. **Exudate** is fluid that oozes out of a wound, also commonly called pus.[5,6]

---

1 This work is a derivative of Clinical Procedures for Safer Patient Care by British Columbia Institute of Technology and is licensed under CC BY 4.0. Access for free at https://opentextbc.ca/clinicalskills/

2 "417 Tissue Repair.jpg" by OpenStax College is licensed under CC BY 3.0. Access for free at https://openstax.org/books/anatomy-and-physiology/pages/1-introduction

3 This work is a derivative of Clinical Procedures for Safer Patient Care by British Columbia Institute of Technology and is licensed under CC BY 4.0. Access for free at https://opentextbc.ca/clinicalskills/

4 This work is a derivative of StatPearls by Grubbs and Mannah and is licensed under CC BY 4.0. Access for free at

5 This work is a derivative of Clinical Procedures for Safer Patient Care by British Columbia Institute of Technology and is licensed under CC BY 4.0. Access for free at https://opentextbc.ca/clinicalskills/

6 This work is a derivative of StatPearls by Grubbs and Mannah and is licensed under CC BY 4.0. Access for free at https://www.ncbi.nlm.nih.gov/books/NBK430685/

My Notes

The **proliferative phase** begins within a few days after the injury and includes four important processes: epithelialization, angiogenesis, collagen formation, and contraction. **Epithelialization** refers to the development of new epidermis and granulation tissue. **Granulation tissue** is new connective tissue with new, fragile, thin-walled capillaries. Collagen is formed to provide strength and integrity to the wound. At the end of the proliferation phase, the wound begins to contract in size.[7,8]

Capillaries begin to develop within the wound 24 hours after injury during a process called **angiogenesis**. These capillaries bring more oxygen and nutrients to the wound for healing. When performing dressing changes, it is essential for the nurse to protect this granulation tissue and the associated new capillaries. Healthy granulation tissue appears pink due to the new capillary formation. It is also moist, painless to the touch, and may appear "bumpy." Conversely, unhealthy granulation tissue is dark red and painful. It bleeds easily with minimal contact and may be covered by shiny white or yellow fibrous tissue referred to as biofilm that must be removed because it impedes healing. Unhealthy granulation tissue is often caused by an infection, so wound cultures should be obtained when infection is suspected. The provider can then prescribe appropriate antibiotic treatment based on the culture results.[9]

During the **maturation phase**, collagen continues to be created to strengthen the wound. Collagen contributes strength to the wound to prevent it from reopening. A wound typically heals within 4-5 weeks and often leaves behind a scar. The scar tissue is initially firm, red, and slightly raised from the excess collagen deposition. Over time, the scar begins to soften, flatten, and become pale in about nine months.[10]

Types of Wound Healing

There are three types of wound healing: primary intention, secondary intention, and tertiary intention. Healing by **primary intention** means that the wound is sutured, stapled, glued, or otherwise closed so the wound heals beneath the closure. This type of healing occurs with clean-edged lacerations or surgical incisions, and the closed edges are referred to as approximated. See Figure 20.2[11] for an image of a surgical wound healing by primary intention.

---

7 This work is a derivative of Clinical Procedures for Safer Patient Care by British Columbia Institute of Technology and is licensed under CC BY 4.0. Access for free at https://opentextbc.ca/clinicalskills/

8 This work is a derivative of StatPearls by Grubbs and Mannah and is licensed under CC BY 4.0. Access for free at https://www.ncbi.nlm.nih.gov/books/NBK430685/

9 This work is a derivative of StatPearls by Alhajj, Bansal, and Goyal and is licensed under CC BY 4.0. Access for free at https://www.ncbi.nlm.nih.gov/books/NBK430685/

10 This work is a derivative of StatPearls by Grubbs and Mannah and is licensed under CC BY 4.0. Access for free at https://www.ncbi.nlm.nih.gov/books/NBK430685/

11 "Ventriculoperitoneal shunt - surgical wound healing - belly - day 12.jpg" by Hansmuller is licensed under CC BY-SA 4.0. Access for free at https://commons.wikimedia.org/wiki/File:Ventriculoperitoneal_shunt_-_surgical_wound_healing_-_belly_-_day_12.jpg

My Notes

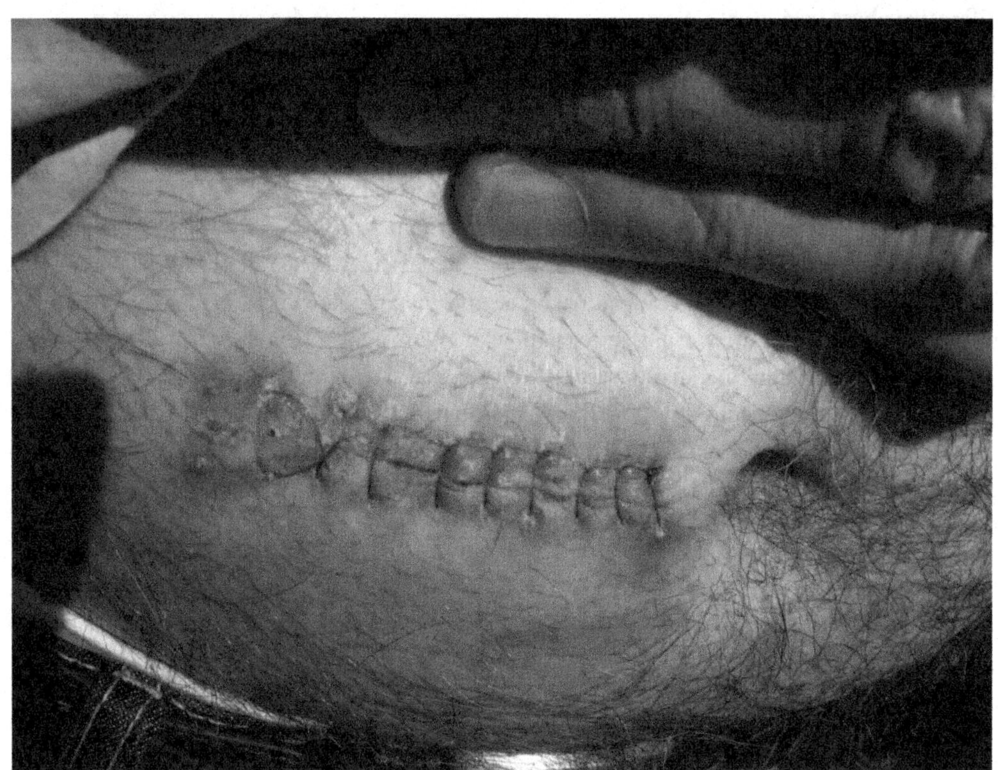

Figure 20.2 Primary Intention Wound Healing

My Notes

Secondary intention occurs when the edges of a wound cannot be approximated (brought together), so the wound fills in from the bottom up by the production of granulation tissue. Examples of wounds that heal by secondary intention are pressure injuries and chainsaw injuries. Wounds that heal by secondary infection are at higher risk for infection and must be protected from contamination. See Figure 20.3[12] for an image of a wound healing by secondary intention.

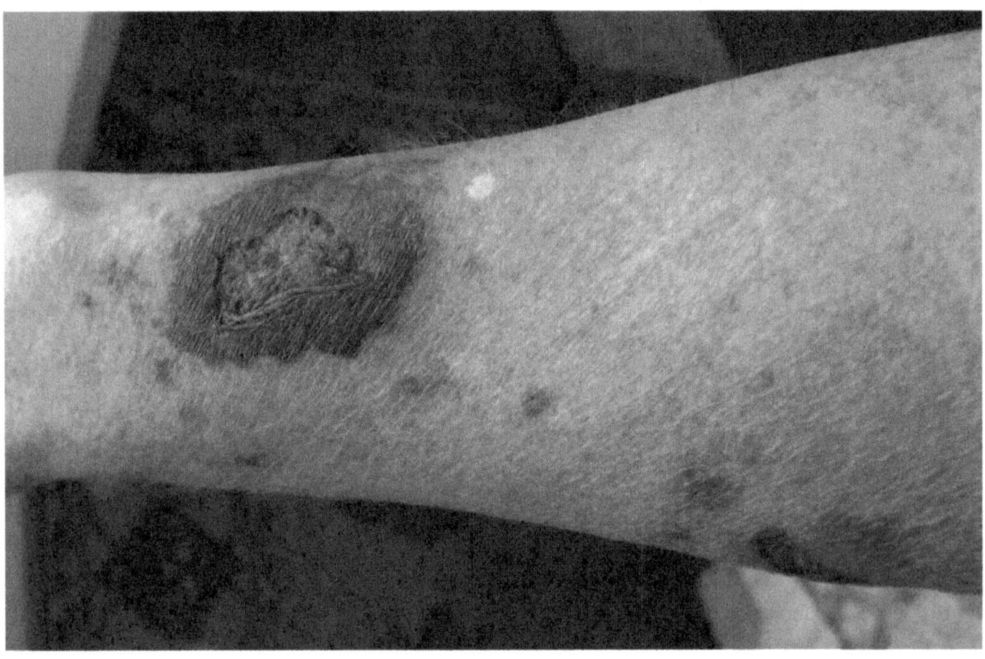

Figure 20.3 Secondary Intention Wound Healing

Tertiary intention refers to a wound that has had to remain open or has been reopened, often due to severe infection. The wound is typically closed at a later date when infection has resolved. Wounds that heal by secondary and tertiary intention have delayed healing times and increased scar tissue.

Wound Closures

Lacerations and surgical wounds are typically closed with sutures, staples, or dermabond to facilitate healing by primary intention. See Figure 20.4[13] for an image of sutures, Figure 20.5[14] for an image of staples, and Figure 20.6[15] for an image of a wound closed with dermabond, a type of sterile surgical glue. Based on agency policy,

12 "Atrophied skin.png" by sansea2 is licensed under CC BY-SA 3.0. Access for free at https://commons.wikimedia.org/wiki/File:Atrophied_skin.png

13 "Wound closed with surgical sutures.jpg" by Wikip2011 is licensed under CC BY-SA 3.0. Access for free at https://commons.wikimedia.org/wiki/File:Wound_closed_with_surgical_sutures.jpg

14 "Surgical staples1.jpg" by Llywrch is licensed under CC BY-SA 2.5. Access for free at https://commons.wikimedia.org/wiki/File:Surgical_staples1.jpg

15 "Incision wound on child's arm, closed with Dermabond.jpg" by ragesoss is licensed under CC BY-SA 3.0. Access for free at https://commons.wikimedia.org/wiki/File:Incision_wound_on_child%27s_arm,_closed_with_Dermabond.jpg

My Notes

the nurse may remove sutures and staples based on a provider order. See Figure 20.7[16] for an image of a disposable staple remover. See the checklists in the subsections later in this chapter for procedures related to surgical and staple removal.

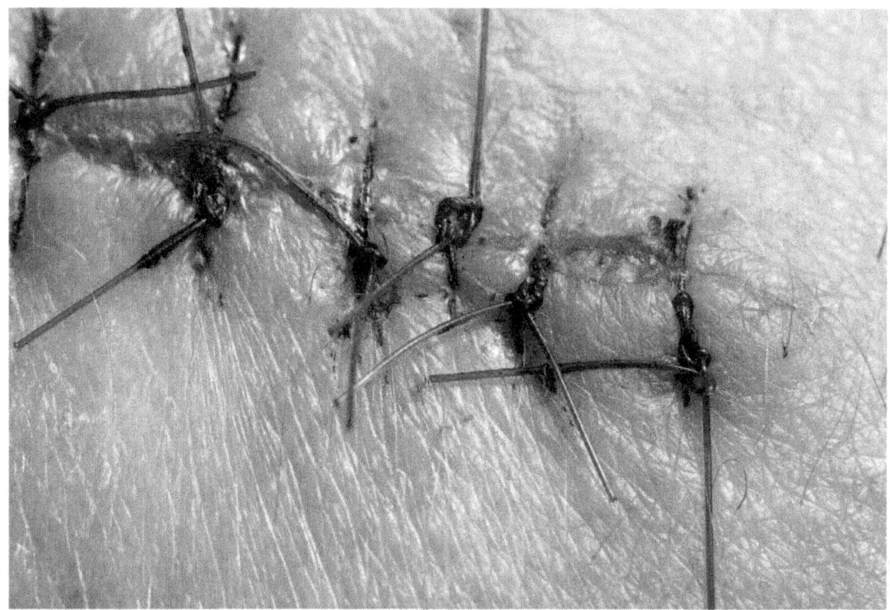

Figure 20.4 Sutures

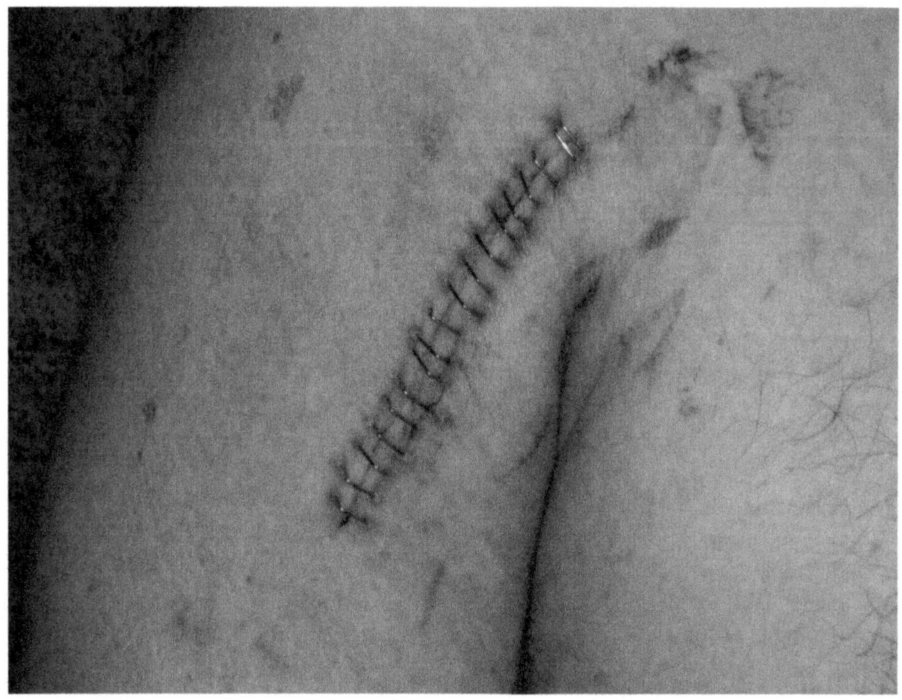

Figure 20.5 Staples

16 "Not quite scissors - TROML - 1366" by Clint Budd is licensed under CC BY 2.0. Access for free at https://www.flickr.com/photos/58827557@N06/24503995344

My Notes

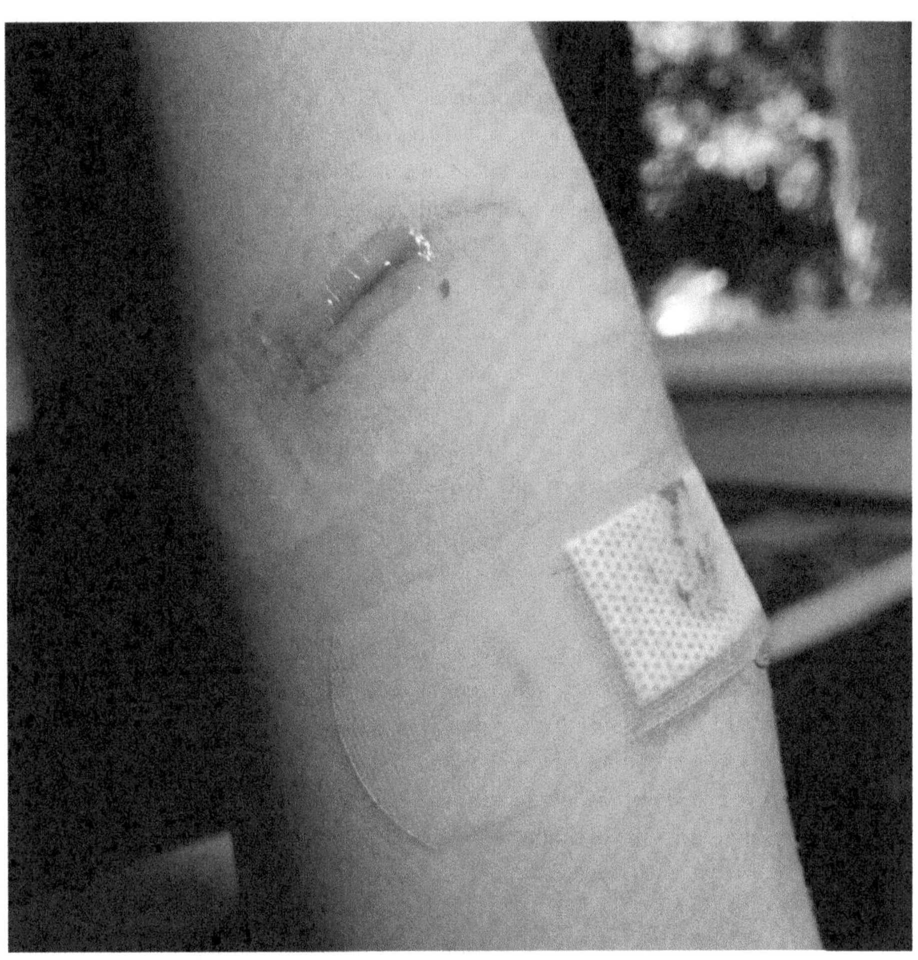

Figure 20.6 Dermabond

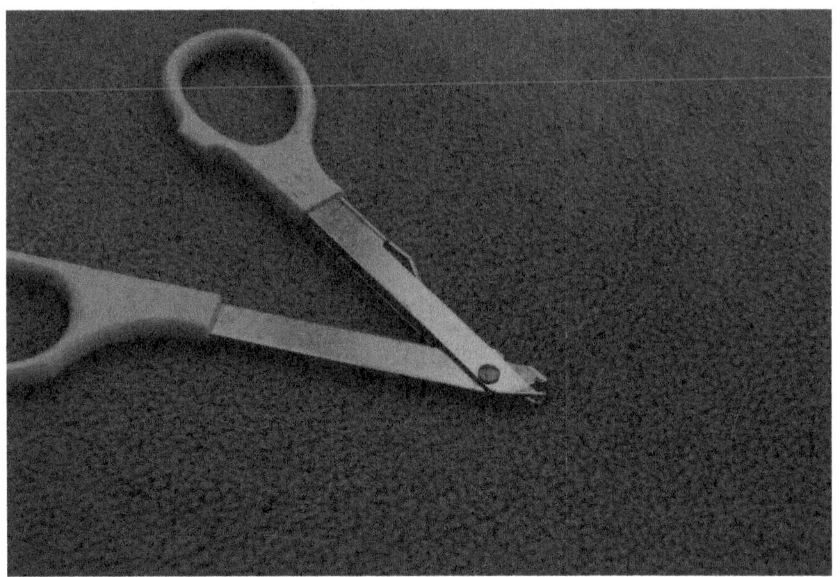

Figure 20.7 Staple Remover

My Notes

Common Types of Wounds

There are several different types of wounds. It is important to understand different types of wounds when providing wound care because each type of wound has different characteristics and treatments. Additionally, treatments that may be helpful for one type of wound can be harmful for another type. Common types of wounds include skin tears, venous ulcers, arterial ulcers, diabetic foot wounds, and pressure injuries.[17]

Skin Tears

Skin tears are wounds caused by mechanical forces such as shear, friction, or blunt force. They typically occur in the fragile, nonelastic skin of older adults or in patients undergoing long-term corticosteroid therapy. Skin tears can be caused by the simple mechanical force used to remove an adhesive bandage or from friction as the skin brushes against a surface. Skin tears occur in the epidermis and dermis but do not extend through the subcutaneous layer. The wound bases of skin tears are typically fragile and bleed easily.[18]

Venous Ulcers

Venous ulcers are caused by lack of blood return to the heart causing pooling of fluid in the veins of the lower legs. The resulting elevated hydrostatic pressure in the veins causes fluid to seep out, macerate the skin, and cause venous ulcerations. **Maceration** refers to the softening and wasting away of skin due to excess fluid. Venous ulcers typically occur on the medial lower leg and have irregular edges due to the maceration. There is often a dark-colored discoloration of the lower legs, due to blood pooling and leakage of iron into the skin called **hemosiderin staining**. For venous ulcers to heal, compression dressings must be used, along with multilayer bandage systems, to control edema and absorb large amounts of drainage.[19] See Figure 20.8[20] for an image of a venous ulcer.

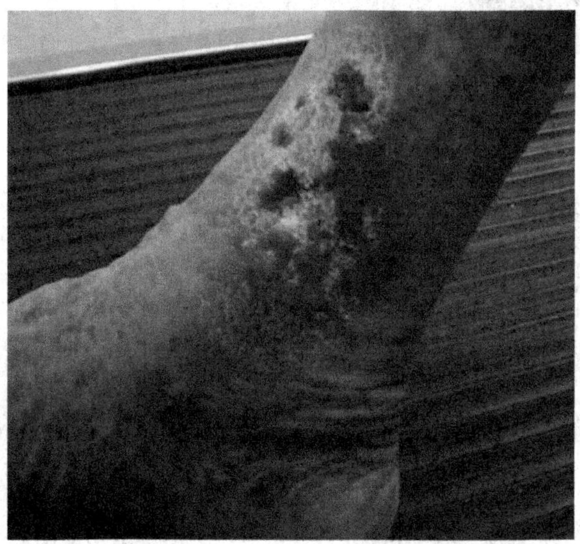

Figure 20.8 Venous Ulcer

---

17 Cox, J. (2019). Wound care 101. *Nursing, 49*(10). https://doi.org/10.1097/01.nurse.0000580632.58318.08

18 Cox, J. (2019). Wound care 101. *Nursing, 49*(10). https://doi.org/10.1097/01.nurse.0000580632.58318.08

19 Cox, J. (2019). Wound care 101. *Nursing, 49*(10). https://doi.org/10.1097/01.nurse.0000580632.58318.08

20 "Úlceras_antes_da_cirurgia.JPG" by Nini00 is licensed under CC BY-SA 3.0. Access for free at https://commons.wikimedia.org/wiki/File:Úlceras_antes_da_cirurgia.JPG

Arterial Ulcers

My Notes

Arterial ulcers are caused by lack of blood flow and oxygenation to tissues. They typically occur in the distal areas of the body such as the feet, heels, and toes. Arterial ulcers have well-defined borders with a "punched out" appearance where there is a localized lack of blood flow. They are typically painful due to the lack of oxygenation to the area. The wound base may become **necrotic** (black) due to tissue death from ischemia. Wound dressings must maintain a moist environment, and treatment must include the removal of necrotic tissue. In severe arterial ulcers, vascular surgery may be required to reestablish blood supply to the area.[21] See Figure 20.9[22] for an image of an arterial ulcer on a patient's foot.

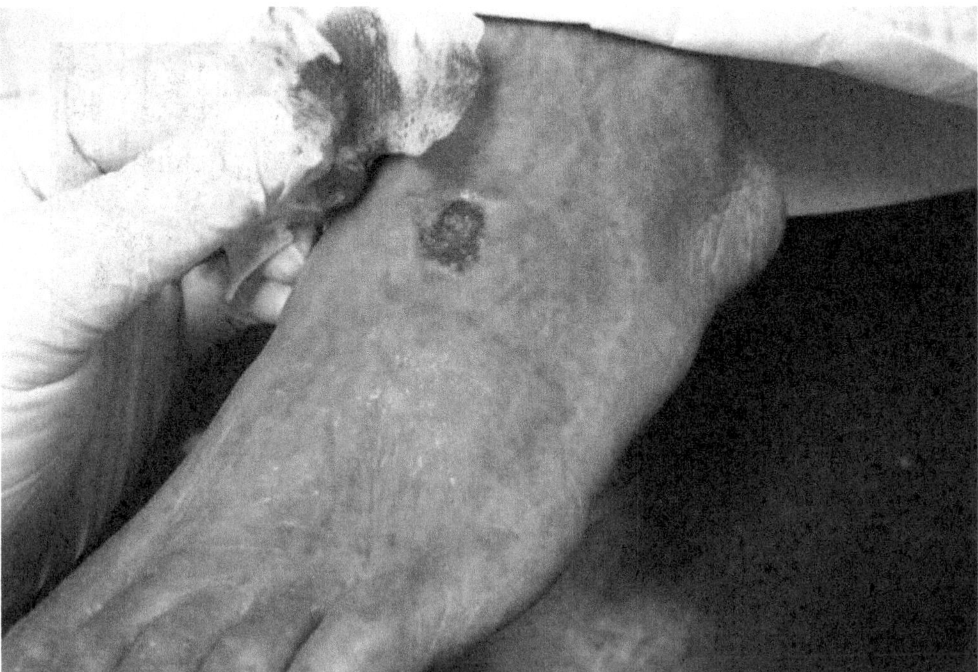

Figure 20.9 Arterial Ulcer

21 Cox, J. (2019). Wound care 101. *Nursing, 49*(10). https://doi.org/10.1097/01.nurse.0000580632.58318.08

22 "Arterial ulcer peripheral vascular disease.jpg" by Jonathan Moore is licensed under CC BY 3.0. Access for free at https://commons.wikimedia.org/wiki/File:Arterial_ulcer_peripheral_vascular_disease.jpg

My Notes

Diabetic Ulcers

Diabetic ulcers are also called neuropathic ulcers because peripheral neuropathy is commonly present in patients with diabetes. **Peripheral neuropathy** is a medical condition that causes decreased sensation of pain and pressure, especially in the lower extremities. **Diabetic ulcers** typically develop on the plantar aspect of the feet and toes of a patient with diabetes due to lack of sensation of pressure or injury. See Figure 20.10[23] for an image of a diabetic ulcer. Wound healing is compromised in patients with diabetes due to the disease process. In addition, there is a higher risk of developing an infection that can reach the bone requiring amputation of the area. To prevent diabetic ulcers from occurring, it is vital for nurses to teach meticulous foot care to patients with diabetes and encourage the use of well-fitting shoes.[24]

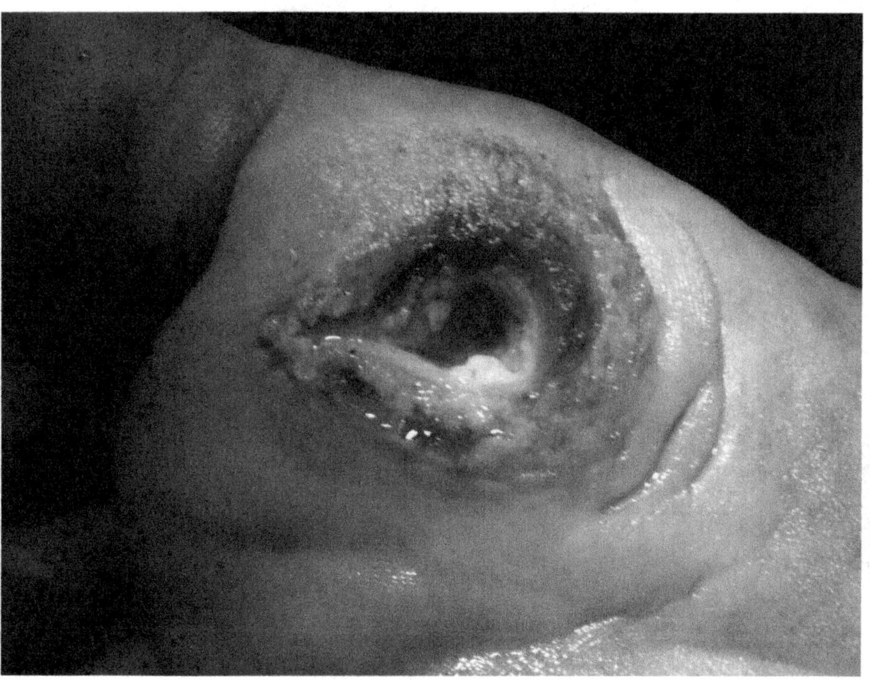

Figure 20.10 Diabetic Ulcer

Pressure Injuries

Pressure injuries are defined as "localized damage to the skin or underlying soft tissue, usually over a bony prominence, as a result of intense and prolonged pressure in combination with shear."[25] **Shear** occurs when tissue layers move over the top of each other, causing blood vessels to stretch and break as they pass through the subcutaneous tissue. For example, when a patient slides down in bed, the outer skin remains immobile because it remains attached to the sheets due to friction, but deeper tissue attached to the bone moves as the patient slides down. This

---

23 "Diabetic Planta ulcer.jpg" by Dr. Lorimer is licensed under CC BY-SA 4.0.

24 Cox, J. (2019). Wound care 101. *Nursing, 49*(10). https://doi.org/10.1097/01.nurse.0000580632.58318.08

25 Edsberg, L. E., Black, J. M., Goldberg, M., McNichol, L., Moore, L., & Sieggreen, M. (2016). Revised national pressure ulcer advisory panel pressure injury staging system: Revised pressure injury staging system. *Journal of Wound, Ostomy, and Continence Nursing: Official Publication of The Wound, Ostomy and Continence Nurses Society, 43*(6), 585–597. https://journals.lww.com/jwocnonline/Fulltext/2016/11000/Revised_National_Pressure_Ulcer_Advisory_Panel.3.aspx

opposing movement of the outer layer of skin and the underlying tissues causes the capillaries to stretch and tear, which then impacts the blood flow and oxygenation of the surrounding tissues.

Braden Scale

Several factors place a patient at risk for developing pressure injuries, including nutrition, mobility, sensation, and moisture. The Braden Scale is a tool commonly used in health care to provide an objective assessment of a patient's risk for developing pressure injuries. See Figure 20.11[26] for an image of a Braden Scale. The six risk factors included on the Braden Scale are sensory perception, moisture, activity, mobility, nutrition, and friction/ shear, and these factors are rated on a scale from 1-4 with 1 being "completely limited" to 4 being "no impairment." The scores from the six categories are added, and the total score indicates a patient's risk for developing a pressure injury. Ranges of scores indicate mild risk for scores 15-19, moderate risk for scores 13-14, high risk for scores 10-12, and severe risk for scores less than 9. Nurses create care plans using these scores to plan interventions that prevent or treat pressure injuries.

For more information about using the Braden Scale, go to the "Integumentary" chapter of the Open RN *Nursing Fundamentals* textbook.

26 The Braden Scale, from Prevention Plus, is included on the basis of Fair Use. http://www.bradenscale.com/

My Notes

BRADEN SCALE – For Predicting Pressure Sore Risk

SEVERE RISK: Total score ≤ 9 **HIGH RISK**: Total score 10-12
MODERATE RISK: Total score 13-14 **MILD RISK**: Total score 15-18

DATE OF ASSESS ➡

RISK FACTOR	SCORE/DESCRIPTION				1	2	3	4
SENSORY PERCEPTION Ability to respond meaningfully to pressure-related discomfort	**1. COMPLETELY LIMITED** – Unresponsive (does not moan, flinch, or grasp) to painful stimuli, due to diminished level of consciousness or sedation, **OR** limited ability to feel pain over most of body surface.	**2. VERY LIMITED** – Responds only to painful stimuli. Cannot communicate discomfort except by moaning or restlessness, **OR** has a sensory impairment which limits the ability to feel pain or discomfort over ½ of body.	**3. SLIGHTLY LIMITED** – Responds to verbal commands but cannot always communicate discomfort or need to be turned, **OR** has some sensory impairment which limits ability to feel pain or discomfort in 1 or 2 extremities.	4. **NO IMPAIRMENT** – Responds to verbal commands. Has no sensory deficit which would limit ability to feel or voice pain or discomfort.				
MOISTURE Degree to which skin is exposed to moisture	1. **CONSTANTLY MOIST**– Skin is kept moist almost constantly by perspiration, urine, etc. Dampness is detected every time patient is moved or turned.	2. **OFTEN MOIST** – Skin is often but not always moist. Linen must be changed at least once a shift.	3. **OCCASIONALLY MOIST** – Skin is occasionally moist, requiring an extra linen change approximately once a day.	4. **RARELY MOIST** – Skin is usually dry; linen only requires changing at routine intervals.				
ACTIVITY Degree of physical activity	1. **BEDFAST** – Confined to bed.	2. **CHAIRFAST** – Ability to walk severely limited or nonexistent. Cannot bear own weight and/or must be assisted into chair or wheelchair.	3. **WALKS OCCASIONALLY** – Walks occasionally during day, but for very short distances, with or without assistance. Spends majority of each shift in bed or chair.	4. **WALKS FREQUENTLY**– Walks outside the room at least twice a day and inside room at least once every 2 hours during waking hours.				
MOBILITY Ability to change and control body position	1. **COMPLETELY IMMOBILE** – Does not make even slight changes in body or extremity position without assistance.	2. **VERY LIMITED** – Makes occasional slight changes in body or extremity position but unable to make frequent or significant changes independently.	3. **SLIGHTLY LIMITED** – Makes frequent though slight changes in body or extremity position independently.	4. **NO LIMITATIONS** – Makes major and frequent changes in position without assistance.				
NUTRITION Usual food intake pattern [1]NPO: Nothing by mouth. [2]IV: Intravenously. [3]TPN: Total parenteral nutrition.	**1. VERY POOR** – Never eats a complete meal. Rarely eats more than 1/3 of any food offered. Eats 2 servings or less of protein (meat or dairy products) per day. Takes fluids poorly. Does not take a liquid dietary supplement, **OR** is NPO[1] and/or maintained on clear liquids or IV[2] for more than 5 days.	**2. PROBABLY INADEQUATE** – Rarely eats a complete meal and generally eats only about ½ of any food offered. Protein intake includes only 3 servings of meat or dairy products per day. Occasionally will take a dietary supplement **OR** receives less than optimum amount of liquid diet or tube feeding.	**3. ADEQUATE** – Eats over half of most meals. Eats a total of 4 servings of protein (meat, dairy products) each day. Occasionally refuses a meal, but will usually take a supplement if offered, **OR** is on a tube feeding or TPN[3] regimen, which probably meets most of nutritional needs.	4. **EXCELLENT** – Eats most of every meal. Never refuses a meal. Usually eats a total of 4 or more servings of meat and dairy products. Occasionally eats between meals. Does not require supplementation.				
FRICTION AND SHEAR	1. **PROBLEM**- Requires moderate to maximum assistance in moving. Complete lifting without sliding against sheets is impossible. Frequently slides down in bed or chair, requiring frequent repositioning with maximum assistance. Spasticity, contractures, or agitation leads to almost constant friction.	2. **POTENTIAL PROBLEM**– Moves feebly or requires minimum assistance. During a move, skin probably slides to some extent against sheets, chair, restraints, or other devices. Maintains relatively good position in chair or bed most of the time but occasionally slides down.	3. **NO APPARENT PROBLEM** – Moves in bed and in chair independently and has sufficient muscle strength to lift up completely during move. Maintains good position in bed or chair at all times.					
TOTAL SCORE	Total score of 12 or less represents HIGH RISK							

ASSESS	DATE	EVALUATOR SIGNATURE/TITLE	ASSESS.	DATE	EVALUATOR SIGNATURE/TITLE
1	/ /		3	/ /	
2	/ /		4	/ /	

NAME-Last	First	Middle	Attending Physician	Record No.	Room/Bed

Form 3166P BRIGGS, Des Moines, IA 50306 (800) 247-2343 www.BriggsCorp.com R304 PRINTED IN U.S.A

Source: Barbara Braden and Nancy Bergstrom. Copyright, 1988. Reprinted with permission. Permission should be sought to use this tool at www.bradenscale.com

BRADEN SCALE

Use the form only for the approved purpose. Any use of the form in publications (other than internal policy manuals and training material) or for profit-making ventures requires additional permission and/or negotiation.

Figure 20.11 Braden Scale. Used under Fair Use.

Staging

My Notes

Pressure injuries commonly occur on the sacrum, heels, ischial tuberosity, and coccyx. The 2016 National Pressure Ulcer Advisory Panel (NPUAP) Pressure Injury Staging System now uses the term "pressure injury" instead of pressure ulcer because an injury can occur without an ulcer present. Pressure injuries are staged from 1 through 4 based on the extent of tissue damage. For example, Stage 1 pressure injuries have reddened but intact skin, and Stage 4 pressure injuries have deep, open ulcers affecting underlying tissue and structures such as muscles, ligaments, and tendons. See Figure 20.12[27] for an image of the four stages of pressure injuries.[28] The NPUAP's definitions of the four stages of pressure injuries are described below:

- **Stage 1** pressure injuries are intact skin with a localized area of nonblanchable erythema where prolonged pressure has occurred. **Nonblanchable erythema** is a medical term used to describe skin redness that does not turn white when pressed.
- **Stage 2** pressure injuries are partial-thickness loss of skin with exposed dermis. The wound bed is viable and may appear like an intact or ruptured blister. Stage 2 pressure injuries heal by reepithelialization and not by granulation tissue formation.[29]
- **Stage 3** pressure injuries are full-thickness tissue loss in which fat is visible, but cartilage, tendon, ligament, muscle, and bone are not exposed. The depth of tissue damage varies by anatomical location. Undermining and tunneling may occur in Stage 3 and 4 pressure injuries. **Undermining** occurs when the tissue under the wound edges becomes eroded, resulting in a pocket beneath the skin at the wound's edge. **Tunneling** refers to passageways underneath the surface of the skin that extend from a wound and can take twists and turns. Slough and eschar may also be present in Stage 3 and 4 pressure injuries. **Slough** is an inflammatory exudate that is usually light yellow, soft, and moist. **Eschar** is dark brown/black, dry, thick, and leathery dead tissue. See Figure 20.13[30] for an image of eschar in the center of the wound. If slough or eschar obscures the wound so that tissue loss cannot be assessed, the pressure injury is referred to as **unstageable**.[31] In most wounds, slough and eschar must be removed by debridement for healing to occur.

---

27 "Wound stage.jpg" by Babagolzadeh is licensed under CC BY-SA 3.0. Access for free at https://commons.wikimedia.org/wiki/File:Wound_stage.jpg

28 Edsberg, L. E., Black, J. M., Goldberg, M., McNichol, L., Moore, L., & Sieggreen, M. (2016). Revised National Pressure Ulcer Advisory Panel Pressure Injury Staging System: Revised pressure injury staging system. *Journal of Wound, Ostomy, and Continence Nursing: Official Publication of The Wound, Ostomy and Continence Nurses Society, 43(6)*, 585–597. https://doi.org/10.1097/WON.0000000000000281

29 Edsberg, L. E., Black, J. M., Goldberg, M., McNichol, L., Moore, L., & Sieggreen, M. (2016). Revised national pressure ulcer advisory panel pressure injury staging system: Revised pressure injury staging system. *Journal of Wound, Ostomy, and Continence Nursing: Official Publication of The Wound, Ostomy and Continence Nurses Society, 43*(6), 585–597. https://doi.org/10.1097/WON.0000000000000281

30 "Inoculation_eschar_Rickettsia_sibirica_mongolitimonae_infection.jpg" by José M. Ramos , Isabel Jado, Sergio Padilla, Mar Masiá, Pedro Anda, and Félix Gutiérrez is licensed under *CC0*. Access for free at https://commons.wikimedia.org/wiki/File:Wound_stage.jpg

31 Edsberg, L. E., Black, J. M., Goldberg, M., McNichol, L., Moore, L., & Sieggreen, M. (2016). Revised national pressure ulcer advisory panel pressure injury staging system: Revised pressure injury staging system. *Journal of Wound, Ostomy, and Continence Nursing: Official Publication of The Wound, Ostomy and Continence Nurses Society, 43*(6), 585–597. https://doi.org/10.1097/WON.0000000000000281

My Notes

- **Stage 4** pressure injuries are full-thickness tissue loss like Stage 3 pressure injuries, but also have exposed cartilage, tendon, ligament, muscle, or bone. **Osteomyelitis** (bone infection) may be present.[32]

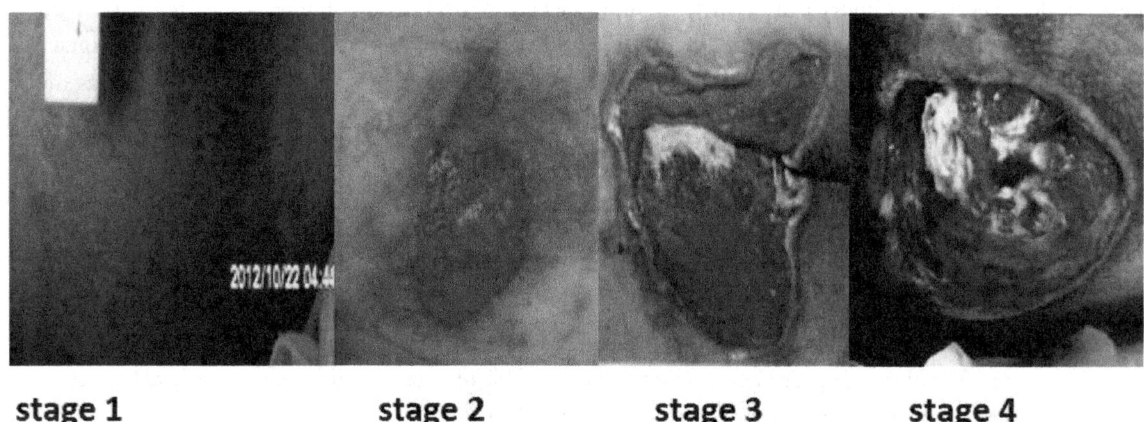

Figure 20.12 Stages of Pressure Wounds

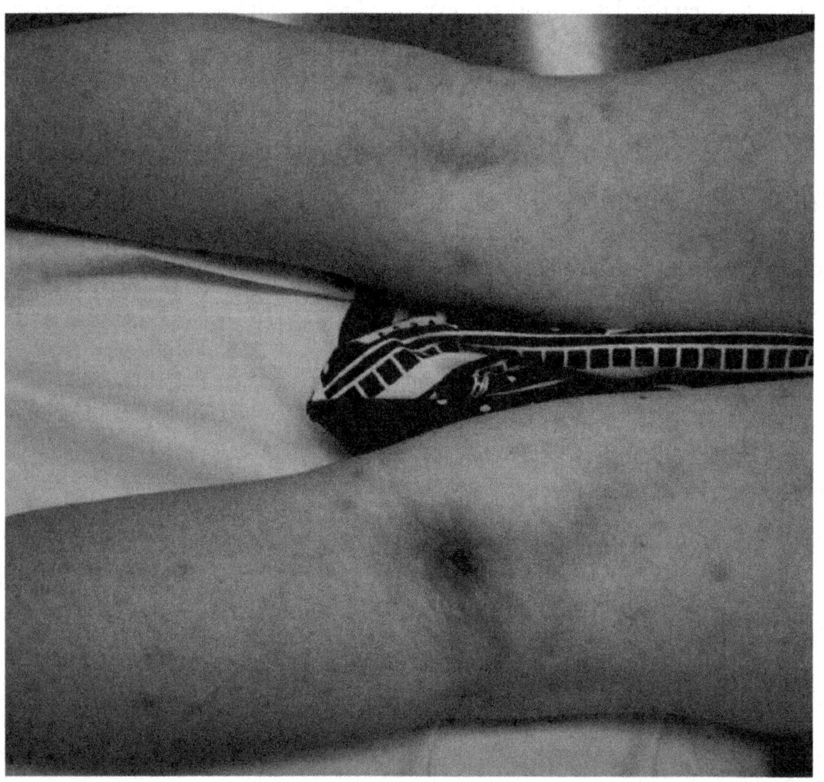

Figure 20.13 Eschar

---

32 Edsberg, L. E., Black, J. M., Goldberg, M., McNichol, L., Moore, L., & Sieggreen, M. (2016). Revised national pressure ulcer advisory panel pressure injury staging system: Revised pressure injury staging system. *Journal of Wound, Ostomy, and Continence Nursing: Official Publication of The Wound, Ostomy and Continence Nurses Society, 43*(6), 585–597. https://doi.org/10.1097/WON.0000000000000281

My Notes

Video Review of Pressure Injuries[33]

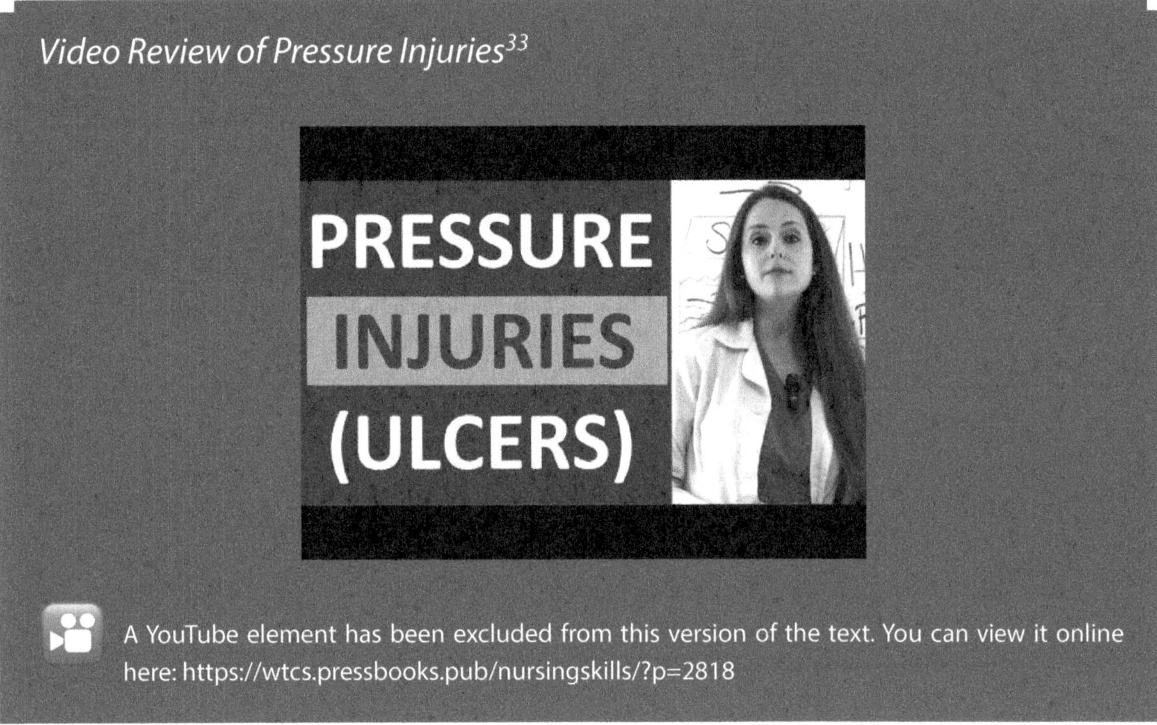

A YouTube element has been excluded from this version of the text. You can view it online here: https://wtcs.pressbooks.pub/nursingskills/?p=2818

Factors Affecting Wound Healing

Multiple factors affect a wound's ability to heal and are referred to as local and systemic factors. Local factors refer to factors that directly affect the wound, whereas systemic factors refer to the overall health of the patient and their ability to heal. Local factors include localized blood flow and oxygenation of the tissue, the presence of infection or a foreign body, and venous sufficiency. **Venous insufficiency** is a medical condition where the veins in the legs do not adequately send blood back to the heart, resulting in a pooling of fluids in the legs.[34]

Systemic factors that affect a patient's ability to heal include nutrition, mobility, stress, diabetes, age, obesity, medications, alcohol use, and smoking.[35] When a nurse is caring for a patient with a wound that is not healing as anticipated, it is important to further assess for the potential impact of these factors:

- **Nutrition.** Nutritional deficiencies can have a profound impact on healing and must be addressed for chronic wounds to heal. Protein is one of the most important nutritional factors affecting wound healing. For example, in patients with pressure injuries, 30 to 35 kcal/kg of calorie intake with 1.25 to 1.5g/kg of protein and micronutrients supplementation is recommended daily.[36] In addition, vitamin C and zinc deficiency have many roles in wound healing. It is important to collaborate with a dietician to identify and manage nutritional deficiencies when a patient is

33 RegisteredNurseRN. (2018, March 7). *Pressure ulcers (injuries) stages, prevention, assessment | Stage 1, 2, 3, 4 unstageable NCLEX.* [Video]. YouTube. All rights reserved. Video used with permission. https://youtu.be/MDtPik1UE6k

34 Guo, S., & Dipietro, L. A. (2010). Factors affecting wound healing. *Journal of Dental Research, 89*(3), 219–229. https://doi.org/10.1177/0022034509359125

35 Guo, S., & Dipietro, L. A. (2010). Factors affecting wound healing. *Journal of Dental Research, 89*(3), 219–229. https://doi.org/10.1177/0022034509359125

36 Cox, J. (2019). Wound care 101. *Nursing, 49*(10). https://doi.org/10.1097/01.nurse.0000580632.58318.08

My Notes

experiencing poor wound healing.[37]

- **Stress.** Stress causes an impaired immune response that results in delayed wound healing. Although a patient cannot necessarily control the amount of stress in their life, it is possible to control one's reaction to stress with healthy coping mechanisms. The nurse can help educate the patient about healthy coping strategies.
- **Diabetes.** Diabetes causes delayed wound healing due to many factors such as neuropathy, atherosclerosis (a buildup of plaque that obstructs blood flow in the arteries resulting in decreased oxygenation of tissues), a decreased host immune resistance, and increased risk for infection.[38] Read more about neuropathy and diabetic ulcers under the "Types of Wounds" section. Nurses provide vital patient education to patients with diabetes to effectively manage the disease process for improved wound healing.
- **Age.** Older adults have an altered inflammatory response that can impair wound healing. Nurses can educate patients about the importance of exercise for improved wound healing in older adults.[39]
- **Obesity.** Obese individuals frequently have wound complications, including infection, dehiscence, hematoma formation, pressure injuries, and venous injuries. Nurses can educate patients about healthy lifestyle choices to reduce obesity in patients with chronic wounds.[40]
- **Medications.** Medications such as corticosteroids impair wound healing due to reduced formation of granulation tissue.[41] When assessing a chronic wound that is not healing as expected, it is important to consider the side effects of the patient's medications.
- **Alcohol consumption.** Research shows that exposure to alcohol impairs wound healing and increases the incidence of infection.[42] Patients with impaired healing of chronic wounds should be educated to avoid alcohol consumption.
- **Smoking.** Smoking impacts the inflammatory phase of the wound healing process, resulting in poor wound healing and an increased risk of infection.[43] Patients who smoke should be encouraged to stop smoking.

---

37 Guo, S., & Dipietro, L. A. (2010). Factors affecting wound healing. *Journal of Dental Research, 89*(3), 219–229. https://doi.org/10.1177/0022034509359125

38 Guo, S., & Dipietro, L. A. (2010). Factors affecting wound healing. *Journal of Dental Research, 89*(3), 219–229. https://doi.org/10.1177/0022034509359125

39 Guo, S., & Dipietro, L. A. (2010). Factors affecting wound healing. *Journal of Dental Research, 89*(3), 219–229. https://doi.org/10.1177/0022034509359125

40 Guo, S., & Dipietro, L. A. (2010). Factors affecting wound healing. *Journal of Dental Research, 89*(3), 219–229. https://doi.org/10.1177/0022034509359125

41 Guo, S., & Dipietro, L. A. (2010). Factors affecting wound healing. *Journal of Dental Research, 89*(3), 219–229. https://doi.org/10.1177/0022034509359125

42 Guo, S., & Dipietro, L. A. (2010). Factors affecting wound healing. *Journal of Dental Research, 89*(3), 219–229. https://doi.org/10.1177/0022034509359125

43 Guo, S., & Dipietro, L. A. (2010). Factors affecting wound healing. *Journal of Dental Research, 89*(3), 219–229. https://doi.org/10.1177/0022034509359125

Lab Values Affecting Wound Healing

My Notes

When a chronic wound is not healing as expected, laboratory test results may provide additional clues regarding the causes of the delayed healing. See Table 20.2 for lab results that offer clues to systemic issues causing delayed wound healing.[44]

Table 20.2 Lab Values Associated with Delayed Wound Healing[45]

Abnormal Lab Value	Rationale
Low hemoglobin	Low hemoglobin indicates less oxygen is transported to the wound site.
Elevated white blood cells (WBC)	Increased WBC indicates infection is occurring.
Low platelets	Platelets are important during the proliferative phase in the creation of granulation tissue and angiogenesis.[46]
Low albumin	Low albumin indicates decreased protein levels. Protein is required for effective wound healing.
Elevated blood glucose or hemoglobin A1C	Elevated blood glucose and hemoglobin A1C levels indicate poor management of diabetes mellitus, a disease that impacts wound healing.
Elevated serum BUN and creatinine	BUN and creatinine levels are indicators of kidney function, with elevated levels indicating worsening kidney function. Elevated BUN (blood urea nitrogen) levels impact wound healing.
Positive wound culture	Positive wound cultures indicate an infection is present and provide additional information including the type and number of bacteria present, as well as identifying antibiotics to which the bacteria is susceptible. The nurse reviews this information when administering antibiotics to ensure the prescribed therapy is effective for the type of bacteria present.

Wound Complications

In addition to delayed wound healing, several other complications can occur. Three common complications are the development of a hematoma, infection, or dehiscence. These complications should be immediately reported to the health care provider.

44 Grey, J. E., Enoch, S., & Harding, K. G. (2006). Wound assessment. *BMJ (Clinical research ed.), 332*(7536), 285–288. https://doi.org/10.1136/bmj.332.7536.285

45 Grey, J. E., Enoch, S., & Harding, K. G. (2006). Wound assessment. *BMJ (Clinical research ed.), 332*(7536), 285–288. https://doi.org/10.1136/bmj.332.7536.285

46 This work is a derivative of StatPearls by Grubbs and Mannah and is licensed under CC BY 4.0. Access for free at https://www.ncbi.nlm.nih.gov/books/NBK430685/

My Notes

Hematoma

A **hematoma** is an area of blood that collects outside of the larger blood vessels. A hematoma is more severe than **ecchymosis** (bruising) that occurs when small veins and capillaries under the skin break. The development of a hematoma at a surgical site can lead to infection and incisional dehiscence.[47] See Figure 20.14[48] for an image of a hematoma.

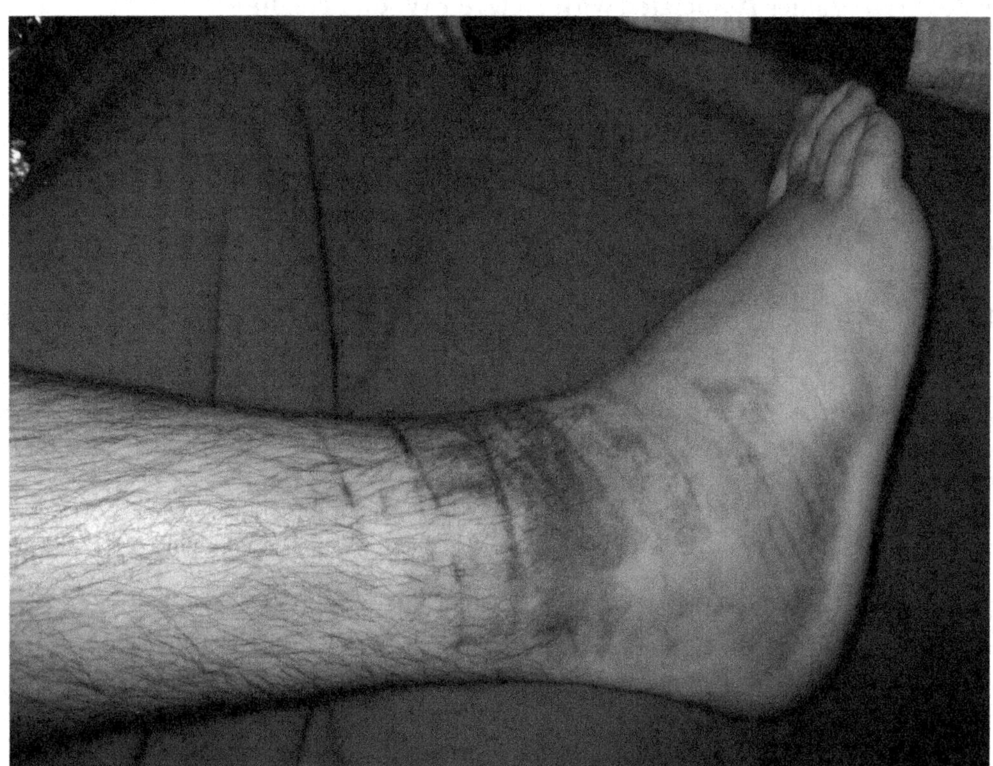

Figure 20.14 Hematoma

Infection

A break in the skin allows bacteria to enter and begin to multiply. Microbial contamination of wounds can progress from localized infection to systemic infection, sepsis, and subsequent life- and limb-threatening infection. Signs of a localized wound infection include redness, warmth, and tenderness around the wound. Purulent or malodorous drainage may also be present. Signs that a systemic infection is developing and requires urgent medical management include the following:[49]

---

47 Edsberg, L. E., Black, J. M., Goldberg, M., McNichol, L., Moore, L., & Sieggreen, M. (2016). Revised national pressure ulcer advisory panel pressure injury staging system: Revised pressure injury staging system. *Journal of Wound, Ostomy, and Continence Nursing: Official Publication of The Wound, Ostomy and Continence Nurses Society, 43*(6), 585–597. https://doi.org/10.1097/won.0000000000000281

48 "Ankle swell and internal bleeding" by Glen Bowman is licensed under CC BY-SA 2.0. Access for free at https://www.flickr.com/photos/glenbowman/3109068066/

49 WoundSource. (2016, October 19). *8 signs of wound infection*. https://www.woundsource.com/blog/8-signs-wound-infection

My Notes

- Fever over 101 F (38 C)
- Overall malaise (lack of energy and not feeling well)
- Change in level of consciousness/increased confusion
- Increasing or continual pain in the wound
- Expanding redness or swelling around the wound
- Loss of movement or function of the wounded area

Dehiscence

Dehiscence refers to the separation of the edges of a surgical wound. A dehisced wound can appear fully open where the tissue underneath is visible, or it can be partial where just a portion of the wound has torn open. Wound dehiscence is always a risk in a surgical wound, but the risk increases if the patient is obese, smokes, or has other health conditions, such as diabetes, that impact wound healing. Additionally, the location of the wound and the amount of physical activity in that area also increase the chances of wound dehiscence.[50] See Figure 20.15[51] for an image of dehiscence in an abdominal surgical wound in a 50-year-old obese female with a history of smoking and malnutrition.

Wound dehiscence can occur suddenly, especially in abdominal wounds when the patient is coughing or straining. Evisceration is a rare but severe surgical complication when dehiscence occurs and the abdominal organs protrude out of the incision. Signs of impending dehiscence include redness around the wound margins and increasing drainage from the incision. The wound will also likely become increasingly painful. Suture breakage can be a sign that the wound has minor dehiscence or is about to dehisce.[52]

To prevent wound dehiscence, surgical patients must follow all post-op instructions carefully. The patient must move carefully and protect the skin from being pulled around the wound site. They should also avoid tensing the muscles surrounding the wound and avoid heavy lifting as advised.[53]

---

50 WoundSource. (2018, March 28). *Complications in chronic wound healing and associated interventions.* https://www.woundsource.com/blog/complications-in-chronic-wound-healing-and-associated-interventions

51 "Bogota bag.png" by Suarez-Grau, J. M., Guadalajara Jurado, J. F., Gómez Menchero, J., Bellido Luque, J. A. is licensed under CC BY 4.0. Access for free at https://commons.wikimedia.org/wiki/File:Bogota_bag.png

52 WoundSource. (2018, March 28). *Complications in chronic wound healing and associated interventions.* https://www.woundsource.com/blog/complications-in-chronic-wound-healing-and-associated-interventions

53 WoundSource. (2018, March 28). *Complications in chronic wound healing and associated interventions.* https://www.woundsource.com/blog/complications-in-chronic-wound-healing-and-associated-interventions

My Notes

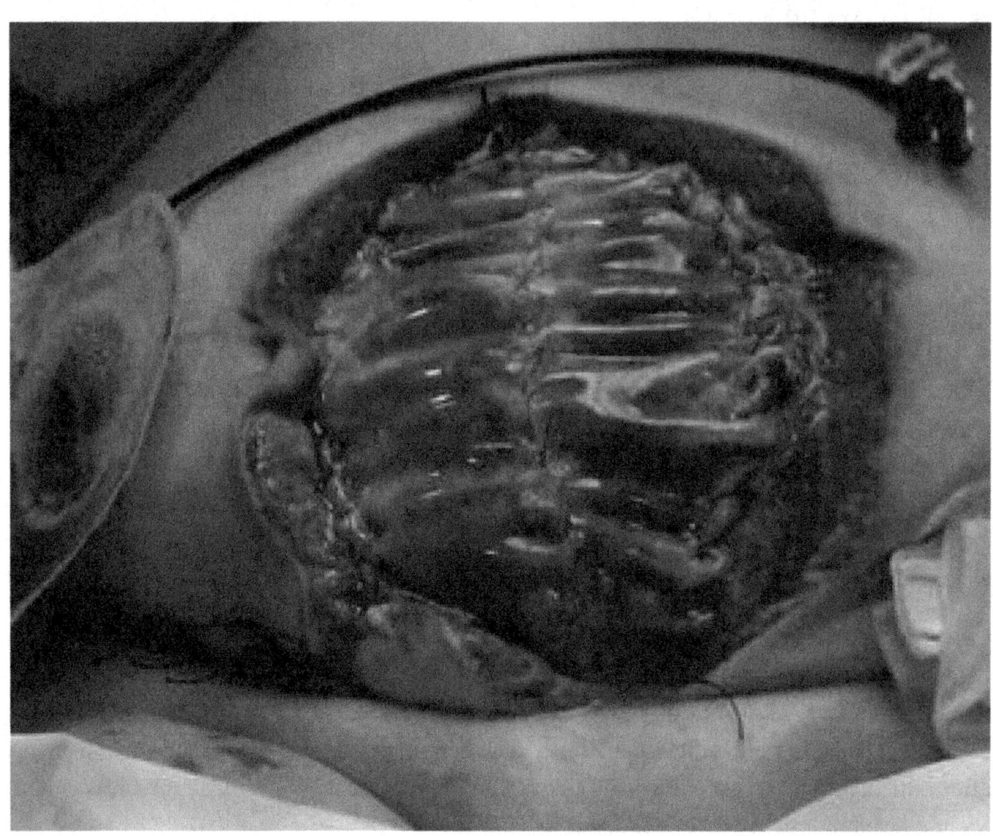

Figure 20.15 Dehiscence

20.3 ASSESSING WOUNDS

My Notes

Wounds should be assessed and documented at every dressing change. Wound assessment should include the following components:

- Anatomic location
- Type of wound (if known)
- Degree of tissue damage
- Wound bed
- Wound size
- Wound edges and periwound skin
- Signs of infection
- Pain[1]

These components are further discussed in the following sections.

Anatomic Location and Type of Wound

The location of the wound should be documented clearly using correct anatomical terms and numbering. This will ensure that if more than one wound is present, the correct one is being assessed and treated. Many agencies use images to facilitate communication regarding the location of wounds among the health care team. See Figure 20.16[2] for an example of facility documentation that includes images to indicate wound location.

The location of a wound also provides information about the cause and type of a wound. For example, a wound over the sacral area of an immobile patient is likely a pressure injury, and a wound near the ankle of a patient with venous insufficiency is likely a venous ulcer. For successful healing, different types of wounds require different treatments based on the cause of the wound.

1 Cox, J. (2019). Wound care 101. *Nursing, 49*(10). https://doi.org/10.1097/01.nurse.0000580632.58318.08

2 "putool7bfig.jpg" by unknown is in the Public Domain. Access for free at https://www.ahrq.gov/patient-safety/settings/hospital/resource/pressureulcer/tool/pu7b.html

My Notes

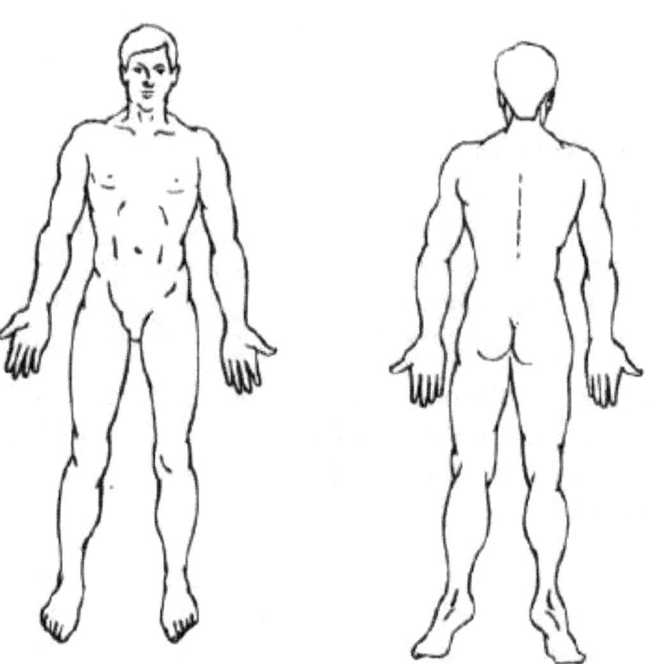

PRESSURE ULCER IDENTIFICATION POCKET PAD

Place the patient's/resident's name on the top of the pad, date it and place an "X" on the area on the body where you see the skin concern. Give this to the nurse and ask him or her to check the patient/resident. They will follow up as needed.

Date: ____________________ Time: ____________________

Patient's/Resident's Name: ____________________

Reporter: ____________________

Figure 20.16 Wound Documentation

Degree of Tissue Damage

It is important to continually assess the degree of tissue damage in pressure injuries because the level of damage can worsen if they are not treated appropriately. Refer to the "Staging" subsection of "Pressure Injuries" in the "Basic Concepts Related to Wounds" section for more information about tissue damage.

Wound Base

Assess the color of the wound base. Recall that healthy granulation tissue appears pink due to the new capillary formation. It is moist, painless to the touch, and may appear "bumpy." Conversely, unhealthy granulation tissue is dark red and painful. It bleeds easily with minimal contact and may be covered with biofilm. The appearance of slough (yellow) or eschar (black) in the wound base should be documented and communicated to the health care provider because it likely will need to be removed for healing. Tunneling and undermining should also be assessed, documented, and communicated.

My Notes

Type and Amount of Exudate

The color, consistency, and amount of exudate (drainage) should be assessed and documented at every dressing change. The amount of drainage from wounds is categorized as scant, small/minimal, moderate, or large/copious. Use the following descriptions to select the appropriate terms:[3]

- **No exudate:** The wound base is dry.
- **Scant amount of exudate:** The wound is moist but no measurable amount of exudate appears on the dressing.
- **Minimal amount of exudate:** Exudate covers less than 25% of the size of the bandage.
- **Moderate amount of drainage:** Wound tissue is wet, and drainage covers 25% to 75% of the size of the bandage.
- **Large or copious amount of drainage:** Wound tissue is filled with fluid, and exudate covers more than 75% of the bandage.[4]

The type of wound drainage should be described using medical terms such as serosanguinous, sanguineous, serous, or purulent.

- **Sanguineous:** Sanguineous exudate is fresh bleeding.[5]
- **Serous:** Serous drainage is clear, thin, watery plasma. It's normal during the inflammatory stage of wound healing, and small amounts are considered normal wound drainage.[6]
- **Serosanguinous:** Serosanguineous exudate contains serous drainage with small amounts of blood present.[7]
- **Purulent:** Purulent exudate is thick and opaque. It can be tan, yellow, green, or brown. It is never considered normal in a wound bed, and new purulent drainage should always be reported to the health care provider.[8] See Figure 20.17[9] for an image of purulent drainage.

---

3 Wound Care Advisor. (n.d.). *Exudate amounts.* https://woundcareadvisor.com/exudate-amounts/#:~:text=Small%20or%20minimal%20amount%20of,than%2075%25%20of%20the%20bandage

4 Wound Care Advisor. (n.d.). *Exudate amounts.* https://woundcareadvisor.com/exudate-amounts/#:~:text=Small%20or%20minimal%20amount%20of,than%2075%25%20of%20the%20bandage

5 Wound Care Advisor. (n.d.). *Exudate amounts.* https://woundcareadvisor.com/exudate-amounts/#:~:text=Small%20or%20minimal%20amount%20of,than%2075%25%20of%20the%20bandage

6 Wound Care Advisor. (n.d.). *Exudate amounts.* https://woundcareadvisor.com/exudate-amounts/#:~:text=Small%20or%20minimal%20amount%20of,than%2075%25%20of%20the%20bandage

7 Wound Care Advisor. (n.d.). *Exudate amounts.* https://woundcareadvisor.com/exudate-amounts/#:~:text=Small%20or%20minimal%20amount%20of,than%2075%25%20of%20the%20bandage

8 Wound Care Advisor. (n.d.). *Exudate amounts.* https://woundcareadvisor.com/exudate-amounts/#:~:text=Small%20or%20minimal%20amount%20of,than%2075%25%20of%20the%20bandage

9 "Purulant knee aspirate.JPG" by James Heilman, MD is licensed under CC BY 3.0. Access for free at https://commons.wikimedia.org/wiki/File:Purulant_knee_aspirate.JPG

My Notes

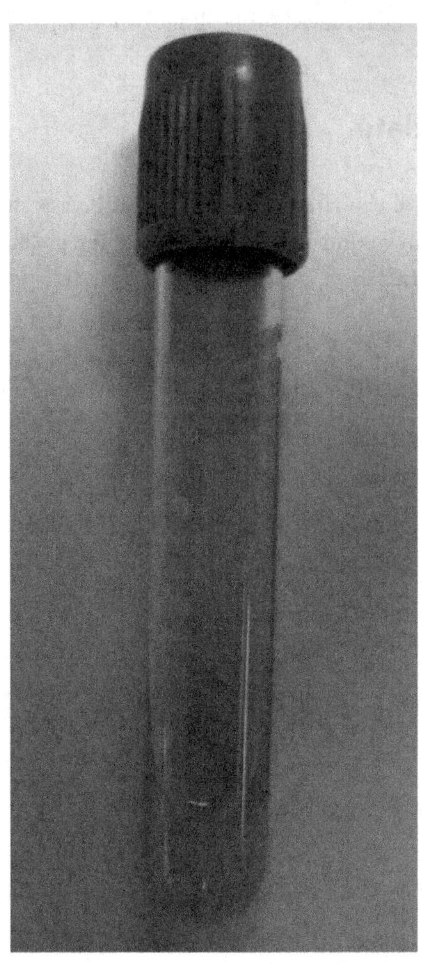

Figure 20.17 Purulent Drainage

Wound Size

Wounds should be measured on admission and during every dressing change to evaluate for signs of healing. Accurate wound measurements are vital for monitoring wound healing. Measurements should be taken in the same manner by all clinicians to maintain consistent and accurate documentation of wound progress. This can be difficult to accomplish with oddly shaped wounds because there can be confusion about how consistently to measure them. Wounds should be described by length by width, with the length of the wound based on the head-to-toe axis. The width of a wound should be measured from side to side laterally. If a wound is deep, the deepest point of the wound should be measured to the wound surface using a sterile, cotton-tipped applicator. Many facilities use disposable, clear plastic measurement tools to measure the area of a wound healing by secondary intention. Measurements are typically documented in centimeters. See Figure 20.18[10] for an image of a wound measurement tool.

10 "Sample Wound Measuring Guide.jpg" by Deanna Hoyord, Chippewa Valley Technical College is licensed under CC BY 4.0. Access for free at https://drive.google.com/file/d/1x_9xpkeTq_f60wsm2QVCc8Bupa6WliXg/view?usp=sharing

My Notes

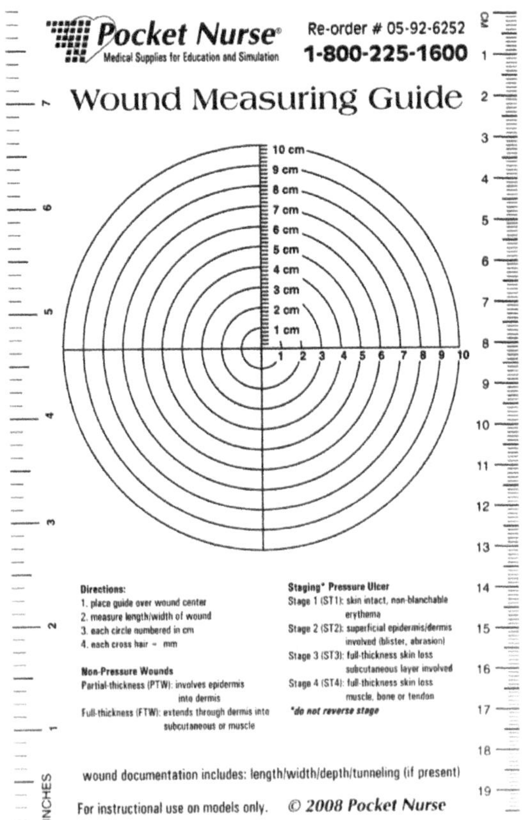

Figure 20.18 Wound Measurement Tool

Tunneling can occur in a full-thickness wound that can lead to abscess formation. The depth of a tunneling can be measured by gently probing the tunnelled area with a sterile, cotton-tipped applicator from the wound base to the end of the tract. When probing a tunnel, it is imperative to not force the swab but only insert until resistance is felt to prevent further damage to the area. The location of the tunnel in the wound should be documented using the analogy of a clock face, with 12:00 pointing toward the patient's head.[11]

Undermining occurs when the tissue under the wound edges becomes eroded, resulting in a pocket beneath the skin at the wound's edge. Undermining is measured by inserting a probe under the wound edge directed almost parallel to the wound surface until resistance is felt. The amount of undermining is the distance from the probe tip to the point at which the probe is level with the wound edge. Clock terms are also used to identify the area of undermining.[12]

11 Cox, J. (2019). Wound care 101. *Nursing, 49*(10). https://doi.org/10.1097/01.nurse.0000580632.58318.08

12 WoundEducators.com. (2016, July 1). *Wound undermining.* https://woundeducators.com/measure-wound-undermining/#:~:text=Wound%20undermining%20occurs%20when%20the,surface%20until%20resistance%20is%20felt

My Notes

Wound Edges and Periwound Skin

If the wound is healing by primary intention, it should be documented if the wound edges are well-approximated (closed together) or if there are any signs of dehiscence. The skin outside the outer edges of the wound, called the **periwound** skin, provides information related to wound development or healing. For example, a venous ulcer often has excess wound drainage that macerates the periwound skin, giving it a wet, waterlogged appearance that is soft and gray white in color.[13] See Figure 20.19[14] for an image of erythematous periwound with partial dehiscence.

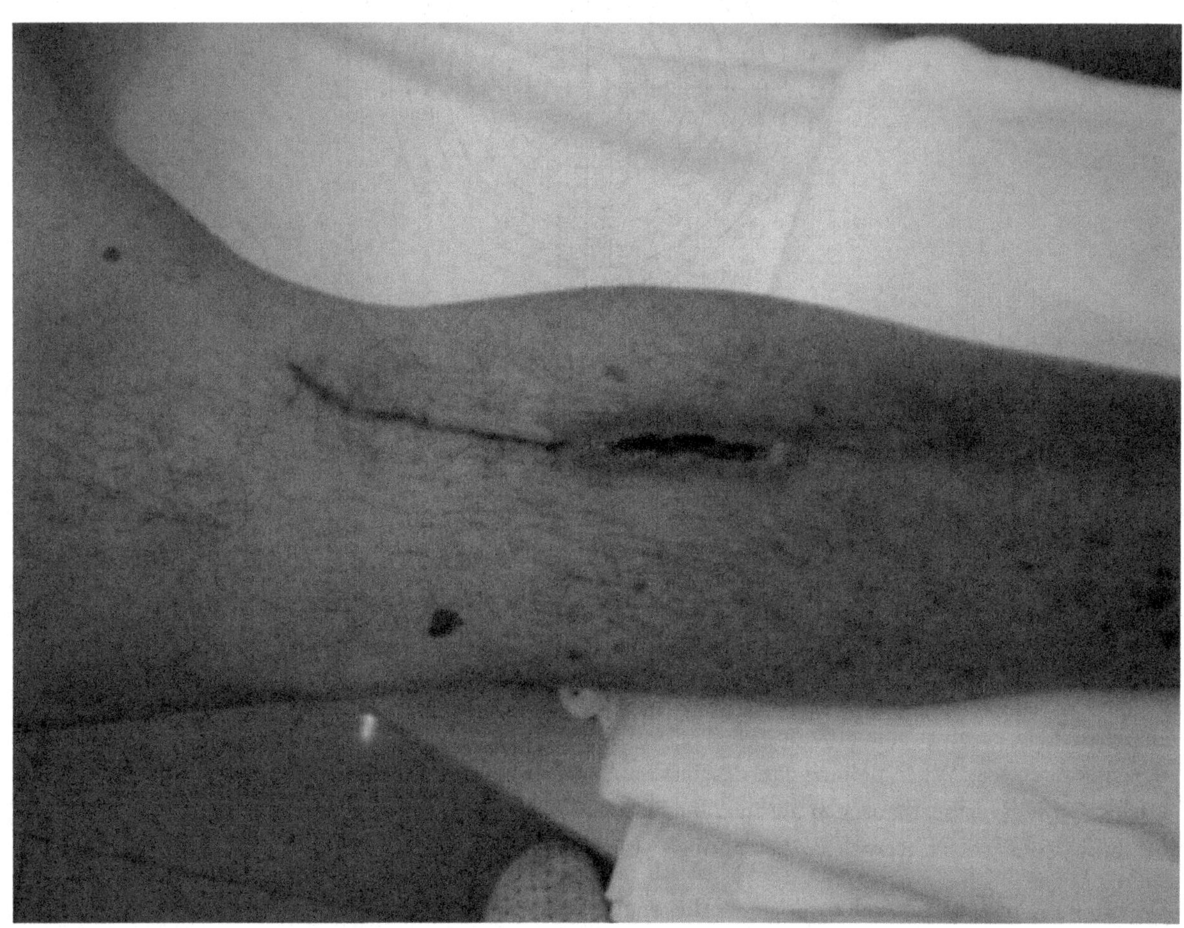

Figure 20.19 Periwound

Signs of Infection

Wounds should be continually monitored for signs of infection. Signs of localized wound infection include **erythema** (redness), **induration** (area of hardened tissue), pain, edema, purulent exudate (yellow or green drainage),

13 Cox, J. (2019). Wound care 101. *Nursing, 49*(10). https://doi.org/10.1097/01.nurse.0000580632.58318.08

14 "Post operative wound.JPG" by Intermedichbo is licensed under CC BY-SA 3.0. Access for free at https://commons.wikimedia.org/wiki/File:Post_operative_wound.JPG

and wound odor.[15] New signs of infection should be reported to the health care provider with an anticipated order for a wound culture.

My Notes

Pain

The intensity of pain that a patient is experiencing with a wound should be assessed and documented. If a patient experiences pain during dressing changes, it should be managed with administration of pain medication before scheduled dressing changes. Be aware that the degree of pain may not correlate to the extent of tissue damage. For example, skin tears are often painful because the nerve endings are exposed in the dermal layer, whereas patients with severe diabetic ulcers on their feet may experience little or no pain because of existing neuropathic damage.[16]

15 Cox, J. (2019). Wound care 101. *Nursing, 49*(10). https://doi.org/10.1097/01.nurse.0000580632.58318.08

16 Cox, J. (2019). Wound care 101. *Nursing, 49*(10). https://doi.org/10.1097/01.nurse.0000580632.58318.08

My Notes

20.4 WOUND THERAPY

Wound therapy is often prescribed by a multidisciplinary team that can include the provider, a wound care nurse, a dietician, and the bedside nurse who performs dressing changes. Topical dressings should be selected that create an environment conducive to healing the specific type of wound and its causes. It is important to perform the following actions when providing wound care:

- Prevent and manage infection
- Cleanse the wound
- Debride the wound
- Maintain appropriate moisture in the wound
- Control odor
- Manage wound pain
- Consider the big picture[1]

Each of these objectives is further discussed in the following subsections.

Prevent and Manage Infection

One of the primary goals of wound dressings is to protect the wound base from bacteria and contaminants (i.e., urine and feces). If new signs of infection are present during a wound dressing change, wound swabs should be taken according to agency policy and the need for a wound culture and possible antibiotic therapy discussed with the primary provider.[2]

Silver sulfadiazine is an example of a common topical antibiotic prescribed for wounds. Topical antibiotics are covered with a secondary dressing.[3]

Cleanse the Wound

Routine cleansing should be performed at each dressing change with products that are physiologically compatible with wound tissue. Normal saline is the most gentle solution and is typically delivered using a syringe or commercial cleansers. See Figure 20.20[4] for an image of wound irrigation with a syringe. Commercial cleansers may be used, but hydrogen peroxide, betadine, and acetic acid should be avoided because these agents can be cytotoxic.[5]

> Visit the journal article in *American Nurse* titled "Is Your Wound-Cleansing Practice Up To Date?" to read more information about wound cleansing (https://www.myamericannurse.com/is-your-wound-cleansing-practice-up-to-date/).

---

1 Cox, J. (2019). Wound care 101. *Nursing, 49*(10). https://doi.org/10.1097/01.nurse.0000580632.58318.08

2 Cox, J. (2019). Wound care 101. *Nursing, 49*(10). https://doi.org/10.1097/01.nurse.0000580632.58318.08

3 Cox, J. (2019). Wound care 101. *Nursing, 49*(10). https://doi.org/10.1097/01.nurse.0000580632.58318.08

4 "DSC_1732-150x150.jpg" by British Columbia Institute of Technology is licensed under CC BY 4.0. Access for free at https://opentextbc.ca/clinicalskills/chapter/4-5-complex-dressing-change/

5 Cox, J. (2019). Wound care 101. *Nursing, 49*(10). https://doi.org/10.1097/01.nurse.0000580632.58318.08

My Notes

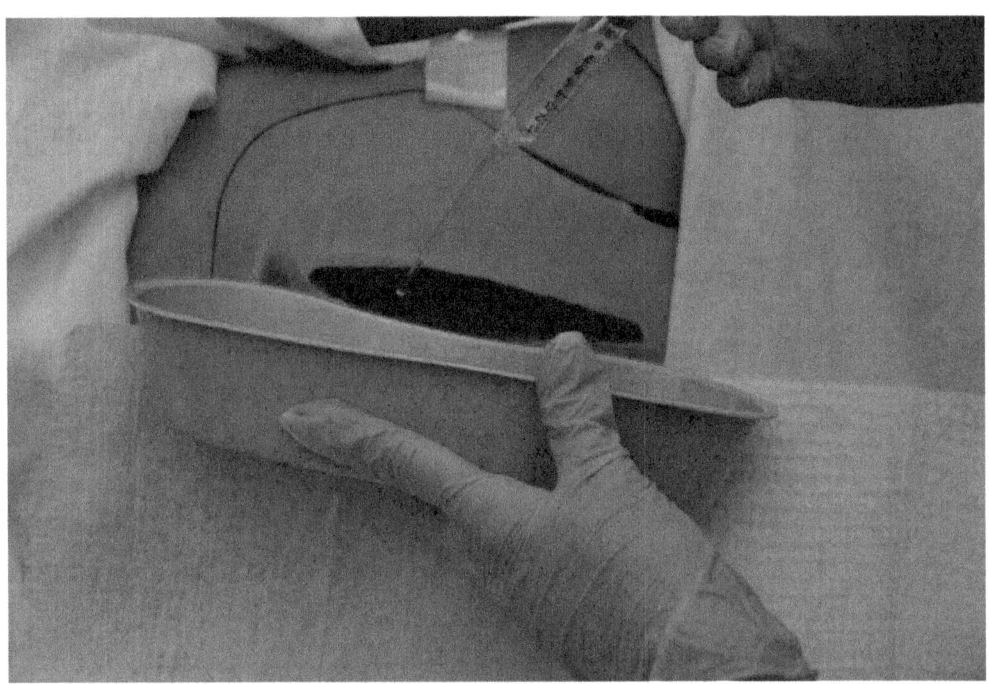

Figure 20.20 Irrigating a Wound

Debride the Wound

Debridement is the removal of nonviable tissue in a wound. If necrotic (black) tissue is present in the wound bed, it must be removed in most circumstances for the wound to heal. However, one exception is stable, dry eschar on a patient's heel that should be left in place until the patient's vascular status is determined.[6]

Wound debridement can be accomplished using several methods, such as autolytic, enzymatic, or sharp wound debridement. Autolytic debridement occurs when moist topical dressings foster the breakdown of necrotic tissue. Enzymatic debridement occurs when prescribed topical agents are directly applied to the wound bed.[7] Collagenase ointment is an example of a topical enzymatic debridement ointment that is applied daily (or more frequently if the dressing becomes soiled) and covered with sterile gauze or a foam dressing.[8] Sharp wound debridement is performed by a trained health care provider and may be at the bedside or in the operating room. Sharp debridement is an invasive procedure using a scalpel or scissors to remove necrotic tissue so that only viable tissue remains. See Figure 20.21[9] for an image of a wound that has been surgically debrided of necrotic tissue.

6 Cox, J. (2019). Wound care 101. *Nursing, 49*(10). https://doi.org/10.1097/01.nurse.0000580632.58318.08

7 Cox, J. (2019). Wound care 101. *Nursing, 49*(10). https://doi.org/10.1097/01.nurse.0000580632.58318.08

8 National Institutes of Health. (2019, May 17). *DailyMed - Collagenase Santyl ointment.* U.S. National Library of Medicine. https://dailymed.nlm.nih.gov/dailymed/drugInfo.cfm?setid=6b6fbfc6-98fa-46aa-88cf-ab00fbb08ffd

9 "Open wound after debridement of NF.jpg" by Morphx1982 is licensed under CC BY-SA 4.0. Access for free at https://commons.wikimedia.org/wiki/File:Open_wound_after_debridement_of_NF.jpg

My Notes

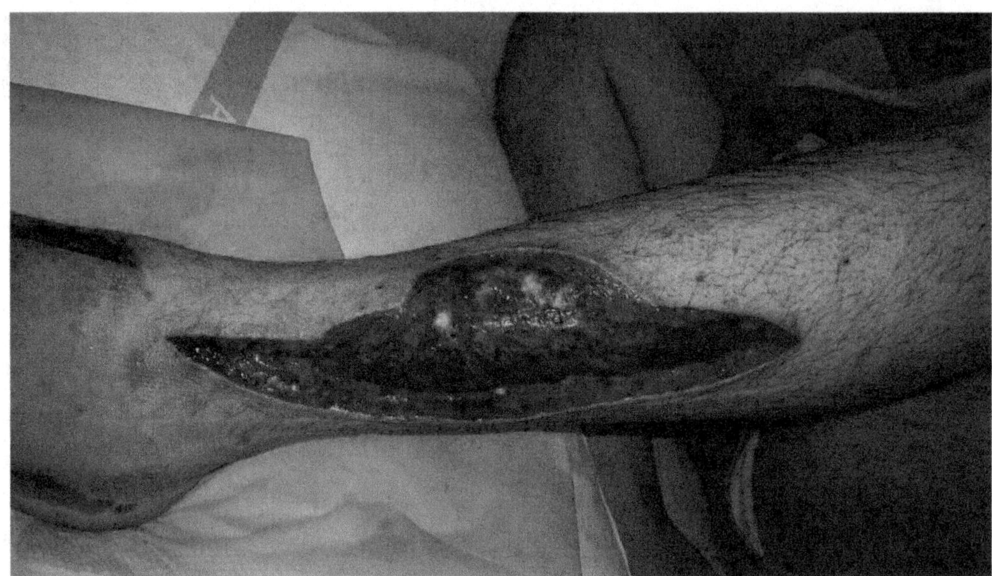

Figure 20.21 Wound Debridement

Maintain Appropriate Moisture in the Wound

Wound dressings should maintain a moist wound environment to facilitate the development of granulation tissue. However, excessive exudate must be managed with dressings that absorb excess moisture to avoid maceration of the surrounding tissue.[10] For example, dressings such as alginate or hydrofiber are used in wounds with large amounts of exudate to maintain an appropriate moisture level but also prevent maceration of tissue. Frequent dressing changes may also be required in wounds with heavy drainage.

Eliminate Dead Space

Deep wounds and tunneling should be packed with dressings to keep the wound bed moist. Sterile gauze dressings moistened with normal saline or hydrogel-impregnated dressings are examples of packing agents used to keep the wound bed moist. Packing material should be easy to remove from the wound base during each dressing change to avoid injuring the fragile granulation tissue. Keep in mind that dressings made of alginate have a slight greenish tint when removed and should not be confused with purulent drainage.

Control Odor

If odor is present in a wound, the nurse should consult with the health care provider about the frequency of dressing changes, wound cleansing agents, and the possible need for topical antimicrobial therapy or debridement. Room deodorants can be obtained for use after dressing changes.[11]

---

10 Cox, J. (2019). Wound care 101. *Nursing, 49*(10). https://doi.org/10.1097/01.nurse.0000580632.58318.08

11 Cox, J. (2019). Wound care 101. *Nursing, 49*(10). https://doi.org/10.1097/01.nurse.0000580632.58318.08

My Notes

Manage Wound Pain

Wounds that are becoming increasingly painful should be assessed for potential infection or dehiscence. The nurse should plan on administering medication to the patient before performing dressing changes on wounds that are painful. If pain medication is not ordered, then the nurse should contact the health care provider for a prescription before performing the dressing change.[12]

Protect Periwound Skin

Heavily draining wounds or the improper use of moist dressings can cause maceration of the periwound skin. The nurse should apply dressings carefully to maintain wound bed moisture yet also protect the periwound skin. Skin barrier creams, skin protective wipes, or skin barrier wafers can also be used to protect the periwound skin.[13]

Consider the Big Picture

Most wounds do not occur in isolation but also have other systemic or local factors that impact wound healing. Be sure to consider the following points when caring for patients with wounds with delayed wound healing:

- Minimize pressure and shear for patients with pressure injuries. For example, a patient with a pressure injury should be repositioned at least every two hours to minimize pressure.
- Educate patients with neuropathy and decreased sensation about preventing further injury. For example, a patient with diabetes should wear well-fitting shoes and never go barefoot to prevent injuries.
- Control edema in patients with venous ulcers through the use of compression dressings.
- Promote adequate perfusion to patients with arterial ulcers. For example, in most cases, the extremity of a patient with an arterial ulcer should not be elevated.
- Protect fragile skin in patients with skin tears to prevent further injury.
- Manage blood sugar levels in patients with diabetes mellitus for optimal healing.
- Promote good nutrition and hydration for all patients with wounds. Consult a registered dietician to assess the patient's nutritional status and develop a nutrition plan if needed.[14]
- Document ongoing assessment findings and wound interventions for good communication and continuity of care across the multidisciplinary health care team.
- Concerns about the healing of a chronic wound or the dressings ordered should be communicated to the health care provider. Referral to a specialized wound care nurse is often helpful.

---

12 Cox, J. (2019). Wound care 101. *Nursing, 49*(10). https://doi.org/10.1097/01.nurse.0000580632.58318.08

13 Cox, J. (2019). Wound care 101. *Nursing, 49*(10). https://doi.org/10.1097/01.nurse.0000580632.58318.08

14 Cox, J. (2019). Wound care 101. *Nursing, 49*(10). https://doi.org/10.1097/01.nurse.0000580632.58318.08

My Notes

20.5 WOUND DRESSINGS

Wound dressings should be selected based on the type of the wound, the cause of the wound, and the characteristics of the wound. A specially-trained wound care nurse should be consulted, when possible, for appropriate selection of dressings for chronic wounds. See Table 20.5 for commonly used wound dressings and associated nursing considerations.[1]

Table 20.5 Wound Dressings[2]

Type of Dressing	Description	Nursing Considerations
Sterile gauze (see Figure 22[3]) **Kerlix** (see Figure 23[4])	Can be used as a primary dressing or moistened wound packing.	■ Least expensive option. ■ Dressings must be changed frequently (at least daily). ■ If unmoistened, the gauze can adhere to the wound base causing injury to granulation tissue.
Nonadherent dressings, nonadherent gauze, or petroleum impregnated gauze **Nonadherent dressing** (see Figure 24[5]) **Petroleum impregnated gauze** (see Figure 25[6])	Applied over open wounds and covered with a secondary dressing. Nontraumatic to skin and wound base. May be applied over skin tears.	■ Change dressing every 24-28 hours to prevent drying and adherence to the wound bed.

1 Cox, J. (2019). Wound care 101. *Nursing, 49*(10). https://doi.org/10.1097/01.nurse.0000580632.58318.08

2 Cox, J. (2019). Wound care 101. *Nursing, 49*(10). https://doi.org/10.1097/01.nurse.0000580632.58318.08

3 "Sterile 4x4 Dressing and Package 3I3A0330.jpg" by Deanna Hoyord, Chippewa Valley Technical College is licensed under CC BY 4.0. Access for free at https://drive.google.com/file/d/1Y7Tbn6w65JgizAn3cNlx6HaeMBr8swIL/view?usp=sharing

4 "Kerlix with Package 3I3A0365.jpg" by Deanna Hoyord, Chippewa Valley Technical College is licensed under CC BY 4.0. Access for free at https://drive.google.com/file/d/1QmFoXfm173lt9xDqfOHdUxnhfmkCiKxp/view?usp=sharing

5 "Nonadherent Dressing and Packaging 3I3A0203.jpg" by Deanna Hoyord, Chippewa Valley Technical College is licensed under CC BY 4.0. Access for free at https://drive.google.com/file/d/1NjRZwOt3GnjhD1s26FUMWGzX5EiGED0i/view?usp=sharing

6 "Vaseline Gauze Package -1 3I3A0296.jpg" and "Vaseline Gauze Dressing 3I3A0299" by Deanna Hoyord, Chippewa Valley Technical College are licensed under CC BY 4.0. Access for free at https://drive.google.com/file/d/12lEhsQsTLK-YY1z2pMVrtmuFg8StUdNC/view?usp=sharing

My Notes

Type of Dressing	Description	Nursing Considerations
Transparent films (see Figure 26[7])	Can be used on wounds with minimal or no exudate to retain moisture. Commonly used to secure other dressing materials such as foam.	■ Do not use on skin tears or fragile skin. ■ Surrounding skin can macerate if the wound has more than minimal drainage.
Hydrocolloids (see Figure 27[8])	Used as an occlusive dressing to prevent contaminants, promote a moist wound environment, and cause autolytic debridement. Thicker hydrocolloids absorb moderate amounts of drainage.	■ Avoid in infected wounds. ■ Commonly used for pressure injuries. ■ Odor may be present on removal due to composition. ■ Change dressing every 3 – 5 days.
Hydrogels	Creates a moist wound environment in wounds with little or no exudate. If in gel form, apply directly to the wound and cover with secondary dressing.	■ Can be soothing for painful wounds. ■ Typically changed daily. ■ Take care to only cover the wound and not the surrounding skin to avoid maceration.
Silicone-based dressings	Nonadherent dressing used on moderately to highly exudative wounds. Nontraumatic to wound bed and promotes a moist wound environment.	■ Can be used for all types of wounds including skin tears. ■ Sacral and heel-shaped silicone dressings can be used to prevent pressure injuries.
Foam (see Figure 28[9])	Nonadherent and absorptive.	■ Can be used as a primary dressing. ■ Can be used under compression dressings for venous ulcers to manage exudate.
Alginate/ hydrofibers (see Figure 29[10])	Nonadherent and highly absorptive for highly exudative wounds. Used for wound packing in full-thickness wounds such as Stage 3 or 4 pressure injuries.	■ Usually changed every 24-48 hours; left in place based on the saturation of wound drainage. ■ Can be used as a primary dressing for exudative wounds like venous ulcers and covered with a secondary dressing such as foam or silicone. ■ Do not use in dry wounds because it may injure the wound bed.

7 "Transparent Film.jpg" by Deanna Hoyord, Chippewa Valley Technical College is licensed under CC BY 4.0. Access for free at https://drive.google.com/file/d/1RjarkghI4E5Rw6xMVmVOfibRBhyRpeos/view?usp=sharing

8 "Hydrocolloid.jpg" by Deanna Hoyord, Chippewa Valley Technical College is licensed under CC BY 4.0. Access for free at https://drive.google.com/file/d/1jEeS3unYDTcOmJRZwVNyXNnrA8bl2JvO/view?usp=sharing

9 "Foam Dressing 3I3A0406.jpg" by Deanna Hoyord, Chippewa Valley Technical College is licensed under CC BY 4.0. Access for free at https://drive.google.com/file/d/1JMMUqA1TDj6Dd0gxXb7DdpA6ooOzkjKv/view?usp=sharing

10 "Alginate Dressing 3I3A0396.jpg" by Deanna Hoyord, Chippewa Valley Technical College is licensed under CC BY 4.0. Access for free at https://drive.google.com/file/d/13U5SEodqegteIO722s79ZBE2oDKyarcn/view?usp=sharing

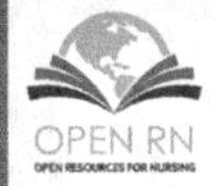

My Notes

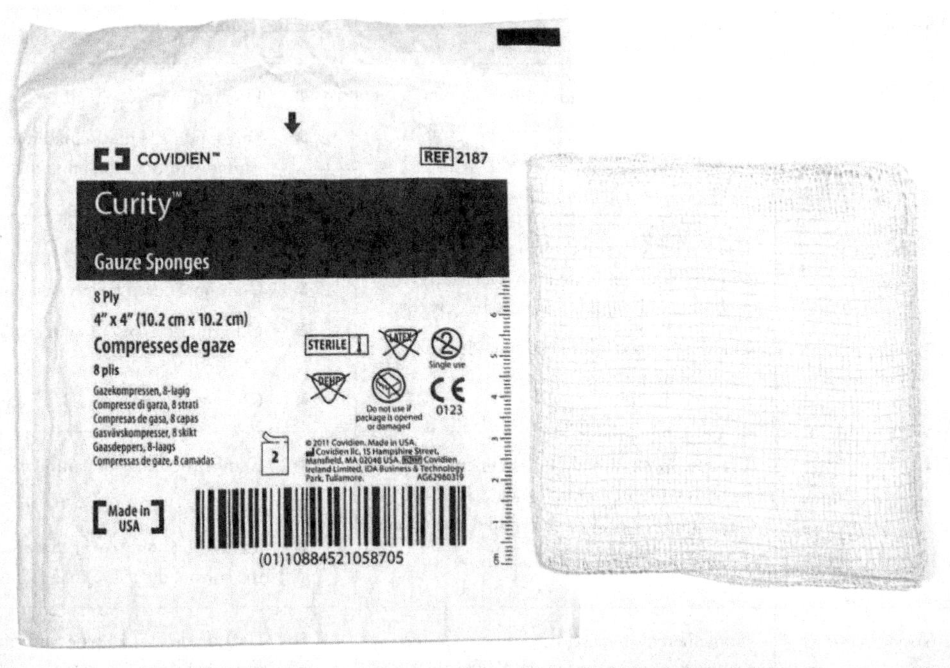

Figure 20.22 Sterile Gauze

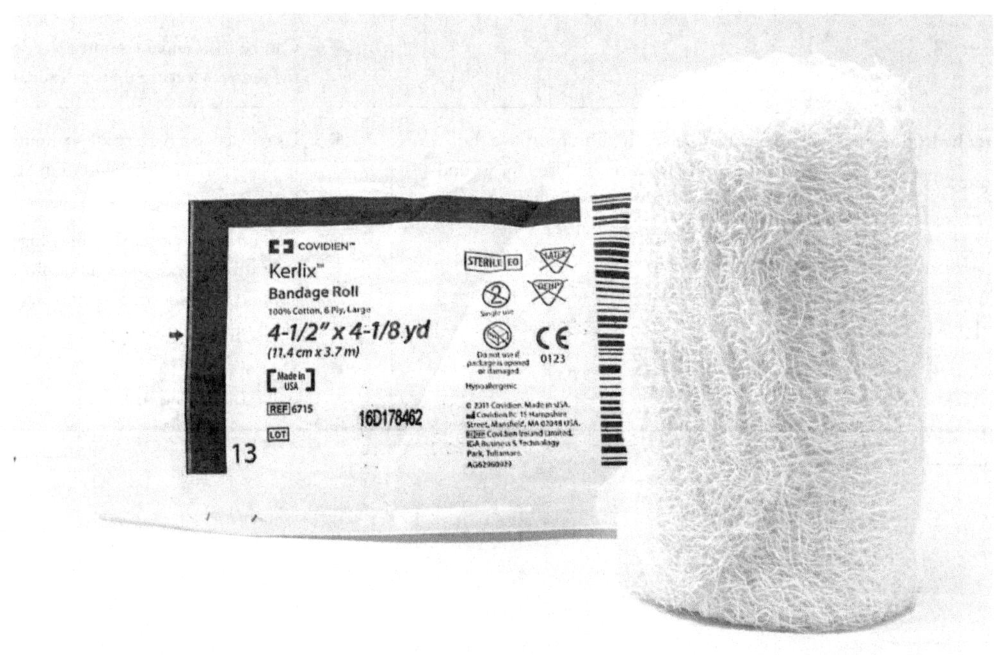

Figure 20.23 Kerlix

My Notes

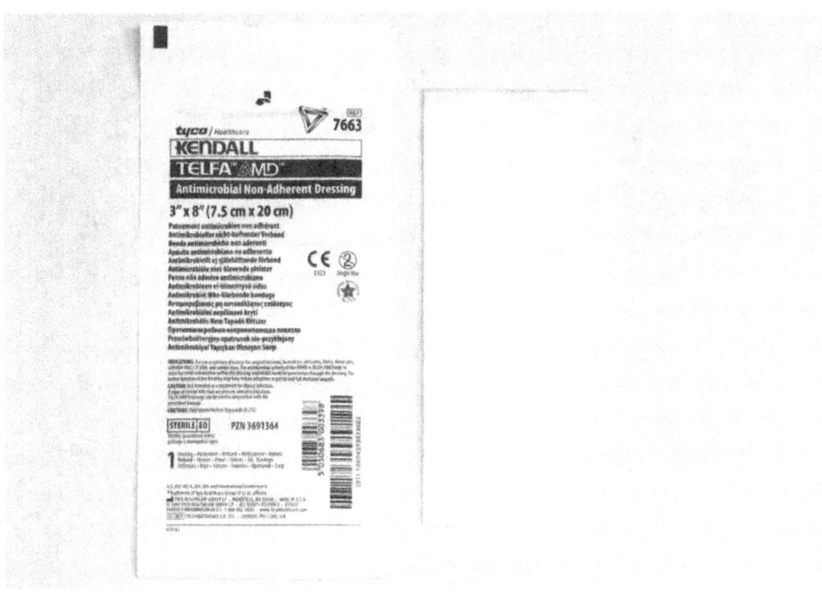

Figure 20.24 Nonadherent Dressing

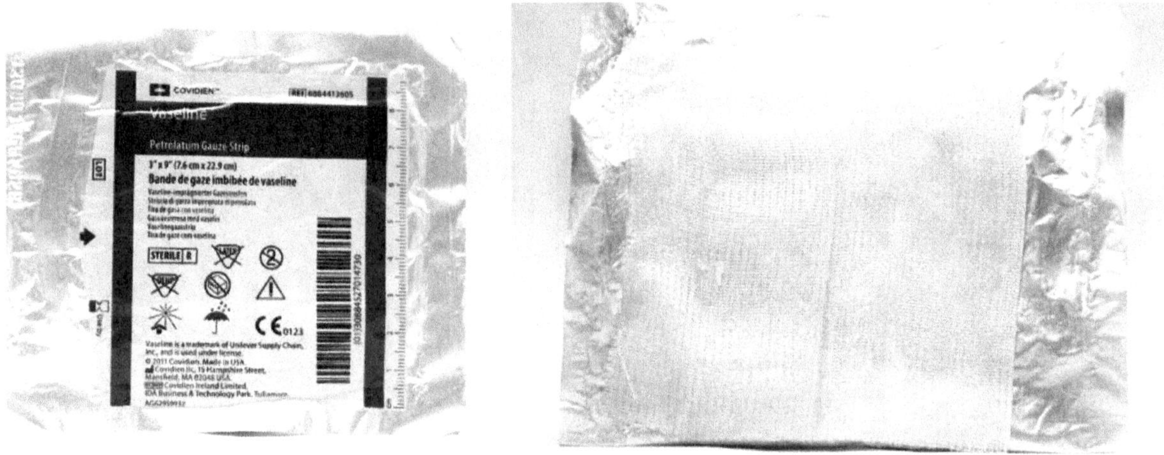

Figure 20.25 Petroleum Gauze

My Notes

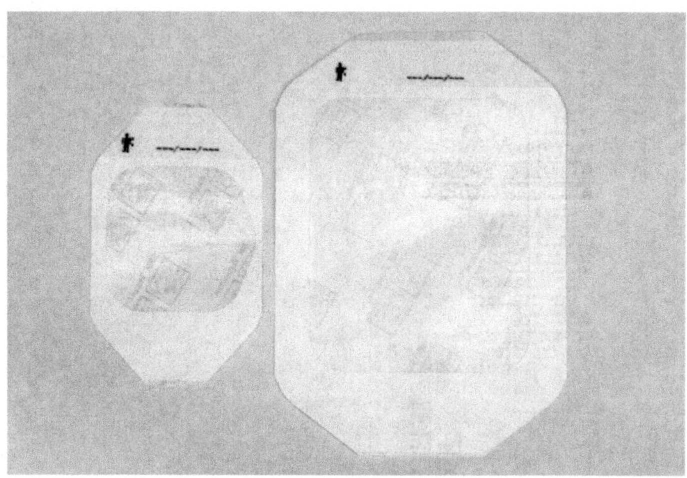

Figure 20.26 Transparent Film

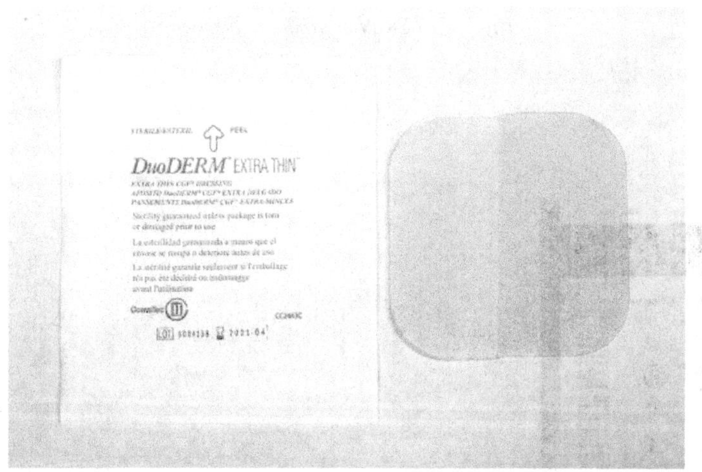

Figure 20.27 Hydrocolloid

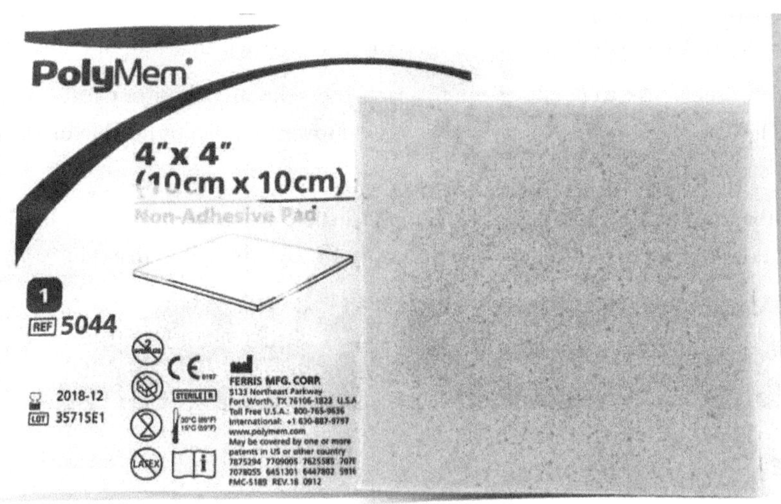

Figure 20.28 Foam Dressing

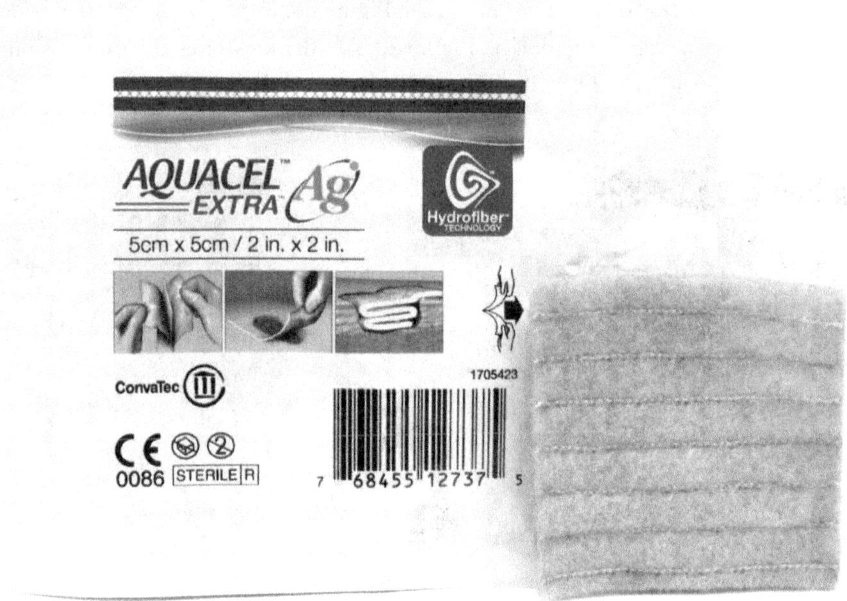

Figure 20.29 Alginate Dressing

Types of Tape

There are several types of tape that can be used to secure dressings. The most commonly used types of tape are medical transpore, micropore paper, cloth, and waterproof tape.

- **Medical transpore tape** (often referred to as "medi-pore") is inexpensive, durable, and very sticky. It has tiny holes in it that allow air to reach the skin underneath and sweat and body fluid to pass through it without causing it to come off. However, it leaves residue and can damage sensitive skin.

My Notes

- **Micropore paper tape** is gentle on skin and doesn't leave residue, but it is not waterproof and doesn't work well on irregular areas. It allows air to reach the skin underneath.
- **Cloth tape** sticks well, allows air to reach the skin, and does not leave a residue. It has high strength so it can be used to secure a splint. However, it is not flexible or waterproof and can be difficult to tear.
- **Waterproof tape** is more expensive but it is flexible and doesn't leave residue. It sticks well to skin but does not stick well to hair. It is waterproof when applied to dry skin.

Read Inside First Aid's webpage about different types of medical tape: "5 Different Types of Medical Tapes and How to Use Them" (https://insidefirstaid.com/first-aid-kit/medical-tape-buy-the-right-kind).

Wound Vacs

The term **wound vac** refers to a device used with special foam dressings and suctioning to remove fluid and decrease air pressure around a wound to assist in healing. During a wound vac procedure, the nurse applies a special foam dressing over an open wound and seals it with a thin film layer. The film has an opening that rubber tubing fits through to connect to a vacuum pump. Once connected, the vacuum pump removes fluid from the wound while also helping to pull the edges of the wound together. A person with a wound vac typically wears the device 24 hours a day while the wound is healing.[11] See Figure 20.30[12] for an image of a wound vac foam dressing attached to suctioning by a wound vac device. Figure 20.31[13] demonstrates the progression of a wound healing with a wound vac from image A to D.

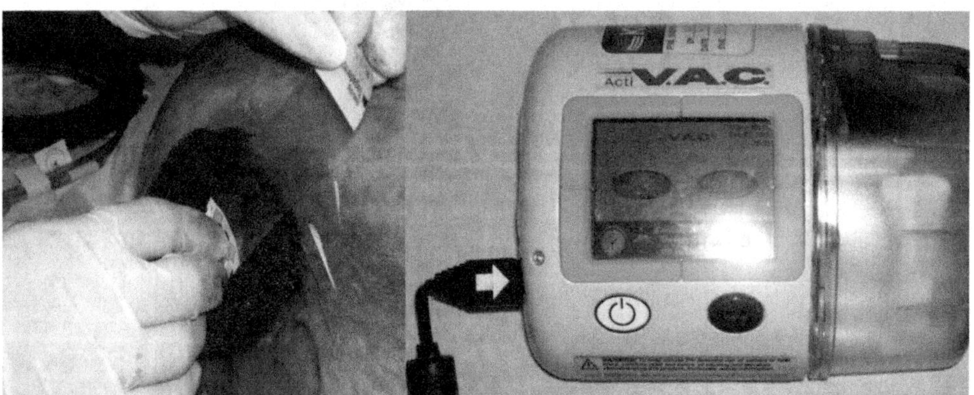

Figure 20.30 Wound Vac

11 Yetman, D. (2020, March 23). *What you need to know about vacuum-assisted wound closure (VAC).* Healthline. https://www.healthline.com/health/wound-vac#how-it-works

12 "KCI Wound Vac01.jpg" and "KCI Wound Vac02.jpg" by Noles1984 at English Wikipedia are in the Public Domain. Access for free at https://commons.wikimedia.org/wiki/File:KCI_Wound_Vac01.jpg

13 "0100-6991-rcbc-44-01-00081-gf1.gif" by unknown is licensed under CC BY 4.0. Access for free at https://www.scielo.br/scielo.php?script=sci_arttext&pid=S0100-69912017000100081#f1

My Notes

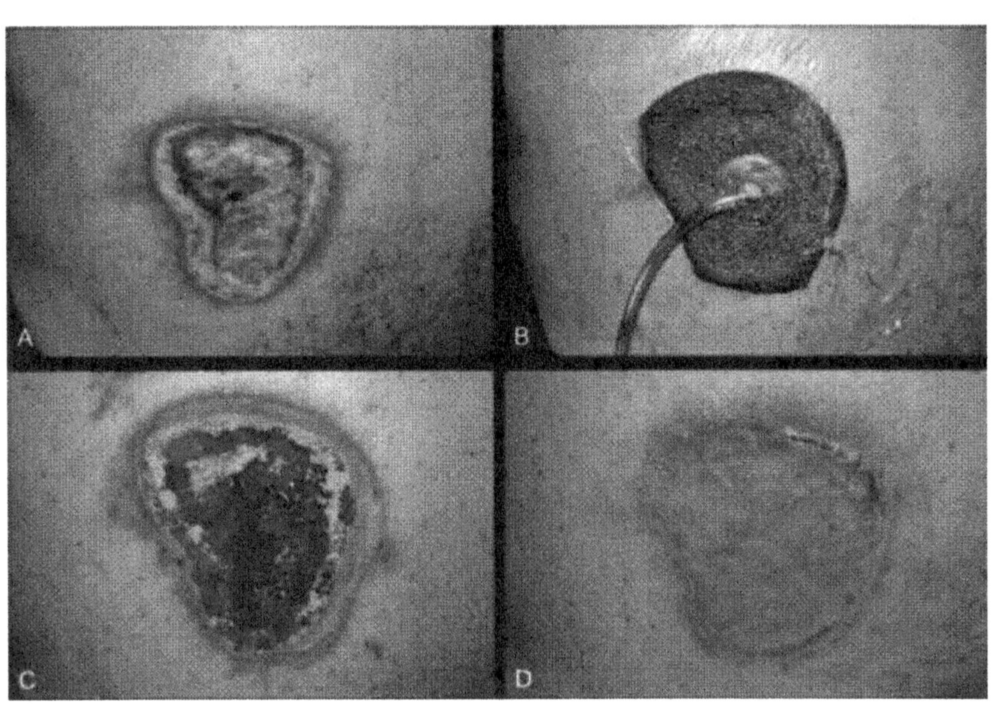

Figure 20.31 Progression of Healing with a Wound Vac

My Notes

20.6 SAMPLE DOCUMENTATION

Sample Documentation of Expected Findings

3 cm x 2 cm Stage 3 pressure injury on the patient's sacrum. Dark pink wound base with no signs of infection. Cleansed with normal saline spray and hydrocolloid dressing applied.

Sample Documentation of Unexpected Findings

3 cm x 2 cm Stage 3 pressure injury on the patient's sacrum. Wound base is dark red with yellowish-green drainage present. Periwound skin is red, warm, and tender to palpation. Patient temperature is 36.8C. Cleansed with normal saline spray and wound culture specimen collected. Hydrocolloid dressing applied and Dr. Smith notified. Order received for wound culture.

20.7 CHECKLIST FOR WOUND ASSESSMENT

My Notes

Use the checklist below to review the steps for completion of "Wound Assessment."

Steps

Disclaimer: Always review and follow agency policy regarding this specific skill.

1. Gather supplies: gloves, wound measuring tool, and sterile cotton-tipped swab.
2. Perform safety steps:
    - Perform hand hygiene.
    - Check the room for transmission-based precautions.
    - Introduce yourself, your role, the purpose of your visit, and an estimate of the time it will take.
    - Confirm patient ID using two patient identifiers (e.g., name and date of birth).
    - Explain the process to the patient and ask if they have any questions.
    - Be organized and systematic.
    - Use appropriate listening and questioning skills.
    - Listen and attend to patient cues.
    - Ensure the patient's privacy and dignity.
    - Assess ABCs.
3. Identify wound location. Document the anatomical position of the wound on the body using accurate anatomical terminology.
4. Identify the type and cause of the wound (e.g., surgical incision, pressure injury, venous ulcer, arterial ulcer, diabetic ulcers, or traumatic wound).
5. Note tissue damage:
    - If the wound is a pressure injury, identify the stage and use the Braden Scale to assess risk factors.
6. Observe wound base. Describe the type of tissue in the wound base (i.e., granulation, slough, eschar).
7. Follow agency policy to measure wound dimensions, including width, depth, and length. Assess for tunneling, undermining, or induration.
8. Describe the amount and color of wound exudate:
    - Serous drainage (plasma): clear or light yellowish
    - Sanguineous drainage (fresh bleeding): bright red
    - Serosanguineous drainage (a mix of blood and serous fluid): pink
    - Purulent drainage (infected): thick, opaque, and yellow, green, or other color
9. Note the presence or absence of odor; noting the presence of odor may indicate infection.

My Notes

10. Assess the temperature, color, and integrity of the skin surrounding the wound. Assess for tenderness of periwound area.

11. Assess wound pain using PQRSTU. Note the need to premedicate before dressing changes if the wound is painful. (Read more about PQRSTU assessment in the "Health History" chapter.)

12. Assess for signs of infection, such as fever, change in level of consciousness, type of drainage, presence of odor, dark red granulation tissue, or redness, warmth, and tenderness of the periwound area.

13. Assist the patient back to a comfortable position, ask if they have any questions, and thank them for their time.

14. Ensure safety measures when leaving the room:

    - CALL LIGHT: Within reach
    - BED: Low and locked (in lowest position and brakes on)
    - SIDE RAILS: Secured
    - TABLE: Within reach
    - ROOM: Risk-free for falls (scan room and clear any obstacles)

15. Perform hand hygiene.

16. Document the assessment findings and report any concerns according to agency policy.

View a supplementary video of a nurse performing a wound assessment in "Wound Care: Assessing Wounds."[1]

1 Phillips, P. (2011, May 17). *Wound care: Assessing wounds.* [Video]. YouTube. All rights reserved. https://youtu.be/s76P1DdtBAA

20.8 CHECKLIST FOR SIMPLE DRESSING CHANGE

My Notes

Use this checklist to review the steps for completion of "Simple Dressing Change."

Steps

Disclaimer: Always review and follow agency policy regarding this specific skill.

1. Gather supplies: nonsterile gloves, sterile gloves per agency policy, wound cleansing solution or sterile saline, sterile 2" x 2" gauze for wound cleansing, 4" x 4" sterile gauze for wound dressing, scissors, and tape (if needed).
    - Use the smallest size of dressing for the wound.
    - Take only the dressing supplies needed for the dressing change to the bedside.
2. Perform safety steps:
    - Perform hand hygiene.
    - Check the room for transmission-based precautions.
    - Introduce yourself, your role, the purpose of your visit, and an estimate of the time it will take.
    - Confirm patient ID using two patient identifiers (e.g., name and date of birth).
    - Explain the process to the patient and ask if they have any questions.
    - Be organized and systematic.
    - Use appropriate listening and questioning skills.
    - Listen and attend to patient cues.
    - Ensure the patient's privacy and dignity.
    - Assess ABCs.
3. Assess wound pain using PQRSTU. Premedicate before dressing changes if the wound is painful.
4. Prepare the environment, position the patient, adjust the height of the bed, and turn on the lights. Ensure proper lighting to allow for good visibility to assess the wound. Ensure proper body mechanics for yourself and create a comfortable position for the patient.
5. Perform hand hygiene immediately prior to arranging the supplies at the bedside.
6. Place a clean, dry, barrier on the bedside table. Create a sterile field if indicated by agency policy.
7. Pour sterile normal saline into opened sterile gauze packaging to moisten the gauze.
    - Normal saline containers must be used for only one patient and must be dated and discarded within at least 24 hours of being opened.
    - Commercial wound cleanser may also be used.
8. Expose the dressing.
9. Perform hand hygiene and apply nonsterile gloves.

My Notes

10. Remove the outer dressing.

11. Remove the inner dressing. Use transfer forceps, if necessary, to avoid contaminating the wound bed.

12. Remove gloves, perform hand hygiene, and put on new gloves.

    - Wrap the old inner dressing inside the glove as you remove it, if feasible, to prevent contaminating the environment.

13. Assess the wound:

    - See "Checklist for Wound Assessment" checklist for details.

14. Drape the patient with a water-resistant underpad, if indicated, to protect the patient's clothing and linen.

15. Apply gloves and other PPE as indicated. Goggles, face shield, and/or mask may be indicated.

16. Cleanse the wound based on agency policy, using moistened gauze, commercial cleanser, or sterile irrigant. When using moistened gauze, use one moistened 2" x 2" sterile gauze per stroke. Work in straight lines, moving away from the wound with each stroke. Strokes should move from a clean area to a dirty area and from top to bottom.

    - Note: A suture line is considered the "least contaminated" area and should be cleansed first.

17. Cleanse around the drain (if present):

    - Clean around the drain site using a circular stroke, starting with the area immediately next to the drain.
    - Using a new swab with each stroke, cleanse immediately next to the drain in a circular motion. With the next stroke, move a little farther out from the drain. Continue this process with subsequent circular swabs until the skin surrounding the drain is cleaned.

18. Remove gloves, perform hand hygiene, and apply new gloves.

19. Apply sterile dressing (4" x 4" sterile gauze), using nontouch technique so that the dressing touching the wound remains sterile.

20. Apply outer dressing if required. Secure the dressing with tape as needed.

21. Remove gloves and perform hand hygiene.

22. Assist the patient to a comfortable position, ask if they have any questions, and thank them for their time.

23. Ensure safety measures when leaving the room:

    - CALL LIGHT: Within reach
    - BED: Low and locked (in lowest position and brakes on)
    - SIDE RAILS: Secured
    - TABLE: Within reach
    - ROOM: Risk-free for falls (scan room and clear any obstacles)

24. Perform hand hygiene.

25. Document the procedure and related assessment findings. Compare the wound assessment to previous documentation and analyze healing progress. Report any concerns according to agency policy.

My Notes

My Notes

20.9 CHECKLIST FOR WOUND CULTURE

Wound cultures are obtained from wounds suspected to be infected. Results are used to determine treatment options. Wound culture results indicate the type and number of bacteria present, as well as the antibiotics to which bacteria are susceptible. When performing a wound culture, it is vital for the nurse to avoid contamination and to use evidence-based techniques to obtain a good specimen that the patient's treatment plan will be based upon.[1]

Use the checklist to review the steps to "Perform a Wound Culture."

Steps

Disclaimer: Always review and follow agency policy regarding this specific skill.

1. Gather supplies: sterile wound swab, sterile normal saline, sterile irrigation kit with 30-60 mL syringe, and sterile 2" x 2" gauze.
2. Perform safety steps:
    - Perform hand hygiene.
    - Check the room for transmission-based precautions.
    - Introduce yourself, your role, the purpose of your visit, and an estimate of the time it will take.
    - Confirm patient ID using two patient identifiers (e.g., name and date of birth).
    - Explain the process to the patient and ask if they have any questions.
    - Be organized and systematic.
    - Use appropriate listening and questioning skills.
    - Listen and attend to patient cues.
    - Ensure the patient's privacy and dignity.
    - Assess ABCs.
3. Prepare the environment, position the patient, adjust the height of the bed, and turn on the lights. Ensure proper body mechanics for yourself and create a comfortable position for the patient. Ensuring proper lighting allows for good visibility to assess the wound. Premedicate if indicated and ensure patient's comfort prior to and during the procedure.
4. Place a clean, dry barrier on the bedside table or create a sterile field per agency policy. Pour sterile saline into the irrigation tray.
5. Perform hand hygiene and apply nonsterile gloves.
6. Remove the dressing and expose the patient's wound. Dispose of the soiled dressing according to agency policy.
7. Remove gloves and perform hand hygiene.

---

1 Wound specimen collection. (2020). Lippincott procedures. http://procedures.lww.com

My Notes

8. Put on a new pair of nonsterile or sterile gloves, depending on the patient's condition and the type, location, and depth of the wound.

9. Irrigate the wound with sterile normal saline solution to remove surface debris or exudate and to prevent specimen contamination. Alternatively, cleanse the wound with a commercial wound irrigation device.

10. Wipe the surface of the wound with a sterile gauze pad moistened with normal saline solution to remove surface contaminants.

11. Gently blot excess normal saline solution from the wound bed with a dry sterile gauze pad.

12. Remove gloves and perform hand hygiene.

13. Put on new nonsterile gloves.

14. Open the swab specimen collection and transport system. Prepare the contents as needed following the manufacturer's instructions.

15. Use the culture swab(s) to collect the specimen according to agency policy.

    - Note that some agencies use swab collection and transport systems that contain specific swabs designed for anaerobic and aerobic specimen collection.

16. If the wound bed appears dry, moisten the swab with normal saline solution.

17. Identify a 1-cm^2 area of viable wound tissue at or near the center of the wound.

    - Note: The culture must be obtained from the cleanest tissue possible and not from pus, slough, eschar, or necrotic tissue.

18. Rotate the tip of the swab over the identified 1-cm^2 area of the wound for 5 seconds, applying sufficient pressure to express fluid from the wound.

19 Remove the swab from the wound.

20. Immediately insert the swab into the appropriate transport system following the manufacturer's instructions for use. Use caution to avoid contaminating the swab when placing it into the transport system:

    - Clinical alert: Note that the culture must come from the cleanest tissue possible and not from pus, slough, eschar, or necrotic material. Never collect exudate from the skin.

21. Remove gloves and perform hand hygiene.

22. Put on a new pair of nonsterile or sterile gloves depending on the patient's condition and the type, location, and depth of the wound.

23. Apply a new sterile dressing to the patient's wound using a sterile, no-touch technique.

24. Assist the patient to a comfortable position, ask if they have any questions, and thank them for their time.

25. Label the specimen in the presence of the patient (such as name, date, time, location of the wound, and site and source of the specimen) to prevent mislabeling:

My Notes

- Note the patient's recent or current antibiotic therapy on the laboratory request form because it might affect test results. If possible, obtain a culture specimen before starting antimicrobial therapy.

26. Ensure safety measures when leaving the room:
    - CALL LIGHT: Within reach
    - BED: Low and locked (in lowest position and brakes on)
    - SIDE RAILS: Secured
    - TABLE: Within reach
    - ROOM: Risk-free for falls (scan room and clear any obstacles)
27. Immediately send the specimen to the laboratory in a laboratory biohazard transport bag with a completed laboratory request form.
28. Document the procedure and related assessments in the patient's chart. Report any concerns according to agency policy.

20.10 CHECKLIST FOR INTERMITTENT SUTURE REMOVAL

My Notes

Sutures are tiny threads, wire, or other material used to sew body tissue and skin together. They may be placed deep in the tissue and/or superficially to close a wound. The most commonly seen suture is the intermittent suture.

Sutures may be absorbent (dissolvable) or nonabsorbent (must be removed). Nonabsorbent sutures are usually removed within 7 to 14 days. Suture removal is determined by how well the wound has healed and the extent of the surgery. See Figure 20.32[1] for an example of suture removal. Sutures must be left in place long enough to establish wound closure with enough strength to support internal tissues and organs. If sutures are removed too early in the wound healing process, dehiscence can occur. The wound line must be observed for separations during the process of suture removal and the procedure stopped if there are any concerns.

The health care provider must assess the wound to determine whether or not to remove the sutures and provide an order for the removal of sutures. Alternate sutures (every second suture) may be removed first, and then the remaining sutures removed after adequate approximation of the skin tissue is determined. If the wound is well-healed, all the sutures may be removed at the same time, but if there are concerns about approximation, the removal of the remaining sutures may be delayed for several days to avoid dehiscence. Steri-Strips may be applied prior to suture removal to lessen the chance of wound dehiscence. See Figure 20.33.[2]

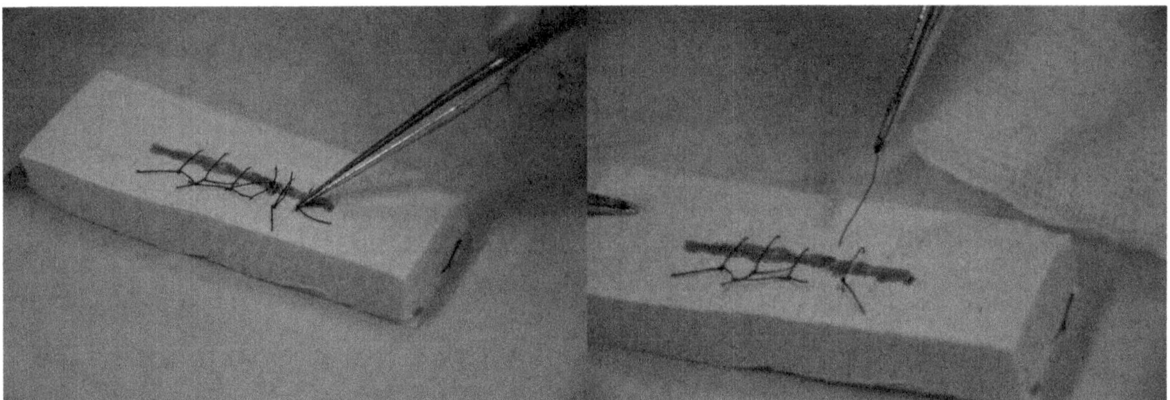

Figure 20.32 Suture Removal from a Simulated Wound

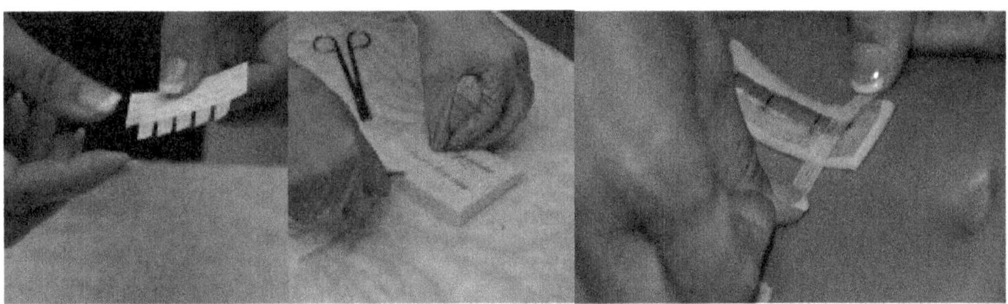

Figure 20.33 Applying Steri-Strips to a Simulated Wound

---

1 "DSC_0262.jpg" and "DSC_0263.jpg" by British Columbia Institute of Technology are licensed under CC BY 4.0. Access for free at https://opentextbc.ca/clinicalskills/chapter/4-3-suture-care-and-removal/

2 "DSC_1658.jpg" and "DSC_09811.jpg" by British Columbia Institute of Technology are licensed under CC BY 4.0. Access for free at https://opentextbc.ca/clinicalskills/chapter/4-3-suture-care-and-removal/

My Notes

Checklist for Intermittent Suture Removal

Use the checklist below to review the steps for completion of "Intermittent Suture Removal."

Steps

Disclaimer: Always review and follow agency policy regarding this specific skill.

1. Gather supplies: sterile suture scissors, sterile dressing tray (to clean incision site prior to suture removal), nonsterile gloves, normal saline, Steri-Strips, and sterile outer dressing.
2. Perform safety steps:
    - Perform hand hygiene.
    - Check the room for transmission-based precautions.
    - Introduce yourself, your role, the purpose of your visit, and an estimate of the time it will take.
    - Confirm patient ID using two patient identifiers (e.g., name and date of birth).
    - Explain the process to the patient and ask if they have any questions.
    - Be organized and systematic.
    - Use appropriate listening and questioning skills.
    - Listen and attend to patient cues.
    - Ensure the patient's privacy and dignity.
    - Assess ABCs.
3. Confirm provider order and explain procedure to patient. Inform the patient that the procedure is not painful but they may feel some pulling of the skin during suture removal.
4. Prepare the environment, position the patient, adjust the height of the bed, and turn on the lights. Ensuring proper lighting allows for good visibility to assess the wound. Ensure proper body mechanics for yourself and create a comfortable position for the patient.
5. Perform hand hygiene and put on nonsterile gloves.
6. Place a clean, dry barrier on the bedside table. Add necessary supplies.
7. Remove dressing and inspect the wound. Visually assess the wound for uniform closure of the wound edges, absence of drainage, redness, and swelling. After assessing the wound, decide if the wound is sufficiently healed to have the sutures removed. If there are concerns, discuss the order with the appropriate health care provider.
8. Remove gloves and perform hand hygiene.
9. Put on a new pair of nonsterile or sterile gloves, depending on the patient's condition and the type, location, and depth of the wound.
10. Irrigate the wound with sterile normal saline solution to remove surface debris or exudate and to help prevent specimen contamination. Alternatively, commercial wound cleanser may be used. This step reduces risk of

infection from microorganisms on the wound site or surrounding skin. Cleaning also loosens and removes any dried blood or crusted exudate from the sutures and wound bed.

11. To remove intermittent sutures, hold the scissors in your dominant hand and the forceps in your nondominant hand for dexterity with suture removal.
12. Place a sterile 2" x 2" gauze close to the incision site to collect the removed suture pieces.
13. Grasp the knot of the suture with the forceps and gently pull up the knot while slipping the tip of the scissors under the suture near the skin. Examine the knot.
14. Cut under the knot as close as possible to the skin at the distal end of the knot:
    - Never snip both ends of the knot as there will be no way to remove the suture from below the surface.
    - Do not pull the contaminated suture (suture on top of the skin) through tissue.
15. Grasp the knotted end of the suture with forceps, and in one continuous action pull the suture out of the tissue and place it on the sterile 2" x 2" gauze.
16. Remove every second suture until the end of the incision line. Assess wound healing after removal of each suture to determine if each remaining suture will be removed. If the wound edges are open, stop removing sutures, apply Steri-Strips (using tension to pull wound edges together), and notify the appropriate health care provider. Remove remaining sutures on the incision line if indicated.
17. Using the principles of no-touch technique, cut and place Steri-Strips along the incision line:
    - Cut Steri-Strips so that they extend 1.5 to 2 inches on each side of the incision.
18. Remove gloves and perform hand hygiene.
19. Assist the patient to a comfortable position, ask if they have any questions, and thank them for their time. Return the patient's bed to the lowest position to help prevent falls and maintain patient safety.
20. Ensure safety measures when leaving the room:
    - CALL LIGHT: Within reach
    - BED: Low and locked (in lowest position and brakes on)
    - SIDE RAILS: Secured
    - TABLE: Within reach
    - ROOM: Risk-free for falls (scan room and clear any obstacles)
21. Document the procedure and related assessment findings of the incision. Report any concerns according to agency policy.

My Notes

20.11 CHECKLIST FOR STAPLE REMOVAL

Staples are made of stainless steel wire and provide strength for wound closure. Staples are strong, quick to insert, and simple to remove, but may cause more scarring than sutures.

Removal of staples is similar to the removal of sutures, but requires a sterile staple extractor instead of forceps and suture scissors. Typically every second staple is initially removed, and then the remaining staples are removed at a later time. In general, staples are removed within 7 to 14 days. See Figure 20.34[1] for an example of staple removal.

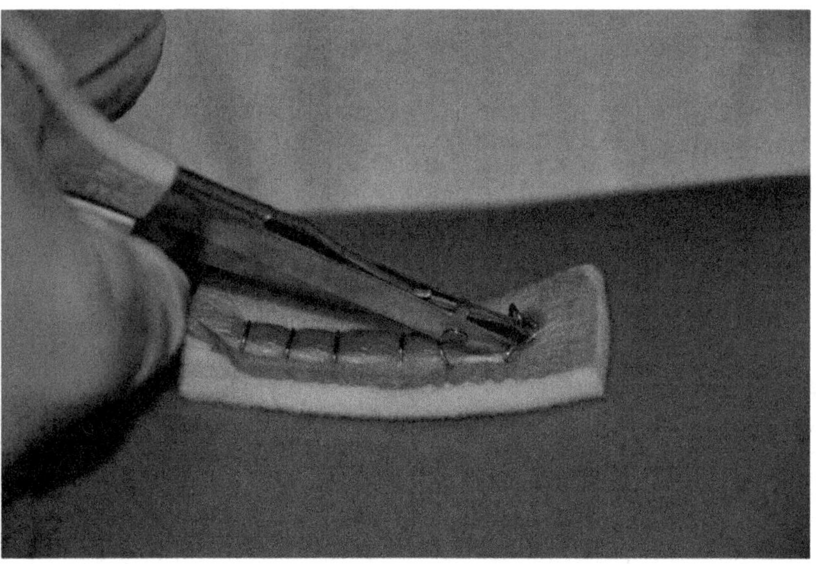

Figure 20.34 Staple Removal from a Simulated Surgical Wound

Checklist for Staple Removal

Please follow the checklist below to review the steps for completion of "Staple Removal."

Steps

Disclaimer: Always review and follow agency policy regarding this specific skill.

1. Gather supplies: sterile staple extractors, sterile dressing tray, nonsterile gloves, normal saline, Steri-Strips, and sterile outer dressing.
2. Perform safety steps:
    - Perform hand hygiene.
    - Check room for transmission-based precautions.
    - Introduce yourself, your role, the purpose of your visit, and an estimate of the time it will take.

1 "DSC_02191.jpg" by British Columbia Institute of Technology is licensed under CC BY 4.0. Access for free at https://opentextbc.ca/clinicalskills/chapter/4-4-suture-care-and-removal/

My Notes

- Confirm patient ID using two patient identifiers (e.g., name and date of birth).
- Be organized and systematic.
- Use appropriate listening and questioning skills.
- Listen and attend to patient cues.
- Ensure the patient's privacy and dignity.
- Assess ABCs.

3. Confirm the provider order and explain the procedure to patient. Explanation helps prevent anxiety and increases compliance with the procedure. Inform the patient the procedure is not painful but they may feel some pulling or pinching of the skin during staple removal.

4. Prepare the environment, position the patient, adjust the height of the bed, and turn on the lights. Ensuring proper lighting allows for good visibility to assess the wound. Ensure proper body mechanics for yourself and create a comfortable position for the patient.

5. Place a clean, dry barrier on the bedside tables and add necessary supplies.

6. Perform hand hygiene and apply nonsterile gloves.

7. Remove the dressing and inspect the wound. Visually assess the wound for uniform closure of the wound edges, absence of drainage, redness, and swelling. After assessing the wound, decide if the wound is sufficiently healed to have the staples removed. If there are concerns, discuss the status of the wound before proceeding with the health care provider. For safety purposes, count the number of staples before beginning the procedure.

8. Irrigate the wound with sterile normal saline solution to remove surface debris or exudate to reduce risk of infection from microorganisms on the wound site or surrounding skin and to help loosen and remove any dried blood or crusted exudate from the sutures and wound bed.

9. Remove gloves, perform hand hygiene, and apply nonsterile gloves.

10. Place a sterile 2" x 2" next to the wound to collect the staples.

11. Remove the staples (start with every second staple).

12. Place the lower tip of the staple extractor beneath the staple. Do not pull up while depressing the handle on the staple remover or change the angle of your wrist or hand. Close the handle, and then gently move the staple side to side to remove. The closed handle depresses the middle of the staple causing the two ends to bend outward and out of the top layer of skin.

13. When both ends of the staple are visible, move the staple extractor away from the skin and place the staple on a sterile piece of gauze by releasing the handles on the staple extractor. This avoids pulling the staple out prematurely and avoids putting pressure on the wound. It also prevents scratching the skin with the sharp staple.

14. Using the principles of no-touch technique, place Steri-Strips on the location of every removed staple along the incision line. Steri-Strips are supplied in pre-cut lengths. Cut the Steri-Strips to allow them to extend 1.5 to 2 cm on each side of the incision. Steri-Strips support wound tension across wounds and eliminate scarring. This allows wounds to heal by primary intention.

My Notes

15. Remove the remaining staples as indicated, followed by applying Steri-Strips along the incision line. Count the number of removed staples and compare to the pre-count to ensure safety.
16. Apply a dry, sterile dressing on the incision site or leave it exposed to the air according to provider orders.
17. Discard the supplies according to agency policies for sharps disposal and biohazard waste:
    - The staple extractor may be disposed of or sent for sterilization according to agency policy.
18. Perform hand hygiene.
19. Complete patient teaching regarding Steri-Strips, bathing, and inspecting wound for separation. Instruct the patient to:
    - Take showers rather than bathe in a tub.
    - Avoid pulling off Steri-Strips but allow them to fall off naturally and gradually (usually takes one to three weeks).
    - Receive adequate rest, fluids, nutrition, and ambulation for optional wound healing
20. Assist the patient to a comfortable position, ask if they have any questions, and thank them for their time.
21. Ensure safety measures when leaving the room:
    - CALL LIGHT: Within reach
    - BED: Low and locked (in lowest position and brakes on)
    - SIDE RAILS: Secured
    - TABLE: Within reach
    - ROOM: Risk-free for falls (scan room and clear any obstacles)
22. Document the procedure and assessment findings regarding the appearance of the incision. Report any concerns according to agency policy.

My Notes

20.12 CHECKLIST FOR WOUND CLEANSING, IRRIGATION, AND PACKING

Cleansing is an important step when changing dressings in wounds healing by secondary intention to remove surface debris and to provide optimal visualization for the wound assessment. See Figure 20.35[1] for removal of dressing and wound assessment.

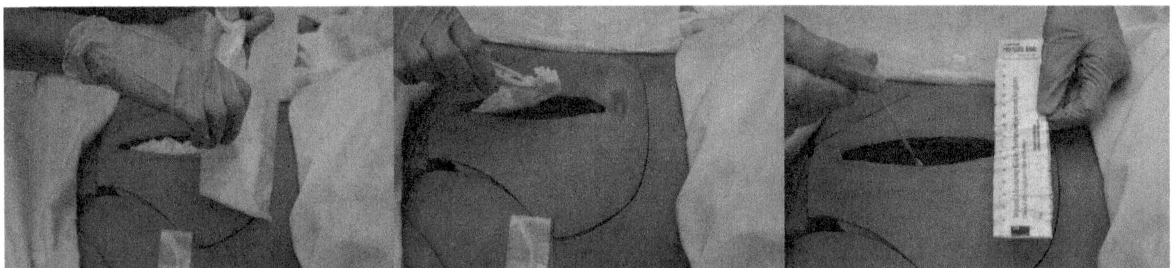

Figure 20.35 Removal of Dressings and Wound Assessment

Follow agency policy and provider orders regarding cleansing solution and method. Many wounds can be cleansed with normal saline. See Figure 20.36[2] for an example of wound irrigation.

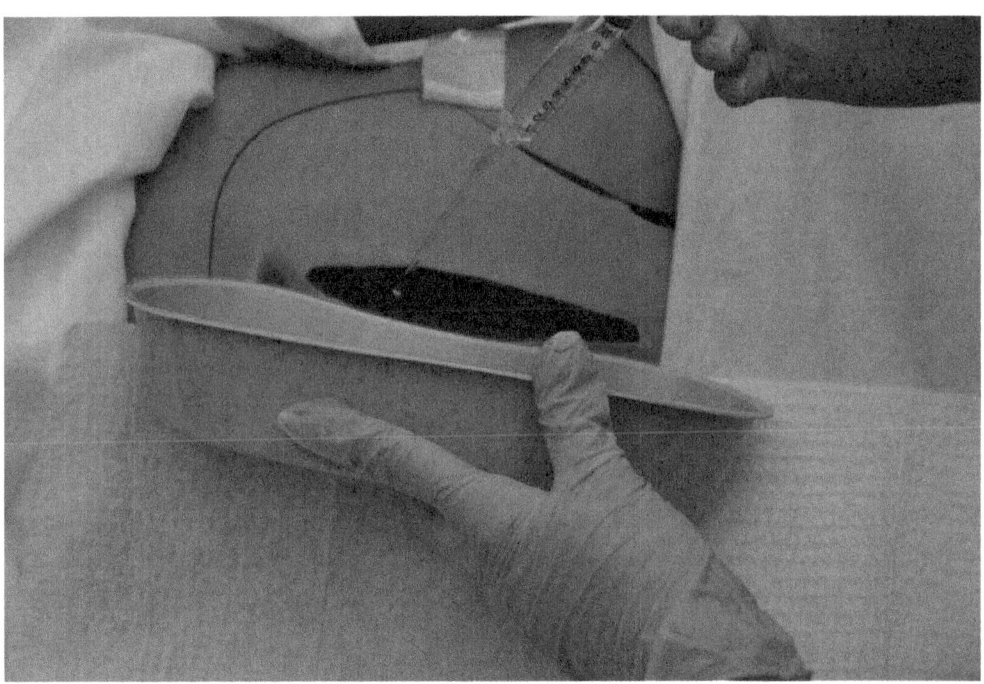

Figure 20.36 Irrigating the Wound

---

1 "DSC_1724.jpg," "SC_1727.jpg," and "DSC_1730.jpg" by British Columbia Institute of Technology are licensed under CC BY 4.0. Access for free at https://ecampusontario.pressbooks.pub/clinicalskills/chapter/4-5-complex-dressing-change/

2 "DSC_1732.jpg" by British Columbia Institute of Technology is licensed under CC BY 4.0. Access for free at https://ecampusontario.pressbooks.pub/clinicalskills/chapter/4-5-complex-dressing-change/

My Notes

Cleansing solution should be applied with sufficient pressure to cleanse the wound without damaging tissue or driving bacteria into the wound.[3] Following cleansing, the wound may be packed to allow for granulation of new tissue. See Figure 20.37[4] for an example of wound packing.

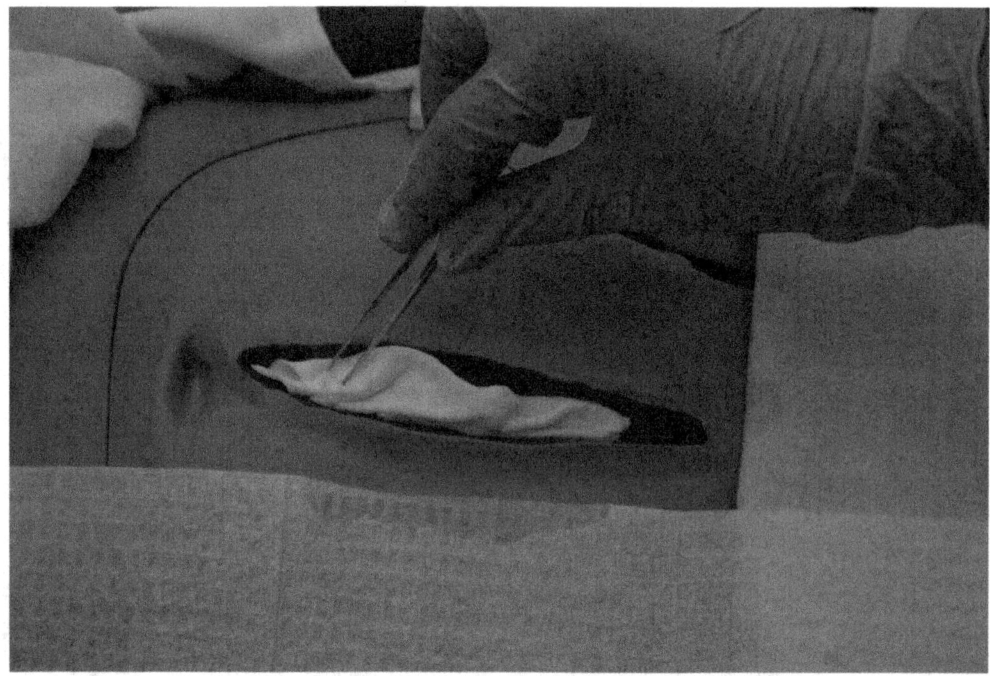

Figure 20.37 Packing the Wound

Checklist for Wound Cleansing, Irrigation, and Packing

Use the checklist below to review the steps for completion of "Wound Cleansing, Irrigation, and Packing."

Steps

Disclaimer: Always review and follow agency policy regarding this specific skill.

1. Gather supplies: syringe, cannula with needleless adaptor, irrigation fluid, basin, waterproof pad, dressing tray with sterile forceps, scissors, skin barrier/protectant, cotton tip applicators, measuring guide, outer sterile dressing, and packing gauze or packing as per physician's orders.
2. Perform safety steps:
    - Perform hand hygiene.
    - Check the room for transmission-based precautions.

---

3 National Pressure Ulcer Advisory Panel, European Pressure Ulcer Advisory Panel and Pan Pacific Pressure Injury Alliance. (2014). *Prevention and treatment of pressure ulcers: Quick reference guide.* Emily Haesler (Ed.). https://www.epuap.org/wp-content/uploads/2010/10/Quick-Reference-Guide-DIGITAL-NPUAP-EPUAP-PPPIA-16Oct2014.pdf

4 "DSC_1742.jpg" by British Columbia Institute of Technology is licensed under CC BY 4.0. Access for free at https://ecampusontario.pressbooks.pub/clinicalskills/chapter/4-5-complex-dressing-change/

My Notes

- Introduce yourself, your role, the purpose of your visit, and an estimate of the time it will take.
- Confirm patient ID using two patient identifiers (e.g., name and date of birth).
- Explain the process to the patient and ask if they have any questions.
- Be organized and systematic.
- Use appropriate listening and questioning skills.
- Listen and attend to patient cues.
- Ensure the patient's privacy and dignity.
- Assess ABCs.

3. Confirm the provider order and verify appropriateness of order according to wound assessment.
4. Prepare the environment, position the patient, adjust the height of the bed, and turn on the lights. Ensure proper lighting to allow for good visibility to assess the wound. Ensure proper body mechanics for yourself and create a comfortable position for the patient. Position the patient so the wound is vertical to the collection basin, if possible, to allow the solution to flow off the patient.
5. Place a waterproof pad under the patient to protect the patient's clothing and bedding from irrigation fluid.
6. Perform hand hygiene and apply clean gloves.
7. Remove outer dressing:
    - Using sterile forceps, remove the inner dressing (packing) from the wound.
    - If the packing sticks, gently soak the packing with normal saline or sterile water and gently lift off the packing. Removing packing that adheres to the wound bed without soaking can cause trauma to the wound bed tissue. If packing material cannot be removed, contact the provider. If packing adheres to the wound, reassess the amount of wound exudate and consider a different packing material. All packing must be removed with each dressing change.
    - Confirm the quantity and type of packing are the same as recorded on previous dressing change.
8. Assess the wound:
    - Note the location and type of wound.
    - Measure the wound's length, width, and depth.
    - If undermining or tunneling are present, note the location and measure the depth.
    - Determine if the level of tissue damage indicates wound healing or worsening.
    - Assess appearance of wound bed, noting color.
    - Note presence of odor after cleansing.
    - Assess appearance of periwound skin.
    - Wound assessment helps identify if the wound care is effective. Always compare the current wound assessment with the previous assessment to determine if the wound is healing, delayed, worsening, or showing signs of infection.
9. Apply nonsterile gloves, gown, and goggles or face shield according to agency policy.

My Notes

10. If irrigation is indicated, fill a 35-mL syringe with sterile saline and attach a needleless cannula to the end of the syringe.
11. Hold the syringe about 1 inch above the wound and flush gently with continuous pressure until returned fluid is clear:
    - Irrigation should be drained into the basin because it is a medium for bacterial growth and subsequent infection.
    - Irrigation should not increase patient discomfort.
12. Dry wound edges with sterile gauze using sterile forceps to prevent maceration of surrounding tissue from excess moisture.
13. Remove goggles or face shield and gloves.
14. Perform hand hygiene and apply sterile gloves (if not using sterile forceps) or nonsterile gloves if using sterile forceps.
15. Apply a skin barrier/protectant on the periwound skin as needed to prevent saturated packing materials and/or wound exudate from macerating or irritating the periwound skin.
16. While maintaining sterility, moisten the gauze with sterile normal saline and wring it out so it is damp but not wet:
    - The wound must be moist, not wet, for optimal healing. Gauze packing that is too wet can cause tissue maceration and reduces the absorbency of the gauze.
    - Normal saline gauze packing needs to be changed at least once daily.
    - Ensure the wound is not overpacked or underpacked as either may diminish the healing process.
17. Open the gauze and gently pack it into the wound using sterile forceps or the tip of a sterile, cotton-tipped swab:
    - Continue until all wound surfaces are in contact with gauze.
    - Do not pack too tightly.
    - Do not overlap wound edges with wet packing.
18. Apply an appropriate outer dry dressing, depending on the frequency of the dressing changes and the amount of exudate from the wound:
    - The dressing on the wound must remain dry on the outside to avoid cross-contamination of the wound. If it becomes saturated before the next dressing change, it must be replaced.
19. Discard the supplies.
20. Remove gloves and perform hand hygiene.
21. Assist the patient to a comfortable position, ask if they have any questions, and thank them for their time.
22. Ensure safety measures when leaving the room:
    - CALL LIGHT: Within reach
    - BED: Low and locked (in lowest position and brakes on)

- SIDE RAILS: Secured
- TABLE: Within reach
- ROOM: Risk-free for falls (scan room and clear any obstacles)

23. Document procedure, wound assessment, irrigation solution, and patient response to the irrigation and dressing change. Report any concerns according to agency policy.

My Notes

20.13 CHECKLIST FOR DRAIN MANAGEMENT

Drain management systems are commonly used during post-operative surgical management to remove drainage, prevent infection, and enhance wound healing. A drain may be superficial in the skin or deep in an organ, duct, or cavity, such as a hematoma. A patient may have several drains depending on the extent and type of surgery. A closed system uses a vacuum system to withdraw fluids and collect them in a reservoir. Closed systems must be emptied and drainage measured routinely according to agency policy.

Drainage tubes contain perforations to allow fluid to drain from the surgical wound site. The drainage is collected in a closed sterile collection system/reservoir, such as a Hemovac or Jackson-Pratt. The amount of drainage varies depending on location and type of surgery. A Hemovac drain (see Figure 20.38[1]) can hold up to 500 mL of drainage. A Jackson- Pratt (JP) drain (see Figure 20.39[2]) is used for smaller amounts of drainage, usually ranging from 25 to 50 mL. Drains are usually sutured to the skin to prevent accidental removal, and the drainage site is covered with a sterile dressing. The site and drain should be checked periodically throughout the shift to ensure the drain is functioning effectively and that no leaking is occurring.

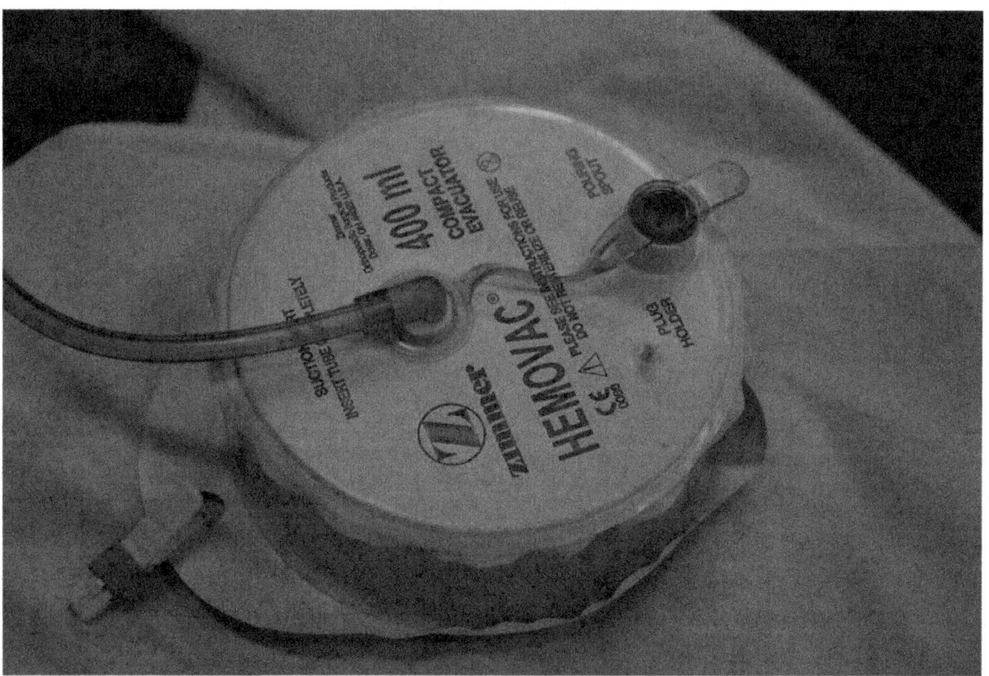

Figure 20.38 Hemovac Drain

1 "DSC_0272-1024x678.jpg" by British Columbia Institute of Technology is licensed under CC BY 4.0. Access for free at https://opentextbc.ca/clinicalskills/chapter/4-8-drain-management-and-removal/

2 "DSC_0285-1024x678.jpg" by British Columbia Institute of Technology is licensed under CC BY 4.0. Access for free at https://opentextbc.ca/clinicalskills/chapter/4-8-drain-management-and-removal/

My Notes

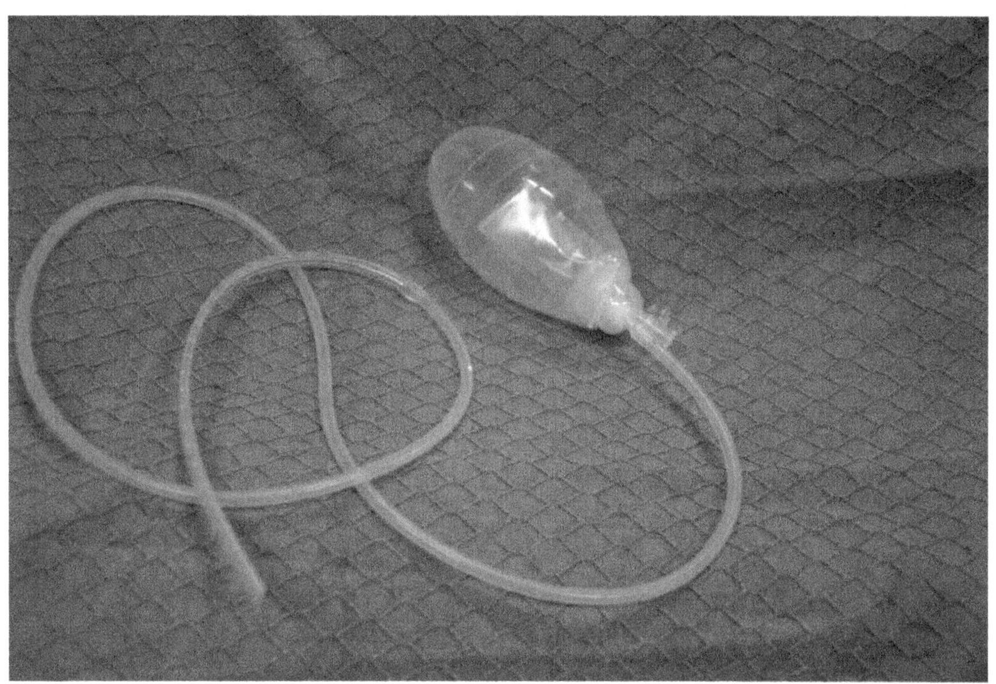

Figure 20.39 Jackson-Pratt Drain

Checklist for Drain Management

Use the checklist below to review the steps for completion of "Drain Management."

Steps

Disclaimer: Always review and follow agency policy regarding this specific skill.

1 Gather supplies: drainage measurement container, nonsterile gloves, waterproof pad, and alcohol swab.

2. Perform safety steps:

- Perform hand hygiene.
- Check the room for transmission-based precautions.
- Introduce yourself, your role, the purpose of your visit, and an estimate of the time it will take.
- Confirm patient ID using two patient identifiers (e.g., name and date of birth).
- Explain the process to the patient and ask if they have any questions.
- Be organized and systematic.
- Use appropriate listening and questioning skills.
- Listen and attend to patient cues.
- Ensure the patient's privacy and dignity.
- Assess ABCs.

My Notes

3. Apply nonsterile gloves and goggles or face shield according to agency policy to reduce the transmission of microorganisms and protect against an accidental body fluid exposure.

4 Maintaining a sterile technique, remove the plug from the pouring spout as indicated on the drain:

    - Open the plug pointing away from your face to avoid an accidental splash of contaminated fluid.
    - Maintain the plug's sterility.
    - Notice that the vacuum will be broken and the reservoir (drainage collection system) will expand.

5. Gently tilt the opening of the reservoir toward the measuring container and pour out the drainage away from you to prevent exposure to body fluids. Do not touch the measuring container with the reservoir opening.

6. Place the drainage container on the bed or hard surface, tilt it away from your face, and compress the drain to flatten it with one hand to remove all the air before closing the spout to establish the vacuum system.

7. Cleanse the plug with the alcohol swab per agency policy. Maintaining sterility, place the plug back into the pour spout of the drainage system to establish the vacuum system of the drainage system.

8. Secure the device onto the patient's gown using a safety pin; check patency and placement of tube. Ensure that enough slack is present in tubing and that the reservoir hangs lower than the wound. Proper placement of the reservoir allows gravity to facilitate wound drainage. Providing enough slack to accommodate patient movement prevents tension of the drainage system and pulling on the tubing and insertion site.

9. Note the characteristics of the drainage: color, consistency, odor, and amount. Drainage counts as patient fluid output and must be documented on the patient chart per agency policy.

    - Monitor and empty drains frequently in the post-operative period to reduce the weight of the reservoir and to assess drainage.

10. Remove gloves and perform hand hygiene.

11. Assist the patient to a comfortable position, ask if they have any questions, and thank them for their time.

12. Ensure safety measures when leaving the room:

    - CALL LIGHT: Within reach
    - BED: Low and locked (in lowest position and brakes on)
    - SIDE RAILS: Secured
    - TABLE: Within reach
    - ROOM: Risk-free for falls (scan room and clear any obstacles)

13. Document the procedure and assessment findings according to agency policy. Report any unusual findings or concerns to the health care provider. If the amount of drainage increases or changes, notify the appropriate health care provider according to agency policy.

    - If the amount of drainage significantly decreases, the drain may be ready to be assessed and removed.

- Notify required health care provider if the wound appears infected.
- Record the number of drains if there is more than one, and record each one separately.

My Notes

My Notes

20.14 LEARNING ACTIVITIES

Learning Activities

(Answers to "Learning Activities" can be found in the "Answer Key" at the end of the book. Answers to interactive activity elements will be provided within the element as immediate feedback.)

Mr. Jones is a 76-year-old patient admitted to the medical surgical floor with complications of a nonhealing foot ulcer. Mr. Jones has a history of diabetes, hypertension, and COPD. He has a BMI of 29. His daily medications include metformin, Lisinopril, and prednisone. His wife has recently passed away and he lives alone.

a. Based upon what is known about Mr. Jones, what factors might be contributing to his nonhealing wound?
b. What other factors that influence wound healing might be important to assess with Mr. Jones?

Interactive Activity

An interactive or media element has been excluded from this version of the text. You can view it online here: https://wtcs.pressbooks.pub/nursingskills/?p=2935

Interactive Activity

An interactive or media element has been excluded from this version of the text. You can view it online here: https://wtcs.pressbooks.pub/nursingskills/?p=2935

Interactive Activity

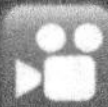

An interactive or media element has been excluded from this version of the text. You can view it online here: https://wtcs.pressbooks.pub/nursingskills/?p=2935

Interactive Activity

An interactive or media element has been excluded from this version of the text. You can view it online here: https://wtcs.pressbooks.pub/nursingskills/?p=2935

XX GLOSSARY

My Notes

Angiogenesis: The development of new capillaries in a wound base.

Arterial ulcers: Ulcers caused by lack of blood flow and oxygenation to tissues and typically occur in the distal areas of the body such as the feet, heels, and toes.

Debridement: The removal of nonviable tissue in a wound.

Dehiscence: The separation of the edges of a surgical wound.

Diabetic ulcers: Ulcers that typically develop on the plantar aspect of the feet and toes of patients with diabetes due to lack of sensation of pressure or injury.

Ecchymosis: Bruising that occurs when small veins and capillaries under the skin break.

Edema: Swelling.

Epithelialization: The development of new epidermis and granulation tissue.

Erythema: Redness.

Eschar: Dark brown/black, dry, thick, and leathery dead tissue in a wound base that must be removed for healing to occur.

Exudate: Fluid that oozes out of a wound; also commonly called pus.

Granulation tissue: New connective tissue in a wound base with fragile, thin-walled capillaries that must be protected.

Hematoma: An area of blood that collects outside of larger blood vessels.

Hemosiderin staining: Dark-colored discoloration of the lower legs due to blood pooling.

Hemostasis phase: The first phase of wound healing that occurs immediately after skin injury. Blood vessels constrict and clotting factors are activated.

Induration: Area of hardened tissue.

Inflammatory phase: The second phase of wound healing when vasodilation occurs so that white blood cells in the bloodstream can move into the wound to start cleaning the wound bed.

Maceration: The softening and wasting away of skin due to excess fluid.

Maturation phase: The final phase of wound healing as collagen continues to be created to strengthen the wound, causing scar tissue.

Necrotic: Black tissue color due to tissue death from lack of oxygenation to the area.

Nonblanchable erythema: Skin redness that does not turn white when pressure is applied.

Osteomyelitis: Bone infection.

Peripheral neuropathy: A condition that causes decreased sensation of pain and pressure, typically in the lower extremities.

Periwound: The skin around the outer edges of a wound.

Pressure injuries: Localized damage to the skin or underlying soft tissue, usually over a bony prominence, as a result of intense and prolonged pressure in combination with shear.[1]

Primary intention: Wound healing that occurs with surgical incisions or clean-edged lacerations that are closed with sutures, staples, or surgical glue.

---

1 Edsberg, L. E., Black, J. M., Goldberg, M., McNichol, L., Moore, L., & Sieggreen, M. (2016). Revised national pressure ulcer advisory panel pressure injury staging system: Revised pressure injury staging system. *Journal of Wound, Ostomy, and Continence Nursing: Official Publication of The Wound, Ostomy and Continence Nurses Society, 43*(6), 585–597. https://doi.org/10.1097/WON.0000000000000281

My Notes

Proliferative phase: The third phase of wound healing that includes epithelialization, angiogenesis, collagen formation, and contraction.

Purulent drainage: Wound exudate that is thick and opaque and can be tan, yellow, green, or brown in color. It is never considered normal in a wound, and new purulent drainage should always be reported to the health care provider.

Sanguineous drainage: Wound drainage that is fresh bleeding.

Secondary intention: Wound healing that occurs when the edges of a wound cannot be approximated (brought together), so the wound fills in from the bottom up by the production of granulation tissue. Examples of wounds that heal by secondary intention are pressure injuries and chainsaw injuries.

Serosanguinous drainage: Wound exudate contains serous drainage with small amounts of blood present.

Serous drainage: Wound drainage that is clear, thin, watery plasma. It is considered normal in minimal amounts during the inflammatory stage of wound healing.

Shear: A mechanical force that occurs when tissue layers move over the top of each other, causing blood vessels to stretch and break as they pass through the subcutaneous tissue.

Skin tears: Wounds caused by mechanical forces, typically in the nonelastic skin of older adults.

Slough: Inflammatory exudate that is light yellow, soft, and moist and must be removed for wound healing to occur.

Tertiary intention: Wound healing that occurs when a wound must remain open or has been reopened, often due to severe infection.

Tunneling: Passageways underneath the surface of the skin that extend from a wound and can take twists and turns.

Undermining: A condition that occurs in wounds when the tissue under the wound edges becomes eroded, resulting in a pocket beneath the skin at the wound's edge.

Unstageable: Occurs when slough or eschar obscures the wound so that tissue loss cannot be assessed.

Venous insufficiency: A medical condition where the veins in the legs do not adequately send blood back to the heart, resulting in a pooling of fluids in the legs that can cause venous ulcers.

Venous ulcers: Ulcers caused by the pooling of fluid in the veins of the lower legs when the valves are not working properly, causing fluid to seep out, macerate the skin, and cause an ulcer.

Wound vac: A device used with special foam dressings and suctioning to remove fluid and decrease air pressure around a wound to assist in healing.

Chapter 21

Facilitation of Elimination

21.1 FACILITATION OF ELIMINATION INTRODUCTION

My Notes

Learning Objectives

- Perform urinary catheterization, ostomy care, and urine specimen collection
- Manage urinary catheters to prevent complications
- Maintain aseptic or sterile technique
- Explain procedure to patient
- Modify assessment techniques to reflect variations across the life span
- Document actions and observations
- Recognize and report significant deviations from norms

Elimination is a basic human function of excreting waste through the bowel and urinary system. The process of elimination depends on many variables and intricate processes that occur within the body. Many medical conditions and surgeries can adversely affect the processes of elimination, so nurses must facilitate their patients' bowel and urinary elimination as needed. Common nursing interventions related to facilitating elimination include inserting and managing urinary catheters, obtaining urine specimens, caring for ostomies, providing patient education to promote healthy elimination, and preventing complications. In this chapter, we will discuss the technical skills used to support bowel and bladder function, as well as the application of the nursing process while doing so.

My Notes

21.2 BASIC CONCEPTS

Before discussing specific procedures related to facilitating bowel and bladder function, let's review basic concepts related to urinary and bowel elimination. When facilitating alternative methods of elimination, it is important to understand the anatomy and physiology of the gastrointestinal and urinary systems, as well as the adverse effects of various conditions and medications on elimination.

For more information about the anatomy and physiology of the gastrointestinal system and medications used to treat diarrhea and constipation, visit the "Gastrointestinal" chapter of the Open RN *Nursing Pharmacology* textbook.

For more information about the anatomy and physiology of the kidneys and diuretic medications used to treat fluid overload, visit the "Cardiovascular and Renal System" chapter in Open RN *Nursing Pharmacology textbook.*

For more information about applying the nursing process to facilitate elimination, visit the "Elimination" chapter in Open RN *Nursing Fundamentals.*

Urinary Elimination Devices

This section will focus on the devices used to facilitate urinary elimination. **Urinary catheterization** is the insertion of a catheter tube into the urethral opening and placing it in the neck of the urinary bladder to drain urine.

There are several types of urinary elimination devices, such as indwelling catheters, intermittent catheters, suprapubic catheters, and external devices. Each of these types of devices is described in the following subsections.

Indwelling Catheter

An **indwelling catheter**, often referred to as a "Foley catheter," refers to a urinary catheter that remains in place after insertion into the bladder for the continual collection of urine. It has a balloon on the insertion tip to maintain placement in the neck of the bladder. The other end of the catheter is attached to a drainage bag for the collection of urine. See Figure 21.1[1] for an illustration of the anatomical placement of an indwelling catheter in the bladder neck.

1 "Foley Catheter.png" by BruceBlaus is licensed under CC BY-SA 4.0. Access for free at https://commons.wikimedia.org/wiki/File:Foley_Catheter.png

My Notes

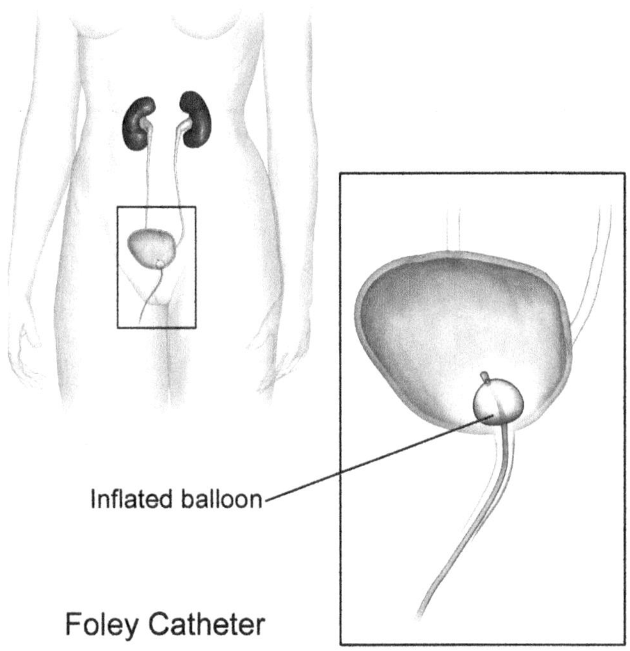

Figure 21.1 Anatomical Placement of an Indwelling Catheter

The distal end of an indwelling catheter has a urine drainage port that is connected to a drainage bag. The size of the catheter is marked at this end using the French catheter scale. A balloon port is also located at this end, where a syringe is inserted to inflate the balloon after it is inserted into the bladder. The balloon port is marked with the amount of fluid required to fill the balloon. See Figure 21.2[2] for an image of the parts of an indwelling catheter.

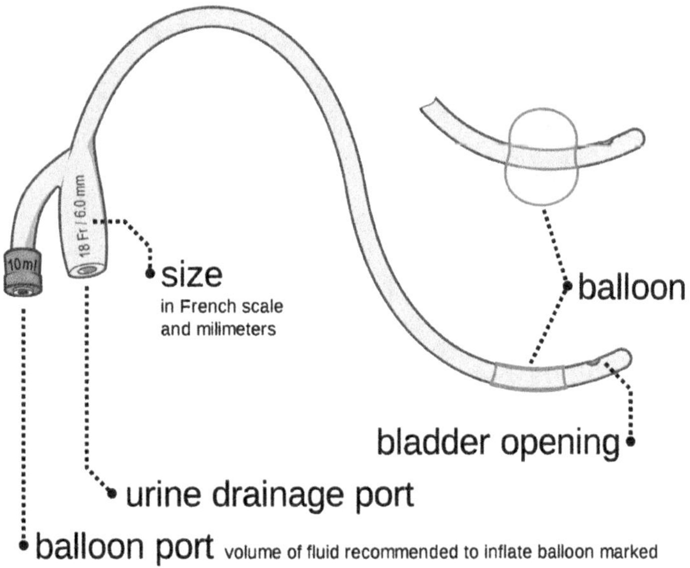

Figure 21.2 Parts of an Indwelling Catheter

2 "Foley catheter inflated and deflated EN.svg" by Olek Remesz (wiki-pl: Orem, commons: Orem) is licensed under CC BY-SA 3.0. Access for free at https://commons.wikimedia.org/wiki/File:Foley_catheter_inflated_and_deflated_EN.svg

My Notes

Catheters have different sizes, with the larger the number indicating a larger diameter of the catheter. See Figure 21.3[3] for an image of the French Catheter Scale.

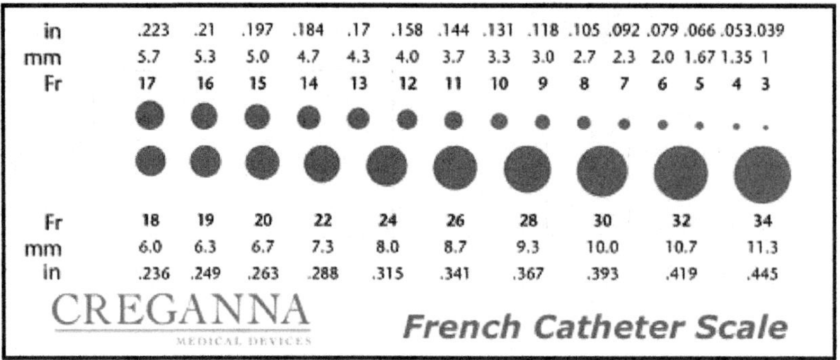

Figure 21.3 French Catheter Scale

There are two common types of bags that may be attached to an indwelling catheter. During inpatient or long-term care, larger collection bags that can hold up to 2 liters of fluid are used. See Figure 21.4[4] for an image of a typical collection bag attached to an indwelling catheter. These bags should be emptied when they are half to two-thirds full to prevent traction on the urethra from the bag. Additionally, the collection bag should always be placed below the level of the patient's bladder so that urine flows out of the bladder and urine does not inadvertently flow back into the bladder. Ensure the tubing is not coiled, kinked, or compressed so that urine can flow unobstructed into the bag. Slack should be maintained in the tubing to prevent injury to the patient's urethra. To prevent the development of a urinary tract infection, the bag should not be permitted to touch the floor.

3 "French catheter scale.gif" by Glitzy queen00 is licensed under CC BY-SA 3.0. Access for free at https://commons.wikimedia.org/wiki/File:French_catheter_scale.gif

4 "DSC_2104.jpg" by British Columbia Institute of Technology is licensed under CC BY 4.0. Access for free at https://ecampusontario.pressbooks.pub/clinicalskills/chapter/2-2-head-to-toe-assessment-checklist/

My Notes

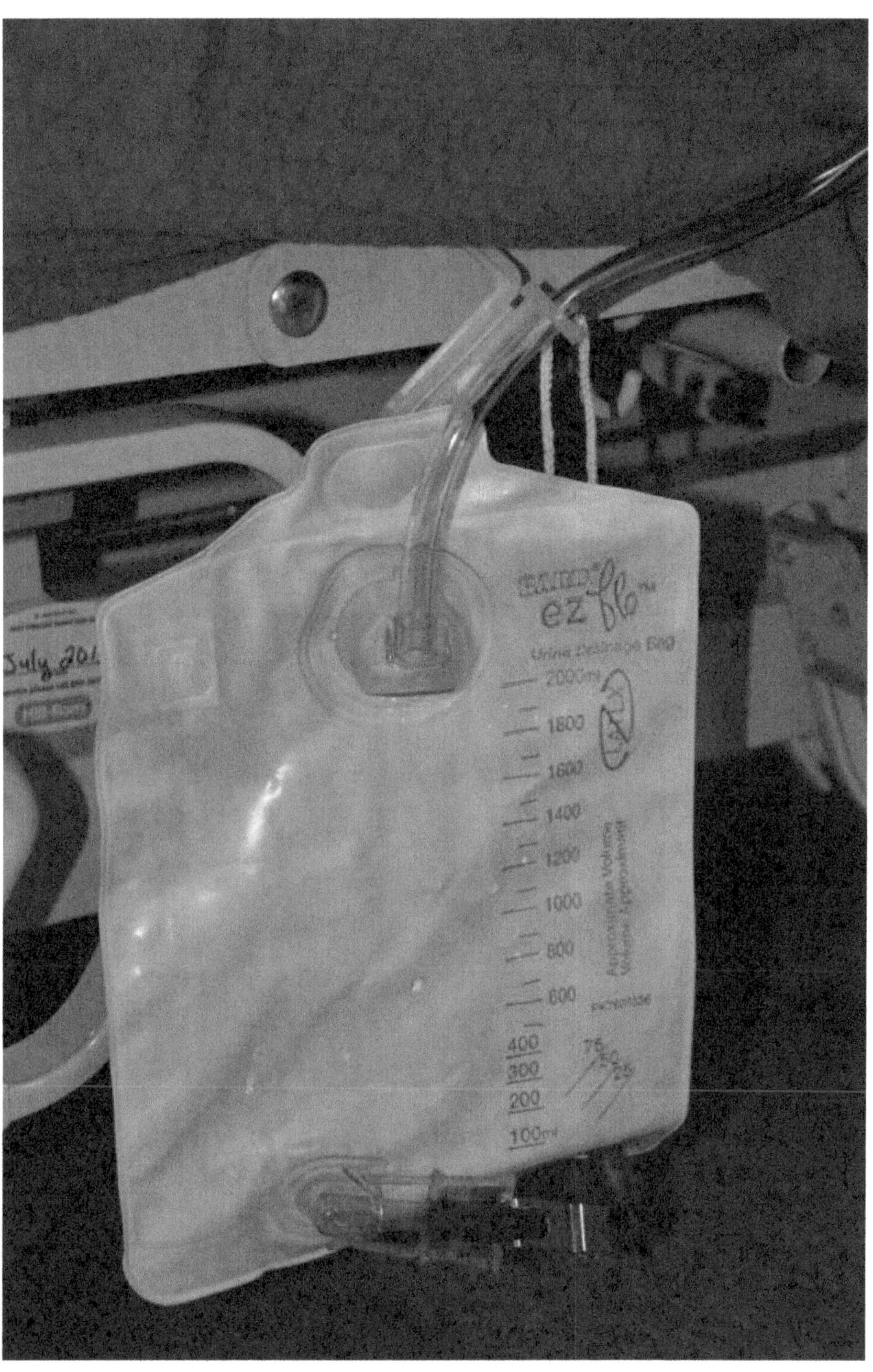

Figure 21.4 Urine Collection Bag

My Notes

See Figure 21.5[5] for an illustration of the placement of the urine collection bag when the patient is lying in bed.

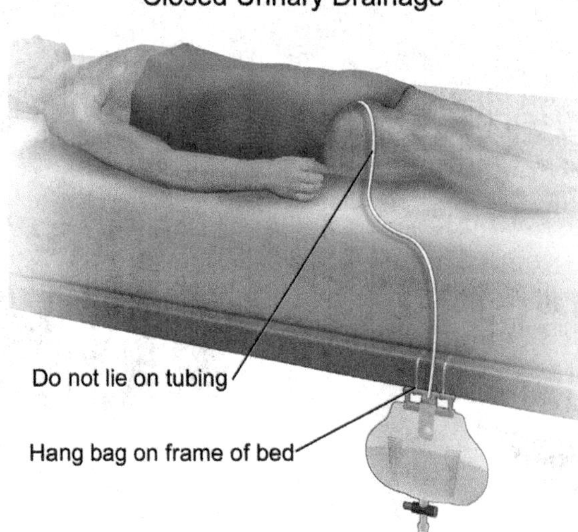

Figure 21.5 Placement of Urine Collection Bag

A second type of urine collection bag is a leg bag. Leg bags provide discretion when the patient is in public because they can be worn under clothing. However, leg bags are small and must be emptied more frequently than those used during inpatient care. Figure 21.6[6] for an image of leg bag and Figure 21.7[7] for an illustration of an indwelling catheter attached to a leg bag.

---

5 "Closed Urinary Drainage.png" by BruceBlaus is licensed under CC BY-SA 4.0. Access for free at https://commons.wikimedia.org/wiki/File:Closed_Urinary_Drainage.png

6 "Leg Bag_3I3A0667.jpg" by Deanna Hoyord, Chippewa Valley Technical College is licensed under CC BY 4.0. Access for free at https://drive.google.com/file/d/10gVnuoWYK9ZlJemjz4nc5aekWFlwEAoI/view?usp=sharing

7 "Foley Catheter Drainage (cropped).png" by BruceBlaus is licensed under CC BY-SA 4.0. Access for free at https://commons.wikimedia.org/wiki/File:Foley_Catheter_Drainage_(cropped).png

My Notes

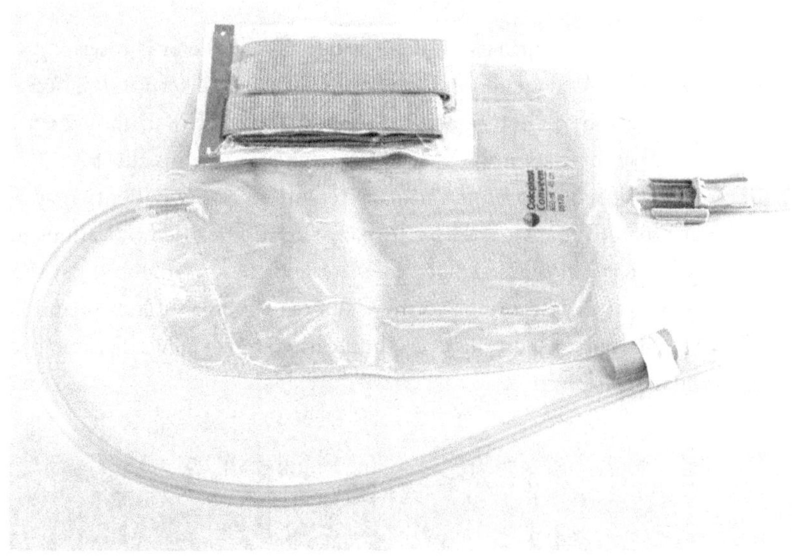

Figure 21.6 Leg Bag

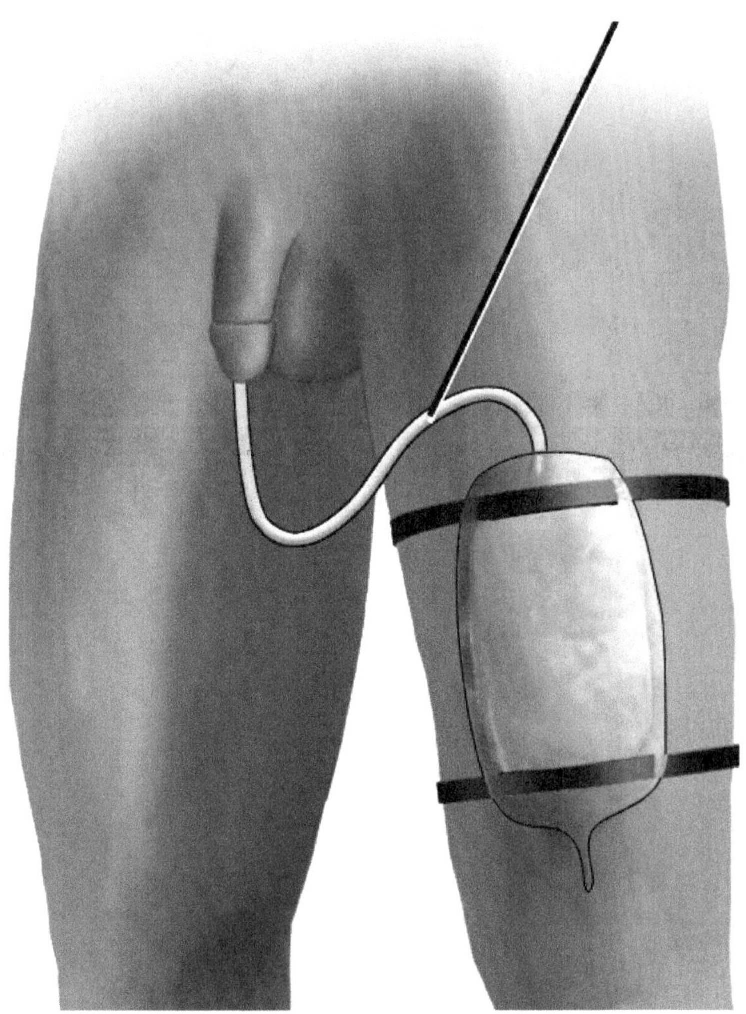

Figure 21.7 Indwelling Catheter Attached to Leg Bag

My Notes

Straight Catheter

A **straight catheter** is used for intermittent urinary catheterization. The catheter is inserted to allow for the flow of urine and then immediately removed, so a balloon is not required at the insertion tip. See Figure 21.8[8] for an image of a straight catheter. **Intermittent catheterization** is used for the relief of urinary retention. It may be performed once, such as after surgery when a patient is experiencing urinary retention due to the effects of anesthesia, or performed several times a day to manage chronic urinary retention. Some patients may also independently perform self-catheterization at home to manage chronic urinary retention caused by various medical conditions. In some situations, a straight catheter is also used to obtain a sterile urine specimen for culture when a patient is unable to void into a sterile specimen cup. According to the Centers for Disease Control and Prevention (CDC), intermittent catheterization is preferred to indwelling urethral catheters whenever feasible because of decreased risk of developing a urinary tract infection.[9]

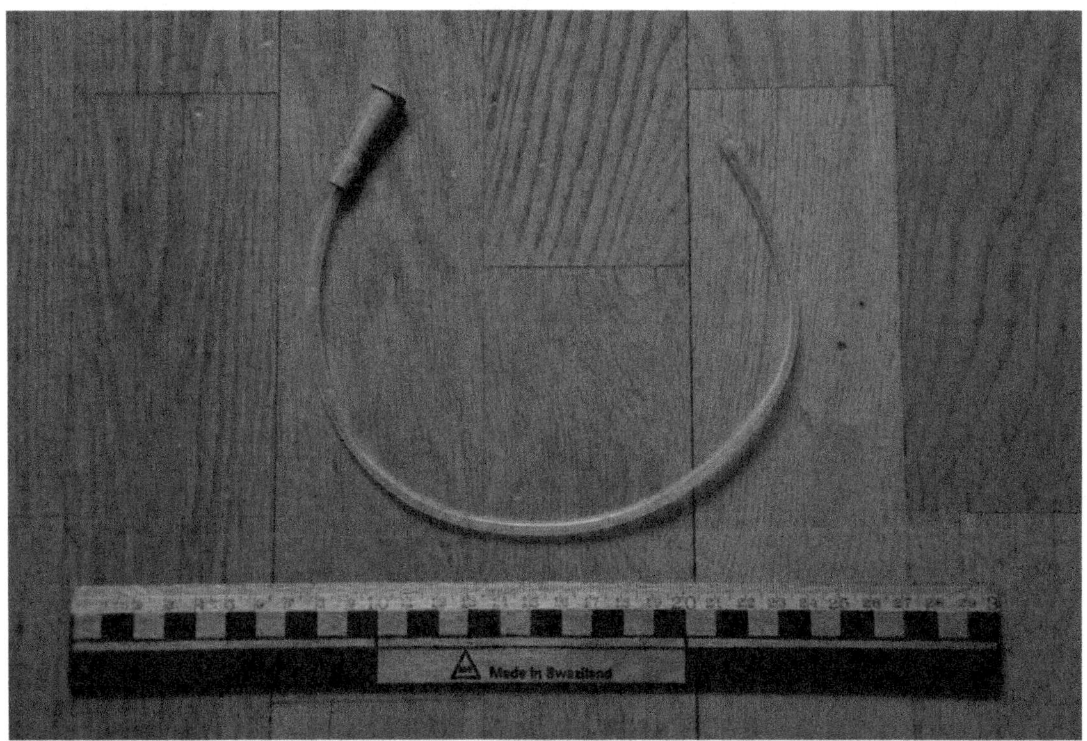

Figure 21.8 Straight Catheter

---

8 "Urinary catheter.JPG" by Bengt Oberger is licensed under CC BY-SA 3.0. Access for free at https://commons.wikimedia.org/wiki/File:Urinary_catheter.JPG

9 Centers for Disease Control and Prevention. (2015, November 15). *Catheter-associated urinary tract infections (CAUTI)*. https://www.cdc.gov/infectioncontrol/guidelines/cauti/

Other Types of Urinary Catheters

My Notes

Coude Catheter Tip

Coude catheter tips are curved to follow the natural curve of the urethra during catheterization. They are often used when catheterizing male patients with enlarged prostate glands. See Figure 21.9[10] for an example of a urinary catheter with a coude tip. During insertion, the tip of the Coude catheter must be pointed anteriorly or it can cause damage the urethra. A thin line embedded in the catheter provides information regarding orientation during the procedure; maintain the line upwards to keep it pointed anteriorly.

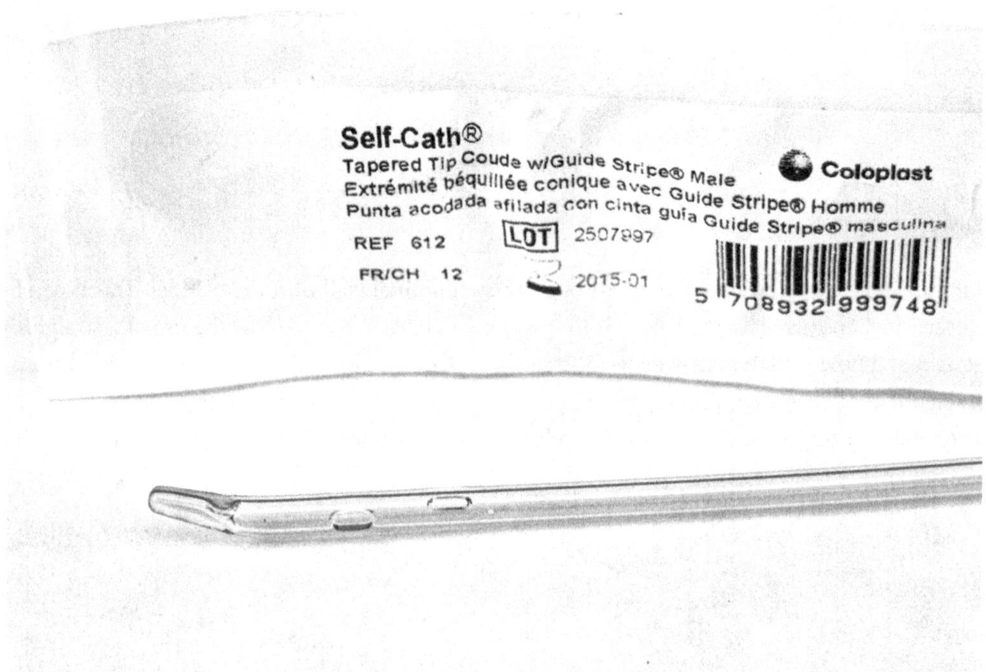

Figure 21.9 Coude Tipped Catheter

10 "Self Cath_3I3A0676.jpg" by Deanna Hoyord, Chippewa Valley Technical College is licensed under CC BY 4.0. Access for free at https://drive.google.com/file/d/1xAvcatjMLa23RK9-mySjO7IkbMNlWGez/view?usp=sharing

My Notes

Irrigation Catheter

Irrigation catheters are typically used after prostate surgery to flush the surgical area. These catheters are larger in size to allow for larger amounts of fluid to flush. See Figure 21.10[11] for an image comparing a larger 20 French catheter (typically used for irrigation) to a 14 French catheter (typically used for indwelling catheters).

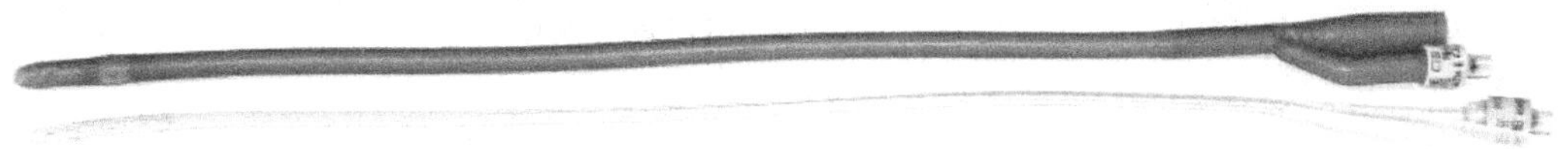

Figure 21.10 Comparison of a 20 French and a 14 French Catheter

Suprapubic Catheters

Suprapubic catheters are surgically inserted through the abdominal wall into the bladder. This type of catheter is typically inserted when there is a blockage within the urethra that does not allow the use of a straight or indwelling catheter. Suprapubic catheters may be used for a short period of time for acute medical conditions or may be used permanently for chronic conditions. See Figure 21.11[12] for an image of a suprapubic catheter. The insertion site of a suprapubic catheter must be cleaned regularly according to agency policy with appropriate steps to prevent skin breakdown.

11 "Irrigation Catheter and a 14 Fr. Catheter - 3I3A0753.jpg" by Deanna Hoyord, Chippewa Valley Technical College is licensed under CC BY 4.0. Access for free at https://drive.google.com/file/d/1OGSOUkX9_70SRUyckVsmMWlbZjxShal7/view?usp=sharing

12 "NewlyPlaceSubprapubic.jpg" by James Heilman, MD is licensed under CC BY-SA 4.0. Access for free at https://commons.wikimedia.org/wiki/File:NewlyPlaceSubprapubic.jpg

My Notes

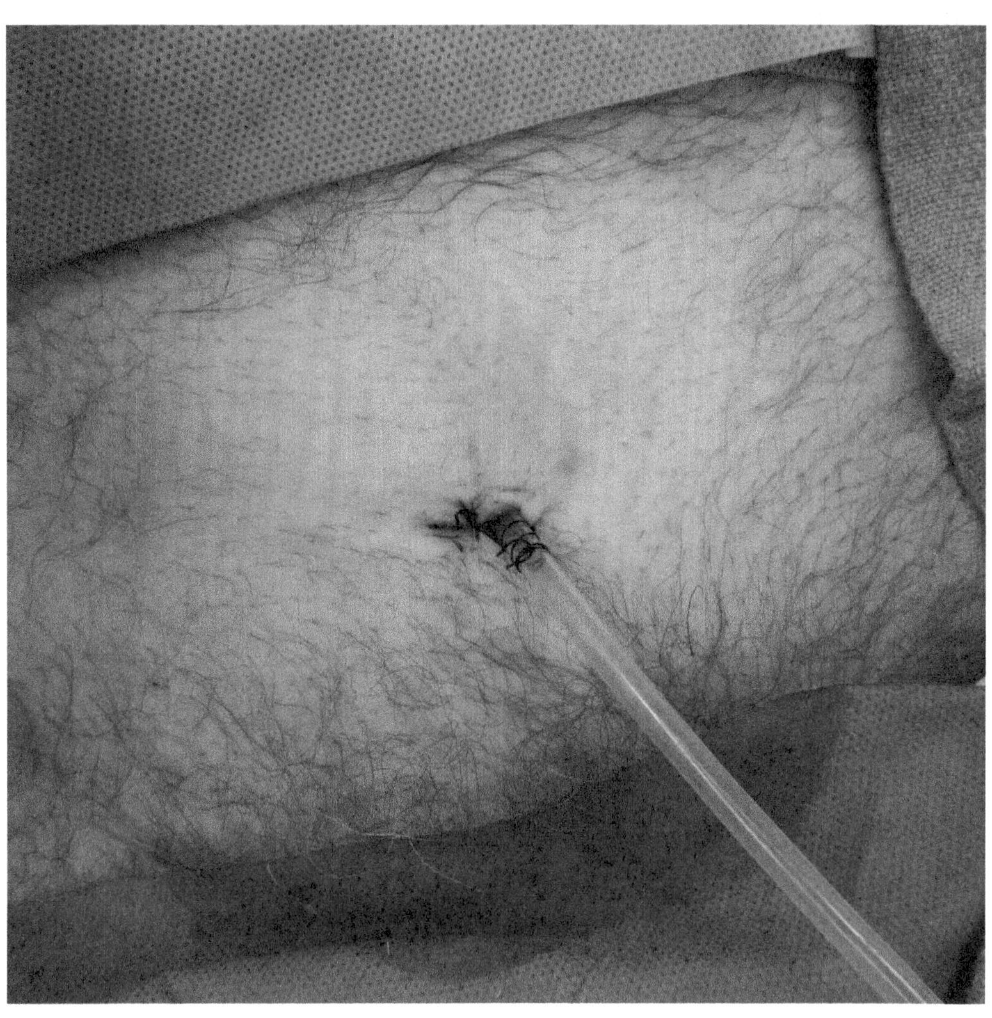

Figure 21.11 Suprapubic Catheter

My Notes

Male Condom Catheter

A condom catheter is a noninvasive device used for males with incontinence. It is placed over the penis and connected to a drainage bag. This device protects and promotes healing of the skin around the perineal area and inner legs and is used as an alternative to an indwelling urinary catheter. See Figure 21.12[13] for an image of a condom catheter and Figure 21.13[14] for an illustration of a condom catheter attached to a leg bag.

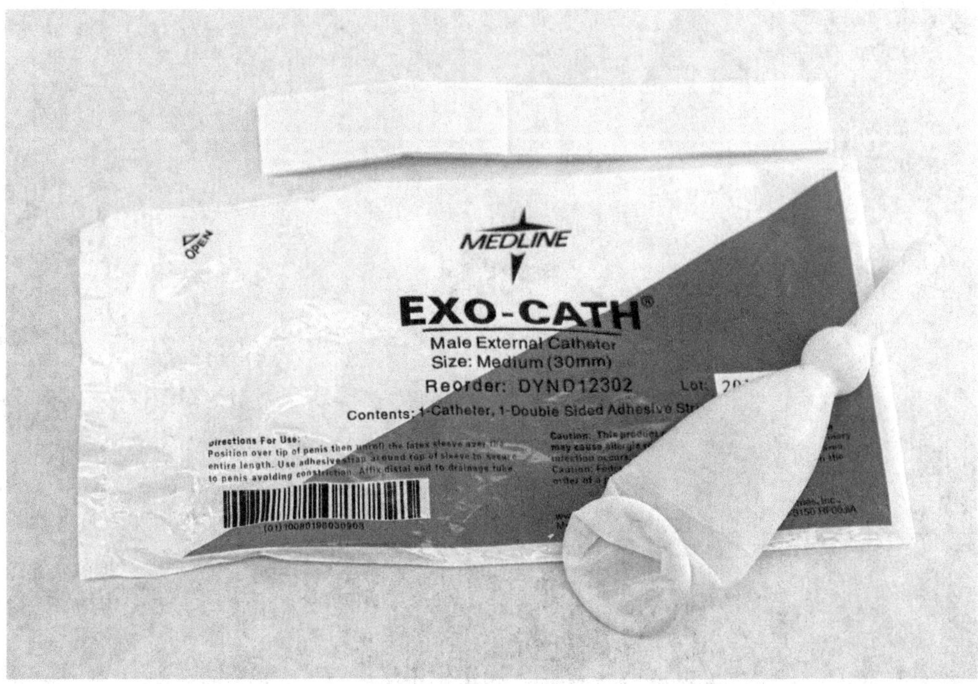

Figure 21.12 Condom Catheter

13 "Male External Cath 1 .jpg" by Deanna Hoyord, Chippewa Valley Technical College is licensed under CC BY 4.0. Access for free at https://drive.google.com/file/d/1bSoD_b3BKvjAvqUrtyoL3Y4NU2haRbTt/view?usp=sharing

14 "Condom Cather Drainage.png" by BruceBlaus is licensed under CC BY-SA 4.0. Access for free at https://commons.wikimedia.org/wiki/File:Condom_Cather_Drainage.png

My Notes

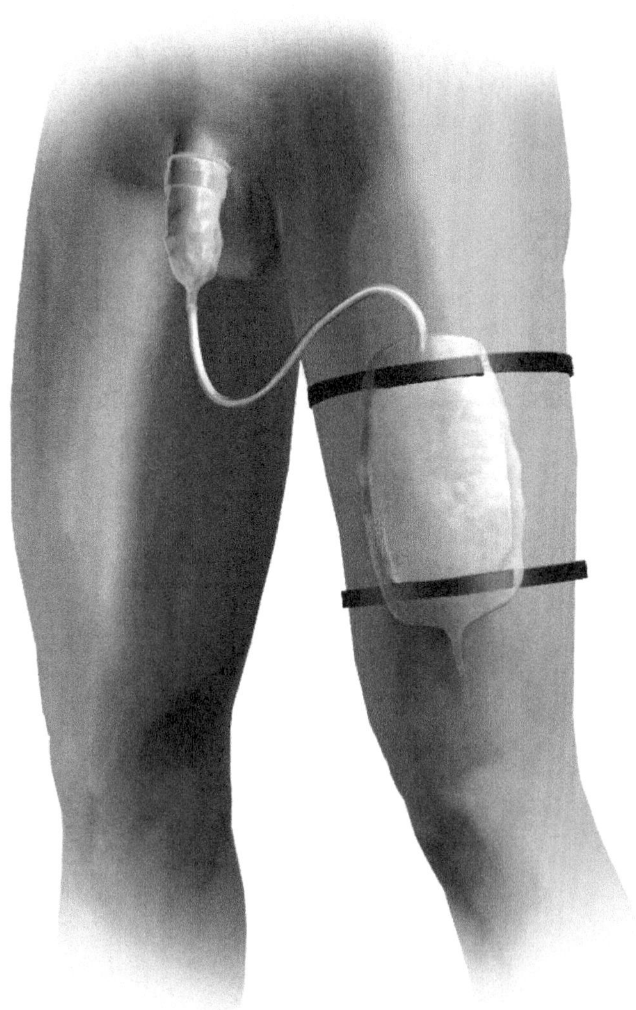
Strap the Drainage
Bag to the Thigh

Figure 21.13 Condom Catheter Attached to Leg Bag

My Notes

Female External Urinary Catheter

Female external urinary catheters (FEUC) have been recently introduced into practice to reduce the incidence of catheter-associated urinary tract infection (CAUTI) in women.[15] The external female catheter device is made of a purewick material that is placed externally over the female's urinary meatus. The wicking material is attached to a tube that is hooked to a low-suction device. When the wick becomes saturated with urine, it is suctioned into a drainage canister. Preliminary studies have found that utilizing the FEUC device reduced the risk for CAUTI.[16,17]

View these supplementary videos on female external urinary catheters:
"Students demonstrate use of Purewick Female External Catheter"[18]
"How to use the use the PureWick – a female external catheter"[19]

---

15 Eckert, L., Mattia, L., Patel, S., Okumura, R., Reynolds, P., & Stuiver, I. Reducing the risk of indwelling catheter-associated urinary tract infection in female patients by implementing an alternative female external urinary collection device: A quality improvement project. *Journal of Wound Ostomy Continence Nursing, 47*(1), 50-53. https://doi.org/10.1097/won.0000000000000601

16 Eckert, L., Mattia, L., Patel, S., Okumura, R., Reynolds, P., & Stuiver, I. Reducing the risk of indwelling catheter-associated urinary tract infection in female patients by implementing an alternative female external urinary collection device: A quality improvement project. *Journal of Wound Ostomy Continence Nursing, 47*(1), 50-53. https://doi.org/10.1097/won.0000000000000601

17 Glover, E., Bleeker, E., Bauermeister, A., Koehlmoos, A., & Van Whye, M. (2018). *External catheters and reducing adverse effects in the female inpatient.* Northwestern College Department of Nursing. https://nwcommons.nwciowa.edu/cgi/viewcontent.cgi?article=1026&context=celebrationofresearch

18 Madrid, S. (2019, June 19). *Purewick.* [Video]. YouTube. All rights reserved. https://youtu.be/1rnQaHvIMBc

19 Newton, C. (2016, August 4). *PureWick User Instructions.* [Video]. YouTube. All rights reserved. https://youtu.be/xSOuvcShikw

21.3 PREVENTING CAUTI

My Notes

A catheter-associated urinary tract infection **(CAUTI)** is a common, life-threatening complication caused by indwelling urinary catheters. The development of a CAUTI is associated with patients' increased length of stay in the hospital, resulting in additional hospital costs and a higher risk of death. It is estimated that 17% to 69% of CAUTI cases are preventable, meaning that up to 380,000 infections and 9,000 patient deaths per year related to CAUTI can be prevented with appropriate nursing measures.[1]

Nurses can save lives, prevent harm, and lower health care costs by following interventions outlined in the document created by the American Nurses Association titled *Streamlined Evidence-Based RN Tool: Catheter Associated Urinary Tract Infection (CAUTI) Prevention.* Review the entire tool in the hyperlink provided below. Key interventions include the following:

- Ensure the patient meets CDC-approved indications prior to inserting an indwelling catheter. If the patient does not meet the approved indications, contact the provider and advocate for an alternative method to facilitate elimination.
    - According to the Centers for Disease Control and Prevention (CDC), appropriate indications for inserting an indwelling urinary catheter include the following[2]:
        - Urinary retention or bladder outlet obstruction
        - Hourly monitoring of urinary output in critically ill patients
        - Perioperative use for selected surgeries
        - Healing of open sacral and perineal wounds in patients with urinary incontinence
        - Prolonged immobilization
        - End-of-life care[3]
    - Inappropriate reasons for inserting an indwelling urinary catheter include the following:
        - Substitution of nursing care for a patient or resident with incontinence
        - A means for obtaining a urine culture when a patient can

      voluntarily void
        - Prolonged postoperative care without appropriate indications[4]
- After an indwelling urinary catheter is inserted, assess the patient daily to determine if the patient still meets the CDC criteria for an indwelling catheter and document the findings. If the patient no longer meets the approved criteria, follow agency policy for removal.

---

1 Centers for Disease Control and Prevention. (2015, November 15). *Catheter-associated urinary tract infections (CAUTI).* https://www.cdc.gov/infectioncontrol/guidelines/cauti/

2 Centers for Disease Control and Prevention. (2015, November 15). *Catheter-associated urinary tract infections (CAUTI).* https://www.cdc.gov/infectioncontrol/guidelines/cauti/

3 Centers for Disease Control and Prevention. (2015, November 15). *Catheter-associated urinary tract infections (CAUTI).* https://www.cdc.gov/infectioncontrol/guidelines/cauti/

4 Centers for Disease Control and Prevention. (2015, November 15). *Catheter-associated urinary tract infections (CAUTI).* https://www.cdc.gov/infectioncontrol/guidelines/cauti/

My Notes

- When an indwelling catheter is in place, prevent CAUTI by following the maintenance steps outlined by the CDC.
- Continually monitor for signs of a CAUTI and report concerns to the health care provider.[5]
    - Signs and symptoms of CAUTI to urgently report to the health care provider include fever greater than 38 degrees Celsius, change in mental status such as confusion or lethargy, chills, malodorous urine, and suprapubic or flank pain. Flank pain can be assessed by assisting the patient to a sitting or side-lying position and percussing the costovertebral areas.[6]

Read a nurse-driven, evidence-based PDF tool to prevent CAUTI from the American Nurses Association:[7] "Streamlined Evidence-Based RN Tool: Catheter Associated Urinary Tract Infection (CAUTI) Prevention."

---

5 American Nurses Association. (n.d.). *Streamlined evidence-based RN tool: Catheter associated urinary tract infection (CAUTI) prevention*. https://www.nursingworld.org/~4aede8/globalassets/practiceandpolicy/innovation--evidence/clinical-practice-material/cauti-prevention-tool/anacautipreventiontool-final-19dec2014.pdf

6 Blodgett, T. J., Gardner, S. E., Blodgett, N. P., Peterson, L. V., & Pietraszak, M. (2015). A tool to assess the signs and symptoms of catheter-associated urinary tract infection: Development and reliability. *Clinical Nursing Research, 24*(4), 341-356. https://doi.org/10.1177/1054773814550506

7 American Nurses Association. (n.d.). Streamlined evidence-based RN tool: Catheter associated urinary tract infection (CAUTI) prevention. https://www.nursingworld.org/~4aede8/globalassets/practiceandpolicy/innovation--evidence/clinical-practice-material/cauti-prevention-tool/anacautipreventiontool-final-19dec2014.pdf

21.4 INSERTING AND MANAGING INDWELLING URINARY CATHETERS

My Notes

Safely and accurately placing an indwelling urinary catheter poses several challenges that require the nurse to use clinical judgment. Challenges can include anatomical variations in a specific patient, medical conditions affecting patient positioning, and maintaining sterility of the procedure with confused or agitated patients. See the checklists on Foley Catheter Insertion (Male) and Foley Catheter Insertion (Female) for detailed instructions.

Nursing interventions to prevent the development of a catheter-associated urinary tract infection (CAUTI) on insertion include the following[1]:

- Determine if insertion of an indwelling catheter meets CDC guidelines.
- Select the smallest-sized catheter that is appropriate for the patient, typically a 14 French.
- Obtain assistance as needed to facilitate patient positioning, visualization, and insertion. Many agencies require two nurses for the insertion of indwelling catheters.
- Perform perineal care before inserting a urinary catheter and regularly thereafter.
- Perform hand hygiene before and after insertion, as well as during any manipulation of the device or site.
- Maintain strict aseptic technique during insertion and use sterile gloves and equipment.
- Inflate the balloon after insertion per manufacturer instructions. It is not recommended to preinflate the balloon prior to insertion.
- Properly secure the catheter after insertion to prevent tissue damage.
- Keep the drainage bag below the bladder but not resting on the floor.
- Check the system to ensure there are no kinks or obstructions to urine flow.
- Provide routine hygiene of the urinary meatus during daily bathing, and cleanse the perineal area after every bowel movement. In uncircumcised males, gently retract the foreskin, cleanse the meatus, and then return the foreskin to the original position. Do not cleanse the periurethral area with antiseptics after the catheter is in place.[2] To avoid contaminating the urinary tract, always clean by wiping away from the urinary meatus.
- Empty the collection bag regularly using a separate, clean collecting container for each patient. Avoid splashing and prevent contact of the drainage spigot with the nonsterile collecting container or other surfaces. Never allow the bag to touch the floor.[3,4]

---

1 American Nurses Association. (n.d.). *Streamlined evidence-based RN tool: Catheter associated urinary tract infection (CAUTI) prevention.* https://www.nursingworld.org/~4aede8/globalassets/practiceandpolicy/innovation--evidence/clinical-practice-material/cauti-prevention-tool/anacautipreventiontool-final-19dec2014.pdf

2 Centers for Disease Control and Prevention. (2015, November 15). *Catheter-associated urinary tract infections (CAUTI).* https://www.cdc.gov/infectioncontrol/guidelines/cauti/

3 Centers for Disease Control and Prevention. (2015, November 15). *Catheter-associated urinary tract infections (CAUTI).* https://www.cdc.gov/infectioncontrol/guidelines/cauti/

4 American Nurses Association. (n.d.). *Streamlined evidence-based RN tool: Catheter associated urinary tract infection (CAUTI) prevention.* https://www.nursingworld.org/~4aede8/globalassets/practiceandpolicy/innovation--evidence/clinical-practice-material/cauti-prevention-tool/anacautipreventiontool-final-19dec2014.pdf

My Notes

Video Review of Thompson Rivers University's Urinary Catheterization:
Urinary Catheterization – Female video[5]
Urinary Catheterization – Male video[6]

---

5 Thomson Rivers Open Learning. (2018). *Urinary catheterization - female.* [Video]. https://barabus.tru.ca/nursing/urinary_catherization_female.html. All rights reserved.

6 Thomson Rivers Open Learning. (2018). *Urinary catheterization - male.* [Video]. https://barabus.tru.ca/nursing/urinary_catherization_male.html. All rights reserved.

21.5 OBTAINING URINE SPECIMEN FOR CULTURE

My Notes

If a small amount of fresh urine is needed for specimen collection for urinalysis or culture, aspirate the urine from the needleless sampling port with a sterile syringe after cleansing the port with a disinfectant.[1] See the "Checklist for Obtaining a Urine Specimen from a Foley Catheter" for more detailed instructions. Do not collect the urine that is already in the collection bag because it is contaminated and will lead to an erroneous test result.

---

1. Centers for Disease Control and Prevention. (2015, November 15). *Catheter-associated urinary tract infections (CAUTI).* https://www.cdc.gov/infectioncontrol/guidelines/cauti/

My Notes

21.6 REMOVING AN INDWELLING URINARY CATHETER

It is the nurse's responsibility to assess for a patient's continued need for an indwelling catheter daily and to advocate for removal when appropriate.[1] Prolonged use of indwelling catheters increases the risk of developing CAUTIs. For patients who require an indwelling catheter for operative purposes, the catheter is typically removed within 24 hours or less. Some agencies have a protocol for the removal of indwelling catheters, whereas others require a prescription from a provider. For additional instructions about how to remove an indwelling catheter, see the "Checklist for Foley Removal."

When removing an indwelling urinary catheter, it is considered a standard of practice to document the time and track the time of the first void. This information is also communicated during handoff reports. If the patient is unable to void within 4-6 hours and/or complains of bladder fullness, the nurse determines if incomplete bladder emptying is occurring according to agency policy. The ANA has made the following recommendations to assess for incomplete bladder emptying:

- The patient should be prompted to urinate.
- If urination volume is less than 180 mL, the nurse should perform a bladder scan to determine the post-void residual. A **bladder scan** is a bedside test performed by nurses that uses ultrasonic waves to determine the amount of fluid in the bladder.
- If a bladder scanner is not available, a straight urinary catheterization is performed.[2]

When a urinary catheter is removed, instruct the patient on the following guidelines:

- Increase or maintain fluid intake (unless contraindicated).
- Void when able with the goal to urinate within six hours after removal of the catheter. Inform the nurse of the void so that the amount can be measured and documented.
- Be aware that there may be a mild burning sensation during the first void.
- Report any burning, discomfort, frequency, or small amounts of urine when voiding.
- Report an inability to void, bladder tenderness, or distension.

---

1 American Nurses Association. (n.d.). *Streamlined evidence-based RN tool: Catheter associated urinary tract infection (CAUTI) prevention.* https://www.nursingworld.org/~4aede8/globalassets/practiceandpolicy/innovation--evidence/clinical-practice-material/cauti-prevention-tool/anacautipreventiontool-final-19dec2014.pdf

2 American Nurses Association. (n.d.). *Streamlined evidence-based RN tool: Catheter associated urinary tract infection (CAUTI) prevention.* https://www.nursingworld.org/~4aede8/globalassets/practiceandpolicy/innovation--evidence/clinical-practice-material/cauti-prevention-tool/anacautipreventiontool-final-19dec2014.pdf

21.7 MANAGING OSTOMIES

My Notes

An **ostomy** is the surgical procedure that creates an opening (stoma) from an area inside the body to the outside of the body. In ostomies related to elimination, a stoma is an opening on the abdomen that is connected to the gastrointestinal or urinary system to allow waste (i.e., urine or feces) to be collected in a pouch. See Figure 21.14[1] for an image of a stoma. A stoma can be permanent, such as when an organ is removed, or temporary, such as when an organ requires time to heal. Ostomies are created for patients with conditions such as cancer of the bowel or bladder, inflammatory bowel diseases, or perforation of the colon.

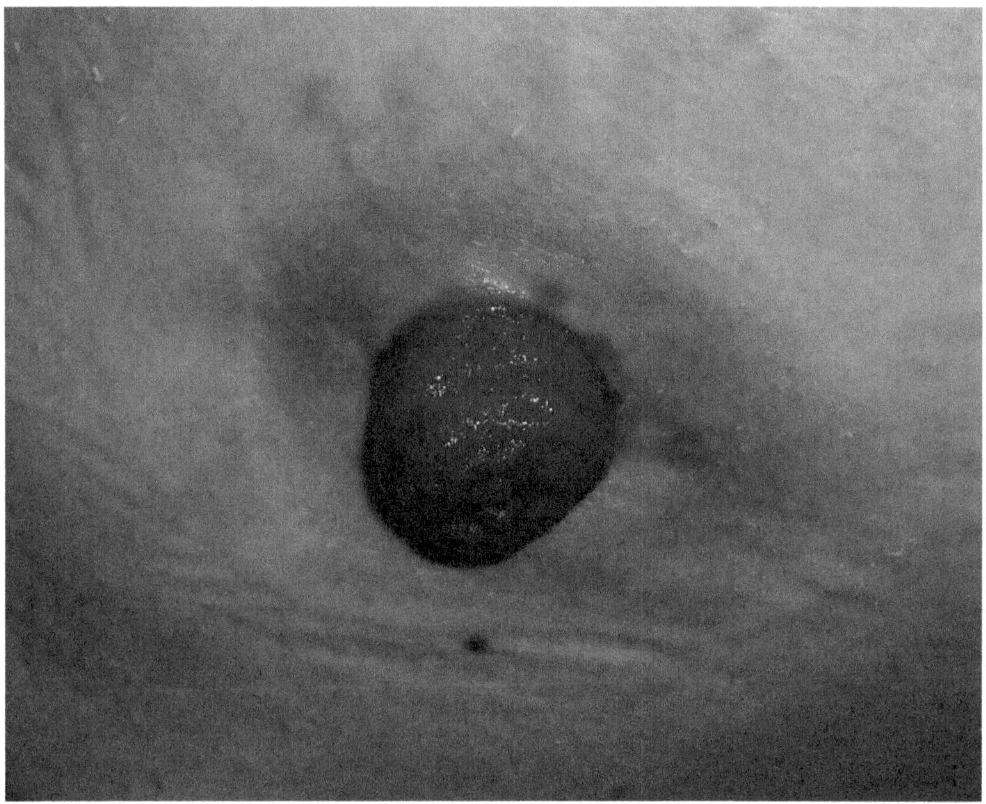

Figure 21.14 Ileostomy Stoma

There are several different kinds of ostomies related to elimination. Common types of ostomies include the following:

- **Ileostomy:** The lower end of the small intestine (ileum) is attached to a stoma to bypass the colon, rectum, and anus.
- **Colostomy:** The colon is attached to a stoma to bypass the rectum and the anus.
- **Urostomy:** The ureters (tubes that carry urine from the kidney to the bladder) are attached to a stoma to bypass the bladder.[2]

---

1 "Ileostomy 2017-02-20 5351.jpg" by Salicyna is licensed under CC BY-SA 4.0. Access for free at https://commons.wikimedia.org/wiki/File:Ileostomy_2017-02-20_5351.jpg

2 MedlinePlus [Internet]. Bethesda (MD): National Library of Medicine (US); [updated 2020, Apr 24]. Ostomy. [reviewed 2014, Jul 3; cited 2020, Nov 17]. https://medlineplus.gov/ostomy.html

My Notes

See Figure 21.15[3] comparing the anatomical locations of ileostomies and various sites of colostomies. It is important for the nurse to understand the site of a patient's colostomy because the site impacts the characteristics of the waste. For example, due to the natural digestive process of the colon and absorption of water, waste from an ileostomy or a colostomy placed in the anterior ascending colon will be watery compared to waste from an ostomy placed in the descending colon.

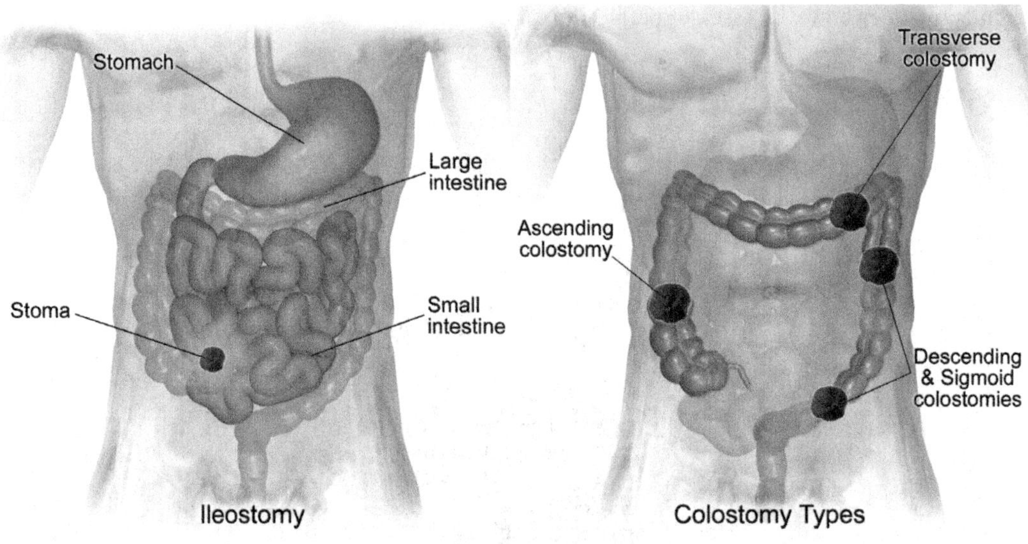

Figure 21.15 Location of an Ileostomy Compared to Colostomies

The tissue of a **stoma** is very delicate. Immediately after surgery, a stoma is swollen, but it will shrink in size over several weeks. A healthy, healed stoma appears moist and dark red or pink in color. Stomas that are swollen; dry; have malodorous discharge; or are bluish, purple, black, or pale should be reported to the provider. The skin surrounding a stoma can easily become irritated from the pouch adhesive or leakage of fluid from the stoma, so the nurse must perform interventions to prevent skin breakdown. Any identified signs of skin breakdown should be reported to the provider.[4]

Stoma appliances are supplied as a one- or two-piece set. A two-piece set consists of an ostomy barrier (also called a wafer) and a pouch. The ostomy barrier is the part of the appliance that sticks to the skin with a hole that is fitted around the stoma. The pouch collects the waste and must be emptied regularly. It attaches to the ostomy barrier in a clicking motion to secure the two parts, similar to how a plastic storage container cover snaps to a container to create a seal. The pouching system must be completely sealed to prevent leaking of the waste and to protect the surrounding peristomal skin. The pouch has an end with an opening where the waste is drained and is closed using a plastic clip or Velcro™ strip.[5] In a one-piece stoma appliance set, the ostomy barrier and the pouch are one

---

3 "Ileostomy.png" by *BruceBlaus* is licensed under CC BY-SA 4.0 and "Blausen_0247_Colostomy.png" by CC BY 3.0. Access for free at https://commons.wikimedia.org/wiki/File:Ileostomy.png

4 A.D.A.M. Medical Encyclopedia [Internet]. Atlanta (GA): A.D.A.M., Inc.; c1997-2020. Ileostomy - caring for your stoma; [updated 2020, Nov 3]. https://medlineplus.gov/ency/patientinstructions/000071.htm

5 A.D.A.M. Medical Encyclopedia [Internet]. Atlanta (GA): A.D.A.M., Inc.; c1997-2020. Ileostomy - caring for your stoma; [updated 2020, Nov 3]. https://medlineplus.gov/ency/patientinstructions/000071.htm

piece. See Figure 21.16[6] for an image of a stoma with an ostomy barrier in place. See Figure 21.17[7] for an image of a patient with an ileostomy appliance with a pouch attached.

Individuals with colostomies, ileostomies, and urostomies have no sensation and no control over the output of the stoma. Depending on the type of system, the ostomy appliance can last from four to seven days, but the pouch must be changed if there is leaking, odor, excessive skin exposure, or itching or burning under the skin barrier. Patients with pouches can swim and take showers with the pouching system on.[8]

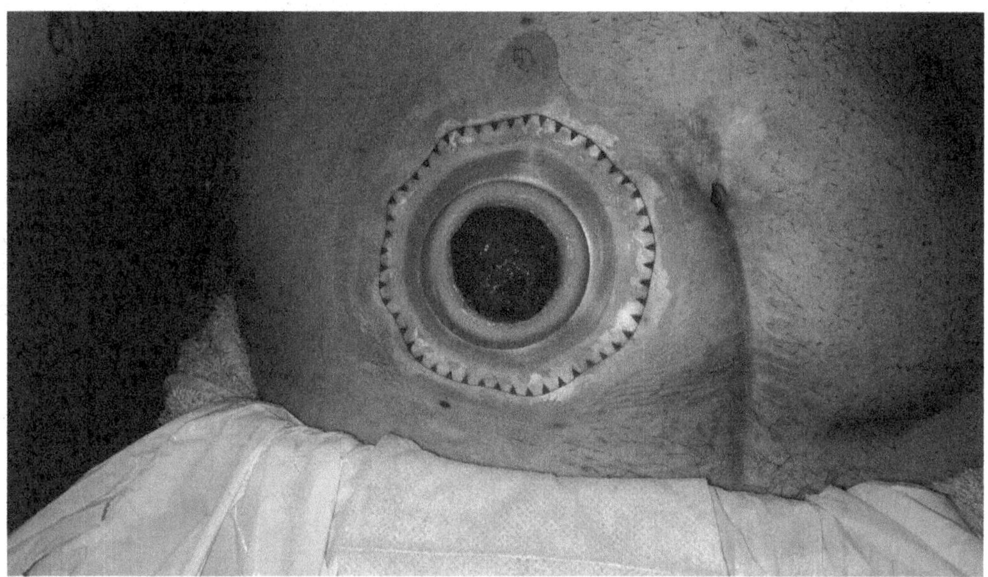

Figure 21.16 Stoma with a Wafer Barrier

6 "Ostomy_wafer_being_worn_by_an_ileostomy_patient.jpg" by Eric Polsinelli (VeganOstomy) is licensed under CC BY 4.0. Access for free at https://commons.wikimedia.org/wiki/File:Ostomy_wafer_being_worn_by_an_ileostomy_patient.jpg

7 "Ileostomy_2016-09-09_4158.jpg" by Salicyna is licensed under CC BY-SA 4.0. Access for free at https://commons.wikimedia.org/wiki/File:Ileostomy_2016-09-09_4158.jpg

8 This work is a derivative of Clinical Procedures for Safer Patient Care by British Columbia Institute of Technology and is licensed under CC BY 4.0. Access for free at https://opentextbc.ca/clinicalskills/

My Notes

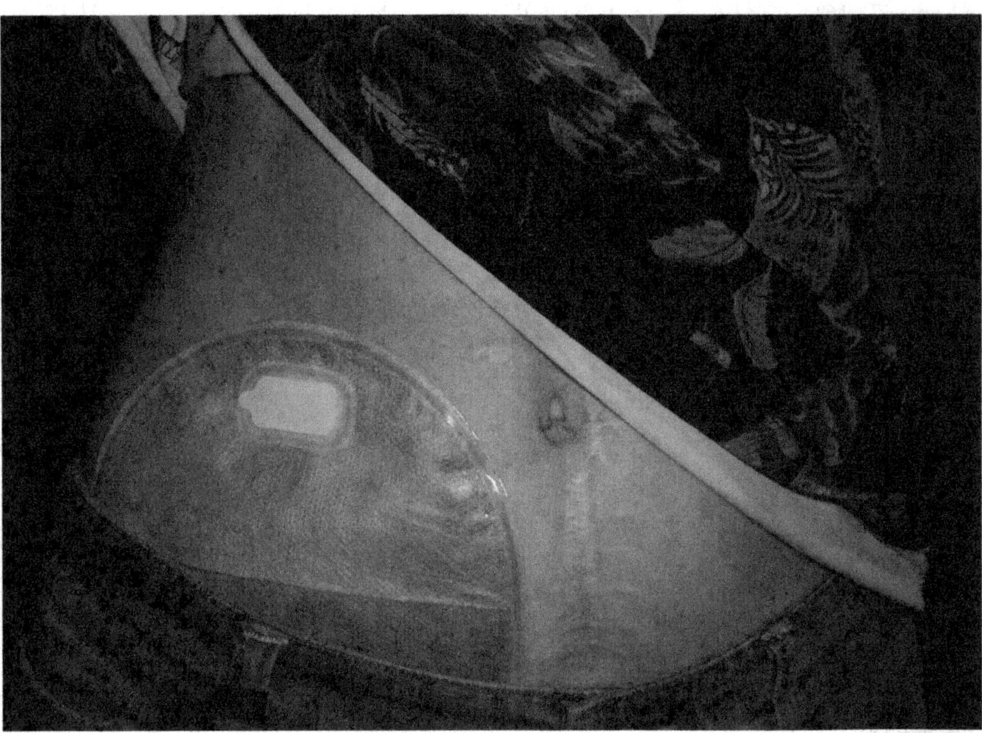

Figure 21.17 Ileostomy Appliance with a Pouch Attached

When changing an ostomy appliance, the ostomy barrier is cut to fit closely around the stoma without impinging on it. See the "Checklist for Ostomy Appliance Change" for detailed instructions. The nurse measures the stoma with a template and then cuts and fits the ostomy barrier to a size that is 2 mm larger than the stoma.[9] See Figure 21.18[10] for an image of a nurse measuring and cutting the ostomy barrier to fit around a stoma.

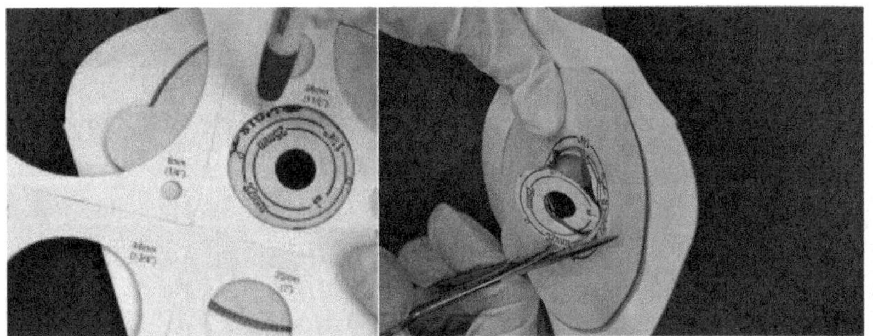

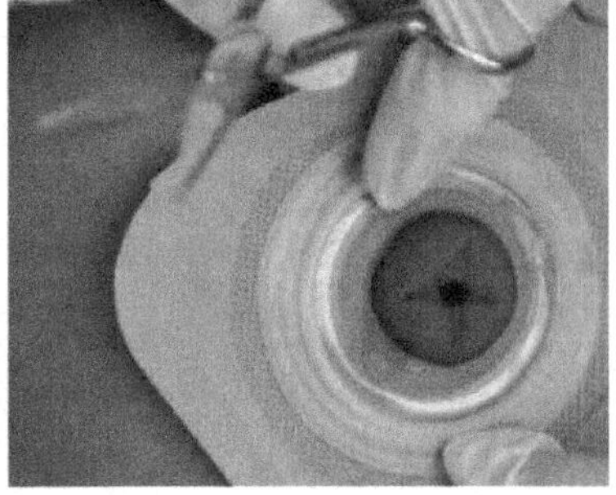

Figure 21.18 Fitting Barrier to Stoma

9 This work is a derivative of Clinical Procedures for Safer Patient Care by British Columbia Institute of Technology and is licensed under CC BY 4.0. Access for free at https://opentextbc.ca/clinicalskills/

10 "DSC_1284-e1442766479432.jpg" and "Assess-if-flange-is-the-correct-size-for-stoma-001.jpg" by British Columbia Institute of Technology are licensed under CC BY 4.0. Access for free at https://ecampusontario.pressbooks.pub/clinicalskills/chapter/10-6-ostomies/

My Notes

After the skin barrier is applied to the skin, the pouch is snapped to the ostomy barrier. See Figure 21.19[11] for an image of applying the pouch.

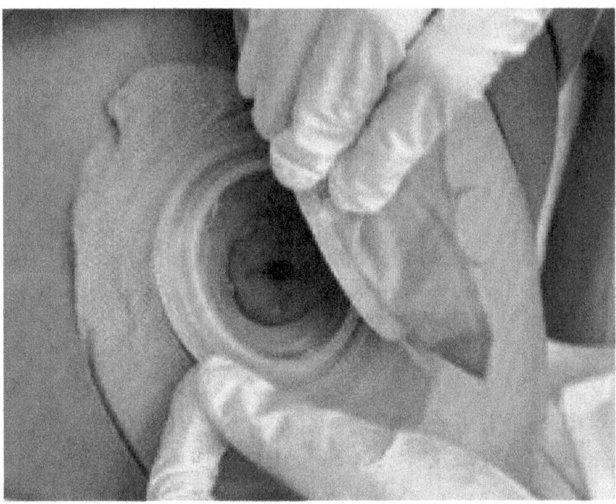

Figure 21.19 Applying an Ostomy Pouch

The ostomy bag may become filled with gas from the intestine. A patient may "burp" the bag through the opening at the top of a two-piece system by opening a corner of the ostomy pouch from the flange to let the air out. As the patient becomes more comfortable with the ostomy appliance, dietary changes can also help reduce the amount of gas produced.

Physical and Emotional Assessment

Patients may have other medical conditions that affect their ability to manage their ostomy care. Conditions such as arthritis, vision changes, Parkinson's disease, or post-stroke complications can hinder a patient's coordination and ability to manage the ostomy. In addition, the emotional burden of coping with an ostomy may be devastating for some patients and may affect their self-esteem, body image, quality of life, and ability to be intimate. It is common for patients with ostomies to struggle with body image and their altered pattern of elimination. Nurses can promote healthy coping by ensuring the patient has appropriate referrals to a wound/ostomy nurse specialist, a social worker, and support groups. Nurses should also be aware of their nonverbal cues when assisting a patient with their appliance changes. It is vital not to show signs of disgust at the appearance of the ostomy or at the odor that may be present when changing an appliance or pouching system.[12]

---

11 "Removing-ostomy-bag-from-flange-001.jpg" by British Columbia Institute of Technology is licensed under CC BY 4.0. Access for free at https://ecampusontario.pressbooks.pub/clinicalskills/chapter/10-6-ostomies/

12 This work is a derivative of Clinical Procedures for Safer Patient Care by British Columbia Institute of Technology and is licensed under CC BY 4.0. Access for free at https://opentextbc.ca/clinicalskills/

My Notes

When a patient is discharged from acute care with a new ostomy, ensure they are able to empty the pouch system independently or with the assistance of the caregiver. Provide enough supplies for two or three days of home care or until ordered supplies are expected to arrive. Evaluate the patient's and caregiver's understanding of the signs of complications. Remind them to call the provider if the stoma becomes swollen, dry, discolored, or develops a malodorous discharge.

Video Review for Changing an Ostomy Pouch[13]

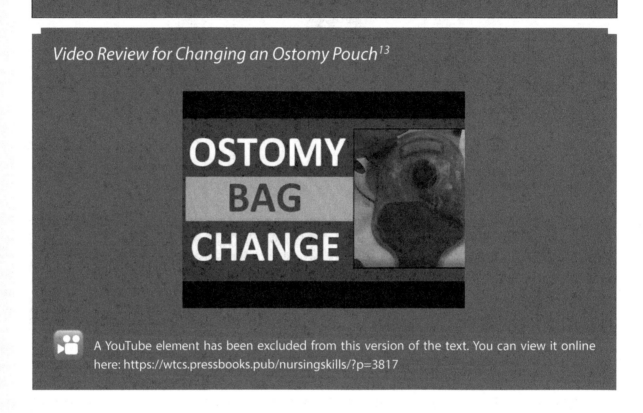

A YouTube element has been excluded from this version of the text. You can view it online here: https://wtcs.pressbooks.pub/nursingskills/?p=3817

Urostomy Care

A urostomy is similar to a colostomy, but it is an artificial opening for passing urine. Urostomies are surgically created due to medical conditions such as bladder cancer, removal of the bladder, trauma, spinal cord injuries, or congenital abnormalities.

A urostomy patient has no voluntary control of urine, so the pouching system must be emptied regularly. Many patients empty their urostomy bag every two to four hours or when the pouch becomes one-third full. The pouch may also be attached to a drainage bag for overnight drainage. Patients with a urostomy are at risk for urinary tract infections (UTIs), so it is important to educate them regarding the signs and symptoms of an infection.

---

13 RegisteredNurseRN. (2017, February 14). *Ostomy bag pouch change | Ostomy care nursing | Colostomy, ileostomy bag change.* [Video]. YouTube. All rights reserved. Video used with permission. https://youtu.be/h8CtsPAaa5Y

My Notes

Some mucous in the urine is normal with a urostomy, but blood is not a normal or expected finding and should be reported to the health care provider.

My Notes

21.8 APPLYING THE NURSING PROCESS TO CATHETERIZATION

When preparing to insert an indwelling urinary catheter, it is important to use the nursing process to plan and provide care to the patient. Begin by assessing the appropriateness of inserting an indwelling catheter according to CDC criteria as discussed in the "Preventing CAUTI" section of this chapter. Determine if alternative measures can be used to facilitate elimination and address any concerns with the prescribing provider before proceeding with the provider order.

Subjective Assessment

In addition to verifying the appropriateness of the insertion of an indwelling catheter according to CDC recommendations, it is also important to assess for any conditions that may interfere with the insertion of a urinary catheter when feasible. See suggested interview questions prior to inserting an indwelling catheter and their rationale in Table 21.8a.

Table 21.8a Suggested Interview Questions Prior to Urinary Catheterization

Interview Questions	Rationale
Do you have any history of urinary problems such as frequent urinary tract infections, urinary tract surgeries, or bladder cancer? For males: Do you have any history of prostate enlargement or prostate problems? For females: Have you had any gynecological surgeries?	Previous medical conditions and surgeries may interfere with urinary catheter placement. Information about a male patient's prostate will assist in determining the size and type of catheter used. (Recall that using a catheter with a Coude tip is helpful when a male patient has an enlarged prostate.) If a patient has a history of previous urinary tract infections, they may be at higher risk of developing CAUTI.
Have you ever had a urinary catheter placed in the past? If so, were there any problems with placement or did you experience any problems while the catheter was in place?	Questioning the patient about placement and prior catheterizations assists the nurse in identifying any problems with catheterization or if the patient has had the procedure before, they may know what to expect.
Do you have any questions about this procedure? How do you feel about undergoing catheterization?	The nurse should encourage patient involvement with their care and identify any fears or anxiety. Nurses can decrease or eliminate these fears and anxieties with additional information or reassurance.
Do you take any medications that increase urination such as diuretics or any medications that decrease urgency or frequency? If so, please describe.	Identifying medications that increase or decrease urine output is important to consider when monitoring urine output after the catheter is in place.
Have you had any orthopedic surgeries that may affect your ability to bend your knees or hips? Are you able to tolerate lying flat for a short period of time?	The patient may not be able to tolerate the positioning required for catheter insertion. If so, additional assistance from other staff may be required for patient comfort and safety.

Cultural Considerations

When inserting urinary catheters, be aware of and respect cultural beliefs related to privacy, family involvement, and the request for a same-gender nurse. Inserting a urinary catheter requires visualization and manipulation of anatomical areas that are considered private by most patients. These procedures can cause emotional distress, especially if the patient has experienced any history of abuse or trauma.

Objective Assessment

In addition to performing a subjective assessment, there are several objective assessments to complete prior to insertion. See Table 21.8b for a list of objective assessments and their rationale.

Table 21.8b Objective Assessment

Objective Data Collection	Rationale
Review the patient's medical record for any documented medical conditions the patient may not have reported, such as urethral strictures, structural problems with the bladder or urethra, or frequent urinary tract infections.	Any type of obstruction or scar tissue within these areas may prevent the catheter from advancing into the bladder.
Analyze the patient's weight and most recent electrolyte values.	Weight is used to determine a patient's fluid status, especially if they have fluid overload. Electrolyte levels are also affected by fluid balance and the use of diuretic medications. Establish a baseline to use to evaluate outcomes after placing the urinary catheter.
Determine the patient's level of consciousness, ability to cooperate, developmental level, and age.	Evaluate the patient's ability to follow directions and cooperate during the procedure and seek additional assistance during the procedure if needed. This data will impact how to explain the procedure to the patient.
Perform physical assessment of the bladder and perineum. Palpate the bladder for signs of fullness and discomfort. (Bladder emptying may also be assessed using a bladder scanner per agency policy). Inspect the perineum for erythema, discharge, drainage, skin ulcerations, or odor. Note the position of anatomical landmarks. For example, in females identify the urethra versus the vaginal opening.	A full bladder produces discomfort and urgency to void, especially on palpation. These symptoms should be relieved with the placement of a urinary catheter. Identify any abnormal physical signs in the perineal area that may interfere with comfort during insertion. Determining the urethral opening improves accuracy and ease of insertion.
When examining the perineal area, note the approximate diameter of the urinary meatus. Choose the smallest, appropriately-sized diameter catheter.	An appropriately-sized catheter is important to avoid unnecessary discomfort or trauma to the urinary tissue. Catheters that are 14 French diameter are typically used in adults.

Life Span Considerations

Children

It is often helpful to explain the catheterization procedure using a doll or toy. According to agency policy, a parent, caregiver, or other adult should be present in the room during the procedure. Asking a younger child to blow into a straw can help relax the pelvic muscles during catheterization.

Older Adults

The urethral meatus of older women may be difficult to identify due to atrophy of the urogenital tissue. The risk of developing a urinary tract infection may also be increased due to chronic disease and incontinence.

My Notes

Expected Outcomes/Planning

Expected patient outcomes following urinary catheterization should be planned and then evaluated and documented after the procedure is completed. See Table 21.8c for sample expected outcomes related to urinary catheterization.

Table 21.8c Expected Outcomes of Urinary Catheterization

Expected Outcomes	Rationale
The patient's bladder is nondistended and not palpable.	Verifies appropriate bladder emptying.
The patient reports no abdominal or bladder discomfort or pressure.	Verifies correct catheter placement by allowing urine flow and relieving discomfort or pressure.
Urine output is at least 30 mL/hr.	Verifies correct catheter placement and appropriate kidney functioning. If urine output is less than 30 mL/hour, check tubing for kinking and obstruction, and notify the provider if there is no improvement after manipulating the tubing.
Patient verbalizes understanding of the purpose of the catheter and signs of a urinary tract infection to report.	Verifies the patient's understanding of the procedure and signs of complications.

Safety is a priority! Acquire additional staff assistance to help support and position patients who are weak, obese, frail, confused, uncooperative, or have a fractured hip or pelvis.

Implementation

When inserting an indwelling urinary catheter, the expected finding is that the catheter is inserted accurately and without discomfort, and immediate flow of clear, yellow urine into the collection bag occurs. However, unexpected events and findings can occur. See Table 21.8d for examples of unexpected findings and suggested follow-up actions.

My Notes

Table 21.8d Unexpected Findings and Follow-Up Actions

Unexpected Findings	Follow-Up Action
Urine flow does not occur when catheterizing a female patient.	The catheter may have entered the vagina and not the urethral meatus. Leave the catheter in the vagina as a landmark to avoid incorrect reinsertion. Obtain a new catheter kit and cleanse the urinary meatus again before reinsertion. If reinsertion is successful into the bladder, remove the catheter that is in vagina after the second attempt.
Sterile field is broken during the procedure.	If supplies or the catheter become contaminated, obtain a new catheter kit and restart the procedure.
Patient reports continued bladder pain or discomfort although urinary flow indicates correct catheter placement.	Ensure there is no tension pulling at the catheter. It may be helpful to advance the catheter another 2-3 inches to ensure it is in the bladder and not the urethra. If these actions do not resolve the discomfort, notify the provider because it is possible the patient is experiencing bladder spasms. Continue to monitor urine output for clarity, color, and amount and for signs of urinary tract infection.
The nurse is unable to advance the catheter on a male patient with an enlarged prostate.	Do not force advancement because this may cause further damage. Ask the patient to take deep breaths and try again. If a second attempt is unsuccessful, obtain a Coude catheter and attempt to reinsert. If unsuccessful with a Coude catheter, notify the provider.
Urine is cloudy, concentrated, malodorous, dark amber in color, or contains sediment, blood, or pus.	Notify the health care provider of signs and symptoms of a possible urinary tract infection. Obtain a urine specimen as prescribed.

Evaluation

Evaluate the success of the expected outcomes established prior to the procedure.

My Notes

21.9 SAMPLE DOCUMENTATION

Sample Documentation for Expected Findings

A size 14F Foley catheter inserted per provider prescription. Indication: Prolonged urinary retention. Procedure and purpose of Foley catheter explained to patient. Patient denies allergies to iodine, orthopedic limitations, or previous genitourinary surgeries. Balloon inflated with 10 mL of sterile saline. Patient verbalized no discomfort or pain with balloon inflation or during the procedure. Peri-care provided before and after procedure. Catheter tubing secured to right upper thigh with stat lock. Drainage bag attached, tubing coiled loosely with no kinks, bag is below bladder level on bed frame. Urine drained with procedure 375 mL. Urine is clear, amber in color, no sediment. Patient resting comfortably; instructed the patient to notify the nurse if develops any bladder pain, discomfort, or spasms. Patient verbalized understanding.

Sample Documentation for Unexpected Findings

A size 14F Foley catheter inserted per provider prescription. Indication was for oliguria with accurate output measurements required. Procedure and purpose of Foley catheter explained to patient. Patient denies allergies to iodine, orthopedic limitations, or previous genitourinary surgeries. As the balloon was being inflated with saline, patient began to report discomfort. Saline removed, catheter further advanced one inch and balloon reinflated with 10 mL of normal saline. Patient denied discomfort after the catheter advancement. Catheter tubing secured to right upper thigh with stat lock. Drainage bag attached, tubing coiled loosely with no kinks, bag is below bladder level. Urine drained with procedure 100 mL. Urine drainage is dark amber, noticeable sediment in tubing, with foul odor. Patient resting comfortably, denies any bladder pain or discomfort. Instructed the patient to notify the nurse if develops any bladder pain, discomfort, or urinary spasms. Patient verbalized understanding. Notify the health care provider of urine assessment. Continue monitoring patient for any new or worsening symptoms such as change in mental status, fever, chills, or hematuria.

21.10 CHECKLIST FOR FOLEY CATHETER INSERTION (MALE)

My Notes

Use the checklist below to review the steps for completion of "Foley Catheter Insertion (Male)."

See Figure 21.20[1] for an image of a Foley catheter kit.

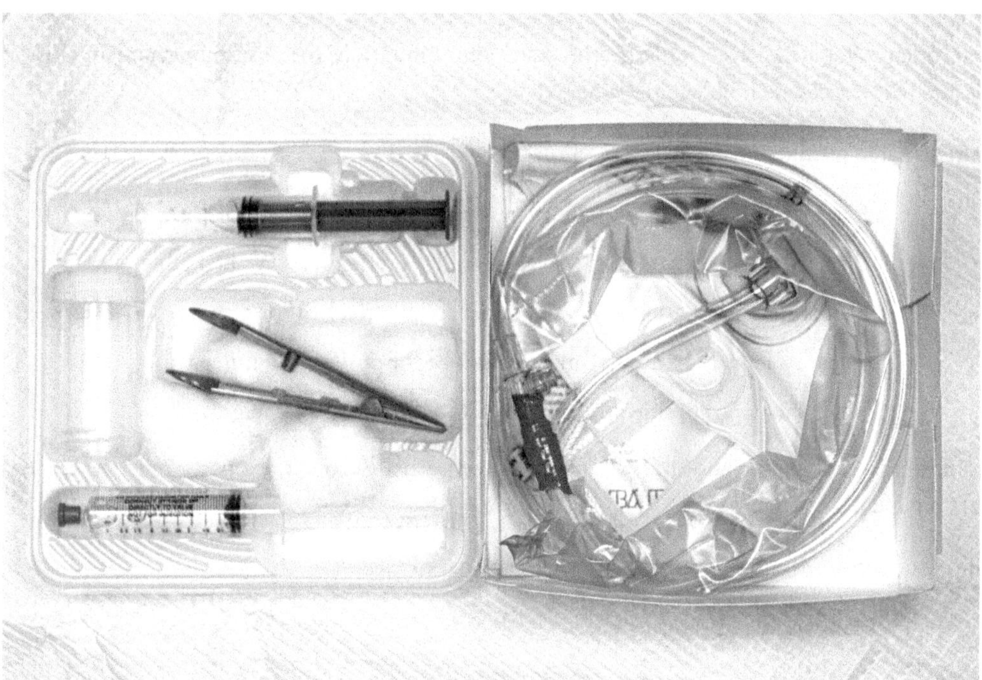

Figure 21.20 Foley Catheter Kit

Steps

Disclaimer: Always review and follow agency policy regarding this specific skill.

1. Gather supplies: peri-care supplies, clean nonsterile gloves, Foley catheter kit, extra pair of sterile gloves, Velcro™ catheter securement device to secure Foley catheter to leg, linen bag, wastebasket, and light source (i.e., goose neck lamp or flashlight).
2. Perform safety steps:
    - Perform hand hygiene.
    - Check the room for transmission-based precautions.
    - Introduce yourself, your role, the purpose of your visit, and an estimate of the time it will take.
    - Confirm patient ID using two patient identifiers (e.g., name and date of birth).
    - Explain the process to the patient.

1 "Open Foley Kit 3I3A0654.jpg" by Deanna Hoyord, Chippewa Valley Technical College is licensed under CC BY 4.0. Access for free at https://drive.google.com/file/d/1JZ5KYxK7kGFyw4oljVMHdpstjy1HdNKT/view?usp=sharing

My Notes

- Be organized and systematic.
- Use appropriate listening and questioning skills.
- Listen and attend to patient cues.
- Ensure the patient's privacy and dignity.
- Assess ABCs.

3. Assess for latex/iodine allergies, enlarged prostate, joint limitations for positioning, and any history of previous issues with catheterization.

4. Prepare the area for the procedure:

   - Place hand sanitizer for use during/after procedure on the table near the bed.
   - Place the catheter kit and peri-care supplies on the over-the-bed table.
   - Secure the wastebasket and linen cart/bag near the bed for disposal.
   - Ensure adequate lighting. Enlist assistance for positioning if needed.
   - Raise the opposite side rail. Set the bed to a comfortable height.

5. Position the patient supine and drape the patient with a bath blanket, exposing only the necessary area to maintain patient privacy.

6. Apply clean nonsterile gloves and perform peri-care.

7. Remove gloves and perform hand hygiene.

8. Open the outer package wrapping. Remove the sterile wrapped box with the paper label facing upward to avoid spilling contents and place it on the bedside table or, if possible, between the patient's legs. Place the plastic package wrapping at the end of the bed or on the side of the bed near you, with the opening facing you or facing upwards for waste.

9. Open the kit to create and position a sterile field (if on bedside table):

   - Open first flap away from you.
   - Open second flap toward you.
   - Open side flaps.
   - Only touch the outer 1" edge of the field to position the sterile field on the table.

10. Carefully remove the sterile drape from the kit. Touching only the outermost edges of the drape, unfold and place the touched side of the drape closest to linen, under the patient. Vertically position the drape between the patient's legs to allow space for the sterile box and sterile tray. Do not reach over the drape as it is placed.

11. Wash your hands and apply sterile gloves.

12. OPTIONAL: Place the fenestrated drape over the patient's perineal area with gloves on inside of the drape, away from the patient's gown, with peri-area visible through the opening. Maintain sterility.

13. Empty the syringe or package of lubricant into the plastic tray. Place the empty syringe/package on the sterile outer package.

14. Simulate application (do not open) of the iodine cleanser to the cotton. Place package on sterile outer package.

My Notes

15. Remove the sterile urine specimen container and cap and set them aside.

16. Remove the tray from the top of the box and place on sterile drape.

17. Carefully remove the plastic catheter covering, while keeping the catheter in the container. Attach the syringe filled with sterile water to the balloon port of the catheter; keep the catheter sterile.

18. Lubricate the tip of the catheter by dipping it in lubricant and replace it in the box. Maintain sterility.

19. If preparing the kit on a bedside table, place the plastic tray on top of the sterile box and carry it as one unit to the sterile drape between the patient's legs, taking care not to touch your gloves on the patient's legs or bed linens.

20. Place the top plastic tray on the sterile drape nearest to the patient. An alternate option is to leave the plastic tray on top of the box until after cleaning is complete.

21. Tell the patient that you are going to clean the catheterization area and they will feel a cold sensation.

22. With your nondominant hand, grasp the penis and retract the foreskin if present; position at a 90-degree angle. Your nondominant hand will now be nonsterile. This hand must remain in place throughout the procedure.

23. With your sterile dominant hand, use the forceps to pick up a cotton ball. Cleanse the glans penis with a saturated cotton ball in a circular motion from the center of the meatus outward. Discard the cotton ball after use into the plastic outer wrap, not crossing the sterile field. Repeat for a total of three times using a new cotton ball each time. Discard the forceps in the plastic bag without touching your sterile gloved hand to the bag.

24. Pick up the catheter with your sterile dominant hand. Instruct the patient to take a deep breath and exhale or "bear down" as if to void, as you steadily insert the catheter, maintaining sterility of the catheter, until urine is noted in the tube.

25. Once urine is noted, continue inserting to the catheter bifurcation.

26. With your nondominant/nonsterile hand, continue to hold the penis, and use your thumb and index finger to stabilize the catheter. With the dominant hand, inflate the retention balloon with the water-filled syringe to the level indicated on the balloon port of the catheter. With the plunger still pressed, remove the syringe and set it aside. Pull back on the catheter slightly until resistance is met, confirming the balloon is in place. Replace the foreskin, if retracted, for the procedure.

If the patient experiences pain during balloon inflation, deflate the balloon and insert the catheter farther into the bladder. If pain continues with the balloon inflation, remove the catheter and notify the patient's provider.

27. Remove the sterile draping and supplies from the bed area and place them on the bedside table. Remove the bath blanket and reposition the patient.

28. Remove your gloves and perform hand hygiene.

29. Apply new gloves. Secure the catheter with the securement device, allowing room to not pull on the catheter.

My Notes

30. Place the drainage bag below the level of the bladder and attach the bag to the bed frame.
31. Perform peri-care as needed; assist the patient to a comfortable position.
32. Dispose of waste and used supplies.
33. Remove your gloves and perform hand hygiene.
34. Assist the patient to a comfortable position, ask if they have any questions, and thank them for their time.
35. Ensure safety measures when leaving the room:
    - CALL LIGHT: Within reach
    - BED: Low and locked (in lowest position and brakes on)
    - SIDE RAILS: Secured
    - TABLE: Within reach
    - ROOM: Risk-free for falls (scan room and clear any obstacles)
36. Perform hand hygiene.
37. Document the procedure and related assessment findings. Report any concerns according to agency policy.

21.11 CHECKLIST FOR FOLEY CATHETER INSERTION (FEMALE)

My Notes

Use the checklist below to review the steps for completion of "Foley Catheter Insertion (Female)."

Steps

Disclaimer: Always review and follow agency policy regarding this specific skill.

1. Gather supplies: peri-care supplies, clean gloves, Foley catheter kit, extra pair of sterile gloves, Velcro™ catheter securement device to secure Foley catheter to leg, linen bag, wastebasket, and light source (i.e., goose neck lamp or flashlight).
2. Perform safety steps:
    - Perform hand hygiene.
    - Check the room for transmission-based precautions.
    - Introduce yourself, your role, the purpose of your visit, and an estimate of the time it will take.
    - Confirm patient ID using two patient identifiers (e.g., name and date of birth).
    - Explain the process to the patient.
    - Be organized and systematic.
    - Use appropriate listening and questioning skills.
    - Listen and attend to patient cues.
    - Ensure the patient's privacy and dignity.
    - Assess ABCs.
3. Assess for latex/iodine allergies, GYN surgeries, joint limitations for positioning, and any history of previous difficulties with catheterization.
4. Prepare the area for the procedure:
    - Place hand sanitizer for use during/after procedure on the table near the bed.
    - Place the catheter kit and peri-care supplies on the over-the-bed table.
    - Secure the wastebasket and linen cart/bag near the bed for disposal.
    - Ensure adequate lighting. Enlist assistance for positioning if needed.
    - Raise the opposite side rail. Set the bed to a comfortable height.
5. Position the patient supine and drape the patient with a bath blanket, exposing only the necessary area for patient privacy.
6. Apply nonsterile gloves and perform peri-care.
7. Remove gloves and perform hand hygiene.
8. Create a sterile field on the over-the-bed table.
9. Open the outer package wrapping. Remove the sterile wrapped box with the paper label facing upward to avoid spilling contents and place it on the bedside table or, if possible, between the patient's legs. Place the

My Notes

plastic package wrapping at the end of the bed or on the side of the bed near you, with the opening facing you or facing upwards for waste.

10. Open the kit to create and position a sterile field:
    - Open the first flap away from you.
    - Open the second flap toward you.
    - Open side flaps.
    - Only touch within the outer 1" edge to position the sterile field on the table.
11. Carefully remove the sterile drape from the kit. Touching only the outermost edges of the drape, unfold and place the touched side of drape closest to linen, under the patient. Vertically position the drape between the patient's legs to allow space for the sterile box and sterile tray.
12. Wash your hands and apply sterile gloves.
13. OPTIONAL: Place the fenestrated drape over the patient's perineal area with gloves on inside of the drape, away from the patient's gown, with peri-area visible through the opening. Maintain sterility.
14. Empty the lubricant syringe or package into the plastic tray. Place the empty syringe/package on the sterile outer package.
15. Simulate application of iodine/antimicrobial cleanser to cotton balls.
16. Remove the sterile urine specimen container and cap and set them aside.
17. Remove the tray from the top of the box and place it on the sterile drape.
18. Carefully remove the plastic catheter covering, while keeping the catheter in the sterile box. Attach the syringe filled with sterile water to the balloon port of the catheter; keep the catheter sterile.
19. Lubricate the tip of the catheter by dipping it in lubricant and place it in the box while maintaining sterility.
20. If preparing the kit on the bedside table, prepare to move the items to the patient. Place the plastic tray on top of the sterile box and carry as one unit to the sterile drape between the patient's legs, taking care not to touch your gloves to the patient's legs or bed linens.
21. Place the plastic top tray on the sterile drape nearest to the patient. An alternate option is to leave the plastic tray on top of the box until after cleaning is complete.
22. Tell the patient that you are going to clean the catheterization area and they will feel a cold sensation.
23. With your nondominant hand, gently spread the labia minora and visualize the urinary meatus. Your nondominant hand will now be nonsterile. This hand must remain in place throughout the procedure.
24. With your sterile dominant hand, use the forceps to pick up a cotton ball. Cleanse the periurethral mucosa with the saturated cotton ball. Discard the cotton ball after use into the plastic bag, not crossing the sterile field. Repeat for a total of three times using a new cotton ball each time. Discard the forceps in the plastic bag without touching the sterile gloved hand to the bag.
25. Pick up the catheter with your sterile dominant hand. Instruct the patient to take a deep breath and exhale or "bear down" as if to void, as you steadily insert the catheter maintaining sterility of the catheter until urine is noted.

My Notes

26. Once urine is noted, continue inserting the catheter 1"-2". Do not force the catheter.

27. With your dominant hand, inflate the retention balloon with the water-filled syringe to the level indicated on the balloon port of the catheter. With the plunger still pressed, remove the syringe and set it aside. Pull back on the catheter until resistance is met, confirming the balloon is in place.

If the patient experiences pain during balloon inflation, deflate the balloon and insert the catheter farther into the bladder. If pain continues with the balloon inflation, remove the catheter and notify the patient's provider.

28. Remove the sterile draping and supplies from the bed area and place them on the bedside table. Remove the bath blanket and reposition the patient.

29. Remove your gloves and perform hand hygiene.

30. Apply new gloves. Secure the catheter with securement device, allowing room as to not pull on the catheter.

31. Place the drainage bag below the level of the bladder, attaching it to the bed frame.

32. Perform peri-care as needed; assist the patient to a comfortable position.

33. Dispose of waste and used supplies.

34. Remove gloves and perform hand hygiene.

35. Assist the patient to a comfortable position, ask if they have any questions, and thank them for their time.

36. Ensure safety measures when leaving the room:

    - CALL LIGHT: Within reach
    - BED: Low and locked (in lowest position and brakes on)
    - SIDE RAILS: Secured
    - TABLE: Within reach
    - ROOM: Risk-free for falls (scan room and clear any obstacles)

37. Perform hand hygiene.

38. Document the procedure and related assessment findings. Report any concerns according to agency policy.

My Notes

12.12 CHECKLIST FOR OBTAINING A URINE SPECIMEN FROM A FOLEY CATHETER

Use the checklist below to review the steps for completion of "Obtaining a Urine Specimen from a Foley Catheter."

Steps

Disclaimer: Always review and follow agency policy regarding this specific skill.

1. Gather supplies: peri-care supplies, nonsterile gloves, 30 – 60 mL Luer-lock syringe for sterile specimen, alcohol wipes/scrub hubs, two preprinted patient labels, clear biohazard bag for lab sample, urinary graduated cylinder, and 10-mL syringe.
2. Perform safety steps:
    - Perform hand hygiene.
    - Check the room for transmission-based precautions.
    - Introduce yourself, your role, the purpose of your visit, and an estimate of the time it will take.
    - Confirm patient ID using two patient identifiers (e.g., name and date of birth).
    - Explain the process to the patient.
    - Be organized and systematic.
    - Use appropriate listening and questioning skills.
    - Listen and attend to patient cues.
    - Ensure the patient's privacy and dignity.
    - Assess ABCs.
3. Verify the order and assemble the supplies on a protective drape on the table: gloves, Luer-lock syringe, alcohol swabs, sterile container, two preprinted patient labels, and clear lab specimen biohazard bag for transport to lab.
4. Perform hand hygiene and put on nonsterile gloves.
5. Check for urine in the tubing and position the tubing on the bed.
6. If additional urine is needed, clamp the tubing below the port for 10-15 minutes or until urine appears.
7. Clean the sample port of the catheter with an alcohol swab.
8. Attach the Luer-lock syringe to the sample port of the catheter and withdraw 10-30 mL of urine; remove the syringe and unclamp the tubing.
9. Open the lid of the sterile container, inverting the lid on the drape and maintaining sterility. Transfer the urine to the sterile container, preventing touching the syringe to the container; place the syringe on the drape; close the lid tightly; clean the outside of the container with germicidal wipes.
10. Remove gloves and perform hand hygiene.

My Notes

11. Add information to the preprinted label: date, time collected, and your initials. Apply gloves. Place the label on the specimen container and put the container inside the biohazard bag. Remove gloves and wash your hands. Place the second label outside of the bag. Transport to the lab immediately.

12. Assist the patient to a comfortable position, ask if they have any questions, and thank them for their time.

13. Ensure safety measures when leaving the room:

    - CALL LIGHT: Within reach
    - BED: Low and locked (in lowest position and brakes on)
    - SIDE RAILS: Secured
    - TABLE: Within reach
    - ROOM: Risk-free for falls (scan room and clear any obstacles)

14. Perform hand hygiene.

15. Document the procedure and related assessment findings. Report any concerns according to agency policy.

My Notes

21.13 CHECKLIST FOR FOLEY REMOVAL

Use the checklist below to review the steps for completion of "Foley Removal."

Steps

Disclaimer: Always review and follow agency policy regarding this specific skill.

1. Verify order.
2. Gather supplies: urinary graduated cylinder, gloves, 10-mL syringe, peri-care supplies, chux/waterproof pad, and wastebasket.
3. Perform safety steps:
    - Perform hand hygiene.
    - Check the room for transmission-based precautions.
    - Introduce yourself, your role, the purpose of your visit, and an estimate of the time it will take.
    - Confirm patient ID using two patient identifiers (e.g., name and date of birth).
    - Explain the process to the patient.
    - Be organized and systematic.
    - Use appropriate listening and questioning skills.
    - Listen and attend to patient cues.
    - Ensure the patient's privacy and dignity.
    - Assess ABCs.
4. Place peri-care supplies, chux, and syringe on the overbed table. Place the wastebasket near the bed and place the urinary graduate on the floor near the Foley bag:
    - Empty urine from the tubing into the catheter bag. Empty the catheter bag into the urinary graduate.
    - Note amount of urine for I & O.
    - Empty graduate in the bathroom.
5. Remove gloves. Perform hand hygiene and then apply clean nonsterile gloves.
6. Uncover the patient so that only the genital area and catheter are exposed.
7. Place a protective pad under the patient.
8. Remove any securement device holding the catheter to the upper thigh.
9. Attach the 10-mL syringe into the balloon port and remove all the fluid from the balloon; while holding the plunger, detach the syringe.
10. Ask the patient to take a deep breath and exhale, as you remove the catheter on expiration. Stop if resistance is met.

My Notes

11. Inspect the catheter to determine if it was removed intact; place it in the wastebasket or facility-approved receptacle.

12. Cleanse the perineal area or allow the patient to cleanse the area.

13. Remove the catheter materials and waste and place them in the wastebasket.

14. Remove gloves and perform hand hygiene.

15. Assist the patient to a comfortable position, ask if they have any questions, and thank them for their time.

16. Ensure safety measures when leaving the room:
    - CALL LIGHT: Within reach
    - BED: Low and locked (in lowest position and brakes on)
    - SIDE RAILS: Secured
    - TABLE: Within reach
    - ROOM: Risk-free for falls (scan room and clear any obstacles)

17. Perform hand hygiene.

18. Document the procedure and related assessment findings. Report any concerns according to agency policy.

My Notes

21.14 CHECKLIST FOR STRAIGHT CATHETERIZATION – FEMALE/MALE

Please follow the checklist below to review the steps for completion of "Straight Catheterization for Female/Male."

Steps

Disclaimer: Always review and follow agency policy regarding this specific skill.

1. Gather supplies: peri-care supplies, nonsterile gloves, straight catheter kit, extra pair of sterile gloves, and preprinted patient label.
2. Perform safety steps:
    - Perform hand hygiene.
    - Check the room for transmission-based precautions.
    - Introduce yourself, your role, the purpose of your visit, and an estimate of the time it will take.
    - Confirm patient ID using two patient identifiers (e.g., name and date of birth).
    - Explain the process to the patient.
    - Be organized and systematic.
    - Use appropriate listening and questioning skills.
    - Listen and attend to patient cues.
    - Ensure the patient's privacy and dignity.
    - Assess ABCs.
3. Assess for latex/iodine allergies, joint limitations for positioning, and history of previous difficulties with catheterization:
    - Female: Ask about previous gynecological surgeries.
    - Male: Ask about previous diagnosis of enlarged prostate.
4. Place the hand sanitizer and other supplies for use during/after procedure off the table near the bed.
5. Place the catheter kit and peri-care supplies on the over-the-bed table.
6. Secure the wastebasket and linen cart/bag near the bed for disposal.
7. Ensure adequate lighting. Enlist assistance for positioning if needed.
8. Raise the opposite side rail. Set the bed to a comfortable height.
9. Position the patient supine and uncover the patient, exposing the patient's groin, legs, and feet for positioning and sterile field (male = supine, legs extended; female = dorsal recumbent; may need assistance to position patient and help support legs).
10. Wash your hands, apply clean gloves, and clean the perineal area.
11. Remove your gloves and perform hand hygiene.

My Notes

12. Open the package. Take out the sterile package and place it on the table. Place the plastic package wrapping at end of the bed or on the side of the bed near you.

13. Open the kit extending the outer wrapping to create a sterile field; position the sterile field on the table to create space for opening gloves at the end of the table.

14. Place the sterile pad/sheet under the patient without contaminating the center of the drape by only holding onto the edges of the drape.

15. Perform hand hygiene and apply sterile gloves.

16. Place the fenestrated drape over the patient's perineal area, keeping your gloves sterile by folding the corners of the sterile drape over the sterile gloves before approaching the patient.

17. Remove the sterile specimen container and remove the lid, if attached. Set the container on the sterile drape and invert the lid to maintain sterility. Position the container on the sterile drape to be within reach during the procedure.

18. Place the plastic tray with cotton balls and forceps on the sterile drape. Simulate opening the iodine solution and simulate pouring on the cotton balls; set the iodine package on the drape. Iodine cannot be used on mannequins.

19. Locate the catheter in the bottom of the tray; leave it in the tray. Open the water-soluble sterile lubricant and empty it into the bottom of the tray.

20. Put the plastic tray with saturated cotton balls horizontally on top of the tray to fit above the catheter and lubricant, which are located in the bottom of the tray.

21. Make sure that the sterile specimen container is within reach of your dominant hand. Then carefully move the tray as a unit with supplies inside to the sterile drape between patient's legs.

22. Tell the patient that you are now going to start the cleaning process and that there will be a cold sensation:

    - Once the nondominant/nonsterile hand touches the patient, the position is held throughout the procedure until the catheter is inserted.

23. Inspect for the urinary meatus:

    - Female: Gently spread the labia minora with your thumb and index finger of your nondominant hand and visualize the urinary meatus.
    - Male: Gently grasp the penis with the nondominant hand and retract the foreskin if present.

24. Cleanse the urinary meatus:

    - Female: Holding the labia apart with your nondominant/nonsterile hand, use your dominant/sterile hand to hold the forceps and pick up a cotton ball soaked in antimicrobial solution and cleanse the urethra with one downward stroke each time, once on each side and then once down the center. Discard each cotton ball after use without crossing the sterile field. With the dominant sterile gloved hand, pick up the lubricated catheter about 4 inches from the end for stability. Hold the catheter loosely in your hand. Place the distal end in the receptacle.

My Notes

- Male: With your sterile dominant hand, use the forceps to pick up a cotton ball. Cleanse the glans penis with the antimicrobial cleanser using a circular motion from the center of the meatus outward to the base of the glans. Discard each cotton ball after use without crossing the sterile field. Continue to hold the penis perpendicular to the body or labia apart with your nondominant hand. With the dominant sterile gloved hand, pick up the lubricated catheter about 4 inches from the end for stability.

25. Steadily insert the catheter, maintaining sterility into the meatus until a return of urine occurs.
26. Continue inserting another 1-2 inches and hold the catheter in place.
27. When urine begins to drain out of the catheter, pinch the catheter with your thumb and index finger of your nondominant/nonsterile hand while continuing to hold the labia apart or penis perpendicular to the body.
28. With your dominant/sterile hand, obtain the sterile specimen container from the table and put it under the catheter.
29. Release clamping/pinching of the catheter, allowing urine to drain into the sterile specimen container.
30. When the container is almost full, use your dominant hand to remove the container from under the stream of urine and set it on the table, maintaining sterility.
31. Allow urine to continue to flow into the receptacle provided until the flow of urine stops.
32. Tell the patient that the catheter will be removed. Instruct the patient to take a deep breath and exhale, and then remove the catheter and place it on the sterile drape on the bed.
33. Carefully remove the urine container full of urine from the bed and place it on the kit wrapper on the table. Do not put the urine container directly on the table.
34. Put the cap on the sterile specimen container, maintaining sterility.
35. Remove the catheter and other supplies from the patient's bed; provide peri-care. For males, replace foreskin if it was retracted for the procedure.
36. Remove your gloves; wash hands and apply new gloves.
37. Assist the patient to a comfortable position.
38. Write the date, time collected, and your initials on the two preprinted patient labels.
39. With an antibacterial wipe, clean the outer surface of the specimen container.
40. Apply one patient label to the specimen container and one patient label to the outside of the clear biohazard bag for transport to the lab.
41. Place the specimen container in the biohazard bag.
42. Measure and dispose of the urine in the bathroom.
43. Remove your gloves and perform hand hygiene.
44. Assist the patient to a comfortable position, ask if they have any questions, and thank them for their time.
45. Ensure safety measures when leaving the room:

My Notes

- CALL LIGHT: Within reach
- BED: Low and locked (in lowest position and brakes on)
- SIDE RAILS: Secured
- TABLE: Within reach
- ROOM: Risk-free for falls (scan room and clear any obstacles)

46. Send the specimen to the lab for processing.

47. Document the procedure and related assessment findings. Report any concerns according to agency policy.

My Notes

21.15 CHECKLIST FOR OSTOMY APPLIANCE CHANGE

Use the checklist below to review the steps for completion of an "Ostomy Appliance Change."

Steps

Disclaimer: Always review and follow agency policy regarding this specific skill.

1. Gather supplies: washcloth and warm water, stoma products/appliances per order/patient preference (wafer, bag, clip), sizing measures, scissors, pen, nonsterile gloves, skin prep or other skin products per patient preference, and wastebasket.
2. Perform safety steps:
    - Perform hand hygiene.
    - Check the room for transmission-based precautions.
    - Introduce yourself, your role, the purpose of your visit, and an estimate of the time it will take.
    - Confirm patient ID using two patient identifiers (e.g., name and date of birth).
    - Explain the process to the patient.
    - Be organized and systematic.
    - Use appropriate listening and questioning skills.
    - Listen and attend to patient cues.
    - Ensure the patient's privacy and dignity.
    - Assess ABCs.
3. Set the bed to a comfortable height; raise the opposite side rail.
4. Ask the patient about preferences, usual practices, care, and maintenance at home.
5. Apply nonsterile gloves.
6. Position the patient according to patient status:
    - Assist the patient to the bathroom and have him/her sit on the toilet to be near the sink for ease of process.
    - If in bed, uncover the patient, exposing only the abdomen. Apply drape/chux under the patient or ostomy pouch. Place the wastebasket near the bed.
7. Empty the pouch depending on the type of the appliance and the location type of procedure:
    - Remove the pouch and empty it into the toilet.
    - Set pouch aside in the basin or receptacle if at bedside.
    - Assess ostomy bag contents, and remove current ostomy appliance (keep clamp if present).
8. Remove adhesive residue from the skin with adhesive remover wipes.
9. Cleanse the stoma and surrounding skin with gauze and room temperature tap water; pat dry the skin.

My Notes

10. Assess the condition of the stoma and peristomal skin.
11. Place the gauze pad over the stoma while you are preparing the new wafer and pouch.
12. Trace the pattern onto the paper backing of the wafer and cut the wafer. No more than 1/8 inch of skin around the stoma should be exposed for correct fit.
13. Apply skin prep and wait until tacky (optional).
14. Remove the gauze pad from the orifice of the stoma.
15. Remove the paper backing from the wafer and place it on the skin with the stoma centered in the cutout opening of the wafer; press gently on the wafer to remove air/seal to the skin.
16. Apply pouch to wafer with clamp on pouch and opening in downward position.
17. Attach and close the pouch clamp.
18. Dispose of old supplies and wrappings.
19. Remove your gloves and perform hand hygiene.
20. Assist the patient to a comfortable position, ask if they have any questions, and thank them for their time.
21. Ensure safety measures when leaving the room:
    - CALL LIGHT: Within reach
    - BED: Low and locked (in lowest position and brakes on)
    - SIDE RAILS: Secured
    - TABLE: Within reach
    - ROOM: Risk-free for falls (scan room and clear any obstacles)
22. Document the procedure and related assessment findings. Report any concerns according to agency policy.

My Notes

21.16 LEARNING ACTIVITIES

Learning Activities

(Answers to "Learning Activities" can be found in the "Answer Key" at the end of the book. Answers to interactive activity elements will be provided within the element as immediate feedback.)

1. Your patient complains of pain while you are inflating the balloon during a urinary catheter insertion. Describe your next steps.
2. Your patient is admitted with a fractured head of the right femur and is scheduled for surgery in the next six hours. You have a prescription to insert a Foley catheter. After you assess the patient's ability for the recommended position to insert the catheter, you note that the patient is unable to move the right leg and should not move the leg. Describe how you will proceed with the procedure.
3. A patient with a new colostomy refuses to look at the stoma or participate in changing the pouching system. What are some suggestions to help your patient adjust to the stoma?
4. The nurse is caring for a female patient who is experiencing inadequate bladder emptying. The nurse obtains an order to determine post-void residual. Which catheter type would the nurse use to evaluate post-void residual?
   a. Coude catheter
   b. Indwelling catheter
   c. Straight catheter
   d. Foley catheter
5. The nurse is caring for a patient who had a colostomy placed two days earlier. The nurse notes that the stoma is moist and beefy red. Which action should the nurse be expected to take based on these findings?
   a. Notify the physician of the findings immediately.
   b. Remove the bag and apply pressure to the stoma.
   c. Document the assessment findings of the stoma.
   d. Change the appliance pouch and clean the skin.
6. The nurse is providing patient education on the care of an ostomy. Which of the following statements by the patient would indicate that further education is necessary?
   a. "I should plan to replace the pouch system every 8-10 days."
   b. "Wafer should be cut 1/16 to 1/8 an inch larger than the stoma."
   c. "It is important to chew all foods completely and slowly."
   d. "I will keep a diary of the foods I eat and my stool pattern."

My Notes

Check your knowledge using this flashcard activity:

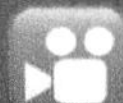

An interactive or media element has been excluded from this version of the text. You can view it online here: https://wtcs.pressbooks.pub/nursingskills/?p=3839

Use this drag and drop activity to check your knowledge about catheters:

An interactive or media element has been excluded from this version of the text. You can view it online here: https://wtcs.pressbooks.pub/nursingskills/?p=3839

Take a quiz on managing catheters:

An interactive or media element has been excluded from this version of the text. You can view it online here: https://wtcs.pressbooks.pub/nursingskills/?p=3839

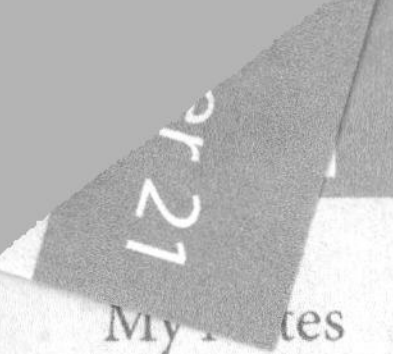

My Notes

XXI GLOSSARY

Bladder scan: A bedside test using a noninvasive tool used to measure the volume of urine in the bladder.

CAUTI: Catheter-associated urinary tract infection.

Colostomy: The colon is attached to a stoma to bypass the rectum and the anus.

Coude catheter: A catheter specifically designed to maneuver around obstructions or blockages in the urethra such as with enlarged prostate glands in males. Coude originates from the French word that means "bend."

Ileostomy: The lower end of the small intestine (ileum) is attached to a stoma to bypass the colon, rectum, and anus.

Indwelling catheter: A device often referred to as a "Foley catheter" that is inserted into the neck of the bladder and remains in place for continual collection of urine into a collection bag.

Intermittent catheterization: The insertion and removal of a straight catheter for relief of urinary retention.

Ostomy: The surgical procedure that creates the opening from the stoma outside the body to an organ such as the small intestine, colon, rectum, or bladder. A stoma can be permanent, such as when an organ is removed, or temporary, such as when an organ requires time to heal.

Prostate hypertrophy: A common medical condition of the enlargement of the prostate gland in males as they age, causing uncomfortable urinary symptoms such as urgency and frequency.

Stoma: An opening on the abdomen that is connected to the gastrointestinal or urinary systems to allow waste (urine or feces) to be collected in a pouch.

Straight catheter: A catheter used for intermittent urinary catheterization; it does not have a balloon at the insertion end.

Urinary catheterization: The insertion of a catheter tube into the urethral opening and placing it in the neck of the urinary bladder to drain urine.

Urinary Tract Infection (UTI): An infection in the urinary system causing symptoms such as burning on urination (dysuria), frequent urination, malodorous urine, fever, and change in level of consciousness.

Urostomy: The ureters (tubes that carry urine from the kidney to the bladder) are attached to a stoma to bypass the bladder.

Chapter 22

Tracheostomy Care & Suctioning

22.1 TRACHEOSTOMY CARE & SUCTIONING INTRODUCTION

My Notes

Learning Objectives

- Safely perform nasal, oral, pharyngeal, and tracheostomy suctioning
- Provide tracheostomy care
- Explain procedure to patient
- Adapt procedure to reflect variations across the life span
- Document actions and observations
- Recognize and report significant deviations from norms

This chapter will discuss tracheostomy care and various types of suctioning (e.g., oral, nasal, pharyngeal, and tracheostomy) performed by nurses. The purpose of respiratory suctioning is to maintain a patent airway and improve oxygenation by removing mucous secretions and foreign material (e.g., vomit or gastric secretions). During oral suctioning, a rigid plastic suction catheter is typically used in a patient's mouth to remove oral secretions. Nasal and pharyngeal suctioning is performed with a sterile, soft, flexible catheter to remove accumulated saliva, pulmonary secretions, blood, vomitus, or other foreign material from nasopharyngeal areas that cannot be removed by the patient's spontaneous cough or other less invasive procedures.[1]

Tracheostomy suctioning uses a sterile catheter that is inserted through a tracheostomy tube into a patient's trachea. A tracheostomy tube is a tube that is inserted through a surgical opening in the neck to the trachea to create an artificial airway. Tracheostomies require routine care to prevent infection and obstruction, as well as frequent suctioning to maintain a patent airway.[2] Tracheostomy care and suctioning are performed collaboratively by nurses and respiratory therapists.

---

1 American Association for Respiratory Care. (2004). AARC clinical practice guideline: Nasotracheal suctioning - 2004 revision & update. *Respiratory Care, 49*(9), 1080-1084. https://www.aarc.org/wp-content/uploads/2014/08/09.04.1080.pdf

2 This work is a derivative of Clinical Procedures for Safer Patient Care by British Columbia Institute of Technology and is licensed under CC BY 4.0. Access for free at https://opentextbc.ca/clinicalskills/

My Notes

22.2 BASIC CONCEPTS RELATED TO SUCTIONING

Respiratory System Anatomy

It is important for the nurse to have an understanding of the underlying structures of the respiratory system before performing suctioning to ensure that care is given to protect sensitive tissues and that airways are appropriately assessed during the suctioning procedure. See Figure 22.1[1] for an illustration of the anatomy of the respiratory system.

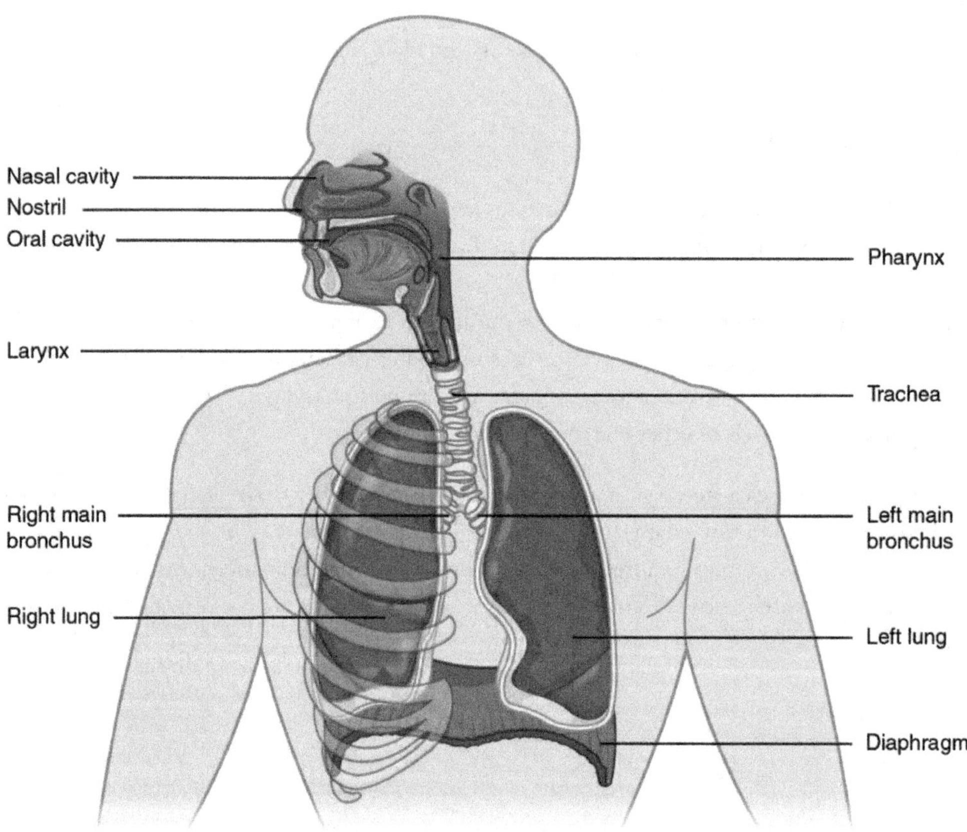

Figure 22.1 Anatomy of the Respiratory System

Maintaining a patent airway is a top priority and one of the "ABCs" of patient care (i.e., Airway, Breathing, and Circulation). Suctioning is often required in acute-care settings for patients who cannot maintain their own airway due to a variety of medical conditions such as respiratory failure, stroke, unconsciousness, or postoperative care. The suctioning procedure is useful for removing mucus that may obstruct the airway and compromise the patient's breathing ability.

To read more details about the respiratory system, see the "Respiratory Assessment" chapter.

---

1 "2301 Major Respiratory Organs.jpg" by OpenStax is licensed under CC BY 3.0. Access for free at https://commons.wikimedia.org/wiki/File:2301_Major_Respiratory_Organs.jpg

Respiratory Failure and Respiratory Arrest

My Notes

Respiratory failure and respiratory arrest often require emergency suctioning. Respiratory failure is a life-threatening condition that is caused when the respiratory system cannot get enough oxygen from the lungs into the blood to oxygenate the tissues, or there are high levels of carbon dioxide in the blood that the body cannot effectively eliminate via the lungs. Acute respiratory failure can happen quickly without much warning. It is often caused by a disease or injury that affects breathing, such as pneumonia, opioid overdose, stroke, or a lung or spinal cord injury. Acute respiratory failure requires emergency treatment. Untreated respiratory failure can lead to respiratory arrest.

Signs and symptoms of respiratory failure include shortness of breath (dyspnea), rapid breathing (tachypnea), rapid heart rate (tachycardia), unusual sweating (diaphoresis), decreasing pulse oximetry readings below 90%, and air hunger (a feeling as if you can't breathe in enough air). In severe cases, signs and symptoms may include cyanosis (a bluish color of the skin, lips, and fingernails), confusion, and sleepiness.

The main goal of treating respiratory failure is to ensure that sufficient oxygen reaches the lungs and is transported to the other organs while carbon dioxide is cleared from the body.[2] Treatment measures may include suctioning to clear the airway while also providing supplemental oxygen using various oxygenation devices. Severe respiratory distress may require intubation and mechanical ventilation, or the emergency placement of a tracheostomy may be performed if the airway is obstructed. For additional details about oxygenation and various oxygenation devices, go to the "Oxygen Therapy" chapter.

2 National Heart, Lung, and Blood Institute. (n.d.). *Respiratory failure*. https://www.nhlbi.nih.gov/health-topics/respiratory-failure

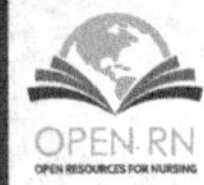

My Notes

Tracheostomy

A **tracheostomy** is a surgically-created opening called a stoma that goes from the front of the patient's neck into the trachea. A tracheostomy tube is placed through the stoma and directly into the trachea to maintain an open (patent) airway. See Figure 22.2[3] for an illustration of a patient with a tracheostomy tube in place.

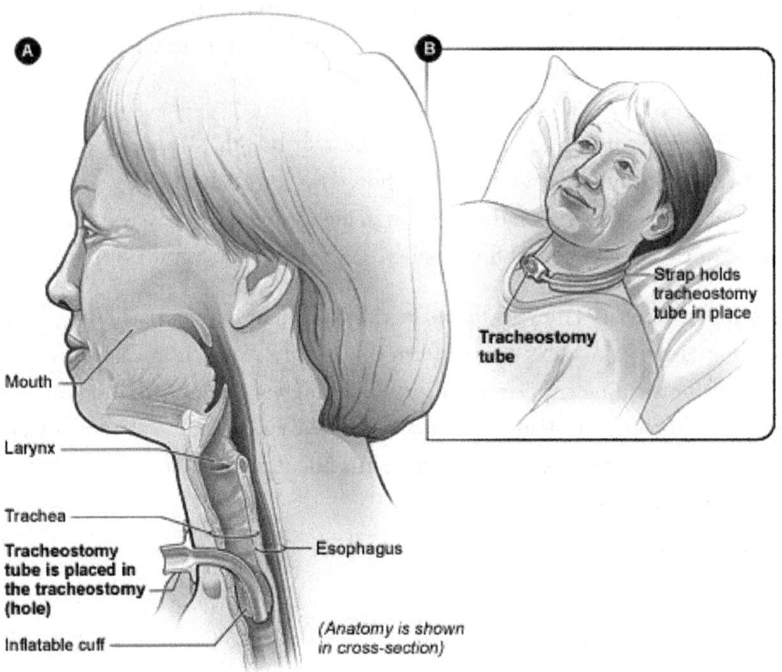

Figure 22.2 Patient with Tracheostomy Tube

Placement of a tracheostomy tube may be performed emergently or as a planned procedure due to the following:

- A large object blocking the airway
- Respiratory failure or arrest
- Severe neck or mouth injuries
- A swollen or blocked airway due to inhalation of harmful material such as smoke, steam, or other toxic gases
- Cancer of the throat or neck, which can affect breathing by pressing on the airway
- Paralysis of the muscles that affect swallowing
- Surgery around the larynx that prevents normal breathing and swallowing
- Long-term oxygen therapy via a mechanical ventilator[4]

---

3 "Tracheostomy NIH.jpg" by National Heart Lung and Blood Institute is in the Public Domain. Access for free at https://commons.wikimedia.org/wiki/File:Tracheostomy_NIH.jpg

4 A.D.A.M. Medical Encyclopedia [Internet]. Atlanta (GA): A.D.A.M., Inc.; c1997-2020. Nail abnormalities; [updated 2020, June 2] https://medlineplus.gov/ency/article/002955.htm

My Notes

See Figure 22.3[5] for an image of the parts of a tracheostomy tube. The outside end of the outer cannula has a flange that is placed against the patient's neck. The **flange** is secured around the patient's neck with tie straps, and a split 4" x 4" tracheostomy dressing is placed under the flange to absorb secretions. A cuff is typically present on the distal end of the outer cannula to make a tight seal in the airway. (See the top image in Figure 22.3.) The cuff is inflated and deflated with a syringe attached to the pilot balloon. Most tracheostomy tubes have a hollow **inner cannula** inside the **outer cannula** that is either disposable or removed for cleaning as part of the tracheostomy care procedure. (See the middle image of Figure 22.3.) A solid obturator is used during the initial tracheostomy insertion procedure to help guide the outer cannula through the tracheostomy and into the airway. (See the bottom image of Figure 22.3.) It is removed after insertion and the inner cannula is slid into place.

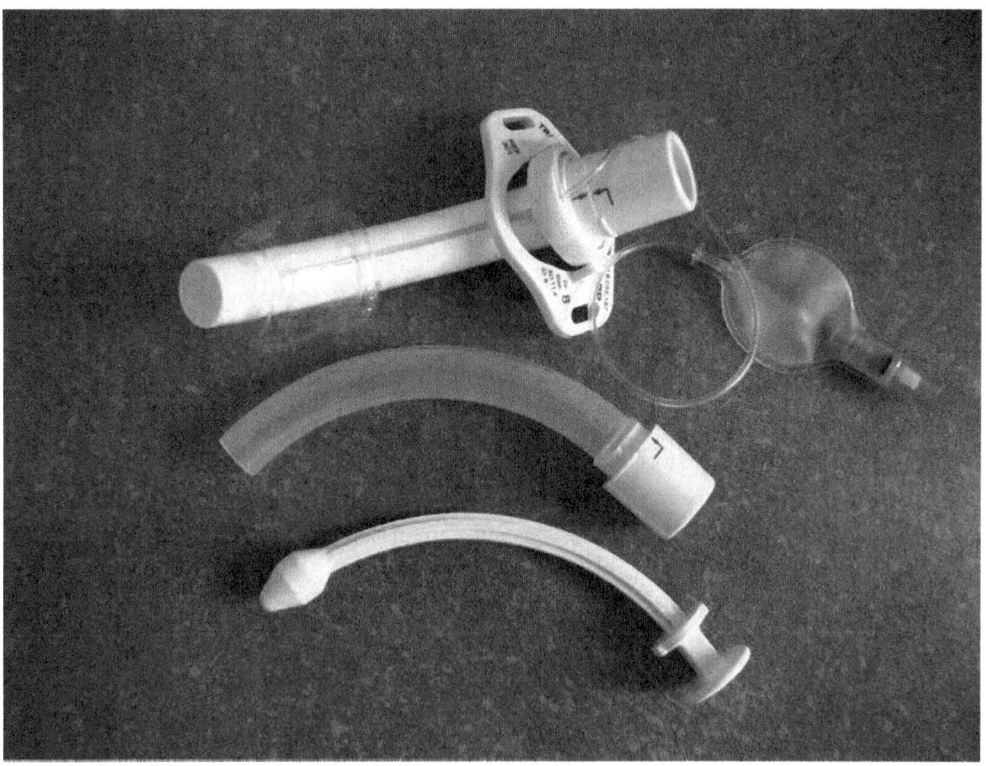

Figure 22.3 Parts of a Tracheostomy Tube

When a tracheostomy is placed, the provider determines if a fenestrated or unfenestrated outer cannula is needed based on the patient's condition. A **fenestrated** tube is used for patients who can speak with their tracheostomy tube in place. Under the guidance of a speech pathologist and respiratory therapist, the inner cannula is eventually removed from a fenestrated tube and the cuff deflated so the patient is able to speak. Otherwise, a patient with a tracheostomy tube is unable to speak because there is no airflow over the vocal cords, and alternative communication measures, such as a whiteboard, pen and paper, or computer device with note-taking ability, must be put into place by the nurse. Suctioning should never be performed through a fenestrated tube without first inserting

5 "Tracheostomy tube.jpg" by Kaluse D Peter, Wiehl, Germany is licensed under CC BY 2.0 DE. Access for free at https://commons.wikimedia.org/wiki/File:Tracheostomy_tube.jpg

My Notes

a nonfenestrated inner cannula, or severe tracheal damage can occur. See Figure 22.4[6] for images of a fenestrated and nonfenestrated outer cannula.

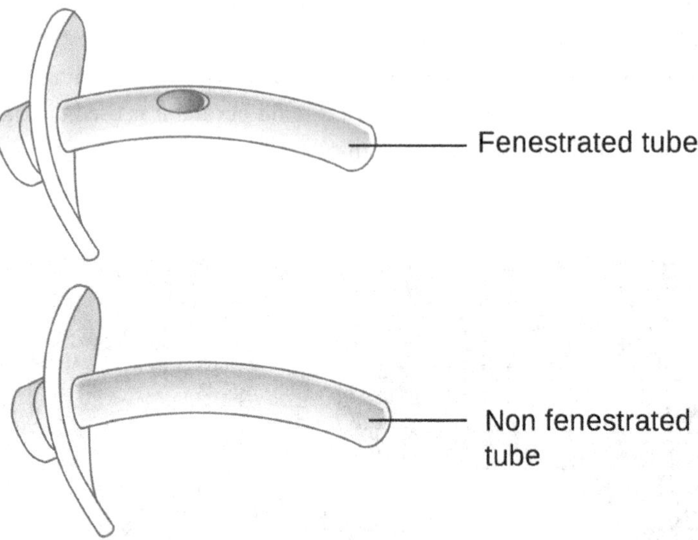

Figure 22.4 Fenestrated and Nonfenestrated Outer Cannula

Caring for a patient with a tracheostomy tube includes providing routine tracheostomy care and suctioning. Tracheostomy care is a procedure performed routinely to keep the flange, tracheostomy dressing, ties or straps, and surrounding area clean to reduce the introduction of bacteria into the trachea and lungs. The inner cannula becomes occluded with secretions and must be cleaned or replaced frequently according to agency policy to maintain an open airway. Suctioning through the tracheostomy tube is also performed to remove mucus and to maintain a patent airway.

When caring for a patient with a tracheostomy tube in the acute care setting, it is important to ensure that proper safety equipment is present at the patient's bedside. Patients with a tracheostomy should have the obturator used for initial tracheostomy placement present and readily available. Many health facilities recommend that obturators be taped to the wall at the head of the bed in case of the need for emergency tracheostomy tube reinsertion. Additionally, there should be spare tracheostomy tubes (same size and one size smaller), lubricant, syringe for cuff inflation, and tracheostomy ties (or means to resecure the tracheostomy tube) if reinsertion is required. A bag valve mask should always be kept at the bedside.

6 "Diagram showing a fenestrated and a non fenestrated tracheostomy tube CRUK 066.svg" by Cancer Research UK is licensed under CC BY-SA 4.0. Access for free at https://commons.wikimedia.org/wiki/File:Diagram_showing_a_fenestrated_and_a_non_fenestrated_tracheostomy_tube_CRUK_066.svg

My Notes

22.3 ASSESSMENTS RELATED TO AIRWAY SUCTIONING

Subjective Assessment

If appropriate, perform a focused interview collecting a brief history of respiratory conditions and assess for feelings of shortness of breath (dyspnea), sputum production, and coughing.

Objective Assessment

Prior to suctioning, a baseline assessment for indications of respiratory distress and the need for suctioning should be obtained and documented, including, but not limited to, the following:

- Secretions from the mouth and/or tracheal stoma
- Auscultation of lung sounds
- Heart rate
- Respiratory rate
- Cardiac rhythm
- Oxygen saturation
- Skin color and perfusion
- Effectiveness of cough[1]

Prepare the patient by explaining the procedure and providing adequate sedation and pain relief as needed. Place the patient in semi-Fowler's position if conscious or in a lateral position facing you if they are unconscious. While suctioning the patient, if signs of worsening respiratory distress occur, stop the procedure and request emergency assistance. The following should be monitored during and following the procedure:

- Lung sounds
- Skin color
- Breathing pattern and rate
- Oxygenation (pulse oximeter)
- Pulse rate
- Dysrhythmias if electrocardiogram is available
- Color, consistency, and volume of secretions
- Presence of bleeding or evidence of physical trauma
- Subjective response including pain
- Cough
- Laryngospasm (spasm of the vocal cords that can result in airway obstruction)[2]

---

1 American Association for Respiratory Care. (2004). AARC clinical practice guideline: Nasotracheal suctioning - 2004 revision & update. *Respiratory Care, 49*(9), 1080-1084. https://www.aarc.org/wp-content/uploads/2014/08/09.04.1080.pdf

2 American Association for Respiratory Care. (2004). AARC clinical practice guideline: Nasotracheal suctioning - 2004 revision & update. *Respiratory Care, 49*(9), 1080-1084. https://www.aarc.org/wp-content/uploads/2014/08/09.04.1080.pdf

My Notes

After completing suctioning, the outcomes from the procedure should be evaluated and documented, including the following:

- Improvement of lung sounds
- Removal of secretions
- Improvement of pulse oximetry
- Decreased work of breathing
- Stabilized respiratory rate
- Decreased dyspnea

Be aware that the patient's lung sounds may not clear completely after suctioning, but the removal of secretions should improve the patency of the patient's airway.

Potential complications resulting from this procedure include nasal irritation/bleeding, gagging/vomiting, discomfort and pain, and uncontrolled coughing. Potential adverse reactions include mucosal hemorrhage, laceration of nasal turbinate, perforation of the pharynx, hypoxia/hypoxemia, cardiac dysrhythmias/arrest, bradycardia, elevated blood pressure, hypotension, respiratory arrest, laryngospasm, bronchoconstriction, bronchospasm, hospital-acquired infection, atelectasis, increased intracranial pressure, and pneumothorax.

22.4 Oropharyngeal and Nasopharyngeal Suctioning Checklist & Sample Documentation

My Notes

Suctioning via the **oropharyngeal** (mouth) and nasopharyngeal (nasal) routes is performed to remove accumulated saliva, pulmonary secretions, blood, vomitus, and other foreign material from these areas that cannot be removed by the patient's spontaneous cough or other less invasive procedures. Nasal and pharyngeal suctioning are performed in a wide variety of settings, including critical care units, emergency departments, inpatient acute care, skilled nursing facility care, home care, and outpatient/ambulatory care. Suctioning is indicated when the patient is unable to clear secretions and/or when there is audible or visible evidence of secretions in the large/central airways that persist in spite of the patient's best cough effort. Need for suctioning is evidenced by one or more of the following:

- Visible secretions in the airway
- Chest auscultation of coarse, gurgling breath sounds, rhonchi, or diminished breath sounds
- Reported feeling of secretions in the chest
- Suspected aspiration of gastric or upper airway secretions
- Clinically apparent increased work of breathing
- Restlessness
- Unrelieved coughing[1]

In emergent situations, a provider order is not necessary for suctioning to maintain a patient's airway. However, routine suctioning does require a provider order.

For oropharyngeal suctioning, a device called a **Yankauer suction tip** is typically used for suctioning mouth secretions. A Yankauer device is rigid and has several holes for suctioning secretions that are commonly thick and difficult for the patient to clear. See Figure 22.5[2] for an image of a Yankauer device. In many agencies, Yankauer suctioning can be delegated to trained assistive personnel if the patient is stable, but the nurse is responsible for assessing and documenting the patient's respiratory status.

---

1 American Association for Respiratory Care. (2004). AARC clinical practice guideline: Nasotracheal suctioning - 2004 revision & update. *Respiratory Care, 49*(9), 1080-1084. https://www.aarc.org/wp-content/uploads/2014/08/09.04.1080.pdf

2 "Yankauer Suction Tip.jpg" by *Thomasrive* is licensed under CC BY-SA 3.0. Access for free at https://commons.wikimedia.org/wiki/File:Yankauer_Suction_Tip.jpg

My Notes

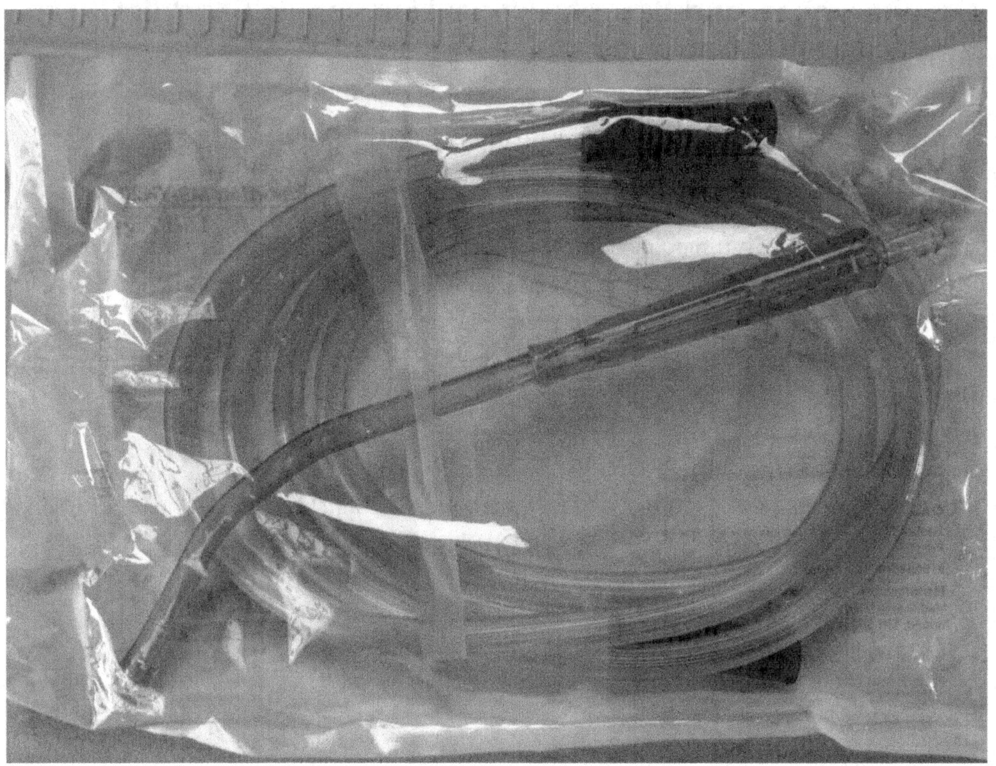

Figure 22.5 Yankauer Suction Tip

Yankauer suction devices are made of rigid firm plastic. The nurse or assistive personnel who performs suctioning with these devices should use care to protect the patient's soft mucous membranes and prevent unnecessary trauma.

Nasopharyngeal suctioning removes secretions from the nasal cavity, pharynx, and throat by inserting a flexible, soft suction catheter through the nares. This type of suctioning is performed when oral suctioning with a Yankauer is ineffective. See Figure 22.6[3] for an image of a sterile suction catheter.

3 "DSC_0210-150x150.jpg" by British Columbia Institute of Technology is licensed under CC BY 4.0. Access for free at https://opentextbc.ca/clinicalskills/chapter/5-7-oral-suctioning/

My Notes

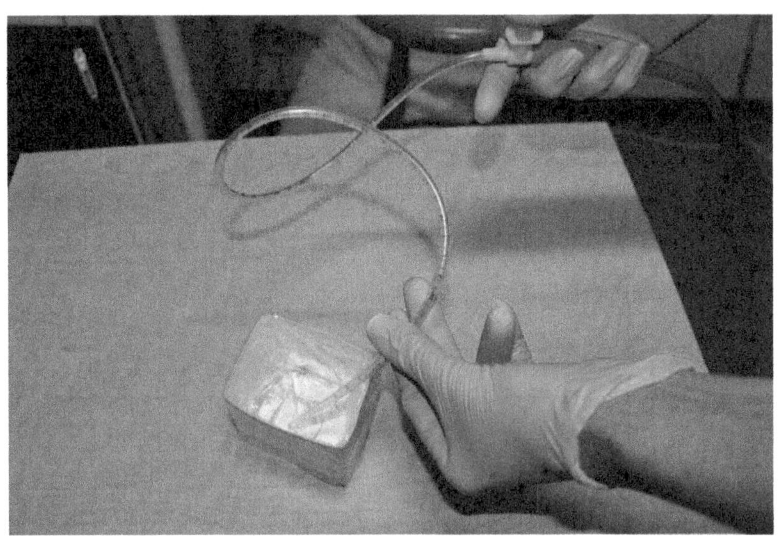

Figure 22.6 Sterile Suction Catheter

Extension tubing is used to attach the Yankauer or suction catheter device to a suction canister that is attached to wall suction or a portable suction source. The amount of suction is set to an appropriate pressure according to the patient's age. See Figure 22.7[4] for an image of extension tubing attached to a suction canister that is connected to a wall suctioning source.

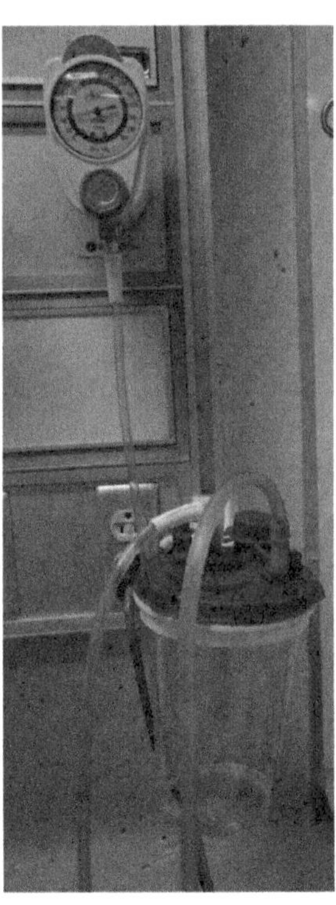

Figure 22.7 Tubing Attaching Suction Canister to Wall Suction Source

4 "DSC_0206-e1437445438554.jpg" by British Columbia Institute of Technology is licensed under CC BY 4.0. Access for free at https://opentextbc.ca/clinicalskills/chapter/5-7-oral-suctioning/

My Notes

Follow agency policy regarding setting suction pressure. Pressure should not exceed 150 mm Hg because higher pressures have been shown to cause trauma, hypoxemia, and atelectasis. The following ranges are appropriate pressure according to the patient's age:

- Neonates: 60-80 mm Hg
- Infants: 80-100 mm Hg
- Children: 100-120 mm Hg
- Adults: 100-150 mm Hg

Suction only when clinically indicated and for up to 15 seconds at a time to decrease the risk of respiratory complications. Hyperoxygenation and hyperventilation should be performed prior to the nasal and tracheal procedures to avoid the most common hazards of suctioning (hypoxemia, arrhythmias, and atelectasis). For nasal suctioning, increase the amount of O2 the patient is receiving for a few minutes prior to the procedure and instruct the patient to take several deep breaths. For tracheal suctioning, do the same. If the patient is on a ventilator, you can either hyperoxygenate and ventilate with the Ambu bag or provide a few extra machine assisted breaths prior to the procedure. Allow the patient to recover and hyperventilate and hyperoxygenate between each passing of the suction catheter. The patient should recover for 30-60 seconds between passes.[5]

When performing nasal suctioning, have the patient lean their head backwards to open the airway. This helps guide the catheter toward the trachea rather than the esophagus.

Checklist for Oropharyngeal or Nasopharyngeal Suctioning

Use the checklist below to review the steps for completion of "Oropharyngeal or Nasopharyngeal Suctioning."

Steps

Disclaimer: Always review and follow agency policy regarding this specific skill.

1. Gather supplies: Yankauer or suction catheter, suction machine or wall suction device, suction canister, connecting tubing, pulse oximeter, stethoscope, PPE (e.g., mask, goggles or face shield, nonsterile gloves), sterile gloves for suctioning with sterile suction catheter, towel or disposable paper drape, nonsterile basin or

---

5 American Association for Respiratory Care. (2010). AARC clinical practice guideline: Endotracheal suctioning of mechanically ventilated patients with artificial airways 2010. *Respiratory Care, 55*(6), 758-764. http://www.rcjournal.com/cpgs/pdf/06.10.0758.pdf

disposable cup, and normal saline or tap water.

My Notes

2. Perform safety steps:
    - Perform hand hygiene.
    - Check the room for transmission-based precautions.
    - Introduce yourself, your role, the purpose of your visit, and an estimate of the time it will take.
    - Confirm patient ID using two patient identifiers (e.g., name and date of birth).
    - Explain the process to the patient.
    - Be organized and systematic.
    - Use appropriate listening and questioning skills.
    - Listen and attend to patient cues.
    - Ensure the patient's privacy and dignity.
    - Assess ABCs.
3. Adjust the bed to a comfortable working height and lower the side rail closest to you.
4. Position the patient:
    - If conscious, place the patient in a semi-Fowler's position.
    - If unconscious, place the patient in the lateral position, facing you.
5. Move the bedside table close to your work area and raise it to waist height.
6. Place a towel or waterproof pad across the patient's chest.
7. Adjust the suction to the appropriate pressure:
    - Adults and adolescents: no more than 150 mm Hg
    - Children: no more than 120 mmHg
    - Infants: no more than 100 mm Hg
    - Neonates: no more than 80 mm Hg

   For a portable unit:
    - Adults: 10 to 15 cm Hg
    - Adolescents: 8 to 15 cm Hg
    - Children: 8 to 10 cm Hg
    - Infants: 8 to 10 cm Hg
    - Neonates: 6 to 8 cm Hg
8. Put on a clean glove and occlude the end of the connection tubing to check suction pressure.
9. Place the connecting tubing in a convenient location (e.g., at the head of the bed).

My Notes

10. Open the sterile suction package using aseptic technique. (NOTE: The open wrapper or container becomes a sterile field to hold other supplies.) Carefully remove the sterile container, touching only the outside surface. Set it up on the work surface and fill with sterile saline using sterile technique.

11. Place a small amount of water-soluble lubricant on the sterile field, taking care to avoid touching the sterile field with the lubricant package.

12. Increase the patient's supplemental oxygen level or apply supplemental oxygen per facility policy or primary care provider order.

13. Don additional PPE. Put on a face shield or goggles and mask.

14. Don sterile gloves. The dominant hand will manipulate the catheter and must remain sterile.

15. The nondominant hand is considered clean rather than sterile and will control the suction valve on the catheter.

    - In the home setting and other community-based settings, maintenance of sterility is not necessary.

16. With the dominant gloved hand, pick up the sterile suction catheter. Pick up the connecting tubing with the nondominant hand and connect the tubing and suction catheter.

17. Moisten the catheter by dipping it into the container of sterile saline. Occlude the suction valve on the catheter to check for suction.

18. Encourage the patient to take several deep breaths.

19. Apply lubricant to the first 2 to 3 inches of the catheter, using the lubricant that was placed on the sterile field.

20. Remove the oxygen delivery device, if appropriate. Do not apply suction as the catheter is inserted. Hold the catheter between your thumb and forefinger.

21. Insert the catheter. For nasopharyngeal suctioning, gently insert the catheter through the naris and along the floor of the nostril toward the trachea. Roll the catheter between your fingers to help advance it. Advance the catheter approximately 5 to 6 inches to reach the pharynx. For oropharyngeal suctioning, insert the catheter through the mouth, along the side of the mouth toward the trachea. Advance the catheter 3 to 4 inches to reach the pharynx.

22. Apply suction by intermittently occluding the suction valve on the catheter with the thumb of your nondominant hand and continuously rotate the catheter as it is being withdrawn.[6]

    - Suction only on withdrawal and do not suction for more than 10 to 15 seconds at a time to minimize tissue trauma.

23. Replace the oxygen delivery device using your nondominant hand, if appropriate, and have the patient take several deep breaths.

---

6 Oronasopharyngeal suctioning. (2020). Lippincott procedures. http://procedures.lww.com

My Notes

24. Flush the catheter with saline. Assess the effectiveness of suctioning by listening to lung sounds and repeat, as needed, and according to the patient's tolerance. Wrap the suction catheter around your dominant hand between attempts:

    - Repeat the procedure up to three times until gurgling or bubbling sounds stop and respirations are quiet. Allow 30 seconds to 1 minute between passes to allow reoxygenation and reventilation.[7]

25. When suctioning is completed, remove gloves from the dominant hand over the coiled catheter, pulling them off inside out.

26. Remove the glove from the nondominant hand and dispose of gloves, catheter, and the container with solution in the appropriate receptacle.

27. Assist the patient to a comfortable position. Raise the bed rail and place the bed in the lowest position.

28. Turn off the suction. Remove the supplemental oxygen placed for suctioning, if appropriate.

29. Remove face shield or goggles and mask; perform hand hygiene.

30. Perform oral hygiene on the patient after suctioning.

31. Reassess the patient's respiratory status, including respiratory rate, effort, oxygen saturation, and lung sounds.

32. Assist the patient to a comfortable position, ask if they have any questions, and thank them for their time.

33. Ensure safety measures when leaving the room:

    - CALL LIGHT: Within reach
    - BED: Low and locked (in lowest position and brakes on)
    - SIDE RAILS: Secured
    - TABLE: Within reach
    - ROOM: Risk-free for falls (scan room and clear any obstacles)

34. Perform hand hygiene.

35. Document the procedure and related assessment findings. Report any concerns according to agency policy.

Sample Documentation

Sample Documentation of Expected Findings

Patient complaining of not being able to cough up secretions. Order was obtained to suction via the nasopharyngeal route. Procedure explained to the patient. Vital signs obtained prior to procedure were heart rate 88 in regular rhythm, respiratory rate 28/minute, and O2 sat 88% on room air. Coarse rhonchi present over anterior upper airway. No cyanosis present. Patient tolerated procedure without difficulties. A small amount of clear, white, thick sputum was obtained. Post-procedure vital signs were heart rate 78 in regular rhythm, respiratory rate 18/minute, and O2 sat 94% on room air. Lung sounds clear and no cyanosis present.

---

7 Oronasopharyngeal suctioning. (2020). Lippincott procedures. http://procedures.lww.com

My Notes

Sample Documentation of Unexpected Findings

Patient complaining of not being able to cough up secretions. Order was obtained to suction via the nasopharyngeal route. Procedure explained to the patient. Vital signs obtained prior to procedure were heart rate 88 in regular rhythm, respiratory rate 28/minute, and O2 sat 88% on room air. Coarse rhonchi present over anterior upper airway. No cyanosis present. After first pass of suctioning, patient began coughing uncontrollably. Procedure was stopped and emergency assistance was requested from the respiratory therapist. Post-procedure vital signs were heart rate 78 in regular rhythm, respiratory rate 18/minute, and O2 sat 94% on room air. Coarse rhonchi continued to be present over anterior upper airway but no cyanosis present. Dr. Smith notified and a STAT order was received for a chest X-ray and to call with results.

22.5 CHECKLIST FOR TRACHEOSTOMY SUCTIONING AND SAMPLE DOCUMENTATION

My Notes

Tracheostomy suctioning may be performed with open or closed technique. Open suctioning requires disconnection of the patient from the oxygen source, whereas closed suctioning uses an inline suctioning catheter that does not require disconnection. This checklist will explain the open suctioning technique.

Indications for tracheostomy suctioning include the following:

- The need to maintain the patency and integrity of the artificial airway
- Deterioration of oxygen saturation and/or arterial blood gas values
- Visible secretions in the airway
- The patient's inability to generate an effective spontaneous cough
- Acute respiratory distress
- Suspected aspiration of gastric or upper-airway secretions
- The need to obtain a sputum specimen[1]

Similar assessments and monitoring apply when performing tracheostomy suctioning compared with other types of suctioning with the addition of assessing the stoma. The stoma should be free from redness and drainage. Hyperoxygenation using a bag mask valve attached to an oxygen source may be required before and during the open suctioning procedure based on the patient's oxygenation status. See Figure 22.8[2] for an image of an example of sterile tracheostomy suctioning kit.

---

1 American Association for Respiratory Care. (2010). AARC clinical practice guideline: Endotracheal suctioning of mechanically ventilated patients with artificial airways 2010. *Respiratory Care, 55*(6), 758-764. http://www.rcjournal.com/cpgs/pdf/06.10.0758.pdf

2 "Example of a Sterile Tracheostomy Kit" by Julie Teeter at Gateway Technical College is licensed under CC BY 4.0. Access for free at https://drive.google.com/file/d/1cIjGbGZznlYvI_JRO1GhRExvvW40WYXK/view?usp=sharing

My Notes

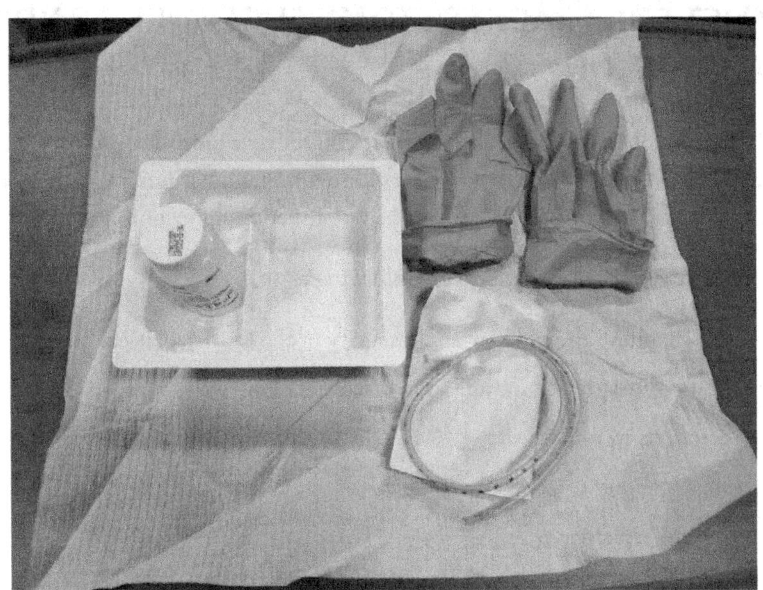

Figure 22.8 Example of a Sterile Tracheostomy Kit

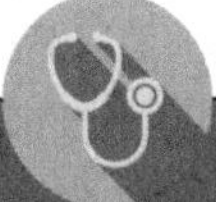

- To ensure patient safety, a replacement tracheostomy tube, an obturator, a bag valve mask (Ambu bag), and suction catheter kit must always be available in the room.
- Communication should be facilitated with the patient using writing when possible.
- Follow agency policy regarding hyperoxygenation and hyperventilation prior to and during suctioning.
- Do not suction for more than 15 seconds per pass.[3]
- During the procedure, it is important to continually monitor the patient's pulse oximetry to determine if the oxygen saturation is maintaining at an adequate level.
- Perform oral care after suctioning according to agency policy.

Checklist for Tracheostomy Suctioning[4]

Use the checklist below to review the steps for "Tracheostomy Suctioning."

3 American Association for Respiratory Care. (2010). AARC clinical practice guideline: Endotracheal suctioning of mechanically ventilated patients with artificial airways 2010. *Respiratory Care, 55*(6), 758-764. http://www.rcjournal.com/cpgs/pdf/06.10.0758.pdf

4 Tracheostomy suctioning. (2020). Lippincott procedures. http://procedures.lww.com

Steps

My Notes

Disclaimer: Always review and follow agency policy regarding this specific skill.

1. Gather supplies: sterile gloves, trach suction kit, mask with face shield, gown, goggles, pulse oximetry, and bag valve device. It is helpful to request assistance from a second nurse if preoxygenating the patient before suction passes.
2. Perform safety steps.
    - Perform hand hygiene.
    - Check the room for transmission-based precautions.
    - Introduce yourself, your role, the purpose of your visit, and an estimate of the time it will take.
    - Confirm patient ID using two patient identifiers (e.g., name and date of birth).
    - Explain the process to the patient and ask if they have any questions.
    - Be organized and systematic.
    - Use appropriate listening and questioning skills.
    - Listen and attend to patient cues.
    - Ensure the patient's privacy and dignity.
    - Assess ABCs.
3. Verify that there are a backup tracheostomy and bag valve device available at the bedside.
4. Assess lung sounds, heart rate and rhythm, and pulse oximetry.
5. Raise the head of the bed to waist level. Place the patient in a semi-Fowler's position and apply the pulse oximeter for monitoring during the procedure.
6. Turn on the suction. Set the suction gauge to appropriate setting based on age of the patient.
7. Perform hand hygiene. Don appropriate PPE (gown and mask).
8. Open the suction catheter package faced away from you to maintain sterility.
9. Don the sterile gloves from the kit.
10. Remove the sterile fluid and check the expiration date.
11. Open the sterile container used for flushing the catheter and place it back into the kit. Pour the sterile fluid into the sterile container using sterile technique.
12. Remove the suction catheter from the packaging. Ensure the catheter size is not greater than half of the inner diameter of the tracheostomy tube.
13. Keep the catheter sterile by holding it with your dominant hand and attaching it to the suction tubing with your nondominant hand. Note that your nondominant hand is no longer sterile.
14. Test the suction and lubricate the sterile catheter by using your sterile hand to dip the end into the sterile saline while occluding the thumb control.

My Notes

15. Ask an assistant to preoxygenate the patient with 100% oxygen for 30 to 60 seconds using a handheld bag valve mask (Ambu bag) per agency protocol. Alternatively, ask the patient to take two or three deep breaths if able.

16. Insert the catheter into the patient's tracheostomy tube using your sterile hand without applying suctioning:

    - For shallow suctioning, insert the catheter the length of the tracheostomy tube before beginning any suctioning.
    - For deep suctioning, insert the catheter until resistance is met (at the carina) and withdraw 1 centimeter before beginning suctioning.
    - Do not force the catheter.
    - Keep the dominant (sterile) hand at least one inch from the end of the trach tube.
    - To apply suction, place your nondominant thumb over the control valve

17. Withdraw the catheter while continually rotating it between your fingers to suction all sides of the tracheostomy tube. Do not suction longer than 15 seconds to prevent hypoxia. Follow agency policy regarding the use of intermittent or continuous suctioning. Do not contaminate the catheter as you remove it from the trach tube.

18. Suction sterile saline each time the suction catheter is removed to flush the catheter and suction tubing of secretions.

19. Assess the patient response to suctioning; hyperoxygenation may be required. If dysrhythmia or bradycardia occur, stop the procedure.

20. Allow the patient to rest. After the patient's pulse oximetry returns to baseline, a second suctioning pass can be initiated if clinically indicated. Encourage the patient to cough and deep breath to remove secretions between suctioning passes.

21. Do not insert the suction catheter more than two times. If the patient's respiratory status does not improve or it worsens, call for emergency assistance.

22. Reattach the preexisting oxygen delivery device to the patient with your noncontaminated hand.

23. Evaluate the effectiveness of the procedure and the patient's respiratory status. Assess patency of the airway and pulse oximetry.

24. Remove the catheter from the tubing and then remove gloves while holding the catheter inside the glove. Perform hand hygiene.

25. Turn off the suction.

26. Perform proper hand hygiene and don clean gloves.

27. Reassess lung sounds, heart rate and rhythm, and pulse oximetry for improvement .

28. Perform patient oral care.

29. Remove gloves and perform proper hand hygiene.

30. Assist the patient to a comfortable position, ask if they have any questions, and thank them for their time.

My Notes

31. Ensure safety measures when leaving the room:

    - CALL LIGHT: Within reach
    - BED: Low and locked (in lowest position and brakes on)
    - SIDERAILS: Secured
    - TABLE: Within reach
    - ROOM: Risk-free for falls (scan room and clear any obstacles)

32. Perform hand hygiene.

33. Document the procedure and related assessment findings. Report any concerns according to agency policy.

Sample Documentation

Sample Documentation of Expected Findings

Mucus present at entrance to tracheostomy tube. Hyperoxygenation provided for 30 seconds before and after suctioning using a bag valve mask with FiO2 100%. Patient's pulse oximetry remained 92-96% during suctioning. Moderate amount of thick, white mucus without odor was suctioned. Post procedure: HR 78, RR 18, O2 sat 96%, and lung sounds clear throughout all lobes. Patient tolerated the procedure without discomfort.

Sample Documentation of Unexpected Findings

Mucus present at entrance to tracheostomy tube. Hyperoxygenation provided for 30 seconds before and after suctioning using a bag valve mask with FiO2 100%. During the first suctioning pass, the ECG demonstrated bradycardia with HR dropping into the 50s. Suctioning was stopped. Trach tube was reattached to the mechanical ventilator and emergency assistance was requested from the respiratory therapist. Moderate amount of thick, white mucus without odor was suctioned. Post procedure, HR 78, RR 18, O2 sat 96% and lung sounds clear throughout all lobes.

My Notes

22.6 CHECKLIST FOR TRACHEOSTOMY CARE AND SAMPLE DOCUMENTATION

Tracheostomy care is provided on a routine basis to keep the tracheostomy tube's flange, inner cannula, and surrounding area clean to reduce the amount of bacteria entering the artificial airway and lungs. See Figure 22.9[1] for an image of a sterile tracheostomy care kit.

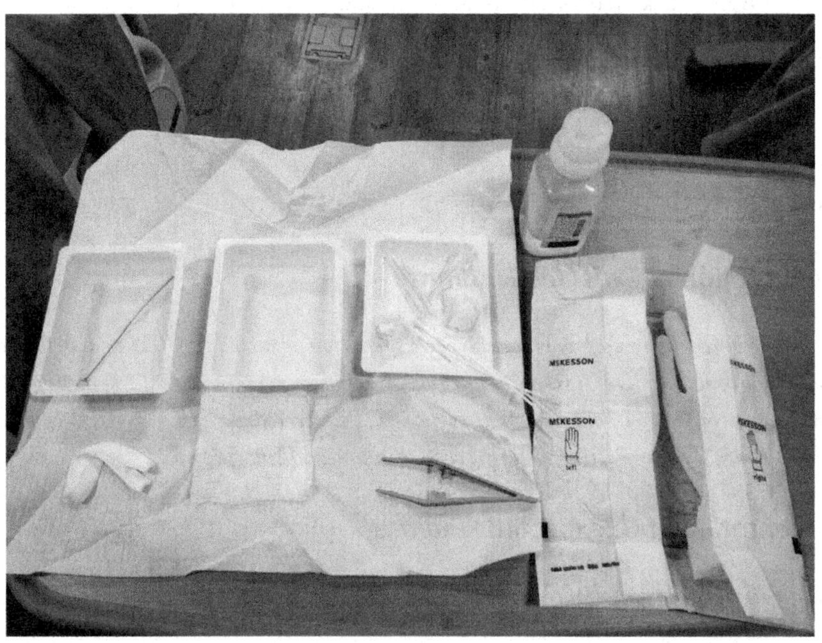

Figure 22.9 Sterile Tracheostomy Care Kit

Replacing and Cleaning an Inner Cannula

The primary purpose of the inner cannula is to prevent tracheostomy tube obstruction. Many sources of obstruction can be prevented if the inner cannula is regularly cleaned and replaced. Some inner cannulas are designed to be disposable, while others are reusable for a number of days. Follow agency policy for inner cannula replacement or cleaning, but as a rule of thumb, inner cannula cleaning should be performed every 12-24 hours at a minimum. Cleaning may be needed more frequently depending on the type of equipment, the amount and thickness of secretions, and the patient's ability to cough up the secretions.

Changing the inner cannula may encourage the patient to cough and bring mucus out of the tracheostomy. For this reason, the inner cannula should be replaced prior to changing the tracheostomy dressing to prevent secretions from soiling the new dressing. If the inner cannula is disposable, no cleaning is required.[2]

1 "Sterile Tracheostomy Care Kit" by Julie Teeter at Gateway Technical College is licensed under CC BY 4.0. Access for free at https://drive.google.com/file/d/1Q81N47BB2cOjgPs5GPpcth2CoXKsajqC/view?usp=sharing

2 This work is a derivative of 12 by British Columbia Institute of Technology and is licensed under CC BY 4.0. Access for free at https://opentextbc.ca/clinicalskills/

Checklist for Tracheostomy Care With a Reusable Inner Cannula

My Notes

Use the checklist below to review the steps for completion of "Tracheostomy Care."

Stoma site should be assessed and a clean dressing applied at least once per shift. Wet or soiled dressings should be changed immediately.[3] Follow agency policy regarding clearing the inner cannula; it should be inspected at least twice daily and cleaned as needed.

Steps

Disclaimer: Always review and follow agency policy regarding this specific skill.

1. Gather supplies: bedside table, towel, sterile gloves, pulse oximeter, PPE (i.e., mask, goggles, or face shield), tracheostomy suctioning equipment, bag valve mask (should be located in the room), and a sterile tracheostomy care kit (or sterile cotton-tipped applicators, sterile manufactured **tracheostomy split sponge dressing,** sterile basin, normal saline, and a disposable inner cannula or a small, sterile brush to clean the reusable inner cannula).
2. Perform safety steps:
    - Perform hand hygiene.
    - Check the room for transmission-based precautions.
    - Introduce yourself, your role, the purpose of your visit, and an estimate of the time it will take.
    - Confirm patient ID using two patient identifiers (e.g., name and date of birth).
    - Explain the process to the patient and ask if they have any questions.
    - Be organized and systematic.
    - Use appropriate listening and questioning skills.
    - Listen and attend to patient cues.
    - Ensure the patient's privacy and dignity.
    - Assess ABCs.
3. Raise the bed to waist level and place the patient in a semi-Fowler's position.
4. Verify that there is a backup tracheostomy kit available.
5. Don appropriate PPE.
6. Perform tracheal suctioning if indicated.
7. Remove and discard the trach dressing. Inspect drainage on the dressing for color and amount and note any odor.
8. Inspect stoma site for redness, drainage, and signs and symptoms of infection.

---

3 Nance-Floyd, B. (2011). Tracheostomy care: An evidence-based guide. *American Nurse*. https://www.myamericannurse.com/tracheostomy-care-an-evidence-based-guide-to-suctioning-and-dressing-changes/

My Notes

9. Remove the gloves and perform proper hand hygiene.
10. Open the sterile package and loosen the bottle cap of sterile saline.
11. Don one sterile glove on the dominant hand.
12. Open the sterile drape and place it on the patient's chest.
13. Set up the equipment on the sterile field.
14. Remove the cap and pour saline in both basins with ungloved hand (4"-6" above basin).
15. Don the second sterile glove.
16. Prepare and arrange supplies. Place pipe cleaners, trach ties, trach dressing, and forceps on the field. Moisten cotton applicators and place them in the third (empty) basin. Moisten two 4" x 4" pads in saline, wring out, open, and separately place each one in the third basin. Leave one 4" x 4" dry.
17. With nondominant "contaminated" hand, remove the trach collar (if applicable) and remove (unlock and twist) the inner cannula. If the patient requires continuous supplemental oxygen, place the oxygenation device near the outer cannula or ask a staff member to assist in maintaining the oxygen supply to the patient.
18. Place the inner cannula in the saline basin.
19. Pick up the inner cannula with your nondominant hand, holding it only by the end usually exposed to air.
20. With your dominant hand, use a brush to clean the inner cannula. Place the brush back into the saline basin.
21. After cleaning, place the inner cannula in the second saline basin with your nondominant hand and agitate for approximately 10 seconds to rinse off debris. Repeat cleansing with brush as needed.
22. Dry the inner cannula with the pipe cleaners and place the inner cannula back into the outer cannula. Lock it into place and pull gently to ensure it is locked appropriately. Reattach the preexisting oxygenation device.
23. Clean the stoma with cotton applicators using one on the superior aspect and one on the inferior aspect.
24. With your dominant, noncontaminated hand, moisten sterile gauze with sterile saline and wring out excess. Assess the stoma for infection and skin breakdown caused by flange pressure. Clean the stoma with the moistened gauze starting at the 12 o'clock position of the stoma and wipe toward the 3 o'clock position. Begin again with a new gauze square at 12 o'clock and clean toward 9 o'clock. To clean the lower half of the site, start at the 3 o'clock position and clean toward 6 o'clock; then wipe from 9 o'clock to 6 o'clock, using a clean moistened gauze square for each wipe. Continue this pattern on the surrounding skin and tube flange. Avoid using a hydrogen peroxide mixture because it can impair healing.[4]
25. Use sterile gauze to dry the area.
26. Apply the sterile tracheostomy split sponge dressing by only touching the outer edges.
27. Replace trach ties as needed. (The literature overwhelmingly recommends a two-person technique when changing the securing device to prevent tube dislodgement. In the two-person technique, one person holds

---

4 Nance-Floyd, B. (2011). Tracheostomy care: An evidence-based guide. *American Nurse*. https://www.myamericannurse.com/tracheostomy-care-an-evidence-based-guide-to-suctioning-and-dressing-changes/

My Notes

the trach tube in place while the other changes the securing device). Thread the clean tie through the opening on one side of the trach tube. Bring the tie around the back of the neck, keeping one end longer than the other. Secure the tie on the opposite side of the trach. Make sure that only one finger can be inserted under the tie.

28. Remove the old tracheostomy ties.

29. Remove gloves and perform proper hand hygiene.

30. Provide oral care. Oral care keeps the mouth and teeth not only clean, but also has been shown to prevent hospital-acquired pneumonia.

31. Lower the bed to lowest the position. If the patient is on a mechanical ventilator, the head of the bed should be maintained at 30-45 degrees to prevent ventilator-associated pneumonia.

32. Assist the patient to a comfortable position, ask if they have any questions, and thank them for their time.

33. Ensure safety measures when leaving the room:

    - CALL LIGHT: Within reach
    - BED: Low and locked (in lowest position and brakes on)
    - SIDE RAILS: Secured
    - TABLE: Within reach
    - ROOM: Risk-free for falls (scan room and clear any obstacles)

34. Perform hand hygiene.

35. Document the procedure and related assessment findings. Report any concerns according to agency policy.

Sample Documentation

Sample Documentation of Expected Findings

Tracheostomy care provided with sterile technique. Stoma site free of redness or drainage. Inner cannula cleaned and stoma dressing changed. Patient tolerated the procedure without difficulties.

Sample Documentation of Unexpected Findings

Tracheostomy care provided with sterile technique. Stoma site is erythematous, warm, and tender to palpation. Inner cannula cleaned and stoma dressing changed. Patient tolerated the procedure without difficulties. Dr. Smith notified of change in condition of stoma at 1315 and stated would assess the patient this afternoon.

My Notes

22.7 SUPPLEMENTARY VIDEOS

View these videos from Santa Fe College for more information on tracheostomy care and suctioning:
"Trach Care Suction"[1]
"Trach Care – Washing the Inner Cannula"[2]

1 SF Educational Media Studio. (2017, August 11). SF Nursing Trach Care 1 Suction. [Video]. YouTube. All rights reserved. https://youtu.be/TNokX_WKCpY

2 SF Educational Media Studio. (2018, March 1). SF Nursing Trach Care Part 2 Change Wash Inner Cannula. [Video]. YouTube. All rights reserved. https://youtu.be/EWAA_saUDSo

22.8 LEARNING ACTIVITIES

My Notes

Learning Activities

(Answers to "Learning Activities" can be found in the "Answer Key" at the end of the book. Answers to interactive activity elements will be provided within the element as immediate feedback.)

1. You are caring for a patient with a tracheostomy. What supplies should you ensure are in the patient's room when you first assess the patient?
2. Your patient with a tracheostomy puts on their call light. As you enter the room, the patient is coughing violently and turning red. Prioritize the action steps that you will take.
   a. Assess lung sounds
   b. Suction patient
   c. Provide oxygen via the trach collar if warranted
   d. Check pulse oximetry

Interactive Activity

An interactive or media element has been excluded from this version of the text. You can view it online here: https://wtcs.pressbooks.pub/nursingskills/?p=817

Interactive Activity

An interactive or media element has been excluded from this version of the text. You can view it online here: https://wtcs.pressbooks.pub/nursingskills/?p=817

Interactive Activity

An interactive or media element has been excluded from this version of the text. You can view it online here: https://wtcs.pressbooks.pub/nursingskills/?p=817

My Notes

XXII GLOSSARY

Fenestrated cannula: Type of tracheostomy tube that contains holes so the patient can speak if the cuff is deflated and the inner cannula is removed.

Flange: The end of the tracheostomy tube that is placed securely against the patient's neck.

Inner cannula: The cannula inside the outer cannula that is removed during tracheostomy care by the nurse. Inner cannulas can be disposable or reusable with appropriate cleaning.

Oropharyngeal suctioning: Suction of secretions through the mouth, often using a Yankauer device.

Outer cannula: The outer cannula placed by the provider through the tracheostomy hole and continuously remains in place.

Suction canister: A container for collecting suctioned secretions that is attached to a suction source.

Suction catheter: A soft, flexible, sterile catheter used for nasopharyngeal and tracheostomy suctioning.

Tracheostomy: A surgically created opening that goes from the front of the neck into the trachea.

Tracheostomy dressing: A manufactured dressing used with tracheostomies that does not shed fibers, which could potentially be inhaled by the patient.

Yankauer suction tip: Rigid device used to suction secretions from the mouth.

Chapter 23

IV Therapy Management

23.1 IV THERAPY MANAGEMENT INTRODUCTION

My Notes

Learning Objectives

- Inspect established IV site for deviations from normal
- Prepare and safely administer primary and secondary IV fluids and medication
- Calculate and ensure designated flow rate
- Change IV tubing
- Change IV site dressing
- Discontinue short-term peripheral IV
- Modify the procedure to reflect variations across the life span
- Document actions and observation
- Report significant deviations from norms

The purpose of intravenous (IV) therapy is to replace fluid and electrolytes, provide medications, and replenish blood volume.

The nurse's responsibilities in managing IV therapy include the following:

- assessing an IV site
- priming and hanging a primary IV bag
- preparing and hanging a secondary IV bag
- calculating IV rates
- monitoring the effectiveness of IV therapy
- discontinuing a peripheral IV

IV medications and fluids enter the patient's bloodstream directly through the vein. They act rapidly within the body to restore fluid volume and deliver medications. Once a medication enters the vein, there is no way to terminate this action. Therefore, it is important to properly prepare the IV medication or fluid, correctly calculate the dosage, and administer it safely to the patient. Additionally, IV fluid administration is considered a medical intervention and requires a medication order prior to the initiation of fluid therapy.

My Notes

23.2 IV THERAPY BASICS

Primary IV Fluid Infusion

Primary IV fluid infusions are prescribed by health care providers to restore or maintain hydration and electrolyte status within the body. When administering IV fluids to a patient, the nurse must continually monitor the patient's fluid and electrolyte status to evaluate the effectiveness of the infusion and to avoid potential complications of fluid overload and electrolyte imbalance.

The most commonly used primary IV fluid bag contains 1,000 mL. There are also 500 mL, 250 mL, 100 mL, and 50 mL bags. The size of the primary fluid bag is based on infusion need, patient condition, and age. Most adult patients receive continuous IV fluids with 1,000 mL bags due to the higher drip (gtt) rate. Many other fluid volume bags are used for intermittent infusions or short-term therapy.

For example, for renal dialysis patients, IV bags smaller than 1,000 mL are used because large amounts of continuous fluids are contraindicated due to their renal impairment. Many institutions will hang smaller volume normal saline continuous infusion bags just to serve as an additional reminder that these patients should not receive large amounts of primary fluids. Another example of patients requiring smaller IV bags are pediatric patients who, due to their smaller anatomical size, do not require large primary fluid infusion volumes.

Primary fluids are typically administered using an IV pump. An IV pump is the safest method of administration to ensure specific amounts of fluid are administered. However, there may be situations when IV pumps are not available and nurses administer primary fluids by gravity using drip tubing. Read more about calculating infusion rates in the "Math Calculation" chapter.

Primary fluids are run at consistent infusion rates for a prescribed period of time. For example, a continuous fluid infusion may be ordered at a rate of 125 mL/hour for 24 hours. Continuous fluids may also be ordered to run until the provider gives a follow-up order to discontinue or decrease the fluid rate.

IV primary fluid bags consist of various types of fluid such as 0.9% normal saline, 0.45% (½) normal saline, lactated ringers solution, and dextrose (5%) preparations. They may also contain replacement electrolytes like potassium chloride. The provider will order primary fluids based on the patient's fluid and electrolyte statuses.

There are three types of intravenous fluid concentrations: isotonic, hypertonic, and hypotonic fluids.

- Isotonic fluids are typically administered for fluid and electrolyte replacement. Isotonic fluids have a similar concentration to the solutes contained in blood, so they do not cause the osmotic movement of fluid into or out of the patient's individual cells. An example of isotonic fluid is 0.9% normal saline.
- Hypertonic fluids have a higher concentration of solutes than blood. They are typically used in critical care situations to treat hyponatremia and avoid pulmonary edema by relying on osmosis to help remove excess fluid. An example of a hypertonic fluid is dextrose 5% in 0.9% normal saline (D5NS).
- Hypotonic fluids have a lower concentration of solutes than blood. The goal of hypotonic fluid administration is to move fluids into a patient's cells due to osmosis. Hypotonic solutions are commonly used when a patient has severe intracellular dehydration such as during diabetic

My Notes

ketoacidosis. An example of hypotonic fluid is 0.45% normal saline (1/2NS). See Figure 23.1[1] for an example of the effects of the administration of hypertonic, isotonic, and hypotonic IV fluids on a patient's red blood cells.

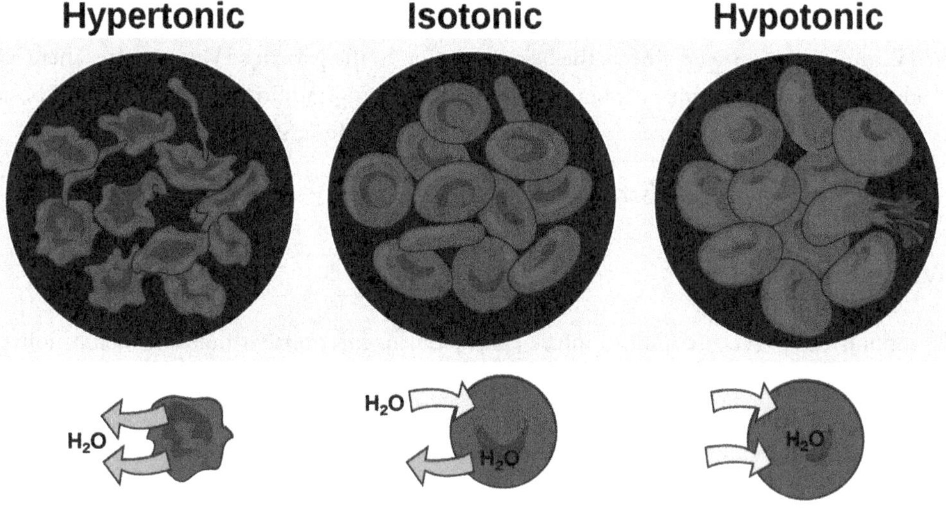

Figure 23.1 Osmotic Effects of Hypertonic, Isotonic, and Hypotonic IV Fluids on Red Blood Cells

Because a patient's fluid and electrolyte statuses are constantly changing when receiving IV fluids, it is important for the nurse to monitor for signs of fluid or electrolyte imbalances and appropriately notify the health care provider of any concerns. For example, primary fluids may be started at a higher rate of infusion when a patient is receiving nothing by mouth (NPO), but should be tapered as they resume normal diet and fluid intake. It is important for the nurse to continually monitor a patient's skin turgor, urinary output, lung sounds, and oxygen requirements and to assess for any new edema to offer important insight into their fluid volume status. A nurse must also evaluate the effects of replacement fluids and discuss their ongoing need with the prescribing provider.

Read more about types of intravenous fluids in the "Fluids and Electrolytes" chapter in Open RN *Nursing Fundamentals*.

Secondary Fluid Infusion

Secondary IV fluid administration is usually an intermittent infusion that infuses at regular intervals (e.g., every 8 hours). This form of IV therapy usually contains medications that are supplied in a smaller infusion bag and mixed with a diluent fluid like saline (e.g., IV antibiotics). Many common preparations come in 25 to 100 mL bags.

Secondary IV therapy is often referred to as "IV piggyback" (IVPB) medication because it is attached to the primary bag of intravenous fluids. In this case, the primary line maintains venous access between drug doses.

It is important to remember that not all IV solutions are compatible with all IV medications. It is vital for the nurse to triple check that the secondary medications/fluids are compatible with primary fluids. If medication and

1 "Osmotic pressure on blood cells diagram.svg" by LadyofHats is in the Public Domain. Access for free at https://commons.wikimedia.org/wiki/File:Osmotic_pressure_on_blood_cells_diagram.svg

My Notes

fluids are not compatible, a precipitate may form when the fluids mix within the line, posing a significant health danger for the patient.

IV Administration Equipment

Intravenous (IV) fluids and medications are administered through flexible plastic tubing called an IV administration set. The IV administration set connects the bag of solution to the patient's IV access site. There are two major types of IV administration sets: primary tubing and secondary tubing. Additionally, IV fluids can be administered by gravity or by infusion pump, and each method requires its own administration set.

Primary and Secondary Administration Sets

Primary IV Administration Sets

Primary IV administration sets are used to infuse continuous or intermittent fluids or medications. Primary IV tubing can be a macro-drip or micro-drip solution set. A macro-drip infusion set delivers 10, 15, or 20 drops per milliliter, whereas a micro-drip infusion set delivers 60 drops per milliliter. The drop factor is located on the packaging of the IV tubing and is important to verify when calculating medication administration rates.

Macro-drip sets are used for routine primary infusions for adults. Micro-drip IV tubing is used in pediatric or neonatal care where small amounts of fluids are administered over a long period of time.

Primary IV administration sets consist of the following parts:

Sterile spike: This part of the tubing must be kept sterile as you spike the IV fluid bag.

Drip chamber: The drip chamber allows air to rise out from a fluid so that it is not passed onto the patient. It is also used to calculate the rate at which fluid is administered by gravity (drops per minute). It should be kept ¼ to ½ full of solution.

Backcheck valve: A backcheck valve prevents fluid or medication from travelling up into the primary IV bag.

Access ports: Access ports are used to infuse secondary medications and to administer IV push medications. These may also be referred to as "Y ports."

Roller clamp: A roller clamp is used to regulate the speed, or stop, an infusion by gravity.

Secondary IV Administration Sets

Secondary IV administration sets are used to intermittently administer a secondary medication, such as an antibiotic, while the primary IV is also running. Secondary IV tubing is shorter in length than primary tubing and is connected to a primary line via an access port or an IV pump. The secondary infusion is hung above the primary infusion and connected at an access port.

Secondary fluids should always be "piggybacked" into primary infusion lines to ensure that the correct amount of medication is infused. By piggybacking a medication, the solution from the primary fluid line is used to prime the secondary tubing. However, if a secondary infusion is run as a primary fluid, there is a risk of losing some of the secondary medication when priming the line, which results in less medication being administered. Loss of medication is considered a medication error because the patient received less active medication than prescribed.

My Notes

See Figure 23.2[2] for an illustration of the set up of a primary and secondary tubing for administration of fluids and a secondary medication by gravity. See Figure 23.3[3] for an example of an IV infusion pump.

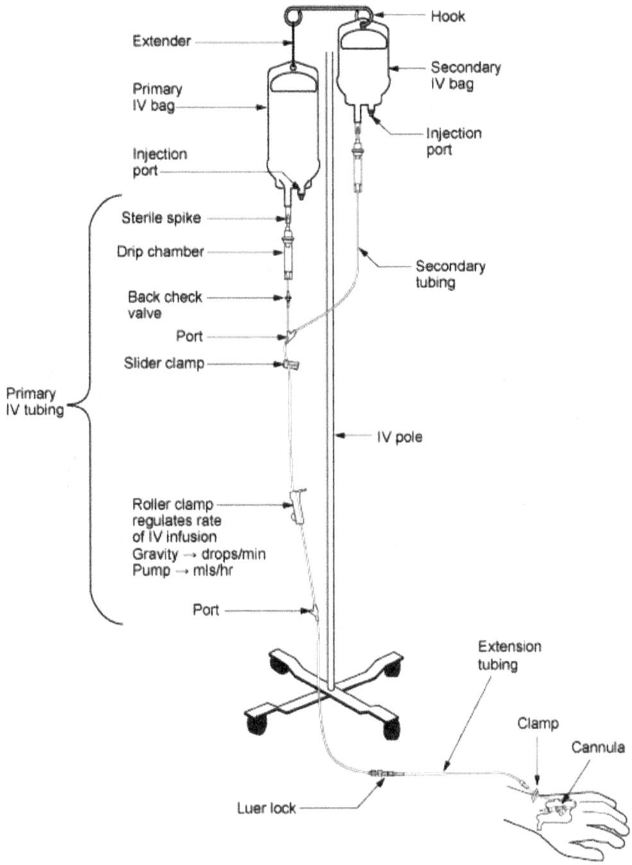

Figure 23.2 Primary and Secondary Tubing Administration Set

2 "intravenous_equipment_labels-2.png" by British Columbia Institute of Technology is licensed under CC BY 4.0. Access for free at https://opentextbc.ca/clinicalskills/chapter/8-2-types-of-iv-therapy/

3 "DSC_0738-e1443533768679-678x1024.jpg" by British Columbia Institute of Technology is licensed under CC BY 4.0. Access for free at https://opentextbc.ca/clinicalskills/chapter/8-2-types-of-iv-therapy/

My Notes

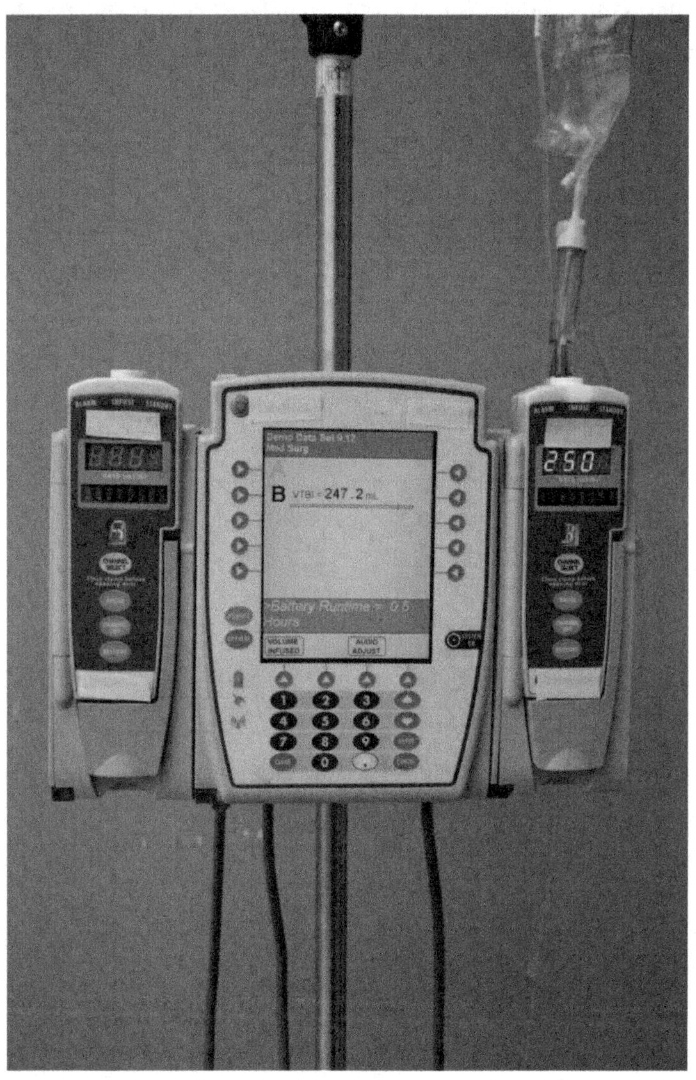

Figure 23.3 Example of an IV Infusion Pump

IV Administration

When initiating or changing an IV bag of fluids or medications, it is important to remember these items:

- IV fluids are a medication. Verify physician orders and check that the patient does not have an allergy to this medication. Perform the six rights of medication administration three times as you would when giving any other medication. Check the type of fluid and the expiration date, and verify the fluid is free of discoloration and sediment. Check the expiration date when obtaining a new tubing administration set.
- Examine the bag to ensure that the bag itself is intact and not leaking. There may be moisture on the inside of the plastic IV bag storage container; this is normal.
- Verify the infusion rate of IV fluids is appropriate based on the patient's age, size, preexisting medical conditions, and prescribed indication. If a manual calculation is needed to set the IV flow rate, calculate the rate and double-check the calculated rate with another registered nurse.

My Notes

- IV tubing administration sets require routine replacement to prevent infection. Follow agency policy regarding initiating tubing change before initiating a new bag of fluid or medications.
- If administration set tubing is present, trace the tubing from the patient to its point of origin to make sure that you're accessing the correct port.
- Assess the IV site. Inspect for redness, swelling, or tenderness that can be a sign of irritation, inflammation, or infection.
- Ensure the IV site is patent when initiating new fluid or medication. Aspirate for blood return and flush the IV catheter according to agency policy.

Complications of IV Therapy

While monitoring a patient receiving IV fluids, it is important to assess for potential complications such as infiltration, extravasation, phlebitis, or infection. If these conditions occur, promptly notify the provider for treatment; the IV catheter will need to be removed and replaced at an alternative site, and additional medication may be prescribed.

Infiltration occurs when the tip of the catheter slips out of the vein. The catheter passes through the wall of the vein, or the blood vessel wall allows part of the fluid to infuse into the surrounding tissue, resulting in the leakage of IV fluids into the surrounding tissue. Infiltration may cause pain, swelling, and skin that is cool to the touch. If you are concerned an IV is infiltrated, follow your facility policy and, as a general guideline, discontinue the site and relocate the IV. If the infiltration is severe, you may consider the application of a compress in addition to elevating the affected limb. Check your institution's policy regarding which type of compress (warm or cold) should be applied.[4,5] Additionally, clinical pharmacists can also be helpful resources for determining the appropriate type of infiltration treatment.

Extravasation refers to infiltration of damaging intravenous medications, such as chemotherapy, into the extravascular tissue around the site of infusion. Extravasation causes tissue injury, and depending on the medication, site, and length of exposure, it can cause tissue death, which is also referred to as necrosis. If detected early, extravasation may be treated with medications that help avoid the complication of necrosis.

Phlebitis is inflammation of a vein. Phlebitis of superficial veins can occur due to trauma to the vein during insertion of the IV catheter. It can cause redness and tenderness along the vein and can lead to infection if not treated appropriately. Treatment may include warm compresses and nonsteroidal anti-inflammatory medications.

Infection can occur whenever the skin barrier is broken by the insertion of an IV catheter. Signs of infection include redness, warmth, tenderness, and possible fever. Vascular catheter–associated infection is considered a hospital-acquired condition because it can be prevented using best practices. Be sure to follow evidence-based infection prevention practices, such as performing hand hygiene, performing a vigorous mechanical scrub of needleless connectors, limiting catheter access, and following sterile no-touch technique during intravenous infusion to reduce the risk of vascular catheter–associated infection.

---

4 Drugs.com [Internet]. IV Infiltration. © 2000-2020 [updated 3 February, 2020; cited 7 August, 2020]. https://www.drugs.com/cg/iv-infiltration-aftercare-instructions.html

5 AMN Healthcare Education Services. (2015). *Know the difference: Infiltration versus extravasation.* https://www.rn.com/nursing-news/know-the-difference-infiltration-vs-extravasation/

My Notes

23.3 INTRAVENOUS THERAPY ASSESSMENT

To prepare for intravenous therapy administration, the nurse should collect important subjective and objective assessment information from the patient.

Subjective Assessment

When performing the subjective assessment, the nurse should begin by focusing on data collection that may signify a potential complication if a patient receives IV infusion therapy. The nurse should begin by identifying if the patient has medication allergies or a latex allergy. The patient's history should also be considered with special attention given to those with known congestive heart failure (CHF) or chronic kidney disease (CKD) because they are more susceptible to developing fluid overload. Additionally, the patient should be asked if they have any pain or discomfort in their IV access site now or during the infusion of medications or fluids.

Life Span Considerations

Children

Safety measures for a child with an IV infusion include assessing the IV site every hour for patency. Infused volumes and signs of fluid overload should be carefully assessed and documented frequently per agency policy. The IV may be wrapped in gauze or an arm board may be used to deter the child from tampering with the IV site or tubing. Additionally, the tubing should be well-secured, and the dressing should remain free from moisture so the IV site is not compromised. Be aware that mobile children will require guidance to ensure that the tubing is not obstructed if they sit or lie on the tubing accidentally.

Older Adults

Older adults with an IV infusion should be frequently monitored for the development of fluid volume overload. Signs of fluid volume overload include elevated blood pressure and respiratory rate, decreased oxygen saturation, peripheral edema, fine crackles in the posterior lower lobes of the lungs, or signs of worsening heart failure. Additionally, older adults have delicate venous walls that may not withstand rapid infusion rates. It is important to monitor the IV site patency carefully when infusing large amounts of fluids at faster rates and appropriately modify the infusion rate.

Every time you interact with the patient, assess the IV site for signs of complications and educate the patient to inform you if there is tenderness or swelling at the IV site.

Objective Assessment

The patient's IV site should be checked for patency before initiating IV therapy and throughout the course of treatment. The IV site should be free of redness, swelling, coolness, or warmth to the touch. The IV infusion should flow freely. The nurse should also be aware of different types of intravenous access that may be used for an infusion. For example, a peripherally inserted central catheter (PICC) looks similar to intravenous access, but requires different assessment and monitoring as a central line. Please review Table 23.3 to consider the expected and unexpected assessment findings that may occur with IV therapy.

My Notes

Table 23.3 Expected Versus Unexpected Findings With IV Therapy		
Assessment	**Expected Findings**	**Unexpected Findings (document and notify provider if a new finding*)**
Inspection	IV site free of redness, swelling, tenderness, coolness, or warmth to touch	IV site with redness, swelling, tenderness, coolness, or warmth to the touch
Patency	IV fluid flows freely	IV fluid does not flow; patient reports pain during flush
***CRITICAL CONDITIONS to report immediately**		Notify the HCP if there is redness, warmth, or blisters at the site

My Notes

23.4 SAMPLE DOCUMENTATION

Sample Documentation of Expected Findings

Initiated IV infusion of normal saline at 125 mL/hr using existing 22 gauge IV catheter located in the right hand. The IV site is free from pain, coolness, redness, or swelling.

Sample Documentation of Unexpected Findings

Attempted to initiate IV infusion in right hand using existing 22 gauge IV catheter. The IV site was free from pain, redness, or signs of infiltration. It infused freely with the normal saline flush. IV fluids were connected to run the normal saline infusion at 200 mL/hr. The infusion was started, but immediate leaking around the infusion site was noted. Swelling was noted superior to the infusion site and the fluids were immediately stopped.

23.5 CHECKLIST FOR PRIMARY IV SOLUTION ADMINISTRATION

My Notes

Use the checklist below to review the steps for completion of "Primary IV Solution Administration." Review the steps to safely administer all types of medication in the "Checklist for Oral Medication Administration" in the "Administration of Enteral Medications" chapter.

Steps

Disclaimer: Always review and follow agency policy regarding this specific skill.

1. Gather supplies: IV fluid, primary tubing, tubing change label, and alcohol pads/scrub hubs.
2. Verify the provider order with the medication administration record (eMAR/MAR).
3. Perform the first check of the six rights of medication administration while withdrawing the IV fluids from the medication dispensing unit. Check expiration date and verify patient allergies.
4. Remove the IV solution from the packaging and gently apply pressure to the bag while inspecting for tears or leaks.
5. Check the color and clarity of the solution.
6. Perform the second check of the six rights of medication administration.
7. Enter the patient room and greet the patient.
8. Perform safety steps:
    - Perform hand hygiene.
    - Check the room for transmission-based precautions.
    - Introduce yourself, your role, the purpose of your visit, and an estimate of the time it will take.
    - Confirm patient ID using two patient identifiers (e.g., name and date of birth).
    - questions.
    - Be organized and systematic.
    - Use appropriate listening and questioning skills.
    - Listen and attend to patient cues.
    - Ensure the patient's privacy and dignity.
    - Assess ABCs.
9. Perform the third medication check of the six rights of medication administration at the patient's bedside.
10. Remove the primary IV tubing from the packaging. If administering IV fluid by gravity, note the drip factor on the package and calculate drops/min. Perform the necessary calculations for the infusion rate.
11. Move the roller clamp so that it is halfway up the tubing and clamp it.
12. Remove the cover from the tubing port on the bag of IV fluid.

My Notes

13. Remove the cap from the insertion spike on the tubing. While maintaining sterility, insert the spike into the tubing port of the bag of IV fluid.
14. Squeeze the drip chamber two or three times to fill the chamber halfway.
15. Loosen the cap from the end of the IV tubing and open the clamp to prime the tubing over the sink:
    - If using multiple port tubing, invert the ports to prime them and to prevent air accumulation in line.
    - If the solution is an antibiotic, take care to not waste solution while priming the tubing to ensure the patient receives the correct dosage.
16. Once primed, clamp the IV tubing and check the entire length of the tubing for air bubbles. Tap the tubing gently to remove any air.
17. Replace or tighten the cap on the end of the tubing.
18. Label the primary IV fluid bag with the date and time. Place the tubing label on the tubing near the drip chamber.
19. Assess the patient's venipuncture site for signs and symptoms of vein irritation or infiltration. Do not proceed with administering fluids at this site if there are any concerns.
20. Vigorously cleanse the catheter cap on the patient's IV port with an alcohol pad/scrub hub (or the agency required cleansing agent) for at least five seconds and allow it to dry.
21. Assess IV site patency according to agency policy. Purge a prefilled normal saline syringe of air. Attach the syringe onto the the saline lock cap. Undo the clamp on the extension tubing. Inject 3 to 5 mL of normal saline using a turbulent stop-start technique. If resistance is felt, do not force the flush and do not proceed with IV solution administration; follow up according to agency policy.
22. Remove the syringe from the IV cap and then clamp the extension tubing.
23. Vigorously cleanse the catheter cap on the patient's IV port with an alcohol pad/scrub hub (or the agency required cleansing agent) for at least five seconds and allow it to dry.
24. Remove the protective cap from the end of the primary tubing and attach it to the IV port while maintaining sterility.
25. Move the slide clamp on the saline lock to open the tubing.
26. Set the infusion rate based on the provider order:
    - For infusion pump: Set volume to be infused and rate (mL/hr) to be administered.
    - For gravity: Calculate drop per minute.
27. Assess the patient's IV site for signs and symptoms of vein irritation or infiltration after infusion begins.
28. Secure the tubing to the patient's arm.
29. Assist the patient to a comfortable position, ask if they have any questions, and thank them for their time.
30. Ensure safety measures when leaving the room:

My Notes

- CALL LIGHT: Within reach
- BED: Low and locked (in lowest position and brakes on)
- SIDE RAILS: Secured
- TABLE: Within reach
- ROOM: Risk-free for falls (scan room and clear any obstacles)

31. Perform hand hygiene.
32. Document the procedure and related assessment findings. Report any concerns according to agency policy. Include IV fluids on patient's input/output documentation.

My Notes

23.6 CHECKLIST FOR SECONDARY IV SOLUTION ADMINISTRATION

Use the checklist below to review the steps for completion of "Secondary IV Solution Administration." This checklist is used when fluids are already being administered via the primary IV tubing and a second IV solution is administered.

Steps

Disclaimer: Always review and follow agency policy regarding this specific skill.

1. Gather supplies: secondary IV fluid/medication, secondary IV tubing, alcohol wipe/scrub hubs, and tubing labels.
2. Verify the provider order with the medication administration record (eMAR/MAR).
3. Perform the first check of the six rights of medication administration while withdrawing the IV solution and tubing from the medication dispensing unit. Check expiration dates on the fluid and the tubing and verify allergies.
4. Verify compatibility of the secondary IV solution with the other IV fluids the patient is concurrently receiving.
5. Remove the IV solution from the packaging and gently apply pressure to the bag while inspecting for tears or leaks. Check the color and clarity of the solution.
6. Perform the second check of the six rights of medication administration.
7. Enter the patient room and greet the patient.
8. Perform safety steps:
    - Perform hand hygiene.
    - Check the room for transmission-based precautions.
    - Introduce yourself, your role, the purpose of your visit, and an estimate of the time it will take.
    - Confirm patient ID using two patient identifiers (e.g., name and date of birth).
    - Explain the process to the patient.
    - Be organized and systematic.
    - Use appropriate listening and questioning skills.
    - Listen and attend to patient cues.
    - Ensure the patient's privacy and dignity.
    - Assess ABCs.
9. Perform the third check of the six rights of medication administration at the patient's bedside.
10. If the patient is receiving the medication for the first time, teach the patient and family (if appropriate) about the potential adverse reactions and other concerns related to the medication.
11. Remove the secondary IV tubing from the packaging.

My Notes

12. Place the roller clamp to the "off" position.

13. Remove the protective sheath from the IV spike and the cover from the tubing port of the IV solution.

14. Insert the spike into the IV bag while maintaining sterility.

15. Compress and release the drip chamber, filling halfway.

16. Prime the secondary IV tubing. Back priming is considered best practice and is performed using an infusion pump with primary fluids attached:

    - Vigorously cleanse the catheter tip on the patient's IV port with an alcohol pad/scrub hub (or the agency required cleansing agent) for at least five seconds and allow it to dry.
    - Connect the secondary tubing to the port closest to the drip chamber. Lower the secondary bag below the primary bag, and allow the fluid from the primary bag to fill secondary tubing. Fill the secondary tubing until it reaches the drip chamber, and then raise the secondary bag above the primary line.

17. Hang the secondary IV solution on the IV pole with the primary bag lower than the secondary bag.

18. Label the secondary tubing near the drip chamber.

19. Set the infusion rate:

    - For infusion pump: Set the volume to be infused and the rate (mL/ hr) to be administered based on the provider order.
    - For gravity: Set the roller clamp to achieve the appropriate number of drops per minute based on the provider order.

Take time to watch the IV fluid or medication to drip into the drip chamber to ensure the medication or fluid is flowing to the patient.

20. Assess the patient's IV site for signs and symptoms of vein irritation or infiltration after infusion begins. Do not proceed with administering secondary fluids if there are any concerns about the site.

21. Assist the patient to a comfortable position, ask if they have any questions, and thank them for their time.

22. Ensure safety measures when leaving the room:

    - CALL LIGHT: Within reach
    - BED: Low and locked (in lowest position and brakes on)
    - SIDE RAILS: Secured
    - TABLE: Within reach
    - ROOM: Risk-free for falls (scan room and clear any obstacles)

23. Perform hand hygiene.

24. Document the procedure and assessment findings. Report any concerns according to agency policy.

My Notes

23.7 SAMPLE DOCUMENTATION

Sample Documentation of Expected Findings

IV catheter on the right hand was discontinued. IV catheter tip was intact. Site is free from redness, warmth, tenderness, or swelling. Gauze applied with pressure for one minute with no bleeding noted. Dressing applied to the site.

Sample Documentation of Unexpected Findings

IV catheter on the right hand was discontinued. IV catheter tip was intact. Site free from redness, warmth, tenderness, or swelling. Gauze applied with pressure for one minute but bleeding was noted to continue around the gauze dressing. Ongoing pressure was held for five minutes until hemostasis was achieved.

23.8 CHECKLIST FOR DISCONTINUING AN IV

My Notes

Use the checklist below to review the steps for completion of "Discontinuing an IV."

Steps

Disclaimer: Always review and follow agency policy regarding this specific skill.

1. Gather supplies: gauze, tape, or a Band-Aid.
2. Perform safety steps:
   - Perform hand hygiene.
   - Check the room for transmission-based precautions.
   - Introduce yourself, your role, the purpose of your visit, and an estimate of the time it will take.
   - Confirm patient ID using two patient identifiers (e.g., name and date of birth).
   - Explain the process to the patient.
   - Be organized and systematic.
   - Use appropriate listening and questioning skills.
   - Listen and attend to patient cues.
   - Ensure the patient's privacy and dignity.
   - Assess ABCs.
3. Prepare the gauze and tape.
4. Place the IV clamp to the "off" position (clamped).
5. Loosen the edges of the transparent dressing and tape in the direction of the IV site.
6. Place a gauze pad over the IV site and gently pull the IV out parallel to the skin in a slow and steady motion.
7. Hold pressure on the IV site for 2-3 minutes. If the patient is on anticoagulant medication, you may need to hold for 5-10 minutes.
8. Inspect the catheter to ensure it is intact and dispose of it in an appropriate container.
9. Remove the gauze pad once bleeding has stopped and assess for any signs of infection at the site, such as redness, swelling, warmth, tenderness, or purulent drainage.
10. Tape the gauze or apply a Band-Aid over the IV site.
11. Assist the patient to a comfortable position, ask if they have any questions, and thank them for their time.
12. Ensure safety measures when leaving the room:
    - CALL LIGHT: Within reach
    - BED: Low and locked (in lowest position and brakes on)
    - SIDE RAILS: Secured

My Notes

- TABLE: Within reach
- ROOM: Risk-free for falls (scan room and clear any obstacles)

13. Perform hand hygiene.

14. Document the procedure and related assessment findings. Report any concerns according to agency policy.

23.9 SUPPLEMENTARY VIDEO RELATED TO IV THERAPY

My Notes

Video Review for Priming IV Tubing and Spiking an IV Bag:[1]

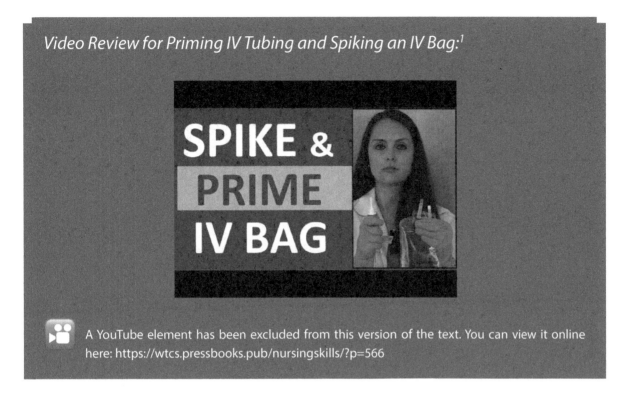

A YouTube element has been excluded from this version of the text. You can view it online here: https://wtcs.pressbooks.pub/nursingskills/?p=566

1 RegisteredNurseRN. (2017, March 10). *How to prime IV tubing line | How to spike a IV bag for nursing.* [Video]. YouTube. All rights reserved. Video used with permission. https://youtu.be/4ntqS_R1r70

My Notes

23.10 LEARNING ACTIVITIES

Learning Activities

(Answers to "Learning Activities" can be found in the "Answer Key" at the end of the book. Answers to interactive activity elements will be provided within the element as immediate feedback.)

The patient's IV site is cool to the touch and swollen. The patient states "it hurts a little." List in order the steps the nurse should take.

a. Discontinue the IV
b. Stop the IV infusion
c. Elevate the affected site
d. Document the findings

Interactive Activity

An interactive or media element has been excluded from this version of the text. You can view it online here: https://wtcs.pressbooks.pub/nursingskills/?p=569

Interactive Activity

An interactive or media element has been excluded from this version of the text. You can view it online here: https://wtcs.pressbooks.pub/nursingskills/?p=569

Interactive Activity

An interactive or media element has been excluded from this version of the text. You can view it online here: https://wtcs.pressbooks.pub/nursingskills/?p=569

XXIII GLOSSARY

My Notes

Extravasation: The infiltration of damaging intravenous medications, such as chemotherapy, into the extravascular tissue around the site of infusion, causing tissue injury and possible necrosis.

Fluid volume overload (hypervolemia): A condition when there is too much fluid in the blood. Patients may present with shortness of breath, edema to the extremities, and weight gain.

Infiltration: Infiltration occurs when the tip of the IV catheter slips out of the vein, the catheter passes through the wall of the vein, or the blood vessel wall allows part of the fluid to infuse into the surrounding tissue, resulting in the leakage of IV fluids into the surrounding tissue.

Necrosis: Tissue death.

Phlebitis: Inflammation of a vein.

Answer Keys

Answer keys for the learning activities in each chapter are provided in the following sections.

My Notes

CHAPTER 1 (GENERAL SURVEY)

Answer Key to Chapter 1 Learning Activities

1. D – Patient is experiencing increased difficulty breathing. (Rationale: The severity of an airway concern and the life threatening nature of the condition neccessitates immediate notification of the provider.)

Answers to interactive elements are given within the interactive element.

CHAPTER 2 (HEALTH HISTORY)

My Notes

Answer Key to Chapter 2 Learning Activities

1. To demonstrate respect for individual culture beliefs, the nurse should use open-ended questions to explore the patient's culture. Demonstrating engagement and interest in learning more about the patient's culture facilitates therapeutic communication and information sharing. Requesting that the patient share cultural background/information that the patient believes is important to their health care demonstrates respect and inclusion for different cultural beliefs and practices.

Answers to interactive elements are given within the interactive element.

My Notes

CHAPTER 3 (BLOOD PRESSURE)

Answer Key to Chapter 3 Learning Activities

1. To safely obtain an individual's blood pressure, it is important to note the size of the patient to select the appropriate blood pressure cuff size. Additionally, it is important to note if the patient has an limb restrictions such as an injury, mastectomy, lymph node removal, fistula placement, etc. Blood pressures should not be taken in any limb with a potential restriction.

Answers to interactive elements are given within the interactive element.

CHAPTER 4 (ASEPTIC TECHNIQUE)

My Notes

Answer Key to Chapter 4 Learning Activities

1. The five moments of hand hygeine occur: 1) before touching a patient, 2) before a procedure, 3) after a procedure/body fluid exposure risk, 4) after touching a patient, 5) after touching a patient's surroundings.

When entering a patient's room to perform the skill of intermittent catheterization, hand hygeine should be performed:

- Upon entry into the room
- After touching the patient's surroundings and preparing for the procedure
- Before touching the patient
- After the procedure/body fluid exposure risk
- After touching the patient's surroundings
- Upon exiting the room

2. B – Patient on *Clostridium Difficile* (C-Diff) contact precautions, D – Hands are visibly soiled

Answers to interactive elements are given within the interactive element.

My Notes

CHAPTER 5 (MATH CALCULATIONS)

Answer Key to Chapter 5 Learning Activities

5.3 Military Time

1. 7:30 PM
2. 12:30 AM
3. 0900
4. 2200

5.4 Household and Metric Equivalents

1. 5 mL
2. 30 mL
3. 500 mg
4. 3636 grams
5. 0.7 cm

5.5 Rounding

1. 6.5
2. 6.5
3. 5.5
4. 5.5
5. 0.19
6. 0.19
7. 0.2
8. 0.2

Answers to interactive elements are given within the interactive element.

CHAPTER 6 (NEUROLOGICAL ASSESSMENT)

My Notes

Answer Key to Chapter 6 Learning Activities

1. D – Remove obstacles when ambulating (Rationale: Cranial nerve II is the optic nerve, which governs vision. The nurse can provide safety for the visually impaired client by clearing the path of obstacles when ambulating.)

2. A – Cerebral function (Rationale: The mental status examination assesses functions governed by the cerebrum. Some of these are orientation, attention span, judgment, and abstract reasoning.)

Answers to interactive elements are given within the interactive element.

My Notes

CHAPTER 7 (HEAD AND NECK ASSESSMENT)

Answer Key to Chapter 7 Learning Activities

1. To alleviate pain and discomfort associated with strep throat, the patient may receive instruction to:
    - Drink soothing liquids such as lemon tea with honey or ice water
    - Gargle several times a day with warm salt water made of 1/2 tsp. of salt in 1 cup of water
    - Suck on hard candies or throat lozenges
    - Use a cool-mist vaporizer or humidifier to moisten the air
    - Try over-the-counter pain medicines, such as acetaminophen
2. B – White patches noted on both tonsils, D – Speech is slurred, E – Thyroid enlarged

Answers to interactive elements are given within the interactive element.

CHAPTER 8 (EYE & EAR ASSESSMENT)

My Notes

Answer Key to Chapter 8 Learning Activities

1. Signs of auditory challenges may be reflected with a patient asking the nurse to repeat instruction, tilting the head to one side or angling an ear forward, inappropriate responses, garbled speech, attempts at lipreading, etc.

Answers to interactive elements are given within the interactive element.

My Notes

CHAPTER 9 (CARDIOVASCULAR ASSESSMENT)

Answer Key to Chapter 9 Learning Activities

1. C – Heart Failure (Rationale: The patient's symptoms indicate fluid volume overload and reflect a clinical diagnosis of heart failure.)
2. B – Stay with the patient and notify the HCP of the ECG results (Rationale: The patient's cardiac rhythm change is reflective of an abnormality. This change should be communicated to the healthcare provider.)

Answers to H5P interactive elements are given within the interactive element.

CHAPTER 10 (RESPIRATORY ASSESSMENT)

My Notes

Answer Key to Chapter 10 Learning Activities

1. B – Sitting upright (Rationale: The patient who is short of breath will experience greatest comfort sitting in an upright position. This position will also allow for comprehensive auscultation of all lung fields.)
2. fluid or mucus
3. A – Assess pulse oximeter probe site to ensure accurate reading (Rationale: If the patient's clinical presentation does not align with collected metrics, it is important confirm the metric prior to implementing additional actio.)

Answers to interactive elements are given within the interactive element.

My Notes

CHAPTER 11 (OXYGEN THERAPY)

Answer Key to Chapter 11 Learning Activities

1.

Answer Key to Chapter 11 Learning Activities	
Priority	**Actions**
First	Assess pulse oximetry
Second	Assess lung sounds
Third	Apply oxygen as ordered
Four	Reassess pulse oximetry
Fifth	Institute actions to improve oxygenation
Sixth	Teach oxygen safety

(Rationale: Priority of actions includes the gathering of assessment information to reflect the patient's respiratory condition. Once you have collected information, intervention can be initiated with application of oxygen if needed and subsequent reassessment of the pulse oximetry reading. Additional actions to improve client oxygenation and lung capacity can then be implemented with coughing, deep breathing, and use of incentive spirometry. Finally, once the patient experiences improvement in oxygenation and breathing status, reinforcement of oxygen education and safety measures would be appropriate.)

Answers to interactive elements are given within the interactive element.

My Notes

CHAPTER 12 (ABDOMINAL ASSESSMENT)

Answer Key to Chapter 12 Learning Activities

1. A – Nausea, B – Vomiting, D – Bloating
2. A – Bowel Sounds
3. B – There are hypoactive bowel sounds in all quadrants, C – Firmness is palpated in left lower quadrant
4. SAMPLE NOTE:

   D (SO): Patient reports ongoing constipation without bowel movement for greater than 24 hours. The patient reports intermittent nausea that is increasing in frequency and has had one episode of vomiting. The patient's abdomen appears bloated and bowel sounds are hypoactive in all quadrants. There is notable firmness present in the left lower quadrant with palpation. The patient denies tenderness.

   A: Provider updated regarding patient's bowel status and assessment. Order received to administer Milk of Magnesia 30 mL PO times one dose. Medication was administered at 0800.

   R (P). Patient reported having a large formed brown stool at 1100. Stool is noted to be soft and brown. Patient reports relief from nausea. Bowel sounds are noted in all quadrants. Will continue to monitor bowel status.

4. Nurse Signature, Credentials, Date/Time

Answers to interactive elements are given within the interactive element.

My Notes

CHAPTER 13 (MUSCULOSKELETAL ASSESSMENT)

Answer Key to Chapter 13 Learning Activities

1. A – It measures muscle strength symmetry.
2. C – 5 out of 5
3. B – Inspection

Answers to interactive elements are given within the interactive element.

CHAPTER 14 (INTEGUMENTARY ASSESSMENT)

My Notes

Answer Key to Chapter 14 Learning Activities

1. A patient admitted with diarrhea is at risk for skin breakdown and dehydration. Assessment of the patient's skin condition and hydration status would be important for assessing the severity of the patient's illness. Hydration status can be assessed through evaluation of skin turgor with this patient due to normal skin elasticity in this age group.

Answers to interactive elements are given within the interactive element.

My Notes

CHAPTER 15 (ADMINISTRATION OF ENTERAL MEDICATIONS)

Answer Key to Chapter 15 Learning Activities

1. Dimensional Analysis:

$$\frac{750\ mg}{x\ mL}\ x\ \frac{1\ g}{1000\ mg}\ x\ \frac{8\ mL}{2\ g} = \frac{6000}{2000} = 3\ mL$$

$$\frac{750\ mg}{X\ mL} = \frac{2000\ mg}{8\ mL}$$

Ratio Proportion:

$$750\ mg\ x\ 8\ mL = 2000\ mg\ x\ X\ mL$$

$$\frac{6000\ mg}{mL} = 2000\ mg\ x\ X\ mL$$

$$\frac{6000\ \cancel{mg}\ mL}{2000\ \cancel{mg}} = X\ mL$$

$$3\ mL = X\ mL$$

2. If an incorrect medication is given, the nurse should promptly take the following actions:
    - Assess the patient given the wrong medication. Assess for adverse effects related to the error.
    - Notify the nurse manager/primary care provider regarding the medication error.
    - Discuss the course of action to be taken.
    - Implement action and continue to monitor the patient for signs of complication or change in condition.
    - Report the incident via institution policy.

Answers to interactive elements are given within the interactive element.

CHAPTER 16 (ADMINISTRATION OF MEDICATIONS VIA OTHER ROUTES)

My Notes

Answer Key to Chapter 16 Learning Activities

1. Patients suffering from nausea or experiencing difficulty swallowing may not tolerate medications administered via the enteral route. For a patient experiencing pain, appropriate alternate methods of medication administration may be transdermal medication administration. Transdermal medications are beneficial in that they provide a consistent level of drug into the bloodstream during distribution.
2. B – When placing a patch, the nurse should press firmly to the skin to ensure adequate adherence, C – Gloves are required for patch application and removal, E – Date and location of patch application should be promptly documented in the medication administration record (MAR).

Answers to interactive elements are given within the interactive element.

My Notes

CHAPTER 17 (ENTERAL TUBE MANAGEMENT)

Answer Key to Chapter 17 Learning Activities

1. D – Slow or stop the infusion based on the patient's response.

Answers to interactive elements are given within the interactive element.

CHAPTER 18 (ADMINISTRATION OF PARENTERAL MEDICATIONS)

My Notes

Answer Key to Chapter 18 Learning Activities

1. The optimal size needle would be 23G 5/8 inch with injection into the deltoid muscle. With the limited amount of fat tissue, a ⅝-inch needle will be sufficient for entering the muscular tissue. Additionally, a 23G diameter needle is adequate for aqueous and water-based medications.
2. The optimal size needle would be 21G 1 1/2inch with injection into the buttock. With the excess amount of adipose tissue, the nurse should ensure that the length of the needle would be appropriate to reach the intramuscular route.
3. A – Injects 5 units of air into the regular insulin vial first and withdraws 5 units of regular insulin

Answers to interactive elements are given within the interactive element.

My Notes

CHAPTER 19 (SPECIMEN COLLECTION)

Answer Key to Chapter 19 Learning Activities

1. When experiencing difficulty in collecting a capillary blood sample, one should consider the location of the lancet puncture. It is best to avoid calloused areas. Additionally, the hand can be placed in a dependent position for a short period of time to facilitate blood collection into the fingertips. The use of a warm pack or heat application can also facilitate vasodilation and increase blood flow.

Answers to interactive elements are given within the interactive element.

CHAPTER 20 (WOUND CARE)

My Notes

Answer Key to Chapter 20 Learning Activities

1. a) Mr. Jones has a history of diabetes, is overweight, takes a corticosteroid, and has had a recent life stressor. These factors may all be contributory to the lack of wound healing.

   b) Other factors that would be important to assess with Mr. Jones would be his current diet and level of dietary protein, smoking, and alcohol consumption.

Answers to interactive elements are given within the interactive element.

My Notes

CHAPTER 21 (FACILITATION OF ELIMINATION)

Answer Key to Chapter 21 Learning Activities

1. Deflate the balloon, ensure flow of urine, advance the catheter, and attempt reinflation.
2. Utilize assistant to help with positioning and holding. Manipulation of the left leg should only occur, and additional personnel may be needed to assist in holding, providing light source, and retracting skin as needed.
3. The patient should be encouraged to verbalize feelings related to the colostomy. Body image issues can be a significant concern with new stoma creation. The nurse should ensure that the patient is allowed to voice their feelings, while also reinforcing the measures required to provide care. Education regarding colostomy management can aid in empowerment and facilitate the beginning of normalization. Additionally, it can be helpful to provide guidance on measures for dress to accommodate the colostomy.
4. C – Straight catheter
5. C – Document the assessment findings of the stoma.
6. A – "I should plan to replace the pouch system every 8-10 days."

CHAPTER 22 (TRACHEOSTOMY CARE & SUCTIONING)

My Notes

Answer Key to Chapter 22 Learning Activities

1. The items that you should have available include the replacement trach, Ambu bag, and suctioning kit.
2. D – Check pulse oximetry, B – Suction patient, C – Provide oxygen via the trach collar if warranted, A – Assess lung sounds

Answers to interactive elements are given within the interactive element.

My Notes

CHAPTER 23 (IV THERAPY MANAGEMENT)

Answer Key to Chapter 23 Critical Thinking Activities

1. Correct Order: 2 – Stop the IV infusion, 1 – Discontinue the IV, 3 – Elevate the affected side, 4 – Document the findings

Answers to interactive elements are given within the interactive element.

Appendix A

Checklists

My Notes

Checklist for Hand Washing

1. Remove rings/watches and push sleeves above wrists.
2. Turn on the water and adjust the flow so that the water is warm. Wet your hands thoroughly, keeping your hands and forearms lower than your elbows. Avoid splashing water on your uniform.
3. Apply a palm-sized amount of hand soap.
4. Perform hand hygiene using plenty of lather and friction for at least 15 seconds:
    - Rub hands palm to palm
    - Back of right and left hand (fingers interlaced)
    - Palm to palm with fingers interlaced
    - Rotational rubbing of left and right thumbs
    - Rub your fingertips against palm of opposite hand
    - Rub your wrists
    - Repeat sequence at least 2 times
    - Keep your fingertips pointing downward throughout
5. Clean under your fingernails with disposable nail cleaner *(if applicable)*.
6. Wash for a minimum of 20 seconds.
7. Keep your hands and forearms lower than your elbows during the entire washing.
8. Rinse hands with water, keeping fingertips pointing down so water runs off fingertips. Do not shake water from your hands.
9. Do not lean against the sink or touch the inside of the sink during the hand washing process.
10. Dry your hands thoroughly from fingers to wrists with a paper towel or air dryer.
11. Dispose of paper towel(s).
12. Use a new paper towel to turn off the water and dispose of the paper towel.

Checklist for Using Hand Sanitizer

1. Remove rings/watches and push sleeves above wrists.
2. Apply enough product into the palm of one hand to cover hands thoroughly.
3. Rub hands together, covering all surfaces of hands and fingers with antiseptic until alcohol is dry (a minimum of 30 seconds):
    - Rub hands palm to palm
    - Back of right and left hand (fingers interlaced)

My Notes

- Palm to palm with fingers interlaced
- Rotational rubbing of left and right thumbs
- Rub your fingertips against the palm of the opposite hand
- Rub your wrists

Checklist for Vital Signs

(See "Blood Pressure" chapter for "Blood Pressure Checklist.")

1. Knock, enter the room, greet the patient, and provide for privacy.
2. Introduce yourself, your role, the purpose of your visit, and an estimate of the time it will take.
3. Perform hand hygiene and clean the stethoscope before approaching the patient.
4. Ask the patient their name and date of birth for the first identifier and verify wristband while the patient is stating information. Then use one of the following for the second identifier:
    - Scan wristband
    - Compare name/DOB to MAR
    - Ask staff to verify patient (LTC setting)
    - Compare picture on MAR to patient
5. Explain the procedure to the patient; ask if he/she has any questions.
6. Obtain temperature using correct technique in Celsius. Inform instructor if temperature is out of range. Normal Range: 98.6 F or 37 C.
7. Obtain accurate pulse using radial artery. Inform instructor if pulse is out of range. Normal range for a pulse in an adult: 60-100 with regular rhythm.
8. Obtain accurate respiratory rate over 60 seconds. Inform instructor if respiratory rate is out of range. Normal range for respiratory rate in an adult: 12-20.
9. Obtain oxygen saturation reading (SpO2) using a pulse oximeter. Inform instructor if SpO2 is out of range. Normal range for SpO2: 94-100%.
10. Ensure five safety measures before leaving the room:
    - CALL LIGHT: Within reach
    - BED: Low and locked (in lowest position and brakes on)
    - SIDE RAILS: Secured
    - TABLE: Within reach
    - ROOM: Risk-free for falls (scan room and clear any obstacles)
11. Perform hand hygiene and clean the stethoscope.
12. Follow the agency policy for following up on vital signs outside of normal range.
13. Document vital signs.

Appendix B

My Notes

Name	Classification	Description	Indication for Use	Instruction for Use	Other
Duoderm	Hydrocolloid	Contains gel-forming agents, impermeable to outside contaminants, promotes autolysis, reduces pain, promotes moist wound healing.	Partial or full-thickness wounds, may be used to hold other dressing in place, avoid use with infections or diabetes.	Cleanse wound, select dressing 1-2 inches larger than wound, apply light pressure to allow body heat to promote adhesion, change 3-5 days and PRN.	Watch for moisture buildup and odor.
Tegaderm	Transparent film	Permeable to oxygen and water vapor, protects from environmental contaminants, nonabsorbent, "second skin."	PICC/IV site covers, dry wounds, contains moisture in wound when desired.	Cleanse wound. Use skin sealant around edges to hold firm. Change 4-7 days.	Use adhesive remover to remove and protect from skin tears in the elderly.
Steri-Strip	Adhesive	Surgical tape	May be used for linear wound closure or placement after removal of staples or sutures on surgical wounds.	Apply adhesive sealant prior to application. Apply perpendicular to wound edges to promote closure.	
Tubigrip	Compression wrap/skin cover	Woven elastic fabric	May be used as compression wrap or protection of skin.	Sizes vary from infant to body wrap.	When used as compression, double layer provides low end compression 15-20mm Hg.
Vaseline Gauze	Occlusive gauze	Woven gauze impregnated with petroleum	May be used as a nonadherent depression or to keep wounds moist.	Frequent changes. Cleanse wound prior to each application.	Watch for bacteria buildup and odor.

My Notes

Name	Classification	Description	Indication for Use	Instruction for Use	Other
Xeroform Gauze	Occlusive gauze	Petrolatum impregnated gauze dressing with 3% bismuth tribromophenate	The bismuth tribromophenate works to reduce wound odor easily. It also has a non-sticking surface and protects the wound from contamination. ■ Surgical incisions ■ Donor sites ■ Skin grafts ■ First- and second-degree burns	Cleanse wound prior to placement. Place dressing directly over wound. Cover with appropriate cover/secondary dressing.	Helps minimize bacterial buildup.
Coban	Elastic wrap	Sticks to itself without need for adhesive, pins, or clips. Wrap stays in place – lightweight, porous, and comfortable for patients. Reduces pain.	Can be used as compression wrap. Holds primary dressing in place. Can be used to protect skin or medical device.	If using wrap as compression, verify pulse first. Do not apply compression to infected area or exposed bone/organ.	Do not tape to skin. If used as compression, check pulse regularly. May be left in place up to 7 days.
Iodosorb Gel	Fiber gel	Absorbing fluids, removing exudate, slough, and debris, and forming a gel over the wound surface. As the gel absorbs exudate, iodine is released, killing bacteria and changing color as the iodine is used up.	For use in cleaning wet ulcers and wounds such as venous stasis ulcers, pressure injuries, diabetic foot ulcers, and infected traumatic and surgical wounds.	Cleanse wound, squeeze gel in shape of wound onto sterile gauze, apply to wound, and hold with secondary dressing.	May be used to eliminate pseudomonas bacteria. Verify allergies prior to use.
2"x2" Gauze	Gauze	Wound cover	Cleaning, coverage	Apply to wound and tape.	Avoid applying tape to skin.
3"x3" 4-ply Nonwoven	Gauze	Wound cover	Cleaning, coverage	Apply to wound and tape.	Avoid applying tape to skin.
4"x4" 8-ply Gauze Sponge	Gauze	Wound cover	Cleaning, coverage, wet-to-dry	Apply to wound and tape.	Avoid applying tape to skin.

My Notes

Name	Classification	Description	Indication for Use	Instruction for Use	Other
4"x4" 6-ply Drain Sponge	Gauze	Wound cover, trachea, PEG tube, drain cover/ protection.	Use to surround trachea, drain, PEG tube for protection and drainage absorption.	Cleanse area surrounding tube; apply surrounding the drain site top and bottom.	If applying tape to hold, use minimal tape to protect skin upon removal.
6"x6" Super Sponge ("fluff")	Gauze	Woven-layered, super absorbent for moderate to large drainage.	Wound cover drainage collection, wet-to-dry.	Cleanse wound, apply and change as prescribed and wound drainage dictates.	Do not allow drainage-filled gauze to remain on wound surface for extended periods. Promotes bacteria and infection.
Abdominal Pad	Gauze	Absorbent of a soft nonwoven outer layer that quickly wicks fluid to a cellulose center. Cellulose quickly absorbs and disperses fluids laterally to prevent pooling.	Wound cover, heavy drainage collection. Keeps moisture off skin. Similar to incontinent pad.	Cleanse wound and apply as prescribed and wound drainage dictates.	Do not allow drainage-filled pad to remain on wound surface for extended periods. Promotes bacteria and infection.
Optilock	Polymer	Super-absorbent polymer core locks in drainage under compression. Adjusts absorption to the amount of drainage. Protects skin from maceration. Nonadherent wound contact layer.	Pressure injuries, partial and full-thickness wounds, leg ulcers, lacerations and abrasions, and wounds under compression.	Cleanse wound, apply to wound bed and hold in place with tape, wrap, etc. May be left in place up to 7 days if drainage is minimal.	Do not allow drainage-filled pad to remain on wound surface for extended periods. Promotes bacteria and infection.
Kerlix 4" 6-ply **Gauze Roll**	Gauze	Prewashed, fluff-dried 100% woven gauze with crinkle-weave pattern for loft and bulk. Provides fast-wicking action, aeration, and absorbency. Comes in large variety of sizes.	Wound cover, wound packing, skin wrap protection, wet-to-dry.	Cleanse wound and apply.	Change as prescribed. Do not allow drainage-filled gauze to remain on wound surface for extended periods. Promotes bacteria and infection.

My Notes

Name	Classification	Description	Indication for Use	Instruction for Use	Other
4" stretch Bandage ("Kling")	Gauze	Nonsterile absorbent gauze roll and stretches and conforms to the body shape and clings to itself as it is wrapped. Conforms to the wound area and offers flexibility to allow for body movement.	May be used to hold dressings in place or wrap for skin protection.	Apply as needed.	Avoid applying tape to skin. Apply tape to Kling to hold. Comes in large variety of sizes.
Adaptic	Contact layer	Nonadhering dressing, primary wound contact dressing designed to minimize wound adherence and prevent maceration, mesh impregnated with a specially formulated petroleum emulsion, and easy to remove, minimize pain.	Dry to heavily exuding wounds for which adherence of dressing and exudate is to be prevented.	Cleanse wound, apply to wound, apply primary dressing, hold with appropriate dressing or tape.	May be used as a contact layer with wound VAC foam, or cover skin tears.
Telfa	Composite	Made of cotton fabric with a perforated seal of polyester resin. This perforated seal acts as a nonadherent, preventing the dressing from sticking to the wound and/or acting as a barrier between the wound and excretions.	Cover cuts and abrasions. It is also used to prevent infection to sutured wounds and as an absorbent dressing for wound secretions.	Cleanse wound and apply as primary or secondary (contact) layer. May be used with topical medications.	Change daily or when saturated.
¼" Plain Packing Strip	Gauze	100% cotton, fine mesh gauze ideal for wet-to-dry packing. Available in plain and iodoform (antiseptic).	Used for packing or as drainage conduits in nasal, sinus, or tunnel packing.	Cleanse wound. Apply as packing or filler in wound tunnel, nasal passage, or sinus cavity.	Change daily or as prescribed. Do not cut in small pieces to avoid not being able to locate them for removal.
Aquacel Ag (also comes as plain hydrofiber with no additives)	Hydrofiber	Primary wound dressing made from sodium carboxymethylcellulose. Textile fiber and presented in the form of fleece held together by a needle bonding process and is available both as a "ribbon" for packing cavities and as a flat nonwoven pad for application to larger open wounds. Fiber turns to gel when moistened by drainage.	Primary wound dressing to absorb large amounts of drainage. Silver component is antimicrobial. The dressing is easy to remove without causing pain or trauma and leaves minimal residue on the surface of the wound.	Cleanse wound. Apply to surface of lightly pack into wound. Cover with secondary dressing.	Some patients may be sensitive to silver. Silver must remain in place for at least 24 hours to be effective. Change frequency as prescribed by physician.

My Notes

Name	Classification	Description	Indication for Use	Instruction for Use	Other
Hydrofera Blue	Antimicrobial foam	Pulls bacteria-laden exudate up and away from the wound, which may facilitate healing. Provides a protective antibacterial cover that inhibits the growth of microorganisms. Foam impregnated with methylene blue.	Pressure injuries, diabetic ulcers, venous stasis ulcers, arterial ulcers, superficial burns, donor sites, post-surgical incisions, trauma wounds, abrasions, and lacerations.	Cleanse wound. Moisten foam with saline or sterile water. Ring out excess moisture. Apply to wound and hold with occlusive cover (Tegaderm, Duoder).	Hydrofera Blue foam is effective against microorganisms commonly found in wounds including MRSA, VRE, and Candida.
Polymem (Pink) **Polymem (Silver)**	Foam	Polymem contains a mild, nonionic, nontoxic, tissue-friendly cleansing agent, activated by moisture that is gradually released into the wound bed. Built-in cleansing capabilities reduce the need to cleanse wounds during dressing changes, which can disrupt the growth of healthy tissue, as the wounds heals. Wicks away up to ten times its weight in exudate. The absorption capability activates only if the material detects exudate. Nonstick surface to reduce pain and tissue loss during removal.	Wounds with small to moderate drainage. Pressure injuries, diabetic ulcers, venous stasis ulcers, arterial ulcers, superficial burns, donor sites, post-surgical incisions, trauma wounds, abrasions, and lacerations.	Cleanse wound. Place uncut foam directly on wound. Hold with nonocclusive dressing to allow for moisture evaporation. May use Kerlix, Kling, or Tubigrip to hold in place.	May be changed daily or weekly depending on drainage amount. Silver is most effective when left in place > 24 hours. Some patients complain of pain with use of silver.
Aquacel Ag Foam	Foam	Absorbs wound fluid and creates a soft gel, maintaining a moist wound environment. Locks in exudates through vertically wicking, reducing the risk of maceration. Helps minimize pain while in place and during dressing changes.	Wounds with small to moderate drainage. Pressure injuries, diabetic ulcers, venous stasis ulcers, arterial ulcers, superficial burns, donor sites, post-surgical incisions, trauma wounds abrasions, and lacerations.	Cleanse wound. Place uncut foam directly on wound. Hold with nonocclusive dressing to allow for moisture evaporation. May use Kerlix, Kling, or Tubigrip to hold in place.	May be changed daily or weekly depending on drainage amount. Sliver is most effective when left in place > 21 hours. Some patients complain of pain with use of silver.

My Notes

Name	Classification	Description	Indication for Use	Instruction for Use	Other
Lyofoam	Foam	Management of moderately to highly exuding wounds. Its high absorbency and fluid-handling capacity, combined with the reduced risk of maceration and leakage, provide a longer wear time. Waterproof backing film acts as a barrier to bacterial and viral penetration. Works under compression.	Moderate to heavy draining wounds. Pressure injuries, diabetic ulcers, venous stasis ulcers, arterial ulcers, superficial burns, donor sites, post-surgical incisions, trauma wounds, abrasions, and lacerations.	Cleanse wound. Place uncut foam directly on wound. Hold with nonocclusive dressing to allow for moisture evaporation. May use Kerlix, Kling, or Tubigrip to hold in place.	Monitor dressing frequently and change when saturated with drainage.
Mepilex Border	Foam	Absorbs and retains exudate and maintains a moist wound environment. The Safetac® layer seals the wound edges, preventing the exudate from leaking onto the surrounding skin, which minimizes the risk for maceration. The Safetac® layer ensures that the dressing can be changed without damaging the wound or surrounding skin or exposing the patient to additional pain.	For moderate to high exuding wounds, such as pressure injuries, leg and foot ulcers, traumatic wounds, and other secondary healing wounds. May also be used for skin and pressure injury protection/prevention.	Clean the wound prior to applying a dressing. The dressing should overlap the wound bed by at least 2 cm onto the surrounding skin.	Adhesive border is designed to be peeled back to view wound and reseal multiple times. Monitor wound frequently. Comes in a variety of sizes.
Mepilex Border Ag	Foam	Silver has been added. Silver kills bacteria and might be used both for preventing infection and also on wounds with signs of local infection. The Safetac® layer ensures that the dressing can be changed without damaging the wound or surrounding skin or exposing the patient to additional pain.	For moderate to high exuding wounds, such as pressure injuries, leg and foot ulcers, traumatic wounds, and other secondary healing wounds.	Clean the wound prior to applying a dressing. The dressing should overlap the wound bed by at least 2 cm onto the surrounding skin.	Adhesive border is designed to be peeled back to view wound and reseal multiple times. Monitor wound frequently. Comes in a variety of sizes. Mepilex surgical dressing has a super adhesive border and remains in place for 7-10 days. Some patients complain of pain with use of silver.

My Notes

Name	Classification	Description	Indication for Use	Instruction for Use	Other
KCI Granufoam Black	Negative Pressure Wound Therapy (NPWT)	Promotes wound healing through Negative Pressure Wound Therapy (NPWT). This helps draw wound edges together, remove infectious materials, and actively promote granulation. By provider order.	Do not place foam dressings directly in contact with exposed blood vessels, anastomotic sites, organs, or nerves.	Detailed instruction for use available online at the myKCI website.	Consider pain control prior to application and removal.

Appendix C

Head-to-Toe Assessment Checklist

This checklist is intended as a guide for a routine, general, daily assessment performed by an entry-level nurse during inpatient care. Students should use a systematic approach and include these components in their assessment and documentation. Assessment techniques should be modified according to life span considerations. Focused assessments should be performed for abnormal findings and according to specialty unit guidelines. Unanticipated findings should be reported per agency protocol with emergency assistance obtained as indicated.

1. Gather supplies: stethoscope, penlight, watch with second hand, gloves, hand sanitizer, and wound measurement tool.
2. Perform hand hygiene before providing care and clean stethoscope. Check the room for transmission-based precautions.
3. Greet the patient, introduce oneself, explain the task, and provide privacy:
    - Knock before entering the room.
    - Greet the patient and others in the room. Ask the patient's preferred way of being addressed. Ask if the patient is comfortable if others are present in the room during the assessment.
    - Introduce your name and role.
    - Explain the planned task and estimate the duration of time to complete it.
    - Provide for privacy.
    - During the assessment, listen and attend to patient cues. Use appropriate listening and questioning skills.
4. Identify the patient with two appropriate identifiers.
5. Perform a primary survey to ensure medical stability. Obtain emergency assistance if needed.
    - **Airway:** Is the airway open? Is suctioning needed?
    - **Breathing:** Is the patient breathing normally?
    - **Circulation:** Are there any abnormal findings in the overall color and moisture of the patient's skin (cyanosis, diaphoresis)
    - **Mental Status:** Is the patient responsive and alert?
6. Perform a general survey while completing the head-to-toe assessment. Include general appearance, behavior, mood, mobility (i.e., balance and coordination), communication, overall nutritional status, and overall fluid status.
7. Address patient needs before starting assessment (toileting, glasses, hearing aids, etc.).
8. Evaluate chief concern using PQRSTU (i.e., ask the patient their reason for seeking/receiving care). Ask, "Do you have any concerns or questions you'd like to talk about before we begin?"
9. Obtain and/or analyze vital signs. (Initiate emergency assistance as needed.)
10. Evaluate for the presence of pain or other type of discomfort. If pain or discomfort is present, perform comprehensive pain assessment using PQRSTU.
11. Perform a neuromuscular assessment:

My Notes

- Perform a subjective assessment. Ask if headache, dizziness, weakness, numbness, tingling, or tremors are present. Inquire if the patient has experienced loss of balance, decreased coordination, previous falls, or difficulty swallowing. Be aware of previously diagnosed neuromuscular conditions and currently prescribed medications and how these impact your assessment findings.
- Assess level of consciousness and orientation to person, place, and time.
- Assess PERRLA using penlight.
- Assess motor strength and sensation:
    1. Bilateral hand grasps
    2. Upper strength and resistance
    3. Lower strength and resistance
    4. Sensation in extremities
- Note unanticipated neurological findings in symmetrical facial expressions, extremity movement, and speech and obtain emergency assistance as needed.
- Assess fall assessment risk per agency policy.
- Perform a focused assessment if neurological or musculoskeletal condition is present.

12. Perform a basic head, neck, eye, and ear assessment:

- Perform a subjective assessment. Be aware of previously diagnosed head, neck, eye, or ear conditions and associated medications and how these impact your assessment findings.
    1. Ask if they are having any problems with their teeth or gums, and if so, has this impacted their ability to eat.
    2. Ask if they use glasses, hearing aids or dentures.
    3. Ask if they have any difficulty seeing or blurred vision.
    4. Ask if they have trouble hearing or experience ringing in their ears.
- Inspect the external eye and the external ear. Inspect the oral cavity for lesions, tongue position, moisture, and oral health. Ask the patient to swallow their saliva and note any difficulty swallowing.
- Palpate the lymph nodes (per agency policy).

13. Perform a cardiovascular system assessment:

- Perform a subjective assessment. Ask if they are having chest pain, shortness of breath, edema, palpitations, calf pain, or pain in their feet or lower legs when exercising. Be aware of previously diagnosed cardiovascular conditions and currently prescribed medications and how these impact your assessment findings.
- Inspect:
    1. The face, lips, and extremities for pallor or cyanosis.
    2. The neck for JVD in upright position or with head of bed at 30-45 degree angle.
    3. The bilateral upper and lower extremities for color, warmth, and sensation.
    4. The lower extremities for hair distribution, edema, and signs of deep vein thrombosis (DVT)
- Palpate:

1. Palpate and compare the radial, brachial, dorsalis pedis, and posterior tibial pulses bilaterally. Note the presence and amplitude of pulses.
2. Palate the nail beds for capillary refill.

- Auscultate:

1. Auscultate with both the bell and the diaphragm of the stethoscope over the five auscultation areas of the heart. Note the rate and rhythm. Identify S1 and S2 and any unexpected findings (i.e., extra sounds or irregular rhythm).
2. Measure the apical pulse for one minute.

14. Perform a respiratory assessment:

- Perform a subjective assessment. Ask if they have shortness of breath or a cough. Ask if the cough is dry or productive. Ask if they smoke, and if so, what products, how many a day, and if they are interested in quitting. Be aware of previously diagnosed respiratory conditions and currently prescribed medications or treatments and how these impact your assessment findings.
- Inspect:

1. Level of consciousness and for signs of irritability, restlessness, anxiety, or confusion
2. Breathing pattern, including rate, rhythm, effort, and depth of breathing. Note signs of difficulty breathing such as nasal flaring, use of accessory muscles, or pursed-lip breathing.
3. Skin color of lips, face, hands and feet for cyanosis and pallor
4. Trachea (midline)
5. Symmetrical chest movement

- Auscultate lung sounds using stethoscope directly on the skin over anterior and posterior auscultation areas. Compare sounds from side to side and note any adventitious sounds such as rhonchi, crackles, wheezing, stridor, or pleural rub.
- If oxygen equipment is prescribed:

1. Note if the patient is using oxygenation devices during the exam or on room air.
2. If the patient is using an oxygenation device, document the name of device and current flow rate and/or fraction of inspired oxygen (FiO2).
3. Inspect for signs of skin breakdown due to the use of oxygenation devices.

- If a tracheostomy is present, document the condition of the tracheostomy site and characteristics of sputum present.

15. Perform an abdominal assessment:

- Perform a subjective assessment:

1. Ask if the patient is having any abdominal pain, cramping, nausea, vomiting, constipation, loss of appetite, or difficulty swallowing. Inquire about the date of the last bowel movement, if there have been any changes in the pattern or consistency of the stool, and if any blood is present or dark stool. Be aware of previously diagnosed gastrointestinal or genitourinary conditions and currently prescribed medications and how these impact your assessment findings.
2.. Ask if the patient has pain or problems with urination or leakage of urine.

My Notes

- Inspect the general contour and symmetry of the abdomen and for distension.
- Auscultate for bowel sounds over four quadrants for one minute, note any hypoactive, high pitched sounds.
- Palpate lightly for tenderness and masses.
- Analyze weight trend and 24-hour input and output, as appropriate for patient status.
- If enteral tube is present, assess tube insertion site, tube placement, and amount of enteral feeding/fluids administered during your shift per agency policy.
- If an indwelling urinary catheter is present, assess urine output and urine characteristics. Document continued need for indwelling catheter per agency policy.
- If an ostomy is present, document the condition of stoma and peristomal skin. Document amount and characteristics of output during your shift.

16. Perform an integumentary assessment:
    - Perform a subjective assessment. Ask if the patient has any skin concerns such as itching, rashes, or an unusual mole or lump. Be aware of previously diagnosed integumentary conditions and currently prescribed medications or treatments and how these impact your assessment findings.
    - Inspect:
        1. Assess overall skin color and note pallor, cyanosis, jaundice, erythema, bruising, mositure, and turgor.
        2. If an intravenous site is present, assess the insertion site for redness, warmth, tenderness, or induration. If intravenous fluids and/or medications are infusing, document the type and amount of fluids during your shift per agency policy.
        3. Assess for skin breakdown in pressure points (behind ears, occipital area, elbows, sacrum, and heels).
        4. If a pressure injury is present, stage from 1 to 4.
        5. If a wound is present, perform a wound assessment.
    - Palpate for temperature, moisture, and texture. If erythema or rashes are present, assess for blanching. If edema is present, document the depth of indentation and the time it takes to rebound to original position and grade on a scale from 1 to 4.
17. When the assessment is completed, assist the patient back to a comfortable position. Thank them and ask if anything is needed before you leave the room.
18. Ensure safety measures before leaving room:
    - Call light is within reach.
    - Bed is low and locked.
    - Side rails are secured.
    - Table and personal items are within reach.
    - Room is risk-free for falls.
19. Remove any PPE before leaving the room. Perform hand hygiene and clean stethoscope.
20. Document assessment findings and report unanticipated findings according to agency policy.